Pakolis

(480) 893-~~2400~~ 6020

# An Alternative Medicine Definitive Guide to CANCER

W. JOHN DIAMOND, M.D.

AND W. LEE COWDEN, M.D.

WITH BURTON GOLDBERG

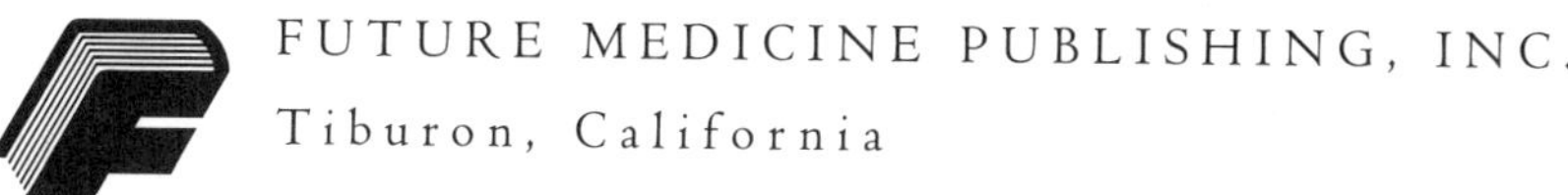

FUTURE MEDICINE PUBLISHING, INC.

Tiburon, California

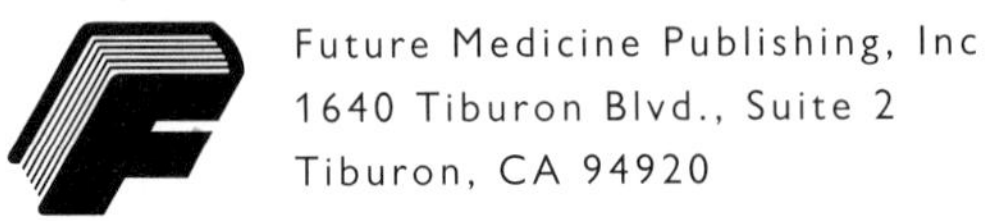

Future Medicine Publishing, Inc.
1640 Tiburon Blvd., Suite 2
Tiburon, CA 94920



Editor: Richard Leviton
Associate Editor: Stephanie Marohn
Editorial Assistants: Nina Giglio, John Anderson
Production Director: Janine White
Cover design, book design and production: Amparo Del Rio Design
Index: Brooke Graves

Manufactured in the United States of America.

10 9 8 7 6 5 4 3 2

Library of Congress Cataloging-in-Publication Data

Diamond, W. John, 1948-
An alternative medicine definitive guide to cancer / W. John Diamond and W. Lee Cowden; with Burton Goldberg.
p. cm.
Includes bibliographical references and index.
ISBN 1-887299-01-7 (hard cover)
1. Cancer—Alternative treatment. I. Cowden, W. Lee, 1952- .
II. Goldberg, Burton, 1926- .
RC271.A62D53 1997
616.99'406—dc21 96-6580
CIP

# Dedication

*For all the cancer doctors who helped with this book and who are helping to make alternative medicine treatments for cancer a reality in North America.*

# DISCLAIMER

This book is intended as an educational tool to acquaint the reader with alternative methods of preventing and treating cancer. Future Medicine Publishing hopes the book will enable you to improve your well-being and to better understand, assess, and choose the appropriate course of treatment. Because the methods described in this book are for the most part alternative methods, by definition, many of them have not been investigated and/or approved by any government or regulatory agency. National, state, and local laws vary regarding the use and application of many of the treatments that are discussed. Accordingly, this book should not be substituted for the advice and treatment of a physician or other licensed health-care professional. Pregnant women in particular are especially urged to consult with their physician before using any therapy. Throughout the book, icons appear in many instances where caution is especially necessary.

Your health is important. Use this book wisely. Discuss the alternative treatment options that are described with your doctor. Ultimately, you, the reader, must take full responsibility for your health and how you use this book. Future Medicine and the authors expressly disclaim responsibility for any adverse effects resulting from your use of the information that is contained in this book.

Future Medicine Publishing and the authors have no financial interest in any of the health-care products discussed in this book, with one exception. Chapter 33 describes the medical practice of co-author, Lee Cowden, M.D. An accurate explanation of Dr. Cowden's practice must include reference to Health Restoration Systems' products in which he has a financial interest.

# About the Authors

## W. JOHN DIAMOND, M.D.

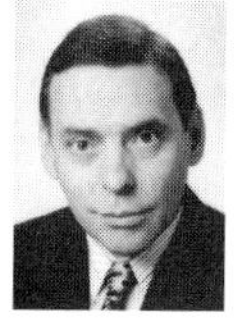

Dr. Diamond earned his M.D. in 1973 from the University of the Witwatersrand in Johannesburg, Republic of South Africa. A board-certified pathologist, Dr. Diamond has extensive training in alternative medicine, including in medical acupuncture, classical homeopathy, and neural therapy. He is currently the medical director of the Triad Medical Center in Reno, Nevada, associate and alternative medicine consultant to the Bakersfield Family Medicine Center and Heritage Physician Network in Bakersfield, California, medical director of Botanical Laboratories, and director of the Associated Complementary Medicine Research Group, both in Ferndale, Washington.

## W. LEE COWDEN, M.D.

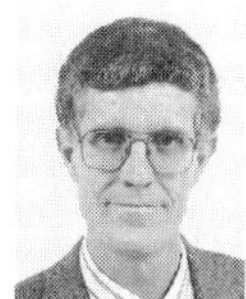

Dr. Cowden received his M.D. from the University of Texas Medical School in Houston in 1978, followed by an internship and residency at St. Louis University in Missouri, and critical care and cardiology fellowships at the same hospital. Dr. Cowden is board certified in internal medicine, cardiovascular disease, and clinical nutrition.

Administering "crisis intervention medicine" convinced Dr. Cowden that to help people he needed to direct his efforts to preventive medicine. Dr. Cowden is accomplished in applied kinesiology, electrodermal screening, homeopathy, reflexology, acupuncture, acupressure, biofeedback, and color, sound, neural, magnetic, electromagnetic, and detoxification therapies. Dr. Cowden now conducts clinical research and teaches alternative medicine at the Conservative Medicine Institute in Richardson, Texas.

## BURTON GOLDBERG

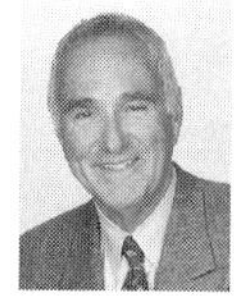

Burton Goldberg was a retired businessman when a friend's daughter attempted suicide. After conventional medicine failed to help, Goldberg took her to a holistic doctor who cured her of a chemical imbalance. Goldberg has been researching alternative medicine worldwide ever since and came out of retirement to publish the best-selling book, *Alternative Medicine: The Definitive Guide*, and the bimonthly magazine, *Alternative Medicine Digest*. Compelling, controversial, and passionate, Goldberg is becoming recognized internationally as the "voice of alternative medicine" and is heard regularly on the subject on TV and radio and through print media.

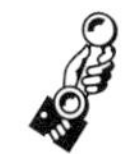

To contact **Dr. Diamond**: Triad Medical Center, 4600 Kietzke Lane, M-242, Reno, NV 89502; tel: 702-829-2277; fax: 702-829-2365. **Dr. Cowden**: Conservative Medicine Institute, P.O. Box 832087, Richardson, TX 75083-2087; fax: 214-238-0327. **Burton Goldberg**, Future Medicine Publishing, 1640 Tiburon Blvd., Suite 2, Tiburon, CA 94920; tel: 415-435-7770; fax: 415-435-7775.

# Contents

## PART II

## Criteria for Successful Cancer Treatment

*Cancer—Its Nature, Causes, Politics, Detection, and Prevention*



## PART III:

## A Complete Guide to Innovative Approaches to Cancer Treatment

*Nutrition, Botanicals, New Pharmacologicals, Immune Stimulators, Metabolic Factors, Physical and Energy Support Therapies*

# Contents

# If it were any good, my doctor would know about it.

**OUR MESSAGE IS SIMPLE**, direct, and lifesaving: cancer can be successfully reversed using alternative medicine. The book you're now holding in your hands shows you how. There has never been a book about cancer like this one and it is desperately needed. No other health topic today has the urgency of cancer because no other health condition is escalating as fast. A century ago, 1 in 33 people had cancer; today, it is more than 1 in 3, and growing.

This book offers clinically proven solutions to reversing that trend: the recommendations of 37 leading cancer physicians who use alternative and complementary therapies to treat cancer and restore life to thousands of cancer patients, including those whom conventional cancer treatments such as surgery, chemotherapy, and radiation failed to help. Read 55 documented patient case histories and see how alternative approaches to cancer can make the difference between life and death.

Although many of the alternative methods for treating cancer have been with us for perhaps 50 years, it is only in the 1990s that these approaches have achieved major clinical breakthroughs and moved into wider public awareness. I wish I had known more about them myself when my sister and my mother were dying of cancer. Seeing them ravaged not only by cancer but by the toxic treatments of conventional medicine made me think there must be a way to treat cancer without poisoning the body and destroying the immune system, and I vowed to find it. The result of that search is in your hands.

By meeting with hundreds of alternative doctors, I learned how they treat hundreds of health conditions using alternative methods. Their recommendations and views became *Alternative Medicine: The Definitive Guide*, a national best-seller that changed the lives of many readers by showing them, as I tell everyone I meet, *you don't have to be sick*. You can get better using safe, effective, inexpensive, and nontoxic methods from the world of alternative medicine. Letters from our readers tell how this information has benefited them by showing them the way to reclaim their health.

Let me give you an example. Stacey Milgrim is a mother who used alternative medicine to reverse her breast cancer. "I knew I would never recover from the stress of surgery and chemotherapy for breast cancer," she told me. "There was information in your book about alternative treatments that enabled me to avoid a mastectomy and keep my breast intact."

Everything we've learned about cancer since doing *Alternative Medicine: The Definitive Guide* is in this new book. A great deal of what you will read will probably be new to you and you may well say, "If alternative medicine for cancer were any good, my doctor would know about it and would have told me." I offer you two reasons for why this is not the case.

First, your doctor may not know about it. Very few physicians are taught in medical school even the rudiments of nutrition or the immune system. Until the mid-1990s, no conventional medical school ever discussed alternative approaches to treating illness. Too often, physicians blindly follow the conventions of their field and never look beyond to see what might work better. Sadly, while a great deal of new information about alternative approaches to cancer actually appears in mainstream medical journals, too few doctors seem to pay any attention.

Second, your doctor may not want you to know about it. Many powerful economic forces—pharmaceutical drug companies, physicians' trade groups, insurance companies, the Food and Drug Administration (FDA) and the National Institutes of Health (NIH), the latter two being taxpayer-funded organizations within the U.S. government—want health care to stay exactly the way it is because they're *thriving* under it. Successful alternative approaches to cancer are a direct financial threat to this system. They are also a serious intellectual threat to the belief systems of conventional medicine. If nutrition and the immune system are so crucial to health and healing and they have never addressed either, this means conventional doctors will have to "go back to school" to catch up.

The 37 doctors profiled in this book were not too proud to go back to school and learn as much as possible about successful alternative approaches. Part of this is learning how to deliver medical treatment scientifically. For all their crowing about science, most conventional doctors are highly unscientific in their practices. They ignore results (in this case, the failure of such accepted treatments as chemotherapy) and refuse to change their methods based on results. The true meaning of being *scientific* is: observing patients and studying what works, then adjusting the therapy accordingly.

Our doctors all have prestigious medical credentials and bring to alternative cancer care decades of careful study and practice—true medical science. Many are oncologists who sought safer, more effective ways of treating cancer; some come from fields such as naturopathy, acupuncture, and homeopathy, long recognized for their nontoxic holistic approach to treating illness.

All of our doctors know that there is no single magic bullet cure for cancer. The message they bring you is this: *many* factors contribute to the development of cancer and *many* modalities and substances must be used to reverse it. To be successful, cancer doctors must become generalists and address the whole person along with the many interdependent factors that contributed to this cancer. Nutrition, diet, the vitality of the immune system, and the emotional life and beliefs of the person with cancer must all be examined.

***Our doctors all have prestigious medical credentials and bring to alternative cancer care decades of careful study and practice—true medical science.***

In this book, you will learn about 33 contributing causes to cancer. You will see how each of these factors can weaken your immune system, start breaking down your health, and make you more susceptible to developing cancer following additional exposure to one or more of the 33 causes. On the other hand, a healthy, strong, and vital immune system can withstand a great deal of such exposure and prevent cancer from ever starting.

Why is there so much cancer today? In simple fact, we are being slowly poisoned to death. The list of poisons includes pollution, pesticides, carcinogens in our food, air, and water, electromagnetic radiation, tobacco smoke, antibiotics, conventional drugs, hormone therapies, irradiated foods, nuclear radiation, mercury toxicity from dental fillings, diet and nutritional deficiencies, parasites, toxic emotions, X rays, and more. Most conventional doctors do not take these factors into consideration when treating cancer.

Here is a remarkable example. A man was diagnosed with prostate cancer. His tumor biopsy was examined by two different types of doctor: one a pathologist, the other a toxicologist. The pathologist saw only clear signs of cancer in the tissue sample, but the toxicologist found something more because she knew what to look for. She found abnormally high levels of a variety of carcinogenic chemicals including arsenic, chlordane, and DDT. In other words, there was evidence of pesticides and other environmental toxins in the tumorous tissue sample itself. If you know the toxin, you can remove it. But first you have to be *looking* for toxins and, here, conventional medicine is inexcusably lax. Most conventional oncologists disregard toxicity as a factor in cancer.

> ***You will quickly see why so few conventional cancer doctors today can honor the Hippocratic Oath to* first, do no harm. *Chemotherapy and radiation are toxic and often do as much damage to the body as the cancer itself.***

The patient was overloaded with toxins and his liver could no longer detoxify his body. The pathologist missed the point entirely: he did not understand that in the tumor itself were the likely causes of the cancer. With this gap in understanding, the treatment he designed for the patient couldn't possibly be effective, because it would fail to address the root cause. This example is typical of the myopia so common in conventional medicine.

In this book, we show you the multiple causes that lead to cancer and take you through all the steps that lead to the removal of these causes. While no doctor offers a simplistic cookbook solution to cancer treatment, instead, emphasizing the unique individuality of each case, you will see a certain uniformity and consistency among their approaches. All of them detoxify the body of its many cumulative poisons; all fortify the body with nutrients; all do everything possible to strengthen the immune system; and all honor the Hippocratic Oath to *first, do no harm*.

You will quickly see why so few conventional cancer doctors today can uphold this vow. Chemotherapy and radiation are toxic and often do as much damage to the body as the cancer itself. Even though conventional medicine presents and often forces these treatments (along with surgery) as the *only* options in existence for cancer, we wrote this book to prove to you that this is a lie. There are many successful alternatives to conventional care that can remove the root causes of cancer and restore you to health without further poisoning or damaging your body. There are also ways to minimize the side effects of chemotherapy, radiation, and surgery. Again, while mainstream medicine ignores this, we tell you how it is done.

I urge you to give your doctors a copy of this book and insist they read it. Alternative medicine *is* good and your doctor should know about it. There is a famous saying I love to quote: Science and medicine advance funeral by funeral. This means old beliefs and practices die out and give way to new approaches only when the older generation of scientists holding them literally die off and leave the field.

We no longer have time to wait for those who swear by conventional medicine to leave the field. The escalation of the rate of cancer demands this urgency. Doctors of all ages must open their minds to new possibilities, to alternative approaches that have been clinically proven to work. Otherwise, the toll of cancer deaths will continue to mount as thousands of cancer patients fail to hear about alternatives that could save their lives.

Let me adapt that previous famous quote to say: Cancer care will advance patient by patient. As each cancer patient recovers their health, thanks to alternative medicine, and tells a friend and the family doctor, this will transform Western medicine. Conventional physicians will *have* to start adopting these new approaches because these approaches are the only ones consistently getting results and saving lives. If they don't, both their patients and more progressive colleagues will leave them behind in the archives of failed medicine. With your help, we can make this change happen quickly and decisively.

God bless.

—BURTON GOLDBERG

# Introduction

## HOW TO MAKE THIS BOOK WORK FOR YOU

**WE HAVE ORGANIZED THIS BOOK** so that you can find lifesaving information as quickly and easily as possible. The chapters are arranged in a slightly unorthodox fashion. Rather than starting with an explanation of cancer and its causes, then moving into treatments, we move you immediately into what 23 pioneering alternative physicians are doing to reverse cancer, devoting a chapter to each. We start with actual treatments. Then in the other 11 chapters, we present more information about other alternative cancer doctors.

Once you are reassured that there are alternative physicians confidently using a multimodal approach to treating cancer and getting clinically proven positive results, then you will probably find the later sections of the book—cancer's nature, causes, politics, detection, prevention, as well as information about dozens of substances, therapies, and remedies—of keener practical interest. In fact, here you will encounter the treatment programs of another 14 physicians. First we tell you how, then we explain why.

Feel free to open the book anywhere. Start reading in the middle or from the back, or jump around from chapter 2 to 20 to 30, as you wish. No matter where you are in the book, we'll be right there with you, clearly guiding you to more information, related topics, or product help elsewhere in the book. Your key to the open-ended use of this book is the icon, of which you will find 12 types in the text.

### A User's Guide to Our Interactive Icons

One of the book's chief features is that it is *interactive*, thanks to these 12 icons.

This means you can turn to the listed pages elsewhere in this book for more information on the topic. For example, if you are reading about toxicity as a contributing cause for cancer in Chapter 25, this icon directs you to Chapter 33 for practical information on detoxification protocols; it also guides you to those cancer doctors in Part I who have detailed programs for detoxification.

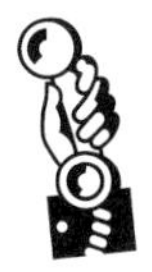

This tells you where to contact a physician, group, or publication, or how to obtain substances mentioned in the text. This is an editorial service to our readers. Most importantly, the use of this icon empowers you right now, by giving you a source to acquire something vital to your health, quickly and easily. Whenever possible, we give you complete contact information for all substances mentioned in the text. All items are based on recommendations from the clinical practice of physicians in this book. The publisher has no financial interest in any clinic, physician, or product discussed in this book.

Many times the text mentions a medical term that requires explanation. We don't want to slow down the text, so instead we put the explanation in the margins under this icon. This gives you the option of proceeding with the text or taking a moment to learn more about an important term. You will find some of the key definitions repeated at different places in the book so you don't have to search for the definition.

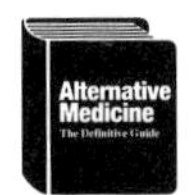


This sign tells you there may be some risks, uncertainties, side effects, or special contraindications regarding a procedure or substance. Pay close attention to these icons.

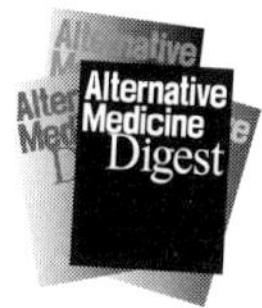


Here we refer you to our best-selling book, *Alternative Medicine: The Definitive Guide*, for more information on a particular topic.

This icon will alert you to an article published in our bimonthly magazine, *Alternative Medicine Digest*, that is relevant to the topic under discussion.

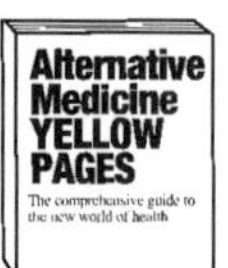


For the name, address, and telephone number of an alternative medicine practitioner near you, consult our *Alternative Medicine Yellow Pages*. Listings are by therapy type and geographical location.

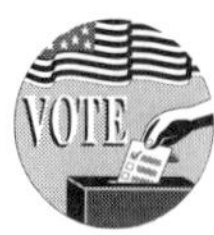


Medicine in the United States is a highly political topic. Often an issue may inspire you to express your views to Congressional representatives. When you see this icon, consider getting involved in the political process to give all citizens the right to choose whatever therapy they deem best for their own health maintenance.

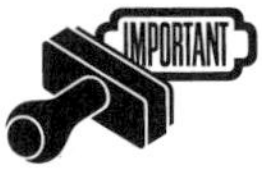


This icon asks you to give a particular point special attention in your thinking. It is important to the overall discussion at hand.

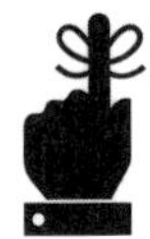

This icon highlights a particularly noteworthy point and bids you to *remember* it.

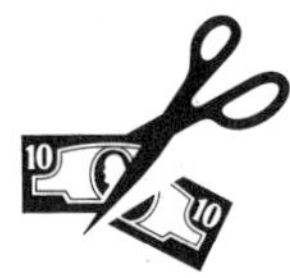


In many cases, alternative medicine is far less expensive than conventional treatments. This icon means that the widespread acceptance of the therapy or substance under discussion could save considerable health-care money.

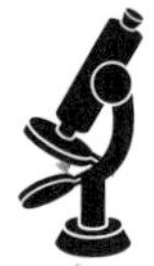

More research on this topic would be valuable and should be encouraged to further substantiate or clinically prove a promising possibility of benefit to many.

## The Success of Alternative Cancer Treatments Is Clinically Proven

You will read 55 patient cases—actual, documented, real case histories—in the chapters about alternative cancer physicians. While the patient's names have been changed, all the medical data is verifiable, based on case records kept by each physician. In many respects, these 55 patient stories are the most important element in this book. They represent clinical proof that alternative cancer therapies can reverse cancer, prevent deaths, and extend lives far better than conventional treatments. If you would like to enter the book by reading about successful patient outcomes, here is a quick reference guide.

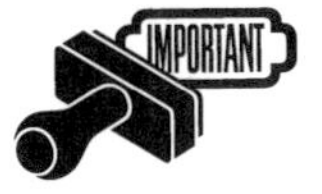


The doctors in this book present information on many therapies, substances, and methods, from nutrition to energy techniques such as Qigong and yoga. The authors and publisher do not specifically or exclusively endorse any single method or belief system, but support all practices that produce clinically verifiable results.

## Interest in Alternative Approaches to Cancer Is Growing Worldwide

Although there is no other book about cancer like this one, the field of alternative cancer treatments is well under way in the U.S., Canada, Europe, and Australia.

Increasingly, new studies and polls in the U.S. indicate a steadily rising acceptance of alternative medicine as a treatment option for disease. The first major indication of this shift appeared in 1993 in a study published in the prestigious *New England Journal of Medicine*. This article reported that, based on interviews with 1,539 Americans in 1990, 34% had used at least one "unconventional" practitioner in 1990, and that one third of these had seen an exclusively alternative physician an average of 19 times in that year. The study also revealed that 72% of those consulting alternative physicians did not tell their conventional doctor of this choice. On the basis of this poll, the researchers estimated that in 1990 Americans made 425 million office visits to alternative practitioners, spending about $13.7 billion, of which $10.3 billion was out of their own pockets.[1]

In 1992, U.S. government data showed that the number of alternative medicine offices grew by 163% over the previous 5 years compared to that of conventional doctors, which grew by only 56%. According to U.S. government data, between 1987 and 1992, the second fastest growing field in U.S. health care was alternative medicine, second only to home health care.[2] In 1994, *Self* magazine reported that 84% of its readers had consulted an alternative medicine physician and 36% said they had more faith in alternative medicine than in conventional.[3] In 1995, 41% of people living in the San Francisco Bay Area tried alternative medicine at least once; 54% said they were "very satisfied" with the results, and 80% said they would do it again.[4]

Confidence in the efficacy of alternative medicine as a treatment option for cancer is similarly growing. The American Cancer Society esti-

# QUICK REFERENCE GUIDE

## Patient Success Stories Found in This Book

| CANCER TYPE | CHAPTER(S) |
|---|---|
| Bladder | 4 |
| Bone | 9, 15 |
| Brain | 15, 26, 34 |
| Breast | 2, 3, 6, 7, 9, 10, 12, 16, 18, 19, 26, 33, 34 |
| Cervical | 11 |
| Colon | 1, 8, 15, 18 |
| Hodgkin's lymphoma | 20 |
| Kidney | 18 |
| Leukemia | 12, 21, 22 |
| Lung | 10, 15, 18 |
| Lymphocytic lymphoma | 14 |
| Lymphoma | 17, 21, 22 |
| Melanoma | 24, 27, 34 |
| Non-Hodgkin's lymphoma | 18 |
| Ovarian | 1 |
| Pancreatic | 18 |
| Prostate | 2, 9, 14, 18, 19, 21, 31, 34 |
| Soft-tissue sarcoma | 14 |
| Testicular | 18, 20 |
| Uterine | 13, 31 |

mated in 1993 that 9% of U.S. cancer patients used complementary therapies,[5] although other researchers placed the figures higher, at 10% to 60%.[6] A study undertaken at New York Hospital revealed that about 30% of breast cancer patients polled said they had consulted an alternative practitioner while 25% were currently receiving some form of "unconventional" therapy such as shark cartilage, medicinal mushrooms, Chinese herbs, or vitamin injections.[7]

Yet another study estimated that from 10% to 50% of cancer patients try some form of alternative or complementary care; the same study reported that 5% of cancer patients abandon conventional treatment in favor of alternative approaches.[8] Estimates by the U.S. government place annual expenditures on alternative cancer treatments for 1992 at $2 billion.[9] Based on the most conservative estimate that 10% of U.S. cancer patients consult alternative practitioners every year, this means that at least 100,000 cancer patients are under alternative care or using alternative substances as part of a cancer treatment program.[10]

***According to U.S. government data, between 1987 and 1992, the second fastest growing field in U.S. health care was alternative medicine, second only to home health care. In 1994,*** **Self** ***magazine reported that 84% of its readers had consulted an alternative medicine physician and 36% said they had more faith in alternative medicine than in conventional.***

The trend toward incorporating more alternative practices in cancer care is growing worldwide. A British survey of 415 cancer patients in 2 London hospitals in 1994 indicated that 16% had used alternative therapies for cancer.[11] A study at the Women's and Children's Hospital in South Australia showed that about 46% of children with cancer had received at least one alternative treatment and that less than 50% of the children's parents discussed their use of alternative methods with their conventional doctors.[12] In the Netherlands, of 949 oncology outpatients polled at several hospitals, 9% said they were presently using alternative medicine in addition to conventional approaches.[13] Of the patients with lymphatic cancer at the Center of Oncology in Krakow, Poland, 25% had received alternative therapies prior to admission.[14] In Germany, out of 160 cancer patients,

53% said they had used alternative medicine at some point in their medical history.[15]

More than anything else, we have designed this book to be an indispensable reference work for you in charting your way through the complex field of cancer research and treatment. Although the book has 34 chapters, do not feel obliged to read from the beginning. There are many themes to explore. Perhaps you are intrigued to learn of anticancer substances entirely new to you, such as laetrile, hydrazine sulfate, or antineoplastons; perhaps you wonder why you have never heard of these before, either in written form or through your physician. You may have already read about them in several doctor's chapters and in the comprehensive A-Z listings in Chapter 30: The New Pharmacology for Treating Cancer. If this is the case, you may wish to turn immediately to our chapter on the politics of cancer, Chapter 26. Here you will be introduced to the many political and economic factors that have managed to suppress lifesaving information about alternative cancer approaches. Or you may feel that it's crucial to understand how other cancer patients have navigated through both the process of cancer and various alternative methods used to reverse it. Here you may participate in and draw inspiration from a living narrative of successful cancer outcomes using alternative medicine.

Our point is simple: Whatever your interest, this book is intensively *reader friendly*. The information is here to work for you, to empower and inspire you, and to show you ways in which you might experience a successful outcome in reversing cancer.

# *Part One*

# Successful Cancer Treatment Plans of 23 Alternative Physicians

## CURRICULUM VITAE

# Robert C. Atkins, M.D.

The Atkins Center, 152 East 55th Street,
New York, NY 10022;
tel: 212-758-2110; fax: 212-754-4284.

Dr. Atkins received his M.D. from Cornell University Medical College and is today a certified member of the American Board of Chelation Therapy and 5 other medical societies. In 1985, he won the National Health Federation Man of the Year Award; in 1990, he won the World Organization of Alternative Medicine Recognition of Achievement. Dr. Atkins has been in private practice in internal medicine, nutrition, and complementary medicine since 1959. He is the host of "Design for Living," a daily radio talk show on WOR-AM in New York City and is the host of "Your Health Choices," a nationally syndicated radio talk show. Dr. Atkins is the author of 6 books, including *Dr. Atkins' Health Revolution* (Houghton-Mifflin, 1988) *Dr. Atkins' New Diet Revolution* (M. Evans, 1992), and is the editor of the monthly newsletter, *Dr. Atkins' Health Revelations.*

***"In my view, cancer is a controllable chronic illness," says Dr. Atkins. "Alternative doctors are not only concerned with attacking the cancer; we're also supporting the body fully, striving to make it stronger so that it can fight cancer for us, rather than just sit on the sidelines, not being allowed to perform its usual cancer-controlling functions."***

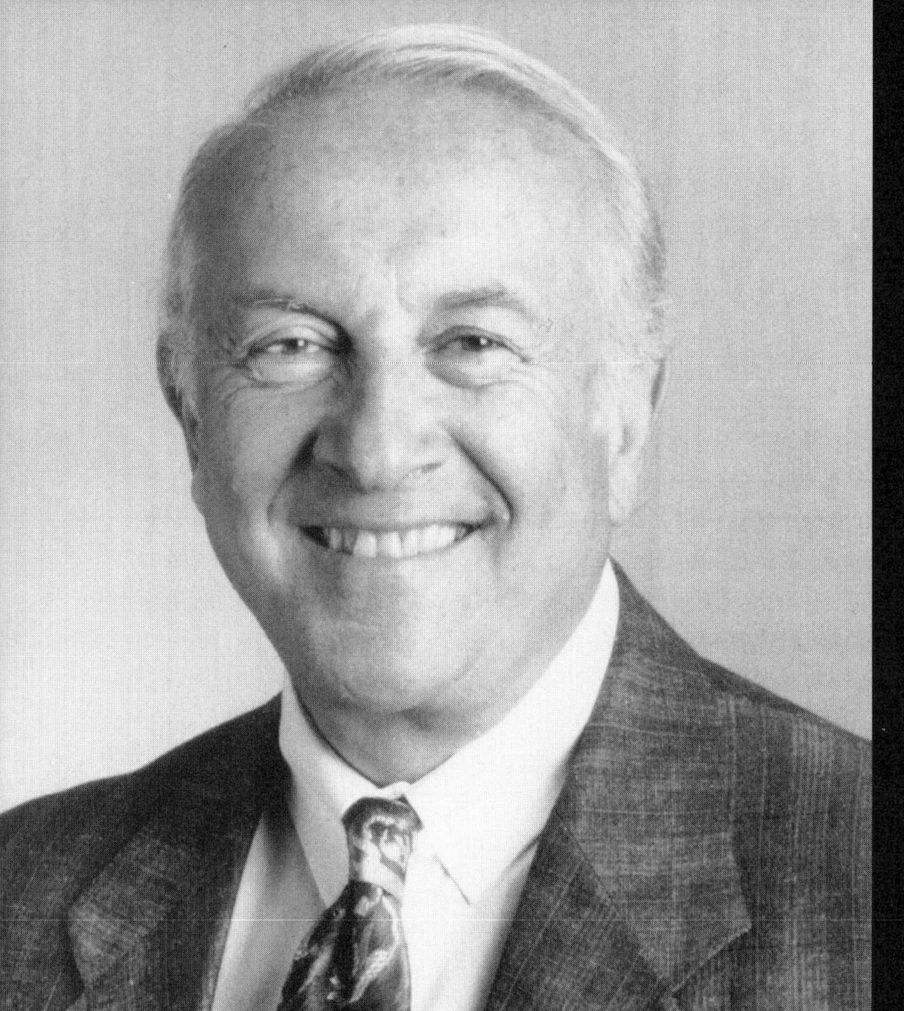

# *Robert C. Atkins, M.D.*

**IF YOU WANT TO REVERSE CANCER** without the person getting sicker, you need to give the body substances that selectively kill the cancer while strongly supporting the body's nutritional and immunological health, says Robert C. Atkins, M.D.

Among the more outspoken proponents of the use of alternative cancer therapies is Robert C. Atkins, M.D. Though originally trained as a cardiologist, Dr. Atkins became interested in cancer management as an offshoot of his interest in nutritional medicine. He became alarmed at the way highly toxic conventional treatments weakened cancer patients, depleting their nutritional reserves, compromising their self-healing resources, and often providing them a lower quality of life than untreated cases. He learned that many cancer patients were malnourished, and that orthodox oncologists were entirely ignoring the role of nutritional support for their cancer patients.

### Destroying the Tumor while Strengthening the Immune System

Orthodox oncology misses the boat by totally ignoring the strengthening of the patient and only focusing on destroying tumors, says Dr. Atkins. "There's no better example of the weaknesses of our dominant medicine than its clearly ineffective war on cancer," he states. "By the same token, there's no better example of the superiority of complementary, alternative medicine than in the management of cancer."[1]

Dr. Atkins has supervised scores of cases in which cancer patients were

# Dr. Atkins' Generalized Model for Cancer Treatment

| STRATEGY | DOSAGE/ KEY COMPONENTS | FOR MORE INFORMATION see page # |
|---|---|---|
| **Dietary Plan** | | |
| Sugar-free; adequate protein, essential fatty acids intake; high phytochemicals from dense uncooked vegetables, | raw or lightly cooked, organically-grown and unprocessed foods, including fresh vegetables and fruits, whole grains and beans; avoid refined sugar, red meat, caffeine, alcohol, tobacco | 749 |
| **Primary Alternatives to Chemotherapy** | | |
| Ukrain | 5-20 mg every other day | 873 |
| 714X | once a day for periods of 21 consecutive days, followed by 2-day break; repeat 2 more 21-day cycles | 871 |
| Iscador (mistletoe) | 10-16 injections given in increasing concentrations | 830 |
| Carnivora | as determined by physician | 860 |
| Shark cartilage | 3 oz powder or 1/2 tbsp of active extract/day | 863 |
| Amygdalin | as determined by physician | 812 |
| Oxygenators: germanium, DC4, Koch's glyoxylide | as determined by physician | 34, 771, 922 |
| **Biological Support from Botanicals and Other Biological Response Modifiers** | | |
| Hoxsey herbs | as determined by physician | 827 |
| Essiac | as determined by physician | 815 |
| Cat's claw | 3-6 g/day; up to 20 g/day in advanced cases | 814 |
| Siberian ginseng | as determined by physician | 821 |
| Tissue extracts | variable, depending on individual | 935 |
| Pancreatic enzymes | variable, depending on individual | 928 |
| **Primary Antioxidants for Reversing Cancer** | | |
| Beta carotene | up to 100,000 IU/day as determined by physician | 764 |

*Continued*

## Dr. Atkins' Generalized Model for Cancer Treatment (cont.)

| STRATEGY | DOSAGE/ KEY COMPONENTS | FOR MORE INFORMATION see page # |
|---|---|---|
| Vitamin C | as determined by physician | 786 |
| Vitamin E | as determined by physician | 790 |
| Selenium | as determined by physician | 783 |
| L-cysteine, N-acetyl cysteine, and glutathione | as determined by physician | 37, 763, 868 |
| L-arginine | as determined by physician | 762 |
| Coenzyme Q10 | as determined by physician | 766 |
| Bioflavonoids | variable, depending on supplement | 817 |
| **Psychosocial Support for Cancer Patients** | | |
| Counseling and ongoing communications | encourage a "fighting spirit" attitude, a more assertive, active, participatory role in healing | 40 |
| Support groups | same as above | |

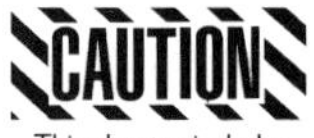


This chapter includes information regarding actual treatments used by Dr. Atkins only after his careful diagnosis of each patient. All cancer patients are unique. **Do not administer these treatments to yourself or others.** Discuss these treatments with your physician or other qualified health-care professional. Readers should not interpret this material as therapeutic advice, but should see a physician in all cases.

getting worse, as indicated by various blood tests (cancer markers), but then improved dramatically when he administered the botanicals and nontoxic medicines central to his program. "In my view, cancer is a controllable chronic illness, rather than an illness that will destroy you unless you totally eradicate it, as conventional medicine considers it," says Dr. Atkins. "Alternative and complementary doctors are not only concerned with attacking the cancer; we're also supporting the body fully, striving to make it stronger so that it can fight cancer for us, rather than just sit on the sidelines, not being allowed to perform its usual cancer-controlling functions."

For the past 10 years Dr. Atkins has investigated a large number of alternative cancer therapies. Today he concludes that these alternative methods are every bit as powerful as their conventional counterparts, and work without the harmful side effects of radiation or chemotherapy. Through his multifaceted program, Dr. Atkins seeks the ideal environment for the body to overcome cancer, emphasizing substances that selectively kill the tumor while encouraging the growth of normal cells and tissues. Chemotherapy has never been able to do this, Dr. Atkins notes.

"Cancer control is a tug of war between you and the disease," Dr. Atkins says. "As the cancer gains strength, it pulls you over the center line and into the pit. The key to winning is to add your own 'power pullers' in this tug of war, that is, natural substances that help your body destroy only the cancer, while strengthening the immune system." Dr. Atkins' "power pullers" include Ukrain, 714X, shark cartilage, Carnivora, mistletoe, and other substances that can help reverse even the most advanced forms of cancer.

***Through his multifaceted program, Dr. Atkins creates the ideal environment for the body to overcome cancer, emphasizing substances that selectively kill the tumor while encouraging the growth of normal cells and tissues.***

Many of these medicinal substances are delivered intravenously or by injection to expose the person to concentrated dosages and to prevent their inactivation that would be caused by digestion. The program also involves the daily oral administration of nutritional and herbal therapies. "The exciting concept that mainstream oncologists do not grasp is that these are nontoxic and that the benefit-to-risk ratio is nearly infinity-to-zero," says Dr. Atkins.

## SUCCESS STORY

### Reversing Ovarian Cancer

At 52, Claudette began having bouts of fatigue, weakness, and depression, and was losing a considerable amount of weight. After visiting her gynecologist for a routine checkup, Claudette was told she had an ovarian cyst and would need an operation. After undergoing surgery to remove both ovaries, she was diagnosed as having ovarian cancer that had spread to the tissues supporting the stomach and adjacent organs.

Claudette's doctors wanted her to begin immediately a 6-month chemotherapy course, telling her that after a year they would do exploratory surgery. But Claudette had decided otherwise and consulted with Dr. Atkins. "I knew that chemotherapy was not for me," says Claudette. "I felt that if I were ever to die from cancer, then let it be from the disease and not the 'cure.' Perhaps I would become a statistic for something I believe in."

When Claudette told her doctors she would be treated by Dr. Atkins instead, they were furious. Phone calls ensued from her oncologist, surgeon, and gynecologist, all telling her she was crazy. "When I met with Dr. Atkins for the first time, I told him that my orthodox doctors told me I couldn't be cured. Dr. Atkins replied, 'You should finish that sentence differently: You can't be cured ... *by them.*'"

Claudette was immediately started on Dr. Atkins' anticancer program. Within 2 weeks of her initial intravenous treatments, Claudette began feeling stronger. "It was a marvelous feeling. I was blossoming like a flower. After a short time, I regained my appetite, went on shopping sprees with my daughter, even went to shows. I began to live again! Can I ever repay Dr. Atkins for giving me the gift of life? Perhaps not. But if I stay well and healthy, I think that will be his greatest reward."

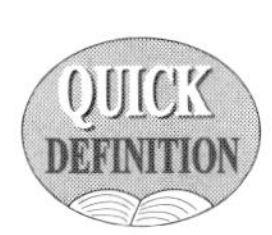


An **intestinal polyp** is a mass of tissue, roughly spherical in shape, at the end of a stalk. The polyp bulges outward from the normal intestinal surface; it may be either benign or malignant, having arisen from the focus of an inflammation or a degenerative lesion.

For the next 2½ years, Claudette came in for regular follow-ups. Her program consisted of a sequence of intravenous treatments using many of the substances discussed below. Claudette has shown no signs of a relapse since. Her treatments are monitored every 4-6 weeks and her results consistently improve. Today, more than 3 years after beginning treatment, Claudette continues to live a normal and fruitful life.

## SUCCESS STORY
### Reversing Colon Cancer

After David, 52, underwent a visual examination of the inner surface of his colon by colonoscopy, which discovered four large polyps, his doctors called him a "grower." For almost a year he had been in and out of hospital for tests, probings, examinations, operations, and countless blood transfusions. At one point, his doctors, short on theories, said that his problem was probably caused by hemorrhoids. During yet another operation, David's surgeons not only found a tumor behind his intestine, but saw that he had an extra 3 feet of intestines. Although they assured him that they saved his life, shortly after his symptoms started returning.

When his doctors told him chemotherapy was the only viable treatment, David asked if there were any alternative treatments. "No such thing," they replied. But because David was a medical equipment supplier, he had seen what chemotherapy patients go through and wanted none of it. "I knew that was not the way I wanted to live my life. "That's also when I knew I had to see Dr. Atkins. I was convinced that Dr. Atkins would be able to treat me because, the way I see it, if his treatment is a natural one with vitamins and minerals, and my body is made up of chemicals, then what harm could he cause me?"

David began Dr. Atkins' nutritional program with oral supplements, immune boosters, and intravenous infusions. The next month, he received the anticancer formula by intravenous infusion once a week along with daily dosages of 714X. "After the first treatment, I was happy there were no side effects," said David. "No fatigue or nausea. By the third and fourth treatment, I started to experience a warmth throughout my body. I was walking more with no more fatigue. I could actually *feel* my body building itself up. I felt reborn!" David regained his formerly hearty appetite and put on 14 pounds. After 7 months, his IV treatments were reduced to once every 2 weeks.

**CT** (computed tomography) scan, formerly CAT scan, is an X-ray technique that provides a detailed cross-section view of tissue structure in the part of the body being scanned; useful for detecting tumors, fluid accumulations, and certain bone and spine abnormalities.

A year after starting treatment, the frequency of David's IVs was reduced to once every 3 weeks, and he continued receiving 714X. His tumor markers remained within the normal range, indicating no growth of cancer. Ten months later, he began a Ukrain protocol; then, 2 months after that, Dr. Atkins conducted a CT scan of his abdomen and pelvis. It came out completely normal.

When David went in for a colonoscopy the next month, the test found nothing significant and he was negative for intestinal polyps. Today, more than 3 years after beginning treatment, David continues his regular visits to the Atkins Center every 2-3 weeks. He lives a normal life and still holds down 2 jobs. "I know there is no more cancer in me," says David. "My energy level is beyond anyone's imagination. I'm looking forward to 60 more years of life, and then some."

## The Importance of Choosing the *Right* Therapy

"The key to success in alternative medicine approaches to cancer is to gather as much data as possible on each patient, then to apply what I call the 'Hippocratic pecking order,'" says Dr. Atkins. This means using the more benign, nontoxic therapies first and saving the riskier, more invasive therapies for last, if ever. Data collection involves studying the patient's immune system and the status of its key T and B cells in detail. Dr. Atkins also uses tumor markers (blood tests that detect the presence and extent of tumors) of every conceivable kind and sonographic or X-ray studies when needed. "The priority is to see whether we are getting a response to our initial treatments," says Dr. Atkins.

Dr. Atkins has observed that, in general, people diagnosed with advanced-stage cancers benefit more from nutrition and other biologic treatments (e.g., enzymes, botanicals, and glandular extracts) than from chemotherapy. For this reason, in most cases he suggests "holding off" on chemotherapy and conventional treatments unless it becomes clear that the safer treatments alone are not getting the job done.

By employing nontoxic strategies first, Dr. Atkins is able to support his patients' immune capacity to reverse cancer *before* the system is ravaged by toxic treatments. Those patients who take this approach, says Dr. Atkins, tend to benefit the most from alternative cancer therapies. As one patient told him, "I've gotten to know about 2 dozen of your patients and the ones who went through chemotherapy before they saw you aren't here or alive anymore."

***In most cases, Dr. Atkins suggests "holding off" on chemotherapy and conventional treatments unless it becomes clear that the safer treatments alone are not getting the job done.***

## The Atkins Injectable Program

**Ukrain—**This substance is derived from a combination of a common weed called celendine (*Chelidonium majus*) and thiophosphoric acid (also called thiotepa, one of the original chemotherapeutic agents). This combination appears to neutralize the toxic effect of the alkaloids contained in the plant. By this method, Ukrain has been rendered almost completely nontoxic. Ukrain does not harm the body's healthy tissues and anticancer defenses; to the contrary, it actually fortifies them.[2]

"Ukrain is clearly a potent anticancer agent and also a very safe and supportive one," says Dr. Atkins. "So it fits into our cancer treatment system very well. Ukrain may soon become recognized as alternative medicine's most effective nontoxic tumor destroyer." According to recent clinical studies, the optimal dosages for Ukrain appear to be 15 to 20 days of 5-20 mg Ukrain per injection, usually given 3 times a week, depending on the individual patient's condition.[3] Dr. Atkins advises doctors who work with advanced cancer patients to find the dose that causes a mild, tolerable febrile reaction, as this seems to provide optimal response.

Dr. Atkins regards Ukrain as the single best anticancer agent he has used to date. "Like chemotherapy, it kills cancer cells very well but, unlike chemotherapy, it spares normal, healthy tissue. If the medical community were willing to give it a try, Ukrain could replace chemotherapy in treating almost all cancers." The majority of terminal cancer patients would benefit from Ukrain through the reduction or stabilization of their cancers as well as through the consistent improvement in their immune cell counts that Ukrain produces, says Dr. Atkins. Of the first 52 people who came to the Atkins Center and were treated with Ukrain, 40 have achieved a significant degree of benefit.

One of Dr. Atkins' patients, a woman with pancreatic cancer, at first showed definite improvement in her condition, then "suffered a relapse when the supply of Ukrain was cut off by officials from the FDA," Atkins says. "Within days of resuming her Ukrain injections, she had dramatic relief from her cancer pain and other symptoms." When a young woman with non-Hodgkin's lymphoma started using Ukrain and various other nontoxic, immune-enhancing therapies, the tumors in her abdomen shrunk consistently after each treatment—without the help of chemotherapy.

***When a young woman with non-Hodgkin's lymphoma started using Ukrain and various other nontoxic, immune-enhancing therapies, the tumors in her abdomen shrunk consistently after each treatment—without the help of chemotherapy.***

At the same time, her energy levels and immune-system profile (numbers and activities of key immune cells) improved weekly for the next two years. This case and many others recorded by Dr. Atkins clearly shows that using Ukrain early in cancer treatment, or soon after the diagnosis, produces the best results.

Despite its potential to target cancer cells, bolster immunity, and prolong life, Ukrain's published cure rate (a statistical measure, based on group studies) is still low. This is in part because inappropriately low dosages have been used in the controlled studies, says Dr. Atkins. Because Ukrain's production costs are very high—$20 per cc administered—and European hospitals conducting the tests have limited funds, many studies limited treatment to 10 of the 10-cc injections. "In actual practice, 50 to 100 of these injections are needed," Dr. Atkins says. "Perhaps once the research is done with these longer treatment regimens, our own National Cancer Institute will stop dragging its feet and designate the funding necessary to investigate Ukrain."[4]

**714X**—Developed by Canadian biologist Gaston Naessens, 714X is composed of ammoniated camphor and other substances. 714X is thought to neutralize a substance produced by tumor cells, one that ordinarily paralyzes the immune system; 714X acts to prevent this substance from protecting cancer cells. "The 714X compound doesn't kill the cancer cells directly but blocks them from feeding themselves," says Dr. Atkins, adding, "Even though it was studied as a single therapy, I find it to be a valuable adjunct to other treatments."

> ***"714X doesn't kill the cancer cells directly but blocks them from feeding themselves," says Dr. Atkins. "I find it to be a valuable adjunct to other treatments."***

Dr. Atkins cautions that patients undergoing the 714X treatment should not take therapeutic doses of vitamin E or vitamin B12 at the same time, as the 2 vitamin supplements may interfere with its therapeutic action. The only side effects from 714X his patients have reported are transient burning sensations at or around the site of injection.

The treatment consists of at least 3 consecutive series of 714X injected directly into the lymphatic nodes of the groin, once a day for at least 21 consecutive days. This is followed by a break of 2 days to allow the patient to rest while the natural defenses of the body are restored. People with advanced cases of cancer can receive more intense and prolonged therapy, since 714X has no harmful side effects.

**Mistletoe**—Fermented extracts of mistletoe, or *Viscum album*, (known by their brand names, Iscador and Helixor) have been used by European physicians since 1920.

European anthroposophical doctors, practicing a type of medicine founded by Rudolf Steiner, who discovered mistletoe as an anticancer remedy, claim the best results overall have been with the treatment of solid tumors before and after surgery and radiation treatment. "We really don't know why mistletoe works, but the German doctors have used it successfully for decades," Dr. Atkins says. "They're the real experts, which is why I tend to follow their programs." Dr. Atkins administers Iscador every other month, when Ukrain is not being given, and usually along with 714X. The typical course of mistletoe treatments consists of 10 to 16 injections given in increasing concentrations.

**Carnivora®—**This substance, derived from Venus flytrap, has been studied primarily by Helmut Keller, M.D., in German cancer treatment clinics, where excellent results have been obtained. "The reason these results are impressive is that they show that the treatment 'works' and is suitable to act as an effective partner to other nontoxic treatments that also work," says Dr. Atkins. "Carnivora may work in a different way from other therapies, by rendering the tumor less malignant rather than by destroying any tissue." After the intravenous program is completed, intramuscular injections of Carnivora may be carried out several times a week until the treatment program is finished. Even more of Atkins' patients take an herbal decoction of Venus flytrap every day.

**Amygdalin/Laetrile—**This substance is highly concentrated in the pits of apricots, peaches, cherries, and berries. As one of a group of substances called nitrilosides, amygdalin has been found to have strong cancer-fighting potential, particularly with regard to secondary cancers, including a 60% reduction in lung metastases.[5] Some research indicates that it can extend the lives of both breast and bone cancer patients.[6] "Amygdalin appears to neutralize the oxidative cancer-promoting compounds such as free radicals," says Dr. Atkins. "It's just one more key component for keeping cancer from growing or spreading. Contrary to what people have said about laetrile, amygdalin's former name, it should be considered an effective, entirely safe treatment for all types of cancer." Amygdalin may be used every month, as an alternative to Ukrain.

**Oxygenating Therapies—**Atkins favors the use of compounds, such as germanium sesquioxide, which enhance the availability of oxygen to both healthy cells and cancer cells. The reason is that cancer cells cannot thrive under oxygen-rich conditions. "These compounds take advantage of cancer's basic inability to use oxygen as a fuel source," says Dr. Atkins. "They reinforce the effects of other therapies for this reason." Germanium sesquioxide blocks or slows the growth of tumors and significantly lengthens survival times, according to studies involving laboratory animals.[7]

In addition to germanium, Dr. Atkins includes other oxygen-providing therapies. Although Dr. Atkins was the first American doctor to treat large numbers of cancer patients with ozone, he now favors the use of chlorine dioxide, also known as DC4. "This compound, like hydrogen peroxide, releases oxygen in the form of ozone into the blood," says Dr. Atkins.

He also uses Koch's Glyoxylide in his injectable treatments. "Koch's Glyoxylide provides a constant oxygenating source and also has a remarkable track record, though it seemed to work better in the 1920s and 1930s," says Dr. Atkins. In the 1920s, William F. Koch, M.D., conducted studies with a compound "glyoxylide," which apparently utilized the oxygen of hydrogen peroxide ($H_2O_2$).[8] Unlike the intravenous methods of $H_2O_2$ administration used today, Dr. Koch preferred to deliver glyoxylide only once or twice in the form of intramuscular injections (2 cc), in a highly diluted (possibly homeopathic) form.[9] Dr. Atkins believes a less polluted environment was the main reason that Koch's Glyoxylide was more effective in those early years; under such conditions, the human body responded more readily to the therapeutic effects of oxygenating compounds.

For more information about **Koch's Glyoxylide**, see Chapter 32: Enhancing Whole-Body Metabolism for Treating Cancer, p. 922.

**Tissue Extracts**—Amazingly, when taken orally or by injection, glandular and organ tissue extracts migrate directly to the gland or organ from which they were derived to provide support to that particular gland or organ and help it fulfill its body-regulating and balancing functions. "We've been using a variety of glandular extracts to strengthen the immune system," says Dr. Atkins. In addition to thymus glandular extract, this includes extracts of liver, pineal gland, and spleen.

Thymus extracts, containing the thymus hormone called thymosin, have demonstrated effectiveness in treating cancers in both human and animal studies. In an animal study of lung cancer, a combination of thymosin and interferon (a natural immune system secretion or "lymphokine") caused a "dramatic and rapid disappearance of tumor burden."[10] The animals treated with thymosin had stronger natural killer (NK) cell activity and lived significantly longer than those receiving standard chemotherapy. In trials involving people with lung cancer, patients receiving thymosin had "significantly prolonged survival times relative to the other treatment groups."[11]

Dr. Atkins often prescribes thymus in the form of Nat Cell T, a frozen extract that can be taken sublingually. Giving thymus by injection is considerably more effective because these complex molecules are broken down easily by the digestive enzymes, says Dr. Atkins.

Using the substances in his injectables program, Dr. Atkins is able to accomplish 2 things at once: tumor destruction and immune support. "My belief is that if you intend to cure cancer, you must do more than just destroy the tumor," Dr. Atkins says. "The destruction of the tumor itself as the sole treatment would only work if the entire disease were localized or confined within the walls of the tumor. The genesis of a tumor is just part of a larger *process*, which is an answer to some internal imbalance."

***"My belief is that if you intend to cure cancer, you must do more than just destroy the tumor," Dr. Atkins says. "The genesis of a tumor is just part of a larger*** **process, *which is an answer to some internal imbalance."***

We next consider some of the ways Dr. Atkins rebalances the body, whether it means getting rid of accumulations of toxins or enhancing the immune response in specific ways. If these more general host-supporting measures are not taken, it is rarely possible to achieve a permanent cancer remission, Dr. Atkins says.

## The Atkins Oral Supplement Program

Let us now consider some of the other herbal and nutritional substances which Dr. Atkins has found effective in treating cancer. Substances such as enzymes, vitamins, minerals, amino acids, trace elements, essential fatty acids, and other products support the body's self-protection process that keeps premalignant conditions from turning into tumors.

"Conventional cancer specialists seem to ignore this by using chemotherapy and radiation, which cripple or destroy the immune system," says Dr. Atkins. "But we need to do everything we can to revitalize and balance this system." In addition to herbs, he recommends the use of supplements made from glandular and organ extracts—those obtained from thymus, pineal gland, liver, spleen, and placenta tissues. Almost all of his thriving cancer patients have taken at least some of these extracts.

**Pancreatic Enzymes—**Perhaps the most valuable of the oral supplements are relatively unprocessed pancreatic enzymes. Dr. Atkins' patients

***Pancreatic enzymes "digest away the protein coating or shell which protects cancer cells from being destroyed by our immune system," explains Dr. Atkins, and remove the "shield" that otherwise enables cancer cells to protect themselves.***

take up to 30 capsules daily of crude pork pancreas extract (from New Zealand) in an around-the-clock dosage system (divided into equal doses throughout the day). These enzymes "digest away the protein coating which protects cancer cells from being destroyed by our immune system," explains Dr. Atkins. In effect, pancreatic enzymes remove the "shield" that otherwise enables cancer cells to protect themselves. "It's fascinating how many of the successful cancer programs that I have studied incorporate pancreatic enzymes," says Dr. Atkins.

**Antioxidants—**"Employing the full spectrum of antioxidants is part of every Atkins Center patient's program, whether for treatment or prevention," says Dr. Atkins. In general, antioxidants help protect the cell's genetic material and membranes from free radical damage, thus preserving normal cell reproduction and overall functioning. Antioxidants are a "huge part of the body's anticancer defenses," says Dr. Atkins. Dosages vary with individual needs.

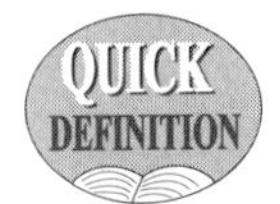


A **free radical** is an unstable molecule with an unpaired electron that steals an electron from another molecule and produces harmful effects. Free radicals are formed when molecules within cells react with oxygen (oxidize) as part of normal metabolic processes. Free radicals then begin to break down cells, especially if there are not enough free radical quenching nutrients, such as vitamins C and E, in the cell. While free radicals are normal products of metabolism, uncontrolled free radical production plays a major role in the development of degenerative disease, including cancer, heart disease, and aging. Free radicals alter important molecules, such as proteins, enzymes, fats, even DNA. Other sources of free radicals include pesticides, industrial pollutants, smoking, alcohol, viruses, most infections, allergies, stress, even certain foods and excessive exercise.

- **Beta carotene:** Beta carotene is the centerpiece of the antioxidant program. "The trick is to use natural beta carotene and to give *all* the supporting nutrients that allow the carotene to be converted to vitamin A," explains Dr. Atkins. When cancer is present, the dosage level approaches 100,000 IU.
- **Vitamin C:** This is the other most commonly used antioxidant. A daily dose of 10 g of vitamin C significantly extended the survival and improved the quality of life in 100 terminal cancer patients.[12] A typical Atkins dose is 10 g daily.
- **Vitamin E:** This vitamin is among the major nutrients required for a strong immune response.[13] A typical Atkins dose is 600 IU daily.
- **Selenium:** This mineral works in concert with vitamin E and has numerous anticancer effects; it is often

deficient in cancer patients.[14] Selenium works synergistically with vitamin E, meaning that the effects of one nutrient greatly enhance the effects of the other. A study by Harvard's Walter Willett, Ph.D., and colleagues in Linxian, China, found that supplementation with selenium, vitamin E, and beta carotene, led to a 13% reduction in cancer deaths. A typical dose is 50 mcg daily.

- **L-cysteine:** Cancer patients receiving amygdalin may require this sulfur-containing amino acid supplement to supply the sulfur necessary to convert cyanide (found in amygdalin) to a harmless compound called thiocyanate.[15] Cysteine assists in various detoxification processes and reduces the toxic side effects of both chemotherapy and radiation treatments.[16]
- **N-acetyl cysteine:** Cysteine needs may be better met by N-acetyl cysteine, since over 80% of the orally ingested dose of cysteine, but not N-acetyl cysteine, is inactivated by stomach acid. Thus N-acetyl cysteine provides more precursor for the production of glutathione, which serves in the key antioxidant system called glutathione peroxidase. Blood levels of glutathione peroxidase tend to decrease after the sixth decade of life and are typically lower in patients with malignant cancers.[17]
- **Lipoic Acid:** Dr. Atkins is enthusiastic about lipoic acid, a recently studied nutritional antioxidant, because of its ability to protect other antioxidants from degradation. "With lipoic acid, moderate doses of antioxidants become equivalent to high doses, and the entire concept of a 'team' of antioxidants becomes a reality," Dr. Atkins states. In other words, lipoic acid evidently increases the effectiveness or potency of other antioxidants. A typical dose is 400 mg daily.
- **Coenzyme Q10:** Also known as CoQ10 or ubiquinone, this substance protects the heart from the toxic effects of chemotherapy and has various immune-enhancing effects. The usual Atkins dose is 200-300 mg daily, dissolved in oil.
- **Bioflavonoids:** These are a group of brightly colored compounds commonly found in food alongside vitamin C; they aid mainly in blood vessel repair and help prevent bruising easily. Among the better known bioflavonoids are citrin, hesperidin, rutin, quercetin,

and pycnogenol. Some bioflavonoids support the cancer-fighting activities of vitamin C, while Japanese research has found that quercetin dramatically inhibits the growth of human stomach cancer cells.[18] Amounts of bioflavonoids will vary depending on the supplement and individual factors, says Dr. Atkins.

Plant-based antioxidants, such as medicinal mushrooms (maitake, reishi, and shiitake), genistein from soybeans, and green tea are also on Dr. Atkins' checklist. "Antioxidants were at one time thought to counteract the effects of chemotherapy and radiation," says Dr. Atkins. "We now know that they actually enhance their positive, cancer-killing effects while protecting the body from their more adverse effects. They are a huge part of the body's anticancer defenses."

**Shark Cartilage**—To grow, all tumors require the development of new blood vessels, a process known as *angiogenesis.* Cartilage is a tough, elastic connective tissue that does not develop a blood supply because it contains various "anti-angiogenic" substances. "Shark cartilage seems to prevent tumors from creating their own blood supply," Dr. Atkins says. "As long as your body receives a hefty daily dose, you can keep tumors from growing." Dr. Atkins recommends 3 ounces of pulverized shark cartilage daily. An interesting alternative is a derivative called Car-T Cell in which one vial containing ½ tablespoon of defrosted frozen active extract is taken daily under the tongue.

**Essiac**—Preferably used as an herbal tea, Essiac has the following benefits: (1) strengthens the immune system; (2) reduces the toxic side effects of many drugs; (3) increases energy levels; and (4) diminishes inflammatory processes.[19] "Essiac is a therapeutic tea that all cancer patients can benefit from," says Dr. Atkins. "Such benefits may be mild in advanced-stage cancer therapy, but they can also contribute to feelings of well-being which in turn influence the patient's quality of life and potential for recovery." Most patients take 2-3 ounces of potent Essiac, added to herbal tea and taken daily, according to Dr. Atkins.

**Cat's Claw (*Uña de Gato*)**—In Dr. Atkins' opinion, the rain forest herb cat's claw has actually surpassed the therapeutic effectiveness of such prominent anticancer herbs as astragalus, *Echinacea*, and goldenseal. "The available research suggests that 3-6 g per day can be used for therapeutic dosages," says Dr. Atkins. "It would not be unthinkable to use doses of up to 20 g a day in initiating treatment on advanced cases."

**Hoxsey Herbs**—Originally developed by herbal healer Harry Hoxsey, this therapy involves a selection of herbal preparations which seem to work well together. The major component of the Hoxsey internal tonic is potassium iodide. The herbs include red clover, buckthorn bark, burdock root (which has known antimutagenic properties[20]), stillingia root, berberis root, poke berries and root, licorice root, *Cascara amarga*, and prickly ash bark. "Although these herbs have never been rigorously studied or tested," says Dr. Atkins, "decades of observation attest to their potential merit. None of my patients have had adverse reactions to the treatment, and many seemed to get better."

**Maitake "D" Fraction**—Medicinal mushrooms have considerable research behind them showing prolongation of life and enhancement of other therapies, says Dr. Atkins. "I was impressed by the animal-based research of maitake 'D' fraction; it looks like the most effective of available medicinal mushrooms."

**Wholesome Diet**—Dr. Atkins recommends following a sugarless diet, based on the recommendations of Nobel Prize winner Otto Warburg, Ph.D., who demonstrated that cancer cells almost always depend upon oxygen-free (anaerobic) nutrition, for which sugar is the primary fuel. Dr. Atkins believes that Dr. Warburg's theories were given major additional significance by an Israeli study showing that cancer cells contain 3 times the amount of insulin as normal cells. "This is silent proof that cancer feeds on glucose," Dr. Atkins notes. He recommends that his patients avoid processed, refined foods and that they use organically grown vegetables (preferably eaten raw) to maximize the absorption of their living enzyme content.

He is reluctant to recommend a low-protein diet because "so much of the biochemistry of the immune system is based on amino acids, found in protein." However, raw foods are emphasized and moderately cooked foods are also included. High-fiber foods, such as lima beans and kale, require cooking to be more palatable and digestible. "Light or moderate cooking is helpful in making nutrients available to the body," says Dr. Atkins. "Both the wholesomeness and unadulterated nature of the food is important. You don't want to cook away the food values nor should you restrict yourself to fresh juices."

## Cultivating the Psyche That Can Overcome Cancer

Dr. Atkins says that illness is either worsened or improved by your frame of mind. His therapies work to enhance the person's mood and attitude thereby facilitating the healing process. In contrast, conventional treatments tend to make people feel ill, so that they are more likely to become depressed and anxious during the therapy. "Being made sick from radiation or chemotherapy then sitting in a waiting room where others seem even sicker certainly won't uplift your spirits," says Dr. Atkins. "It might even lead you to believe the situation is hopeless."

> ***"Cancer patients beginning our program stop feeling they're all alone," Dr. Atkins says. "They begin to acquire more of a 'fighting spirit' attitude toward their cancer, which is the strongest psychological component of all for promoting survival."***

Dr. Atkins insists that his patients receive the IV program not just for its biological benefits, but also for the psychological support derived from interactions with the Atkins Center staff. During the IV treatments, newcomer cancer patients have an opportunity to talk with staff and patients who have overcome their cancer, and to cultivate a winner's attitude. "Many of these patients come from Memorial Sloan-Kettering and other conventional cancer treatment institutions which give them very poor prognoses," says Dr. Atkins. "They're told they have 4 to 9 months to live, and unfortunately, this often becomes a self-fulfilling prophecy."

At the Atkins Center, everyone expects the patient to get well and stay well. Their attitude is this: "You don't have to 'buy' the gloomy prognosis given by conventional medicine, because you have chosen not to be a part of their world. Rather, you are a survivor; you are beating this cancer; you are turning it around through these treatments and the changes you have made in your life." On most occasions, people who have clearly improved through the treatment or who have already recovered make themselves available to the Atkins Center to provide positive reinforcement for struggling patients.

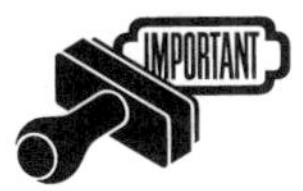


"Cancer patients who are beginning our program stop feeling that they're all alone," Dr. Atkins says. "They also begin to feel that they are special, and that they're doing things in a special way. It's important for their self-esteem and overall attitude to feel this way." At the same time, the cancer patients begin to feel fortunate that they have made the *correct* choice—a choice that would have been denied them had they stayed under conventional care. They begin to acquire more of a "fighting spirit" attitude toward their cancer, which is the strongest psychological component of all for promoting survival, explains Dr. Atkins.

In many cases, on the basis of his initial interview, Dr. Atkins can predict who will and who will not survive cancer. "Survival is not based so much on the severity of the disease as on the patient's *attitude*," says Dr. Atkins. "This is why we're more concerned with knowing the person than the disease, its symptoms, mechanisms, or complications." In Dr. Atkins' experience, cancer survivors almost invariably have the following characteristics: (1) they do not succumb to the destructive intimidation of orthodox medicine; and (2) they adopt a fundamental this-is-not-my time-so-cancer-I'm getting-rid-of-you attitude. On the whole, the act of choosing a therapy and believing strongly in its therapeutic value are keys to successful cancer treatment.

## Alternative Therapies Plus Limited, Careful Use of Conventional Means

Although Dr. Atkins believes strongly that the first line of therapy for cancer patients should be nontoxic natural medicine, he will take patients whose immune systems have been dangerously suppressed by conventional drug and radiation treatments. "As a consequence, their ability to recover is virtually obliterated by the drugs and radiation, and then they turn up in the very last stages and say, 'Help me out—conventional medicine isn't working,'" says Dr. Atkins.

Yet the either-or question many patients ask—"should I go with orthodox treatment or alternative treatment?"—is off the mark. This question is like asking which half of the card deck a person wants to play with, says Dr. Atkins. "As long as both halves are there, let's play with the whole deck," he says. "Patients with cancer who seek either orthodox or alternative approaches are entrusting their lives to doctors who are playing with half a

## Did Conventional Cancer Medicine Kill Jackie Kennedy before Her Time?

Jackie Kennedy's fight with cancer is one of Dr. Atkins' favorite examples of how conventional medicine mistreats cancer. "From the very beginning, orthodox oncologists take an illness which has a 50/50 chance of reversal and by their actions they seem to say, we're either going to cure her or kill her. Early in the course of her treatment, they began pouring chemotherapy into her brain." When this intensely toxic treatment failed, the illness was able to run away like a brushfire. It led to the rapid demise of Jackie Kennedy, which is virtually unheard of in an untreated case of lymphoma.

Dr. Atkins points out that the same kind of mistreatment nearly occurred with the late baseball player, Mickey Mantle, who died from lung cancer and complications related to conventional treatment. "As weak as Mantle was in the final weeks, some of his doctors wanted to give him even more chemotherapy," Dr. Atkins says. "They were absolutely determined to use every toxic weapon in their arsenal, without really understanding how his body's natural defenses would be compromised." In Dr. Atkins' view, modern oncology still has a long way to go before it learns to adhere to the Hippocratic dictum of "first, do no harm."

deck."[21] In most cases of cancer, Dr. Atkins says that a *complementary* approach is needed, one which emphasizes alternative therapies along with limited and judicious use of conventional methods.

Although Dr. Atkins contends it is a fallacy to think all cancer resides within the boundaries of a tumor, he does find a role for surgery on a case-by-case basis. He finds it rarely appropriate in prostate cancer, but in breast cancer, for example, surgery can be appropriate, where possible. "Surgical removal of breast tumors can lead to a complete remission of breast cancer," says Dr. Atkins. "Chemotherapy and radiation are completely unwarranted in this situation, and surgery alone, when combined with our integrated immune-enhancement and detoxification program, is almost always sufficient for curing breast cancer."

Dr. Atkins regards chemotherapy as otherwise dangerous and best avoided in treating the majority of cancers. "Only in situations in which chemotherapy is proven to be effective and curative would I recommend it," he says. "In general, this might be testicular cancer, many children's tumors, and extreme cases of Hodgkin's lymphoma. On the other hand, Ukrain can do everything chemotherapy does but without any side effects, so it renders chemotherapy largely unnecessary."

Radiation treatments are typically futile, too, says Dr. Atkins. "In some cases, however, we need to shrink tumors if they're encroaching or impinging on more vital parts of the body. In that case, a combination of radiation and hyperthermia [heat treatment delivered by ultrasound or microwave] can be effective." Dr. Atkins was among the first doctors in the U.S. to successfully combine radiation with hyperthermia (heat treatment) to help treat prostate cancer.

For more information about **heat therapy** (hyperthermia), see Chapter 33: Physical Support Therapies, pp. 996-1000.

Another option for localized tumor destruction that Dr. Atkins prefers to radiation is called Accelerated Charge Neutralization (ACN). The principle of ACN is to locate the skin area of greatest electrical differential (the difference between negative and positive charges) caused by the tumor, then to administer electrical current of the opposite charge. "This modality is perfectly safe, can destroy tumors, and works synergistically with heat therapy (hyperthermia)," says Dr. Atkins.

***In most cases of cancer, Dr. Atkins says that a complementary approach is needed, one which emphasizes alternative therapies along with limited and judicious use of conventional methods.***

## CURRICULUM VITAE

# Keith I. Block, M.D.

Block Medical Center, 1800 Sherman Avenue,
Suite 515, Evanston, IL 60201;
tel: 847-492-3040; fax: 847-492-3045.

Dr. Block received his M.D. from the University of Miami School of Medicine. In addition to his private practice, Dr. Block is medical director of the Cancer Institute Program at Edgewater Medical Center in Chicago, Illinois; he is also research assistant professor of nutrition and medical dietetics at the University of Illinois and clinical instructor at the University of Illinois College of Medicine in Chicago. Dr. Block is a member of 7 medical societies and author of numerous medical papers on cancer treatment. He lectures frequently on complementary and alternative medicine topics to scientific groups and the public. From 1987-1990, Dr. Block served as medical consultant on nutrition oncology research to the Office of Technology Assessment (OTA) for the U.S. Congress during which time he wrote a key paper on nutrition as an essential tool in cancer care. Dr. Block was also a member of the committee assessing alternative therapies for OTA.

***"I've seen many people overcome illness even when nobody thought they had a chance," says Dr. Block. "I help my patients cultivate the ability to take charge of their health and well-being. Physicians need to propose a treatment plan that the cancer patient can psychologically, culturally, and socially accept."***

Chapter 2

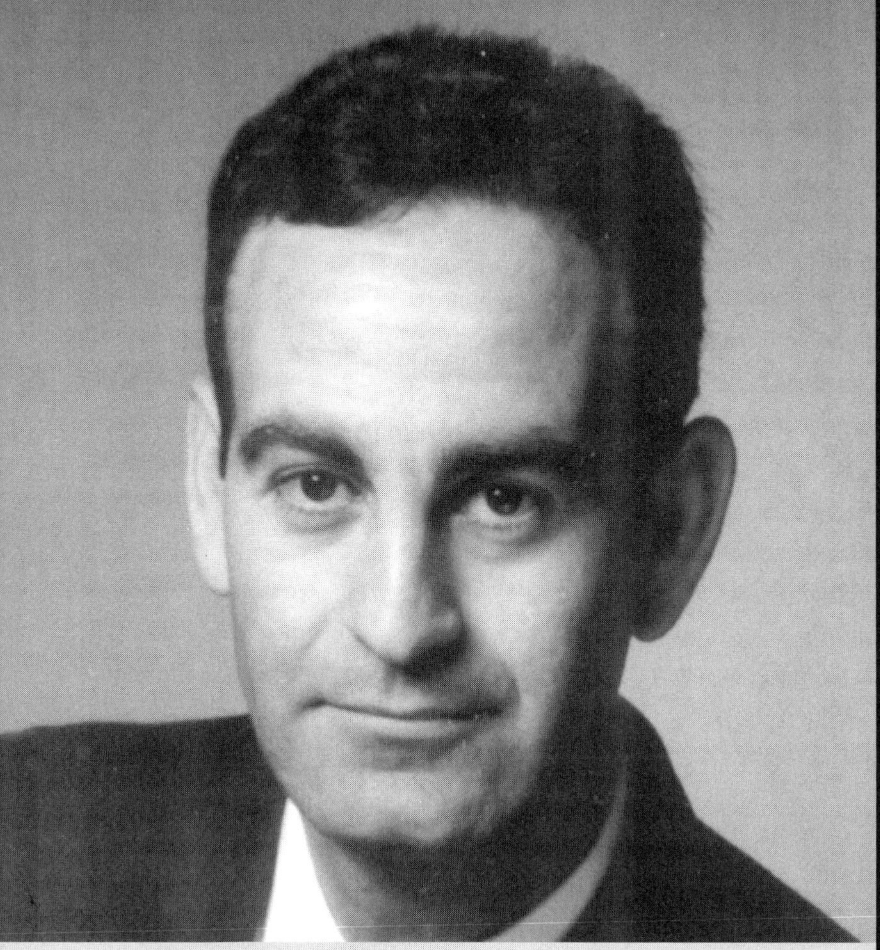

# *Keith I. Block, M.D.*

**NO MATTER WHAT KIND OF CANCER** you're treating, for the most successful outcome, Keith Block, M.D., considers it essential to flush all the toxins out of the body through major dietary changes and a multifaceted detoxification program that "cleans" the liver, kidneys, lung, lymph, and skin.

Keith I. Block, M.D., is fast becoming to cancer care what Dean Ornish, M.D., now is to the field of cardiovascular care—a highly regarded bridge-builder between conventional and alternative medicine. Dr. Block, who directs the Block Medical Center in Evanston, Illinois, is a pioneering practitioner with an impressive background in scientific research and clinical work, who embraces an integrated, no-nonsense approach to cancer treatment.

Since the 1970s, when he began exploring nutrition as a cancer treatment and as a component of both noninvasive and conventional therapies, Dr. Block has treated many thousands of cancer patients. He believes that in some cases a blending of both conventional and alternative treatments may be the only way to keep patients alive.

Dr. Block's staff includes professionals trained in oncology, nursing, psychology, physical care, biofeedback, lifestyle therapy, dietetics, herbal medicine, functional food and phytonutrient research, laboratory analyses, and clinical research.

## Medical Gradualism: Fortifying the Body So Treatments Can Succeed

Dr. Block calls the philosophy that guides his approach to cancer "medical gradualism." In his view, treatment should generally begin with the least invasive therapies, moving only incrementally up the stepladder toward more invasive therapies, and even then only as absolutely needed and as the informed *patient*, not the physician, chooses (though with the physi-

# Dr. Block's Generalized Model for Cancer Treatment

| STRATEGY | DOSAGE/ KEY COMPONENTS | FOR MORE INFORMATION see page # |
|---|---|---|
| **Nutritional Support** | | |
| Diet: grains, fruits, vegetables, proteins and fats | determined by body composition, food grouping exchange lists | 749 |
| Multivitamin, antioxidant, and other recommended supplements | determined on an individual basis | 784 |
| Cruciferous vegetables | 2-3 servings daily | 58 |
| Onion group vegetables | 1-2 servings daily | 58 |
| Sea vegetables (for radiation patients, optional for others) | 2-3 servings per week or 1-2 kelp tablets daily | 809 |
| Caffeine, alcohol, refined sugar, junk food | avoid all | 58 |
| **Liver/Digestive System Support** | | |
| MDS Fiber supplement | 1 scoop mixed with water or juice, either with or apart from meals | 58 |
| MDS Botanical supplement | 2 tablets, 3x/day with meals | 58 |
| MDS Enzyme supplement | 2 tablets, 3x/day with meals | 59 |
| MDS Antioxidant supplement | 1 tsp, 3x/day with meals | 59 |
| **Kidney Support** | | |
| Pure water (spring water) | 60-64 ounces daily | 791 |
| Diluted fruit juice, vegetable juices, herb teas (ginger, goldenrod, chamomile, passionflower), kukicha tea (noncaffeine variety) | up to half of your daily fluid intake (60-64 oz) may consist of these liquids | 60 |
| **Lung and Skin Support** | | |
| Deep breathing | 10 minutes, 2x/day | 60 |
| Aerobic exercise | 30 minutes daily, longer or shorter as tolerated | 60 |
| Saunas (with added fluid and electrolyte intake) | as physical condition allows | 60 |

*Continued*

## Dr. Block's Generalized Model for Cancer Treatment (cont.)

| STRATEGY | DOSAGE/ KEY COMPONENTS | FOR MORE INFORMATION see page # |
|---|---|---|
| Baths | 20 minutes, 3x/week; may include sea salt or Dead Sea salt mixtures | 61 |
| **Blood and Lymph Support** | | |
| Diet as outlined | see "Nutritional Support" | |
| Goldenseal (MDS botanical supplement) | see "Liver/Digestive System Support" | |
| *Gingko biloba* extract (for radiation patients) | 40-mg tablets, 3x/day, for at least 2 months after radiation therapy | 820 |
| **Other Components of Dr. Block's Approach** | | |
| Physical care | gentle, centering exercises such as yoga, tai chi, Qigong, focused breathing, and walking. Mild aerobic activities, muscle and maintenance regimens, all individually tailored | 65, 1003, 1005 |
| Psychosocial and psychotherapeutic support | support groups, individualized counseling, cognitive restructuring, guided imagery, meditation, self-hypnosis, biofeedback | 66 |
| Reasonable alternative cancer treatments | selections are variable, depending on individual perceptions of efficacy as well as on research, safety, and clinical observation | 64 |
| Medical care | conventional approaches are utilized in a "gradualistic" plan combined with complementary strategies intended to diminish side effects while enhancing efficacy. | 62 |

cian's input). To make this work, Block encourages his patients to undergo 3-14 days of special education, including options for therapy, how to follow a balanced therapeutic diet, maintain a tailored fitness program, cope effectively with stress, and use imagery, brain-wave biofeedback, and cognitive restructuring to activate the brain and immune system.

This strategy gives patients confidence and breathing space within which to select a treatment plan that satisfies not only their physical needs, such as a stronger immune system, but their emotional, personal, and social needs. With the doctor's coaching, each patient then chooses whatever treatment and lifestyle changes they find most appropriate. This tack enables cancer patients to become more engaged in their own care—an invaluable aspect of accessing their inner healing resources.

Dr. Block routinely has his patients undergo an extensive series of biochemical, nutritional, immune, and detoxification analyses. He advocates the cautious and highly selective use of conventional therapy with a precise and innovative complementary system of care. Highly invasive procedures are avoided whenever possible, but when a person is faced with an aggressive cancer, Dr. Block and his extended staff (which includes surgeons and other specialists) may recommend surgery or even chemotherapy.

**CAUTION**

This chapter includes information regarding actual treatments used by Dr. Block only after his careful diagnosis of each patient. All cancer patients are unique. **Do not administer these treatments to yourself or others.** Discuss these treatments with your physician or other qualified health-care professional. Readers should not interpret this material as therapeutic advice, but should see a physician in all cases.

If such procedures are used, however, he then does everything possible to prevent adverse side effects through the use of a carefully and individually tailored complementary approach. This includes a substance-specific and disease-specific detoxification system, including selective foods, oral and intravenous supplementation, botanicals, phytonutrients, and body fitness strategies.

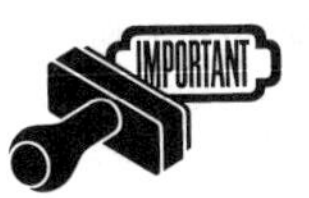


Dr. Block acknowledges that cancer patients may die not from the cancer as such, but from the side effects of conventional treatment. "Chemotherapy, radiation, and surgery can be extremely harsh on the body," Dr. Block says. "Not only do they have direct negative effects on immunity, but often the body becomes overly toxic and malnourished as a result of the treatment." Most patients are not offered the option by oncologists of receiving these treatments in *smaller* doses and *slower* infusion rates or of taking steps to protect their immune systems.

Dr. Block's complementary strategy uses conventional therapy to reduce the tumor burden (the volume of the tumor, which determines how much of a toxic and immune-suppressive effect it has) while fortifying the body to fight the cancer at the cellular level. Dr. Block's use of chemotherapy is cautious and individualized, generally based on fractionated or smaller infusing dosages administered over an extended period. His program not only protects the body but actually *enhances* the intended effects of conventional treatment.

"I've seen time and again how much better cancer patients tolerate and respond to chemotherapy and radiation with the right support," Dr. Block says. "This seems related to the ability of nutrients, phytochemicals, and other substances to reduce or even reverse the free-radical damage and toxicities that result from radiation and chemotherapy."

To stimulate immune function and further counteract specific problems resulting from toxic cancer therapies, Dr. Block recommends a variety of "Innovative Low-Invasive Therapies," or ILITs, as he calls them. These include the individually tailored use of agents such as omega-3 fatty acids, garlic, *Echinacea*, astragalus, *Gingko biloba*, Siberian or Panax ginseng, antioxidant vitamins, minerals, and *Acidophilus*. More selective use of compounds such as DHEA, melatonin, genistein (soybean derivative), and others are considered as well, says Dr. Block.

***"Most patients are not offered the option by oncologists of receiving [radiation or chemotherapy] in*** **smaller** ***doses and*** **slower** ***infusion rates or of taking steps to protect their immune systems," says Dr. Block.***

Before determining which supplements are most suitable, Dr. Block evaluates patients extensively in terms of many key parameters. These include their pro-oxidant levels (a measure of how much free-radical damage they may be incurring), DNA damage and repair status, hormonal and immune status, toxic levels and detoxification capacities, nutrient balances, phytochemical levels, body composition (analyzing body fat relative to lean tissue, which in turn relates to immune function), and other key factors that influence recovery. Additionally, ear (auricular) acupuncture and micro-electrical stimulation therapy (a technique used primarily for drug-free pain relief) are part of Dr. Block's program.

Such tests enable Dr. Block to individually tailor a treatment program in primary areas, such as nutrition, body and mind fitness, supplements, stress management, and medical care. The supplement program includes antioxidants, detoxifiers, gut wall enhancers (substances that help maintain the integrity of the digestive tract, thereby reducing potential stress on the immune system), immune stimulators, adaptogens (substances that make the body more resilient to stress), and hormonal agents. All the supplements, which were designed by Dr. Block and his staff, contain a unique phytochemical-rich base, rapidly dissolve in the digestive tract (within 5-15 minutes), and are readily absorbed.

## SUCCESS STORY

### Reversing Breast Cancer

Lisa, aged 44, was a chemist with a lifelong habit of eating high-fat foods and pushing herself to workaholic extremes. In addition to working full time, she was a single mother raising 3 children. When she was diagnosed with breast cancer, she agreed to the orthodox strategy of surgery and chemotherapy.

Following these treatments, Lisa decided to forgo the radiation treatment her surgeon had recommended because, as she put it, "the chemotherapy had already left me feeling so weak. To have radiation on top of this felt like too much for my system to handle. I figured the chemotherapy was better than nothing." Three years later, the cancer returned with a vengeance, this time metastasizing to Lisa's bones.

A new bone scan revealed that cancer had permeated both sides of her rib cage and seemed to be moving into her spine. Several specialists told her nothing could be done and that she probably had less than a year to live. At this point, Lisa had arrived at a crossroads of decision: Should she receive the same treatments as before and hope for the best? Or should she look for ways to support her body's self-healing abilities?

The next month, Lisa visited Dr. Block and found that his integrated system of nutrition, botanicals, phytochemicals, tailored exercise, and personalized stress management appealed to her. She was also attracted by his limited and judicious use of chemotherapy with the support of a variety of noninvasive or low-invasive methods intended to diminish side effects while attempting to boost effectiveness.

Within days of beginning Dr. Block's program, Lisa began to feel more energized and enthusiastic. Ten months into the program, her bone cancer was markedly reduced. Though for several months she continued to take an anti-estrogen drug (Tamoxifen, a drug that blocks estrogen's effects on tumor growth), she later discontinued it, with Dr. Block's approval, due to unrelenting side effects.

Lisa followed his dietary and lifestyle advice, even attending his intensive health-education seminars in nutrition, cooking, therapeutic fitness, medicinal herbs, and stress reduction, along with training sessions in nutrition, detoxification, meditation, imagery, cognitive restructuring (reorienting self-destructive values and belief systems), and personally tailored fitness techniques to fortify her immune system.

Eager to do anything further that might help her recover her health, Lisa participated in a 3-day seminar offered by Dr. Block and his staff. The first step in bolstering her immune system was diet. "The biggest change for me was the new diet," Lisa says. "In the past, I was always skinny and wanted to gain weight, so I ate a lot of rich food, especially high-fat dairy products."

Exercise and relaxation were vital aspects of Lisa's recovery as well. She practiced a series of slow, contemplative movements which Dr. Block taught her, and she engaged in regular bicycling and walking. "These activities were very relaxing to me," Lisa recalls. "I did them a lot, especially during the first couple of years." Lisa's efforts paid off in a big way. After 16 months on the Block program, new CT and bone scans and blood tests revealed that all of Lisa's cancer had disappeared. More than 13 years later, she feels better than ever. "My life feels much more balanced now," Lisa says.

## SUCCESS STORY

### Reversing Prostate Cancer

Ethan, aged 66, was a retired sales administrator with a lifelong "junk food" habit and a "couch-potato" existence that left him overweight. The impetus to change all this started when he was diagnosed with prostate cancer. During the first 2 years after learning he had cancer, Ethan followed the standard hormone therapy (estrogen) as suggested by his doctor, taking 3 diethylstilbestrol pills daily. Every 6 months Ethan underwent a bone scan and a prostate exam, both of which showed little or no improvement in his condition.

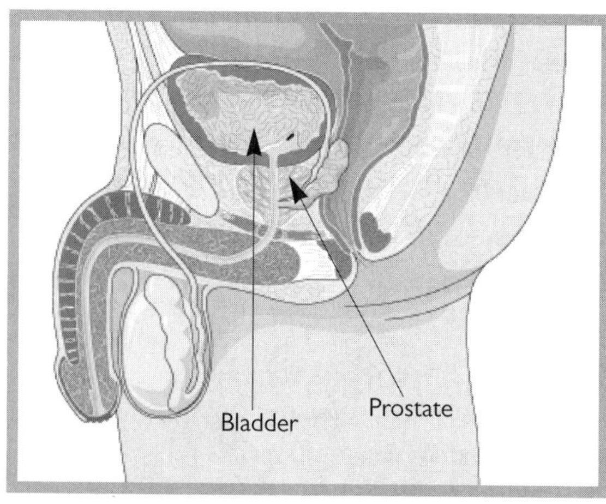


**Figure 2.1—The prostate gland**

At the end of the first 2 years, the severity of his condition was driven home to him when a bone scan showed that the cancer in his prostate gland had spread to the bones in his pelvis, forehead, ribs, spine, and thoracic area. According to his oncologist, Ethan's prognosis was extremely poor. Serendipitously, he happened on a *Saturday Evening Post* story of Anthony Sattilaro, M.D., who recovered from metastatic prostate cancer using the macrobiotic diet. Soon Ethan began his own macrobiotic diet, cutting out all meats, dairy foods, refined sugars and flours, caffeine, and alcohol. He immediately began to feel much better. Upon the advice of his doctor, Ethan stopped taking hormones.

When Ethan consulted Dr. Keith Block for the first time, Dr. Block discovered that Ethan's health was on the downswing. Based on his analysis of current and previous CT scans, Dr. Block saw that Ethan now had progressive bone metastases. At Dr. Block's suggestion, Ethan used the Block program to make adjustments in his health recovery. He took up the dietary adjustments, aerobic exercises, and relaxation techniques. About 6 months later, all of Ethan's bone scans were clear of cancer. A biopsy also showed no evidence of cancer cells in the prostate.

Seven years later, Ethan remained active both physically and socially, and during a visit to Dr. Block, no signs of cancer could be found. A total of 16 years after his initial diagnosis of prostate cancer, Ethan says: "I'm well aware of what eating a proper diet has done for me. It not only cured me of cancer, but controlled my weight and relieved my hypertension, for which I had been on medication for 42 years."

## Individually Tailored Cancer Treatment Programs

Lisa's recovery from breast cancer and Ethan's from prostate cancer are among many long-term, cancer survival success stories achieved by Dr. Block. Speaking before an audience of doctors and researchers at a cancer symposium called Adjuvant Nutrition for Cancer Treatment, Dr. Block described results from his pilot study of 10 long-term cancer survivors. The study was designed to assess his patients' adherence to the program, such as the foods they ate most often, how much they exercised, and how well they handled stress.

**_Developing a positive attitude and a life-affirming conviction are the starting points for Dr. Block's approach._**

"We certainly aren't claiming any grand answer to cancer," Dr. Block said. But the 10 patients whose cases he recounted all had metastatic cancer—it had spread to other sites and had become more aggressive—and most had been given less than a year to live. Under Dr. Block's care, they continue to thrive, on average, 8 years beyond their previous doctors' predictions.

Developing a positive attitude and a life-affirming conviction are the starting points for Dr. Block's approach. "I've seen many people overcome illness even when nobody thought they had a chance," he says. "I help my patients cultivate the ability to take charge of their health and well-being." For example, before entering the Block Medical Center, patients complete an 18-page attitude-and-behavior questionnaire which enables Dr. Block's team to steer people toward an individually tailored regimen that recognizes as much who the patient is as what condition they have. "Physicians need to propose a treatment plan that the cancer patient can psychologically, culturally, and socially accept," says Dr. Block.

## Two Keys to Cancer Reversal

- A 15-year study by Steven Greer, M.D., found that women who show a "fighting spirit" or a spirited, combative attitude may have a significant survival advantage compared to those who succumb to emotional passivity and helplessness.[1]
- Cancer patients treated in Japan, where low-fat diets are the norm, survived twice as long as a comparable group of cancer patients in the U.S.[2] Swedish researchers have found that raising the fat-calorie content of the diet by just 10%, the rate of breast cancer recurrence increases 4 to 8 times.[3]

By definition, Dr. Block's individually tailored program does not apply to every person with cancer. His recommendations, as presented here, are based on interviews with half a dozen of his patients, each with a different treatment plan determined by their specific conditions, previous diet and medication histories, activity levels, social and personal considerations, environmental factors, and lab test results.

Thus, the overview here is a generic representation or composite of the variety of Dr. Block's guidelines. "Recommendations will differ markedly from patient to patient, obvious examples including differences from bedridden patients to someone who is able to exercise regularly," Dr. Block comments. "Similarly, cancer patients who practice daily meditation or prayer may benefit more from participating in support groups. In every case, it's essential to determine what programs or activities the patient feels most *supported* by and to emphasize these."

Most cancer patients have received substantial doses of toxic drugs and most have been exposed to high levels of toxic contaminants in their food, air, and water. These toxins, still residing in the body's tissues, should be removed to enhance the cancer patient's ability to recover. One part of Dr. Block's basic treatment program includes his Metabolic Detoxification System (MDS) and calls for clinical work in 5 areas: (1) diet and nutritional support; (2) liver and digestive support; (3) kidney support; (4) lung and skin support; and (5) blood and lymph support.

Dr. Block considers this scientifically formulated detoxification program essential for cancer patients, particularly for those receiving toxic conventional therapies. In fact, he believes that much of the side effects and lack of effectiveness of conventional treatments are due to the buildup of toxic by-products (metabolites) from these drug therapies.

## MDS #1: DIET AND NUTRITIONAL SUPPORT

For information on **diet and nutritional support**, see Chapter 28: Nutrition as Cancer Medicine.

While attitude and medical care are fundamental, food is the foundation of Dr. Block's cancer treatment program and changing one's diet is a first step toward healing. "You can't compromise on a healing diet when it comes to cancer, nor can you cancel out harmful dietary habits with supplements," Dr. Block says. His dietary approach has several goals: (1) to maintain adequate nutritional support in order to improve patients' quality of life and "to help them retain a sense of self-empowerment" or personal autonomy; (2) to enhance patients' resistance to cancer by bolstering immunity and inhibiting tumor growth; and (3) to diminish the side effects of conventional treatments.

Dr. Block spent 3 years developing a scientific and practical set of food-exchange lists, which are food groupings organized by nutrient and calorie content. This system allows people to quantify their food intake according to their specific nutritional needs. The Block diet is a medically sound, modified-macrobiotic approach (a diet centered around whole grains, fruits and vegetables, adequate protein from beans, soy products, and fish, and various naturally fermented products).

Dr. Block's version of this well-known dietary system consists of five groups of foods: whole grains; protein foods (legumes and fish); vegetables (broccoli, kale, collards, as well as yellow, orange, and red vegetables such as carrots, squashes, and peppers); fruits (minimal use of citrus); and specified use of type and quantity of fats (classified as a separate category).

***People who have advanced or aggressive forms of cancer are particularly vulnerable to the ill effects of high-fat foods, says Dr. Block.***

In the diet, 50 to 60% of calories are derived from complex carbohydrates (mainly grains), 12 to 25% of calories from fat, and the remainder from protein sources. Adjustments according to individual needs is determined by ongoing composition analyses using an infrared device that helps gauge the amount of body fat relative to lean tissue (the latter being more important to cancer resistance). Dr. Block advocates the regular use of various "power foods"—broccoli and other cruciferous vegetables, sea vegetables, maitake and shiitake mushrooms, and soy products—that are particularly rich in cancer-repelling phytochemicals (anticancer substances derived from plants).

For more on **omega 3 and 6 oils**, see Chapter 28: Nutrition as Cancer Medicine, pp. 768-771; for **soy**, see Chapter 29: Botanicals as Cancer Medicines, pp. 824-825.

For pragmatic reasons, Block classifies fat as a food group. If you don't do this, he says, cancer patients will allow their fat intake (both quantity and type) to get seriously out of hand. High-fat diets not only predispose people to cancer—recall Lisa's penchant for high-fat foods prior to being diagnosed with breast cancer—they also greatly limit the cancer patient's chances of recovery. People who have advanced or aggressive forms of cancer are particularly vulnerable to the ill effects of high-fat foods.

"Dietary fat is definitely a factor in cancer," Dr. Block says. "In advanced breast cancer, as you increase the amount of dietary fat, you greatly increase the progression of disease and risk of death. A person on a mainly vegan [no animal or dairy products] diet tends to repel cancer far more successfully than someone on a high-fat diet." In fact, Dr. Block's research shows that vegans have 2.5 times the cancer-killing potential as omnivores.

The fat content of the Block diet is quite low, representing only 12 to 25% of the diet's total caloric value, depending on need, treatment, and stage of disease. A fat content of about 15% is Dr. Block's general advice to most patients. A pure vegan diet is encouraged for those who are able and willing; however, Dr. Block also provides a modified, semi-vegetarian diet for patients desiring an easier transition.

In any case, the low-fat content does not put them at greater risk of lean tissue loss which would worsen the cancer patient's prognosis. Instead, as noted by an independent reviewer, few of Dr. Block's patients "experience weight loss, except those with anorexia in late stages of disease, or experience hair loss during chemotherapy."[4]

As indicated, Dr. Block regards the type of fat to be as important as the quantity of fat. Dietary fat intake should be primarily of the omega-3 variety (named according to a convention of biochemisty; the number three refers to the position of the first double bond along the carbon chain of the fatty acid molecule), since these fats inhibit tumor promotion and may prolong survival; omega 9 in the form of olive oil is also acceptable.

Corn oil, safflower oil, and other oils higher in omega-6 fatty acids are strictly avoided, since these oils enhance the production of certain cancer-promoting substances, or "bad eicosanoids," such as prostaglandin E2. Canola, sesame, and olive oil are recommended—in moderation—while flax and walnut oils (both excellent sources of omega-3 fats, sources of "good eicosanoids" or cancer-repelling substances) are good as well.

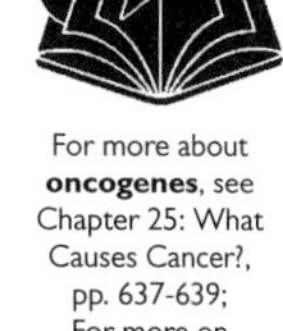

For more about **oncogenes**, see Chapter 25: What Causes Cancer?, pp. 637-639; For more on **detoxification**, see Chapter 33: Physical Support Therapies for Reversing Cancer, pp. 949-980.

**Phase I/Phase II liver detoxification** is the natural two-step process the liver conducts to rid the body of toxins. During Phase I, the liver converts toxic compounds into intermediate toxins. In Phase II, the liver converts these intermediate toxins into substances that can be eliminated from the body, delivering them to the colon (via the gallbladder) or bladder for excretion.

Soy products are among the staples of the Block diet. The long-term survivors' study revealed that all the patients consumed soy products on a regular basis. According to Dr. Block, soy contains numerous cancer-fighting compounds, including the isoflavone genistein (a potent antioxidant and inhibitor of estrogen's tumor-promoting ability). Both compounds may confer protection against breast cancer, osteoporosis, heart disease, and premenopausal symptoms, and both have been shown to induce differentiation, or the conversion of cancer cells to normal cells.

Dr. Block explains that these substances actually *inhibit* the body's own estrogen activity, thus offering potential protection against breast cancer. The genistein in soy products is a potent antioxidant, and, like certain anticancer drugs, it impedes the action of estrogen and the formation of new blood vessels that would otherwise feed a tumor's growth.[5] Researchers now report that genistein blocks the expression of several oncogenes, believed to program the production of cancer cells.[6]

In addition to the mainly vegetarian diet, Dr. Block's nutritional supplement program calls for, at a minimum, a multivitamin and antioxidant formula containing vitamins C and E and beta carotene. These antioxidants help protect liver cells from the free radicals produced by the liver's first phase of detoxification (carried out by "Phase I enzymes") that converts toxic substances to an intermediate (but not necessarily less toxic) form.

Along with these supplements, Dr. Block emphasizes additional servings of specific "power foods," such as broccoli and brussel sprouts (cruciferous vegetables) and members of the onion family (*Allium*), as these contain compounds that increase the activity of Phase II enzymes. The function of the Phase II enzymes is to convert the intermediate toxins into excretable substances and deliver them to the organs that flush them out of the body.

The recommendation is 2-3 servings a day of cruciferous vegetables, including broccoli, cauliflower, cabbage, Brussels sprouts, kale, mustard greens, collards, turnips, bok choy, broccoli rabe, and sprouting broccoli. Also important are onion group vegetables (1-2 servings daily), including onions, garlic, shallots, green onions, and pearl onions; sea vegetables (2-3 servings per week, or 1-2 kelp tablets daily), particularly recommended for radiation patients. Specific foods and substances to be avoided include all red meats, dairy foods, and white flour products, alcohol, caffeine (in both foods and beverages), additives (in all junk foods), and refined sugar.

## MDS #2: LIVER AND DIGESTIVE SUPPORT

MDS supplements, formulated specifically by Dr. Block for his program, support numerous liver and digestive functions which, when healthy, work in a complementary fashion to help detoxify the body and bolster its ability to ward off cancer.

**Metabolic Detox with Fiber—**Dr. Block's fiber supplement contains oat and beet fiber, which help cleanse the intestines and sweep toxins out of the body. It also contains pectin to nourish intestinal cells, and the amino acids glutamine and glycine which play integral roles in intestinal and liver functioning, respectively. Finally, a dose of *Lactobacillus* bacteria is included in each serving to help promote healthy intestinal flora.

The usual dosage is one scoop mixed with water or juice, taken 2 times daily. The supplement is taken at least 2 hours after breakfast and after dinner, or after breakfast and after lunch, if preferred.

**Metabolic Detox with Botanicals—**Some of the herbs included in Dr.

Block's botanical supplements are silymarin (milk thistle), dandelion, ginger, turmeric, and goldenseal (which contains the bitter component berberine, a powerful immune stimulator). These herbs enhance the liver's detoxification processes and balance the intestinal flora, while also serving to weaken the effects of inflammatory and free-radical activities within the body. Typically, 2 capsules are taken 3 times a day with meals.

Those who have problems with the gallbladder or bile duct, or cancer of the gallbladder or bile duct, are advised against using these herbs because of their choleretic effects (they increase the flow of toxin-rich bile from the gallbladder). If you have these problems, leave this supplement out of your MDS regimen, Dr. Block advises.

**Metabolic Detox with Enzymes—**The MDS enzyme supplement, which includes amylase, lipase, and bromelain, supports the digestive functions. Thorough digestion, facilitated by digestive enzymes, helps ensure that large, potential allergy-triggering food particles do not enter the blood circulation through a "leaky gut." Antigens (foreign substances that produce an allergic response) from foods can further burden the immune system at a time when the need is strongest to restore it, says Dr. Block. These enzymes may reduce the antigenic burden that many cancer patients face, says Dr. Block. Patients are usually advised to take 2 tablets 3 times per day with meals.

**Metabolic Detox with Antioxidants—**The main component of this supplement is superoxide dismutase, an antioxidant enzyme that targets free radicals in the liver. Most often, patients take one teaspoon 3 times per day mixed with juice or food. Another key component is glutathione, which serves in the antioxidation pathway as a cofactor for the enzyme glutathione peroxidase.

Blood levels of glutathione peroxidase are typically low in older people and in patients with malignant cancers.[7] Glutathione reduces free-radical damage to DNA and prevents depletion of other antioxidants. It also helps metabolize various carcinogens, activates certain immune cells, helps synthesize and repair DNA, and may inhibit angiogenesis, a blood vessel-forming process required for tumor growth.[8] Glutathione has been shown to reduce the toxic side effects of conventional cancer treatments.[9]

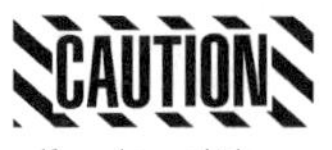

If you have a kidney disorder and/or are unable to manage fluid balance (as with edema), discuss the best ways to achieve adequate fluid levels with a clinical expert, Dr. Block advises.

## MDS #3: KIDNEY SUPPORT

The kidneys act as powerful filters of the blood, removing many toxic metabolites and residues from various chemicals including drugs, environmental pollutants, chemotherapy agents, and others. According to Dr. Block, the single most important way to support the kidneys, especially during chemical or toxic treatments, is by maintaining adequate fluid intake—60 to 64 ounces per day, preferably of purified water.

Adequate fluid intake is important during all phases of treatment. Other than purified water, Dr. Block advises that about half of the fluid intake may consist of the following: fruit juices diluted with 50% water; vegetable juices; noncaffeine *kukicha* tea (also known as *bancha* tea); and noncaffeine herbal teas (especially ginger, chamomile, goldenrod, or passionflower, all of which support various aspects of detoxification).

Here are practical ways to achieve adequate fluid intake of 60-64 ounces per day): drink one 6-ounce glass of water every hour for 10 hours; one 8-ounce glass of water every hour for 8 hours; or use a large plastic water container with an attached straw, fill it up as necessary, and sip throughout the day until you have taken your full 60 to 64 ounces.

## MDS #4: LUNG AND SKIN SUPPORT

The lungs and skin are integral parts of the body's detoxification system. "While detoxification processes in the lung and skin are not well-understood scientifically," says Dr. Block, "it is clear that they detoxify chemicals not processed by the liver or kidneys." For the lungs, Dr. Block recommends trying to do a minimum of 10 minutes of quiet deep-breathing practice twice a day.

For aerobic exercise, 30 minutes a day is usually optimal, says Dr. Block, but if you are healthy, you may exercise longer by walking or through other exercise in moderation. If you feel weak or ill, you may do 3-6 sessions lasting 5-10 minutes each daily or devise a schedule in which you do not become fatigued or strained. Avoiding exhaustive activity is critical if you are seriously ill, cautions Dr. Block.

Support for skin detoxification can be accomplished with saunas, baths, and skin brushing, says Dr. Block. Low-temperature saunas help remove toxins from the skin by stimulating sweating; with proper supervision, these can be taken once or twice a week if you are in good physical condition.

Patients who have taken anticancer drugs, particularly those affecting the heart (e.g., adriamycin), or patients with high blood pressure or heart disease of any sort, should not do a sauna without first consulting with their physician, and then only under the knowledgeable direction of an expert, advises Dr. Block.

If you have undergone chemotherapy in past months, you may take a low-temperature (98 to 102° F) sauna session lasting 10-15 minutes with an attendant present. Exit the sauna if you begin to feel faint; if you feel strong, you may take a longer session. In either case, Dr. Block says to be sure to drink at least 4 cups of pure water before entering the sauna, and use replacement minerals and electrolytes as needed following the sauna.

If saunas are unavailable or inappropriate for your physical condition, Dr. Block recommends taking baths at home 3 times a week. Warm baths in which you remain immersed for 20 minutes or more are advisable. "You should drink 2 cups of water before the bath if you plan to use salt mixtures in the bath. You can use Dead Sea salts, seaweed-salt mixtures, or a mixture of 1 cup of baking soda and 1 cup salt dissolved in the bathwater to help draw toxins and sweat from the skin; then shower after the bath to remove the salt, " Dr. Block says.

Brushing your skin with a natural bristle brush helps to remove flakes of dead skin that may contain toxins, and stimulates circulation of both lymph and blood to the skin, says Dr. Block. Skin brushing should be done every day before the bath; natural bristle brushes with long handles work best.

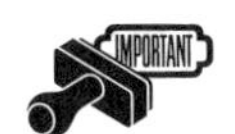


If you have received radiation treatments, particular supplements should be considered. One supplement you should add to your detoxification regimen after the radiation treatments have ended is *Gingko biloba*, says Dr. Block. Radiation makes the body form oxidizing compounds which attach to various cancer-related factors (e.g., tumor necrosis factor). These factors circulate in the blood and, because of their oxidizing activity, damage chromosomes. To counteract these factors, Dr. Block recommends taking *Gingko biloba* extract (40-mg tablets ) 3 times per day for at least 2 months after radiation therapy.

## MDS #5: BLOOD AND LYMPH SUPPORT

The blood and lymph help transport your body's nutrients and necessary life-supporting factors. They also transport toxins coming from both inside and outside the body. Cleansing the blood is a primary function of the liver, so supporting liver function is an effective way to detoxify the blood. Another effective way is to maintain a careful diet, avoiding most (or ideally all) animal products, fatty foods, pesticides, and additives.

The blood's companion system is the lymph system, which filters toxins from the tissues and the blood and directly supports the immune system. Focused breathing (paying attention to the in-and-out movement of the breath) and moderate exercise (particularly systems such as Qigong, tai chi, or yoga) are also effective ways to support lymphatic functioning, particularly since, unlike the heart and circulatory system, the lymphatic system lacks a "pump" to move the lymph fluid. This fluid requires the movement of muscles to maintain its flow, especially leg muscles and the muscles involved in breathing.

After completing their MDS program, Dr. Block recommends that patients continue with the general dietary recommendations. "You should still take at least 5 servings a week of cruciferous and onion group vegetables," he says. "But you may diversify your other vegetable servings. You should also continue to take *Acidophilus* supplements containing healthful *Lactobacillus* [intestinal bacteria] for at least one month after finishing detoxification."

For more information on **detoxification** (pp. 949-980), **friendly bacteria** (pp. 962-964), and **lymph** (pp. 965-971), see Chapter 33: Physical Support Therapies.

For more information about **FOS** and **NutraFlora®**, contact: GTC Nutrition Company, 1400 W. 122nd Avenue, Suite 110, Westminster, CO 80234; tel: 303-254-8012; fax: 303-254-8201.

In addition, Dr. Block notes that patients may benefit from eating foods containing fructo-oligosaccharides (FOS), a naturally occurring form of carbohydrate found in certain foods in minute amounts. Foods with FOS stimulate the growth of helpful intestinal bacteria. FOS is present in garlic, Jerusalem artichokes, soybeans, burdock, chicory root, asparagus, banana, rye, barley, tomato, onions, and triticale.

Japanese researchers determined that FOS was a perfect food for "friendly" bacteria (probiotics), such as *Lactobacilli* and *Bifidobacteria*, because it acts like an intestinal "fertilizer," selectively feeding the friendly microflora in the large intestine so that their numbers can usefully increase. *Bifidobacteria* work to lower the pH (acidity/alkalinity balance) in the large intestine to a slightly more acidic condition, which discourages the growth of unfriendly bacteria and encourages the growth of other friendly bacteria.

## Integrating the MDS Program into Conventional Cancer Treatments

Regardless of the type of cancer, if you are not suffering from cancer-related lean tissue loss (clinically called cachexia) and have not received any conventional treatment, Dr. Block recommends undertaking two 30-day detoxification periods, separated by a 30-day interval during which you simply eat a low-fat, high-fiber diet (described in the next section).

Another option during this period is to fast for 1-2 days—eating no solid food and drinking only diluted fruit juices, vegetable juices, or water. Break fasts by eating lightly, as this causes the body to draw on fat reserves, liberating toxins stored in fat and delivering them to the liver for detoxification, explains Dr. Block. Longer fasts are ill-advised without expert knowledge and supervision, he says. Loss of proteins can have deleterious immune and clinical consequences.

For cancer patients who have undergone surgery, or a combination of surgery and radiation, Block recommends that once you have recovered (in 2-3 months), you can begin the same two 30-day periods of detoxification, separated by a 30-day interval of basic health maintenance. Because of the nutritional problems facing cancer patients (e.g., lean tissue loss), Dr. Block advises against fasting as an adjunct to the detoxification program in these cases, as well as in those who have undergone chemotherapy.

## The Importance of Herbs and Support Groups

- A recent study of workers at Chernobyl nuclear power station in Russia found that *Gingko biloba,* taken over a 2-month period, caused a two-thirds decrease in their chromosome damage.[10] Such damage can eventually lead to the development of cancer.
- Breast cancer patients who underwent supportive/expressive group therapy lived on average twice as long as those who did not (control group).[11] In another study, patients with malignant melanoma assigned to a series of six 90-minute support group meetings were less anxious and depressed than controls, and had significantly lower rates of recurrence and mortality a full 6 years later.[12]

For those considering chemotherapy, Dr. Block generally encourages a fractionated dosage approach, i.e., one in which small infusion doses are spread out over time. Chemotherapy treatments require more careful timing of the MDS program because the administration of the drug takes place in cycles. These phases—treatment, delayed cytotoxicity (destruction of cancer cells), detoxification, and rebuilding—must be adjusted by practitioners experienced in this approach, cautions Dr. Block.

For information on **low-dose chemotherapy**, see Chapter 30: The New Pharmacology for Treating Cancer, pp. 849-850.

In the treatment phase, which lasts 1-5 or 7 days, the cancer patient receives chemotherapy drugs along with agents intended to improve circulation as a way to provide better access to the tumor site. Dr. Block notes that angiogenic inhibitors (substances that block new blood vessel formation) should be stopped entirely for 3-4 days prior to this phase, and resumed only after this phase and the second phase are over.

During the second phase, the drugs remain in the body and kill more cancer cells (cytotoxicity); this lasts about 7 days and concludes as the liver converts the drugs into an inactive form. "The patient during this period is considerably more vulnerable on account of having lowered immune defenses," says Dr. Block. "If more immune and detoxification stimulants are employed during this phase, it is of critical importance that caution be used, that they be tailored to the patient, the type of disease, treatment, and biological variability."

In the third phase, or detoxification, the cancer patient accelerates removal of toxic metabolites left over from the liver's enzymatic breakdown of the drugs. This phase can last from 5-10 days, depending on many variables; it may overlap with the second phase or be separate, again depending on the particulars of the patient's biochemical and digestive status as well as the timing of conventional interventions.

***Dr. Block emphasizes the importance of finding an exercise, or a set of physical activities, that the patient will consistently carry out.***

The fourth phase is followed by a buildup phase, which can last from 5-10 days. During this time, the cancer patient is encouraged to increase the intake of calories, complex carbohydrates, protein, and healthful fats (sesame or olive oil, soy products, nuts and seeds) to rebuild the body before the next chemotherapy treatment while encouraging cell division, making cancer cells more vulnerable to the chemotherapy drugs.

## A Willingness to Pursue Reasonable Alternatives

Dr. Block emphasizes the value of pursuing "reasonable alternatives" in cancer treatment. This is Dr. Block's way of referring to therapeutic interventions that lie outside the medical mainstream but, unlike conventional approaches, do not carry a high price tag or produce serious side effects. "In general, I steer away from recommending things that don't have solid research behind them yet, but I recognize that until funding is made available for such research, we must rely almost entirely on our clinical experience. So I remain open to alternatives that work."

None of the modalities described here carry a high price tag or produce any serious side effects. For example, Dr. Block's research team is working on several unique formulations. One such formula is their own version of Essiac, which Dr. Block considers a rather weak combination of anticancer herbs. Charlotte Gyllenhaal, Ph.D., Dr. Block's botanical expert, helped reformulate a Chinese herbal system which she and Block call "anticancer botanical agents" or ACBA, which is Dr. Block's preferred substitute for Essiac. He says their preliminary research indicates that ACBA has stronger anticancer ability than either Hoxsey or Essiac.

Over the course of 3 years, Dr. Block's staff has also created and tested 4 formulas for detoxifying cancer patients—both those who need to eliminate chemical and environmental toxins and those who underwent either chemotherapy or radiation. The innovative low-invasive therapies, or ILITS, are also among Dr. Block's "reasonable alternatives" which include botanicals, supplements, and various body-oriented therapies such as acupuncture and massage. Dr. Block also uses electroacupuncture, ear acupuncture, acupressure, and other methods to enhance whole-body functioning and assist in his use of chemotherapy when appropriate, as well as micro-electrical stimulation therapy for pain relief.

For more information about **Qigong** as part of a cancer therapy (pp. 1005-1017), and **exercise and massage** (pp. 1000-1005), see Chapter 33: Physical Support Therapies.

## A Program of Physical Care for Cancer Patients

Another key aspect of Dr. Block's approach is *physical care*, which focuses on a comprehensive program to assure muscle mass maintenance, aerobic competence, and flexibility—key factors in helping people resist cancer. The goal is to reduce body fat while maintaining or rebuilding lean tissue (muscle); overweight cancer patients have poorer prognoses than people of normal weight. Dr. Block emphasizes the importance of finding an exercise, or a set of physical activities, that the patient will consistently carry out.

**Qigong** is an aspect of traditional Chinese medicine involving numerous exercises that combine physical movement, breathing, and concentration. In practicing Qigong, one makes a series of slow, rhythmic, meditative movements, with careful attention to the breath and posture. Qigong is also used on patients by doctors of Chinese medicine to stimulate and raise *Qi*, the body's internal "life force."

Rather than high-impact aerobics, Dr. Block advocates more balanced forms of exercise, such as walking and Qigong (pronounced *chee-GUNG*). For bedridden patients, Dr. Block and colleagues developed a set of these gentle exercises that doubles as a meditation and rejuvenative movement discipline. According to Dr. Block, vigorous walking, whenever possible, should be practiced for 30 minutes at least 5 days a week. A brisk walk is not only good for the circulation and lymph systems, but it boosts natural killer cell activity. "Cancer patients who already suffer from a defect in energy metabolism should avoid overdoing to the point of exhaustion. This can lead to either adrenal exhaustion or immune suppression, or both," Dr. Block cautions. "This could have harmful consequences to those patients fighting for their lives."

Massage is offered to Dr. Block's patients as a way to relax and accelerate the detoxification process at the same time. Massage clearly enhances the cancer patient's quality of life and may even promote survival, states Dr. Block. He challenges the speculation that massage may tend to increase the spread of cancer. "I just don't buy it," Dr. Block says. "There is no hard evidence suggesting this whatsoever. My patients seem to do better, not worse, with massage."

*In Dr. Block's long-term survivors study, the successful techniques for reducing stress and improving emotional health included meditation, guided imagery, self-hypnosis, biofeedback, and support groups.*

For people seeking an even gentler approach to physical care, Dr. Block's clinic offers orthobionomy, a relaxing form of bodywork. Orthobionomy works on the principle of finding the easiest range of movement for different body parts. The orthobionomist assists the client in making those simple movements, gradually bringing the body into ever deeper levels of relaxation.

## A Program of Psychosocial Support for Cancer Patients

Psychosocial interventions are an integral part of Dr. Block's program. In his long-term survivors study, the successful techniques for reducing stress and improving emotional health included meditation, guided imagery, self-hypnosis, biofeedback, and support groups. Patients are encouraged to be selective and find the approach that works best for them, Dr. Block says. Once again, the use of well-run support groups has been shown to improve not only the quality of life of cancer patients, but also their actual survival time, according to Dr. Block.

Attention to the mind-body realm is often overlooked in cancer treatment programs, suggests Dr. Block. A combination of psychotherapy and support groups (depending on the patient's affinity or comfort level with either one) is often an effective means to guide cancer patients toward recovering a sense of meaning and fulfillment—a reason to go on living, Dr. Block explains. Cultivating and sustaining this attitude is key to recovery—and a major goal of the Block program.

As is obvious, a fundamental premise of Dr. Block's approach is that giving patients a sense of personal power and responsibility regarding their care is as important as prescribing the right medications. When they begin to enhance their own emotional and physical vitality, this sense of empowerment begins to grow quickly. Dr. Block's insight in this area derives from his personal experience as a patient. His introduction to alternative medicine began at the other end of the stethoscope when a personal health crisis led him to explore dietary and botanical therapies.

In the course of working through his own experience, Dr. Block became acutely sensitized to the emotional needs of patients. "I try to help people discover the chords in their being that connect them to a desire to live more fully," Dr. Block says. "If I can help them identify with that zest for life and tap into their own inner resources, then deeper healing of their inner being can occur."

***"If I can help patients identify with that zest for life and tap into their own inner resources, then deeper healing of their inner being can occur," says Dr. Block.***

## CURRICULUM VITAE

# Douglas Brodie, M.D.

309 Kirman Avenue, #2, Reno, NV 89502;
tel: 702-324-7071; fax: 702-324-7639.

A graduate of the University of Michigan Medical School, Dr. Brodie completed his residency training in internal medicine, finishing as chief medical resident at Highland-Alameda County Hospital in Oakland, California. Now based in Reno, Nevada, Dr. Brodie has developed alternative methods aimed at stengthening the immune system against cancer and other degenerative diseases, with an emphasis on natural and humane approaches to these conditions. Dr. Brodie is licensed in both homeopathy and allopathy, and has served on the Nevada State Board of Homeopathic Medical Examiners by appointment of the governor of Nevada.

***The preventive focus is essential for long-range cancer care, Dr. Brodie says. "Many patients tend to believe that if they get rid of a tumor, then they have succeeded and nothing more needs to be done. However, it's precisely at this point that diet and supplements play their most profound role, helping to keep the cancer from recurring."***

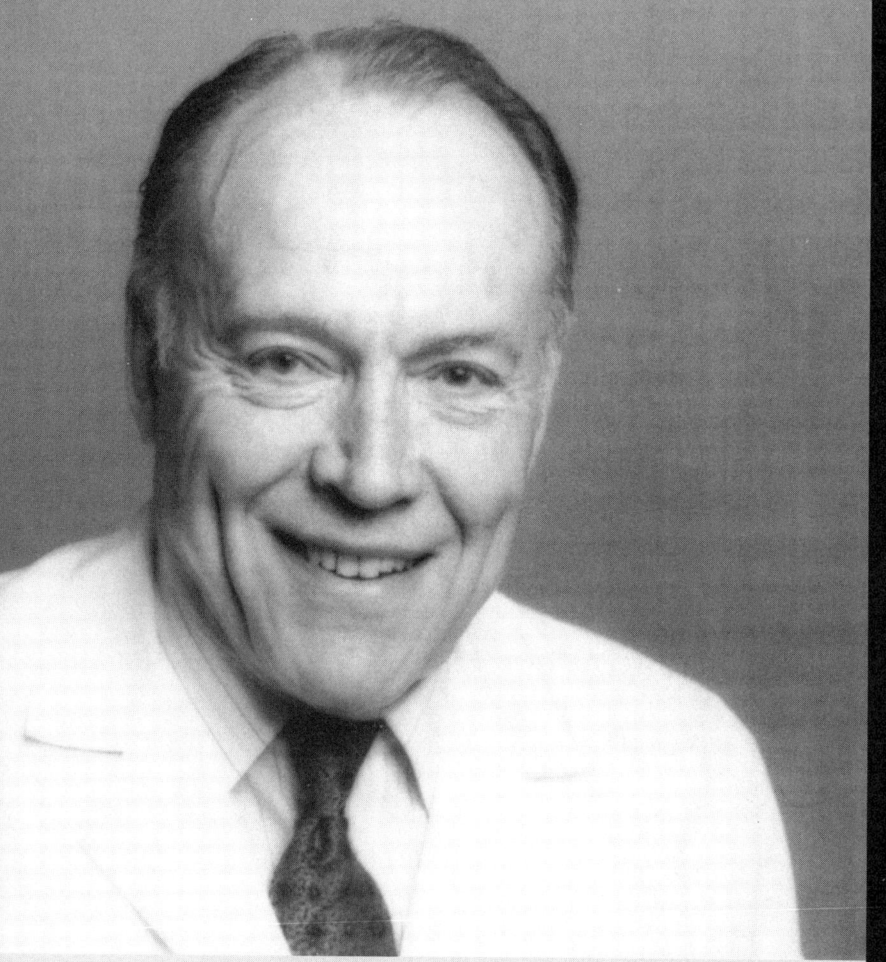

# *Douglas Brodie, M.D.*

**WHEN YOU INCLUDE** nutritional and herbal supplements along with strong physical and psychological support as part of an intensive cancer treatment plan, the chances of beating cancer are markedly improved, says Douglas Brodie, M.D.

Cancer cells are a natural part of human life, but it is only a weakened or unhealthy immune system that makes the body cancer-prone, states Dr. Brodie. "Each one of us produces several hundred thousand cancer cells every day of our lives. Whether we develop clinical cancer or not depends upon the ability of our immune systems to destroy these cancer cells. That's because cancer thrives in the presence of a deficient immune system." Dr. Brodie adds that the long-established notion of cancer existing independently of the host's "immune competence" is no longer tenable and must be rejected.

## Bolster the Body's Natural Immune Defenses against Cancer

The main thrust of Dr. Brodie's approach, therefore, is to bolster the body's natural immune defenses against cancer through optimum nutrition, supplements, and a variety of special nontoxic substances. Many of the cancer-fighting substances he uses are known to biochemists as Biological Response Modifiers (BRMs). These include nutrients and other food factors, as well as hormones and special immune-modulating substances. "My main objective over the past 2 decades has been to find those natural substances that most effectively enhance the immune system in its battle against cancer," says Dr. Brodie. "When these substances are included

# Dr. Brodie's Generalized Model for Cancer Treatment

| STRATEGY | DOSAGE/ KEY COMPONENTS | FOR MORE INFORMATION see page # |
|---|---|---|
| **Lifestyle Plan** | | |
| Balanced vegetarian diet | raw and unprocessed foods, including fresh fruits and vegetables, whole grains and beans; avoid refined sugars, red meat, caffeine, chemically preserved foods | 749 |
| Moderate, regular exercise | one-half hour of brisk walking 3 times a week or 15 minutes of brisk walking daily | 74 |
| **Oral and Intravenous Supplement Program** | | |
| Vitamin A | 10 drops emulsified vitamin A (125,000 IU per day) | 784 |
| Vitamin C | 15-25 g intravenously, followed by 5-10 g orally, per day, depending on patient's condition | 786 |
| Thymus extracts | 2 cc daily | 935 |
| Digestive enzymes | variable, depending on individual condition | 928 |
| Amygdalin (laetrile) | 9 g (three 3-g vials) intravenously daily for up to 3 weeks; then 500 mg 3x/day, taken orally | 812 |
| Germanium sesquioxide | 500 mg intravenously per day, followed by 100-150 mg orally per day | 771 |
| Antioxidants: vitamin E, selenium, zinc, cysteine, glutathione, and others | selenium, 200 mcg daily (intravenously at first, orally later); vitamin E, 400 IU, 3x/day | 790, 783, 793, 37, 868 |
| B-complex vitamins | tailored to individual needs, but often 1 B-complex tablet daily, plus 400 mg B6 | 784 |
| Bovine cartilage | 9 g daily (3 grams 3x/day) | 861 |
| Phytochemicals | 1 cup soy powder daily | 80 |
| **Homeopathy to Support the Recovery Process** | | |
| Dozens of remedies | tailored to individual needs | – |

*Continued*

## Dr. Brodie's Generalized Model for Cancer Treatment (cont.)

| STRATEGY | DOSAGE/ KEY COMPONENTS | FOR MORE INFORMATION see page # |
|---|---|---|
| **Alternative Therapies with More Specific Applications** | | |
| Ukrain | 5-20 mg injection every other day | 873 |
| Carnivora | variable dosage, depending on cancer type/stage, as well as individual factors | 860 |
| Polypeptides | variable dosage, depending on cancer type/stage, as well as individual factors | 936 |
| Interferon | same as above | 82 |
| Melatonin/IL-2 | same as above | 941 |
| **Psychological Maintenance** | | |
| Psychotherapy | tailored by therapist to meet individual needs | 82 |
| Deep relaxation techniques | same as above | — |
| Support groups | same as above | — |

**CAUTION**

This chapter includes information regarding actual treatments used by Dr. Brodie only after his careful diagnosis of each patient. All cancer patients are unique. **Do not administer these treatments to yourself or others.** Discuss these treatments with your physician or other qualified health-care professional. Readers should not interpret this material as therapeutic advice, but should see a physician in all cases.

as part of a comprehensive cancer treatment plan, which includes strong physical *and* psychological support, the chances of beating cancer are markedly improved."

Dr. Brodie notes that a weakened or suppressed immune system may result from a deficiency of a single nutrient or, more often, multiple nutrients. Most cancer patients, he says, are so deficient nutritionally they require relatively high doses of many nutrients at once. "Because of this widespread malnutrition and because cancer patients also appear to have problems with insufficient absorption and utilization of nutrients, they respond best when certain of these special nutrients are given intravenously at first," Dr. Brodie says. "This approach also helps alleviate some of the body's usual energy requirements for digesting food and extracting individual nutrients."

Giving the body the fair chance to heal itself is the main thrust of Dr. Brodie's treatment strategy for cancer. His program is not intended to replace whatever conventional treatment may be indicated. "Our immune enhancement program is often administered in conjunction with conventional therapy," Dr. Brodie says. "It has been our experience that this combination usually reduces and sometimes eliminates the toxic effects of chemotherapy or radiation. Not only does our program make conventional treatment more tolerable, but it usually makes it more effective as well." His immune support program is complementary to conventional methods, Dr. Brodie notes.

For more information about **BRMs**, see Chapter 29: Botanicals as Cancer Medicine, pp. 808-836.

***"Our immune enhancement program is often administered in conjunction with conventional therapy," Dr. Brodie says. "This combination usually reduces and sometimes eliminates the toxic effects of chemotherapy or radiation."***

## SUCCESS STORY
### Reversing Breast Cancer

Here's a case history from Dr. Brodie's files about a strong-willed woman who kept her breasts and beat her cancer. When she was 49, Rebecca, a switchboard supervisor, noted a lump in her left breast. When a needle-guided excision biopsy indicated a tumor was present, Rebecca's doctor planned a mastectomy for her. When she insisted that he perform a simple excision instead and he refused, Rebecca started looking for an alternative. She found it in Douglas Brodie, M.D.

This was quite bold on Rebecca's part because, first, the breast cancer was highly malignant, and second, both her mother and a cousin had died of breast cancer at an early age. Rebecca told Dr. Brodie that if she must have conventional treatment she wanted to at least build herself up in preparation. She still had a small cancerous mass in her breast, and her immune function was very poor, based on an analysis of live blood cells with a darkfield microscope.

For more information about the **AMAS test**, see Chapter 27, Early Detection and Prevention, pp. 700-706.

Dr. Brodie started Rebecca on his program of immune system augmentation, using intravenous infusions of high doses of numerous nutritional substances, along with injections into the muscles of thymus peptides (several amino acids joined together). To complement the injections, Rebecca took oral supplements and glandular extracts. This phase took 3 weeks. During this time, Rebecca's immune system vitality improved from 20% of normal to 100%, as evidenced by white blood cell activity viewed through darkfield microscopy. Dr. Brodie sent her home with a self-care supplement program.

She managed to persuade her surgeon to remove only 25% of her left breast where the tumor resided. He had wanted to cut it all off including the lymph nodes. The surgical pathology indicated that this 25% portion actually contained no cancer at all. About 10 weeks later, an AMAS test, which quite accurately measures levels of antibodies to cancer cells, came back normal, indicating no trace of cancer.

***"Some patients, after successfully subduing their cancer, become lulled into a false sense of security and stop taking the supplements," says Dr. Brodie. "The consequence of returning to their old dietary and other habits is often disastrous. The cancer comes back with a vengeance. We need to recognize that treating cancer is a lifelong endeavor."***

About 8 months later, Rebecca saw Dr. Brodie again, reporting that stress from obstacles she was facing in her life had weakened her system. Tests indicated she had no return of cancer but that her immune system had dropped in vitality. Dr. Brodie put her on a 7-day intravenous supplementation program and gave her stress-management counseling. In one week, her immune system had regained its vitality.

Back home, once she dealt with the personal stress in her life, her mood, energy level, and sense of well-being rapidly improved. About 2 years after her initial visit with Dr. Brodie, Rebecca told him that all her cancer markers were normal and that she was in an "excellent state of mind and health."

## Making Diet and Exercise Lifelong Healing Strategies

The practical starting point for Dr. Brodie's program is to educate his patients about the importance of supporting the body's built-in mechanisms for cancer resistance. The initial focus is on diet and exercise, two lifestyle components that serve as the foundation for bolstering the body's cancer-repelling ability.

A balanced, health-promoting diet reinforces the supplement program as well as the other aspects of Dr. Brodie's approach to cancer. In designing his dietary plan, Dr. Brodie drew upon research from such medically conservative organizations as the National Cancer Institute showing definitive relationships between diet and cancer. "A diet high in animal fat and low in fiber, such as the typical American diet, leads to a higher incidence of cancer, especially breast, colon, pancreas, and prostate," Dr. Brodie says. "We also know that vegetarians have substantially lower rates of cancers, which is why most of our patients are encouraged to follow a mainly vegetarian diet."

A preventive focus is essential for long-range cancer care, Dr. Brodie says, since those who successfully undergo cancer treatment must then strive to ward off cancer for the rest of their lives. "Many patients tend to believe that if they get rid of a tumor, then they have succeeded and nothing more needs to be done. However, it's precisely at this point that diet and supplements play their most profound role, helping to keep the cancer from recurring."

Dr. Brodie's diet emphasizes raw and unprocessed foods, including fresh fruits and vegetables and whole grains and beans, and avoids refined sugars, red meat, caffeine, and chemically preserved foods. The diet is always modified to satisfy individual requirements. For example, some people are more physically active and require more starches, vegetable oils, and other energy-rich foods; while others may have a fondness for sweet-tasting foods, so healthful substitutes (e.g., fruits and fruit juices) must be identified to keep the person from resorting to soft drinks, candies, and other "junk foods."

Dr. Brodie encourages his patients to engage in moderate, regular exercise. Walking for 30 minutes 3 times a week, or 15 minutes a day, is excellent for cancer patients. However, whatever form of physical activity is pursued, it should not unduly strain or stress the body, cautions Dr. Brodie. "The person with cancer needs to conserve energy as much as possible. Move as much as possible, but don't overdo it."

One of the primary advantages of exercise, in Dr. Brodie's view, is that it increases the body's oxygen supply. Since cancer operates in an oxygen-

## Preventing Cancer with Diet

Dr. Brodie acknowledges that, for the most part, the research supporting his dietary plan focused on ways to prevent cancer. For example, numerous studies have found that people who eat plenty of fruits and vegetables have a lower risk of developing cancers of the stomach, pancreas, colon, rectum, pharynx, esophagus, oral cavity, larynx, lung, bladder, endometrium, cervix, and ovary.[1] In a recent review of 156 studies of dietary influences on these cancers, 128 of the studies, or 80%, showed a statistically significant protective effect from fruit and vegetable consumption.[2]

***Since cancer operates in an oxygen-poor environment, the well-exercised body is far more likely to repel cancer cells or keep them from propagating.***

poor environment, the well-exercised body is far more likely to repel cancer cells or keep them from propagating. In a large-scale study of Harvard alumni, men who burned as few as 500 calories a week in exercise—the equivalent to about an hour's worth of brisk walking—had death rates about 20% lower than men who rarely exercised.[3]

More avid exercisers experienced even fewer cancer-related deaths: men who walked about 4 hours each week (about 2,000 calories burned) were 35% less likely to die of cancer than their less active counterparts. People who follow an inactive or sedentary lifestyle are more likely to develop colon cancer, the second leading cause of cancer-related death in the U.S., according to research; conversely, the more one exercises, the lower one's risk for colon cancer;[4] and in helping to ward off cancer, exercise tends to benefit men more than women.[5]

## Dr. Brodie's 3-Week Intensive Supplementation Program

Dr. Brodie uses an array of supplements to treat cancer. His initial procedure is to administer over a 3-week period intravenous (IV) infusions of many substances (giving high doses of the appropriate vitamins and minerals) along with intramuscular injections of polypeptides (protein fragments, or chains of amino acids) and other BRMs. This program is accompanied by certain detoxification procedures, using glutathione, selenium, and other supplements (such as vitamins A, C, and E) aimed at helping the body rid itself of toxins that may be impairing the immune system's ability to attack cancer cells. The IV program is then followed by a less intensive oral supplement program that the cancer patient carries out at home.

Before making any recommendations for supplements, Dr. Brodie uses either **darkfield microscopy** or **live blood analysis** to evaluate a patient's nutritional imbalances and immune system function and to monitor progress. For more information on both subjects, see Chapter 27: Early Detection and Prevention of Cancer.

The supplements should be continued for several years after the cancer has presumably disappeared, Dr. Brodie emphasizes.

**Vitamin A**—This vitamin is essential to strong immunity and provides added resistance to cancer by stimulating the activity of immune cells against tumor cells.[6,7,8] Some research indicates that vitamin A inhibits the *promotion* of cancer, whereas beta carotene (the precursor to vitamin A) inhibits the *initiation* of cancer. This, in turn, suggests that vitamin A plays a more active role in cancer therapy compared to beta carotene.[9] Dr. Brodie believes this vitamin works best with cancers involving the lungs, skin, and other epithelial surfaces. He prefers to use an emulsified, oil-based form of vitamin A, 10 drops per day, or more, depending on the patient's condition.

**Vitamin C—**According to Dr. Brodie, vitamin C has an ability to inhibit the invasiveness of cancer cells "by neutralizing the toxins produced by those cancer cells." This vitamin can selectively kill tumor cells in a manner similar to the chemotherapeutic drugs used by conventional doctors.[10] Unlike chemotherapy, however, vitamin C actually *enhances* those parts of the immune system that are highly active against cancer, notably the natural killer (NK) cells.[11]

"People who are under a high level of stress or who are sick, whether from cancer or some other disease, have a much higher requirement for vitamin C than those not under such stress or illness," says Dr. Brodie. "Cancer patients not supplementing with vitamin C are frequently deficient in the vitamin. Giving ascorbic acid in high doses along with other nutrients brings about almost immediate improvement in the feeling of well-being in these patients."

***"People who are under a high level of stress or who are sick, whether from cancer or some other disease, have a much higher requirement for vitamin C than those not under such stress or illness," says Dr. Brodie.***

Dr. Brodie's usual strategy is to use 15-25 g of vitamin C intravenously (higher in some cases), with 5-10 g taken orally at night. If you are particularly ill, Dr. Brodie says you should lean toward the higher end of the oral C range at night. After the initial intravenous therapy is completed, the oral vitamin C is continued; the amount may actually be increased, since the body is no longer receiving the intravenous form.

**Thymus Extract—**The thymus gland is the activator of T-lymphocytes (the "T" stands for thymus), cells that play an essential role in the body's defenses against cancer as well as viral infections. The thymus produces some 60 different hormone-like proteins called peptides or polypeptides which act as chemical messengers, instructing T cells to fight cancer cells. "As we grow older, our thymus becomes smaller and less active," Dr. Brodie says. "Cancer patients appear to be particularly deficient in this area." Dr.

Brodie notes that the thymus gland is also adversely affected by stress and by severe or prolonged illness. Dr. Brodie's thymus extract contains thymosin and numerous peptides from the thymus; his patients usually receive 2 cc per day of this extract.

**Digestive Enzymes—**These protein-digesting (proteolytic) enzymes produced by the pancreas are essential to the body's anticancer defenses. "This is because they act to digest the protective protein coating or shell which encases all tumors," Dr. Brodie says. "Cancers are somehow able to surround themselves with a shield of protective armor which keeps the body's defenders at bay."

Enzymes also appear to prevent cancer from gaining a foothold in the body in the following way: precancerous cells become attached to body tissues by means of fibrin, a protein component necessary for blood clotting. However, enzymes digest the fibrin and prevent the attachment of precancerous cells to body tissues, thereby releasing these cells into the blood where they are normally destroyed, Dr. Brodie explains. Research shows that protein-digesting enzymes (proteases such as bromelain) can induce the transformation of cancer cells into normal cells.[12] Dr. Brodie uses a combination of pancreatic enzymes from animal sources and a range of vegetable-derived enzymes; dosages vary greatly depending on individual factors.

QUICK DEFINITION

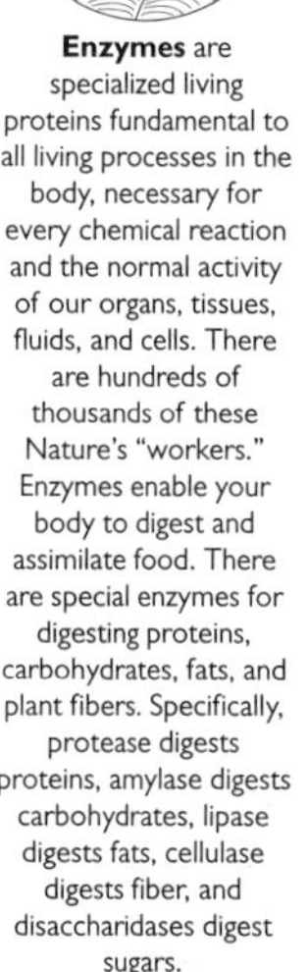

**Enzymes** are specialized living proteins fundamental to all living processes in the body, necessary for every chemical reaction and the normal activity of our organs, tissues, fluids, and cells. There are hundreds of thousands of these Nature's "workers." Enzymes enable your body to digest and assimilate food. There are special enzymes for digesting proteins, carbohydrates, fats, and plant fibers. Specifically, protease digests proteins, amylase digests carbohydrates, lipase digests fats, cellulase digests fiber, and disaccharidases digest sugars.

**Amygdalin (Laetrile)—**"After years of observing patients using amygdalin, we can say with complete assurance that it is neither toxic nor worthless," Dr. Brodie says. "Nor do we find it to be a cure or panacea for cancer. The experience of our clinic, like that of many clinics worldwide, is that amygdalin has the ability to improve the patient's sense of well-being, relieve the pain of cancer, and reduce the requirement for pain medication."

When amygdalin is used in conjunction with other nutritional substances such as vitamin A and enzymes, its anticancer effects become more pronounced, Dr. Brodie notes.

Dosage levels depend on the stage of cancer. Dr. Brodie prefers administering the substance intravenously for up to 3 weeks, 9 g per IV per day. After the intravenous treatment, he has his patients switch to oral amygdalin—500 mg taken 3 times a day, continuing with this dosage even after the physical evidence of cancer has disappeared.

**Germanium Sesquioxide**—This natural element helps the body to activate and use oxygen, says Dr. Brodie. Cancer thrives in an oxygen-poor environment which is probably one of the ways germanium bolsters the body's resistance to cancer; it also enhances natural killer cell activity against cancer cells.[13] Germanium sesquioxide is the nontoxic form of the mineral. Dr. Brodie administers it intravenously, 500 mg per day during initial therapy, then orally, 100-150 mg per day.

**Antioxidants**—Antioxidants act as scavengers of free radicals, highly unstable molecules created from electrons that are released in the course of the millions of chemical reactions occurring in the body throughout the day. Free radicals are especially prevalent following exposure to toxic chemicals and are thought to play a key role in the conversion of normal cells to cancer cells, as well as in the growth of tumors. "Antioxidants protect the cell's DNA and membranes from free-radical damage, thus preserving normal cell reproduction and overall functioning," says Dr. Brodie.

***"Antioxidants protect the cell's DNA and membranes from free-radical damage, thus preserving normal cell reproduction and overall functioning," says Dr. Brodie.***

Dr. Brodie usually prescribes a daily supplement of multiple antioxidants that combines cysteine, methionine, glutathione, zinc, beta carotene, and other antioxidants. Selenium (200 mcg per day) is first given intravenously, later by oral supplementation; vitamin E is given in 400 units, 3 times a day.

**B-Complex Vitamins**—The B vitamins (B1, B2, B3, B6, folic acid, and pantothenic acid) work in concert with each other, acting as agents that help speed up chemical reactions. In this way, they plug into the body's enzyme systems and energy metabolism, Dr. Brodie explains. Deficiencies of one or more of the B vitamins inhibit the immune system's ability to fight cancer.[14] Both pantothenic acid and vitamin B6 have been shown to impede the development of tumors.[15] Dr. Brodie notes that vitamin B6 is also essential in the production of prostaglandin E1, which is necessary for normal thymus function and regulation of T cells. Folic acid inhibits the growth of chemically induced tumors, and cancer patients are frequently deficient in this B vitamin.[16,17]

"Many people in the U.S. may be deficient in various B vitamins, notably vitamin B6, because of overconsumption of refined carbohydrate foods," says Dr. Brodie. "This may not only increase their risk of cancer, but diminish their chances of recovery." In addition to the B-complex supplement in standard doses, Dr. Brodie recommends taking extra vitamin B6 (400 mg) each day.

**Shark and Bovine Cartilage**—The main scientific rationale for using cartilage to treat cancer is that compounds in cartilage appear to "turn off" the growth of new blood vessels feeding tumors. Ordinarily, as tumors grow, their surrounding blood vessels continue to expand and multiply to meet the nutritional needs of the tumors—a process known as angiogenesis.

"In no way should cartilage be considered a cure for cancer, or by itself to be sufficient to control cancer," says Dr. Brodie. "However, when combined with other immune-enhancing agents, it has been a welcome addition to our arsenal." Although Dr. Brodie uses the cartilage from both sharks and cows (bovine), he says the bovine form is "equally effective while considerably less expensive, requiring much smaller dosages than the shark material."

**Phytochemicals**—These natural chemicals found only in plants (hence the term, "phyto") have many cancer-repelling properties.[18] Examples include allyl sulfides (found in garlic, leeks, and onions), dithiolthiones (in broccoli and cabbages), and indoles (most members of the cabbage family). Allyl sulfides increase the production of an enzyme that helps the body excrete carcinogens and inhibit the tumor cells' ability to reproduce. Dithiolthiones help produce enzymes that block carcinogens from damaging a cell's DNA. Indoles stimulate the activity of enzymes that can detoxify carcinogens and may make estrogen less potent, thus lowering the risk of breast cancer. Other phytochemicals include saponins, flavonoids, coumarins, protease inhibitors, thiocyanates, and isothiocyanates.[19]

In addition to green concentrates or "green drinks" based on concentrated plant-derived preparations that are high in phytochemicals, Dr. Brodie recommends the use of soy products, such as tofu and soy powder, which are among the richest sources of phytochemicals. One cup of soy powder per day, mixed into beverages (soups, juices, etc.) or vegetable dishes, provides an ample amount of phytochemicals, according to Dr. Brodie.

## Innovative Patented Anticancer Substances

Dr. Brodie is studying other substances, such as Ukrain, Carnivora, and melatonin, for possible inclusion in his anticancer program. These have been developed outside the United States, chiefly owing to the restrictive attitude of the FDA toward natural and nontoxic methods for treating disease.

**Ukrain**—This compound, derived from a plant called chelidonium, has shown powerful immune-stimulating effects in people with a variety of cancers.[20] The main advantage of Ukrain, Dr. Brodie says, is that apparently it *selectively* kills cancer cells, and not only does it do no harm to the body's defenses, it actually fortifies them.[21] Based on studies of 70 cancer patients, the most appropriate dosages for Ukrain appear to be 20 days of 5, 10, 15, or 20 mg of Ukrain per injection, each day or every other day, depending on the condition of the cancer patient.[22]

***The main advantage of Ukrain, Dr. Brodie says, is that apparently it* selectively *kills cancer cells, and not only does it do no harm to the body's defenses, it actually fortifies them.***

**Carnivora®**—This unique substance is derived from Venus flytrap, a carnivorous plant. "Like Ukrain, Carnivora seems to attack tumor cells while at the same time strongly enhancing the immune system," says Dr. Brodie. The Carnivora solution is typically placed in 500-cc bottles (5 mg) and given intravenously 3-4 times a week for 1-3 months. Even higher doses have afforded better results in some cases, Dr. Brodie notes, adding that after the intravenous program is completed, intramuscular injections may be carried out 2-3 times a week for several more months.

**Melatonin and Interleukin-2 (IL-2)**—Melatonin is a powerful immune-enhancing hormone produced naturally by the brain as well as by many plants, which are the source of most melatonin supplements on the market today. When combined with IL-2, another immune-stimulating compound, mela-

***Dr. Brodie explains that making the appropriate adjustments in the psychological realm, however difficult this may be, can profoundly affect the course of the disease.***

tonin has substantial cancer-repelling power. "There are literally thousands of chemical messengers in the body, many of which participate in the body's orchestrated attack on tumor cells," says Dr. Brodie. "Melatonin is unique because it is both a messenger and a powerful antioxidant, which probably helps protect the brain from toxins that contribute to disease and aging."

Dr. Brodie recommends using 3 million units daily of interleukin-2 (a synthetic version of a naturally-occurring cytokine found in the human immune system). The exact dosage depends on the patient's cancer and overall condition. The typical IL-2 dose (as embraced by conventional medicine) is 90 million units a day, but this amount carries with it toxic effects that can even be deadly, cautions Dr. Brodie. The smaller dose of 3 million units can be used to "tonify" or give a moderate degree of stimulation to the immune system, adding to the overall immune enhancement provided by other supplements and modalities. Melatonin should always be taken at night, since the substance promotes natural sleep.

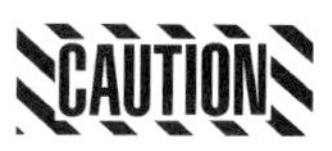


Megadoses of the alpha-interferon compound can be extremely toxic, which is why Dr. Brodie and his colleagues prefer to use it in relatively small amounts, combined with other key modalities.[23] The standard dose in his practice is 3 million units a day, says Dr. Brodie.

**Alpha-Interferon**—This other immune system secretion, or lymphokine, is increasingly used by conventional and alternative doctors alike as an immune-stimulating agent. Interferon is produced naturally by the body but is also available as a genetically engineered compound.

## Psychological Keys for Helping Cancer Patients

Emotional stress, certain personality traits, and other psychological factors can deeply influence the origin, development, and outcome of almost every disease, including cancer, says Dr. Brodie. How one deals with stress plays a vital role in the development of cancer as well as in the body's ability to battle the disease. Dr. Brodie explains that making the appropriate adjustments in the psychological realm, however difficult this may be, can profoundly affect the course of the disease.

Among the psychological features that may actually promote cancer, says Dr. Brodie, is a profound sense of loss, perhaps over a loved one, a home, or a business. He has observed hundreds of cases in which the person with cancer had suffered an intense emotional loss in the decade preceding the diagnosis. In many cases, however, the individual never effectively "processed" the grief, guilt, anguish, and other heavy emotions associated with the loss of an important relationship. Psychotherapy may provide a way to work through these emotions and arrive at a place of inner harmony.

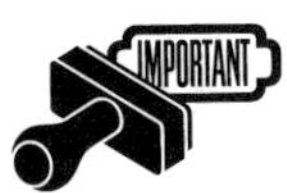


Certain personality characteristics correlate with cancer susceptibility, says Dr. Brodie. "Cancer patients are typically conscientious, caring, intelligent, and hard-working. They tend to take on other people's burdens and accept extra obligations to such an extent that they have little time for themselves or for relaxation and pleasurable pursuits." Another feature of the cancer-prone psyche is that these individuals usually prefer to suffer in silence, bearing their burdens without complaint or even acknowledgment.

Burdens of their own as well as of others weigh heavily, sometimes subconsciously, upon these individuals because they tend to internalize their cares, concerns, and problems, Dr. Brodie explains. "The carefree extrovert seems to be invulnerable, or at least far less likely to develop cancer than the caring introvert. Also, stress causes a suppression of the immune system, but it does so more overwhelmingly in the cancer-susceptible individual. Thus, personal tragedies and excessive levels of stress combine with the underlying personality to promote the immune deficiency which allows cancer to thrive."

To improve the prognosis of cancer patients, Dr. Brodie's counseling sessions are designed to help them establish a sense of personal control, an optimistic, positive outlook, greater facility for expressing their feelings, and a solid support system of immediate family members, extended family, and health professionals. "These psychological and social changes correlate with a better prognosis. Negative emotions such as guilt, animosity, bitterness, and pessimism must be purged from the patient who has been victimized by them, and replaced with love and optimism."

Dr. Brodie encourages his patients to maintain good dietary and exercise habits, since these help them begin to feel better about themselves and their lives, he points out. Dr. Brodie also encourages his patients to become active participants in their medical care and to learn as much as possible about the alternative methods available.

***"We try to help them cope with this disease, both physically and psychologically, to replace hopelessness with hope," says Dr. Brodie.***

Initially, however, when patients are feeling distressed or depressed, they tend to neglect their self-care. "It is difficult to bring about major change in one's lifestyle, and many patients find it too hard, too unpleasant, or just too inconvenient to make such sacrifices and alterations in their settled way of life, even in the face of a life-threatening illness," says Dr. Brodie. "For this reason, we counsel our patients to address these problems and to make adjustments to the best of their ability. We try to help them cope with this disease, both physically and psychologically, to replace hopelessness with hope."

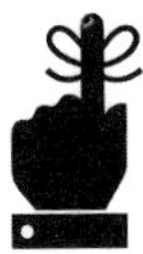

*Natural killer (NK) cells can stop the spread of cancer cells (micrometastases). Research has shown that NK activity is amplified by supplementation with selenium, germanium, and ascorbic acid. Vegetarians may have double the NK activity of their meat-eating counterparts.*

## CURRICULUM VITAE

# Etienne Callebout, M.D.

10 Harley Street, London, England W1N1AA;
tel: 44-171-467-8300; fax: 44-171-467-8312
or 44-1582-769832.

Etienne Callebout, M.D., (pronounced AY-tee-enn CAL-a-boo), a native of Belgium, received his medical training at the Free University of Brussels in Belgium in tropical medicine, and later in acupuncture, homeopathy, and naturopathy. While serving as a general practitioner in Brussels, he cofounded the group Arnica, which provides "non-toxic, alternative emergency care" for Brussels and surrounding areas. The turning point in Dr. Callebout's career occurred in 1987 when he was assisting the surgeon operating on his father, who had pancreatic cancer.

> ***"Rather than administer all the therapies at one time, I alternate and rotate the protocols so that the malignancy gets hit from different angles at different times," says Dr. Callebout. "Although it's not 'politically correct' to say this, this kind of biological 'guerrilla warfare' is our most effective way to combat cancer."***

Despite the operation and the intensive medical attention that followed, his father died 3 weeks later. Dr. Callebout then started studying the problem of cancer in greater depth. He began traveling and interviewing doctors around the world in an effort to learn about new and effective treatments for cancer. In 1983, he completed a year of study and clinical work at the Royal Homeopathic Hospital in London, becoming a faculty member in homeopathy; in 1990, he received a certificate in craniosacral osteopathy.

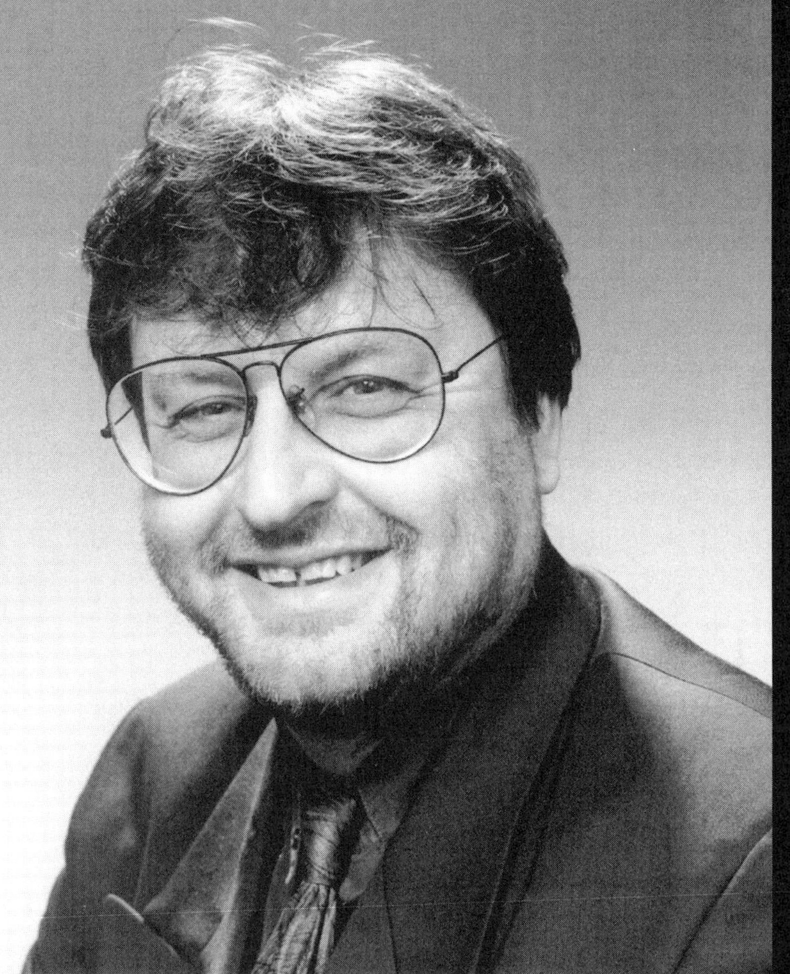

# *Etienne Callebout, M.D.*

**TO ATTEMPT TO SUCCESSFULLY** reverse cancer, Dr. Callebout employs numerous herbs, nutritional supplements, enzymes, and substances uniquely tailored to fight cancer, plus a comprehensive detoxification regimen, a thorough overhaul of the patient's diet and lifestyle, and psychological tips for "healthy survivorship."

For alternative cancer therapies to be effective, they should be rotated frequently, Etienne Callebout, M.D., contends. This way, the cancer process has less of a chance to adequately adjust or adapt to the anticancer therapy in use and thus become unresponsive. "Rather than administer all the therapies at one time, I alternate and rotate the protocols so that the malignancy gets hit from different angles at different times," says Dr. Callebout. "Although it's not 'politically correct' to say this, this kind of biological 'guerrilla warfare' is our most effective way to combat cancer."

Even more intriguing, he finds that some people show better responses to certain treatments when they're administered at specific times of the day, or when the treatments are spread out over time, from several days to weeks or months. "In some instances, I give a treatment then give the body a break for 5 days to allow the treatment to take hold," says Dr. Callebout. "If you don't do this, the treatments are often not as effective." In the interim between treatments, he prescribes detoxification of the liver, colon, or skin. Dr. Callebout also finds that the evening administration of immune system modulators is more effective than at any other time.

# Dr. Callebout's Generalized Model for Cancer Treatment

| STRATEGY | DOSAGE/ KEY COMPONENTS | FOR MORE INFORMATION see page # |
|---|---|---|
| **Nutritional Program** | | |
| Fresh organic vegetables; emphasize the following groups: (1) cruciferous vegetables: cauliflower, Brussels sprouts, broccoli, and cabbage; (2) green leafy vegetables: beet tops, carrot tops, kale, dark lettuce, cress, and spinach; and (3) root vegetables: beets, carrots, radishes and Japanese radishes (daikon), sweet potatoes, turnips, yams, and asparagus | variable | 749 ↓ |
| Fresh organic fruits: apples, apricots, currants, nectarines, peaches, plums, prunes, papayas, mango, kiwi, pineapple, and honeydew melon. Also apricot kernels (2-4 per day), blackberries, raspberries, cranberries, gooseberries, and elderberries | juice 2 oranges, 1 grapefruit, 1 lemon, 3X/day | |
| Sprouted and cooked cereal grains: brown rice, millet, rye, barley, buckwheat, corn, and oats | variable | |
| Seafood if advised: younger, faster swimming fish are preferable. Avoid shellfish. | N/A | |
| Vegetable protein: Legumes include lentils (as sprouts), chickpeas, kidney beans, lima beans, green peas (not split peas), and mung beans (as sprouts). Nuts and seeds are okay. | variable | |
| Other proteins: For some patients, organically produced meats in moderation, on an occasional basis. Live yogurt, organic buttermilk, and low-fat cottage cheese are acceptable on a limited basis. | variable | |
| Supplemental plant foods, seasonings and beverages: (1) a sea-vegetable salad, which may include dulse, kelp, hiziki, kombu, and alaria; (2) generous seasoning of dishes with fresh garlic and fresh ginger every day; (3) light seasoning with turmeric (1 g/day), cumin seeds and fresh basil; (4) liberal use of shiitake, reishi, and maitake mushrooms; and (5) Japanese green tea every day | variable | 809, 818, 823, 833, |
| Fat: Use only cold-pressed (usually labeled as "unrefined") olive and flaxseed oils; Essential Balance Oil® | 1-2 tbsp/day | 768 |

*Continued*

# Dr. Callebout's Generalized Model for Cancer Treatment (cont.)

| STRATEGY | DOSAGE/ KEY COMPONENTS | FOR MORE INFORMATION see page # |
|---|---|---|
| Bee pollen granules, non-heat-treated | 1 tbsp/day | 98 |
| Drink pure or filtered water | 10 cups/day | 791 |
| Avoid:<br>(1) foods high in saturated fats (sausages,pork, ham, cream, lard, etc.);<br>(2) refined oils (olive, sunflower, etc.), using only cold-pressed or unrefined oils;<br>(3) fried or roasted foods;<br>(4) stimulants (coffee, tea, alcohol, etc.);<br>(4) canned food and carbonated drinks;<br>(5) all preservatives and colorings (read labels);<br>(6) foods cooked in aluminum cookware or with aluminum utensils (use stainless steel, ceramic, or glassware);<br>(7) microwaved foods (which change many L-form amino acids into their D-form, are nonusable and promote free-radical production);<br>(8) cakes, jams, chocolate, and ice cream; and<br>(9) poultry and dairy products. | N/A | — |

## Other Daily Life Considerations

| | | |
|---|---|---|
| Spend time in natural surroundings, such as a park, field, forest, river or by the ocean. | at least 1/2 hour per day | 107 |
| Avoid EMF exposure. Turn off all electrical equipment in the bedroom when sleeping. Stop wearing a digital watch. Keep at least 6 feet (two meters) from the television, and do not watch it for more than 3 hours per day. | N/A | 108 |
| Adequate sleep and rest | 7-8 hours per night | 108 |
| Daily walking, yoga, tai chi, or Qigong | 1/2 hour per day | 1003 |
| Invigorating cold bath | 5 to 20 minutes, increase over time | 109 |

## Psychological Healing Strategies

| | | |
|---|---|---|
| Psychotherapy | depending on individual | 117 |
| Autogenic training | depending on individual | 118 |
| Meditation | daily | 117 |
| Self-reflection statements | daily | 118 |

| STRATEGY | DOSAGE/ KEY COMPONENTS | FOR MORE INFORMATION see page # |
|---|---|---|
| **Dr. Callebout's Detoxification Program** | | |
| Coffee enema | 3-4 times per week | 103, 964 |
| Liver flush | once every 3-5 weeks | 102 |
| Clean sweep (colon cleanse) | once every 3-5 weeks | 103 |
| Whole-body purge | once every 6 weeks if advised | 104 |
| Cleansing the skin | daily | 105 |
| Russian steam bath | according to advice | 105 |
| Salt and soda baths | according to advice | 106 |
| Mustard foot soaks | according to advice | 106 |
| Cold-pressed castor oil compresses | daily | 107 |
| **Alternative Cancer Care Strategies** | | |
| 714X | depending on individual | 871 |
| Aloe vera (Aloe Gold, whole leaf) | depending on individual | 812 |
| Amygdalin (Krebs) | depending on individual | 812 |
| Bovine cartilage | 9 g per day | 861 |
| Cat's claw | 3-6 g/daily | 814 |
| Chlorella, green barley grass, Pure Synergy | depending on individual | 809 |
| DMSO | depending on individual | 866 |
| Enzymes (modified Kelly-Taylor) and Wobe-Mugos® | depending on individual | 928 |
| Glandulars (including thymus and thyroid), New Zealand lamb origin | depending on individual | 935 |
| Green tea | 3 cups every day | 823 |
| Herbal medicines | red clover, 10 drops; goldenseal, 5 drops; pokeroot, 5 drops; wild indigo, 5 drops; thuja, 5 drops; figwort, 5 drops | 112 |
| Homeopathic 2LC1 & 2LCL1 | 1 capsule per day | 113 |
| Indocin (indomethacin) | 50 mg, 4X/day | 869 |
| Iscador | depending on individual | 830 |

*Continued*

## Dr. Callebout's Generalized Model for Cancer Treatment (cont.)

| STRATEGY | DOSAGE/ KEY COMPONENTS | FOR MORE INFORMATION see page # |
|---|---|---|
| Flaxseed (linseed) oil, cold-pressed | depending on individual | 768 |
| Maitake mushroom (Grifola), caplets and D-Fraction Liquid | depending on individual | 833 |
| MRV (Mixed Respirator Vaccine, contains staphage lysate) | injection 3 times a week | 872 |
| N-acetyl cysteine | 600 mg daily | 762 |
| Potassium | depending on individual | 783 |
| Shark cartilage | depending on individual | 863 |
| Tagamet® | 300 mg, 4X/day | 873 |
| Urea | depending on individual | 874 |

**CAUTION**

This chapter includes information regarding actual treatments used by Dr. Callebout only after his careful diagnosis of each patient. All cancer patients are unique. **Do not administer these treatments to yourself or others.** Discuss these treatments with your physician or other qualified health-care professional. Readers should not interpret this material as therapeutic advice, but should see a physician in all cases.

### SUCCESS STORY
### Reversing Bladder Cancer

When John, aged 73, was diagnosed with bladder cancer he underwent an intensive round of chemotherapy, but 18 months later his condition was basically unchanged. A few months after this, he went through a 6-month period of radiotherapy; after another 2 years had passed, when laboratory tests could not detect any signs of bladder cancer, John's doctors were confident that he would remain stable and, in effect, not be bothered by the cancer.

But only 2 months after that supposedly definitive prognosis, a biopsy revealed a tumor in the same location on the bladder. John's oncologist wanted to perform a rather mutilating procedure (called cystectomy) that involves removing the urinary bladder. After discussing options with Dr. Callebout, John was also to be treated with the Bacillus Calmette-Guérin vaccine (BCG) which, according to research, is effective against bladder cancer.

For reasons of his own, John refused to adopt Dr. Callebout's complete program. "John was reluctant to take large amounts of supplements or to undergo a drastic dietary and lifestyle change," Dr. Callebout says. "As a compromise, I placed him on a few key supplements for general support. It wasn't the optimal strategy, but it was the most he was willing to do."

***This strategy calls for a considerable amount of knowledge and intuition on the physician's part regarding the cancer process, the individual's physiological and biochemical status, and the effects of different therapeutic modalities, explains Dr. Callebout.***

Despite John's lack of full compliance, about 5 months into Dr. Callebout's partial program, a biopsy revealed that his bladder tumor had disappeared. Then 6 months later, the cancer returned for which John received mitomycin (a conventional cancer drug) and this apparently eliminated the cancer, according to biopsies performed 2 months later. But in another 6 months, John experienced his fourth cancer recurrence. The mitomycin was tried again, but caused such discomfort and other serious side effects that John decided to stop all conventional treatment. Once again, he went to see Dr. Callebout.

For more information about the **Bacillus Calmette-Guérin vaccine** (BCG), see Chapter 31: New Approaches to Immune Stimulation for Reversing Cancer, pp. 891-893; for more information on **enzymes**, see Chapter 32: Enhancing Whole-Body Metabolism for Treating Cancer, pp. 928-934.

This time, John was far more open to making major changes in his diet and lifestyle. He tried to adopt a primarily vegan diet, taking small amounts of dairy products and various supplements, but had difficulty complying with the overall lifestyle, which included regular exercise and various self-care detoxification measures. However, John was meticulous in taking his supplements which included high doses of antioxidants, a mixture of Western and Chinese herbs, garlic, magnesium orotate, organic sulphur, quercetin, coenzyme Q10, enzymes, shark cartilage, and various medicinal mushrooms.

Six months later, a new biopsy revealed that John's body was clear of cancer. All subsequent biopsies performed every 6 months thereafter revealed the same result. Given the persistence of John's cancer under conventional treatment and the fact that recurrences are typically more aggressive with each successive episode, John's complete recovery from bladder cancer under Dr. Callebout's alternative regimen is impressive.

## Changing the Diet to Help Cancer Recovery

Central to Dr. Callebout's dietary plan is his advice not to overeat, as this can result in poor digestion and an overly acidic blood condition. Ideally, the blood should always be slightly alkaline. When we overeat or consume high-protein or high-sugar foods, the blood becomes temporarily acidic. The reason this effect is transient is that the kidneys quickly excrete the acids and release "buffers" into the bloodstream, thereby neutralizing the blood pH. Frequent increases in blood acidity (pH readings below 7.0) tend to favor tumor growth and metastasis, as the immune system is less active under these conditions; however, some tumors seem to be inhibited by an acidic environment, notes Dr. Callebout. For this reason, clinical observation on an individual basis is imperative, he adds.

QUICK DEFINITION

In Chinese medicine, the **pulse** can be felt or "read" at 3 different positions and 3 different depths on the wrist of each hand. A total of 28 different energy qualities may be discerned from reading a patient's pulse, including wiry, thready, choppy, tight, knotted, intermittent, rapid, slow, deep, floating, large, slippery, or empty. The quality of the pulse indicates a specific energy state or disharmony of the body and its organs. In conventional Western medicine, the pulse is simply the rhythmic rate of an artery as blood moves through it, pumped by the heart.

Vary the proportion of raw and cooked plant foods, according to your condition, says Dr. Callebout. He relies on the diagnostic system of Chinese medicine (using the pulses, condition of the tongue and skin tone, and other indications) to determine whether a patient should consume more raw or cooked foods. "If you leave the dinner table with a slight hungry feeling, your energy levels, mood, and frame of mind the next morning will be much more conducive to healing," says Dr. Callebout.

Raw or lightly cooked foods are suitable for people who have a history of heavy meat-eating, whereas less raw foods are appropriate for those with a vegan or raw-foods background. Raw foods are best in warmer climates or during the warmer times of the year, when the body's caloric needs are reduced, says Dr. Callebout. All starches, especially grains, should be chewed thoroughly to the point where it seems you are essentially drinking it, says Dr. Callebout. The longer food remains in the mouth, the larger the body's production of digestive enzymes.

Here are additional dietary guidelines from Dr. Callebout:

**Organic Vegetables—**Whenever possible, eat only fresh, organically-grown, chemical-free vegetables, says Dr. Callebout. "With organic foods, you avoid or minimize your exposure to chemicals that may promote cancer, either directly or indirectly, by overloading the immune system." Organically-grown crops contain more protein[1] and vitamin C[2] than conventionally-grown crops. According to a 1993 study, the mineral content of organically-grown foods is 2-4 times higher than their conventionally-grown counterparts.[3]

**Anticancer Vegetables**—Among the recommended anticancer vegetables are the following groups: (1) cruciferous vegetables: cauliflower, Brussels sprouts, broccoli, and cabbage; (2) green leafy vegetables: beet tops, carrot tops, cress, kale, dark lettuce, and spinach; and (3) root vegetables: beets, carrots, radishes and Japanese radish (daikon), sweet potatoes, turnips, yams, and asparagus. Squash is also excellent. Potatoes tend to tax the pancreas, but are allowed on some occasions. Vegetables can be steamed, baked, or stir fried, but never boiled, as too many nutrients will leach into the water, says Dr. Callebout.

He recommends drinking 2 pints per day of freshly made vegetable juice, including combinations of endive, lettuce, parsley, spinach, carrot, or beet root. Dr. Callebout often advises his cancer patients to eat the following foods, seasonings, and beverages on a daily basis: (1) a sea-vegetable salad, including dulse, kelp, hiziki, kombu, or alaria; (2) fresh garlic and ginger; (3) turmeric (1 g/day), cumin seeds, and/or fresh basil; (4) liberal use of shiitake, reishi, and maitake mushrooms; and (5) Japanese green tea. These substances contain copious amounts of phytochemicals, or anticancer factors that are naturally present in vegetables.

***"With organic foods, you avoid or minimize your exposure to chemicals that may promote cancer, either directly or indirectly, by overloading the immune system," says Dr. Callebout.***

**Fresh Organic Fruits**—Fruit, either in whole form or as freshly squeezed juice, provides valuable nutrients and can be consumed in moderation. Avoid tinned, processed, and sweetened fruits or fruit juices; all fruits and juices must be consumed separately from meals, within 1 hour of mealtime. Dr. Callebout advises his cancer patients to eat the following fresh organic fruits on a regular but moderate basis: apples, apricots, currants, nectarines, peaches, plums, prunes, papayas, kiwi, pineapple, mango, and honeydew melon. As long as these foods are eaten close to mealtime (within 1 hour), the potentially detrimental impact of the sugar they contain will be greatly reduced, says Dr. Callebout.

Apricot kernels (2-4 per day) are recommended to provide amygdalin or laetrile. Unsulphured dried fruits are also acceptable, says Dr. Callebout, along with blackberries, raspberries, cranberries, gooseberries, and elderberries. If he recommends citrus fruits to a patient, he advises drinking the freshly squeezed juice of 2 oranges, one grapefruit, and one lemon, 3 times a day. "Take the juice in between meals—do not eat or drink one-half to one hour before and after the meal and do not consume the fruit juice (except for lemon) with vegetable juice. The overall majority of the fruits (and foods in general) recommended must have a low glycemic index, as excess insulin has been linked to increased tumor growth." For example, berries, cherries, honeydew, lemon, kiwi, and pineapple have a low glycemic index, meaning the blood sugar (glucose) levels they are likely to produce are low, thereby minimally stimulating the pancreas to release more insulin.

Dr. Callebout sometimes recommends adding the juice of ⅓ to ½ a lemon to each meal. The juice is poured over the meal, or consumed directly, diluted in water, to aid digestion. Lemon juice has long been known to be a superb source of citric acid and potassium, and their combined form, potassium citrate, is among the strongest blood alkalizers there is. By raising alkalinity, the bloodstream is less likely to show excessive levels of free calcium ions, which tend to encourage tumor growth.[4] Citric acid, found in citrus fruits, is essential to the basic process of metabolism, whereby energy for the body is generated from foods.

***By raising alkalinity, the bloodstream is less likely to show excessive levels of free calcium ions, which tend to encourage tumor growth.***

**Sprouted and Cooked Cereal Grains—**Dr. Callebout advises his patients to consume, either in sprouted or cooked form: brown rice, millet, rye, barley, buckwheat, corn, and oats, avoiding wheat because hybridization of this grain has compromised its nutritional attributes. The best sprouts are mung beans, lentils, millet, pea, and red clover.

Dr. Callebout's specific instructions are to mix equal amounts of the following uncooked, organically grown whole foods: buckwheat, rye, barley, oats, millet, sesame seeds, wheat berries, brown rice, fresh linseeds, (pop)corn, alfalfa seeds, lentils, mung beans, raw almonds. Store the unground mixture in a cool, dry place each night, then grind several tablespoons of it in a coffee grinder or food mill. Cover with water or apple juice and soak overnight at room temperature. In the morning, add fruit to make the mixture tasty, but keep it raw.

**Dietary Fats—**The adverse effects of excessive fat are, first, that it promotes free-radical production, which enhances tumor growth and, second, that it weakens the immune system by altering the physical functioning of the cell membranes. Fats can concentrate environmental pollutants, which, in turn, take their toll on the immune system and stimulate the proliferation of cancer cells. Dr. Callebout recommends using only cold-pressed (usually labeled as "unrefined") olive and flaxseed oils, consumed at a daily rate of 1-2 tablespoons, or more if advised. Dr. Callebout advises against the use of margarine since the hydrogenated fats it contains may promote cancer. (Hydrogenated fats have been saturated with hydrogen, which causes their structure to be rigid and unnaturally shaped.)

**Animal Protein—**"Protein is essential but must be used in moderation," according to Dr. Callebout—"that is, not more than 2 ounces or 60 g daily in general, and often less. To avoid stress on digestive organs, use only one type of protein at a meal." Protein should be consumed in proportion to one's lean body mass and according to temporary therapeutic restrictions, says Dr. Callebout. His recommendation is to eat the big meal in the morning and consume high-protein sources earlier in the day, either at breakfast or lunch.

Excess protein consumed in the evening will not be adequately broken down (catabolized) and used by the body, and that can result in toxicity and in the *promotion* of cancer because the whole elimination process of the body is shortened and delayed by several hours each day. "In the morning, you have 45% more hydrochloric acid in the stomach than later on, which is why you can better digest protein-rich foods earlier in the day." Drink lukewarm water or tea with foods, as these stimulate digestive enzymes.

On occasion, depending on the person's condition and previous diet, Dr. Callebout will recommend they eat organically raised meats. Most dairy products should be avoided, excepting live yogurt, organic buttermilk, and low-fat cottage cheese, but these should be consumed no more than 2-3 times per week. Under his regimen, seafood is permissible, but never shellfish, which is invariably contaminated to some degree. Poultry, even organically raised, is too contaminated for human consumption, so the optimal amount he recommends is none.

**Vegetable Protein from Legumes—**Dr. Callebout's legumes of choice for cancer patients include lentils (as sprouts), chickpeas, kidney beans, lima beans, green peas (not split peas), and mung beans (as sprouts). Many of these legumes are highly concentrated in certain substances (the isoflavones diadzein and genistein), which may block the action of estrogen and thereby impede the growth of hormonally-dependent tumors.[5]

**Nuts and Seeds**—Almonds in raw or sprouted form (not roasted or salted) are an excellent source of protein for cancer patients. If difficulties arise with chewing, patients may grind or blend them to make almond butter. All peanuts or dishes containing peanuts are to be avoided for their possible aflatoxin contamination; aflatoxin is a harmful mold found on peanuts. Seeds, including sesame (unhulled), pumpkin, and sunflower, should be eaten raw; sprinkle them over food and eat as much as you like unless instructed otherwise, says Dr. Callebout.

**Bee Pollen Granules**—Dr. Callebout recommends taking 1 tablespoon per day of non-heat-treated bee pollen granules.

**Food Combining**—The various nutrients in food tend to interact in complex ways, sometimes inhibiting and at other times enhancing the process of digestion. Therefore, careful attention to food combinations will greatly enhance the digestibility of food, particularly when chewed thoroughly as well.

## SPECIFIC DIETARY RESTRICTIONS

- Except for lemon, all the acid fruits should be eaten only on their own.
- Tomato and cucumber are best eaten separate from other foods because they both behave as acidic fruits; melon can be eaten only on its own.
- If salt is allowed, use sea salt only. Limit the intake of salt and salt-containing foods (i.e., hard cheese, sausages, pork, ham, lard, cream, chips, peanuts).
- Avoid sugar and sugar-containing products such as cakes, jams, chocolate, and ice cream. "If sweets are eaten, never consume them by themselves, as this practice tends to destabilize blood sugar levels and promote cancerous conditions," Dr. Callebout says.

## Dr. Callebout's Generalized Model for Cancer Treatment—Dietary Principles

**Easy to digest:**

Sprouted beans + vegetables
Sprouted beans + sweet or sub-acid fruits
Sprouted grains + vegetables
Vegetables + low-starch foods
High-starch foods + low-starch foods

**Relatively easy to digest:**

Protein + leafy greens (or vegetables)
Avocado + leafy greens or sub-acid or sweet fruits
Soaked or sprouted seeds, nuts or grains + sweet/sub-acid fruits
Vegetables + high-starch foods

**Hard to digest; promotes putrefaction and fermentation:**

Protein + starches
Oil + protein
Protein + sweet/sub-acid fruit
Fruit + vegetables

## A Quick Guide to Food Groups

Protein Foods: meat, fish, dairy, beans, tofu, eggs, nuts, seeds
Vegetables: all vegetables except low-starch ones (see below)
High-Starch Foods: all cereals: buckwheat, wheat, oats, rye, barley, millet, brown rice; potatoes, sweet potatoes, yams
Low-Starch Foods: carrot, parsnip, squash, pumpkin, artichoke, corn
Acid Fruit: grapefruit, lemon, lime, orange, pineapple, plum, prune, all berries, sour apples; consider tomato and cucumber acid fruits as well
Sub-Acid Fruit (fresh or dried): apples, apricot, sweet cherry, mango, nectarine, peach, grape, raisin
Sweet Fruit (fresh or dried): papaya, banana, dates, figs

> Sugar stimulates the production of prostaglandin E2 and other "bad eicosanoids" which may contribute to the growth of tumors.[6]

According to Dr. Callebout, other foods to avoid include: (1) foods high in saturated fats (sausages, pork, ham, cream, lard, chips, full-cream yogurt and cow's milk); (2) refined oils (use only cold-pressed or unrefined and in the case of olive oil, "extra virgin"); (3) fried or roasted foods; (4) stimulants (coffee, tea, alcohol); (4) canned food and carbonated drinks; (5) all preservatives and colorings; (6) foods cooked in aluminum cookware or with aluminum utensils (use stainless steel, ceramic, or glassware); and (7) microwaved foods (which change many L-form amino acids into their D-form, which are nonusable and promote free-radical production).

### SUPPORTIVE DIETARY MEASURES

Specific habits and food rituals may reinforce the cancer patient's dietary practice, explains Dr. Callebout.

- Maintain regular and consistent mealtimes.
- Light a candle before a meal, look at the flame for 10 seconds, then begin eating. This practice will put you in a more relaxed state.
- Avoid alternating between hot and cold foods on a frequent basis.
- Avoid taking hot baths and saunas up to 3 hours after your meal, as the digestive system requires an adequate blood supply, which heat immersion will divert to the skin.
- Drink pure water (a minimum of 10 cups per day) to help the body flush out poisons to be excreted in the urine. Don't drink tap water as it often contains herbicides, pesticides, chlorine, fluoride, and other chemicals.[7]

## A 6-Phase Detoxification Program Is Essential

Detoxification is essential to any cancer treatment program, says Dr. Callebout. If a patient does not attempt to relieve the body of toxins, the chances of recovery from cancer may be seriously diminished. "Detoxification can be a difficult and uncomfortable process, so it must be carried out with a clear understanding of what patients can tolerate and what they find difficult or not worth doing."

For information on **detoxification** (pp. 949-980) and **coffee enemas** (pp. 964-965), see Chapter 33: Physical Support Therapy; for more information on **Max Gerson, M.D.**, see Chapter 28: Nutrition as Cancer Medicine, pp. 771-776.

Dr. Callebout's program detoxifies the liver according to its natural physiological function of removing toxins. That is, in Phase I, the liver converts toxic compounds into intermediate toxins, some of them more toxic than the original toxin. (If this phase is not well monitored, an unnecessary "healing crisis" can result, which means the patient can temporarily feel worse as toxins are mobilized and removed from the body as part of the healing process.) In Phase II, the liver converts the intermediate toxins into substances that can be eliminated from the body, delivering them to the colon (via the gallbladder) or bladder for excretion.

Both phases of liver cleansing must be completed for the detoxification program to be successful; for this reason, Dr. Callebout supports both phases simultaneously. "When liver functioning is poor, the rest of the body is more prone to fatigue and illness. There are many vitamins and minerals that stimulate Phase I detoxification, but if the patient doesn't also attend to Phase II, the toxins can build up internally and cause free-radical damage to the cells."

***If a patient does not attempt to relieve the body of toxins, the chances of recovery from cancer may be seriously diminished, says Dr. Callebout.***

Both phases of detoxification are supported and enhanced by the following four detoxifying activities, as described below: coffee enema; liver flush; colonic sweep; cleansing drinks; and miscellaneous detoxification strategies.

A **free radical** is an unstable molecule with an unpaired electron that steals an electron from another molecule and produces harmful effects. Free radicals are formed when molecules within cells react with oxygen (oxidize) as part of normal metabolic processes. Free radicals then begin to break down cells, especially if there are not enough free-radical-quenching nutrients, such as vitamins C and E, in the cell. While free radicals are normal products of metabolism, uncontrolled free-radical production plays a major role in the development of degenerative disease, including cancer, heart disease, and aging. Free radicals alter important molecules, such as proteins, enzymes, fats, even DNA. Other sources of free radicals include pesticides, industrial pollutants, smoking, alcohol, viruses, most infections, allergies, stress, even certain foods and excessive exercise.

**Coffee Enema**—The coffee enema helps to purge the colon and liver of accumulated toxins, dead cells, and waste products. The enema is prepared by brewing organic caffeinated coffee and letting it cool to body temperature, then delivering it via an enema bag.

Coffee contains choleretics, substances that increase the flow of toxin-rich bile from the gallbladder. The coffee enema may be among the only pharmaceutically effective choleretics noted in the medical literature that can be safely used many times daily without toxic effects.[8] After the last enema at night, Dr. Callebout recommends an anal injection of 50 cc of cold-pressed sunflower oil (or a mixture of sunflower and flaxseed oil) before bedtime to preserve cell membrane integrity and improve impaired intestinal absorption.[9]

Early research by Max Gerson, M.D., founder of the Gerson Institute and Gerson Diet Therapy, recognized that the coffee enema is effective in stimulating a complex enzyme system involved in liver detoxification (called the glutathione-S-transferase enzyme system).[10] The increased activity of these enzymes ensures that free-radical activity is greatly diminished and that the activity of carcinogens is blocked.

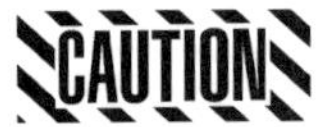

Dr. Callebout advises that the detoxification programs described here should only be conducted under the supervision of a qualified health practitioner.

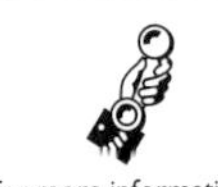

For more information about **Phosphodrops** and **Calc-Acid** (Calcium phosphate), contact: Nutri-West, P.O. Box 950, Douglas, WY 82633; tel: 800-443-3333 or 307-358-5066; fax: 307-358-920

"The coffee enema is capable of purging toxins and partial metabolites [products formed and released during metabolism, or the extraction of energy from foods] because the enema dilates the bile ducts and stimulates an enzyme system that is capable of removing numerous toxins from the blood," says Dr. Callebout. "The activity of the glutathione enzyme system is increased by at least 600% above normal." Caffeine also stimulates dilation of blood vessels and relaxation of smooth muscles, which further increases bile flow; this effect does not happen when the coffee is consumed orally.

**Liver Flush**—Under a physician's supervision, Dr. Callebout recommends assembling the following ingredients: (a) 8 pints of apple juice (unsweetened, preferably organic); (b) 1 ounce of ortho-phosphoric acid (OPA: this stimulates liver function and bile flow), or Phosphodrops; (c) Calcium phosphate (Calc-Acid); (d) Epsom salts; (e) whipping cream; (f) olive oil; and (g) white clay, medicinal green clay, or Bentonite, which is purified for human consumption. Then follow these procedures:

1) Add 1 ounce of OPA to the 8 pints of apple juice and mix well. Over the next 4 days, drink all the juice between meals at the rate of 3-4 glasses per day. Keep the apple juice chilled to avoid fermentation, but let it warm to room temperature first before drinking it. Rinse your mouth out using 1 teaspoon of baking soda in 1 glass of water, or brush your teeth after drinking the juice to prevent the acid from damaging your teeth. Otherwise, eat normally and take your coffee enemas as usual.
2) On the fourth day, while still taking the OPA, take 2 Calc-Acid immediately before breakfast, and 2 immediately before lunch. Drink about 2 pints of pure water that morning.
3) 2 hours after lunch, take 1 tablespoon of Epsom salts dissolved in warm water; add juice, if desired.
4) 5 hours after lunch, take 1 tablespoon of Epsom salts dissolved in warm water; add juice, if desired.
5) 6 hours after lunch, eat a dinner of whipping cream and fruit; the whipping cream contracts the gallbladder; any fruit is acceptable, but berries are a good choice, either fresh or frozen. Take 1 Calc-

Acid with your meal.

6) Half an hour before bedtime, put 1 tablespoon of medicinal green clay (or white clay or Bentonite) in 1 glass of water, mix well (start by adding water slowly), and drink up.
7) At bedtime, drink ½ cup of cold-pressed olive oil; a small amount of orange, grapefruit, or lemon juice may be added, if desired. Immediately after finishing the oil, get into bed and lie on your right side with your knees drawn up; hold this position for 30 minutes. You may feel nauseated during the night due to the release of stored toxins from the gallbladder and liver; this is normal and will pass.
8) On the following day, eat normally. Take 2 Calc-Acid with breakfast, 2 with lunch, and 1 with your evening meal.

**Clean-Sweep Colon Cleanse—** Keeping the large intestine in good working order, without excessive buildup of putrefying protein, fermenting sugars, or other forms of "rotting waste," is highly beneficial to overall health and especially to the cancer patient. To cleanse the colon, Dr. Callebout generally recommends the following strategy:

1) Add 1 tablespoon of psyllium

## How to Administer the Coffee Enema

Here is the regimen generally recommended by Dr. Callebout for administering the coffee enema:

1) Add 3 tablespoons of ground organic coffee (not instant or decaffeinated) to 2 pints of distilled water. Boil for 5 minutes uncovered to drive off oils, then cover, lower heat, and simmer for an additional 15 minutes.
2) Strain and allow to cool to body temperature. Lubricate rectal enema tube with K-Y Jelly (a lubricant widely available at U.S. pharmacies). Hang enema bag above you, but not more than 2 feet from your body. The best level is approximately 6 inches above the intestines. Lying on your right side, draw both legs close to the abdomen.
3) Insert tube several inches into rectum. Open the stopcock and allow fluid to run in very slowly to avoid cramping. Relax and breathe deeply, to let coffee flow in. Retain the solution for 12-15 minutes. If you have trouble retaining or taking the full amount, lower the bag; if you feel spasms, lower the bag to the floor to relieve the pressure.
4) After about 20 seconds, slowly start raising the bucket toward the original level. You can also pinch the tube to control the flow.
5) With symptoms of toxicity such as headache, fever, nausea, intestinal spasms, and drowsiness, one may increase the frequency of enemas. Take in 1-2 pints each time for these conditions.
6) Upon waking the next morning, if you experience headache and drowsiness, an additional enema is recommended that night. Eat a piece of fruit before the first coffee enema of the day to activate the upper digestive tract. Keep all equipment clean.

husks to 8 ounces of water; shake thoroughly in a jar, then drink immediately as the mixture will solidify if allowed to sit. Follow with an another 8-ounce glass of water.

2) Next, drink 4 ounces of the clay solution, mixing at the rate of 2 ounces of powder with 2 pints of water. Prepare the mixture the night before, as it must sit for 12 hours.
3) Repeat these 2 steps 2 more times a day for 5 days—a total of 15 doses, 3 doses daily. During the "clean sweep," follow the regular healing diet outlined below. Take the doses of psyllium and white clay between meals and continue daily coffee enemas.
4) When you finish your 15 doses, eat yogurt 2-3 times a day to replenish your bacterial flora; only use brands with active cultures.
5) A lot of stored wastes will be excreted in this process. You may feel discomfort and bloating the first day or two due to the expansion of psyllium in the intestinal tract. "You may pass a lot of exotic particles and substances similar to snakeskin," says Dr. Callebout. "This is actually dried mucus and dead cells from the surface of your intestines. These wastes can accumulate over a period of many years and seriously interfere with intestinal function."

**Whole-Body Purge—**The purge puts the body at rest and helps in the rapid removal of wastes, says Dr. Callebout. It also pushes the body into an alkaline state (that is, it realkalinizes a system that is on the acidic side of the pH scale), in which repair and rebuilding of damaged tissues occur rapidly, he adds. "But again, to blindly alkalinize is not indicated."

1) Juice 6 grapefruits, 6 lemons, and 6 oranges, pour the juice into a gallon jug, and add purified water until the jug is full.
2) Upon arising the next day, drink a blend of 1 tablespoon of Epsom salts dissolved in 4 ounces of water. Thirty minutes later take another tablespoon of Epsom salts in 4 ounces of water; after another 30 minutes, take another tablespoon of Epsom salts in 4 ounces of water. You will be taking 3 doses over a 1-hour period.
3) Two hours after the last dose of Epsom salts, drink a glass of the 3-fruit punch; thereafter, take a glass every hour. Eat no food that day except, if you wish, an orange for dinner.
4) Take 1 Calc-Acid 3 times, spread out over the course of the day.
5) During the purge, you may experience a variety of symptoms such

as nausea, headaches, muscle aches, and pains. These indicate the body is mobilizing stored wastes in preparation for eliminating them from the body. Gentle exercise and increased consumption of pure water can help alleviate these symptoms.

6) On day 2 of the purge, repeat all the steps in the Whole-Body Purge.

**Skin Cleansing**—During the detoxification procedures, breakdown products of toxins and the cancer itself (tumor cells release toxins into the blood) and other metabolic debris tend to accumulate and can produce skin eruptions.

The following procedure has shown considerable effectiveness in cleansing the skin of these traces of detoxification:

1) Once a week, rub your skin from head to foot with a mixture of equal parts of olive and cold-pressed castor oil.
2) Then, with the oil still coating the skin, immerse yourself in a hot bath for 15 minutes. The bath allows the oil to penetrate to the deepest levels of the skin, but take care entering and leaving the tub as the oil will make everything slippery.
3) After the bath, go to bed under heavy covers for 1 hour to sweat out poisons; then shower. Follow this routine every day for 3 months or as indicated (e.g., 3 times weekly).

Dr. Callebout says it is important to perspire heavily for 15 minutes each day and that aerobic activities can help encourage such sweating. "Exercise is preferable as a detoxification practice," he says, "because it accomplishes so many benefits at once. Rebounding (bouncing on a mini-trampoline) is especially recommended.

**Russian Steam Bath**—The following items are needed for this procedure: an old wooden chair, teakettle, plastic cover (a shower curtain is suitable), 3 towels (one to wear around the neck, one for the shoulders, and one for the knees to keep the plastic from touching the skin), footbath, ice bag, watch with a second hand, and lukewarm drinking water.

1) Take a hot footbath (104°-110° F) to pre-warm yourself, then apply a cold compress to your head; maintain the temperature of the

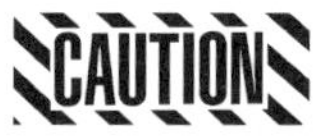

Contraindications for the steam bath include severe heart disease, high blood pressure, and diabetes. If you have any of these conditions, do not perform this procedure unattended.

footbath.

2) Wrap yourself in a sheet and sit on the chair.
3) Fill the teakettle, boil water, then put the steaming kettle under the wooden chair. The spout of the kettle should point away from your legs.
4) Remove the sheet from around your body, then place the towels around your shoulders, neck, and over your knees, but leave your head exposed.
5) Drape the plastic cover around your neck and over the chair, covering your body like a tent from the neck down to the footbath.
6) Put the ice bag over your heart area and keep it there; change the cold compress if necessary.
7) Check your pulse frequently (at the temple if someone else is attending). Stop this treatment if your pulse goes above 130 beats/minute. To check your pulse, place either your index or middle finger about one inch from the wrist, just below the bone running along the top of your forearm. Feel around temporarily for the pulsation. Count the number of beats every 20 seconds, then multiply that number by 3; repeat your measurement 3 times immediately to make sure the results are consistent.
8) Drink hot water if necessary to hasten sweating, but don't sweat for more than 6 minutes.
9) Have a cooling shower afterwards, gradually lowering the temperature of the water so that it's progressively colder; then rest for at least ½ hour afterwards.

## ADDITIONAL DETOXIFICATION ROUTINES

**Salt and Soda Baths—**If you have a history of "toxic habits," such as heavy meat-eating, smoking, or alcohol consumption, Dr. Callebout generally recommends taking salt and soda baths several times a week. Fill tub with warm water and add 1 cup of baking soda (sodium bicarbonate) and 1 cup of sea salt or 1 pound of Epsom salts. Stay in the bath for 20-30 minutes to mobilize toxins out of the body through the skin.

**Mustard Foot Soaks—**"This soak can help eliminate toxic headaches, generalized toxic symptoms, muscle aches and pains, and water retention in the ankles or other parts of the body," Dr. Callebout says. Add 1 tablespoon of mustard seeds and 1 teaspoon of ground cayenne pepper to a basin of warm water. Sit in a comfortable chair and soak your feet for 20-30 minutes in this mixture; repeat 2-3 times daily and especially during periods of intense toxicity.

To prepare a **castor oil pack** for the abdomen, lightly heat enough castor oil to thoroughly wet but not soak a 10" x 12" flannel cloth. Immerse the flannel in the hot oil, then fold to make 3-4 layers and place against the skin. The oil will help to draw out toxins, release tension, and improve blood circulation in the area, such as the lower abdomen where such packs are often used for relief of menstrual cramps, or at joints to relieve pain. Place a heating pad or hot water bottle (wrapped in a towel) over the pack, then cover pack and bottle with another towel to retain heat. Keep in place for 1-2 hours, then store flannel wrapped in plastic in a refrigerator for later use. After the flannel has been used 20 times, discard it.

**Castor Oil Compresses**—These compresses are particularly useful when applied to areas of pain, sites where tumors might be dissolving, says Dr. Callebout. Warm cold-pressed castor oil gently in a stainless steel pan so that the oil is warm, not hot. Soak a wash cloth in the oil, then remove the excess oil so that it does not drip. Apply this oil-soaked cloth over the tumor area or areas of pain or inflammation; keep the compress in place for 20-30 minutes and apply as often as you need relief. Do not reuse the compress; use different flannel each time. Castor oil can also be massaged into the skin in areas surrounding a tumor; use cold-pressed castor oil only. The compress may be applied over the liver, thymus, or spleen areas to stimulate the lymph system, says Dr. Callebout.

## Other Changes in Your Daily Life to Help Reverse Cancer

**Air Quality**—According to the American Lung Association, the typical indoor air in the U.S. is up to 20 times more polluted than outdoor air and people now spend, on average, 90% of their time indoors. Each day the average person has to excrete from the body an estimated 2 tablespoons of particulate matter (including dust, pollen, tar, smoke, acids, bacteria, rubber, carbon, metals, etc.), says Dr. Callebout. Therefore, it is crucial to reduce your exposure to polluted air.

***"The mustard foot soak can help eliminate toxic headaches, generalized toxic symptoms, muscle aches and pains, and water retention in the ankles or other parts of the body," Dr. Callebout says.***

**Natural Environment**—Whenever possible, spend time in natural surroundings, such as a park, field, forest, river, or by the ocean—barefoot is ideal—for the invigorating contact with the ground. In many hospitals in Japan and China, Dr. Callebout notes, cancer patients are encouraged to walk in the park or in other natural settings because this relaxing and rejuvenating activity is considered part of their cancer therapy. Intervention studies have demonstrated increased survival among cancer patients indicating a direct connection between improved quality of life, as typified by the above example, and the ability to overcome cancer.[11,12]

**Electromagnetic Field Exposure—**Electromagnetic fields (EMFs) are generated by electrical currents, including those that run the lights and appliances in your home. The EMFs generated by appliances, including computers, televisions, and kitchen appliances, are considerable, even if you stand or sit a few yards away from them.[13] Low-frequency EMFs can alter gene expression, enzymes involved in growth regulation, cellular calcium balance, and the brain's metabolism of melatonin;[14] some researchers speculate that EMFs may disrupt hormonal processes and tumor-fighting mechanisms.[15]

***Studies have demonstrated increased survival among cancer patients indicating a direct connection between improved quality of life and the ability to overcome cancer.***

To minimize your exposure to EMFs, Dr. Callebout advises that all electrical equipment in the bedroom be switched off when you're sleeping; that it's prudent to stop wearing a digital watch as this emits a field as well; that you sit at least 6 feet away from the television set; that you do not watch television for more than 3 hours a day; and that if you live near (within 1,500 feet) of high-voltage power lines, you should consider relocating, at least temporarily.

For more information about **air quality** (pp. 559-561) and **electromagnetic fields** (pp. 552-556), see Chapter 25: What Causes Cancer? For more information about **cold baths** and **hydrotherapy** (pp. 989-996), **exercise** (pp. 1003-1005), and **Qigong** (pp. 1005-1017), see Chapter 33: Physical Support Therapies.

**Movement and Rest—**Regular physical movement offers numerous benefits for cancer patients; it appears to protect against prostate cancer,[16] colon cancer,[17] and cancers of the breast, ovary, cervix, vagina and uterus.[18] "I recommend exercise primarily as a way to oxygenate the blood, which then helps repel tumor growth," Dr. Callebout says. He encourages people to do any sport or physical activity they like, "if their condition permits and unless instructed otherwise." For example, patients might run or jog for 15-20 seconds at a time, or less, for up to 20 times a day; or they may jump on a trampoline, or practice yoga or Qigong.

**Invigorating Cold Bath**—This cold bath may be done every morning, but only if advised by the physician. Begin with a short bath (5-10 minutes) then gradually increase it to 20 minutes. "Sit in your bathtub before filling it, then fill it with a strong energetic jet of water up to your neck. This stimulates your immune system." Do not follow this with a hot shower afterwards, Dr. Callebout cautions.

## A Roster of Dr. Callebout's Alternative Cancer Care Strategies

Before prescribing specific supplements, Dr. Callebout first assesses his patient's overall health by using both Chinese diagnosis (pulse reading and tongue analysis) and Western methods of health assessment, which typically include blood tests to determine the levels of vitamins A and C, lycopene, glutathione peroxidase, glutathione-S-transferase, primary and secondary bile acids, essential fatty acids, and other parameters. These tests help Dr. Callebout understand how strong the patient's biological resources are for the task of cancer recovery. Other tests include an analysis of the mineral content of hair and perspiration, both of which are helpful in detecting accumulations of heavy metals.

Based on the test results, Dr. Callebout determines specific adjustments that need to be made in his nutritional and botanical applications, most of which are described below. A central concern with respect to cancer is the relative supply of antioxidant nutrients, namely vitamins C, A, and E, plus zinc and selenium, Gold Stake® (a 22-mineral supplement derived from a seabed deposit), or EAP-2 minerals. "I use mainly Selenase (orally or by injection), obtained from Germany, or orally, with a specifically designed selenium for use in cancer."

**Aloe Vera**—Aloe is a garden succulent that is widely used medicinally for cuts, burns, skin problems, infections, and constipation. The antitumor activity of aloe vera gel seems partly due to its ability to inhibit formation of new cancer cells (angiogenesis) and the clumping together of platelets (called platelet aggregation, a blood chemistry change that can promote metastasis), hence, potentially blocking metastasis.[19] Dr. Callebout uses aloe vera in the whole leaf, liquid form, at a dosage of 1 to 9 tablespoons per day.

**Amygdalin/Laetrile**—"Amygdalin deserves to have a regular place in cancer therapy," says Dr. Callebout. "It is nontoxic and water-soluble, and there is considerable evidence that it works against cancer." For example, it has been found to have strong cancer-fighting potential, particularly with regard to secondary cancers, including a 60% reduction in lung metastases;[20] other research indicates amygdalin can extend the lives of both breast and bone cancer patients.[21] Dr. Callebout combines amygdalin with emulsified vitamin A, zinc, the previously mentioned enzymes, B15 (pangamic acid), and niacin.

**Cartilage (Bovine)**—This product, derived from the windpipe (trachea) of cattle (bovine), seems to contain compounds that inhibit the growth of new blood vessels, especially in cancers. Ordinarily, as tumors grow, their surrounding blood vessels continue to expand and multiply to meet the nutritional needs of the tumors.

Dr. Callebout's recommended dosage is 9 g per day (taken as 3 g, 3 times a day). Cartilage products should not be used around the time of surgery, says Dr. Callebout, since their antiangiogenic properties (preventing new blood vessels from forming) might interfere with recovery, which requires the body to produce new blood vessels or repair old ones in the process of healing. Dr. Callebout uses Benefin shark cartilage at the rate of 1 g/kg body weight/day.

For more information about **Lysolyph-Forte**, **Similase**, and **Enteropan**, contact: Euronutri, Buxton Road, New Mills, Stockport, Cheshire SK12 3JU, England, tel: 44663-742753. For more information about **Carbozyme**, **EAP-2 minerals** and **Lipozyme**, contact: Biocare, 54 Northfield Road, Kings Norton, Birmingham B30 1JH England; tel: 44121-433-3727. For more information about **Phytozyme**, contact: NF Formulas, 805 SE Sherman, Portland, OR 97214; tel: 800-325-9326; fax: 503-232-5710. For more information about **Gold Stake**®, contact: Gold Stake Inc., P.O. Box 2510, Cupertino, CA 95015; tel: 800-523-4653 or 408-864-4000; fax: 408-864-4004.

**Cat's Claw (*Uña de Gato*)**—Recent studies indicate that the plant, *Uncaria tomentosa*, contains substances that have immune- and digestion-enhancing properties.[22] Dr. Callebout often advises his cancer patients to take between 3 and 6 g of cat's claw per day. For more advanced cases of cancer, he may double or triple the dosage.

**Chlorella**—Dr. Callebout often recommends chlorella (single-celled algae) in combination with other "green foods," such as spirulina, barley greens, and wheat grass, which have similar properties. The recommended dosage is 3 heaping teaspoons a day. Dr. Callebout also uses Pure Synergy: 1-3 tbsp per day.

**DMSO (Dimethylsulfoxide)**—Dr. Callebout uses DMSO both topically and orally, often combined with aloe vera. DMSO often produces bad breath and skin odor similar to that produced by garlic; other potential side effects include occasional nausea, headaches, dizziness, and localized skin rashes (when DMSO is applied directly to the skin). Never mix DMSO with any chemical or drug and then apply it to the skin, as the proper DMSO dosage for such a combination is unknown and could be harmful, cautions Dr. Callebout. The dosage is variable and can be very diverse, says Dr. Callebout.

**Enzyme Therapy**—Dr. Callebout prescribes "massive amounts" of enzymes on a daily basis. For example, he may recommend that patients take 4 Wobe-Mugos® tablets with water 4-5 times per day; the dosage begins at one tablet the first 5 days, then increases to 2 tablets for the next 5 days, then 4 tablets 5 days later, and maintained at this level thereafter. Other enzyme preparations used by Dr. Callebout include: Lysolyph-Forte, Enteropan, Carbozyme, Lipozyme, Phytozyme, and Similase. He also uses Mannitol, a simple carbohydrate concentrate, to hasten absorption of the enzymes and nutrients through the gastrointestinal tract.

**Flaxseed Oil**—About 60% of the composition of flaxseed (also known as linseed) oil is alpha-linolenic acid (ALA), one of the omega-3 essential fatty acids our bodies need for good health, thus making flaxseed one of the richest source of ALA. A recent study found that linseed oil, but not corn oil, reduced the growth of breast cancers and metastases in animals.[23]

According to Dr. Callebout, cold-pressed and unrefined flaxseed oil should not be heated under any circumstances, since heating will cause the rapid formation of harmful (cancer-promoting) free radicals. Instead, flaxseed should be mixed directly with sulfur-rich protein foods only, i.e., legumes (beans, peas, lentils) or, if allowed, low-fat cottage cheese. If cottage cheese is allowed, Dr. Callebout advises adding 2 tablespoons of pure virgin, cold-pressed, unprocessed flaxseed oil to ½ cup of the low-fat cottage cheese.

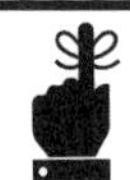

The safe and effective dosage of supplements and other substances suitable to the individual patient may be determined through electrodermal screening. For more information, see Chapter 34: Energy Support Therapies, pp. 1021-1032.

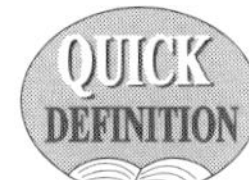


**Enzymes** are fundamental to all living processes in the body, necessary for every chemical reaction and the normal activity of our organs, tissues, fluids, and cells. There are hundreds of thousands of these Nature's "workers." Enzymes are specialized living proteins that enable your body to digest and assimilate food. There are special enzymes for digesting proteins, carbohydrates, fats, and plant fibers. Specifically, protease digests proteins; amylase digests carbohydrates; lipase digests fats; cellulase digests fiber; and disaccharidase digests sugars.

CAUTION

Dr. Callebout advises that since flaxseed oil is highly unsaturated, it readily oxidizes (produces free radicals) when exposed to the open air. For this reason, it has a short shelf life and must be bought as fresh as possible. Always keep flaxseed oil tightly sealed in the refrigerator; never heat or cook the oil. If these guidelines are not followed, the resulting rancidity makes the oil unfit for human consumption; further, if the oil becomes highly oxidized, it can be dangerous for cancer patients.

**Lipid** is a biochemist's term for a fat, which is one of the 6 basic food groups. Fats and oils are made of building blocks called fatty acids. Of these long-chain molecules (comprising atoms of carbon, hydrogen, and oxygen) the "fatty" end does not dissolve in water, while the "acid" end does. Fats are also called triglycerides as they consist of 3 (tri) fatty acid molecules joined to one molecule of glycerol, a kind of sugar. Unsaturated fats required in the diet are called essential fatty acids, and include linoleic acid (an omega-6 oil), found in corn and beans, and alpha linolenic acid (an omega-3 oil), found in fish, flaxseed, and walnuts.

Patients might also add cayenne or garlic, parsley, radish, and other herbs, or 2 tablespoons of the ground grain mixture described on page 96. The recommended amount of pure virgin, cold-pressed, unprocessed flaxseed oil per day is generally 1-2 tablespoons (more, if advised), says Dr. Callebout, but dosages will vary depending on the cancer patient's condition.

**Green Tea—**"As a warm beverage taken with meals, green tea is unrivaled," Dr. Callebout says, noting that this is a highly popular beverage in both China and Japan, countries which tend to have much lower rates of lung and breast cancers compared to Americans. Take 1-2 cups with each meal, advises Dr. Callebout. "Green tea may not have the appeal of popular herbal teas, but its subtle flavors become more enjoyable over time."

**Herbal Medicines—**Among the botanicals Dr. Callebout recommends on a regular basis are goldenseal, pokeroot, wild indigo, thuja (*Arbor vitae*), figwort, red clover, Essiac, and astragalus. Pokeroot has antimicrobial and immune-stimulating properties while red clover aids in detoxification. Astragalus (*Astragalus membranaceus*) has become popular as an immune-system stimulant and as a way to inhibit chemotherapy-induced suppression of the immune system; it has also demonstrated antitumor activity and may indirectly inhibit metastasis.[24] Another herb, *Rauwolfia vomitoria*, is effective in inhibiting neoplastic cell replication; in addition, 70% is absorbed through the intestinal lymphatic system, thus bypassing liver filtration.

The specific choice of these herbs and amounts Dr. Callebout prescribes varies widely depending on the individual and what other treatments are being administered at the same time. As a general rule, he offers the following dosages of liquid extracts to be taken 1 to 3 times daily:

- red clover, 10 drops
- goldenseal, 5 drops
- pokeroot, 5 drops
- wild indigo, 5 drops
- thuja, 5 drops
- figwort, 5 drops

**Homeopathic Nucleic Acids (2LC1 and 2LCL1)**—"I regard 2LC1 and 2LCL1 as among the most significant contributions of homeopathy to have hit the field of cancer management in quite some time," says Dr. Callebout. "They have shown no toxicity and appear to help cancer patients regain their vitality, and the treatments can be used alone or in combination with conventional therapy." 2LC1 and 2LCL1 are taken as encapsulized powder under the tongue. The treatment consists of one capsule per day in the morning on an empty stomach, at least 15 minutes before eating.

"Open the capsule carefully and empty the powder under the tongue, mixing it with the saliva," he suggests. "Once the contents of the capsule are completely dissolved, swallow your saliva." For more advanced or aggressive cancers, which demand intensive treatment, 2 capsules may be taken at different times during the day, advises Dr. Callebout.

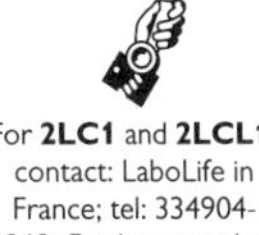

For **2LC1** and **2LCL1**, contact: LaboLife in France; tel: 334904-2212. For Immunoplex-N, contact: Distri-Pharma in Switzerland; tel: 4122-301-0820.

Another homeopathic remedy, Immunoplex-N (natural alpha-interferon in a 4X dilution), can be used as an immune modulator.

**Indocin (Indomethacin)**—By inhibiting the production of prostaglandin E2, the "bad eicosanoid," indocin effectively slows tumor growth while permitting more key immune system cells (macrophages) to enter the tumor.[25] According to Dr. Callebout, this therapeutic agent is most effective when given in dosages of 50 mg, 4 times per day.

**Iscador**—"Here in Europe the use of mistletoe as an adjunctive cancer treatment has been well established for some time," says Dr. Callebout. "The results of using Iscador have been particularly impressive with breast cancer."

**Maitake Mushroom**—Unlike other mushroom extracts, the maitake extract shows strong anticancer activity even when administered orally. Dr. Callebout usually recommends taking 10 drops of Grifron-Pro-D brand 3 times a day to obtain therapeutic amounts of maitake mushroom. Reishi and shiitake mushrooms are also useful.

**N-Acetyl Cysteine (NAC) and Glutathione**—N-acetyl cysteine (NAC) is an amino acid precursor for the production of glutathione which reduces free-radical damage to DNA and prevents depletion of other antioxidants.

> ***"I regard the homeopathic nucleic acids 2LC1 and 2LCL1 as among the most significant contributions of homeopathy to have hit the field of cancer management in quite some time," says Dr. Callebout.***

In addition, it helps metabolize various carcinogens, activates certain immune cells, helps synthesize and repair DNA, and may inhibit the blood vessel-forming process required for tumor growth.[26] Glutathione supplements diminish the toxic side effects of conventional treatments.[27] Dr. Callebout typically recommends patients take 600 mg of NAC daily. Dr. Callebout does not use NAC if the patient's liver is toxic (which can be determined by blood testing). If the liver is unable to convert NAC to glutathione, NAC inhibits T-cell activation.

Dr. Callebout also gives taurine, an amino acid that helps eliminate toxins from the cells via the bile; it also has antioxidant properties, maintains homeostasis in cells, stabilizes cell membranes, and protects the cell from an excess or deficiency of calcium.

**Potassium—**One of the most valuable lessons Dr. Callebout learned from studying Gerson Diet Therapy (developed by Max Gerson, M.D., 1881-1959) is the emphasis on potassium supplementation and sodium restriction. "Dr. Max Gerson found that potassium supplementation in the form of potassium gluconate, phosphate, iodide, or chloride is an effective way to restore the salt-and-water balance inside cells," says Dr. Callebout. "Elevating the potassium level appears to counteract tumor formation." Potassium is not a supplement to be taken lightly or at random. Dr. Callebout's view is that patients should be under strict medical supervision while they are taking potassium so their blood levels can be monitored.

According to Dr. Callebout, potassium gluconate (or phosphate or chloride) should be taken at the beginning of a meal. "From the beginning of the meal, you begin to raise your blood sugar level [glucose] and therefore your insulin level as well; this may make it easier for the potassium to get into the cells. One must be careful to avoid patients taking overdoses of potassium."

In another case, prostate cancer had spread to a man's bones but, after intensive potassium supplementation, the bone pain suddenly and completely disappeared. Yet another patient, on her own initiative, took an excessive dose of potassium chloride and on a CT scan one week later, her 6 brain tumors (which had spread to her ovaries) had all disappeared. "The cancer since then has reoccurred. However, the importance of further research into cell membrane potential and ion flux across that cell membrane needs to be highlighted."

For more information on **Gerson Diet Therapy**, see Chapter 28: Nutrition As Cancer Medicine, pp. 771-776.

**714X**—Dr. Callebout recommends giving 3 consecutive series of injections of 714X directly into the lymphatic nodes of the groin. The injections are given once a day for 21 consecutive days, followed by a break of 2 days to allow the patient to rest. People with advanced cases of cancer can receive more intense and prolonged therapy, since 714X has shown no harmful side effects, he says. In general, patients undergoing the 714X treatment should not take vitamin E or vitamin B12 at the same time to avoid interference with the effects of 714X, cautions Dr. Callebout.

***Numerous case reports exist demonstrating "spontaneous remission" of cancers in people practicing meditation in the absence of conventional treatment. "When we enjoy ourselves we are more conscious, we feel more alive. At the same time, we can learn to discover deeper joys as we change our entire state of health and our way of engaging with life," Dr. Callebout says.***

**Staphage Lysate/MRV (Mixed Respirator Vaccine)**—This is a vaccine consisting of remnants of a common bacterium called *Staphylococcus aureus* as well as viruses that attack this bacterium. It is useful as a general immune booster, as a stimulator of macrophage production, and as an inducer of interferon production. Dr. Callebout gives injections on an every-other-day schedule or 3 times a week, beginning with a dosage of 0.05 cc. The injection, to be effective, should leave an area of redness about 1½ to 2 inches in diameter, as measured 24 hours after administration; the dosage may be adjusted up or down, in 0.05-cc increments, to produce the desired area of redness, he explains. Dosages as small as 0.03 cc or as large as 0.75 cc are also within normal ranges for this medication, says Dr. Callebout.

**Tagamet®**—"The main benefit of this substance seems to be its enhancement of the immune system, thereby aiding in the host's ability to repel cancer," says Dr. Callebout, who often recommends that patients take 1

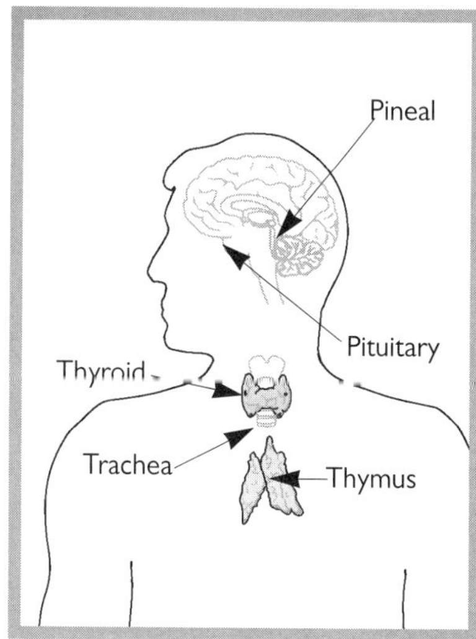


**Figure 4.1—The thyroid gland is the body's metabolic thermostat, controlling body temperature, energy use, and, for children, the body's growth rate.**

tablet (300 mg) 4 times per day.

**Thymus Extracts—**Thymosin and other thymus extracts stimulate immune function and are best combined with enzyme treatment. The thymus is a tiny gland located just above the collarbone at the base of the neck. A combination of thymosin and interferon (an immune system product or lymphokine) can produce a dramatic and rapid disappearance of lung tumors;[28] in these experiments, animals receiving thymosin had stronger natural killer cell activity and lived significantly longer than those receiving standard chemotherapy.

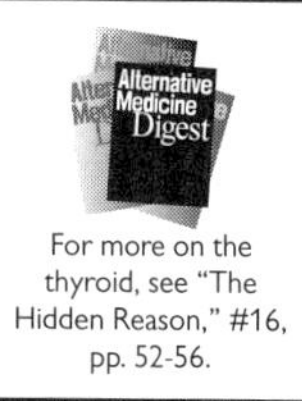


For more on the thyroid, see "The Hidden Reason," #16, pp. 52-56.

**Thyroid Extract—**The thyroid gland regulates metabolism by releasing hormones that control energy production in all the body's cells. Thyroid extract helps the cells eliminate waste and speeds up their restorative functions; thus, a healthy thyroid increases the body's cancer-resisting ability. If the cancer patient is deficient in various nutrients that support the thyroid (such as iodine, chromium, copper, L-carnitine, and selenium[29]), this gland's function becomes depressed and the functioning of the immune system declines accordingly, Dr. Callebout explains.

Dr. Callebout evaluates a patient's metabolic rate by checking the "basal body temperature." A relatively constant (basal) body temperature of less than 97.8° F may indicate low thyroid function, even when thyroid hormone levels appear to be normal in the blood. If the basal temperature is low, Dr. Callebout may recommend thyroid-supporting supplements and thyroid extract. A combination of kelp and cayenne—cayenne should be at least 40,000 HTU (heat thermal units)—can also be used to increase body temperature. He explains that there are different kinds of cayenne, ranging from virtually no heat thermal units, as with paprika, to over 100,000 HTU, as with African cayenne. Dr. Callebout notes that there is some evidence indicating that broccoli, Brussels sprouts, cabbage, and turnips may depress thyroid function.[30]

Dr. Callebout believes that thyroid stimulation needs to be monitored (by temperature and blood tests) in the individual patient. Again, relaxation and relieving stress have a direct effect on our enzymes and cell membranes. Further, elevated cortisol levels inhibit thyroid hormone action at the cellular level and, thus, stimulating thyroid function may overstimulate the cortisol-producing adrenals, leading to even more exhaustion, says Dr. Callebout. Working on the adrenal glands may restore thyroid action, he adds.

***"Psychotherapy and meditation can diminish these negative emotions [fear, guilt, self-blame] or render them less toxic to the individual," says Dr. Callebout.***

**Urea—**This substance is produced naturally by the liver as a waste product of protein metabolism, and it has strong antioxidant properties. Since the liver is the only organ that shows high concentrations of urea after oral administration of the substance, urea therapy may not be effective against cancers other than liver, says Dr. Callebout. For his patients, he generally recommends using about 20 g of urea in powder form, dissolved in a quart of water or juice, and consumed in at least 4 divided doses over the course of the day.

## Psychological Healing Supports Cancer Treatment

Mind/body medicine can greatly reinforce the cancer patient's process of recovery. The intense fear and anxiety evoked by the diagnosis of cancer can adversely affect both body and mind. Uncertainty about the future and not knowing what may be happening inside one's body tend to ignite and magnify such fears. In some cases, people become fixated on past behaviors, believing they may have contributed to the cancer, and this leads to feelings of guilt or self-blame. "Psychotherapy and meditation can diminish these negative emotions or render them less toxic to the individual," says Dr. Callebout.

The primary value of psychotherapy and psychosocial support is to enable the individual to explore past traumas, heal the emotional wounds resulting from those traumas, and deal with negative emotions such as anger, fear, resentment, and guilt, which may be obstructing the process of recovery, says Dr. Callebout. "In many cases, if an individual does not work

## ART THERAPY

# Draw Your Cancer Away

Visual imagery is among the most potent ways by which the subconscious mind communicates thoughts and feelings to the body, says Dr. Callebout. Here's how to put it to work.

Imagine your cancer as weak and your immune system as strong; meditate on whatever images arise.

Choose 2-3 colors, then, based on your imaginative understanding of the process, use them to illustrate how the cancer can be overcome.

"Sometimes the most powerful forms of mind/body communication are evoked through unconscious thoughts and feelings conveyed through imagery," says Dr. Callebout. "When cancer patients go through a guided meditation, in which I describe the cancer process to them in simple terms, they then can begin to form pictures in their minds regarding the interaction between cancer and the immune system. The drawings help amplify the mind's creative capacity to guide and control the immune processes involved in reversing the cancer."

Patients may show healing rays or creatures killing or shrinking the tumors or they may insert words like "Pow!" or "Zap!" into their drawings, emphasizing their immune system's power. Dr. Callebout cites a case in which a young man with colon cancer had drawn two pictures. In the first frame, he depicted the cancer as an ominous, dark, tangled growth consuming a garden of flowers in the colon wall. In the next picture, he drew his version of the immune system, as the Sun, pouring down golden rays that made the garden glow in brilliant pinks and greens; the dark cancer growth had disappeared.

through these traumatic memories or emotional blocks, they will not be able to unleash their inner healing resources."

To cope with their emotions, the cancer patient must be given a structured program of self-care including, for example, meditation, guided imagery, Qigong or yoga, or autogenic training—a combination of imagery and autosuggestion, including the use of self-statements, such as: "My legs and arms are becoming warm and heavy, all the muscles in my body are softening and melting, deep relaxation flows through my body." Numerous case reports exist demonstrating "spontaneous remission" of cancers in people practicing meditation in the absence of conventional treatment.[31] "I try to guide my patients in developing ways to induce present-moment awareness, a state of relaxed yet focused attention, a peaceful, nonjudgmental frame of mind."

Dr. Callebout cautions that psychological work must be done in tandem with biochemical adjustments. "No amount of psychotherapy, support groups, or stress management will help the cancer patient if the body is not receiving adequate biological support at the same time. You can have the best talk therapy in the world without creating any fundamental changes at the most crucial level of living cells."

## Insights for Healthy Cancer Survivorship

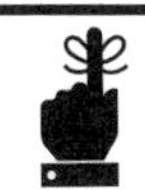

As an example of mind/body holistic medical thinking, Dr. Callebout states that psychological work must be done in tandem with biochemical adjustments.

Survivorship is not simply a matter of outliving the prognosis. As Dr. Callebout points out, "healthy survivorship" is a matter of working through the suffering and other psychophysical challenges posed by the cancer experience. His main advice is simple: "Stop doing things that make you sick—smoking, overeating, not getting enough rest—and start doing the things that make you well, such as a wholesome diet, adequate sleep, and increased fresh air and water."

Dr. Callebout is sensitive to the fact that many of his patients may tend to view his recommendations for lifestyle changes as difficult. As physical health changes, people often begin to relish the changes, he says. "After a while, you will notice that your senses of smell and taste are enhanced, and you are feeling much healthier," he says. "Many people find that after a while, they redevelop their sense for natural tasty food. As their energy levels increase and they feel more relaxed in their bodies, they become more confident and at ease in their treatment program."

While he encourages his patients to find other areas in their lives to enjoy besides food, Dr. Callebout also urges them to observe the effects of food on their health and well-being. He urges a long-range perspective when viewing one's dietary changes: "Once better, and with your rediscovered food instincts, you will be able to eat and drink what your body wants, but that is not now." His parting message to cancer patients is to find a balance of joy and moderation in daily life. "Life is to enjoy, and I am sure you can find other areas in your life to enjoy besides food," he tells his patients. "When we enjoy ourselves we are more conscious, we feel more alive. At the same time, we can learn to discover deeper joys as we change our entire state of health and our way of engaging with life." In that discovery of "deeper joy," says Dr. Callebout, people often come to realize the gifts of healing that are paradoxically an integral part of the cancer experience.

## CURRICULUM VITAE

# Ernesto R. Contreras, M.D.

Oasis Hospital, Organizacion Avanzada en
Sistemas Integrales Para la Salud, S.C.,
Paseo Playas de Tijuana No. 19,
Apartado Postal No. 179, Playas de
Tijuana, B.C. 22700 Mexico;
tel: 5266-80-18-50; fax: 5266-80-18-55.
U.S. address: P.O. Box 43-9045, San Ysidro,
CA 92143, or 4630 Border Village Road,
Suite 203, San Ysidro, CA 92173;
tel: 800-700-1850.

Dr. Contreras graduated as a surgeon and physician in 1939 from the Army Medical School in Mexico City, Mexico. In the 1940s, Dr. Contreras was a general practitioner with a specialty in clinical pathology; from 1949-1963, he worked as a pathologist in Mexico City and Tijuana. Dr. Contreras has held various academic and professional positions, including professor of histology and pathology in the Army Medical School (1946-1955), sub-chief, Pathology Department, Children's Hospital and General Army Hospital, both in Mexico City (1946-1953), then chief, Pathology Department at General Army Hospital (1953-1955). In 1963, Dr. Contreras founded the Hospital Ernesto Contreras R. (Oasis Hospital) in Tijuana and has served since then as chief oncologist and general director.

***"A person's positive attitude and faith bring about favorable chemical changes in the body that ward off offending cancer-causing chemical messengers." As Dr. Contreras sees it, there is no false hope—all hope is therapeutic, which is why optimists live longer.***

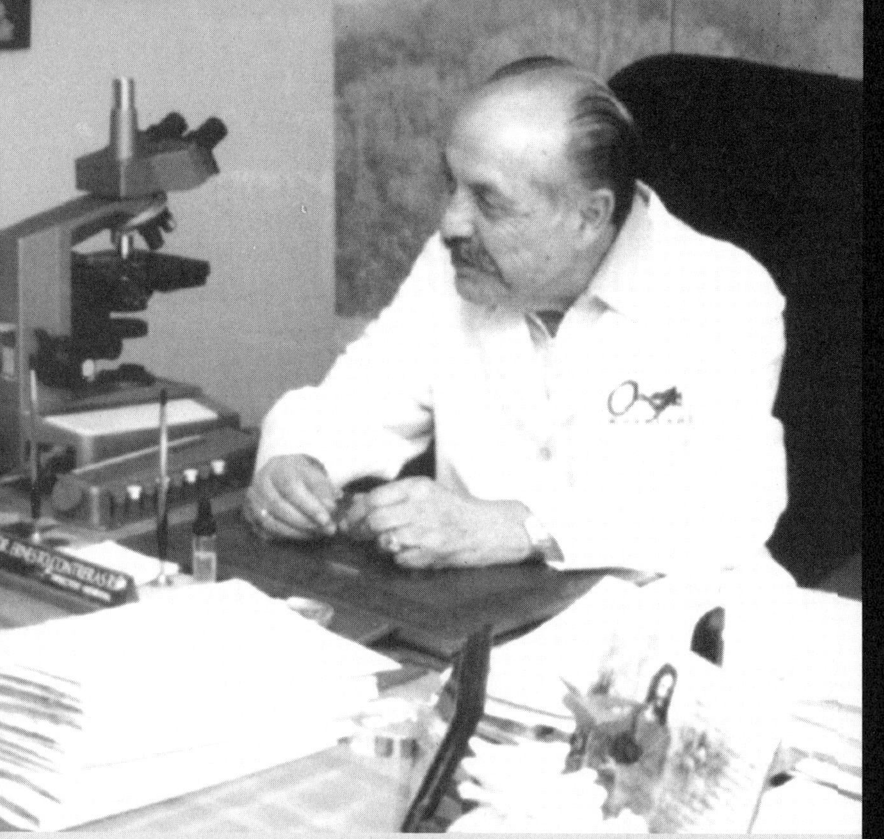

## Chapter 5

# *Ernesto R. Contreras, M.D.*

**SINCE 1963,** Dr. Contreras has used a clinically proven blend of nutrients, herbs, intravenous laetrile, enzymes, detoxification, dietary change, counseling, and a resolute message of hope and optimism to help over 80,000 patients at the Oasis Hospital in Tijuana, Mexico.

Since 1963, Ernesto R. Contreras, M.D., founder and medical director of Oasis Hospital in Tijuana, Mexico, and his staff have treated over 80,000 cancer patients with a high degree of success using nontoxic alternative methods. In fact, Dr. Contreras was the first in Mexico to introduce the multimodal alternative approach to cancer.

In the course of 33 years of treating cancer, Dr. Contreras (originally trained as a pathologist) has never wavered from his commitment to "total care," addressing the whole patient, in body, mind, emotions, and spirit. "This approach is made possible only when physicians are willing to use a special blend of science, medicine, faith, and compassion to make a vital and lasting connection with the patient," says Dr. Contreras.

An essential aspect of this connection is to strongly encourage the attitude of hope. "A person's positive attitude and faith bring about favorable chemical changes in the body that ward off offending cancer-causing chemical messengers." As Dr. Contreras sees it, there is no false hope—all hope is therapeutic, which is why optimists live longer.

## Helping the Patient Become an Active Participant in Healing

For lasting success, the cancer patient must become an active participant in the selection and administration of the treatment program, says Dr. Contreras. In conjunction, "because it is so crucial for a patient's emotional state to be positive," Oasis staff form patient-physician partnerships that include the patient in "every part of the healing process," Dr. Contreras explains.

"Our staff advise patients, listen to them compassionately, even pray actively with and for them because we believe that in doing so we can max-

# Dr. Contreras' Generalized Model for Cancer Treatment

| STRATEGY | DOSAGE/ KEY COMPONENTS | FOR MORE INFORMATION see page # |
|---|---|---|
| **Dietary Plan** | | |
| Eat "living" foods | organic fruits and vegetables, whole or as juices | 749 |
| Avoid | frozen and canned foods; foods with preservatives, additives, or colorings; white flour, salt, white sugar, caffeine, alcohol, shellfish, and red meat | ↓ |
| **15-Day Metabolic Program** | | |
| Laetrile | individually determined | 812 |
| Preven-Ca (*Cardus marianus*, apricot flour, carrot root, shark cartilage, garlic, alfalfa, and boldo) | 1 tablet before each meal | 127 |
| Warburg/Cone cancer therapy | low-fat, high complex carbohydrate diet (3000 calories daily, largely whole grains); taking lente insulin, thyroid hormone, and quercetin | 128 |
| **Supplements** | | |
| Vitamin A | high doses; not to exceed 300,000 IU daily in cases of liver cancer or dysfunction | 784 |
| Vitamin C | intravenous, up to 50 g daily, followed by a 10-g daily oral maintenance dose | 786 |
| Proteolytic enzymes (formula contains pancreatin, papain, bromelain, trypsin, chymotrypsin, lipase, amylase, and rutin) | initially given as suppositories (1-2 daily), then as pills (6-9 daily) for an indefinite period | 928 |
| **Other Therapies** | | |
| Detoxification | organic foods diet; intravenous solutions of vitamin C, potassium, and others; 2 high-colonic enemas and 6 coffee enemas | 949 |
| Chelation | intravenous solution of selected vitamins, minerals, heparin, and EDTA | 973 |
| Counseling | emotional and spiritual | 129 |

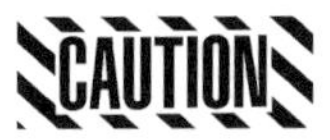

This chapter includes information regarding actual treatments used by Dr. Contreras only after his careful diagnosis of each patient. All cancer patients are unique. **Do not administer these treatments to yourself or others.** Discuss these treatments with your physician or other qualified health-care professional. Readers should not interpret this material as therapeutic advice, but should see a physician in all cases.

imize the possibility of realizing complete healing and remission in each patient." Dr. Contreras's staff includes 8 other M.D.s (including his son) who work in a modern 80-bed facility, complete with an intensive care unit, radiology department (for CT scans, X rays, and ultrasound), and a high-tech laboratory for producing several of their special medicines. The average length of stay is 2-3 weeks.

Most often, patients arrive at Oasis Hospital after having tried conventional treatments which failed to help them. A woman in her thirties arrived from California with a grim prognosis of imminent death from bone marrow cancer. Chemotherapy had made no improvement in her condition.

***"Our staff advise patients, listen to them compassionately, even pray actively with and for them because we believe that in doing so we can maximize the possibility of realizing complete healing and remission in each patient," says Dr. Contreras.***

"Cancer treatment in the U.S. is somewhat primitive with its looming doomsday feeling over your head all the time compared to Oasis where the care is humane," she remarks. "We're treated with hope, smiles, and lots of optimism."

Dr. Contreras is firmly committed to the belief that a cancer approach more in accord with the Hippocratic oath to "first, do no harm" to the patient is not only advisable but gets better results. This means a radically reduced clinical dependency on the highly aggressive forms of treatment such as chemotherapy, surgery, and radiation, and a greater reliance on methods that support the immune system.

"Over the years, we have been able to prove by our statistics that it is true our patients have longer survival rates and a better quality of life than those taking only conventional treatments," says Dr. Contreras. A statistical analysis of 5-year survival outcomes for 863 Oasis Hospital patients with prostate cancer tracked over a 15-year period came out at 83% compared to 73% under conventional care, according to 1993 figures. (See "Laetrile/Metabolic Therapy for Prostate Cancer," on page 125.) "We believe that metabolic therapy is a good alternative to treat cancer of the prostate in all stages," says Dr. Contreras.

Dr. Contreras analyzed the results of using his laetrile/metabolic program on 257 patients with inoperable bronchogenic carcinoma (a form of lung cancer). The program included laetrile, enzymes, vitamins A and C, and selenium; for 20% of patients, moderate doses of radiation therapy were given. The quality of life improved in 60% of cases; the 12-month survival was 55.25% of cases; and the mean survival was 50.4 weeks. In contrast, results obtained using strictly conventional treatments were as follows: quality of life improved in 30% of cases; 12-month survival was 23%; mean survival was 31.8 weeks. "According to these results," says Dr. Contreras, "metabolic therapy is a good alternative to treat this type of cancer when conventional treatments fail or the patients cannot tolerate them."

For Stage 4 cancers (the most serious in which cancer has spread throughout the body), Oasis Hospital gets on average 35% objective improvement, meaning the tumor shrinks by at least 50%, and 60% subjective improvement, meaning the patient feels better without a change in tumor size.

## Laetrile/Metabolic Therapy for Prostate Cancer: Statistical Results for 863 Patients at Oasis Hospital

Protocol: Patients received intravenous amygdalin at the rate of 6 g daily for 3-4 weeks; Wobe-Mugos enzyme suppositories (1 daily for 3-4 weeks); vitamin C (25 g intravenously, daily for 3-4 weeks). In the presence of bone metastases, a 12-day course of intravenous calcium (4 g per dose) plus calcitonin was given provided there was normal calcium in the blood and patients were not receiving digitalis.

**RESULTS:**

Complete remission: 4.5% (39 patients)

Partial remission: 37.3% (322 patients)

Stabilization: 41.3% (356 patients)

Failure: 16.9% (146 patients)

5-Year Survival: 83.1%

## SUCCESS STORY

### Reversing Breast Cancer

Jennifer, aged 68, came to Oasis Hospital after receiving a modified radical mastectomy of her left breast. She had been diagnosed with highly invasive breast cancer that had already spread to 5 out of 14 nearby lymph nodes. Her conventional physicians said this cancer had an exceptionally high risk of recurrence or of spreading widely through her body. Jennifer declined radiation and chemotherapy and traveled from Illinois to Oasis Hospital in Tijuana, Mexico, instead.

Dr. Contreras started Jennifer on his multifaceted metabolic therapy program, emphasizing high doses of intravenous laetrile, enzymes, vitamins A and C, and other substances to improve her immune system. Dr.

Contreras also administered tamoxifen, a conventional cancer drug often given to prevent recurrences of breast cancer. His reason was that Jennifer's tumor was an "estrogen receptor" and would respond well to tamoxifen, which has direct effects on the hormones.

Jennifer completed the 3-week metabolic program with no adverse reactions, then returned home with a 3-month supply of oral nutrients. That was in 1987. "We have been following Jennifer regularly and she had no cancer recurrence for 8 years," says Dr. Contreras. In mid-1996, 2 small tumors just beneath the skin were removed from her left chest wall, for which she received a short course of local radiation.

***For Stage 4 cancers (the most serious in which cancer has spread throughout the body), Oasis Hospital gets on average 35% objective improvement, meaning the tumor shrinks by at least 50%, and 60% subjective improvement, meaning the patient feels better without a change in tumor size.***

"Her general health is excellent," says Dr. Contreras. "The fact that we could keep this patient tumor-free for 8 years using exclusively metabolic therapy, when this case was considered originally as highly aggressive, makes the outcome very successful. The fact that lately she developed 2 small metastases does not reduce the effectiveness of our nontoxic therapy. We will continue protecting her health indefinitely."

## Intensive Laetrile Therapy to Stimulate Immune Health

"The 15-day metabolic program is a treatment based on the use of laetrile, proteolytic enzymes, immuno-stimulants, vitamin and mineral supplements, and other nontoxic anticancer agents," says Dr. Contreras.

**Laetrile**—Also known as amygdalin, this is a natural substance extracted from any of 1200 plants but primarily apricot pits. Oasis Hospital manufactures its own laetrile for use with its patients; typically, it is given intravenously. "For the prevention of cancer and the maintenance of remission, there is nothing as effective as laetrile," comments Dr. Contreras who has used it since 1963 as a cornerstone of his metabolic therapy for cancer. "Its nontoxicity permits its use indefinitely while surgery, radiation, and chemotherapy can only be administered for a limited time."

According to Dr. Contreras, laetrile is not suitable for certain cancers, including primary brain cancer, sarcomas of the muscles, connective tissues, fat tissue, and bone tissue. "All of these are highly resistant to laetrile, so we have to use other alternatives," says Dr. Contreras. "But the majority of the cancers that occur more frequently, such as cancers of the lung, breast, colon, ovaries, stomach, esophagus, prostate, and the lymphomas, are much helped by laetrile."

In the case of metastatic liver cancer (which tends to originate in the colon), Dr. Contreras implants a porta-cath catheter in a branch of the portal vein leading to the liver, a practice he first started in 1984. Through this catheter, he introduces a conventional chemotherapy drug called 5-fluoracil (5 FU, commonly used for colon cancer with about a 5% success rate) over a 4-6 hour period. Dr. Contreras performs this infusion monthly for 5 days in a row; then he introduces laetrile through the catheter daily for 3 weeks.

***"Warburg/Cone cancer therapy is designed to selectively destroy malignant cells without harming the normal cells of the body," Dr. Contreras explains.***

This cycle of 5 FU infusion and laetrile is repeated every month and blood counts (leukocytes and platelets) are monitored for progress. If there is evidence of a positive response, Dr. Contreras continues this for 3-6 more cycles "until a good stabilization or remission is accomplished." At the same time, the patient receives Wobe-Mugos enzyme suppositories, high doses of vitamin C, and several immune-enhancing nutrients. Of the types of cancer for which Dr. Contreras performs this approach, about 80% are rectal or colon cancer.

"When we introduce this directly into the liver with laetrile, in about 30% of the cases, the results are very good. This demonstrates that laetrile can and should be combined with chemotherapy for this kind of liver cancer. With lymphomas, the combination of laetrile with chemotherapy works much better than using either alone."

**Preven-Ca—**This is a blend of medicinal herbs and shark cartilage (produced at the hospital) that helps to stop tumors from creating new blood vessels and thereby growing; it also acts as a detoxifying agent and an antioxidant. Preven-Ca contains *Cardus marianus*, apricot flour, carrot root, shark cartilage, garlic, alfalfa, and boldo (a bitter liver-cleansing herb), and is taken in tablet form, usually 1 before each meal. "Preven-Ca contains most of the nutrients that our daily diet does not contain but that are necessary for our body to work at its highest potential," says Dr. Contreras.

**Warburg/Cone Cancer Therapy—**This approach is based on metabolic principles as developed by Clarence D. Cone, Ph.D., and named to honor Otto Warburg, M.D., who won 2 Nobel prizes for his research on cancer in the late 1800s. Metabolism refers to the processes by which the body extracts energy from foods. "The therapy is designed to selectively destroy malignant cells without harming the normal cells of the body," Dr. Contreras explains.

***"We believe that the main stimulants we can use for our patients, in addition to the metabolic program, are emotional and spiritual. That really helps, believe me, better than the injections," says Dr. Contreras.***

Patients go on a low-fat, high complex carbohydrate diet (3000 calories daily, largely from whole grains) while receiving 3 nontoxic medications: lente insulin (a common prescription drug), thyroid hormone, and the bioflavonoid quercetin (delivered orally).

"The 3 substances work together synergistically producing a blockage around the cancer cells such that they cannot breathe or get nourishment, so they starve to death." Patients receive this therapy for 1-3 weeks at Oasis, then continue it at home, usually for 3 months.

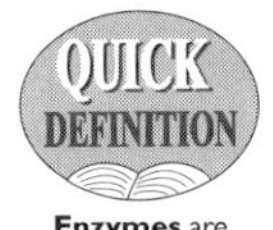


**Enzymes** are specialized living proteins fundamental to all living processes in the body, necessary for every chemical reaction and the normal activity of our organs, tissues, fluids, and cells. There are hundreds of thousands of these Nature's "workers." Enzymes enable your body to digest and assimilate food. There are special enzymes for digesting proteins, carbohydrates, fats, and plant fibers. Specifically, protease digests proteins, amylase digests carbohydrates, lipase digests fats, cellulase digests fiber, and disaccharidases digest sugars.

**Nutrients—**Vitamin C is given intravenously in high doses, often up to 50 g daily, followed by a 10-g daily oral maintenance dose at home. High-dose vitamin A is given, although in cases of liver cancer or dysfunction, the dosage does not exceed 300,000 I.U. daily.

**Enzymes—**Dr. Contreras administers Wobe-Mugos enzymes (from Germany) derived from both vegetable and animal sources. Proteolytic (protein-digesting) enzymes are the body's first defense against tumors. This formula contains pancreatin, papain, bromelain, trypsin, chymotrypsin, lipase, amylase, and rutin (a bioflavonoid). Initially, the enzymes are given as suppositories (1-2 daily), then as pills (6-9 daily) for an indefinite period.

**Diet**—The Contreras dietary plan has both general and patient-specific requirements. Among the general recommendations, Dr. Contreras advises his patients to avoid the following: frozen and canned foods; foods with preservatives, additives, or colorings; white flour, salt, white sugar, caffeine, alcohol, shellfish, and red meat. On the positive side, patients are urged to eat "living" foods such as organic fruits and vegetables, whole or as juices.

Depending on the laetrile dosage prescribed, the specific dietary recommendations may be stricter or looser, says Dr. Contreras. "The nutritional programs are designed to release patients from the harmful effects that certain foods have on them and to encourage the consumption of foods that have beneficial effects."

**Detoxification**—Oasis Hospital administers a 5-10 day detoxification program that includes a complete physical examination, laboratory tests, an organic foods diet, intravenous solutions of vitamin C, potassium, and other natural substances to improve the immune system, and 2 colonic enemas and 6 coffee enemas. The goal is to help the body collect and drain its numerous toxins.

In addition, Oasis physicians administer intravenous nutritional solutions by way of a subclavian catheter inserted into a vein that passes under the clavicle in the chest. According to Dr. Contreras, this helps to reduce inflammation from using smaller veins and makes it easier to administer the solution.

**Chelation Therapy**—By giving an intravenous solution containing selected vitamins, minerals, heparin (a blood thinner), and EDTA (a synthetic amino acid that binds up or "chelates" heavy metals), a patient's circulation is greatly improved and toxicity load is reduced. The solution acts as a magnet, pulling positively charged calcium and other metal ions out of the cells of the arterial walls.

**Counseling**—Oasis patients receive regular counseling sessions with both a staff psychologist and a pastoral adviser. "We believe that the main stimulants we can use for our patients,

For more information about **detoxification protocols**, see Chapter 33: Physical Support Therapies, pp. 949-980. For more information about **enzymes**, see Chapter 32: Enhancing Whole-Body Metabolism, pp. 928-934.

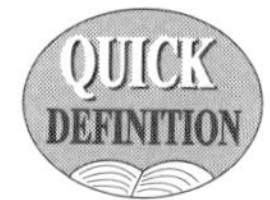


**Chelation therapy** refers to a method of binding ("chelating") an organic substance known as a chelating agent to a metallic ion with a positive electric charge (e.g., a heavy metal) and removing it from the body. One type of chelation therapy involves the chelating agent disodium EDTA given as an intravenous infusion over a 3 1/2-hour period. Usually 20 to 30 treatments are administered at the rate of 1 to 3 sessions per week. Chelation therapy is especially beneficial for all forms of atherosclerotic cardiovascular disease including angina pectoris and coronary artery disease.

in addition to the metabolic program, are emotional and spiritual. Every Thursday afternoon, I get together with my patients, not as a doctor, but as a spiritual advisor. We have a full hour of good humor, laughter, spiritual readings, music, and singing together. That really helps, believe me, better than the injections. It deeply relaxes the patients and improves their immune systems tremendously."

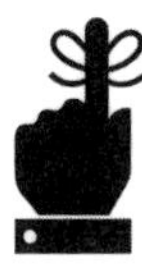

*Each of us is constantly exposed to carcinogens in our food, air, and water, resulting in the production of cancer cells within the body. Normally, the immune system recognizes and destroys these cells before they have a chance to multiply. This means that having abnormal cells develop is probably not the critical factor in determining the course of cancer. The primary threat of cancer may result instead from the body's inability to eliminate the abnormal cells even when they are few in number.*

## CURRICULUM VITAE

# W. John Diamond, M.D.

Triad Medical Center, 4600 Kietzke Lane,
M-242, Reno, NV 89502;
tel: 702-829-2277; fax: 702-829-2365.

W. John Diamond earned his M.D. in 1973 from the University of the Witwatersrand in Johannesburg, Republic of South Africa. He is a board-certified pathologist and received his training in pathology from the University of Capetown and Groote Schuur Hospital, Republic of South Africa, as well as Montefiore Hospital and Medical Center of the Albert Einstein College of Medicine in the Bronx, New York, the Clinical Center of the National Institutes of Health in Bethesda, Maryland, and the State University of New York at the Upstate Medical Center in Syracuse, New York.

Dr. Diamond's training in alternative medicine is extensive, including medical acupuncture at the University of California at Los Angeles, classical homeopathy at the Pacific Academy of Homeopathic Medicine in Berkeley, California, and neural therapy at the American Academy of Neural Therapy in Seattle, Washington.

In addition to being medical director, since 1989, of the Triad Medical Center in Reno, Nevada, Dr. Diamond is an associate and alternative medicine consultant to the Bakersfield Family Medicine Center and Heritage Physician Network in Bakersfield, California.

***Every cancer carries various levels of meaning with regard to the patient's biology. In other words, every symptom has a logical set of reasons for its existence. The symptom itself was created through biological processes, but those processes could have been triggered and propelled by psychological or emotional factors. Every cancer is therefore a collage of symptoms.***

Chapter 6

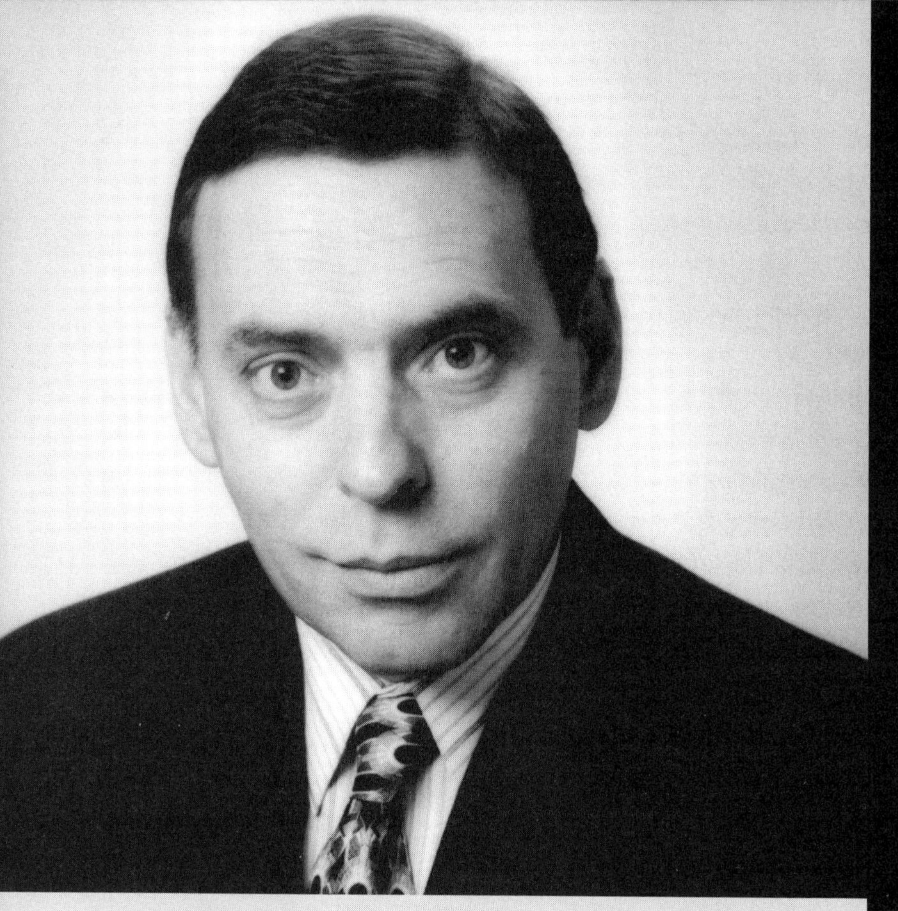

# *W. John Diamond, M.D.*

**FOR THE CANCER PATIENT,** homeopathic remedies, combined with detoxification strategies, major dietary changes, nutritional supplementation, biological dentistry, and neural therapy make a highly effective therapy for treating the whole person and not just the cancer, says homeopathic physician W. John Diamond, M.D.

Cancer is a chronic disease that develops slowly, usually over many years. As such, it is a process involving many factors, beginning with inherited weaknesses in a person's physical condition, conditions that prevailed during the mother's pregnancy, dietary and environmental insults, and the process of forming one's personality. It is this adverse flowing together of conditions and processes that eventually leads to cancer.

Every cancer carries various levels of meaning with regard to the patient's biology. In other words, every symptom has a logical set of reasons for its existence. The symptom itself was created through biological processes, but those processes could have been triggered and propelled by psychological or emotional factors. Every cancer is therefore a collage of symptoms.

In counseling my patients, I try to see what the cancer signifies at a personal and spiritual level. Questions such as the following can be usefully pursued by the person with cancer: Is the tumor an ominous monster coming to consume me? Is the cancer a challenge to change my way of life? Is the metastasis regarded as a punishment for my having lived a "life of sin"? Am I angry at this cancer or do I feel love and appreciation for it? What or whom does the cancer represent? What is the lesson associated with it? The emotions attached to these issues will affect the biological aggressivness of the tumor and its relationship with its "host."

The process of comprehensive cancer therapy begins with peeling back the layers of a person's body/mind as if it were, metaphorically, an onion. Deciphering the many levels of meaning that cancer poses is one of the essential goals of comprehensive treatment.

# Dr. Diamond's Generalized Model for Cancer Treatment

| STRATEGY | DOSAGE/ KEY COMPONENTS | FOR MORE INFORMATION see page # |
|---|---|---|
| **Dietary Plan** | | |
| Balanced, easily assimilated, high-energy, low-fat, high-fiber diet | in general: whole grains, legumes, vegetables, and fruits or macrobiotic diet<br>for individual: determine optimal combination of carbohydrates, proteins, and fats, based on blood groupings, ethnic background, and oxidation status | 749 |
| Avoid most red meat | elk, buffalo, or other extremely lean and hormone-free meat allowable, especially if blood type O | 144 |
| **Alternative Cancer Therapies** | | |
| Homeopathic remedies | single or complex including drainage remedies, depending on individual | 148 |
| Electrodermal screening | for information about individual's cancer and most appropriate homeopathic remedies | 1021 |
| Chinese herbal medicine | for chemotherapy and radiation support: *Quiet Digestion* for nausea; *Astra Essence* for blood deficiency and balancing kidney; *Clear Heat* for high body temperature; *Marrow Plus* for bone marrow suppression | 152 |
| Neural therapy | to rebalance energy flow thrown out of balance by scars and disturbed autonomic nervous system | 602 |
| Biological dentistry | for clearing up dental infections and foci (e.g., from root canal) and removal of mercury amalgams if necessary | 980 |
| **Supplements** | | |
| Vitamin A | 10,000 IU daily | 784 |
| Beta carotene | 20,000 IU daily | 764 |
| Vitamin B complex | balanced supplement, daily | 784 |
| Flaxseed oil | 1 capsule, 3 times daily | 768 |
| Vitamin C | 1-8 g daily | 786 |

# Dr. Diamond's Generalized Model for Cancer Treatment (cont.)

| STRATEGY | DOSAGE/ KEY COMPONENTS | FOR MORE INFORMATION see page # |
|---|---|---|
| Vitamin E | 800 IU daily | 790 |
| Selenium | 300 mcg once daily | 783 |
| Probiotics | 2 capsules with each meal | — |
| Multivitamin/mineral | Multiplex 2 without iron (Tyler Encapsulations) | — |

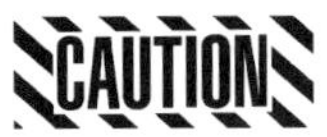


This chapter includes information regarding actual treatments used by Dr. Diamond only after his careful diagnosis of each patient. All cancer patients are unique. **Do not administer these treatments to yourself or others.** Discuss these treatments with your physician or other qualified health-care professional. Readers should not interpret this material as therapeutic advice, but should see a physician in all cases.

The first imperative for the clinician, then, is to understand biologically where the cancer comes from—what combination of emotional, biochemical, structural, and energy components are involved. Then, doctor and patient together can develop a treatment plan that does not just include trying to kill the cancer—that is a simplistic way of working—but supporting and balancing the person whose body and mind ultimately determine whether the cancer will reverse or advance itself.

A rather hard question must be posed: Is it the patient's personal priority to eliminate the cancer? This may sound absurd at first glance, but it isn't. In some instances, people actually may not want treatment at all despite the fact that they are sitting in the physician's office. They may desire to pass on to another reality; they may wish to weather the storm using their own resources; they may be seeking encouragement and ways to reduce their pain and suffering. To answer such questions, an understanding of the individual's psychological and psychospiritual issues is necessary.

***The process of comprehensive cancer therapy begins with peeling back the layers of a person's body/mind as if it were, metaphorically, an onion.***

The patient's needs must actually precede the doctor's objective analysis of what is required for successful treatment. We must move away from the mindset of obliterating the cancer and move towards treating and healing the *whole* person.

## SUCCESS STORY
### Reversing Breast Cancer

Andrea, aged 58, came to me for treatment of recurrent breast cancer, or what had been diagnosed as intraductal carcinoma of the left breast. She had undergone a radical mastectomy and had 3 positive nodes (lymph nodes with cancer present); in addition, she had had 8 courses of chemotherapy (involving the drugs Cytoxan, 5-FU, and Methotrexate).

After this, Andrea was disease free for 6 years; then she had a positive bone scan (indicating cancer in the bone) and evidence of cancer having spread to the liver. Andrea was treated with tamoxifen (an estrogen-blocking drug found to be of some benefit in treating breast cancer) for 8 weeks, but it produced no positive effect and it increased the size of the liver metastases; her oncologist next started her on a different chemotherapy formula. At this point she came to me. Andrea wanted to take control of her disease and use support measures to help her with the nausea, lethargy, and recurrent metastases (meaning her cancer had spread to other parts of her body).

***We must move away from the mindset of obliterating the cancer and move towards treating and healing the whole person.***

During my initial interview with Andrea, she told me she had been exposed to diazinon and other unknown pesticides as a child. As far as her dental history went, Andrea had had a root canal filling removed from a tooth, and she had received extensive dental care (such as crowns and treatment for gingivitis). She had experienced dizziness, facial pain and earache on the left side of her head just prior to the cancer recurrence. Electrodermal screening revealed inflammations of the lymph channels, teeth, nerve points and several acupuncture meridians that passed through her feet, including Liver, Stomach, Gallbladder, and

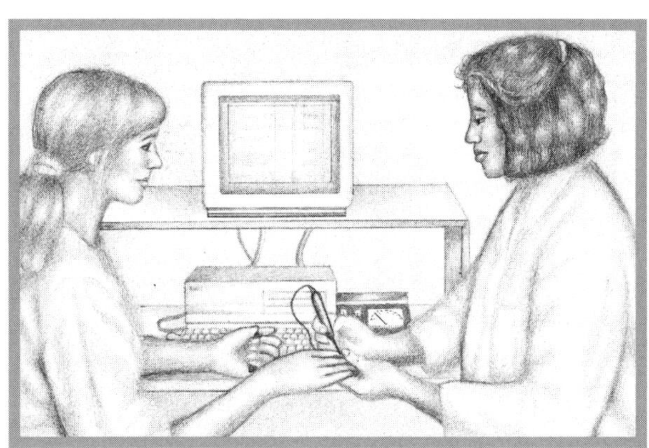

**Figure 6.1—Electrodermal Screening**

## A Primer on Homeopathy

**Homeopathy** was founded in the early 1800s by German physician Samuel Hahnemann. Today, an estimated 500 million people worldwide receive homeopathic treatment; in Britain, homeopathy enjoys royal patronage. Homeopathy is now practiced according to two differing concepts. In classical homeopathy, only one single-component remedy is prescribed at a time in a potency specifically adjusted to the patient; the physician waits to see the results before prescribing anything further. In complex homeopathy, typified by *Hepar compositum*, a prescription involves multiple substances given at the same time, usually in low potencies.

A **homeopathic nosode** is a super-diluted remedy made as an energy imprint from a disease product, such as bacteria, tuberculosis, measles, bowel infection, influenza, and about 200 others. The nosode, which contains no physical trace of the disease, stimulates the body to remove all "taints" or residues it holds of a particular disease, whether it was inherited or contracted in person. Only qualified homeopaths may administer a nosode.

A **homeopathic miasm**, as originally described by Hahnemann, is a subtle taint or energy residue of previous illness, even across the generations. As an inherited predisposition for chronic disease that is far more subtle than anything genetic, miasms are broad-focused, predisposing individuals and families to specific illnesses, such as tuberculosis or cancer. According to Hahnemann, 3 miasms underlie all chronic illness and parallel broad stages in the history of human experience with primary disease states. They are the *Psoric* miasm (from psora, meaning "itch"), the *Syphilitic* miasm (deriving from syphilis), and the *Sycotic* miasm (which arose as a residue of gonorrhea). Some homeopaths add a fourth *Cancer* miasm, and a fifth *Tuberculinum* miasm.

Kidney. Screening of nosodes showed resonance with tooth infection, pesticides, and Coxsackie virus.

The positive resonance of tooth infection, pesticides, and Coxsackie virus indicates that these factors are disturbing the energy balance of the organism. Specifically, they are producing the abnormal readings of acupuncture meridians or energy lines in Andrea's body. For these conditions, application of homeopathic nosodes will correct the energetic imbalance and restore the immune system to a more efficient and functioning entity. If left untreated, however, these imbalances could hinder Andrea's ability to fight the cancer.

I gave Andrea liver and lymphatic detoxification formulas in the form of *Hepeel* drops for the liver and *Lymphomyosot* drops for the lymphatic detoxification. Both were given for 2 weeks in the dose of 10 drops taken 3 times daily, sublingually (under the tongue) for faster absorption. I gave

Andrea these 2 remedies together with homeopathic nosodes to clear the energy taints of the tooth infection and residual pesticides. Andrea also took homeopathic *Carcinocin* 200C twice weekly for 4 weeks; this is a homeopathic preparation made from cancerous tissue cells that are effective in removing the energy preconditions underlying cancer.

***I do not treat cancer so much as I treat patients who have cancer as a prime physical manifestation.***

Next I gave Andrea a single dose 1 month later of *Causticum* 200C. This is a homeopathic "polycrest," which means a remedy with widespread biological effects. It was originally formulated by Samuel Hahnemann, the 19th-century German founder of homeopathy, as a solution of slaked lime and potassium sulfate. Among other symptoms, Andrea's left-sided facial neuralgia was an indicator of the appropriateness of this remedy. Andrea also received 3 acupuncture treatments for muscle spasm related to her liver imbalance and for chronic nausea. She elected to use her own Western herbs including *Echinacea*, silymarin, and pycnogenol (an antioxidant from Maritime pine bark) which she obtained over the counter from a health foods store.

For more information and a source for **Hepeel**, **Lymphomyosot**, **Engystol**, **Carcinocin**, **Causticum**, **nosodes** and other complex homeopathic formulas cited here, physicians may contact: Biologic Homeopathic Industries, 11600 Cochiti S.E., Albuquerque, NM 87123; tel: 800-621-7644 or 505-293-3843; fax: 505-275-1672. For more information about **Pueraria "N" Formula**, (**Qing Bi Tang**, "**Clear Nose Decoction**," for nasal and sinus congestion), contact: McZ and Herbal Formulas, P.O. Box 5312, Santa Monica, CA 90409; tel: 310-822-0500; fax: 310-822-1050.

During the course of treatment, Andrea had an episode of Coxsackie myalgia (involving pain in the voluntary muscles of the chest wall) for which I prescribed the nosode and a homeopathic antiviral. Specifically, I treated her with injectable *Engystol*, a good general homeopathic viral infection remedy, along with the nosode for Coxsackie virus. Around the same time, I treated Andrea's sinusitis with Chinese herbs, relying on a classical Chinese combination called *Purearia "N" Formula*; this included ephedra, ligusticum, glycerrhiza, and magnolia. Following her last course of chemotherapy, Andrea was reevaluated by her oncologist a year later; no evidence of liver or bone metastases was found and she remains disease free.

For information on **electrodermal screening**, see Chapter 34: Energy Support Therapies, pp. 1021-1032.

This case is a good demonstration of the use of multiple alternative modalities in a complicated cancer case that has interrelated emotional, biochemical, and energy imbalances. Andrea is an example of a positively motivated individual who took responsibility for her disease process and turned a potentially negative outcome into a personal victory, even a transformation.

## Assessing the 4 Components of Cancer

I do not treat cancer so much as I treat patients who have cancer as a prime physical manifestation. This is the essential distinction between an orthodox approach to cancer treatment, which seeks to destroy the tumor, and the approach of the alternative physician, who treats the patient and enables the patient's system to destroy the tumor. To accomplish this task, I try to empower the patient at all levels of being, knowing that one's state of health is the ability of the body/mind to balance out the stresses that confront one every day.

If the stresses and our body's response are evenly balanced, then we are in a state of homeostasis or good health. If the stresses are too strong or our response is too weak, then we are in an imbalance which can lead to illness and disease. The disease can be subclinical and hidden at first, not showing any symptoms, but if it continues, it will eventually manifest as physical symptoms. It may start with a disorder of the body's biochemistry, then the cells, organs, and finally the whole body begins to self-destruct and produce a cancer.

From this simple explanation of our biology we can show that every disease, including cancer, has 4 major components to it:

**1) Emotional/Mental—**These are the most important components and are least addressed by conventional medicine. As children, sometimes even as babies or in the womb, we are wounded by circumstances (parental attitudes, relationships with siblings, and the overall family environment). To survive, we produce a response—many call it a wall—to maintain emotional and biological balance and protect ourselves. For example, if you were always told by your father that you were no good and would never amount to much, your response could either be to become passive, believing the lie and fulfilling the dire prophecy, or you could become active, an overachiever, always trying to prove your father wrong.

Either way, you will have trouble later in life as you continue responding to this old imprint—producing a mask of behavior behind which you hide your potential and destiny. In the case of the passive responder, repressed emotions, if not vented or expressed, will seek *physical* expression, such as functional bowel disease, fibromyalgia, or even cancer. In the case of the over-responder, the tendency is to burn out because they never get the approval they seek no matter how well they perform. Heart attack and ulcer are the typical physical expressions. Against either scenario, the physician's role is to make the patient aware of the issues and patterns and to aid them in changing these patterns to produce emotional balance.

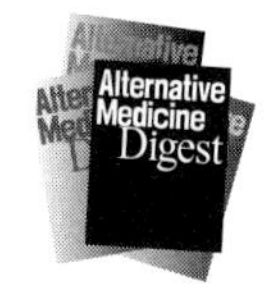


For more information on **Dr. Diamond's protocols** for treating illness, see "Curing Chronic Fatigue with Homeopathy," #16, pp. 72-76.

The emotional balance that we seek may be accelerated and simplified by counseling, hypnosis, classical homeopathy, or time and experience. Once emotional balance is obtained, the organism no longer needs to manifest symptoms in a physical way to reach balance, and the person may then go on to evolve still further. The essence of existence, one might suggest from a homeopathic viewpoint, is to evolve beyond childhood trauma and our primitive protective responses to an understanding, acceptance, and, finally, resolution of the tensions imposed by early emotions and feelings.

After all, if everything in life were the same or if it were perfect, there would be nothing to struggle *against* and no improvement would be possible. Illness also can be seen from this philosophical viewpoint. It is the struggle to balance the opposites that leads to our advancement—these are natural laws.

**2) Biochemical—**This component may be detected by sophisticated biochemical analysis such as analysis of detoxification, metabolic and energy pathways, hormonal, heavy metal, terrain, and mineral status. This information enables the physician to best advise the patient regarding appropriate nutritional supplementation, therapeutic dietary changes, and/or hormonal and glandular support. Detoxification of organ, lymphatic, and gastrointestinal systems can be accomplished by diet, supplements, and homeopathy.

**3) Structural—**This component relates to the musculoskeletal system of the body as disease often has a muscular or pain factor. Consider the tension headache or migraine which are expressed as a spasm of the trapezius and temporalis muscles connecting the neck and head. We treat the myofascial (muscles and the fascia or fibers enclosing the muscles) and skeletal system with acupuncture, chiropractic, osteopathy, craniosacral therapy, trigger point therapy (also known as myotherapy), and neural therapy, among others.

QUICK DEFINITION

**Craniosacral therapy** refers to correcting imbalances in the relationship among breathing, the sacrum (hip bone), and the bones of the skull (cranium), especially the occiput. The sacrum acts as a pump to propel cerebrospinal fluid up the spine to the brain; the cranial bones contract and pump it back down. Health depends on a smoothly functioning sacro-occipital pump. Craniosacral therapy, as delivered by a chiropractor or other trained practitioner, restores the sacrum to full motion and balance with respect to the cranial bones. **Myotherapy** is a technique of pain relief developed by physical fitness and exercise therapy expert Bonnie Prudden. The myotherapist applies deep manual pressure, usually with the fingertips on the skin for 5-7 seconds, to precise sites of muscular pain, called "trigger points." Prudden found that this technique can relieve pain for about 90% of all muscle-related pain conditions, making it unnecessary to use painkilling injections. **Neural therapy** uses localized injections of anesthetics, such as lidocaine or procaine, to remove interferences in the body's electrical network and thus relieve chronic pain, reverse injury, and clear energy blockages. The anesthetics are injected into nerve bundles in the autonomic nervous system, acupuncture points, scars, glands, and other tissues. By clearing the local site of interference, neural therapy helps to regulate energy throughout the body.

**4) Energy—**This component is usually the most difficult to understand—on the part of doctors and patients alike. It relates to the electrical and electromagnetic energy that flows through the body in the various energy pathways, called "meridians" by acupuncturists. Disturbances of these electrical energy channels causes internal organ dysfunction and decreases the overall function of our immune system. We treat and balance this system with acupuncture, Chinese herbs, and homeopathy.

For more information about **Chinese herbs** for cancer, see Chapter 29: Botanicals as Cancer Medicines, pp. 801-805; for more on **homeopathy** in cancer treatment, see Chapter 20: Vincent Speckhart, M.D.

The acupuncturist "reads" the patient's pulse at the wrist—up to 28 different energy qualities can be read—and thereby determines which energy pathways are out of balance. Based on this information, the acupuncturist places acupuncture needles at selected points on the body to correct the energy conditions. Acupuncture can be used both as a preventive measure as well as a curative art. Done regularly, it can keep the immune system and all organs operating at maximum efficiency.

In the cancer patient, acupuncture can be used to improve energy levels and strengthen the immune system, to create a sense of well-being, and to symptomatically treat the side effects of radiation and chemotherapy. It is also effective as a treatment for cancer-associated pain.

Chinese herbs have been shown to affect the energy meridians much like acupuncture, and are often used to augment the activity of acupuncture and to prolong its effects. They can be used specifically as antivirals and energy and immune boosters, as well as support for stressed organs during chemotherapy and radiation. These herbs are especially useful in aiding the bone marrow to produce new immune cells. Chinese ointments are used to lessen the skin burns and pain caused by radiation therapy.

Homeopathy is the modality used to energetically change the emotional patterns that we adopt in childhood that have contributed most to the eventual manifestation of cancer. If we change these patterns early enough in the course of cancer, there is a real chance of reversing this process. Homeopathy can also be used to help clear the emotions of fear, hopelessness, and depression that can accompany the diagnosis of cancer. Lastly, homeopathy can be used symptomatically to decrease the nausea and side effects of chemotherapy and radiation.

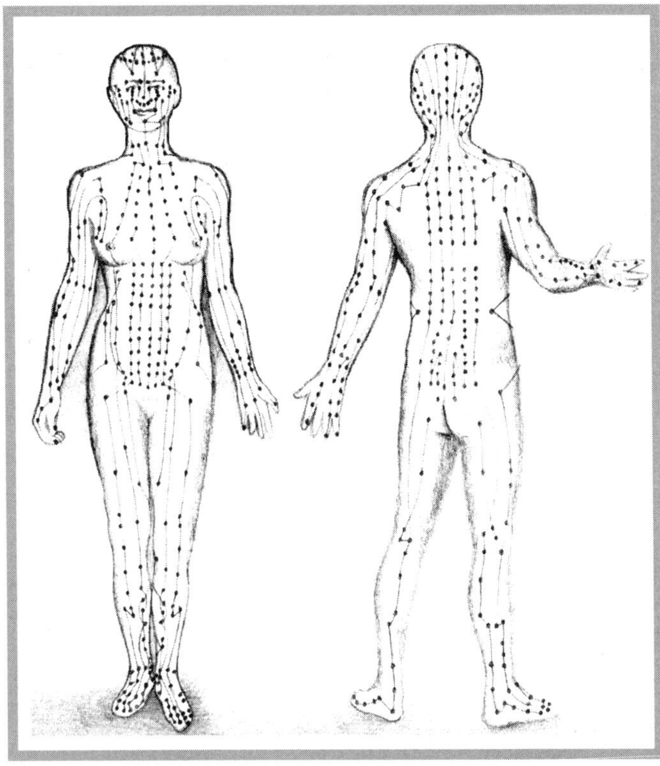

**Figure 6.2—Acupuncture meridians are specific pathways in the human body for the flow of life force or subtle energy, known as Qi (pronounced CHEE). In most cases, these energy pathways run up and down both sides of the body, and correspond to individual organs or organ systems, designated as Lung, Small Intestine, Heart, and others. There are 12 principal meridians and 8 secondary channels. Numerous points of heightened energy, or Qi, exist on the body's surface along the meridians and are called acupoints. There are an estimated 1000 acupoints, each of which is potentially a place for acupuncture treatment.**

## Designing a High-Energy Nutritional Program

Cancer as a biological entity is extremely inefficient in the way it uses energy. It uses up excessive amounts of energy, which is why many patients with cancer tend to lose weight so quickly. My nutritional objective is to provide a balanced, easily assimilated *high-energy* diet. In general, the careful selection of whole grains, vegetables, legumes, and fruits will meet these requirements.

The first task for the physicians is to test for allergies or abnormal sensitivities to food since these reactions will burden the patient's immune system and interfere with the assimilation of food. Common offenders are dairy and wheat allergies which is why I recommend taking all dairy out of the diet immediately. Even for those who don't have a sensitivity to dairy, it should be removed from the diet because the foreign proteins (antigens) in cow's milk tend to burden the immune system.

**Macrobiotics** is a specialized diet and food philosophy roughly based on Chinese medicine and filtered through contemporary Japanese culture and American representatives such as Georges Ohsawa and Michio Kushi. The diet emphasizes balancing the energy qualities of fresh, whole foods to maximize their delivery of *Qi*, or vital life force, to the body. The diet comprises cooked whole grains, beans and bean products, vegetables, fruits, nuts, seeds, small amounts of saltwater fish (salmon), fermented soybean products (miso), seaweeds, shiitake mushrooms, and special pickles and condiments. Macrobiotics has been used successfully when clinically prescribed as a curative and restorative diet in treating chronic and serious illness, including cancer; as a health maintenance diet, it has produced excellent results for many people.

By our evolutionary design, humans are unable to digest winter wheat. Wheat protein (especially the gluten), for example, may add substantially to the immunological burden. Winter wheat is easier to grow, produces more of a yield, and is pest resistant as compared to other kinds of wheat (such as spelt, amaranth, and quinoa) and so has become the dominant wheat in commercial food products.

Second, we must determine which combinations of carbohydrates, proteins, and fats are optimal for the patient. Most of the patients I see are carbohydrate sensitive, which means they fail to utilize the carbohydrates efficiently for energy. In these individuals, the level of carbohydrates in their diet should be decreased, and refined carbohydrates like sugar, white flour, and white rice should be avoided altogether. Until the carbohydrate sensitivity has lessened, starchy foods such as bread, pasta, rice, and other grains should be reduced as well. Most cancer patients are protein deficient and they may need to increase their consumption of dietary protein, primarily from fish and legumes.

For more information about the health hazards of **excessive animal protein intake,** see Chapter 25: What Causes Cancer? pp. 605-607; for more information about **detoxification** and **"friendly" bacteria** (pp. 949-980) and **lymph** (pp. 965-970), see Chapter 33: Physical Support Therapies; for more information on **blood types**, see Chapter 17: Geronimo Rubio, M.D., p. 341.

Though no standard diet applies to all cancer patients, the macrobiotic diet may serve as a reliable model or compass for directing one's dietary practices. Some of my patients have done extremely well on macrobiotic diets.

Though most forms of red meat are ill-advised for the cancer patient, the major problem with meat is the fat marbling as occurs in domesticated beef. High concentrations of fat clearly suppress immune-system function and promote the growth of tumors. Meat-eating as such is not an issue if you can lower meat's fat content, as with elk or buffalo which are extremely lean and hormone free. There are exceptions to every rule, of course; it has been well demonstrated that patients with type O blood require meat in their diet or they may become anemic.

*To enable the immune system to function effectively, all possible routes of toxic exposure must be comprehensively addressed and dealt with aggressively.*

## Detoxifying the Colon, Liver, Kidneys, Lymphatics, and Skin

Detoxification strategies can help cancer patients reverse the accumulation of toxins which otherwise suppress the immune system and promote the proliferation of cancer. Simple avoidance of toxic sources in the air, food, and water is a first step. Some toxic exposures are unique to certain professions or geographic areas. For example, professional golfers can absorb cancer-causing herbicides from the fairways. Among residents of industrial areas, petroleum-based products and manufacturing by-products are carcinogens that pose a cumulative risk to the body; people who work in smoke-filled bars or casinos are similarly at risk.

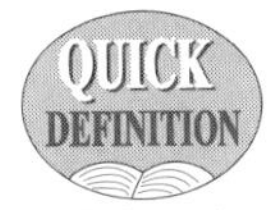


**Friendly bacteria,** or probiotics, refer to beneficial microbes inhabiting the human gastrointestinal tract where they are essential for proper nutrient assimilation. The human body contains an estimated several thousand billion beneficial bacteria comprising over 400 species, all necessary for health. Among the more well known of these are *Lactobacillus acidophilus* and *Bifidobacterium Bifidium*. Overly acidic bodily conditions, chronic constipation or diarrhea, dietary imbalances, overly processed foods, and the excessive use of antibiotics and hormonal drugs can interfere with probiotic function and even reduce their numbers, setting up conditions for illness.

Other toxic sources include viruses, which interfere with portions of the genetic material and, in turn, can trigger cancer development. Molds produce carcinogenic substances. Certain bacteria and parasites may produce cancer-promoting chemicals within the digestive tract.

To enable the immune system to function effectively, all possible routes of toxic exposure must be comprehensively addressed and dealt with aggressively. Five organ systems are intimately involved in detoxification: colon, liver, kidneys, lymphatics, and skin.

First, it's necessary to evaluate colon function, since constipation is a common problem among cancer patients. Constipation not only interferes with the proper assimilation of nutrients, but it also tends to leak toxins into the blood. The intestines are an integral part of the immune system as they contain more immune (lymphoid) tissue than any other organ in the body and produce more hormones and neurochemicals than any other organ. You can reestablish healthy bowel functioning with a high-fiber, low-fat diet, as well as with the use of homeopathics and probiotic supplementation (to support the beneficial,

***Generally, the process of finding the appropriate homeopathic remedy tends to be far more labor-intensive than the process of determining the right drug or allopathic procedure, but then, whoever said that understanding a human being was a simple task?***

health-promoting bacteria in the digestive tract).

The homeopathics that I use in my practice are *Nux Vomica* and *Berberis Homaccord* with *Hepeel.* These are taken at a dosage of 10 drops 3 times daily. For probiotic "seeding" of the intestines, I use *Enterogenic* at the dosage of 2 capsules with each meal. Walking, moderate exercise, or abdominal massage are additional ways of rectifying stagnated intestines.

Second, I examine the condition of the liver, kidneys, and lymphatic system, organs and tissues that must constantly deal with the body's toxic load. In conditions of health, these systems work together to keep the body's toxic load to a minimum. I use "drainage" remedies made up of low-potency homeopathics and tinctures (alcohol extractions) of both Chinese and Western herbs.

The concept of drainage is fairly new to homeopathy. It derives from the work of French homeopaths in the mid-20th century who were more interested in applying homeopathy at a grosser, physiological level than at the level of "mentals," the psychological, emotional, and spiritual plane. These homeopaths developed a system using low-potency homeopathics (even herbal tinctures) to encourage the lymphatic system, liver, kidneys, blood, tissues, intercellular spaces, fat, and skin to eliminate, or drain, their toxins. If drainage is not done when homeopathic remedies are to be used to mobilize toxic substances out of the body (such as mercury from dental amalgams), then the toxic substances will circulate in the body and deposit themselves in another area. The best known drainage remedies are *Solidago* and *Berberis* for the kidney; *Taraxacum*, *Silymarin*, and *Carduus* for the liver; *Hydrastis* as a general drainage; and *Myosotis* for the lymphatic system.

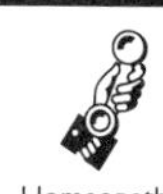

Homeopathic **drainage remedies** are available from Marco Pharma International, 15810 West 6th Avenue, Golden, CO 80401; tel: 303-277-9621; fax: 303-277-9623. **Enterogenic™ Concentrate** (intestinal microflora such as *Lactobacillus acidophilus* and *Bifidobacterium bifidum* with fructo-oligosaccharides, in powder form) is available from Tyler Encapsulations, 2204-8 N.W. Birdsdale, Gresham, OR 97030; tel: 800-869-9705 or 503-661-5401; fax: 503-666-4913.

## Effective Supplementation for Cancer Patients

Nutritional supplementation for cancer patients is particularly important because cancer tends to deplete the body's nutritional supply, and the cancer-ridden body may require more of certain nutrients to maximize its ability to fight cancer. Having said this, I still favor relatively moderate supplementation rather than megadosing with vitamins and minerals. In some cases, massive doses of micronutrients can overwhelm the normal biological processes, including those of the immune system that are involved in repelling cancer.

My patients may receive large doses of vitamins C and E, but not at the inordinately high dosage levels seen in some alternative cancer clinics. High doses of micronutrients carry high biological potency and can throw the body out of balance. Other doctors, including several in this book (e.g., Drs. Block, Brodie, Donovan, Rountree, and Simone), share this view.

The supplements I prescribe vary depending on the individual and his or her specific physical needs. Part of the difficulty in assessing dosage is that scientific research on the physiological effects of specific nutrients is only beginning to catch up with clinical reality. For example, it is known that vitamin B3 (as niacin or niacinamide) increases the blood flow to tumors. If a doctor is also trying to restrict blood flow with substances known as angiogenesis inhibitors, such as shark or bovine cartilage, the B3 will tend to counteract this effect. Niacin may be more effective in delivering substances that are selectively toxic to the tumor such as vitamin C and the D-fraction compound of maitake mushroom. Knowing these interactions, we can either increase or decrease the dosages of the various nutrients depending on whether the interaction is supportive or antagonistic.

CAUTION

As many of my patients already take supplements they have heard about, I urge them to consider abandoning their self-styled program and to consult with a doctor well-versed in nutrition. Particularly in the case of trace elements, arbitrary supplementation can be extremely detrimental. For example, large doses of both zinc and copper are immune-suppressive and an excess of zinc can offset the body's supply of selenium, an essential part of the body's cancer resistance.

Along similar theoretical lines, certain types of cancer may warrant the use of additional supplementation whereas others may call for smaller amounts of certain single nutrients. In cases of squamous cell carcinoma (a type of skin cancer), for example, I typically supply more vitamin A and beta carotene since the research has shown a clinical benefit associated with these vitamins. Women with early-stage cervical dysplasia, a condition that can potentially lead to cervical cancer, can benefit from higher doses of folic acid, vitamin A, and selenium.

## Homeopathy Is an Effective Anticancer Medicine

As a low-cost, nontoxic system of medicine, many physicians, including my-

## Conventional Science Validates Homeopathy

Before struggling to define the mechanism(s) that might explain homeopathy, consider the powerful scientific evidence that homeopathy actually works. In a landmark study reported in *The Lancet*, researchers gave 14 asthmatic patients a placebo, and 14 others a homeopathic treatment. None of the 28 individuals knew whether they had the real remedy or the placebo, which is why this study's design is called a "double-blind, placebo-controlled trial." One month later, those patients who had received homeopathy showed a marked improvement in their symptoms compared to the placebo group.

Researchers reporting in *Pediatrics* focused on a randomized, double-blind, placebo-controlled clinical trial—again, the gold standard of medical research. The study, which was conducted by U.S. public health researchers in Nicaragua, compared homeopathic medicine with a placebo in the treatment of acute childhood diarrhea. Those children who received homeopathic treatment had a statistically significant decrease in the duration of diarrhea, compared to those children in the placebo group.

According to a recent survey published in the *British Medical Journal*, out of 107 such studies of homeopathy, 77% showed positive outcomes for illnesses such as influenza, migraines, and rheumatoid arthritis.

self, have found homeopathy to be particularly effective in treating chronic illnesses that fail to respond to conventional treatment. A number of published case reports have demonstrated the effectiveness of homeopathy against arthritis, inflamed pancreas, chronic sinusitis, hay fever, and other, seemingly intractable medical problems.

Homeopathy is among the best examples of the axiom that we should treat the person rather than the disease. Prescribing homeopathic remedies is a highly individualized science, based on the doctor's assessment of the *totality* of the patient's symptoms. The evaluation covers major symptoms as well as minor complaints, physical signs as well as psychological tendencies. Generally, the process of finding the appropriate homeopathic remedy tends to be far more labor-intensive than the process of determining the right drug or allopathic procedure, but then, whoever said that understanding a human being was a simple task?

Among the more profound benefits of homeopathy is its ability to change the "terrain" of the body—that is, the biochemical environment of the cells that determines a person's susceptibility to disease. When the terrain is improved, the immune responsiveness of the individual can be profoundly strengthened. It is also possible to change some of the hereditary weaknesses, called *miasms* in homeopathy, which make some people more susceptible to cancer. In my practice, I use both types of homeopathy, classical and complex. Classical homeopathy focuses on changing the patient at an emotional and spiritual level. The patient comes into the world with a "disturbing frequency," or *miasm*, which makes them more susceptible to cancer. Often by giving a single homeopathic dose, the miasm can be changed or modulated.

Another important feature of homeopathy are the nosodes, by which we can manipulate the biochemistry and physiology of the body using energy rather than physical substances. Nosodes can be used singly as in classical homeopathy, or in mixtures, as in complex homeopathy. Complex homeopathy even enables us to pull heavy metals out of a cell's mitochondria. With respect to homeopathic remedies, the body recognizes the energy of the diluted substance as information with which to change its biology. In effect, they are biological response modifiers. Specific cancer nosodes are made from dilutions of carcinogens and actual cancer tissue that can change the body's tendency to develop cancer. Homeopathic medicines can be successfully used to treat cancer.

## Nosodes Commonly Used in Homeopathic Practice

- Viruses: Influenza, Enteroviruses, Coxsackie Type B, Epstein Barr, Cytomegalovirus, Herpes group
- Bacteria: *Salmonella typhi, E. Coli, Streptococcus, Staphylococcus, Streptococcus pneumonia, Helicobacter pylorii, H. influenza, Mycoplasma,*
- Parasites and Fungi: *Giardia,* Pinworms, *Candida albicans*

***In my experience, cancer can be reversed by a combination of deep-acting homeopathic remedies and other nontoxic modalities.***

Many reports by homeopathic physicians have confirmed my own experiences that some cancers can be effectively treated—either halted or reversed—with homeopathic treatment. In many cases, homeopathy can also provide symptomatic relief, reducing pain, alleviating nausea, increasing energy levels, and even enhancing mental outlook.

What medical science can no longer deny is that homeopathic remedies, despite containing no detectable amount of medicinal substances, have definite therapeutic activity. We can infer from this that their properties lie outside the domain of classical physics, the mechanical view of the universe that has dominated scientific thinking since the days of Isaac Newton. Instead, homeopathy may be more accurately understood within the domain of quantum physics and within the emerging field of energy medicine.

We now have reasonable grounds for making such a statement. A study using nuclear magnetic resonance (NMR) imaging demonstrated distinctive readings of subatomic activity in 23 different homeopathic remedies, a potency that was not demonstrated in placebos. Italian physicist Emilio del Guidici proposes that water molecules form structures capable of storing minute electromagnetic signals.

If del Giudici's model is accurate, a homeopathic remedy may work by conveying an electromagnetic "message" to the body that matches the specific electromagnetic frequency or pattern of an illness in order to stimulate that body's natural healing response. Research in Germany has shown that homeopathic substances do emit measurable electromagnetic signals; the existence of such signals indicates that specific frequencies are dominant in each remedy. What early homeopathic doctors may have been doing in their empirical research was to unwittingly match the frequencies or "resonance patterns" of the plant or animal extracts with those of the patient's illness.

The subject of biological manipulation of DNA-associated cancer regulating genes should be an area of intensive research in homeopathy.

***With respect to homeopathic remedies, the body recognizes the energy of the diluted substance as information with which to change its biology.***

In my experience, cancer can be reversed by a combination of deep-acting homeopathic remedies and other nontoxic modalities. Among the wide variety of homeopathic applications effective in treating cancer are the drainage remedies. These low-potency remedies aid in detoxification, draining toxins out of the liver, lymphatics, and kidneys and thus enabling these organs to support more effectively the body's disease-fighting ability.

In the case of microbes believed to be associated with a condition, I first identify the particular microbe by means of electrodermal screening and laboratory antibody tests. Viruses, for example, have been shown to be strongly associated with lymphomas and leukemias.[1] I then prepare homeopathic nosodes of the actual viruses, fungi, bacteria, or parasites. Nosodes corresponding to suspected toxins or disease agents are tested with respect to the patient's energy field and organs; if there is electrical resonance with this nosode and the patient, then the nosode is selected for therapeutic use.

In other words, nosodes from the bacteria, viruses, yeasts, and parasites demonstrated to be suppressing the patient's immune function are given to the patient to neutralize the biological activity of these organisms. By removing these organisms, you remove a major toxic load, which, in turn, allows your body to maintain good health and strong resistance to disease.

I use many Chinese herbal medicines, mostly to provide organ support by increasing blood circulation and oxygenation. In China, traditional doctors combine conventional cancer treatment with the use of various botanicals to detoxify the body and reduce the toxic load created by chemotherapy and radiation. Here is an indication of typical Chinese herbs I use in my cancer practice:

***In China, traditional doctors combine conventional cancer treatment with the use of various botanicals to detoxify the body and reduce the toxic load created by chemotherapy and radiation.***

### Liver

- *Relaxed Wanderer* (K'an Herbals): 2 tablets (750 mg each), 3 times daily
- *Ecliptex* (Health Concerns): 3 tablets, 3 times daily
- LD-477 (ProBotanixx): 3 tablets, 3 times daily

### Kidney

- *Quiet Contemplation* (K'an Herbals): 2 tablets, 3 times daily
- *Rehmannia 6* or *Astra Essence* (Health Concerns): 3 tablets, 3 times daily
- *Rehmannia 6* or *Rehmannia 8* (ProBotanixx): 1/2 teaspoon, 3 times daily

### General

- Various combinations of ginseng to act as an adaptogen for the patient, such as *Arouse Vigor* (K'an Herbals) or *Three Ginsengs* (ProBotanixx), each at 2-3 tablets, 2-3 times daily

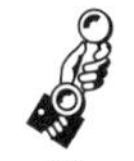

For more information about **ProBotanixx** brand LD-477, *Rehmannia 6* or *Rehmannia 8*, or *Three Ginsengs*, contact: Sun Ten Labs, 9250 Jeronimo Road, Irvine, CA 92718; tel: 714-587-0509; fax: 714-457-6039; for more information about **K'an Herb** products, *Relaxed Wanderer, Quiet Contemplation*, and *Arouse Vigor*, contact: K'an Herb Company, 6001 Butler Lane, Scotts Valley, CA 95066; tel: 800- 543-5233 or 408-438-9450; fax: 408-438-9457; for more information about **Health Concerns** brand *Ecliptex* and *Rehmannia 6* or *Astra Essence*, contact: Health Concerns, 8001 Capwell Drive, Oakland, CA 94621; tel: 510-639-0280; fax: 510-639-9140.

## Dental Problems May Contribute to Cancer

The jaws and teeth can be thought of as the "fuse box" of the body because all of the major acupuncture meridians pass through this area. Any disturbance of the teeth and jaws will cause a short circuit of the energy moving through these channels and create electrical disturbances in the organ associated with that tooth. Many cases of cancer seem related to poorly per-

## Chinese Medicine for Chemotherapy and Radiation Support

Chemotherapy and radiation can cause many imbalances, as described in traditional Chinese medicine, particularly affecting the kidneys, blood, and spleen. The physician must be able to assess which energy imbalance the patient has and to administer acupuncture and prescribe herbs accordingly.

**Herbal Formulas**

*Quiet Digestion* —nausea
*Astra Essence* —kidney yin, yang and blood deficiency
*Astra 8* —weak spleen and lung energy
*Clear Heat* —for hot flashes felt with chemotherapy
*Marrow Plus* —for bone marrow suppression

**Acupuncture Points**

These points can help tonify (put energy into the system) through needle manipulation, moxibustion, or electrical stimulation and disperse (remove energy from the system) by allowing the needle to stand in place without manipulation.

Nausea—tonify Pericardium 6, CV12, Stomach 36.
Kidney deficiency—tonify Kidney 3, 6, 7, 10.
Spleen/Lung deficiency—tonify Spleen 2, 6, 9 and Lung 9
Rising heat—disperse Liver 2
Stimulate marrow—tonify Gallbladder 39

**Homeopathy**

Nausea—*Ipecacuana* 12C, *Nux Vomica* 12C, or *Sepia* 12C
Fever—*Belladonna* 12C
Detoxify kidney—*Solidago* 12C
Detoxify liver—*Taraxacum* 12C

Bone Marrow Suppression—isode of the chemotherapeutic drug at 30C. An isode is a homeopathic preparation made from the substance (in this case, a chemotherapy drug) that is causing the problem in the patient. The patient takes the homeopathic preparation at the same time as taking the actual drug. The homeopathic isode will usually remove the unwanted side effects of the chemotherapy drug without affecting the primary chemical effect of that drug.

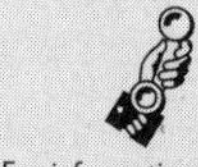

For information about ***Quiet Digestion, Astra Essence, Clear Heat,*** and ***Marrow Plus,*** contact: East West Herbs, 6400 Hollis Street, Suite 10, Emeryville, CA 94608; tel: 800-575-8526 or 510-652-2807; fax: 510-652-2812.

formed root canals as well as circulatory lesions in the jawbone (maxilla and the mandible). Most of the information supporting this connection is anecdotal, yet it is very compelling.

Let's consider the problems with a root canal. The dentist removes the live, but bacterially infected, pulp of the tooth then fills this cavity (the roots of the tooth, usually 3-4) with an inert substance. It is extremely difficult to get the area completely sterile once the tooth pulp has been removed. Bacteria become entrenched inside the structure of the teeth in the dentin tubules. These microbes then may spread locally, affecting other teeth; they may also migrate throughout the body.

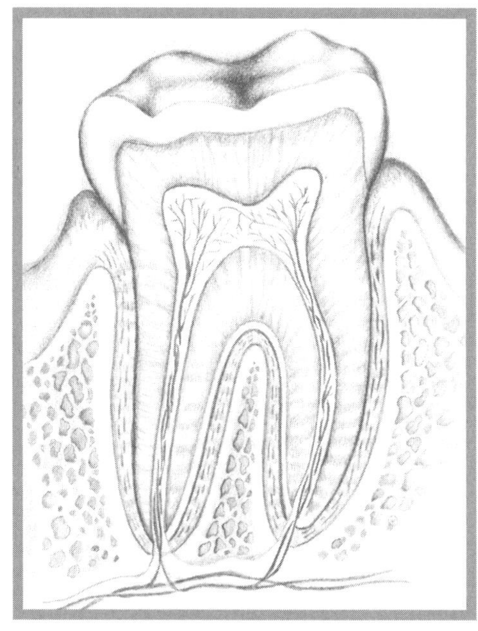

**Figure 6.3—Biological dentistry stresses the use of nontoxic restoration materials for dental work and focuses on the unrecognized impact that dental toxins and hidden dental infections can have on overall health. Typically, a biological dentist will emphasize the safe removal of mercury amalgams; in many cases, either the avoidance or removal of root canals; the investigation of possible jawbone infections (cavitations) as a "dental focus" or source of bodywide illness centered in the teeth; and the health-injuring role of misalignment of teeth and jaw structures.**

Root canal filled teeth, infected teeth, and dry sockets are a potentially large source of toxicity and electrical irritation and may contribute to a host of degenerative conditions. I have a number of patients with breast cancer, all of whom had root canals on the tooth related to the breast area on the associated energy meridian. Poorly performed root canals contain remnants of dead or decayed tissue that cause an energetic irritation or "focus" which interferes with the unobstructed flow of electrical energy through the body's meridians. Similarly, an infected tooth or dry socket acts as an electrical interference field in the head, again, disturbing the free flow of electrical energy. Mixed metals in the mouth—nickel and mercury—produce electrical microcurrents that cause the associated meridians to short-circuit, thereby blocking the flow of *Qi*, or life force energy, through these pathways.

The presence of mercury dental amalgam and nickel may, in some patients, be the irritating focus that depresses the immune system just enough to give cancer the edge. Metal-sensitive patients are encouraged to remove their dental amalgams and root canals under a strict protocol that will pro-

For more information about **dental factors** in cancer, see Chapter 25: What Causes Cancer?, pp. 594-602; and Chapter 33: Physical Support Therapies, pp. 980-989. For information on **neural therapy**, see Chapter 25: What Causes Cancer?, pp. 602-604.

tect the rest of the body from mercury exposure during removal. It is now conclusively proven that the mercury that leaches from dental amalgams can have an adverse impact on the immune system, including, for example, a reduced functioning of lymphocytes and monocytes, cells that play a role in protecting us against cancer.[2] In addition, mercury is known to inhibit the cell's production of glutathione peroxidase, an enzyme pathway essential to the body's detoxification and antioxidant systems.[3] Without adequate functioning of these systems, cancer cells are more likely to form and existing cancer cells are far more likely to proliferate and contribute to tumor growth.

## Removing the Harmful Influence of Old Scars

Neural therapy is a technique developed in Germany that uses injections of local anesthetics to remove an irritating energy focus in the body—root canals, sinus problems, scars, appendix, bowel and pelvic infections, and adhesions that can block the flow of electrical energy. All cancer patients should be carefully inspected for any scars that cross acupuncture meridians. When these scars are injected with lidocaine or novocaine, the electrical activity of the energy lines can be reestablished.

Scar tissue anywhere in the body is composed of electrically impervious, thickened collagen. The scar acts as an electrical insulator and blocks the flow of energy along the meridians and leads to symptoms and energy imbalances that are distant from the scar. For example, I had a patient with intractable chest pain sent to me by a cardiologist; he experienced immediate and permanent relief when I injected a 2-mm scar on the inner aspect of the tip of his left little finger. This is the site of the acupuncture point Heart 9; this means his scar was connected to the energy of his heart through the meridian network.

The scars typical to hysterectomy block many of the meridians that course up the front of the body and may produce symptoms such as headaches or leg pain.[4]

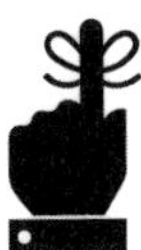

*I do not treat cancer so much as I treat patients who have cancer as a prime physical manifestation. This is the essential distinction between an orthodox approach to cancer treatment, which seeks to destroy the tumor, and the approach of the alternative physician, who treats the patient and enables the patient's system to destroy the tumor.*

—W. JOHN DIAMOND, M.D.

## CURRICULUM VITAE

# Patrick Donovan, N.D.

University Health Clinic,
5312 Roosevelt Way NE, Seattle, WA 98105;
tel: 206-525-8015; fax: 206-525-8014.

Patrick Donovan, R.N., N.D., graduated in 1985 from Bastyr University School of Naturopathic Medicine and did his residency at the university's outpatient clinic. He served on the clinical, research, and academic faculty for 2 years before moving to Philadelphia, where he worked for 5 years while his wife attended medical school at Hahnemann University. While in Philadelphia, Dr. Donovan practiced at a preventive medicine clinic with Steven Halpert, M.D., and also worked as a physician's consultant for Serammune Physicians Laboratory in Reston, Virginia.

Dr. Donovan now practices in Seattle, Washington, at the University Health Clinic and at the King County Alternative Medicine Clinic in Kent, Washington, the first government-funded integrated-medicine clinic in the United States. In addition, he is on the faculty of Bastyr University and teaches rheumatology, gastroenterology, and clinical case management.

***"Generally speaking, it is crucial to consciously transform negative thoughts and emotions, because they can be extremely toxic to the body's anticancer defense system," says Dr. Donovan. "My major job with cancer patients is to help them discover who they are and their new, higher order of living. However, I'm not the dictator of their care but only the navigator; the patient is the pilot."***

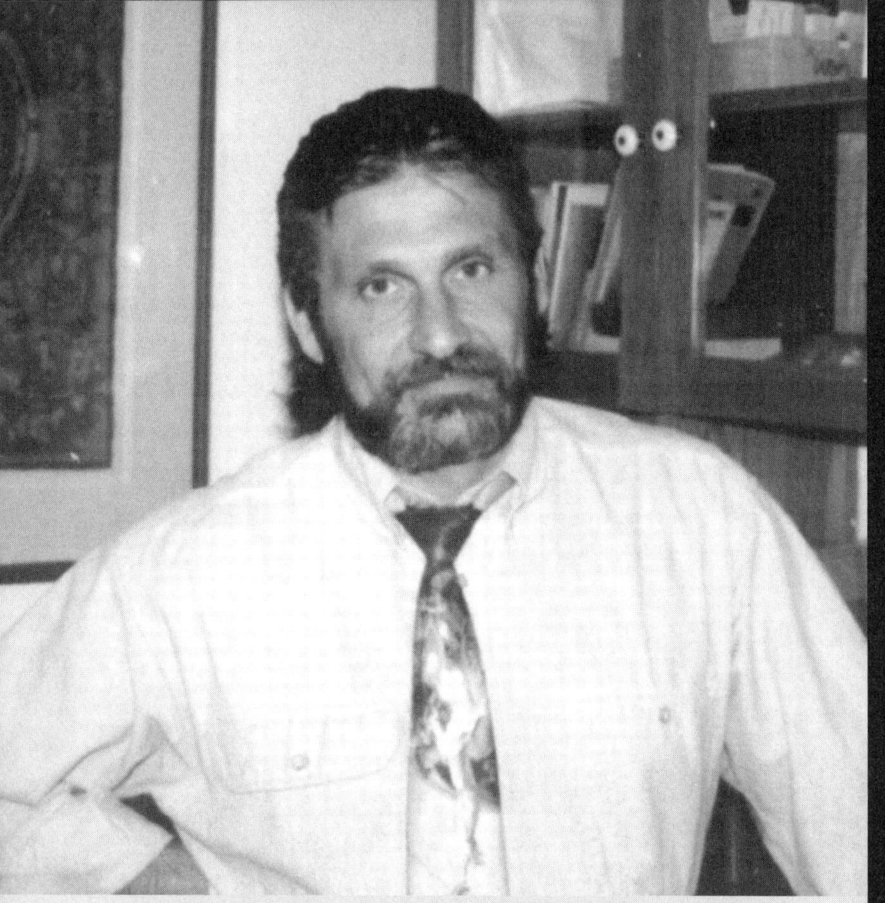

# *Patrick Donovan, N.D.*

**STARTING AN INTENSIVE** program of dietary changes and nutritional/herbal supplementation is crucially important, but equally so is the need for the cancer patient to understand the psychological side of the disease process, says naturopathic physician Dr. Donovan.

For naturopath Patrick Donovan, R.N., N.D., personal growth is as essential a component of successful alternative cancer therapy as the correct supplementation program. Dr. Donovan helps to lay out a psychological road map for each cancer patient "to find out who you are and why this disease has come into your life." The person with cancer must realize that the disease is a process of personal transformation, not a static event. "It is a dynamic movement of their own being, not 'a thing' they have."

"Chaos is inherent in the process of change," Dr. Donovan says. "To move from one level of order to a new level of order (change) entails passing through a phase of chaos. In this case, the cancer experience is the chaotic process. People with cancer need to learn to be patient and attend simply to their own needs, including treatment priorities, in a focused but relaxed way. When you can accept this chaotic element as a natural part of your personal growth process and allow it to fullfill itself, this becomes a major step toward healing."

## A Treatment Plan That Addresses the Patient's Mind and Body

Research indicates that the mind/body connection works both ways. Not only can mind affect immunity, but, since immune cells can send chemical messages to the brain, immunity can affect mind, explains Dr. Donovan.

# Dr. Donovan's Generalized Model for Cancer Treatment

| STRATEGY | DOSAGE/ KEY COMPONENTS | FOR MORE INFORMATION see page # |
|---|---|---|

## Goal and Principles

| | | |
|---|---|---|
| Main goal of program | define relationships to self, source, companions, family, friends, coworkers, and larger community | |
| Principle #1 | reduce or remove obstacles to growth and self-expression as they occur on all levels | |
| Principle #2 | support and nurture the process of growth and the reestablishment of order on all levels | |
| Principle #3 | stimulate growth and accept change and your new order, your new direction of service | |
| Key technique | reframing: adjust frame of reference toward an emotional experience or source of distress | |

## Supplements and Botanicals

| | | |
|---|---|---|
| Multivitamin/mineral complex | without folate is best | 164 |
| Vitamin E | 400-600 IU/day | 790 |
| Mixed carotenes (carotenoids) | 100,000-300,000 units/day (increase the dosage until carotenemia is produced, then decrease) | 764 |
| Vitamin C, buffered ascorbate | start at 1 g, 4X/day, then increase until bowel tolerance is attained | 786 |
| Vitamin K | 1 mg/day | 790 |
| Vitamin B6 | 25-300 mg/day, never exceeding 500 mg/day | 786 |
| Selenium | 200-300 mcg/day | 783 |
| EPA | 2-4 g (2000 to 4000 mg)/day | 768 |
| GLA | 600-1000 mg/day | 770 |
| Amino acid (N-acetyl cysteine) | 500 mg, 2-3X/day | 762, 868 |
| Coenzyme Q10 | 200-400 mg/day | 766 |
| Modified citrus pectin | up to 10 g or more/day | 834 |

*Continued*

## Dr. Donovan's Generalized Model for Cancer Treatment (cont.)

| STRATEGY | DOSAGE/ KEY COMPONENTS | FOR MORE INFORMATION see page # |
|---|---|---|
| Flavonoids | "dosing" with the flavonols (mixed from green tea, grape seeds, berry skins, milk thistle, gingko leaf), 200 mg/day | 817 |
| Green tea extracts | several cups daily, as tea (it does contain caffeine) | 823 |
| Medicinal mushrooms | 2-6 droppersful/day | 833 |
| Hoxsey formula | 1 tsp 3-4X/day | 827 |

**CAUTION**

This chapter includes information regarding actual treatments used by Dr. Donovan only after his careful diagnosis of each patient. All cancer patients are unique. **Do not administer these treatments to yourself or others.** Discuss these treatments with your physician or other qualified health-care professional. Readers should not interpret this material as therapeutic advice, but should see a physician in all cases.

"Therefore stress or disorder occurring on any level—physical, psycho-emotional, or spiritual—can affect all other levels of human functioning, either creating disease, preventing disease, or healing disease." Certain personality traits or behavioral coping styles may make people more susceptible to the types of stress that contribute to cancer, Dr. Donovan adds.

People who tend to develop cancer often are those who are plagued by depression, indecision, hopelessness, low self-esteem, chronic fatigue, and physical weakness.[1] Anxiety, grief, loneliness, or isolation can also depress immune function, possibly increasing one's susceptibility to cancer, contends Dr. Donovan. Fear is "the primary toxin" from which stem all other "toxic" emotions, such as anxiety, hostility, resentment, bigotry, and selfishness.

To begin reversing cancer and to eventually achieve optimal health, Dr. Donovan emphasizes 2 important principles that must be woven into the treatment and all activities.

First, avoid, reduce, or remove obstacles to growth and self-expression. Numerous factors can create obstacles, including: genetic/metabolic disorders, functional/structural disabilities, dysfunctional belief systems, negative or destructive attitudes, emotional distress, anxiety, toxic metabolic by-products, allergies, nutritional deficiencies, overnutrition (excessive fat, sugar, protein), environmental poisons, heavy metals, infectious agents, smoking, poor hygiene, lack of sleep, and dysfunctional relationships.

When these factors are not effectively avoided, minimized, eliminated, or transformed, says Dr. Donovan, they can cause an increase in free radical activity resulting in "oxidative stress" and immune-system problems which, in turn, can lead to many disease-related processes: (1) a breakdown or lapse in the functioning of routine self-repair mechanisms that protect tissue integrity; (2) a depletion of the buffering reserves that ordinarily maintain the body's acid/alkaline balance (which in turn maintains normal biochemical processes); and (3) metabolic alterations that lead to a decreased production or utilization of high-energy compounds the body needs for optimal functioning.[2]

***Certain personality traits or behavioral coping styles may make people more susceptible to the types of stress that contribute to cancer, Dr. Donovan says.***

On the level of psychological and emotional functioning, the continuing presence of these factors can lead to a loss of: (1) hope or a vision of a positive future; (2) faith in oneself or in a higher power; (3) purpose, or a sense of personal meaning; (4) control, or the feeling of having choices and influence in one's life; (5) enthusiasm; and (6) a sense of being part of a greater plan.

Second, the patient must nurture order and balance on all levels. To achieve this goal, Dr. Donovan suggests that the cancer patient needs to: (1) consume a wholesome diet of natural, unrefined whole foods; (2) provide all the nutrients, cofactors and biological substances, especially the trace elements, antioxidants and phosphatides, that are needed to build reserves and encourage repair; (3) maintain proper levels of exercise; (4) get adequate amounts of rest, relaxation, and sleep; (5) use relaxation techniques such as massage and biofeedback; (6) practice good hygiene; (7) practice proper breathing (consciously inhaling and exhaling in times of distress); (8) spend time relaxing with family and friends; (9) express feelings and emotions; (10) undertake creative projects; and (11) practice meditation, visualization, or prayer according to one's beliefs.

For information on **emotions and cancer**, see Chapter 25: What Causes Cancer?, pp. 615-619.

"Generally speaking, it is crucial to consciously transform negative thoughts and emotions, because they can be extremely toxic to the body's anticancer defense system," says Dr. Donovan. "My major job with cancer patients is to help them discover who they are and their new order of living."

## SUCCESS STORY
### Reversing Inflammatory Breast Cancer

Soon after she noticed a lump in her left breast, Joan, aged 66, was diagnosed with breast cancer and promptly underwent a lumpectomy. This revealed that the cancer had already spread to her lymph nodes; out of 26 lymph nodes removed, 3 were malignant. Joan began receiving radiation treatments but stopped them due to the severe reactions she experienced. They made her feel extremely ill, as if she had been "burned alive."

Joan said no to chemotherapy, fearing more terrible reactions. Instead she consulted naturopathic physician Patrick Donovan, N.D., whom she had seen 6 months previously for diabetes. He had put her on a supplement, exercise, and diet program, after which her blood sugar levels stabilized.

This time, Dr. Donovan prescribed nutritional supplements, homeopathic remedies, herbs (notably Siberian ginseng and the Hoxsey formula), and medicinal mushrooms, complemented by psychological and social support strategies. By these means, Dr. Donovan was able to maintain Joan's immune system and prevent the severe side effects of conventional treatments she eventually chose 2 years after her first diagnosis.

After some months, a breast biopsy indicated that the type of cancer Joan had was inflammatory carcinoma. Inflammatory breast cancer is one of the most aggressive forms of cancer known and it is extremely difficult to treat it when metastases are involved; most patients usually survive only a few months, but that's according to conventional thinking.

At this point, Joan's oncologist persuaded her to try radiation again, but this time a rash appeared on the breast, even with the lowest possible X-ray strength. "Her tissues became intensely inflamed and Joan realized she could no longer continue with the radiation," says Dr. Donovan. Joan's oncologist suggested that the reaction was so intense that it may have helped to clear the cancer.

"This doctor expressed surprise that her immune system was producing such a strong inflammatory reaction," Dr. Donovan comments. "Radiation treatment usually has the *opposite* effect on patients, causing suppression of the immune system, but in this case our alternative treatment program had sufficiently bolstered her immune system to enable such a healthy reaction."

Joan's cancer markers remained well within normal range, meaning that her cancer was not progressing. More months passed, then Joan finally agreed to chemotherapy but this proved entirely ineffectual. "I sacrificed all my hair, but it didn't stop the cancer from growing," Joan recalls. Meanwhile, Dr. Donovan gave her intramuscular injections of folate and vitamin B-complex following the chemotherapy; as a result, her fatigue levels and mental functions improved significantly.

About 3 years after her original diagnosis, Joan's doctors performed a complete mastectomy of the left breast and took out more lymph nodes. Though Joan's conventional doctors had predicted that she had only a 20% chance of surviving for one year—based on early pathology reports—she clearly defied the odds. "I wanted to make sure my *real* survival odds were 100%," she notes.

"Dr. Donovan's methods supported my immune system and overall health throughout this entire process. I would have never succeeded in reversing this cancer with standard treatments alone." One of the most remarkable benefits of Dr. Donovan's therapy was that Joan did not experience the bleeding, bruising, chills, or fever that typically result from conventional treatments.

Joan's oncologist was so impressed with her functional improvement and with the fact that she is still alive after 3 years that he called Dr. Donovan to ask what he had done. In fact, he now refers patients to Dr. Donovan and calls him regularly regarding Joan's case to confirm his opinions and discuss treatment options.

## The Role of Nutrition in Supporting the Cancer Reversal Process

Most of Dr. Donovan's cancer patients come to his naturopathic clinic *after* having received extensive conventional treatments. This is unfortunate, he says, because the blood-producing system and immune-system damage caused by intensive chemotherapy and radiation treatments may be beyond repair in many cases. "I have seen chemotherapy-related anemia last for years. If you get the patient *before* they go through chemotherapy and assist them, they can avoid or greatly reduce the long-term side effects, such as fatigue, which can often last for 1 to 2 years."

Dr. Donovan uses nutritional and botanical treatments to help cancer patients obtain far greater benefit with less damage from conventional treatments. "These patients heal much faster and come out of the hospital much quicker, feeling stronger and more energetic. Anemia and the other usual side effects of chemotherapy are turned around far more quickly this way." Given the solid clinical evidence supporting this approach, Dr. Donovan says it is negligent to omit what's called "adjuvant" or complementary-supportive nutrition from any cancer treatment protocol.

**Naturopathy** is an umbrella term to describe the original basis of natural, holistic, and alternative medicine, as first formulated by 19th-century European physicians. In essence, it understands that Nature heals, that the body is inherently self-healing, given the appropriate support therapies, such as diet, herbs, nutritional supplementation, exercise, heat and water therapy, massage, bodywork, counseling, and relaxation. Naturopathy emphasizes disease prevention and health promotion. It is currently licensed as a medical profession in 11 states. In a few states, naturopaths function as primary care physicians, and insurance companies cover their services.

Those who habitually use high-fat foods as "comfort food" in times of stress sometimes respond negatively to dietary suggestions. For this reason, Dr. Donovan explores alternative ways of coping with stress before dietary adjustments are made. He regards it as important to give patients sufficient information about the consequences of making or not making changes in their behaviors and lifestyles. The goal is always to educate them about their options and to give them a sense of power.

Dr. Donovan has found the following nutritional and botanical program to be highly beneficial in resolving the problem of cancer:[3]

**Multivitamin-Mineral Complex—**Dr. Donovan favors the use of a high-potency multivitamin-and-mineral formula to ensure that a broad spectrum of basic nutritional needs are simultaneously met. "The high-potency formulas contain all the essential nutrients except copper and iron, which can be potent free-radical promoters," says Dr. Donovan. "There is some evidence that copper supplementation can rapidly deplete one's zinc reserves; on the other hand, if a copper deficiency exists, suppementation is warranted to avoid the suppressed immunity caused by this deficiency."

When the tumor is more advanced or aggressive, the multivitamin formula is often *without* folate, a B vitamin also known as folic acid. "We know that high folate can suppress early cancer formation and neoplastic changes in tissues," says Dr. Donovan. "Some controversial data suggests, however, that once you have an actively growing tumor, excess folate may stimulate more cell proliferation. This is why some of the orthodox anticancer drugs are antifolate drugs."

**Vitamin E—**Vitamin E plays a major role in protecting cell membranes and supporting the immune system's ability to respond to cancer and infection.[4] Vitamin E also bolsters the effectiveness of chemotherapy agents on tumors,[5] and *lack* of vitamin E increases the toxic effects of adriamycin (a common chemotherapy agent) on heart tissue.[6]

Dr. Donovan is extremely careful in determining the amount of vitamin E to use with the patient. At high doses (any level greater than 600 IU per day), vitamin E can actually stop the oxidation or cell-killing (cytotoxic) mechanisms of neutrophils and macrophages, which are a part of the body's anticancer defenses. For this reason, Dr. Donovan does not recommend taking more than 400-600 IU, even though toxicity studies have found no side effects from vitamin E at levels up to 3,200 mg per day (3,200 IU/day).

***Given the solid clinical evidence, it is negligent to omit complementary-supportive nutrition from any cancer treatment protocol, Dr. Donovan says.***

**Mixed Carotenes**—Carotenes, classified as carotenoids, are the dominant plant pigments in most fruits and vegetables, accounting for much of the orange and yellow colors in the plant world.

There are over 500 naturally occurring carotenoids, of which a large number have been found to be pharmacologically active—beta carotene, phycotene, lycopene, and others. "I prefer to use mixed carotenoids in high doses, but not beta carotene by itself," says Dr. Donovan. "This way you can get the benefit of the whole combination, which is the way we were designed by nature." Dr. Donovan favors the use of a natural carotenoid complex, often prescribing in the range of 100,000-300,000 IU per day. "If the palm of the hand begins to become mildly yellow [indicating carotenemia, or excessive blood levels of carotenoids] decrease the dosage," he suggests. Otherwise, he continues to increase the dosage until carotenemia occurs.

**Vitamin C**—Dr. Donovan uses both oral and intravenous methods of administering vitamin C, but he prefers to use a buffered vitamin combined with magnesium, calcium, zinc, and potassium-ascorbate. He usually starts a patient on vitamin C at 1 g 4 times a day, then increases it until bowel tolerance (resulting in diarrhea) is attained; then he reduces the dosage to just below that level and maintains it there for several months.

**Vitamin K**—This vitamin's primary function is as a coagulating factor, a nutrient that aids in blood clotting. There is some evidence that vitamin K, probably in the form of vitamin K-3 (menadione), is effective as an anticancer agent; this form of the vitamin can be toxic, however, in contrast to the preferred nontoxic form, vitamin K-1 (phylloquine or phytonadione). A growing body of evidence indicates that vitamin K-1 supplements enhance the antimetastatic effects of anticoagulant factors in the body.[7] Severe vitamin K deficiency has been found in cancer patients receiving antimicrobial therapy. A 1 mg-per-day dosage of vitamin K-1 (phytonadione) will not represent any hazard to patients receiving anticoagulant therapy.

**Vitamin B6 (Pyridoxine)**—The immune and nervous systems are heavily influenced by the supply status of this vitamin which aids in DNA/RNA synthesis, fat and protein metabolism, hemoglobin function, and tryptophan metabolism (which in turn affects mood and level of alertness).[8]

Dr. Donovan uses the active form of vitamin B6 (known as pyridoxal 5 phosphate, P5P). His recommended dosage range for B6 is 25-300 mg per day; to avoid toxicity, daily dosages should never exceed 500 mg. Some people on high doses of vitamin B6 experience severe insomnia, an early sign of toxicity; therefore, be sure to take this vitamin early in the day or take smaller doses later in the day, Dr. Donovan advises.

"In an already established tumor, excessive folate intake may promote more tumor growth," says Dr. Donovan. "However, research suggests that it can suppress early cancer formation. For example, in the early stages of cervical metaplasia, high folate levels can reverse and prevent cancer, but it depends on the patient's medical history and profile. I'm cautious in the use of folate."

**Selenium**—This trace element works with vitamin E to reinforce the antioxidant system which is essential to the body's anticancer defenses. Beyond helping to squelch harmful free radicals, selenium enhances NK cell activity against tumors;[9] this element is often deficient in cancer patients.[10] Dr. Donovan's preferred dosage range is 200-300 mcg per day.

**Eicosapentaenoic Acid (EPA)**—This omega-3 fatty acid is the primary fatty acid found in most fish oils. Dr. Donovan states, "EPA is one of the 'good fats' we should consume on a regular basis for optimal health, particularly to prevent and arrest the growth of cancer." He recommends supplementation in the range of 2-4 g of EPA daily, primarily through organic flaxseed oil.

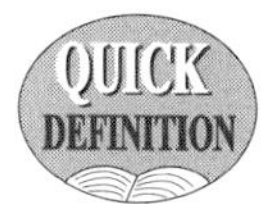

**Lipid** is a biochemist's term for a fat or oil, which is one of the 6 basic food groups. Fats and oils are made of building blocks called fatty acids. Of these long-chain molecules (comprising atoms of carbon, hydrogen, and oxygen) the "fatty" end does not dissolve in water, while the "acid" end does. Fats are also called triglycerides as they consist of 3 (tri) fatty acid molecules joined to one molecule of glycerol, a kind of sugar. Unsaturated fats required in the diet are called essential fatty acids, and include linoleic acid (an omega-6 oil), found in corn, beans, and some nuts and seeds, and alpha linolenic acid (an omega-3 oil), found in fish, flaxseed, and walnuts.

**Amino acids** are the basic building blocks of the 40,000 different proteins in the body, including enzymes, hormones, and the key brain chemical messenger molecules called neurotransmitters. Eight amino acids cannot be made by the body and must be obtained through the diet; others are produced in the body but not always in sufficient amounts. The body's main "amino acid pool" consists of: alanine, arginine, aspargine, aspartic acid, carnitine, citrulline, cysteine, cystine, GABA, glutamic acid, glutamine, glycine, histidine, isoleucine, leucine, lysine, methionine, ornithine, phenylalanine, proline, serine, taurine, threonine, trytophan, tyrosine, and valine.

**Gamma Linolenic Acid (GLA)**—This fatty acid encourages the production of "good eicosanoids" such as PGE1, which in turn impedes the growth of tumors. The richest sources of GLA are evening primrose oil and mother's milk.

According to Dr. Donovan, therapeutic benefits result from supplementing with 600-1000 mg daily, particularly when taken in conjunction with omega-3 oils. The transformation of omega-3 oil into the "good eicosanoids" (such as PGE3) is promoted by zinc, vitamin C, and vitamins B3 and B6.[11] "These nutrient cofactors should accompany any therapy that involves flaxseed oil supplementation," says Dr. Donovan. "In addition, an unrefined, low-fat, mainly vegetarian diet will promote the body's utilization of GLA and omega-3 oil."

**Amino Acids**—Amino acids, the building blocks of protein, can have specific applications for cancer therapy. Cysteine (as N-acetyl cysteine) assists in various detoxification processes and reduces the toxic side effects of both chemotherapy and radiation treatments.[12] Cysteine also helps raise the levels of glutathione which diminishes the toxic side effects of conventional treatments. [13] Dr. Donovan's recommended dosages for N-acetyl cysteine is 500 mg, 2-3 times per day.

**Coenzyme Q10**—CoQ10 is essential for generating energy in the form of adenosine triphosphate (ATP) in living organisms that use oxygen. The body produces its own coQ10, but dietary sources, such as fish, soybean, and rapeseed oils, are important sources of this coenzyme. CoQ10 plays an important part in the body's antioxidant system. When combined with vitamin E, selenium and beta carotene, coQ10 can significantly reduce free-radical damage in the liver, kidney, and heart tissues.[14] Dr. Donovan's recommended intake for coQ10 is 200-400 mg a day, taken with a little flaxseed oil to help absorption.

**Modified Citrus Pectin**—This is an altered form of citrus pectin, a type of fiber that lowers blood cholesterol levels, whose "therapeutic potential for helping prevent cancer metastases is quite strong," says Dr. Donovan. Dr. Donovan recommends up to 10 g or more daily.

**Flavonoids**—This class of plant chemicals (also known as flavonols) include citrin, hesperidin, rutin, pycnogenol, and quercetin. Dr. Donovan recommends "dosing" with the flavonols, usually at the rate of 200 mg per day. "By dosing, I mean increasing the dosages to get pharmacological effects; that is, until they affect the body's mechanisms in much the same way medications affect these mechanisms," he says. "For example, with cancers of the connective tissues, I tend to use the flavonols in high doses (400-500 mg of pycnogenol and green tea extracts daily) since the flavonols exert most of their beneficial effects at the level of connective tissues."

***"Confidence in the therapeutic benefits of medicinal mushrooms is based on 3,000 years of clinical observation by traditional doctors in the Far East," says Dr. Donovan.***

**Green Tea Extracts**—"The green tea flavonols may provide a vital new element in the successful prevention and treatment of liver cancer," Dr. Donovan says, "which is why I recommend taking a few cups of organic green tea daily, preferably before meals."

**Medicinal Mushrooms**—Dr. Donovan uses two kinds: (1) maitake mushroom and its extracts (D-fraction), and (2) a combination of reishi and shiitake. "I have a patient who began using the maitake D-fraction and has had dramatic regression of her breast tumor," says Dr. Donovan. "This mushroom appears to be even more powerful than reishi and shiitake. Confidence in the therapeutic benefits of medicinal mushrooms is based on 3,000 years of clinical observation by traditional doctors in the Far East." Dr. Donovan recommends 2-6 droppersful daily of maitake liquid extract.

**Hoxsey Formula**—This patented herbal therapy is usually combined with balanced diet, vitamin and mineral supplements, and personal counseling. Cancers that have responded favorably to the Hoxsey combination include lymphoma, melanoma, and skin cancer. Dr. Donovan uses the classic Hoxsey formula, with the potassium iodide base; he recommends a teaspoon 3-4 times per day, specifically where there may be lymphatic metastases. Individuals taking the tonic are cautioned to avoid tomatoes, alcohol, processed flour, and vinegar, because of their ability to negate the tonic's effects.

## Accepting the Responsibility to Start Healing

With the intensive program of dietary changes and nutritional supplementation under way, Dr. Donovan begins working with the cancer patient on the psychological level. The goal is to show them ways to accept responsibility for healing through greater self-knowledge. He believes, as his colleague Dr. Leanna Standish once stated, "A patient comes to the healer not to be cured but to be known." Discovering and reestablishing one's *true* identity is at the heart of healing.

***The goal is always to educate patients about their options and the consequences of the consequences of making or not making changes in their behaviors and lifestyles—to give them a sense of power, Dr. Donovan says.***

When Dr. Donovan begins working with a patient, through his counseling techniques, he holds up a "mirror" in which they can see their life, identity, and patterns of relating. He asks them such basic questions as the following: "What was your life like while you were growing up? Tell me about your relationships with your parents and who they were. Tell me about your relationship with your spouse, your family, friends, coworkers, and your creator/God (according to your belief)."

As Dr. Donovan sees it, "To help them see who they are, I have to be as clear and empty as possible, so that I can just reflect back to them what they need to know. I can't tell them who they are; they can only discover this themselves. People need to understand how they live their life and who they are as expressed by the way they live their life."

One of Dr. Donovan's patients, diagnosed with stomach cancer, told him that when she was growing up, her brother used to tease her all the time. "I just couldn't *stomach* it anymore," she told Dr. Donovan. "Then I became an accountant and my boss used to treat me the same way, and I couldn't *stomach* that any more either." The repetition suggests that there may be a psychosomatic connection between the somatic signal (the stomach cancer) and her inability to express the anger within her. "When the expression doesn't happen, anger has to ground itself through the body. In this case, it was grounded in the stomach, as her language indicated."

While Dr. Donovan attempts to unravel the psychological reasons for his patients' health-related behaviors, he lays out all their treatment options. He usually does not advocate chemotherapy or radiation as a first-stage treatment for cancer unless the cancers are extremely advanced or aggressive. Even then, if the patient has made an educated and informed decision to avoid chemotherapy and radiation as much as possible, Dr. Donovan will support this choice.

Conversely, "If the patient chooses to receive these toxic treatments, my nutritional and botanical program will enable them to have much more success and much less toxicity," says Dr. Donovan. "I only advise cancer patients to do chemotherapy when *they* think it's going to help them. I'm not the dictator of their care but the navigator; the patient is the pilot." This approach instills in the patient a sense of hope, optimism, an assertive, fighting-spirit attitude, and personal empowerment.

## Reframing the Cancer Process for Patients

"Reframing" is a term used by psychotherapists to describe adjusting a person's *frame of reference* toward an emotional experience or source of distress. In the case of cancer, unresolved feelings about traumatic life events may affect the way people see themselves and their world and engage with their present circumstances. These feelings are often unconsciously triggered by figures of speech or by everyday objects, such as articles of clothing; the triggers then become the metaphors for the experiences that created the emotional wounds in the first place.

Here is an example of how reframing can help someone with cancer. A lymphoma patient named John came to Dr. Donovan for medical advice. John had suppressed the intense anger, frustration, and other childhood emotions he felt about his father who had beaten him and his siblings. "The rage John felt was so deep and had been suppressed so often, that it grounded through his body," says Dr. Donovan.

"The psychological impulse to rebel turned into a biological one. As much as he wanted to rebel against his father, he could not bring himself to it, so his cells rebelled on his behalf against their normal physiologic restrictions inside his body. The cancer mirrored John's own process." Dr. Donovan's reframing strategy begins with discovering one's personal metaphor, then finding the object (or other key) embodied in the metaphor.

For example, the moment John touched the leather belt his father had used to beat him, he cried profusely, yet he emerged from the experience with a profound sense of relief.

Next, Dr. Donovan has the patient place the "metaphor" on a chair and talk to it, allowing feelings to come to the surface as the therapist sits by. In addressing the belt on the chair before him, "John's profane language reflected the anger and hatred in him," says Dr. Donovan. As a follow-up exercise, a patient sits in the chair, holding the metaphorical object in his lap. In John's case, Dr. Donovan asked him to wear his father's belt and identify with its former owner. "He had to answer questions he had been asking, such as 'What are you [John's father or the cancer] doing here?' John sat for a long time in silence before starting to talk—then all the deeper levels of meaning began to emerge."

As with many others, Dr. Donovan witnessed a wise, compassionate voice coming through John—not the harsh or malicious voice John had associated with his father's voice or the cancer speaking. Often the voice says something like: "I'm here to wake you up and to help you transform yourself. I'm here to remind you that you don't need to succumb to pain and agony. You have the opportunity now to live a fuller, richer, more meaningful existence."

Some time later, when patients feel prepared to be mindfully present, they listen to a tape recording of them speaking to their metaphor and the metaphor speaking back. "They come to learn *why* the process is here," Dr. Donovan says. "They always see a new level of meaning and a new direction. For example, they may get the message that they haven't been paying enough attention to their children or family, and from this they derive a new meaning from their disease process. They see their new order or identity emerging and, through this, their new way to serve."

Finally, patients make a contract with themselves to work harder to improve certain parts of their life, to define a purpose for their life, and to affirm the insights they have gleaned from the experience. The contract embodies the sense of reconciliation the person now feels in relationship to the metaphor, and more importantly, to the *event* represented by the metaphor—the cancer. "John came to realize what his father meant to him and why he was beaten," Dr. Donovan observes. "Of course it's wrong to beat your kids, but John had to realize *why* he was placed in that environment and what he had to learn from it all."

As the last step, the patient takes a copy of this contract and burns it. "The person invariably realizes that in the fire of that contract and those metaphors the contract has been sealed," says Dr. Donovan. "John gave away his leather belt to a homeless person, knowing, as Dr. Donovan suggested, that giving the cancer metaphor away has a healing power of its own."

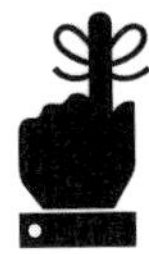

*Many physicians now believe that treating an individual's mental and emotional states is as important as treating any cancerous tumors that may be a result of such conditions. Preliminary studies of biofeedback, meditation, yoga, guided imagery, and other relaxation techniques suggest the mind can enhance immunity against cancer.*

## CURRICULUM VITAE

# Stephen B. Edelson, M.D.

3833 Roswell Road, Suite 110, Atlanta, GA 30342;
tel: 404-841-0088; fax: 404-841-6416.

Dr. Edelson received his M.D. from Tulane University School of Medicine in New Orleans, Louisiana, and he is now licensed to practice medicine in 5 states. He is a Fellow of the American Academy of Family Physicians (F.A.A.F.P.) and the American Academy of Environmental Medicine (F.A.A.E.M.) and a member of 18 other medical societies. His articles have appeared in *Townsend Letter for Doctors* and *The Journal of Applied Nutrition* and he was the host of the Advanced Medicine Radio Show on WQXI-AM in Atlanta, Georgia. Among his other distinctions Dr. Edelson is a diplomate on the American Board of Chelation Therapy, a consultant and visiting professor in Environmental Medicine to the Almaty State Medical Institute in Kazakhstan, on the advisory board of the Cure Autism Now (CAN) Organization, and on the advisory board of directors for Ascent Corporation, a nonprofit organization involved with the study of autism.

***The main problem with today's oncologists, says Dr. Edelson, is that they rarely consider the adverse effects of the toxins produced by the therapies they use. "They wonder why their patients get sick and not well. It's because they're not dealing with the most critical aspect of therapy—detoxification."***

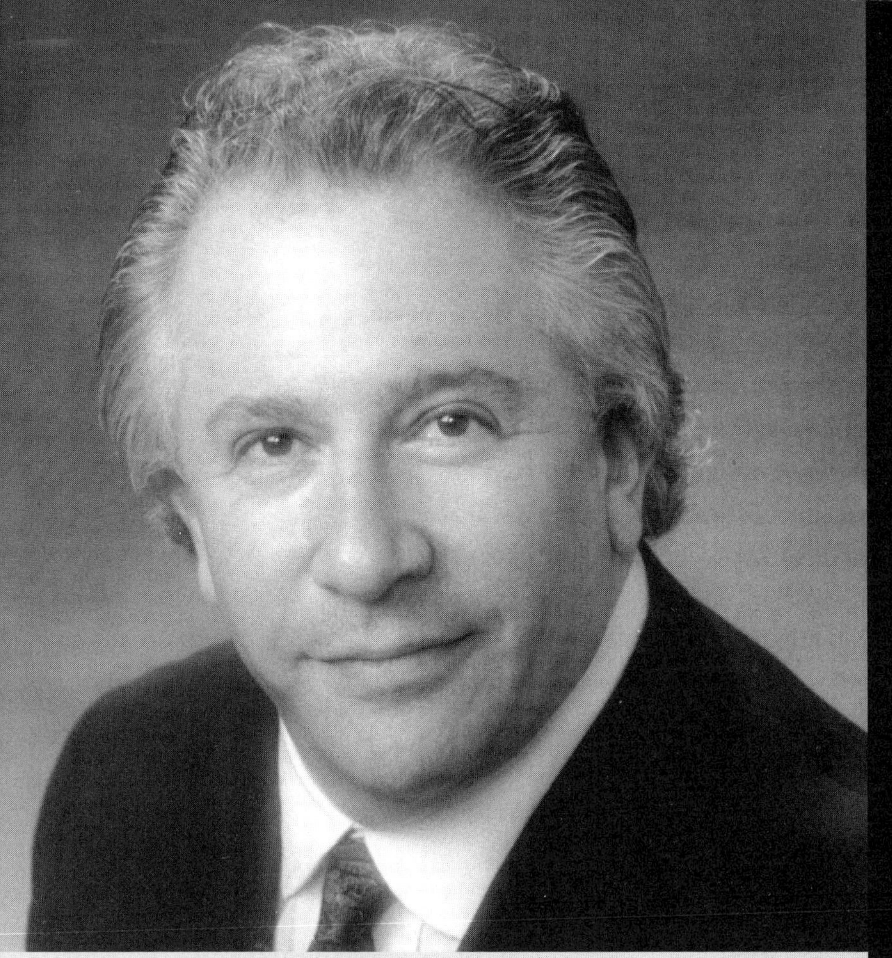

Chapter 8

# *Stephen B. Edelson, M.D.*

**TWO KEYS TO REVERSING** cancer are detoxifying the body and strengthening the immune system, but to do this you need to use many nutrients and alternative therapies together for the best results, says Stephen B. Edelson, M.D.

When Dr. Edelson lost his wife to breast cancer when she was only 40, the experience drove home for him the destructive nature of radiation and chemotherapy, in particular, their immune-suppressive and DNA-damaging effects. Many people receiving conventional care are setting themselves up for cancer recurrence because of these treatments, he says. Since 1991, as director of the Environmental and Preventive Health Center of Atlanta, Georgia, Dr. Edelson has incorporated many alternative cancer therapies into his practice. He believes they hold long-range promise for his patients.

Preventive nutrition and various nontoxic strategies are the major focus of Dr. Edelson's approach, which he calls "environmental oncology," that is, cancer treatment based on the overall condition—mind, body, biochemistry—of the patient, always in relation to the outer world and its conditions. Dr. Edelson's environmental oncology is part of a larger medical field called environmental medicine. "In environmental medicine, we look at how the individual's biochemistry responds to one's environment, at how well the person can detoxify, and how well their organs and systems work to maintain health."

In Dr. Edelson's view, the successful approach to treating cancer lies in

# Dr. Edelson's Generalized Model for Cancer Treatment

| STRATEGY | DOSAGE/ KEY COMPONENTS | FOR MORE INFORMATION see page # |
|---|---|---|
| **Dietary Plan** | | |
| Emphasize plant foods | (1) steamed and raw vegetables, raw fruit and fresh juices; (2) whole grains; (3) legumes ; (4) nuts and seeds; (5) Japanese products (e.g., miso, seaweed and shiitake mushrooms). All fruits and most vegetables should be eaten raw to keep the enzymes in whole, active form. | 749 |
| Avoid animal products | (1) red meats, poultry and most fish; (2) fatty, smoked, and cured meat; (3) butter, cream, and cheeses; (4) commercial whole milk | 184 |
| Avoid certain processed and refined foods | (1) margarine and commercial oils; (2) vegetable shortening (hydrogenated compounds); (3) tropical oils, such as palm and coconut; (4) deep-fat-fried foods; (5) rich desserts (high sugar, fat, white flour); (6) white bread, rolls, buns, pasta cakes, cookies, pies, etc.; and (7) highly processed foods | 184 |
| **Alternative Cancer Therapies** | | |
| Ultraviolet Blood Irradiation (UBI) | amount of blood removed from patient varies according to weight but never exceeds 1 1/2 cc per pound, up to 300 cc of blood; done daily | 185 |
| Melatonin and Interleukin-2 (IL-2) | 50 mg melatonin/day; 3 million units IL-2/day | 941 |
| Hydrogen peroxide ($H_2O_2$) | 0.0375% intravenous solution in 500-cc bottle, 1-3 X/week | 919 |
| Carnivora® | 500-cc bottles, intravenously 5X/week for 1 month; then intramuscular injections | 860 |
| Vitamin C | up to 150 g intravenously | 786 |
| Amygdalin | dosage depends on stage of cancer; intravenously for up to 3 months, then use oral amygdalin | 812 |
| Alpha-interferon | 3 million units daily by intramuscular injection | 187 |

*Continued*

# Dr. Edelson's Generalized Model for Cancer Treatment (cont.)

| STRATEGY | DOSAGE/ KEY COMPONENTS | FOR MORE INFORMATION see page # |
|---|---|---|
| Thymosin | 11 mg of peptides from thymus extract (equivalent to 200 mg of glandular thymus dried) | 944 |
| Soy powder (or Haelan, liquid soy concentrate) | 40 g of soy powder daily; Haelan dosage is variable | 824 |
| Coffee enema | once daily several days a week | 964 |
| Omega-3 fatty acids from flaxseed and fish oils | half flaxseed oil, half fish oil; 2 capsules of each with meals, 3X day | 768 |
| Shark cartilage | 60-70 g/day, orally or rectally by enemas | 863 |
| Tagamet® | 800 mg, taken at bedtime daily for 1 month | 873 |
| Garlic | 6-8 capsules of Kyolic® garlic daily | 818 |
| Hydrazine sulfate | 60 mg gelatin capsules, 3-4X/day, after meals | 868 |
| Modified citrus pectin | 15 g daily | 834 |
| DHEA | 25 mg 2X/day (men); 10 mg 2X/day (women) | 939 |
| Vitamin A (beta carotene) | 150,000-300,000 IU daily | 764,784 |
| Vitamin D | 3000 IU daily | 789 |
| Vitamin E | 1200-2000 IU daily | 790 |
| Vitamin K | 150 mcg daily | 790 |
| Vitamin B1 (thiamine) | 100 mg daily | 784 |
| Vitamin B2 (riboflavin) | 50 mg daily | 784 |
| Vitamin B3 (niacinamide) | 200 mg daily | 785 |
| Vitamin B6 (pyridoxine) | 50 mg daily | 786 |
| Folic acid | 800 mcg daily | 784 |
| Vit B12 (hydroxycobalamin) | 2500 mcg daily | 784 |
| Biotin | 300 mcg daily | — |
| Pantothenic acid (vit. B5) | 500 mg daily | 784 |
| Calcium | 1000-1500 mg daily | 765 |
| Iodine | 200 mcg daily | 776 |
| Magnesium | 500-1000 mg daily | 765 |
| Zinc | 50 mg daily | 793 |
| Selenium | 200-2000 mcg daily | 783 |

| STRATEGY | DOSAGE/ KEY COMPONENTS | FOR MORE INFORMATION see page # |
|---|---|---|
| Manganese | 3 mg daily | 780 |
| Chromium | 400 mcg daily | 766 |
| Molybdenum | 100-1000 mcg daily | 780 |
| Potassium | individually determined, if deficiency exists | 783 |
| Choline | 150 mg daily | — |
| Inositol | 100 mg daily | 776 |
| PABA (para-aminobenzoic acid) | 50 mg daily | — |
| Bioflavonoids | 200 mg daily | 817 |
| Vanadium | 50 mcg daily | — |
| Boron | 15 mg daily | — |
| Silica | 50 mcg daily | — |
| L-carnitine | 250 mg daily | 762 |
| N-acetyl cysteine | 2400 mg daily | 762,868 |
| L-taurine | 250-500 mg daily | 762 |
| Chemo-Arginine (L-Arginine) | 30 g daily (equivalent of 6 tsps of arginine) | — |
| Chemo-Chlor (Chlorella) | 3 capsules, 3X/day | — |
| Chemo-EPA (fish oil) | 3 capsules with meals | — |
| Chemo-Ester-c (vitamin C) | dosage is determined by bowel tolerance, the point at which diarrhea develops | — |
| Chemo-GLA (Gamma Linolenic Acid) | one capsule, 2X/day | — |
| Chemo-Garlic | 6 daily | — |
| Chemo-Glutathione | 8 capsules daily | — |
| Chemo-Sily (Silymarin) | 2 capsules, 3X/day | — |
| Chemo-Veggies | 2 capsules, 3X/day | — |

## Detoxification Strategies

| | | |
|---|---|---|
| Phase I & II detox strategy | "upregulate" the liver using various botanical and nutritional supplements | 190 |
| Phase II detox strategy | use caffeine enemas, since the esters in caffeine appear to stimulate phase II detoxification | 190 |

*Continued*

# Dr. Edelson's Generalized Model for Cancer Treatment (cont.)

| STRATEGY | DOSAGE/ KEY COMPONENTS | FOR MORE INFORMATION see page # |
|---|---|---|
| **Lifestyle Considerations** | | |
| Important points | (1) filter tap water; (2) keep green plants in the house; (3) engage in mild (non-strenuous) physical activity such as walking; and (4) avoid chronic exposure to electromagnetic radiation from power lines, electrical appliances, computers, or poorly insulated electrical wires, particularly when you sleep at night | 791, 191, 1003, 552-556 |

**CAUTION**

This chapter includes information regarding actual treatments used by Dr. Edelson only after his careful diagnosis of each patient. All cancer patients are unique. **Do not administer these treatments to yourself or others.** Discuss these treatments with your physician or other qualified health-care professional. Readers should not interpret this material as therapeutic advice, but should see a physician in all cases.

For more information about **oncogenes,** see Chapter 25: What Causes Cancer? pp. 637-639.

identifying those environmental factors that ruin a patient's genetic integrity, and thus set in motion the preconditions for cancer. For example, the incidence of breast cancer has risen from 1 in 50 women in the early 1900s to 1 in 8 women in 1995, says Dr. Edelson. "Nothing has fundamentally changed about our genetic makeup in the last century; what has fundamentally changed is our environment. The toxic environment causes the oncogenes [cancer-triggering genes] to become activated, damaging DNA and stimulating excessive cell growth. That's why we're seeing more cancer today than ever before."

According to Dr. Edelson, doctors can best help the body rid itself of cancer by employing 2 strategies. First, remove all potential stressors or factors that either contribute to disease or interfere with the healing process. These include toxic chemicals and metals, occult infections (hidden or latent), nutritional imbalances, emotional and spiritual problems, and structural or physical stressors, such as excessive exercise, being overweight, trauma, and postural misalignments. Removal is accomplished through liver detoxification, sauna therapy, treatments of multiple chemical sensitivities, and heavy metal removal through chelation and biological dentistry.

Second, improve the body's internal resistance through preventive nutrition that bolsters the immune system and enhances the overall functioning of cells. Dr. Edelson's anticancer program includes the use of megadoses of vitamin C, intravenous amygdalin and hydrogen peroxide, nutritional supplements (both oral and intravenous), melatonin therapy, Ukrain, Carnivora, immunotherapy with tumor-derived natural killer cells, systemic enzyme therapy, acemannan, and many other nontoxic modalities.

## SUCCESS STORY

### Reversing Colon Cancer

Betsy, aged 44, had been in good health most of her life, except for occasional bouts of constipation, abnormal menstrual periods, and a uterine fibroid which was eventually treated with a hysterectomy. Two years later, when she began experiencing intense cramps and bloating in her abdomen, at first she thought it was constipation; after about 4 months when it had not gone away, she visited a gastroenterologist. He diagnosed colon cancer and found that the cancer had already spread from Betsy's colon to adjacent lymph nodes.

***Dr. Edelson calls his approach "environmental oncology," that is, cancer treatment based on the overall condition—mind, body, biochemistry—of the patient, always in relation to the outer world and its conditions.***

Betsy's oncologist told her she had a 60% chance of dying in the next 5 years from this cancer. Radiation treatments were recommended but Betsy declined. Having read about alternative cancer treatments, she told her doctors she wanted to explore nutritional therapies for enhancing her immune system. To see her plan through, she consulted Stephen B. Edelson, M.D., who immediately started her on a program that included oral and intravenously delivered nutritional supplements, shark cartilage, glandulars, hydrogen peroxide, amino acids, and other substances. Betsy also decided to receive both chemotherapy and radiation therapy during the first part of her program with Dr. Edelson.

Within the first month of receiving the conventional treatments, Betsy was feeling highly nauseated and fatigued. Her white blood cell count had dropped although her liver appeared to be improving. During the treatment period, Dr. Edelson monitored her cancer markers and blood biochemical changes. Then about 6 months later, though still receiving the chemotherapy, Betsy began taking 100 g of vitamin C intravenously on a daily basis. Several months later, she began taking 50 mg of melatonin as well as large doses of beta carotene, acemannan (a form of fiber), and other nutritional supplements.

As a result of Dr. Edelson's program, Betsy's immune system and energy levels markedly improved and her overall condition stabilized. In Dr. Edelson's estimation, Betsy is doing well, and according to all tests (scans, colonoscopy, CEA, and AMAS) she is cancer free. Dr. Edelson notes that, as many therapies were involved in Betsy's treatment program, it is not possible to tell which element had the greatest effect or to what degree the chemotherapy contributed to her recovery.

For more information on the **AMAS test,** see Chapter 27: Early Detection and Prevention, pp. 700-706.

## Tests That Assess the Patient's Cancer-Fighting Potential

Cancer patients at Dr. Edelson's clinic receive a wide range of diagnostic tests to determine which treatment approach may be most appropriate. Dr. Edelson orders the usual biochemical profiles and cancer markers (tests that indicate the presence and extent of cancer), as well as the AMAS test, which measures anti-malignan antibodies in serum (portion of the blood containing immune bodies) and reflects the immune system's response to cancer. By following the results of the AMAS test as repeated over time, the physician can actually monitor the development or regression of a cancer,[1] notes Dr. Edelson.

***"If cancer patients have their lymph nodes or a breast tumor removed, AMAS allows you to know in some cases whether the cancer is still in the body," says Dr. Edelson.***

The greatest value of the AMAS test is in diagnosing cancer at its early stages. The AMAS test is about 95% effective in picking up cancer of all kinds in the earliest stages.[2] This test does not tell which type of cancer a person has—that calls for other blood tests and sometimes CT scans and X rays. "The AMAS test is a sensitive tool," says Dr. Edelson. "If cancer patients have their lymph nodes or a breast tumor removed, AMAS allows you to know in some cases whether the cancer is still in the body. When the test comes back negative, you feel somewhat more convinced that there is no more cancer."

Dr. Edelson believes strongly in baseline scanning procedures such as X rays, CT scans, ultrasound, and various blood tests because they help him determine the stage of the cancer in the patient's body, a necessary foundation for monitoring patient progress and assessing the effectiveness of his therapies. For example, several blood tests provide Dr. Edelson with a detailed picture of the relative strength or "competence" of the patient's immune system by measuring natural killer cell activity, the presence of T-cell subsets (specific types of lymphocytes or white blood cells), and the level of lymphocyte mitogen stimulation (to assess how well a person produces lymphocytes). "I try to establish a baseline measurement for these cancer-fighting cells to see where they're at now in order to compare this level to where they'll be 3 months from now. By doing this, I can alter therapy if needed."

Thyroid hormone evaluation and other endocrine studies are employed for patients with advanced-stage cancers. If the patient is deficient in nutrients that support the thyroid, this gland's function becomes depressed and the functioning of the immune system declines accordingly. For example, the trace elements selenium and copper are needed to help convert a certain form of thyroid hormone (T4) into another more active form (T3). Dr. Edelson uses laboratory tests to evaluate vitamin and mineral levels, antioxidant status, and nutrient imbalances in his cancer patients. On the basis of their results, he recommends dietary adjustments to both treat the cancer and prevent recurrences.

## An Insider's View of the Thyroid

The thyroid gland is located just below the larynx in the throat with interconnecting lobes on either side of the trachea. Of the hormones synthesized in and released by the thyroid, the 2 that concern us here are T3 (triiodothyronine), representing 7%, and T4 (thyroxine), accounting for almost 93% of thyroid hormones active in all of the body's processes.

The secretion of both these hormones is regulated by thyroid-stimulating hormone, or TSH, secreted by the pituitary gland in the brain.

Iodine is essential to forming normal amounts of thyroxine; as long as one consumes about 50 mg per year of iodine, the thyroid gland should be able to make all the T4 it needs.

In the early 1970s, U.S. health authorities referred to the "goiter belt," meaning those regions in the U.S., mostly in the Midwest, in which the incidence of goiter (enlarged thyroid gland) was unusually high.

This problem was later traced to iodine deficiency; since that time, most people in the U.S. use iodized table salt from which they obtain the miniscule amount of iodine needed to keep their thyroid gland theoretically healthy and functional.

I say "theoretically" because in the 1990s, we are seeing a high incidence of thyroid problems, or what I call hidden hypothyroidism, despite dietary fortification with iodized salt.

For a variety of reasons, the thyroid gland of an increasing number of people is becoming dangerously *under*active, upsetting systems throughout the body and mind.

SOURCE: Stephen Langer, M.D., "The Hidden Reason," *Alternative Medicine Digest* 16 (1997), 52-56.

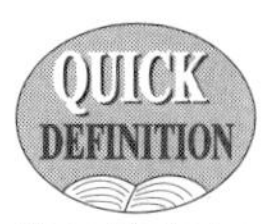

**Macrobiotics** is a specialized diet and food philosophy roughly based on Chinese medicine and filtered through contemporary Japanese culture and American representatives such as Georges Ohsawa and Michio Kushi. The diet emphasizes balancing the energy qualities of fresh, whole foods to maximize their delivery of Qi, or vital life force, to the body. The diet comprises cooked whole grains, beans and bean products, vegetables, fruits, nuts, seeds, small amounts of saltwater fish (salmon), fermented soybean products (miso), seaweeds, shiitake mushrooms, and special pickles and condiments. Macrobiotics has been used successfully when clinically prescribed as a curative and restorative diet in treating chronic and serious illness, including cancer; as a health maintenance diet, it has produced excellent results for many people.

**Lipid** is a biochemist's term for a fat or oil, which is one of the 6 basic food groups. Fats and oils are made of building blocks called fatty acids. Of these long-chain molecules (comprising atoms of carbon, hydrogen, and oxygen) the "fatty" end does not dissolve in water, while the "acid" end does. Fats are also called triglycerides as they consist of 3 (tri) fatty acid molecules joined to one molecule of glycerol, a kind of sugar. Unsaturated fats required in the diet are called essential fatty acids, and include linoleic acid (an omega-6 oil), found in corn, beans, and some nuts and seeds, and alpha linolenic acid (an omega-3 oil), found in fish, flaxseed, and walnuts.

## Changing the Diet Is a Foundation of the Cancer Treatment Program

To repel cancer most effectively, Dr. Edelson often prescribes a strict macrobiotic diet and refers many people to macrobiotic experts for counseling on the diet. According to Dr. Edelson, the optimum foods for cancer resistance are the following: (1) fresh, pure vegetables, fruit, and fresh juices (rich in vitamins, minerals, and enzymes); (2) whole grains (high in B vitamins and complex carbohydrates); (3) legumes (for protein); and (4) nuts and seeds (rich in essential oils).

If a patient is resistant to following a strict macrobiotic diet, Dr. Edelson offers a similar but less austere diet, which has the following composition: no animal products, 65% organic whole grains, 30% organic vegetables and fruit, and 5% Japanese products (e.g., miso, seaweed, and shiitake mushrooms). The main difference between this and the standard macrobiotic diet is that in this diet all fruits and most vegetables are eaten raw to keep their enzymes in whole active form. With either diet, Dr. Edelson steers his cancer patients away from animal products because these foods tend to concentrate many harmful environmental chemicals. The following animal foods are particularly detrimental: (1) fatty, smoked, and cured meats, because they contain harmful nitrites and nitrates; (2) butter, cream, and cheeses, because they contain non-essential saturated fat and toxins; and (3) commercial whole milk, because it contains excess fat, allergenic sources, and sometimes synthetic hormones.

In addition, he recommends strictly avoiding: (1) margarine and commercial oils, for their harmful, hydrogenated compounds; (2) vegetable shortening (hydrogenated compounds); (3) tropical oils, such as palm and coconut (both contain fatty acids that are not nutritionally essential); (4) deep-fat-fried foods, as they are free-radical promoters; (5) rich desserts, because they're high in sugar, fat, and white flour; (6) white bread, rolls, buns, pasta, cakes, cookies, and pies, as they lack nutrients and fiber; and (7) highly processed foods, which have too many potentially harmful chemicals and coloring agents as well as excess sugar and salt.

Dr. Edelson also expresses concern about the status in the body of 2 food substances that may affect one's recovery from cancer. The first is essential fatty acids (EFAs), which are required to mount an effective immune response against cancer. EFAs are deficient in our food supply because of flour milling technology (which causes rancidity and the loss of EFAs), mass food production (EFAs have limited shelf life), meat-eating practices (cattle and chicken are often given feed laced with pesticides and antibiotics), lack of breast-feeding (breast milk is a key source of EFAs as well as immune system components), increased use of pharmaceutical drugs, and elevated levels of toxins in our air, water, and food (which also deplete EFAs).

The second food substance is foreign protein (protein from a source outside the body) which acts as an antigen, overstimulating and burdening the immune system. Such proteins are highly concentrated in dairy and wheat products, which is why these foods are often associated with allergic reactions. "With dairy in particular, you're dealing with peptides [protein fragments] that are more difficult for the body to handle," Dr. Edelson says. "The casein and lactalbumin compounds found in cow's milk are poorly digested and, because all the cancer patients I've seen have a leaky gut, these peptides invariably enter the body and must be neutralized by the immune system." The body's effort to neutralize these "immune complexes" diverts energy needed to resist cancer.

## An Effective Blend of Nontoxic Alternative Therapies

Dr. Edelson's approach blends immune-enhancing and detoxification methods whose anticancer effectiveness has been validated by scientific studies and clinical practice.

**Ultraviolet Blood Irradiation (UBI) Therapy—**Also known as photoluminescence (which differs from photopheresis[3]), UBI therapy involves exposing a small quantity of the cancer patient's blood to ultraviolet light. "Among the more dramatic effects is UBI's ability to activate various parts of the immune system to attack cancer cells and to stimulate key enzyme systems," says Dr. Edelson. A small amount of the patient's blood (varies according to weight) is removed from the patient; the amount never exceeds 1 ½ cc per pound of body weight up to a maximum of 300 cc of blood.

After irradiating the blood with ultraviolet light, it is then returned intravenously to the patient. This procedure may be done daily and takes usually between 1 and 2 hours. Dr. Edelson notes that using UBI as a cancer therapy is still experimental.[4]

**Melatonin and Interleukin-2 (IL-2)**—Melatonin is an immune-enhancing hormone produced by the pineal gland in the human brain. Melatonin has shown considerable cancer-fighting potential, particularly when combined with IL-2 (a naturally-occurring immune system chemical, or lymphokine). "Although we now have clear evidence that this combination causes regression of metastatic cancer, many oncologists don't know that melatonin can do this," Dr. Edelson says. He generally recommends cancer patients take 50 mg of melatonin and 3 million units of IL-2, daily.

For more information about **photoluminescence** and different types of light therapy, see Chapter 34: Energy Support Therapies, pp. 1046-1051.

CAUTION

The typical IL-2 dose is 90 million units a day, which carries considerable toxic effects and can even be deadly. Dr. Edelson uses it to "tonify" the immune system, adding to the overall immune stimulation provided by other supplements and therapies.

**Hydrogen Peroxide ($H_2O_2$)**—Hydrogen peroxide ($H_2O_2$) is formed from the combination of water ($H_2O$) and oxygen ($O_2$). $H_2O_2$ therapy is performed 1-3 times a week intravenously, with each treatment lasting 1-3 hours. The *clinical* dose of $H_2O_2$ is very dilute: only 0.0375% solution in a 500-cc bottle—100 times more dilute than most drugstore preparations, which are about 3% $H_2O_2$. "This [low dose] may explain why I have never seen any side effects with hydrogen peroxide," Dr. Edelson says. "Instead, at this dosage level, people with cancer seem to improve. Hydrogen peroxide apparently works by stimulating the immune system and the system of antioxidant enzymes, including glutathione peroxidase, superoxide, and catalase."

**Carnivora® (Venus' Flytrap)**—"Carnivora is an excellent addition to any cancer treatment program," says Dr. Edelson. The physician places the Carnivora solution in 500-cc bottles and gives it intravenously 5 times a week for 1 month, after which it is administered by intramuscular injection for an indefinite period.

**Megadose Vitamin C**—Dr. Edelson favors the approach pioneered by Robert Cathcart, M.D., who has treated hundreds of cancer and AIDS patients with intravenous vitamin C. High doses may be given intravenously, but not orally, Dr. Edelson notes. "For example, I will give up to 150 g intravenously over a 4 ½ hour period, but I usually don't exceed this amount. The frequency of treatment depends on how often patients can visit our center."

**Amygdalin (Laetrile)**—"Until someone shows me negative studies, I will continue to use amygdalin because it's harmless and potentially very beneficial. In fact, I take some myself every day," says Dr. Edelson. Dosage levels depend on the stage of cancer, but Dr. Edelson prefers administering the substance intravenously for up to 3 months, then having his patients switch to oral amygdalin.

**Alpha-Interferon**—This immune-stimulating chemical is produced naturally by the body, but is also available as a genetically engineered compound. As megadoses of interferon can be extremely toxic, Dr. Edelson uses the substance in small amounts by intramuscular injection and in combination with other key modalities. "Small doses of interferon, such as 3 million units daily, which I often prescribe, can give the immune system an additional boost," Dr. Edelson says. "Large dosages are unnecessary when other immune-enhancing agents are included in a cancer treatment program."

***"Until someone shows me negative studies, I will continue to use amygdalin because it's harmless and potentially very beneficial," says Dr. Edelson.***

**Thymus Extract (Thymosin)**—This active ingredient from the thymus has demonstrated a moderate degree of effectiveness in treating cancer, and yet, "much of the research on this substance has been suppressed," Dr. Edelson notes. His typical dosage is 11 mg of thymus extract, which has a potency equivalent of about 200 mg of dried thymus gland.

**Soy Powder**—Dr. Edelson recommends taking 45 g of soybean powder daily, mainly for its genistein content. Genistein is an antioxidant and may also inhibit the formation of new blood vessels (angiogenesis), thereby inhibiting tumor growth. "The genistein's antioxidant and anti-angiogenesis properties can help stop and perhaps even reverse cancer," says Dr. Edelson. For example, studies of commercial liquid soy concentrates called Haelan

851 (and *wang zhenhua* 851) indicate significant increases in survival among laboratory animals with liver cancer when Haelan is combined with chemotherapy.[5]

For more information on **coffee enemas** and how to perform them, see Chapter 33: Physical Support Therapies, pp. 964-965.

**Coffee Enema—**Dr. Edelson recommends that patients receive a coffee enema once daily several days a week. "It's a great way to support liver detoxification for a variety of reasons," Dr. Edelson says. One reason is that coffee contains choleretics, substances that increase the flow of toxin-rich bile from the gallbladder. This, in turn, means that more toxins are shunted away from the liver, the gallbladder's partner organ, thus assisting in liver detoxification.

In addition, some of the active constituents in coffee enhance the antioxidant glutathione enzyme system, promoting liver detoxification.[6] The coffee enema is among the only pharmaceutically effective choleretic noted in the medical literature that can be safely used many times daily without toxic effects.[7]

**Omega-3 Fatty Acids—**These fatty acids come primarily in the form of alpha-linolenic acid from flaxseed oil. "Taking flaxseed oil will quickly replenish a long-standing omega-3 deficiency," Dr. Edelson notes. "Anyone with cancer or inflammatory disorders needs to use the omega-3 fatty acids more heavily." A dozen 8-ounce bottles of good quality flaxseed oil consumed over the course of a few months will suffice, he adds. Another prime source of omega-3 fatty acids is fish oil, which is why Dr. Edelson's preferred strategy for supporting the cancer patient is to use 50% flaxseed and 50% fish oil.

**Cartilage—**Dr. Edelson's recommended dosage for shark cartilage is 60-70 g a day, delivered either orally or rectally by enema. "I'm not completely sold on this treatment because no quality studies have come out yet," Dr. Edelson says. "However, if my patients report some benefit, I'll help them administer it." Regarding bovine cartilage, Dr. Edelson notes that Dr. John Prudden has done "a significant amount of research showing the anti-angiogenesis as well as immune-stimulation effects. He has a great deal of positive clinical experience as well as having used it for 20 years. I don't think the final answers are in as to the effectiveness, but it is certainly worthy of additional further research and current use in a comprehensive alternative approach in treating malignant disease."

**Tagamet®—**This common over-the-counter medication is widely used for alleviating stomach pain. According to Dr. Edelson, this conventional prescription drug stimulates the immune system, mainly by increasing the number of white blood cells and their ability to incorporate the minerals zinc and magnesium;[8] it also increases natural killer cell activity.[9] Tagamet should not be taken any longer than 1 month (daily) because it shuts down stomach acid production, resulting in various nutritional deficiencies, specifically of zinc and magnesium. But since Dr. Edelson's cancer patients usually receive nutritional supplements intravenously, this side effect can be prevented. His typical dosage is 800 mg, taken at bedtime daily for 1 month.

***"Hydrazine sulfate can decrease pain, stabilize tumor growth, and even promote survival by preventing the terrible wasting process which often occurs in the final stages of cancer," says Dr. Edelson.***

**Garlic—**Garlic has many proven anticancer properties, which is why Dr. Edelson recommends it for both prevention and treatment at the rate of 6-8 capsules of Kyolic® garlic a day.

**Hydrazine Sulfate—**This experimental cancer drug may improve appetite, stabilize weight, decrease lean tissue losses (cachexia), and help "starve" tumors by blocking the tumor's supply of newly formed glucose (gluconeogenesis) from the liver. Favorable results with hydrazine sulfate have been reported for treating cancers of the breast, lung, and larynx, as well as Hodgkin's disease, and other difficult cancers.[10,11] "Hydrazine sulfate can decrease pain, stabilize tumor growth, and even promote survival by preventing the terrible wasting process which often occurs in the final stages of cancer," says Dr. Edelson. His recommended dosage consists of 60 mg gelatin capsules, 3-4 times a day, generally after meals.

**Modified Citrus Pectin—**Modified citrus pectin is plant fiber that seems to provide added protection against cancer by helping to inhibit the spread of cancer cells. Dr. Edelson generally recommends 15 g per day.

**DHEA**—DHEA is an adrenal hormone that helps generate the sex hormones estrogen and testosterone. Some clinical observations suggest that it may be helpful in stimulating the immune system and helping to prevent a recurrence of cancer. "The individual must first have blood drawn to assess his or her DHEA-sulfate level [the sulfate-bound form of DHEA is the form naturally found in the body]," Dr. Edelson says. "If there's a deficiency, I recommend starting at 25 mg twice a day for men, 10 mg twice a day for women." He does not recommend the hormone if a person has an estrogen-sensitive cancer, such as ovarian or breast cancer.

## Detoxification Is an Essential Component of the Cancer Reversal Strategy

Chemo-Prev™ is the trade name Dr. Edelson uses for a line of nutritional supplements he developed specifically to help people prevent and fight cancer and other chronic diseases. The Chemo-Prev™ formulations help improve the cancer patient's antioxidant potential. Chemo-Prev™ Basic F (for women) and Chemo-Prev™ Basic M (for men) are designed differently because each gender has somewhat different biochemical needs.

**Phase I/Phase II liver detoxification** is the natural two-step process the liver conducts to rid the body of toxins. During Phase I, the liver converts toxic compounds into intermediate toxins. In Phase II, the liver converts these intermediate toxins into substances that can be eliminated from the body, delivering them to the colon (via the gallbladder) or bladder for excretion.

For information on **detoxification**, see Chapter 33: Physical Support Therapies, pp. 949-980.

The dosage levels in the Chemo-Prev™ formula are based on *optimum* daily allowances calculated to give the individual the nutrient levels necessary to ensure that all biochemical systems function at optimal efficiency. See the accompanying chart for a review of how Dr. Edelson employs this second phase of his cancer treatment program.

Dr. Edelson uses aggressive detoxification strategies, contending that cancer patients need to keep detoxifying their systems every day. All drugs, chemicals, pesticides, herbicides, and numerous other pollutants must be "biotransformed" in order to be excreted from the body. These processes take place in 2 phases: Phase I, in which the foreign compounds are converted to a form that makes them ready for further processing and eventual excretion; Phase II, in which the by-products (metabolites) of Phase I are combined with various molecules and become less toxic for excretion in the urine. For treating cancer, the Phase II aspect of detoxification requires special attention. "If you don't find a way to strengthen Phase II detoxification, you're going to make things much worse," Dr. Edelson says. "The liver accumulates rather than eliminates toxins, and the cancer patient can eventually die from this excessive buildup of toxins and from severe malnutrition and lean tissue losses."

The Phase II aspect is supported by stimulating (upregulating) the enzyme systems of the liver using various botanical and nutritional supplements and by using coffee enemas, since the esters in caffeine appear to stimulate phase II detoxification. Enzymes, taken as supplements, can "help break down the protein coat around cancer cells and degrade the toxic materials that come from the cancer cells," says Dr. Edelson.

Once you understand the importance of detoxification, you see why Dr. Edelson encourages his patients to change their entire lifestyle so as to reduce all toxic burdens on the body. "The more you can reduce the total burden on the immune system and detoxification system from the unnatural levels we're now forced to handle every day, the more power you put behind your ability to fight cancer." Macrobiotics, for example, work effectively as an anticancer diet because they relieve the body of a large load of toxins, thus allowing the body to devote its energies to healing the disease.

Among the most serious yet most overlooked sources of toxic burden in humans is mercury. Dr. Edelson says that "mercury may well be one of the biggest culprits in damaging DNA and setting the body up for various types of diseases." Many studies have shown, for example, that mercury from silver amalgam dental fillings promotes free-radical damage[12] as well as immune system dysfunction.[13] Dr. Edelson refers many of his patients to biological dentists who focus particular attention on silver amalgam removal and mercury detoxification. Besides dental fillings, other sources of mercury include seafood, polluted air and water, pesticides, fertilizers, auto exhaust, bleached flour, processed foods, fabric softeners, calomel (talc), paint pigments and solvents, cinnabar (used in jewelry), laxatives, and cosmetics.

For more information on the health hazards of **mercury**, (pp. 594-600), polluted, chlorinated, or fluoridated **water** (pp. 577-582), and **electromagnetic energy,** (pp. 552-556), see Chapter 25: What Causes Cancer. For more discussion on the benefits and liabilities of **exercise** in the context of cancer, see Chapter 33: Physical Support Therapies, pp. 1003-1005.

Urban air and tap water often contain unhealthy amounts of pollutants as well. To improve your indoor air quality, grow green plants in different rooms of your home, and for cleaner drinking water, Dr. Edelson recommends a reverse osmosis-carbon filter system; otherwise, good quality spring water can be obtained. To further reduce the toxic burden, Dr. Edelson also recommends that patients stay away from strong

*"Most oncologists have no idea that their chemotherapy patients will do far better with supportive nutritional therapy," says Dr. Edelson.*

sources of electromagnetic radiation, such as power lines and electrical appliances (hair dryers, electric shavers, computers, TVs, radios, etc.).

Mild physical activity such as walking may be helpful to a cancer patient. Strenuous exercise, however, should be strictly avoided since it tends to increase the body's production of free radicals. "The last thing you need when you're treating someone with cancer is *more* free radicals," Dr. Edelson says. "When you engage in vigorous aerobic exercise, you produce extra quantities of free radicals and thus the nutrients that should be supporting the immune system are instead used for quenching the additional free radicals." Running, swimming, and intense aerobic exercise are therefore avoided in Dr. Edelson's program.

## Conventional Treatments Selectively Used, If Necessary

Since treating cancer is a multifaceted process, Dr. Edelson grants the occasional use of conventional cancer therapies as an adjunct to his program. "For advanced cancers, it's best to have a conventional oncologist work alongside someone with a grasp of alternative therapies. The treatment is far more effective when you use the poisons contained in chemotherapy agents together with the natural substances that will improve the immune system and detoxify the body."

For many cases of advanced cancer, surgery is not an option or is only partially effective. As Dr. Edelson sees it, these cases can be effectively reversed by destroying the tumor with chemotherapy drugs while protecting normal cells and tissues with antioxidants and other biological response modifiers. By lowering the tumor burden (overall cost to the body posed by the presence of a tumor), chemotherapy can help the body overcome the immune-suppressive effects of the tumor.

It is critical to consider the type of chemotherapy used, as well as the kinds of agents used to counteract its toxic effects. The main problem with today's oncologists, Dr. Edelson contends, is that they rarely consider the adverse effects of the toxins produced by their therapies. "They wonder why their patients get sick and not well. It's because they're not dealing with the most critical aspect of therapy—detoxification. Most of them have no idea that their chemotherapy patients will do far better with supportive nutritional therapy."

Among the clearest benefits of alternative medicine is its capacity to improve the quality of life and extend the survival of cancer patients. "You can lengthen your life span on our program," Dr. Edelson says. "We can not yet predict who will beat cancer and who will not, but what's clear is that it takes a considerable amount of commitment to see your healing process through." But once his patients make this commitment, Dr. Edelson supports them every step of the way with every aspect of his alternative cancer treatment program.

## CURRICULUM VITAE

# James W. Forsythe, M.D., H.M.D.

Cancer Screening and Treatment Center of Nevada,
Hematology-Oncology, Ltd., 75 Pringle Way, Suite 909,
Reno, NV 89502; tel: 702-329-5000; fax: 702-329-6219.
Also: Century Wellness Center, 380 Brinkby Avenue,
Reno, NV 89509; tel: 702-826-9500; fax: 702-329-6219.

Dr. Forsythe has been practicing oncology in Reno, Nevada, for 22 years. Currently, he manages 2 clinics: Cancer Screening and Treatment Center of Nevada, for conventional cancer treatment; and Century Wellness Center, for alternative medicine, including his speciality, homeopathy, in which he holds a state license. The Century Wellness Center also offers Chinese herbal medicine, acupuncture, hyperbaric oxygen, and intravenous immunotherapy. Conventionally trained, Dr. Forsythe is board certified in Medical Oncology and Internal Medicine, and board eligible in Pathology and Gerontology. He has been an associate professor of medicine at the University of Nevada at Reno and has served as chief of oncology at Washoe Medical Center and Sparks Family Hospital, both in Reno, Nevada. He has also been on the faculty of the University of Nevada Medical School at Reno, Nevada. Dr. Forsythe initially trained at the University of California in San Francisco, but in the early 1980s, became interested in alternative approaches to cancer treatment, including naturopathic and homeopathic protocols.

***"There aren't a lot of doctors out there who want to discuss both sides. Patients have to go to their medical oncologist for one story and then their alternative practitioner, either a homeopath or naturopath, for the other side, says Dr. Forsythe. "They are seldom able to get the full story in one place, which is unfortunate."***

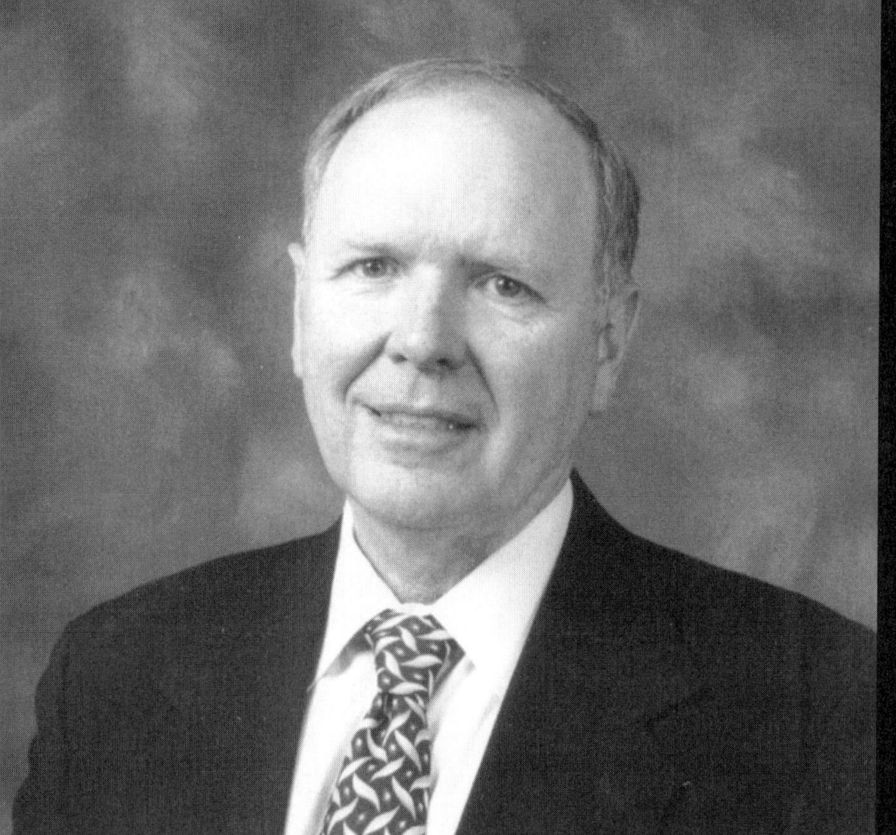

Chapter 9

# *James W. Forsythe, M.D., H.M.D.*

**DRAWING ON HIS** conventional oncology training, Dr. Forsythe's integrated regimen demonstrates the principle that effective cancer care can and should include many different types of therapeutic support from the intelligent, careful, and safe use of chemotherapy to innovative applications of homeopathic remedies, intravenously delivered nutrients, herbs and dietary measures, and immune-stimulating therapies.

As the era of the "kill or cure" approach to conventional cancer therapy draws to a close, the era of biologically supportive therapies is already making profound inroads into mainstream oncology. In sharp contrast with cell-killing chemotherapy and radiation, these new therapies bolster the body's self-healing mechanisms, including the liver's ability to detoxify the body of harmful chemicals and the immune system's capacity to identify and remove cancer cells. A proponent of this shift in focus is James W. Forsythe, M.D., H.M.D.

The new breed of oncologists views cancer not as a localized phenomenon, but as a systemic, whole-body phenomenon; they see cancer not as a static entity, but as a growth process favored by specific biological conditions. As an analogy, just as the fungus on a tree is supported by darkness, warmth and moisture, cancer in the body is supported by toxins, lack of oxygen, poor nutrition, and other specific factors. In addition, just as a fungus can no longer thrive in sunlight and dry conditions, cancer cells will die when the "soil" or biological terrain no longer supports their survival and when the immune system is strong enough to recognize and eliminate them. The person, not the tumor, is the new oncology's focus.

# Dr. Forsythe's Generalized Model for Cancer Treatment

| STRATEGY | DOSAGE/ KEY COMPONENTS | FOR MORE INFORMATION see page # |
|---|---|---|
| **Dietary Plan** | | |
| Nutrient- and phytochemical-rich diet | fruits, vegetables, juices, and whole grains; regularly eat cauliflower, broccoli, Brussels sprouts, lentils, apricots, peaches, and carrots | 749 |
| Low in animal fats and proteins | avoid cured meat products (bologna, salami, sausage, cured hams, bacon, pepperoni, and hot dogs); avoid cholesterol-rich fats; limit, if not avoid, whole milk products, eggs, butter, cheese, red meats, and fried foods; avoid excessive amounts of shellfish | 749 |
| **Detoxification** | | |
| Homeopathic drainage remedies | individually determined | — |
| **Homeopathic Potencies of Anticancer Agents** | | |
| Shark cartilage | 12X to 15X | — |
| *Echinacea purpurea* | 12X to 15X | — |
| **Homeopathic nosodes** | | |
| *Tuberculinum, Medorrhinum* | both 30X, single dose | — |
| Homeopathic thyroid | 6X | — |
| Germanium | 8X | — |
| Laetrile (amygdalin) | 12X to 15X | — |
| Alpha interferon | usually 6X to 12X | — |
| Thymus gland | 7C | — |
| **Supplements** | | |
| Beta carotene | 20,000-40,00 IU daily | 764 |
| Vitamin C | 5-10 g (to bowel tolerance) over the day | 786 |
| Vitamin E | 800-1200 IU daily in divided doses | 790 |
| Calcium/magnesium/zinc | take as combined supplement, in a ratio of 500:250:10 mg, 3X/day | 765, 793 |
| Selenium | 100-200 mcg 3x/daily | 783 |

*Continued*

## Dr. Forsythe's Generalized Model for Cancer Treatment (cont.)

| STRATEGY | DOSAGE/ KEY COMPONENTS | FOR MORE INFORMATION see page # |
|---|---|---|
| Pycnogenol | daily minimum of 1 mg/lb of body weight (e.g., 150-pound person would take 150 mg per day) | 822 |
| Coenzyme Q10 | 100 mg, 2x/day | 766 |
| Pancreatic enzymes | 2 tablets before meals and at bedtime | 928 |
| *Gingko biloba* | 50 mg, 2x/day | 820 |
| Super Blue-Green Algae | 600 mg, 2x/day | 809 |
| Barley grass extract | 500 mg, 2x/day | — |
| *Echinacea* | 400 mg, 2x/day | 815 |

**CAUTION**

This chapter includes information regarding actual treatments used by Dr. Forsythe only after his careful diagnosis of each patient. All cancer patients are unique. **Do not administer these treatments to yourself or others.** Discuss these treatments with your physician or other qualified health-care professional. Readers should not interpret this material as therapeutic advice, but should see a physician in all cases.

### SUCCESS STORY

### Reversing Breast Cancer

Roberta, aged 65, a highly successful realtor, investor, and developer, was diagnosed with cancer of the left breast, Stage II, Grade 3, for which she underwent lumpectomy. At the time she refused radiation but accepted chemotherapy, and had 2 cycles of Cytoxan, methotrexate, and 5-FU. Roberta decided on her own, based on her research, that she did not want any more chemotherapy; she believed it was doing her body more harm than good.

"She was feeling quite awful, very tired and weak, having some hair loss and nausea, and decided she wanted to go on her own," says Dr. Forsythe, who helped her design a program that included vitamins, minerals, herbs, and other substances. This program included germanium, 2X daily; DHEA, 25 mg, 3X daily; bovine cartilage, 4 g daily (500 mg capsules); thymus glandular extract, 200 mg, 3X daily; evening primrose oil gelatin capsules, 2 daily; red clover, 300 mg, 3X daily; vitamin C, 10 g daily, divided into 2.5 g, 4X daily; garlic capsules, 3X daily; glucosamine, 500 mg, 3X daily; Armour natural thyroid glandular extract, 2 grains daily; calcium citrate, 1,500 mg daily, taken as 500 mg, 3X daily; chlorella, 3X daily; pau d'arco, 200 mg, 2X daily; barley greens (barley grass), 500 mg, 3X daily; and Essiac tea, 3 cups daily. She used cat's claw and glutathione for a while, but discontinued them as they did not agree with her system.

Roberta began this program immediately after discontinuing chemotherapy and remained on it faithfully for 3 ½ years, says Dr. Forsythe. Her cancer markers, which had been elevated before, became normal. "Here is a woman with a Stage II cancer who didn't take the prescribed radiation and chemotherapy. She did not have what we call a complete cancer surgery, yet she is doing beautifully, extremely well. Roberta is a very assertive person who runs her own business. She really took charge of her disease and did the healing her own way. She's been very successful."

## SUCCESS STORY
### Reversing Prostate Cancer

Millard, aged 82, was a retired contractor who remained vigorous and active into his eighties. He had fathered 14 children and was still happily married to his wife. Millard came to Dr. Forsythe with prostate cancer; previously he had undergone surgery for prostate enlargement, but no signs of cancer were detected at that time. But 2 years later, a biopsy revealed poorly differentiated prostatic cancer. "This means that under the microscope, the cells look highly malignant as opposed to more benign in appearance," says Dr. Forsythe. Millard's prostate specific antigen (PSA, a prostate cancer marker) was 30, quite high compared to a normal of 0 to 4.

Millard's conventional oncologist offered him the treatment options of radiation therapy, radical prostatectomy, or castration, but he declined all 3. By removing his testicles, the oncologist believed all androgen, a male hormone believed to be involved in prostate cancer, would be removed from Millard's body. "He came to me and said he wanted to take therapy he can live with, that won't be toxic to him, and that will meet his lifestyle. Millard is a pretty healthy, vigorous guy: he maintains

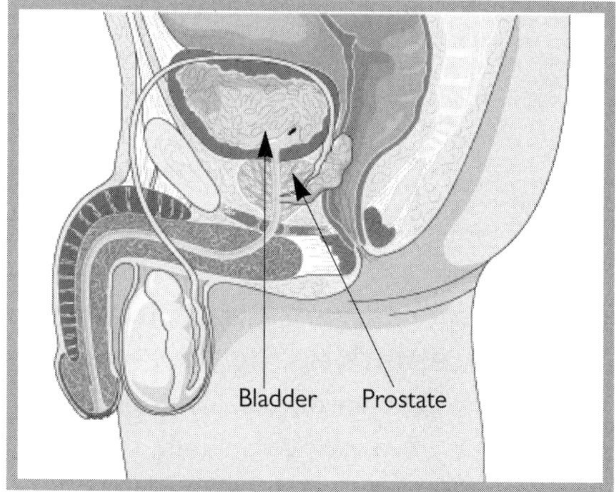


**Figure 9.1—The prostate gland**

a garden and every year he and his wife travel."

Even so, at the time of examination, Dr. Forsythe found that Millard's cancer was spreading to his right hip joint. Dr. Forsythe started Millard on anti-androgen therapy with an injection of Zolodex. "It's a conventional medication which he received once a month to 'turn off' the body's androgen," Dr. Forsythe explains. Androgen, or testosterone, is the primary male sex hormone; conventional oncologists believe that prostate cancer cells need testosterone to grow, so that, therefore, by removing or blocking its action, the prostate cancer should begin to shrink and reverse.

In addition, Dr. Forsythe started Millard on a nutritional supplementation program including: vitamin A (as beta carotene), 40,000 IU daily; vitamin C, 4 g daily, as 1 g taken 4X; vitamin E, 800 IU, in 2 divided daily doses; selenium, 200 mcg daily; calcium, 1 g daily; magnesium, 500 mg daily; zinc, 50 mg daily; flaxseed oil, 2 tablespoons daily; vitamin B complex, 2X daily; pycnogenol grape seed extract, 200 mg, 2X daily; *Echinacea*, 3 capsules daily; and barley grass, 500 mg, 3X daily. Millard also started a vegetarian diet that emphasized fruit juices.

**Homeopathy** was founded in the early 1800s by German physician Samuel Hahnemann. Today an estimated 500 million people worldwide receive homeopathic treatment; in Britain, homeopathy enjoys royal patronage. Homeopathy is now practiced according to 2 differing concepts. In classical homeopathy, only one single-component remedy is prescribed at a time in a potency specifically adjusted to the patient; the physician waits to see the results before prescribing anything further. In complex homeopathy, typified by *Hepar compositum*, a prescription involves multiple substances given at the same time usually in low potencies.

This program brought Millard's PSA down to 4 and after only 2 months of treatment, the cancer was "under good control," says Dr. Forsythe. However, about 4 months after beginning treatment, Millard started having blood in his urine, which turned out to be a sign of bladder cancer that was obstructing his right kidney. Millard went on radiation therapy for 3 weeks and did a small dose of chemotherapy for 4 months for this large tumor, but he refused surgery.

The combined treatment was successful, says Dr. Forsythe. "The man today looks 12 years younger. He is without prostate or bladder cancer activity, and his chemistry panel is completely normal."

## Blending Conventional Oncology with Alternatives Such as Homeopathy

Dr. Forsythe began working with alternative approaches to cancer in the early 1980s. "There was definitely a bias and prejudice against alternative doctors at that time; there still is to some degree, but less so. I became very interested in and amazed by the kinds of reactions and results the homeopaths and naturopaths were getting using alternative methods. I was just used to using chemotherapy or radiation or surgery. With the alternative methods, I saw prolonged remissions in patients with breast, colon, lung and prostate cancer. Through that exposure I became more and more involved in alternative medicine, particularly in nutrition, vitamins, supplements, dietary changes, and more recently in homeopathy and naturopathy."

Dr. Forsythe's approach to cancer tends to be multimodal. As such, he will sometimes combine chemotherapy in *safe* doses with homeopathic remedies and nutritional, herbal, and immune-stimulating therapies. Dr. Forsythe advocates a shift away from the "kill-or-cure" mentality to cancer in favor of an approach centered around respect for the wisdom of the human body. Dr. Forsythe's integrated regimen demonstrates the principle that effective cancer care can and should include many different types of therapeutic modalities. Each of his modalities, either alone or in combination, can have a direct impact on those mechanisms that bolster a person's anticancer defenses.

***Dr. Forsythe's approach to cancer tends to be multimodal. As such, he will sometimes combine chemotherapy in safe doses with homeopathic remedies and nutritional, herbal, and immune-stimulating therapies. Each of his modalities, either alone or in combination, can have a direct impact on those mechanisms that bolster a person's anticancer defenses.***

"We don't claim to treat cancer itself," Dr. Forsythe explains. "I tell patients that the conventional therapy I offer them, including chemotherapy, will be given in such a way that it's not taxing to their immune system. We try not to make the treatment worse than the disease; we try not to overtreat patients. We give chemotherapy, if we have to give it, in a way that will be easy on their system with minimal side effects and minimal toxicities."

For example, often Dr. Forsythe will give the chemotherapy followed immediately by the patient receiving intravenous nutritional supplements, including high-dose vitamin C, while germanium and other antioxidants, plus shark and bovine cartilage, are given orally. Homeopathic remedies may be given intravenously, as can immune-stimulating therapies in homeopathic doses such as intravenous interferon, "which has been a conventional treatment, but it's good for all types of cancers and immune diseases."

Dr. Forsythe sees himself "walking a fine line" between conventional therapy and alternative therapy. "As you know, insurance usually will not cover alternative therapy or homeopathy, but I incorporate them into my conventional practice, so a patient's insurance usually does cover the treatment. This is important because chemotherapy drugs are extremely expensive. A single course of chemotherapy may cost anywhere from $400-$2,000 just for the drugs themselves."

As Dr. Forsythe explains, the patient gets to decide which elements will be part of their treatment program. "If they want to have immune-boosting therapy along with their chemotherapy, that's offered. There's no duress involved: it's simply offered as an alternative. Many patients come to me because they've discussed using nutritional therapy along with chemotherapy with their conventional oncologists. Not infrequently, I hear this story: The doctor asked me to leave the office and find another doctor who would do that. Conventional oncologists are very intolerant of natural approaches. Dr. Forsythe treats many patients who have refused surgery, radiation, or chemotherapy, from the beginning. "They want *only* alternative therapies. They don't want anything to do with chemotherapy. If that's their wish, then we try to build up their immune system."

Dr. Forsythe points to a number of patients he's treated who had primarily breast or lung cancer, had either alternative therapy with or without chemotherapy, and are alive after 5 to 10 years. "I find it's usually a combination of therapies that works best. That's why I'm such a believer in using combination therapies. In my opinion, you have to use some conventional and some alternative or complementary therapies together. Hopefully medicine will evolve in that direction because now we know that alternative therapy either by itself or with conventional therapies can be very helpful in prolonging the disease-free interval and causing cures."

Dr. Forsythe asks patients not to turn a deaf ear to the conventional side of treatment. "Sometimes patients tend to write it off completely and totally ignore the good parts of it. They have to keep an open mind. There aren't a lot of doctors out there who want to discuss both sides. Patients have to go to their medical oncologist for one story and then their alternative practitioner, either a homeopath or naturopath, for the other side. They seldom get the full story, which is unfortunate."

## Tailoring the Treatment Program to the Individual Patient

Before therapy is given, Dr. Forsythe initiates an extensive laboratory work-up to identify toxic chemical, viral (CMV, Herpes I & II, EBV, HHV-6), and allergic (both chemical and inhalant allergies) substances to determine the full scope and nature of all immunosuppressant factors responsible for individual immune system failure in the patient. Dr. Forsythe also screens for toxoplasmosis (a parasital infection from *Toxoplasma gondii* usually transmitted from human contact with infected cats), Lyme disease, and high titers of polio or diphtheria virus.

"We try to find what has been impinging on or harming the patient's immune system," Dr. Forsythe explains. "Then we go after that using homeopathic remedies to desensitize the patient's system. Very small doses of homeopathic preparations are given intravenously over a number of days to make the immune system *recognize* the disease or virus or allergy and respond to it."

On the basis of these results, Dr. Forsythe tailors the overall remedies, including homeopathic remedies, to the individual case. Dr. Forsythe is convinced that in the coming years there will be a "rebirth of enlightenment among oncologists and a greater acceptance of natural forms of healing combined with conventional forms of therapy. After all, a patient with a life-threatening disease wants the full armamentarium of 'weapons' used against the disease, and not one to the exclusion of the other."

The foundation of Dr. Forsythe's program is a diet replete with nutrients and phytochemicals, rich in fruits, vegetables, juices and whole grains, and low in animal fats and proteins. His advice to patients is to regularly consume cauliflower, broccoli, Brussels sprouts, lentils, apricots, peaches, and carrots. "These contain large amounts of anticancer phytochemicals which have been found in many nutritional studies throughout the world's literature to have strong anticancer effects."

For example, broccoli and cabbage contain substantial amounts of specific substances that activate enzymes involved in the liver's detoxification of cancer-causing chemicals, states Dr. Forsythe. He also counsels patients to avoid cured meat products—bologna, salami, sausage, cured hams, bacon, pepperoni, and hot dogs—which have high nitrous urea content. "I ask my patients to avoid cholesterol-rich fats and greatly limit, if not avoid, the use of whole milk products, eggs, butter, cheese, red meats, fried foods, and excessive amounts of shellfish."

The supplements most often prescribed by Dr. Forsythe for cancer patients include the following:

- Beta Carotene: "This is a safe form of vitamin A, which should be ingested anywhere from 20,000 to 40,000 IU per day. I never advise going above 150,000-200,000 units per day," Dr. Forsythe says.
- Vitamin C: "The best and most manageable doses appear to be in the range of 5 to 10 g per day. Bowel tolerance is often the limiting factor, and this is to the point just prior to triggering diarrhea. The vitamin should be spread out through the day and not taken in a single lump dose."
- Vitamin E: 800-1200 IU per day in divided doses
- Pycnogenol: a minimum dose of 1 mg per pound of body weight (e.g., a 150-pound person would take 150 mg per day)
- Calcium, Magnesium, Zinc: As a combined mineral, this should be taken in a ratio of 500:250:10 mg, 3 times per day
- Selenium:100-200 mcg per day
- Coenzyme Q10: 100 mg, twice daily
- Pancreatic Enzymes: 2 tablets before meals and at bedtime
- *Gingko Biloba:* 50 mg, twice daily
- Super Blue-Green Algae: 600 mg, twice daily
- Barley Grass Extract: 500 mg, twice daily
- *Echinacea*: 400 mg, twice daily.

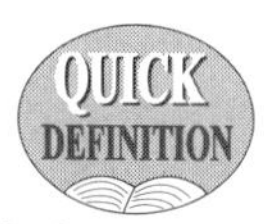


**Drainage remedies** comprise low-potency homeopathic substances and tinctures (alcohol extractions) of both Chinese and Western herbs. The concept of drainage derives from French homeopaths who were interested in applying homeopathy at a grosser, physiological level rather than at the level of "mentals," the psychological, emotional, and spiritual factors. Drainage remedies encourage the lymphatic system, liver, kidneys, blood, tissues, intercellular spaces, fat, and skin to eliminate, or "drain," their toxins and to keep them from circulating in the body and depositing themselves in other areas. The best known drainage remedies are *Solidago* and *Berberis* for the kidney; *Taraxacum, Silymarin* and *Carduus* for the liver; *Hydrastis* as a general drainage; and *Myosotis* for the lymphatic system.

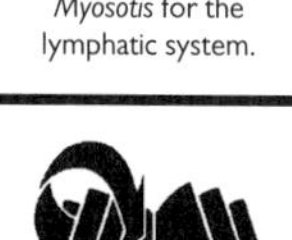

For more information on **homeopathic treatments for cancer**, see Chapter 6: W. John Diamond, M.D., and Chapter 20: Vincent Speckhart, M.D.

Dr. Forsythe is experimenting with formulas of diluted homeopathic potencies of known anticancer agents, including:

- Shark cartilage, 12X to 15X
- *Echinacea purpurea*, 12X to 15X solution, for stimulation of the T-cell system
- Homeopathic nosodes, *Tuberculinum* (made from the disease product of tuberculosis) and *Medorrhinum* (made from gonorrheal virus), both at 30X, single dose
- Homeopathic thyroid, 6X dilution

- Germanium, 8X
- Laetrile (amygdalin), 12X to 15X dilution, for its antitumor effects
- Alpha interferon at various homeopathic potencies, usually 6X to 12X.

A homeopathic **nosode** is a super-diluted remedy made as an energy imprint from a disease product extracted from bacteria, tuberculosis, measles, bowel infection, influenza, and about 200 others. The nosode, which contains no physical trace of the disease, stimulates the body to remove all "taints" or residues it holds of a particular disease, whether it was inherited or contracted. Only qualified homeopaths may administer a nosode.

Dr. Forsythe will often recommend thymus gland in a 7C (homeopathic) dilution for immune dysfunction. The use of drainage remedies which help specific excretory organs enhance their function may be helpful; for instance, the administration of *Solidago* in a 2X potency for clearing of the kidney, or *Sabadilla* or *Potassium Iodine* for mucosal drainage in the case of congested lungs secondary to bronchogenic carcinoma in a 2X potency, given at a dose of 50-75 drops per day. For liver metastases or liver failure, *Rosmarinus officinalis* in a 2X potency for periods up to 2 months in a dose of 50 drops per day may also be helpful, says Dr. Forsythe.

In cancer patients who are malnourished or losing lean tissue, the use of bowel nosodes such as the "Gaertner" nosode is often recommended in a single 30C dosage to help restore appetite and promote weight gain, according to Dr. Forsythe. The Gaertner is a nosode made out of bacteria that inhabit the intestines; administering it can help stop destructive catabolic processes. In addition, Dr. Forsythe will occasionally recommend the use of "sarcodes" which involve the administration of glands, organs, or tissues from healthy animals in homeopathic potencies. These are often from the thymus, spleen, and bone marrow.

"Patients may have low thyroid function and be exhausted metabolically from the tumor itself and thus the homeopathic thyroid in a 5C or 7C dilution is often helpful," Dr. Forsythe explains. "This can be an excellent way to help restore thyroid function. If the patient is anemic, they may require a bone marrow sarcode such as *Medulla* suis (pig bone marrow) in a 7C dilution."

## SUCCESS STORY

### Reversing Bone Metastases

Elizabeth, aged 75, first came to Dr. Forsythe in her 50s with metastatic bone cancer that had spread to her spine and chest wall. It was diagnosed as Stage IV breast cancer, a serious condition. Although Elizabeth received conventional treatment in the early days of her cancer, she moved on to alternative treatments, including homeopathy, and is alive 16 years later, says Dr. Forsythe.

Every 3 months, Dr. Forsythe gave Elizabeth homeopathic remedies or homeopathic preparations of medicinal substances including, in part, the following: *Hydrastis* 30X; *Chelidonium* 100X; *Calcium Carbonate* 30X; Shark embryo 1M; *Lachesis* 30X; drainage remedies; and interferon and shark cartilage. Dr. Forsythe also put Elizabeth on a comprehensive nutrient supplementation program, including a progesterone formula.

"Elizabeth had bone pain with her bone metastasis, but after this was treated and arrested, she became better and has stayed at a plateau of wellness since that time, within the first 5 years of her diagnosis," says Dr. Forsythe. "We used the homepathic preparations to strengthen her immune system as she had a number of allergies and viral infections that were uncovered through our testing. Elizabeth is now living a vigorous life for a woman in her mid-70s who has had this disease for 16 years. She is at home; she's not on any pain medicine; and she's had no spread of her tumor to other bones."

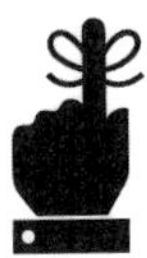

*Prevention is the most important and reliable cancer-fighting tool that exists today. The fact that cancer can be treated and reversed and that it can be detected early and prevented are the most important messages of this book.*

## CURRICULUM VITAE

# Abram Hoffer, M.D., Ph.D.

2727 Quadra, Suite 3, Victoria,
British Columbia, Canada V8T 4E5;
tel: 250-386-8756; fax: 250-386-5828.
Dr. Hoffer's Internet address is:
**http://www.islandnet.com**
(at Member's Mall, Health & Medicine,
Hoffer on schizophrenia).

Dr. Hoffer received his Ph.D. from the University of Minnesota and his M.D. from the University of Toronto. He has held many university positions and has been in private clinical practice since 1967. He is the author of over 500 medical articles and a member of 12 medical societies; his books include *Orthomolecular Medicine for Physicians* (Keats, 1989); *Common Questions on Schizophrenia* (Keats, 1988), and *Hoffer's Laws of Natural Nutrition* (Quarry Press, 1996); Dr. Hoffer is the coauthor of an additional 9 books including *Smart Nutrients* (with Morton Walker; Avery, 1994), *Putting It All Together: The New Orthomolecular Nutrition* (with Morton Walker, Keats, 1996), and is the editor of the *Journal of Orthomolecular Medicine.*

***"The combination of nutritional therapy plus standard approaches is a highly promising, comprehensive approach to cancer treatment," says Dr. Hoffer. "Patients who follow this combined approach for at least 2 months have a significantly better outcome than patients on the standard therapy alone."***

Chapter 10

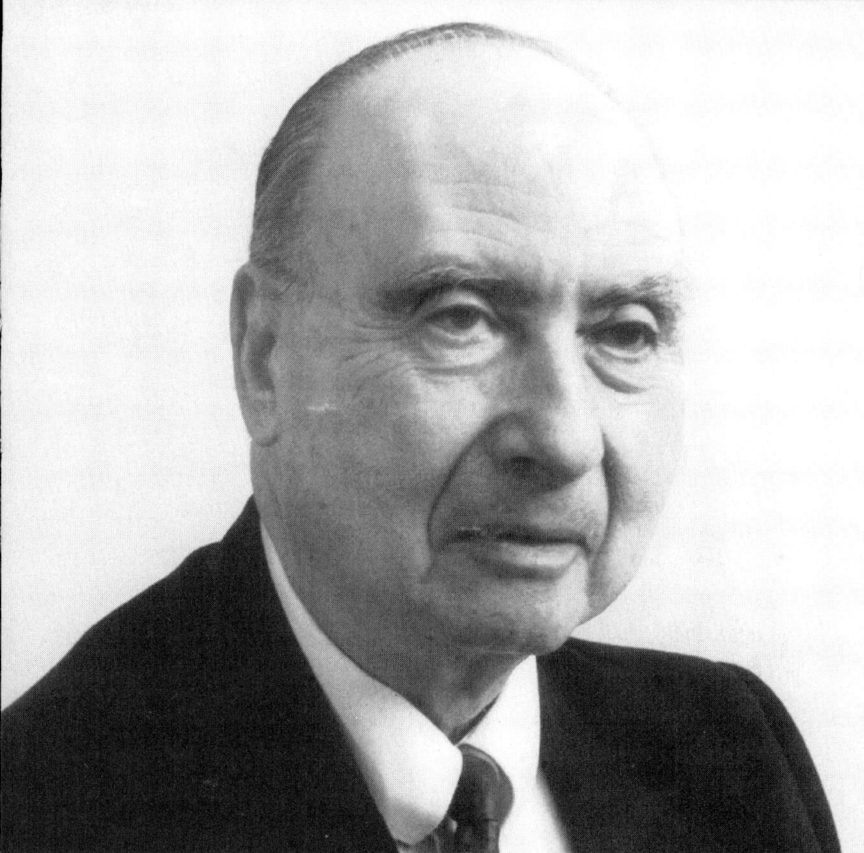

# *Abram Hoffer, M.D., Ph.D.*

**FOR ABRAM HOFFER, M.D.,** a pioneer in the scientific or orthomolecular use of nutritional substances for healing, high sustained doses of vitamin C are a cornerstone in his cancer treatment plan, supplemented by a wide range of supportive nutritional substances and a low-fat, low-sugar, dairy-free diet.

Of the hundreds of cancer patients Abram Hoffer, M.D., has seen since 1979—specifically, 770 to date—almost all have been referred by their doctors and most have received conventional treatment. Dr. Hoffer's preliminary (and striking) success with 2 cancer patients confirmed his belief that high doses of nutritional supplements could prevail against cancer. One patient, a 16-year old girl with osteogenic sarcoma, was about to have a limb amputated. Dr. Hoffer started her on vitamin B3 (niacinamide) and vitamin C (ascorbic acid), 3 g of each. Her tumor regressed, her surgery was canceled, and she has continued to thrive.

That case was in 1962; in 1979, a woman, aged 59, came to Dr. Hoffer with a pancreatic tumor that was blocking the bile duct. She had surgery to relieve the blockage (by installing a substitute duct), then started taking vitamin C at a dosage of 10 g daily. Dr. Hoffer increased this to 40 g daily and added vitamin B3 and other nutrients. After 6 months, medical scans revealed no trace of the tumor and her original bile duct had reopened. She told all her friends that vitamins had saved her from cancer, and soon Dr. Hoffer was taking many new cases (up to 100) each year.

## Dr. Hoffer's Generalized Nutritional Program for Cancer Patients

| STRATEGY | DOSAGE/ KEY COMPONENTS | FOR MORE INFORMATION see page # |
|---|---|---|
| **Dietary Plan** | | |
| Vitamin C | start at 12 grams of oral vitamin C, and adjust the level of intake either upward or downward, depending on bowel tolerance (6 to 40 grams of oral vitamin C). In general, he recommends only the intravenous form of vitamin C for cancer patients who cannot tolerate more than 10 grams of vitamin C orally. | 786 |
| Vitamin B3 | 500 mg 3X/day | 785 |
| Vitamin B complex | 1 tablet/day | 784 |
| Beta carotene | 25,000 IU/day | 764 |
| Vitamin A | starting dosage is usually 25,000-50,000 IU daily | 784 |
| Vitamin E | 25,000 IU/day, preferably with a form called d-alpha tocopherol succinate | 790 |
| Selenium | 200-1000 mcg day | 783 |
| Zinc | 30-60 mg/day | 793 |
| Coenzyme Q10 | 300 mg/day | 766 |
| Essiac tea | 3-4 cups per day | 815 |
| Low-fat, low-sugar, dairy-free, mainly vegetarian diet | no specific proportions, but emphasize high-fiber foods such as grains, legumes, and vegetables | 749 |

Dr. Hoffer has carefully studied his patients to determine the effects of nutritional therapy on cancer outcomes. "Early on, we saw some striking benefits," Dr. Hoffer says. "After following 45 cancer cases, it appeared that patients who followed our orthomolecular program had a better outlook and lived a lot longer than those who remained on the standard treatment alone. Our patients appeared to be not only feeling better but also living longer."[1]

Dr. Hoffer says that his nontoxic treatments do not interfere with conventional treatments, but reinforce or

**CAUTION**

This chapter includes information regarding actual treatments used by Dr. Hoffer only after his careful diagnosis of each patient. All cancer patients are unique. **Do not administer these treatments to yourself or others.** Discuss these treatments with your physician or other qualified health-care professional. Readers should not interpret this material as therapeutic advice, but should see a physician in all cases.

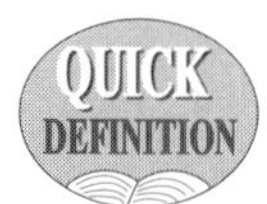

**Staging** in cancer terminology is a relative index of how much cancer exists in the body, its size, location, and containment or metastasis. Stage I, the earliest, most curable stage, shows only local tumor involvement. Stage II indicates some spreading of cancer to the surrounding tissues and perhaps to nearby lymph nodes. Stage III involves metastasis to distant lymph nodes. Stage IV, the most advanced and least easily cured, means the cancer has spread to distant organs.

complement such treatments. "By reducing side effects and boosting my patients' regenerative abilities, my approach simply *completes* their treatment program. The combination of nutritional therapy plus standard approaches is a highly promising, comprehensive approach to cancer treatment. Patients who follow this combined approach for at least 2 months have a significantly better outcome than patients on the standard therapy alone."

Breast and prostate cancer respond very well to Dr. Hoffer's approach. "The majority of my breast cancer patients were Stages III and IV. However, with my Stage I and II patients, most of them have done really well, and all of them have done very much better than the control group, who were patients with the same degree of illness but who did not follow any nutritional program involving vitamins. Of the Stage III and IV cases I saw, and this is perhaps 90% of my series, 50% have already reached a 5-year cure rate. In general, I have found that if they survive 4 years, they automatically would get another 10. Also, the earlier a cancer is caught, the better, though even some cancers at Stage III can be helped. Sarcomas [tumors arising in the connective tissues of the bone, muscle, cartilage and lymph system] have also responded extremely well to treatment."

Regarding lymphoma, Dr. Hoffer treated 19 patients between 1984 and 1993 and had an 80% success rate for 5-year survivals. Of 13 males with lymphoma, 10 survived 2 years, 8 survived 4 years, and 6 lived at least 5 years. One patient with small-cell lymphocytic malignant lymphoma—"one of the worst types of lymphoma," says Dr. Hoffer—who was given 3 months to live by his conventional oncologists, survived for 14 years under Dr. Hoffer's orthomolecular nutrition program in conjunction with chemotherapy and radiation. Dr. Hoffer gave this patient high doses of vitamin C (12-15 g daily on average, but sometimes, 40 g) as well as daily amounts of selenium (400 mcg), vitamin E (400 IU), vitamin A (50,000 IU), zinc citrate (50 mg), niacin (2 g) and magnesium oxide (840 mg).[2]

In contrast, cancers of the lung, liver, and ovary have proven more difficult to treat. Dr. Hoffer believes the use of nontoxic nutritional therapies, referred to as orthomolecular medicine, is crucial for the more aggressive or advanced forms of cancer. "No matter what type of tumor is involved, whether it's a lung or pancreatic tumor, the patient is going to need intensive nutritional support. It makes no medical or scientific sense whatsoever to ignore this vital aspect of treatment."

A recent report on the nutritional treatment of cancer patients attests to the cancer-fighting potential of vitamin and mineral supplements as advocated by Dr. Hoffer. Out of 134 patients, those with cancers of the breast, ovary, uterus, and cervix lived 20 times longer than their conventionally treated counterparts in the control group. For people with other cancers, life expectancy was 12 times higher in the supplement-treated group. In 1993, 16 years after the study began, 34 of those patients who took the supplements were still alive, while all those who had received only conventional cancer treatment had died.[3]

***Dr. Hoffer believes the use of nontoxic nutritional therapies called orthomolecular medicine is crucial for the more aggressive or advanced forms of cancer. "It makes no medical or scientific sense whatsoever to ignore this vital aspect of treatment."***

One of the coauthors of this landmark study was Linus Pauling, M.D., the Nobel prize-winning biochemist who put the efficacy of vitamin C squarely on the medical map. The other author was Dr. Hoffer, who continues to use vitamin C (ascorbic acid or ascorbate) as an integral part of his approach to "orthomolecular oncology."

Orthomolecular medicine involves the scientific use of vitamin and mineral supplements to treat disease. The quantities of nutrients are carefully measured and adjusted to meet the individual metabolic and nutritional needs of the patient. In general, the dosages exceed the basic nutritional requirement (also known as the recommended daily allowance, or RDA), thereby enabling the nutrients to deliver a powerful "pharmacologic effect." Such megadoses are only used on a temporary basis to help reverse illness and are not meant for regular health maintenance.

For more information on **orthomolecular medicine,** see Chapter 28: Nutrition as Cancer Medicine, pp. 780-783.

## SUCCESS STORY

### Reversing Breast Cancer

When Martha found she had a large tumor and two smaller tumors in her left breast, she refused surgery and chemotherapy. The tumors continued to grow. She tried a variety of dietary treatments, including the raw foods diet (the Living Diet) designed by Ann Wigmore, Ph. D., N.D., of Boston, Massachusetts. For 3 months she felt well, but her tumors showed no sign of reversal.

When Dr. Hoffer saw her 5 months later, she was extremely ill and emaciated (she weighed only 85 pounds). Conventional physicians considered her to be a "terminal" case and expected her to die within 2 weeks. "One doctor refused to give her another appointment in a week, telling her she would be dead before then," says Dr. Hoffer. "I could see how he could arrive at this decision, but I could not comprehend his unwillingness to provide her any support."

Under Dr. Hoffer's guidance, Martha began taking vitamin C (4 g, sodium ascorbate) 3 times a day. One month later, she consulted a naturopath, who recommended organ extracts and vitamins in small doses, as well as large doses of vitamin A (1 million units per day), and Martha took these as well.

After 3 months on this program, Martha began to gain weight. More metastases were found and she was told her prognosis was still very bleak. She might live 6 months at best. Because the cancer was still progressing, Martha received an experimental preparation of intravenous collagen (a connective tissue that helps hold bone together) for 2 weeks, after which she took it orally.

Only 1 month later, having gained a few pounds, Martha felt upbeat and more energetic. For the next few months, she received vitamin C in both the oral and intravenous forms. However, the cancer had ulcerated, which means, it had risen and broken out on the skin of her breasts.

Several months later, and a little under 1 year since being diagnosed, Martha's hair fell out and her liver became enlarged. She was still on high doses of vitamin A. Fluid had entered her lungs and abdomen, and she was diagnosed as anemic. Dr. Hoffer immediately had her discontinue the vitamin A and within a month her hair began to grow back. Martha's liver was still enlarged.

Yet after another 3 months, Martha was showing clear signs of recovery. Her energy levels were substantially higher, she weighed 102 pounds, her liver tests were improved, and her hair was growing. The breast pains she had experienced were gone. After another 6 months, with her condition not showing any further signs of substantial improvement, following Dr. Hoffer's recommendation, Martha opted for chemotherapy without radiation.

The results were immediately apparent. The tumor began to recede, new skin began to cover up the previously ulcerated part of her breast (lesion), and the painful swelling that had affected her arm for months was gone. "She experienced very little nausea or discomfort during the chemotherapy treatment, probably because of the nutritional program we placed her on," says Dr. Hoffer.

After about 15 months on Dr. Hoffer's orthomolecular program, Martha could no longer tolerate vitamin C, so Dr. Hoffer placed her on bioflavonoids instead at a dosage of 1 g taken 3 times daily. After a month, the lesion on the breast surface was healing well, with only 1 small sign of cancer on the surface of her breast; after 3 more months, Martha's hair was growing back, she weighed 111 pounds, and the tissue on her breast had returned to normal. There was no sign of cancer upon visual examination and palpation. By all indications, says Dr. Hoffer, Martha was in remission.

## SUCCESS STORY

### Reversing Lung Cancer

Sandra, who also suffered from anorexia, experienced a severe bout of depression. Around the same time, she was found guilty of defrauding her employer and sent to prison. A few days later she entered a coma that would last several weeks. She lost a great deal of weight and recovered only gradually. About 5 years later, Sandra was operated on for lung cancer with metastases to the bone.

After she was released from prison, Sandra went to see Dr. Hoffer when she was experiencing memory loss, depression, and other psychological problems. He started her on a vitamin program that included 9 grams of vitamin C per day. One month later, her memory became normal, but she remained depressed; 2 months later, the pain in her chest and bones had diminished substantially. Sandra received 1 last series of radiation treatments at this time. After 2 years with Dr. Hoffer, she had recovered her normal mental functioning and was no longer depressed. Years later, Sandra was still alive and well, according to Dr. Hoffer.

## The Therapeutic Power of Vitamin C

In 1993, Drs. Hoffer and Pauling published a study they had conducted of 170 patients referred to Hoffer between April 1988 and December 1989.

Most followed his nutritional program, outlined below. Only 10% of the control group, which received only conventional treatment, were alive at the end of the study; in contrast, nearly 40% of the 138 patients who followed the nutritional program were alive. As in another study, patients with cancers of the breast, cervix, ovary, and uterus benefited the most from Dr. Hoffer's nutritional program. Half of these patients remained alive at the end of the study, as did about one third of those with other types of cancer.[4]

In one of Dr. Pauling's early studies, a daily dose of 10 grams of vitamin C was found to significantly increase the life span and enhance the quality of life in 100 terminal cancer patients.[5] Further, vitamin C demonstrates an ability to selectively kill tumor cells in a manner similar to other chemotherapy drugs.[6] Dr. Pauling never stated that vitamin C should be used alone, but rather as an adjunct to other types of therapy, either conventional or alternative. Dr. Hoffer considers oral vitamin C to be the most essential part of his approach to cancer. Before an optimal level of vitamin C intake can be reached, the patient's bowel tolerance must be established, which means the maximum amount that does not produce diarrhea. The temporary diarrhea that results from too much vitamin C can lead to large losses of valuable nutrients, including vitamin C itself.

***"After establishing the highest tolerable dosage of vitamin C, I supply all the other nutrients simultaneously to make sure the individual receives the full range of anticancer benefits," Dr. Hoffer says.***

To establish the optimal oral intake, Dr. Hoffer recommends taking 12 g (a large dose) of vitamin C in divided doses throughout the day, preferably 4 g 3, times a day. Pure crystalline vitamin C can be dissolved in water or juice. If no laxative action results at this dosage, Dr. Hoffer suggests increasing it by 2 g on each successive day, with careful observation of one's bowel movements. Once a laxative action, or mild diarrhea, develops, reduce the dose by 1 or 2 g below this bowel tolerance level and maintain the dose for several months with appropriate medical monitoring.

This approach differs from the protocol for oral vitamin C ingestion used by the Linus Pauling Institute, which recommends beginning with 1 or 2 g (not 12 g) dissolved in water or juice; the cancer patient then increases the intake by 1 or 2 g each day until a laxative action develops. According to Dr. Hoffer, patients with advanced cancers are often severely deficient in vitamin C and can therefore begin immediately at the 12 g level and increase their dosage upwards.

The use of high-dose vitamin C, either orally or intravenously, should be discontinued only gradually, since the body's enzymes become "programmed" or conditioned to the higher ascorbate levels, says Dr. Hoffer. If one's intake is abruptly discontinued, a sudden drop in the blood ascorbate level results—a kind of "rebound effect" analogous to the bouncing of a ball (the harder you force the ball down, the higher it bounces). Thus, all Dr. Hoffer's patients start at 12 g of oral vitamin C and adjust the level of intake either upward or downward, depending on bowel tolerance, which varies in the range of 6-40 g of oral vitamin C. If they can tolerate more, Dr. Hoffer will increase the dosage up to 40 g. In general, he recommends only the intravenous form of vitamin C for cancer patients who cannot tolerate more than 10 g of vitamin C orally.

One of Dr. Hoffer's cancer patients, a man diagnosed with metastatic bone cancer, was told by his oncologists that nothing more could be done for him. "When we started him on the program, he could not tolerate oral vitamin C," Dr. Hoffer says. "I then arranged for him to receive 10 g of intravenous vitamin C 3 times a week." Three months later, the man was completely free of bone cancer and went on to live another 10 years, eventually dying of heart disease but not cancer, says Dr. Hoffer.

**CAUTION**

Although vitamin C has extremely low toxicity even at high doses, certain side effects may occur. In addition to temporary diarrhea, a small percentage of people experience gastric distress, such as gas and bloating. According to nutritional biochemist Ross Pelton, this problem can be alleviated by switching to the less acidic calcium ascorbate salt.[7] If intravenous sodium ascorbate is used, transient fluid retention will occasionally result from the sodium overload; this can be problematic for people with hypertension or heart problems.

## An Orthomolecular Supplement Program

Over the years, Dr. Hoffer learned that vitamin C is an essential component among the many used in comprehensive treatment programs for advanced cancers. Other key nutrients are needed to give the patient's body cancer-fighting ability. In one study by Drs. Hoffer and Pauling, high-dose supplementation with oral vitamin C led to excellent responses in about 10% of 170 cancer patients; however, the addition of other nutrients increased this response rate to about 40%.[8] "After establishing the highest tolerable dosage of vitamin C, I supply all the other nutrients simultaneously to make sure the individual receives the full range of anticancer benefits," Dr. Hoffer says. "Once they have begun the program, I can begin to adjust the amounts of the individual components."

**Vitamin B3 (Niacin)**—"Vitamin B3 may increase the therapeutic efficacy of cancer treatment," says Dr. Hoffer. "In mice, it has been shown to increase the toxicity of radiation treatment for tumors. It also enhances blood flow to the tumor and protects the heart muscle against the toxic effects of adriamycin (a chemotherapy drug), which may explain why the vitamin works well with chemotherapy." Max Gerson, M.D., the developer of the Gerson diet for cancer patients, successfully treated many cancer patients with a dietary regimen that included 50 mg of niacin 8 to 10 times per day.[9]

The only major side effect of niacin or niacinamide supplementation at this level is a tingling or flushing in the skin, beginning in the forehead. If the sensation becomes too intense, Dr. Hoffer recommends switching to the ester form of the vitamin, inositol hexaniacinate. This form is expensive but produces only minimal flushing and provides inositol. "Inositol is an important messenger molecule which may add to the therapeutic properties of niacin," says Dr. Hoffer, who generally recommends cancer patients take vitamin B3 at 500 mg 3 times per day.

**B Complex**—This group of B vitamins, which includes vitamin B1, B2, B3, B6, folic acid, and pantothenic acid, acts as a biochemical team to help speed up chemical reactions (catalysts) and support overall metabolism. Deficiencies of any one or more of the B vitamins inhibit the immune system's ability to fight cancer.[10] "The B complex is needed for overall health whether or not you have cancer," Dr. Hoffer says. "This vitamin complex also reinforces the positive effects of vitamin B3, which is a more specific priority for cancer treatment."

**Beta Carotene**—Dr. Hoffer typically recommends taking 25,000 IU per day of this precursor to vitamin A because it has repeatedly been shown to bolster the activity of natural killer cells and other immune cells against tumors.[11,12,13]

**Vitamin A**—Dr. Hoffer will occasionally recommend a vitamin A supplement if there is some indication, based on dietary records and blood tests, that the individual may be deficient. The starting dosage is usually between 400 and 1200 IU daily.

**Vitamin E**—Dr. Hoffer generally recommends taking 25,000 IU per day of vitamin E, preferably in a form called d-alpha tocopherol succinate. The succinate form is preferred because it is most effective in reducing growth and enhancing the differentiation of cancer cells, says Dr. Hoffer, perhaps because "tumor cells pick up this form of vitamin E more readily than they do other forms. As with vitamin C, the vitamin E research points to a blatant *under*utilization of nutritional therapies for cancer patients." At the very least, he adds, this vitamin should be used to enhance the effects of conventional treatments and to reduce their toxic side effects.

**Selenium—**A range of 200 to 1000 mcg is desirable as a daily supplementation strategy for cancer patients, says Dr. Hoffer, who uses 2 forms of selenium: sodium selenite and a yeast preparation. "I do not think there is any basic difference, but a few patients are allergic to yeast preparations and they prefer to use the selenite preparation." This trace element enhances the effects of vitamin E and works more powerfully as an anticancer agent in the presence of vitamin E.[14]

**CAUTION**

Gerhard Schrauzer, Ph.D., a German scientist known for his research on selenium, reports that high zinc levels in the blood are associated with higher mortality rates from cancers of the colon, breast, ovary, lung, bladder, prostate, and oral cavity. For this reason, caution should be exercised whenever using zinc as part of a cancer treatment program.

**Zinc—**Dr. Hoffer does not always recommend zinc because it is a known antagonist to selenium. However, he will use it as a temporary supplement, at 30-60 mg per day only if the person shows definite signs of a zinc deficiency. Like selenium, zinc supports many aspects of the immune system and its deficiency can potentially make one more vulnerable to certain cancers.[15] Zinc has a close relationship with copper, which is essential to proper functioning of a wide range of immune cell types, including antibody-forming cells, T helper cells, and macrophages, all of which may help the body defend against cancer.[16]

**Coenzyme Q10—**Dr. Hoffer's recommended dosage of coQ10 is 300 mg a day. "This coenzyme is one of the unique additions to our anticancer arsenal," he says. "It is especially important for people who have been involved for long periods of time in vigorous athletics or occupations requiring excessive physical exertion."

**Essiac—**Many of Dr. Hoffer's patients take Essiac tea and have reported more energy as a result. "I'm not sure what Essiac does to extend cancer survival, and for all we know it may not have this effect," says Dr. Hoffer. "On the other hand, it's not toxic and my patients have reported feeling good while taking it, so why not support them?"

## The Benefits of a Low-Fat, Low-Sugar, Dairy-free Diet

Dr. Hoffer finds that many of his patients recover faster when their diets are low in fat and sugar and devoid of dairy products. All 3 factors—fat, sugar, and dairy products—seem to reduce the cancer patient's ability to survive. Dietary fat has been found to significantly depress the immune system.[17] Similarly, excessive amounts of sugar from white flour products, tropical fruits, and fruit juices, may suppress the activity of white blood cells (lymphocytes) for up to 2 hours.[18]

***A clear benefit to increasing hope and encouraging attitudes of faith and positivism, says Dr. Hoffer, is that it increases compliance to treatment. The combination of this compliance to a carefully designed treatment program and the considerable positive impact that enhanced hope can have on the immune system can contribute to a much more favorable outcome.***

The role of dairy products is more elusive. Some researchers assert that the foreign proteins from dairy products lead to chronic stimulation of the lymph system, which could be one factor in the development of lymphomas.[19] Since beef and dairy products also contain fat, increased intake of such foods might further influence the development of various cancers.

In Dr. Hoffer's experience, the incidence of cold, flu, and allergy symptoms tends to decrease when people avoid dairy products and follow a nutritionally balanced diet centered around complex carbohydrates and high-fiber foods (grains, legumes and vegetables). This in turn could reduce the burden on the immune system, freeing up the body's resources to more effectively fight cancer. In theory, says Dr. Hoffer, the allergies and other stresses may exhaust the immune system over time. A study found that allergy sufferers had a highly significant risk of developing certain cancers, namely leukemias, lymphomas, and myelomas.[20]

"I don't know whether allergies or milk-related congestion can make people more susceptible to cancer, but certainly having repeated colds, flus, and allergies taxes the immune system and draws from nutrient stores it needs," says Dr. Hoffer. "I have strong concern that dairy products may also contain estrogens or trigger estrogen production, which could in turn promote hormone-sensitive cancers such as breast and ovarian cancers."

## The Therapeutic Power of Informed Hope

Patients who are fully informed about their medical condition and prospects under alternative care are able to marshal the invaluable and therapeutically potent power of hope, says Dr. Hoffer. "One of the most important psychotherapeutic variables, hope is generated by discussing cases of patients with similar cancers and outlining how they have dealt with their tumor and results of treatment."

A clear benefit to increasing hope and encouraging attitudes of faith and positivism, says Dr. Hoffer, is that it increases compliance to treatment. The combination of this compliance to a carefully designed treatment program and the considerable positive impact that enhanced hope can have on the immune system can contribute to a much more favorable outcome.

***Dr. Hoffer finds that many of his patients recover faster when their diets are low in fat and sugar and devoid of dairy products.***

## CURRICULUM VITAE

# Tori Hudson, N.D.

A Woman's Time—Menopause Options and Natural Medicine, 2067 N.W. Lovejoy, Portland, OR 97209; tel: 503-222-2322; fax: 503-222-0276.

Tori Hudson, N.D., received her naturopathic degree from the National College of Naturopathic Medicine in Portland, Oregon, in 1984 and has been in practice and teaching for 12 years. Dr. Hudson completed premed studies at Portland State University, Portland Community College, and Portland's Lewis and Clark University. She also studied at the Pacific Academy of Homeopathic Medicine and completed the International Foundation for Homeopathy Doctors' Course in Seattle, Washington. From 1989-1993, she was medical director of the Portland Naturopathic Clinic. From 1993-1994, Dr. Hudson was a professor and then academic dean at the National College of Naturopathic Medicine. Dr. Hudson is the author of *Gynecology and Naturopathic Medicine: A Treatment Manual* (TK Publications, Aloha, Oregon, 1992) and since 1992 has been a regular contributor on women's health issues to *Townsend Letter for Doctors and Patients.*

***"Each year, there are over 62,000 cases of cervical cancer, with at least 9,000 women dying from the disease," Dr. Hudson says. "Naturopathic treatment could help lower the death toll considerably, as long as early treatment is emphasized."***

# Chapter 11

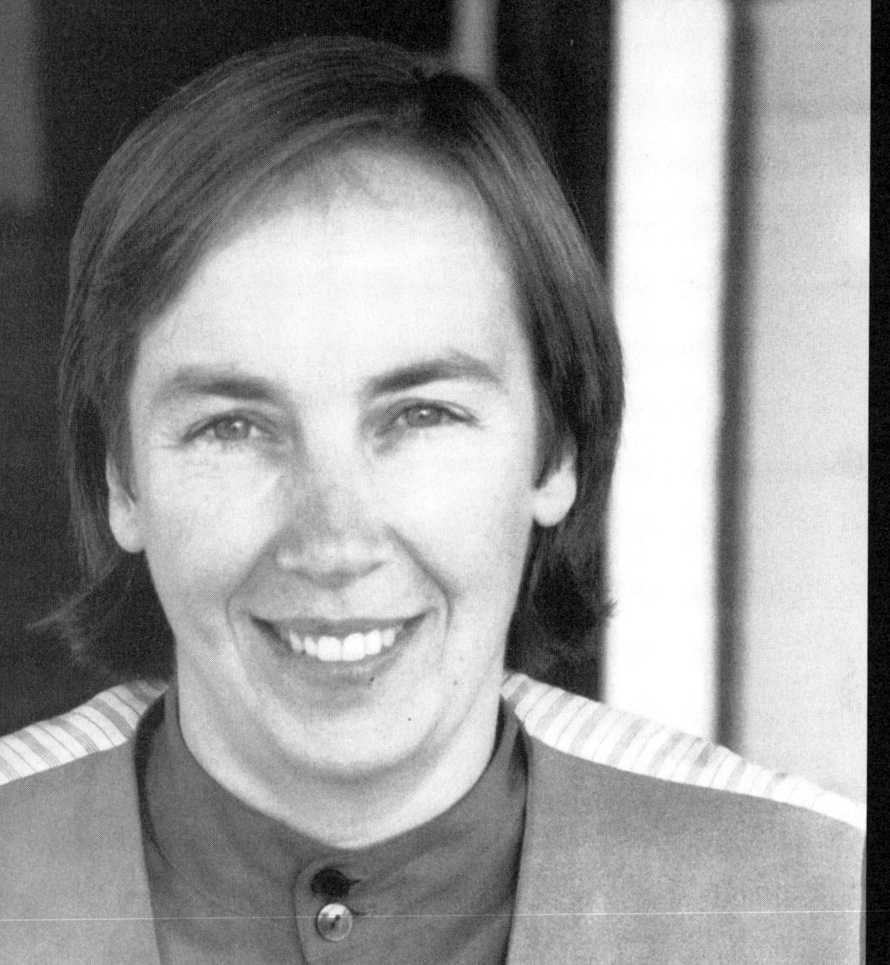

# *Tori Hudson, N.D.*

**THE APPEARANCE OF** cervical cancer is most often preceded by precancerous disturbances in the cervix. Using a precise program of herbs, nutrition, dietary change, and special nontoxic suppositories, naturopathic treatment can often prevent these changes from becoming cancerous, says Dr. Hudson.

As a naturopathic physician specializing in women's health issues, Tori Hudson, N.D., is keenly interested in treating female-specific cancer before it starts. That means reversing the known preconditions and earliest stages of cancer, as manifested by cervical dysplasias, carcinoma in situ of the cervix, and early-stage cervical cancer. While dysplasias do not necessarily constitute cancer, they may develop into cervical cancer if they are allowed to progress.

Uterine fibroids are not precancerous, but they represent a dysfunction in the hormonal system and the uterine tissue that is a sign of a weakened reproductive system. "Each year, there are over 62,000 cases of cervical cancer, with at least 9,000 women dying from the disease," Dr. Hudson says. "Naturopathic treatment could help lower the death toll considerably, as long as *early* treatment is emphasized."

Dr. Hudson's main contribution has been the formulation of effective treatment for early-stage carcinoma in situ of the cervix and cervical dysplasia. Cervical dysplasia is generally regarded as a precancerous lesion with risks factors similar to those of cervical cancer. "Though it does not necessarily lead to cancer," Dr. Hudson says, "it is important for women diagnosed with this condition to be treated and monitored for the possible development of cancer."

Risk factors for cervical cancer are many. They include multiple sex partners, sexual exposure to men who carry the human papilloma virus, and first intercourse at an early age, Dr. Hudson says. There are also numerous cofactors such as smoking, poor diet, folic acid deficiency, oral contraceptive use, immune suppression, and, perhaps, exposure to environmental carcinogens.

## SUCCESS STORY
### Reversing Carcinoma In Situ of the Cervix

Marilyn, aged 36, had suffered from chronic diarrhea, occasional lack of sphincter control, flatulence, and painful bowel movements accompanied with nausea for 6 months before seeing Dr. Hudson. Her health history included a previous abortion and two Pap smears with subnormal results; about 4 months previous, her menstrual cycle had become irregular, alternating

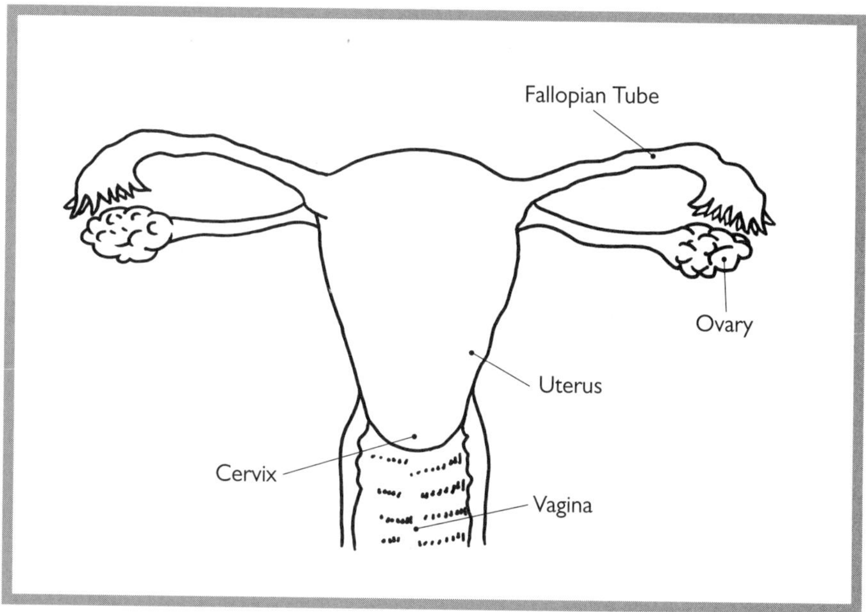


**Figure 11.1—Cervical dysplasia is the abnormal development or change (as in shape or size) of cells, and thus tissues, of the cervix caused by the human papilloma virus (HPV). Carcinoma in situ of the cervix refers to a small cluster of malignant cells that occupy a superficial layer of the cervix but have not penetrated the deeper tissue layers or spread to other body areas; hence, it is called preinvasive. A fibroid is a benign tissue growth, or noncancerous tumor, in the uterus, typically occurring in women beginning at age 35. An estimated 25%-50% of women of child-bearing age have fibroids. The fibroid itself is composed of hard, white tissue. One woman, after examining her fibroid following its surgical removal, compared its appearance to "a piece of high-density polyethylene plastic, the stuff cutting boards are made of." Fibroids (which are also called uterine leiomyomas) lead to an estimated 33% of all gynecological hospital admissions, including surgery (called myomectomy); they are almost never cancerous and often dissolve spontaneously at menopause.**

between 21 and 35 days' onset. Marilyn's maternal grandmother had had uterine cancer.

Marilyn's eating habits were highly unhealthy—15 cups of coffee every day, doughnuts, fast foods, frozen dinners, and processed foods. Technically, Marilyn's condition earned her a diagnosis of diverticulosis, but Dr. Hudson wanted more medical information about the state of her cervix. After another abnormal Pap smear, Marilyn underwent a colposcopy (special microscopic examination of the vagina and cervix, see pages 227-228) and a punch biopsy which revealed carcinoma in situ of the cervix but without any microinvasion. In other words, she was in the early stages of a disturbance that could lead to cervical cancer.

Dr. Hudson immediately recommended sweeping changes in Marilyn's diet. She was to avoid coffee, practice a vegan diet (no eggs, dairy products, poultry, fish, or meat), take vitamin C (10 g daily), beta carotene (150,000 IU daily), selenium (200 mcg, 3 times daily), and a digestive enzymes supplement called Opti-Gest (twice daily, with meals). Within a few weeks of instituting major dietary changes, Marilyn reported an 80% improvement in her primary gastrointestinal symptoms.

Dr. Hudson treated Marilyn twice weekly for the next 5 weeks. During the office visits, Dr. Hudson performed a special naturopathic technique called local escharotic treatment, which involved topical application to the cervix of a tincture of zinc chloride and a sanguinaria and calendula herbal mixture as well as bromelain enzymes and different nontoxic suppositories. An "eschar" is a scab formed by a burn and the term "escharotic" refers to a treatment that is mildly caustic, corrosive, cauterizing, or burning. Escharotic treatment could be considered herbal minor surgery.

During the 5 weeks of escharotic treatment, Marilyn's cervix became eroded, inflamed, and raw, notes Dr. Hudson. Near the end of the treatments, it started to show signs of healing, at which point Dr. Hudson prescribed homeopathic *Sepia* 6C (from squid or cuttlefish ink), taken 4 times daily. About 6 weeks after Dr. Hudson concluded her treatment, Marilyn returned to her conventional gynecologist for another colposcopy and biopsy. The test revealed no cervical abnormalities and her Pap smear was normal.

Dr. Hudson then put Marilyn on a nutritional maintenance program including vitamin C (3 g daily), beta carotene (50,000 IU daily), selenium (200 mcg daily), homeopathic *Sepia* 6C (4 times daily), and had her maintain the vegan diet. As this was a case Dr. Hudson concluded some years ago, she is able to present information on its long-term follow-up. Over the next year, Marilyn's Pap smears were normal, and annual Pap smears have remained that way for 10 years, she reports.

> ***"Though it does not necessarily lead to cancer," Dr. Hudson says, "it is important for women diagnosed with [cervical dysplasia] to be treated and monitored for the possible development of cancer."***

## Early Detection of a Cervical Cancer Is Critical

If the earliest stage of cervical cancer goes undetected and untreated, the cancer cells tend to move into deeper layers of the cervix and glands of the uterus, then spread to nearby organs such as the bladder, rectum, or vagina. Eventually, these cells spread (metastasize) to other parts of the body; in fact, up to 70% of cases of carcinoma in situ will develop into invasive or metastatic cancer over a period of 10 to 12 years, if left untreated.[1] In a small percentage of patients, the in situ carcinoma can develop into invasive cancer in under a year.

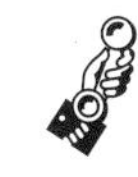

**Opti-Gest** is a broad-spectrum, natural digestive enzymes supplement, available from Eclectic Institute, 14385 Southeast Lusted Rd., Sandy, OR 97055; tel: 800-332-4372 or 503-668-4120; fax: 503-668-3227.

In the development of cervical cancer, cervical cells presumably go through a series of changes, from normal to abnormal (dysplasia) to precancerous (carcinoma in situ). "There's a fine line between severe cervical dysplasia and carcinoma in situ," says Dr. Hudson. "The chances of a cure are excellent when cervical cancer is caught before it becomes actual microinvasive cancer, the in situ phase." In this context, the phrase "in situ" means that the abnormal cells are confined to their original site in the cervical epithelium and have not invaded the basement membrane of the cell. Once invasion of the basement membrane occurs, then there is cancer, says Dr. Hudson.

In most cases, abnormal changes in the cervical tissue are detected by a Pap smear. However, Dr. Hudson cautions, Pap smears are screening tests only, not diagnostic tests. "Colposcopy and biopsy provide the definitive diagnostic workup," Hudson says. "In some cases, loop excision or cone biopsy and hysteroscopy are also used."

In many cases, it is possible to identify the area of abnormal tissue from the Pap smear, and this tissue can easily be removed with a biopsy; otherwise, the colposcopy can provide confirmation. In a colposcopy, the physician uses a special microscope called a colposcope to see whether there is an abnormal pattern to the blood vessels of the cervix and whether a lesion is present.

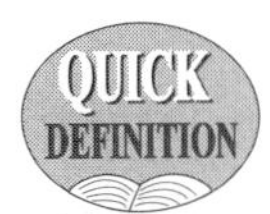

**Colposcopy** is a procedure whereby the vagina and cervix are examined by means of an endoscope. This is usually done when a Pap smear has indicated abnormality. The endoscope affords a magnification of 5 and 50X, enabling the physician to visually inspect the tissue for signs of cervical dysplasia or abnormal cell growth. The endoscope (or colposcope) is a low-powered microscope with a built-in light source designed for examining the interior of a hollow space or canal in the body. It is inserted into the body cavity and relays magnified images back to the physician—something akin to the way a periscope works.

If the Pap smear is normal but the cervix is grossly abnormal, and other known risk factors have been identified, Dr. Hudson advises that the Pap smear be repeated in 3 months, depending on the doctor's judgment. "If there is a discrepancy between the Pap results and what the doctor sees, the possibility of a colposcopy and biopsy should be considered in situations of 1 or more risk factors, and in cases of higher-grade lesions, such as moderate and severe dysplasia, or worse," Dr. Hudson says. She also suggests that doctors refer only to labs that use the Bethesda-Maryland Classification System because it is the most up-to-date system of recording, using the newest terminology.

For more information on **early detection of cervical cancer,** see Chapter 27: Early Detection and Prevention, pp. 712-716.

## Naturopathy Keeps Cervical Cancer at Bay

In 1990, Dr. Hudson reported on a preliminary study of 7 patients who were diagnosed at her clinic with carcinoma in situ. Technically, they had high-grade squamous intra-epithelial lesions, also called CIN III, and formerly indicating cervical cancer according to standard diagnostic procedures. Dr. Hudson treated the 7 women with her naturopathic protocols (described below) then followed their progress for 1 year. Four of the women were disease free after 1 year; 1 woman improved and her carcinoma eventually reverted to mild dysplasia; the 2 remaining women experienced milder improvements.[2]

Next, Dr. Hudson and her colleagues were able to completely reverse 38 out of 43 cases of cervical dysplasia, with 3 patients showing some improvement and only 2 showing no change.[3] In the same study, 7 out of 10 women with carcinoma in situ experienced a total remission.

"Our results with this naturopathic protocol for treating cervical dysplasia and cervical carcinoma in situ are excellent and offer patients a reliable choice in the treatment of one of the most troublesome and common diseases of women," says Dr. Hudson. "In addition to the successful results, the treatment is less costly in most cases, as well as safe and nontoxic. Women who follow our program also experience significant improvements in their overall health."

Conventional doctors report that cancer of the cervix is 100% curable if discovered early as carcinoma in situ.[4] However, their recommended treatments include cryosurgery (freezing), loop excisional electrosurgical procedure (LEEP), cone biopsy, and sometimes removal of the uterus (hysterectomy). All of these are more expensive and more invasive procedures. "In some cases, however, conventional treatment is appropriate because of the seriousness of the condition. A second opinion from a qualified naturopathic physician along with a gynecologist is the ideal approach to determine whether the case is appropriate for alternative treatment, conventional treatment, or an integration of both. And again, prevention and treatment of the earlier phases of cervical dysplasia cannot be overemphasized."

**Naturopathy** is an umbrella term to describe the original basis of natural, holistic, and alternative medicine, as first formulated by 19th-century European physicians. In essence, it understands that Nature heals, that the body is inherently self-healing, given the appropriate support therapies, such as diet, herbs, nutritional supplementation, exercise, heat and water therapy, massage, bodywork, counseling, and relaxation. Naturopathy emphasizes disease prevention and health promotion. It is currently licensed as a medical profession in 11 states. In a few states, naturopaths function as primary care physicians, and insurance companies cover their services.

Dr. Hudson's approach improves the health of the cervical tissues, which means her strategy is intrinsically *preventive.* Preventive measures, almost by definition, are less expensive and less physiologically demanding than crisis intervention procedures typical of conventional medicine. The preventive approach may also lower the risk of an eventual return of the cancer, Dr. Hudson adds. Many people diagnosed with later stages of cervical cancer elect chemotherapy and radiation, which tend to be minimally successful for this particular condition.

***Dr. Hudson and her colleagues were able to completely reverse 38 out of 43 cases of cervical dysplasia, with 3 patients showing some improvement and only 2 showing no change.***

The protocol devised by Dr. Hudson for use at the National College of Naturopathic Medicine in Portland, Oregon, emphasizes nutritional and herbal supplements, enzymes, and herbal paste applied locally to the cervix. In accordance with the holistic treatment philosophy of naturopathy, Dr. Hudson's plan consists of 3 phases, each addressing a layer or aspect of the person and the medical condition:

1) Local treatment of the cervix with enzymes, herbal and nutritional suppositories, herbal pastes, and irrigation (performed by a doctor, the area is swabbed with herbs or enzymes)
2) Systemic treatment of the immune system with oral supplements

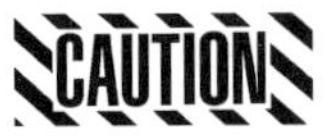


Dr. Hudson's guidelines are formulated for physicians and are not intended for use by other individuals unless they are under the supervision of a naturopathic or other physician cognizant of these types of modalities and their intended therapeutic effects.

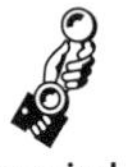

For **vaginal suppositories,** contact Bezwecken, 12525 SW 3rd, Beaverton, OR 97005; tel: 800-743-2256; tel: 503-644-7800; fax: 503-646-9936. Available only through licensed practitioners. For **Lomatium Isolate,** contact Eclectic Institute: 14385 Southeast Lusted Rd., Sandy, OR 97055; tel: 800-332-4372 or 503-668-4120; fax: 503-668-3227.

of vitamin C, beta carotene, selenium, folic acid and botanical preparations

3) Constitutional treatment for overall health and disease resistance, with dietary and lifestyle changes and risk and exposure reduction.

Dr. Hudson says that this treatment program is designed to improve dietary and lifestyle habits, enhance digestion and elimination, and identify sources of stress that can impede the process of recovery. Not just women suspecting early-stage cervical problems, but anyone who has received any form of immunosuppressive therapy must be treated with the appropriate detoxification and immune-enhancing therapies, Dr. Hudson notes.

In the following pages, Dr. Hudson takes us through 8 naturopathic, nontoxic protocols for addressing different stages of the cervical problem, from the mildest almost preclinical stage to severe dysplasia.

## 1. Atypia (Abnormal cells, earliest stages of dysplasia

### I. Initial Naturopathic Plan

**Topical**

**Week 1**—Vitamin A suppository nightly for 6 nights

**Week 2**—Herbal vaginal suppository (Herbal-C suppositories from Bezwecken) nightly for 6 nights: myrrh, *Echinacea*, usnea, hydrastis, althea, geranium, yarrow

**Week 3**—Vitamin A suppository (from Bezwecken) nightly for 6 nights

**Week 4**—Herbal vaginal suppository (as in Week 2) nightly for 6 nights

**Systemic**

**Daily**—Vitamin C (6 g per day) and natural beta carotene (150,000 IU per day). Botanical formula to be taken ½ teaspoon twice daily: Trifolium (¼ oz); Taraxacum root (⅜ oz); Glycerrhiza root (¼ oz);

Hydrastis (1/8 oz). Use systemic treatment for 3-6 months until follow-up.

**Constitutional**

**Daily**—Vegan diet (whole grains, vegetables, beans, fruits, nuts and seeds) for 3-6 months until follow-up

II. Alternate Naturopathic Plan (next phase)

**Topical**

**Week 1**—Vitamin A suppository nightly for 6 nights. One Vaginal Depletion Pack with vitamin A (Vaginal Pack suppositories from Bezwecken)

**Week 2**—Herbal vaginal suppository nightly for 6 nights: myrrh, *Echinacea*, usnea, hydrastis, althea, geranium, yarrow. One Vag Pack suppository with vitamin A

**Week 3**—Vitamin A suppository nightly for 6 nights. One Vag Pack suppository

**Week 4**—Herbal vaginal suppository nightly for 6 nights. One Vaginal Depletion Pack with vitamin A

**Systemic**

**Daily**—Vitamin C (6 g per day) and natural beta carotene (150,000 IU per day); folic acid (10 mg per day for 3 months, then 2.5 mg per day). Botanical formula to be taken 1/2 teaspoon twice daily: Trifolium (1/4 oz); Taraxacum root 3/8 oz); Glycerrhiza root (1/4 oz); Hydrastis (1/8 oz). Use systemic treatment for 3-6 months until follow-up.

**Constitutional**

**Daily**—Vegan diet (whole grains, vegetables, beans, fruits, nuts and seeds) for 3-6 months until follow-up

## Hysterectomies and Heart Attack Risks

Studies show that for a 35-year old woman who has a hysterectomy the risk of heart attack or angina increases by 7 times. Premenopausal women who have a hysterectomy without ovary removal begin menopause typically 5 years earlier, because one long-term effect of the surgery is accelerated aging of the ovaries, according to *Family Practice News*, November 1995.

***Dr. Hudson's approach improves the health of the cervical tissues, which means her strategy is intrinsically preventive.***

***If the Pap smear is normal but the cervix is grossly abnormal, and other known risk factors have been identified, Dr. Hudson advises that the Pap smear be repeated in 3 months, depending on the doctor's judgment.***

III. Additional therapies to consider

Alternating sitz baths twice a week for 4 weeks

IV. Maintenance plan for 3 months

Vegan diet (whole grains, vegetables, beans, fruits, nuts and seeds), with vitamin C (2 g per day) and natural beta carotene (150,000 IU per day)

### 2. Mild Dysplasia (CIN 1, Low-grade SIL)

I. Initial Naturopathic Plan

**Vegetarian diet**

**Week 1**—Vitamin A suppository nightly for 6 nights. One Vag Pack suppository; follow with apple cider vinegar douche (4 tablespoons per quart of water)

**Week 2**—Herbal vaginal suppository nightly for 6 nights: myrrh, *Echinacea*, usnea, hydrastis, althea, geranium, yarrow. One Vag Pack suppository; follow with apple cider vinegar douche (4 tablespoons per quart of water)

**Week 3**—Vitamin A suppository nightly for 6 nights. One Vaginal Depletion Pack with vitamin A for 24 hours; follow with apple cider vinegar douche (4 tablespoons per quart of water)

**Week 4**—Herbal vaginal suppository (as in Week 2) nightly for 6 nights. One Vag Pack suppository; follow with apple cider vinegar douche (4 tablespoons per quart of water)

**Systemic**

**Daily**—Vitamin C (6 g per day) and natural beta carotene (150,000 IU per day). Botanical formula to be taken 1/2 teaspoon twice daily: Trifolium (1/4 oz); Taraxacum root (3/8 oz); Glycerrhiza root (1/4 oz); Hydrastis (1/8 oz). Use systemic treatment for 3 to 6 months until follow-up.

**Constitutional**

**Daily**—Vegan diet (whole grains, vegetables, beans, fruits, nuts and seeds) for 3-6 months until follow-up

### II. Alternate Naturopathic Plan (next phase)

**Topical**

Escharotic treatment twice a week for 3 weeks (see below). After the last escharotic treatment:

**Week 1**—Vitamin A suppository nightly for 6 nights

**Week 2**—Herbal vaginal suppository nightly for 6 nights: myrrh, *Echinacea*, usnea, hydrastis, althea, geranium, yarrow. One Vag Pack suppository

**Week 3**—Vitamin A suppository nightly for 6 nights

**Week 4**—Herbal vaginal suppository nightly for 6 nights

Systemic

**Daily**—Vitamin C (6 g per day) and natural beta carotene (200,000 IU per day); folic acid (10 mg per day for 3 months, then 2.5 mg per day); selenium (400 mcg per day). Use systemic treatment for 3 months until follow-up.

**Constitutional**

**Daily**—Vegan diet (whole grains, vegetables, beans, fruits, nuts and seeds) for 3 months until follow-up.

### III. Additional therapies to consider

Alternating sitz baths twice per week for 4 weeks during suppository routine

### IV. Maintenance plan for 3 months

Vegan diet (whole grains, vegetables, beans, fruits, nuts and seeds) Supplement with vitamin C (2 g per day), natural beta carotene (150,000 IU per day), and folic acid (2.5 mg per day)

## 3. Mild Dysplasia and Condyloma (CIN 1, Low-grade SIL)

### I. Initial Naturopathic Plan

**Local**

Escharotic treatment twice per week for 3 weeks (see below). After the last escharotic treatment:

**Week 1**—Vitamin A suppository nightly for 6 nights

**Week 2**—Herbal vaginal suppository nightly for 6 nights: myrrh, *Echinacea*, usnea, hydrastis, althea, geranium, yarrow

**Week 3**—Vitamin A suppository nightly for 6 nights

**Week 4**—Herbal vaginal suppository (as in Week 2) nightly for 6 nights

### Systemic

**Daily**—Vitamin C (6 g per day) and beta carotene (150,000 IU per day); Lomatium Isolate (5 drops, twice daily). This specially prepared extract of the herb lomatium is available from Eclectic Institute. Botanical formula to be taken 1/2 teaspoon twice daily: Thuja (1/4 oz); Hydrastis (1/8 oz); *Echinacea* (3/8 oz); Ligusticum (1/4 oz). Use systemic treatment for 3 months until follow-up.

### Constitutional

**Daily**—Vegan diet (whole grains, vegetables, beans, fruits, nuts and seeds) for 3 months until follow-up

## II. Alternate Naturopathic Plan (next phase)

### Topical

Escharotic treatment twice per week for 5 weeks (see below). After the last escharotic treatment, follow with 4 weeks of suppositories as follows:

**Week 1**—Vitamin A suppository nightly for 6 nights

**Week 2**—Herbal vaginal suppository nightly for 6 nights: myrrh, *Echinacea*, usnea, hydrastis, althea, geranium, yarrow

**Week 3**—Vitamin A suppository nightly for 6 nights

**Week 4**—Herbal vaginal suppository nightly for 6 nights

### Systemic

**Daily**—Vitamin C (6 g per day) and natural beta carotene (200,000 IU per day); folic acid (10 mg per day for 3 months); Lomatium Isolate (5 drops, twice daily). Botanical formula to be taken 1/2 teaspoon twice daily: Thuja (1/4 oz); Hydrastis (1/4 oz); *Echinacea* (3/8 oz); Ligusticum (1/4 oz). Use systemic treatment for 3 months until follow-up.

**Constitutional**

**Daily**—Vegan diet (whole grains, vegetables, beans, fruits, nuts and seeds) for additional 3 months

III. Additional therapies to consider

Condyloma suppository instead of herbal suppository: Vitamin A, Thuja, and Lomatium, called Papillo suppository (from Bezwecken). Add Lomatium to end of Vag Pack suppository. Alternating sitz baths twice weekly for 4 weeks during suppository routine

IV. Maintenance plan for 3 months

Vegan diet (whole grains, vegetables, beans, fruits, nuts and seeds)

Supplement with vitamin C (3 g per day), natural beta carotene (150,000 IU per day), folic acid (2.5 mg per day), and Lomatium Isolate (5 drops, twice daily)

Botanical formula as above: Alternating 1 month on, 1 month off

Vitamin A and Condyloma suppositories every other week every 3 months: Week 1, Vitamin A suppository nightly for 6 nights; week 3, Condyloma suppository nightly for 6 nights

## 4. Moderate Dysplasia (CIN 2, High-grade SIL)

I. Initial Naturopathic Plan

**Vegan diet**

**Week 1**—Vitamin A suppository nightly for 6 nights. One Vag Pack suppository; follow with apple cider vinegar douche (4 tablespoons per quart of water)

**Week 2**—Herbal vaginal suppository nightly for 6 nights: myrrh, *Echinacea*, usnea, hydrastis, althea, geranium, yarrow. One Vag Pack suppository; follow with apple cider vinegar douche (4 tablespoons per quart of water)

**Week 3**—Vitamin A suppository nightly for 6 nights. One Vag Pack suppository; follow with apple cider vinegar douche (4 tablespoons per quart of water)

**Week 4**—Herbal vaginal suppository (as in Week 2) nightly for 6

## Women's Health Perceptions vs. the Facts

A recent Gallup survey involving 505 women and 300 physicians revealed that while 40% of the women believed breast cancer to be the leading cause of death for women and that all cancers account for 60% of women's deaths, it actually accounts for only 4% and all cancers represent only 23% of female deaths. Instead, heart disease is the cause of 35% of women's deaths, even though the women polled believed it accounts for only 19%, according to *American Health* (June 1996).

nights. One Vag Pack suppository; follow with apple cider vinegar douche (4 tablespoons per quart of water)

**Week 5**—Vitamin A suppository nightly for 6 nights. One Vag Pack suppository; follow with apple cider vinegar douche (4 tablespoons per one quart water)

**Week 6**—Herbal vaginal suppository (as in Week 2) nightly for 6 nights. One Vaginal Depletion Pack for 24 hours; follow with apple cider vinegar douche (4 tablespoons per quart of water)

**Systemic**

**Daily**—Vitamin C (6 g per day) and natural beta carotene (150,000 IU per day). Botanical formula to be taken ½ teaspoon twice daily: Trifolium (¼ oz); Taraxacum root (⅜ oz); Glycerrhiza root (¼ oz); Hydrastis (⅛ oz). Use systemic treatment for 3 months until follow-up.

**Constitutional**

**Daily**—Vegan diet (whole grains, vegetables, beans, fruits, nuts and seeds) for 3 months until follow-up

II. Alternate Naturopathic Plan (next phase)

**Topical**

Escharotic treatment twice a week for 5 weeks (see below). After the last escharotic treatment, follow with 4 weeks of suppositories as follows:

**Week 1**—Vitamin A suppository nightly for 6 nights

**Week 2**—Herbal vaginal suppository nightly for 6 nights: myrrh, *Echinacea*, usnea, hydrastis, althea, geranium, yarrow

**Week 3**—Vitamin A suppository nightly for 6 nights

**Week 4**—Herbal vaginal suppository nightly for 6 nights

**Systemic**

**Daily**—Vitamin C (6 g per day) and natural beta carotene (200,000 IU per day); folic acid (10 mg per day for 3 months); and selenium (400 mcg per day). Use systemic treatment for 3 months until follow-up.

**Constitutional**

**Daily**—Vegan diet (whole grains, vegetables, beans, fruits, nuts and seeds) for 3 months until follow-up

### III. Additional therapies to consider

Zinc (30 mg per day) and vitamin E (800 IU per day). Alternating sitz baths twice weekly for 4 weeks during suppository routine.

### IV. Maintenance plan for 3 months

Vegan diet (whole grains, vegetables, beans, fruits, nuts and seeds)

Supplement with vitamin C (2 g per day), beta carotene (150,000 IU per day), and folic acid (2.5 mg per day)

## 5. Moderate Dysplasia and Condyloma (CIN 2, High-grade SIL)

### I. Initial Naturopathic Plan

**Local**

Escharotic treatment twice a week for 3 weeks (see below). After the last escharotic treatment:

**Week 1**—Vitamin A suppository nightly for 6 nights

**Week 2**—Herbal vaginal suppository nightly for 6 nights: myrrh, *Echinacea*, usnea, hydrastis, althea, geranium, yarrow

**Week 3**—Vitamin A suppository nightly for 6 nights

**Week 4**—Herbal vaginal suppository (as in Week 2) nightly for 6 nights

**Systemic**

**Daily**—Vitamin C (6 g per day); beta carotene (150,000 IU per day); and Lomatium Isolate (5 drops, twice daily). Botanical formula to be taken 1/2 teaspoon twice daily: Thuja (1/4 oz); Hydrastis (1/8 oz); *Echinacea* (3/8 oz); Ligusticum (1/4 oz). Use systemic treatment for 3 months until follow-up.

Constitutional

**Daily**—Vegan diet (whole grains, vegetables, beans, fruits, nuts and seeds) for 3 months until follow-up

***Risk factors for cervical cancer are many. They include multiple sex partners, sexual exposure to men who carry the human papilloma virus, and first intercourse at an early age, Dr. Hudson says. There are also numerous cofactors such as smoking, poor diet, folic acid deficiency, oral contraceptive use, immune suppression, and, perhaps, exposure to environmental carcinogens.***

II. Alternate Naturopathic Plan (next phase)

**Topical**

Escharotic treatment twice a week for 5 weeks (see below). After the last escharotic treatment, follow with 4 weeks of suppositories as follows:

**Week 1**—Vitamin A suppository nightly for 6 nights

**Week 2**—Herbal vaginal suppository nightly for 6 nights: myrrh, *Echinacea*, usnea, hydrastis, althea, geranium, yarrow

**Week 3**—Vitamin A suppository nightly for 6 nights

**Week 4**—Herbal vaginal suppository nightly for 6 nights

**Systemic**

**Daily**—Vitamin C (6 g per day); natural beta carotene (200,000 IU per day); folic acid (10 mg per day for 3 months); and selenium (400 mcg per day). Botanical formula to be taken 1/2 teaspoon twice daily: Thuja (1/4 oz); Hydrastis (1/8 oz); *Echinacea* (3/8 oz); Ligusticum (1/4 oz). Use systemic treatment for 3 months until follow-up.

**Constitutional**

**Daily**—Vegan diet (whole grains, vegetables, beans, fruits, nuts and seeds) for additional 3 months

### III. Additional therapies to consider

Condyloma suppository (instead of herbal): Vitamin A, Thuja, and Lomatium. Add Lomatium to end of Vag Pack suppository.

Zinc (30 mg per day) and Vitamin E (800 IU per day)

Alternating sitz baths twice weekly for 4 weeks during suppository routine

### IV. Maintenance plan for 3 months

Vegan diet (whole grains, vegetables, beans, fruits, nuts and seeds)

Supplement with vitamin C (3 g per day), natural beta carotene (150,000 IU per day), folic acid (2.5 mg per day), and Lomatium Isolate (5 drops, twice daily)

Botanical formula as above: alternating 1 month on, 1 month off

Vitamin A and Condyloma suppositories every other week every 3 months: Week 1, vitamin A suppository nightly for 6 nights; week 3, Condyloma suppository nightly for 6 nights.

## 6. Severe Dysplasia (CIN 3, High-grade SIL)

### I. Initial Naturopathic Plan

**Local**

Escharotic treatment twice a week for 5 weeks (see below). After the last escharotic treatment, follow with 4 weeks of suppositories as follows:

**Week 1**—Vitamin A suppository nightly for 6 nights

**Week 2**—Herbal vaginal suppository nightly for 6 nights: myrrh, *Echinacea*, usnea, hydrastis, althea, geranium, yarrow

**Week 3**—Vitamin A suppository nightly for 6 nights

**Week 4**—Herbal vaginal suppository (as in Week 2) nightly for 6 nights

**Systemic**

**Daily**—Vitamin C (6 g per day) and natural beta carotene (150,000 IU per day). Botanical formula to be taken 1/2 teaspoon twice daily: Trifolium (1/4 oz); Taraxacum root (3/8 oz); Glycerrhiza root (1/4 oz); Hydrastis (1/8 oz). Use systemic treatment for 3 months until follow-up.

### Constitutional

**Daily**—Vegan diet (whole grains, vegetables, beans, fruits, nuts and seeds) for 3 months until follow-up

## II. Alternate Naturopathic Plan (next phase)

### Topical

Escharotic treatment twice per week for 5 weeks (see below). After the last escharotic treatment, follow with 4 weeks of suppositories as follows:

**Week 1**—Vitamin A suppository nightly for 6 nights

**Week 2**—Herbal vaginal suppository nightly for 6 nights: myrrh, *Echinacea*, usnea, hydrastis, althea, geranium, yarrow

**Week 3**—Vitamin A suppository nightly for 6 nights

**Week 4**—Herbal vaginal suppository nightly for 6 nights

### Systemic

**Daily**—Vitamin C (6 g per day), natural beta carotene (200,000 IU per day), folic acid (10 mg per day for 3 months), and selenium (400 mcg per day). Use systemic treatment for 3 months until follow-up.

### Constitutional

**Daily**—Vegan diet (whole grains, vegetables, beans, fruits, nuts and seeds) for 3 months until follow-up. Botanical formula to be taken 1/2 teaspoon twice daily: Trifolium (1/4 oz); Taraxacum root (3/8 oz); Glycerrhiza root (1/4 oz); Hydrastis (1/8 oz). Use systemic treatment for 3 months until follow-up.

## III. Additional therapies to consider

Zinc (30 mg per day); vitamin E (800 IU per day); vitamin B6 (pyridoxine, 50 mg, 3 times a day). Alternate sitz baths twice weekly for 4 weeks during suppository routine.

## IV. Maintenance plan for 3 months

Vegan diet (whole grains, vegetables, beans, fruits, nuts and seeds)

Supplement with vitamin C (3 g per day), natural beta carotene (150,000 IU per day), folic acid (2.5 mg per day), and vitamin E (400 IU per day)

Botanical formula as above: alternating 1 month on, 1 month off

## 7. Severe Dysplasia and Condyloma (CIN 3, High-grade SIL)

### I. Initial Naturopathic Plan

**Local**

Escharotic treatment twice per week for 5 weeks (see below). After the last escharotic treatment:

**Week 1**—Vitamin A suppository nightly for 6 nights

**Week 2**—Herbal vaginal suppository nightly for 6 nights: myrrh, *Echinacea*, usnea, hydrastis, althea, geranium, yarrow

**Week 3**—Vitamin A suppository nightly for 6 nights

**Week 4**—Herbal vaginal suppository (as in Week 2) nightly for 6 nights

***Although an estimated 200,000 hysterectomies are performed every year to remove fibroids, naturopathic protocols can often eliminate the need for this surgery, says Dr. Hudson.***

**Systemic**

**Daily**—Vitamin C (6 g per day), natural beta carotene (180,000 IU per day), selenium (400 mcg), and Lomatium Isolate (8 drops, twice daily). Botanical formula to be taken 1/2 teaspoon twice daily: Thuja (1/4 oz); Hydrastis (1/8 oz); *Echinacea* (3/8 oz); Ligusticum (1/4 oz). Use systemic treatment for 3 months until follow-up.

**Constitutional**

**Daily**—Vegan diet (whole grains, vegetables, beans, fruits, nuts and seeds) for 3 months until follow-up.

### II. Alternate Naturopathic Plan (next phase)

**Topical**

Escharotic treatment twice per week for 5 weeks (see below). After the last escharotic treatment, follow with 4 weeks of suppositories as follows:

**Week 1**—Vitamin A suppository nightly for 6 nights
**Week 2**—Herbal vaginal suppository nightly for 6 nights: myrrh, *Echinacea*, usnea, hydrastis, althea, geranium, yarrow
**Week 3**—Vitamin A suppository nightly for 6 nights
**Week 4**—Herbal vaginal suppository nightly for 6 nights

### Systemic

**Daily**—Vitamin C (10 g per day) and natural beta carotene (200,000 IU per day), folic acid (10 mg per day for 3 months), selenium (400 mcg per day), and Lomatium Isolate (8 drops, twice daily) Botanical formula to be taken 1/2 teaspoon 4 times daily: Thuja (1/4 oz); Hydrastis (1/8 oz); *Echinacea* (3/8 oz); Ligusticum (1/4 oz). Use systemic treatment for 3 months until follow-up.

### Constitutional

**Daily**—Vegan diet (whole grains, vegetables, beans, fruits, nuts and seeds) for additional 3 months

## III. Additional therapies to consider

**Condyloma suppository (instead of herbal):** Vitamin A, Thuja, and Lomatium

Zinc (30 mg per day), vitamin E (800 IU per day), and vitamin B6 (pyridoxine, 50 mg per day). Alternating sitz baths twice weekly for 4 weeks during suppository routine.

## IV. Maintenance plan for 3 months

Vegan diet (whole grains, vegetables, beans, fruits, nuts and seeds)

Supplement with vitamin C (3 g per day), natural beta carotene (150,000 IU per day), and Lomatium Isolate (5 drops, twice daily)

Botanical formula as above: alternating 1 month on, 1 month off

Vitamin A and Condyloma suppositories every other week every 3 months: Week 1, vitamin A suppository nightly for 6 nights; week 3, Condyloma suppository nightly for 6 nights.

## 8. Carcinoma in Situ (CIN 3, High-grade SIL)

### I. Initial Naturopathic Plan

**Local**

Escharotic treatment twice per week for 5 weeks (see below). After the last escharotic treatment:

**Week 1**—Vitamin A suppository nightly for 6 nights

**Week 2**—Herbal vaginal suppository nightly for 6 nights: myrrh, *Echinacea*, usnea, hydrastis, althea, geranium, yarrow

**Week 3**—Vitamin A suppository nightly for 6 nights

**Week 4**—Herbal vaginal suppository (as in Week 2) nightly for 6 nights

**Systemic**

**Daily**—Vitamin C (6 g per day), beta carotene (180,000 IU per day), selenium (400 mcg). Botanical formula to be taken 1/2 teaspoon twice daily: Trifolium (1/4 oz); Taraxacum root (3/8 oz); Glycerrhiza root (1/4 oz); Hydrastis (1/8 oz). Use systemic treatment for 3 months until follow-up.

**Constitutional**

**Daily**—Vegan diet (whole grains, vegetables, beans, fruits, nuts and seeds) for 3 months until follow-up

### II. Alternate Naturopathic Plan (next phase)

**Topical**

Escharotic treatment twice per week for 5 weeks (see below). After the last escharotic treatment, follow with 4 weeks of suppositories as follows:

**Week 1**—Vitamin A suppository nightly for 6 nights

**Week 2**—Herbal vaginal suppository nightly for 6 nights: myrrh, *Echinacea*, usnea, hydrastis, althea, geranium, yarrow

**Week 3**—Vitamin A suppository nightly for 6 nights

**Week 4**—Herbal vaginal suppository nightly for 6 nights

### Systemic

**Daily**—Vitamin C (10 g per day), natural beta carotene (200,000 IU per day), folic acid (10 mg per day for 3 months), and selenium (400 mcg per day). Botanical formula to be taken ½ teaspoon twice daily: Trifolium (¼ oz); Taraxacum root (⅜ oz); Glycerrhiza root (¼ oz); Hydrastis (⅛ oz). Use systemic treatment for 3 months until follow-up.

### Constitutional

**Daily**—Vegan diet (whole grains, vegetables, beans, fruits, nuts and seeds) for additional 3 months.

### III. Additional therapies to consider

Zinc (30 mg per day), vitamin E (800 IU per day), and vitamin B6 (pyridoxine, 50 mg 3 times per day). Alternate sitz baths twice weekly for 4 weeks during suppository routine.

### IV. Maintenance plan for 3 months

Vegan diet (whole grains, vegetables, beans, fruits, nuts and seeds)

Supplement with vitamin C (3 g per day), natural beta carotene (150,000 IU per day), folic acid (2.5 mg per day), and vitamin E (400 IU per day). Botanical formula as above: alternating 1 month on, 1 month off.

## The Problem of Uterine Fibroids as a Potential Cancer Precondition

Uterine fibroids (uterine leiomyomata) are noncancerous tumors comprising fibers or fibrous tissue that arise in the uterus, an organ integral to the reproductive system. Fibroids arise from the uterine muscle and connective tissue, but almost all cases are benign. Less than 1% of uterine fibroids are cancerous. Since these tumors develop following the onset of menstruation, enlarge during pregnancy, and decrease, and often disappear, after menopause, fibroids are thought to be estrogen-dependent (i.e., estrogen stimulates their development). For this reason, it is possible that estrogen-like compounds in the environment may contribute to the problem of uterine fibroids, says Dr. Hudson.

While a fibroid in itself does not usually lead to cancer or become cancerous, it does indicate a potentially serious imbalance in a woman's reproductive and hormonal system. As such, it might reflect a systemic imbalance that can be favorable to the emergence of precancerous or actual cancer conditions in the breast, uterus, cervix, or vagina. For that reason, preventive steps and early intervention are highly advisable, says Dr. Hudson. Fibroids can also continue to grow, cause heavy bleeding, pelvic pain, constipation, low back pain, and more.

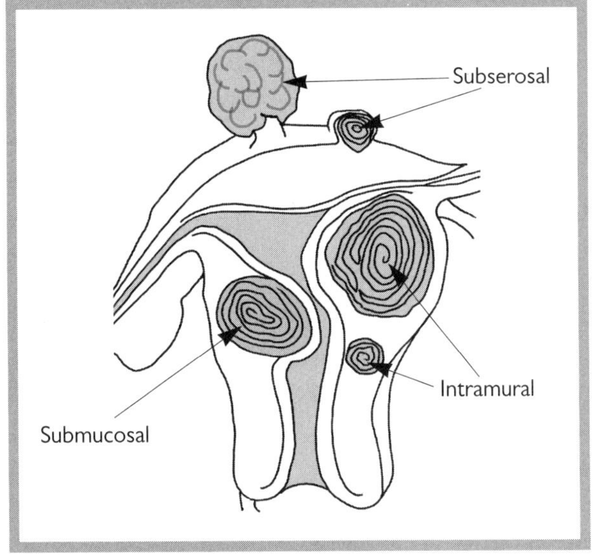


**Figure 11.2—Fibroids in the uterine area**

One in 5 women in the U.S. has at least some evidence of fibroids, with most occurring in women in their thirties and forties.[5] Fibroids are much more common among black women than among white women, although the reason for this difference is not known.[6] Fibroids are usually firm, spherical lumps that occur in groups. The tumors are of varying sizes, usually described in terms of vegetables and fruits—a pea, lemon, apple, or cantaloupe. They can grow near the outer surface of the uterus and in the muscle wall of the uterus, where they are easily detected during a pelvic examination, as well as near the inner lining of the uterus, where ultrasound is required to detect them.

Though most women have no symptoms from fibroids, some experience lower abdominal pain, a feeling of fullness and pressure in the lower abdomen, and frequent urination, which is caused by pressure of the tumor on the bladder. The woman with a fibroid may also experience heavy menstrual periods, bleeding between periods, and increased menstrual

To obtain a copy of Dr. Hudson's *Gynecology and Naturopathic Medicine: A Treatment Manual,* contact: TK Publications, 2067 NW Lovejoy, Portland, OR 97209; tel: 503-222-2322. To contact the **National College of Naturopathic Medicine** where Dr. Hudson teaches: 11231 SE Market Street, Portland, OR 97216; tel: 503-255-4860.

CAUTION

Dr. Hudson's guidelines are formulated for other physicians and are not intended for use by other individuals unless they are under the supervision of a naturopathic or other physician cognizant of these types of modalities and their intended therapeutic effects.

cramps. If a fibroid grows rapidly, it may outstrip its nutrition supply from nearby blood vessels, resulting in the degeneration and death of the oxygen-deprived tissue; severe abdominal pain may also result. Rapid fibroid growth is more likely in pregnancy, when estrogen levels are high.

To reduce the risk of developing fibroids, Dr. Hudson generally recommends that women avoid birth control pills (with estrogen) and estrogen-replacement therapy for menopause symptoms; both can accelerate fibroid tumor growth. "Fibroids are promoted by persistently high estrogen production, so the diet and lifestyle should be oriented toward keeping estrogen at more moderate levels," Dr. Hudson explains. "Antiestrogenic substances and nutritional substances can play a big role in this regard."

For example, reducing consumption of animal proteins and foods grown with pesticides can lower the estrogen load on a woman's body. The effect on the uterus of phytoestrogens, such as soybeans, is unclear, says Dr. Hudson. "It currently appears that one could not eat enough soybeans to cause a problem. Also it may be that phytoestrogens actually block estrogen binding sites and, in effect, protect the uterus."

According to Dr. Hudson, "The choice of intervention is based on the size and position of the fibroids, their rate of growth, the woman's discomfort level and symptomatology, her fertility desires, and her menopausal status." Although an estimated 200,000 hysterectomies are performed every year to remove fibroids, naturopathic protocols can often eliminate the need for this surgery, says Dr. Hudson. These natural approaches can also prevent serious health complications often associated with hysterectomies.

To help reverse fibroids, Dr. Hudson recommends supplementing with large amounts of the following nutrients: vitamin C (6-8 g per day), beta carotene (150,000-200,000 IU per day), selenium (300-400 mcg per day), and zinc (30-50 mg per day). In addition, citrus bioflavonoids such as rutin and hesperidin (a total of 1,000 mg daily) and various botanical medicines such as burdock root, chasteberry (*Vitex agnus*), dandelion root, milk thistle, club moss, corn ergot, rye ergot, tiger lily, and pokeroot may be helpful, says Dr. Hudson. It is also important to improve the liver's metabolism and breakdown of estrogens by using liver restorative herbs and lipotropic factors, such as choline and methionine.

Dr. Hudson emphasizes that these strategies for reversing fibroids and any of the 8 stages of cervical dysplasia and its precursors not only lower a woman's risk of developing more serious problems affecting her reproductive system, but also bolster immunity and improve overall health.

## Clinical Instructions for Cervical Escharotic Treatment

The escharotic treatment was originally used for various tumors, not only of the cervix. Dermatologists used it for skin cancer until some time in the 1950s; it is still employed for that purpose in cancer clinics in Mexico. Naturopaths are trained in and continue to use the technique.

The intent is to burn/slough off the top few millimeters of the cervix. Then, vitamin A and herbal suppositories are used to regenerate normal, healthy tissue and stimulate the lymphoid (immune) tissue in the vagina.

***Dr. Hudson emphasizes that these strategies for reversing fibroids and any of the 8 stages of cervical dysplasia and its precursors not only lower a woman's risk of developing more serious problems affecting her reproductive system, but also bolster immunity and improve overall health.***

Dr. Hudson offers the following clinical protocol for physicians, as adapted from her monograph *Gynecology and Naturopathic Medicine: A Treatment Manual:*

1. Before beginning the treatment, the practitioner needs the following items:
   - Zinc chloride/Sanguinaria mixture. Take 1/4 teaspoon ZnCl2 solution and place in an empty cup. Add 3/4 teaspoon of Sanguinaria tincture to the same bottle. This will now be the mixture used for one treatment.
   - 1 cup distilled water
   - 1/3 cup Calendula succus (A calendula extraction using less alcohol than the customary tincture)
   - A cup containing 2 powdered bromelain enzyme capsules. (The enzymes help "digest" the superficial layer of cells and begin the sloughing process.)
2. Insert speculum and examine the cervix.
3. Blot the cervix dry with a large cotton swab or cotton ball attached to the end of a ring forceps.
4. Dip a large cotton swab into the distilled water and then squeeze out the water with your gloved fingers. Place the damb swab into the Bromelain, then thickly cover the face of the cervix with the

powder. You will probably have to repeat this 2-4 times to cover the surface adequately. Repeat this step for the endocervical canal, this time using a small cotton-tip applicator. Here you must dampen it, place it in the bromelain, then apply it to the endocervix 1-3 times. For each application, use a new cotton-tip applicator.

5. Leave the bromelain on the cervix and in the endocervical canal for 15 minutes. Position the GYN lamp (a regular lamp used during pelvic exams) to face the vagina. The gentle heat from the lightbulb warms the vagina during the procedure and thereby accelerates the enzyme action.
6. Remove the bromelain by placing a large cotton swab in the Calendula succus, then apply it to the cervix to wash off the Bromelain. Do this also to the endocervical canal using a small cotton-tip applicator. Repeat 2-4 times. Take a large dry swab and absorb the washings that have collected in the vagina.
7. Next soak a large swab in the ZnCl2/Sanguinaria mixture already prepared. Apply this once to the cervix. Then repeat this procedure using a small cotton-tip applicator inserted into the endocervical canal; leave in place for 1 minute. If pain arises, wash the cervix with a small amount of distilled water. Avoid contact of the ZnCl2/Sanguinaria mixture with the vaginal wall.
8. Wash off the ZnCl2/Sanguinaria mixture with swabs of calendual solution. Wash the endocervical canal with a cotton-tip applicator. Using a dry cotton swab, absorb the liquid that has pooled in the vagina.
9. Insert 2 "Vag Pack" suppositories. Using either forceps or other appropriate instruments; try to position the suppositories to lie lengthwise across the cervix. Ask the patient to leave these in place for 24 hours. A small Kotex pad may be used to absorb leakage. Follow this procedure with an apple cider vinegar douch using 4 tablespoons vinegar to 1 quart of water.
10. After the last escharotic treatment: during week 1, use a vitamin A suppository nightly for 6 nights; during week 2, use the herbal vaginal suppository nightly for 6 nights, or if the patient has human papilloma virus (HPV), use a condyloma ("Papillo") suppository; during week 3, use a vitamin A suppository nightly for 6 weeks;

during week 4, use an herbal vaginal or condyloma suppository nightly for 6 nights.

As a final note, Dr. Hudson advises that the escharotic treatment is best done twice weekly leaving 2 full days between treatments. She has prepared a special clinician's kit called the "Cervical Escharotic Treatment Kit." Enough for 10 treatments, it contains all the materials described in this protocol and is available through her office.

## CURRICULUM VITAE

# Dan Labriola, N.D.

P.O. Box 99157, Seattle, WA 98199;
tel: 206-285-4993; fax: 206-285-0085.

Dr. Labriola is a graduate of Syracuse University in New York and Bastyr University in Seattle, Washington, where he received his degree as a naturopathic doctor (N.D.). He is the chair of the State of Washington Department of Health Naturopathic Advisory Committee; before this, he was president of the Washington Association of Naturopathic Physicians, past director of the American Association of Naturopathic Physicians, and a member of the State of Washington Health Personnel Resource Plan.

Dr. Labriola has also served as a faculty member at Bastyr University, and has been a leader in the introduction of botanical and nutritional medicine to the public, government bodies, and medical facilities both in the United States and internationally. Dr. Labriola opened a new cancer alternative care and prevention center in 1997; its focus, he says, is to bring alternative and conventional care together with "optimum synergy."

***"Naturopathic, conventional, and osteopathic physicians are learning to work in concert within a multidisciplinary context," says Dr. Labriola. "This represents a giant step forward for the cancer patient. Patients who get the best of what everyone has to offer appear to fare consistently better than those forced to choose one side or the other."***

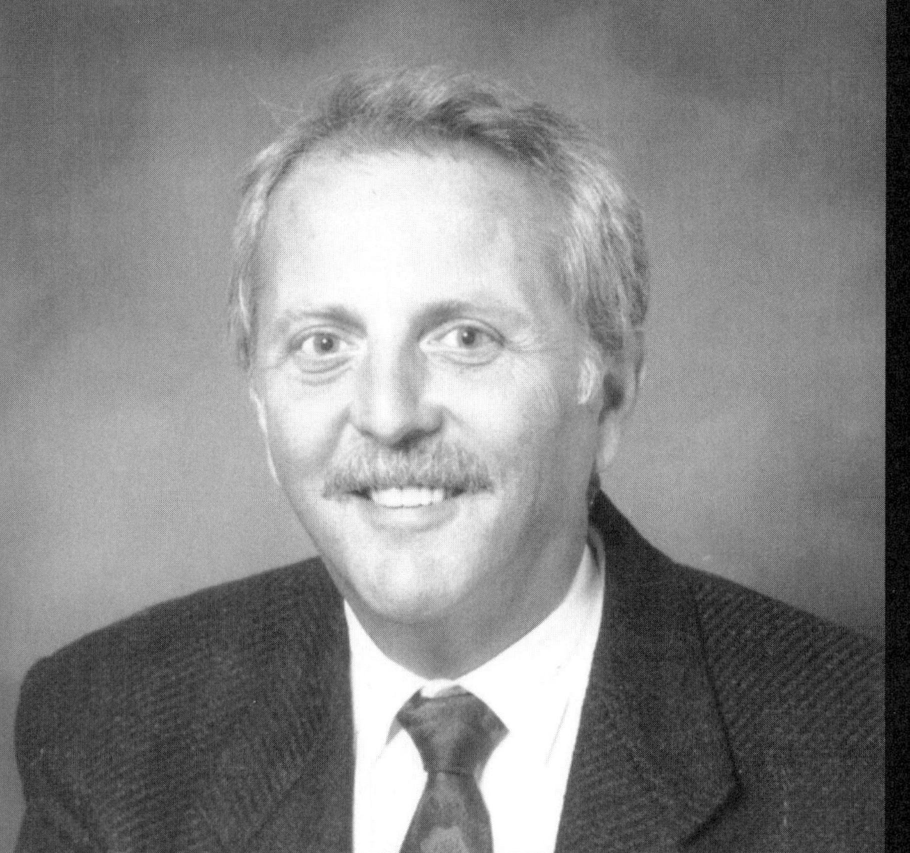

# Chapter 12

# *Dan Labriola, N.D.*

**FOR THE CANCER PATIENT** who needs or wants to stay with conventional treatments, naturopathic medicine can expertly provide nutritional supplementation to dramatically reduce the side effects of chemotherapy and other harsh treatments, says Dr. Labriola.

According to Washington State naturopathic physician Dan Labriola, N.D., it is a mistake to assume that naturopathy and conventional medicine cannot work together in cancer treatment. For years, Dr. Labriola has been encouraging naturopathic physicians and conventional oncologists to embrace a more complementary approach to cancer, blending alternative and conventional therapies when appropriate.

In fact, Dr. Labriola is a consulting physician for several Seattle-area hospitals where he specializes in the appropriate use of alternative care modalities for patients using conventional medical treatments to fight cancer and other diseases. For those cancer patients who do not wish to work exclusively with alternative practitioners or for those already undertaking complex conventional treatments (such as bone marrow transplants), Dr. Labriola's bridge-making efforts are beneficial.

## Blending Naturopathy and Conventional Oncology

"Naturopathic, conventional, and osteopathic physicians are learning to work in concert within a multidisciplinary context," says Dr. Labriola. "This represents a giant step forward for the cancer patient. Patients who get the best of what everyone has to offer appear to fare consistently better than those forced to choose one side or the other."

After graduating from the preeminent naturopathic medical school, John Bastyr University in Seattle, Washington, Dr. Labriola became president of the Washington Association of Naturopathic Physicians. In this capacity, he developed an interest in treating cancer patients who were also using conventional treatments. "At the time, it was obvious that this large group of cancer patients had been grossly neglected by alternative care providers," says Dr. Labriola. "Alternative care providers were saying that chemotherapy, radiation, and surgery created too much interference for natural medicine to have any effect, so they just gave up on those patients, even though they comprised—and still comprise—the majority of cancer patients."

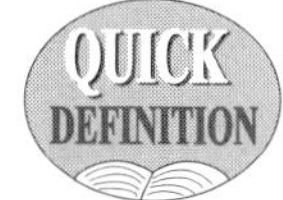


**Naturopathy** is an umbrella term to describe the original basis of natural, holistic, and alternative medicine, as first formulated by 19th-century European physicians. In essence, it understands that Nature heals, that the body is inherently self-healing, given the appropriate support therapies, such as diet, herbs, nutritional supplementation, exercise, heat and water therapy, massage, bodywork, counseling, and relaxation. Naturopathy emphasizes disease prevention and health promotion. It is currently licensed as a medical profession in 11 states. In a few states, naturopaths function as primary care physicians, and insurance companies cover their services.

One unfortunate side effect of this tendency was that many people came to perceive allopathic physicians as the exclusive cancer experts, and naturopathy as best reserved for milder health problems, says Dr. Labriola. In his view, the belief that naturopathy and allopathy cannot combine forces is a mistake, in part because it forces many laypeople to self-prescribe treatments, while others undergo conventional treatment without the benefit of alternative medicine. A problem with self-prescribing vitamins, herbs, and other substances is that often the layperson, especially a sick person, lacks objectivity and clinical guidance in the correct use of these substances.

An additional problem is that in Dr. Labriola's view, "most herbal and other supplemental preparations are not sterile. Most of them are obviously clean enough for you and me to take because we have healthy immune systems. But people who are receiving cancer treatments or who are otherwise immune-suppressed are at risk for infection and must take care regarding what they take while receiving chemotherapy. For some patients, especially those with leukemia and those whose disease is directly affecting the immune system, they need to be *very* careful."

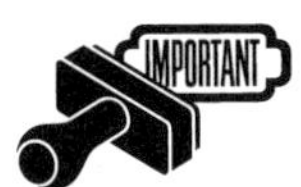


"Many cancer patients are anxious to do everything they can do, and often tend to do more than the body is actually going to make use of," says Dr. Labriola. "In my experience, if you overtreat with too many substances and protocols, you tend to lose their therapeutic value, and you may fail to choose those that will have the best effect." Many of the available substances are powerful and can create specific biochemical and physiological changes, including ones not desired. In some cases, taking alternative substances "can interfere with the potential benefits of standard treatment to the extent that they may cancel each other out," says Dr. Labriola.

Therefore, it is crucial that the physician be exceedingly careful about using chemotherapy drugs and natural substances at the same time, Dr. Labriola explains. "We try to do as little as possible while the patient is receiving chemotherapy. We try to time the serum half lives [duration of action of a drug] (and other factors) so that nothing we do nutritionally will interfere with the action of the drug on the tumor. We make certain that nutritional supplements are not active in the blood at a time when it can interfere with the drug's antitumor action."

For example, the chemotherapy drug methotrexate interferes with an enzyme that converts folate (folic acid, a nutrient essential to B12 assimilation) from its inactive to active form, Dr. Labriola explains. To supplement with folic acid during chemotherapy could be counterproductive. It is more advisable to allow sufficient time to elapse between the administration of chemotherapy and folic acid supplementation, Dr. Labriola says.

***"My basic warning is that if you have cancer, get help from somebody who knows cancer and knows both sides of the fence, both conventional and alternative approaches," says Dr. Labriola.***

The classical case of inadvertent interference is the cancer patient who informs his physician that he had almost no effects during chemotherapy because a clerk at his natural foods store gave him a list of herbs and supplements to take, Dr. Labriola comments. "Sadly, you see those patients a year later with an unpredicted cancer recurrence partly because they interfered with the chemotherapy drug the first time around. They never got the intended benefit."

Similar interference problems may occur with vitamin C, says Dr. Labriola. "High doses of vitamin C (particularly oral doses) during the administration of chemotherapy can not only interfere with the drug, but can actually worsen some of chemotherapy's usual side effects. I am a great believer in vitamin C and think it is one of the great natural miracles of this century. But when you use it in *high* doses like a drug than you must treat it as you would a drug. When you use vitamin C at biological levels (bowel tolerance dose, but much less than a 'high' dose), then it's a different story again."

In general, Dr. Labriola believes that there is no single magic bullet when it comes to treatment. "From my experience, the best outcomes come with people who pay close attention to the basics and use good science. My basic warning is that if you have cancer, get help from somebody who *knows* cancer and knows both sides of the fence, both conventional *and* alternative approaches."

## SUCCESS STORY
### Using Naturopathic Support during Conventional Treatment of Breast Cancer

Ellen, aged 43, who had breast cancer, underwent conventional treatment including high-dose chemotherapy, radiation, and a mastectomy, which brought on numerous side effects. Ellen lost much of her hair, had unpleasant mouth sores, and was highly uncomfortable. Her liver enzymes became very high, indicating probable liver damage from the chemotherapy, and her white blood cell count went very low, as the drugs she received are known to suppress the immune system, explains Dr. Labriola. Over the course of about 1 year, her physicians had to continually interrupt her treatment to enable her white blood cell count to restore itself.

Then about 3 years after the start of her conventional treatment, Ellen experienced a recurrence at the surgical incision point on her breast. It was classified as a Stage III cancer, meaning her lymph nodes were involved but the cancer had not yet spread to any other body region. "This is not uncommon but it can be devastating," comments Dr. Labriola. "Once you have recurrence at the incision point, that is not a good sign, and this cancer was growing quickly."

**Staging** in cancer terminology is a relative index of how much cancer exists in the body, its size, location, and containment or metastasis. Stage I, the earliest, most curable stage, shows only local tumor involvement. Stage II indicates some spreading of cancer to the surrounding tissues and perhaps to nearby lymph nodes. Stage III involves metastasis to distant lymph nodes. Stage IV, the most advanced and least easily cured, means the cancer has spread to distant organs.

Ellen was obese, maintained a very poor diet, and had many emotional issues at play, all of which tended to act as obstacles to her commitment to healing, he adds. When she learned of the tumor recurrence, she decided she would not undergo chemotherapy or radiation again. On her own, she investigated certain alternative approaches, such as herbalism, but had not received benefit. She underwent radiation again for the small tumor on her breast and in doing so suffered greatly from the burning. "She had the worst of side effects," notes Dr. Labriola. "Not all chemotherapy or radiation patients do this badly, but Ellen had a really tough time. She decided she was going to give up at this point."

An oncologist recommended stem cell replacement plus high-dose chemotherapy as a way to address the cancer at a systemic level, then the herbalist Ellen had consulted referred her to Dr. Labriola. He decided to help Ellen through the chemotherapy by providing naturopathic support. Even so, Ellen had prepared herself to die, putting her will in order. However, she agreed to try Dr. Labriola's approach.

In the 4 weeks before chemotherapy began, Dr. Labriola undertook to shore up Ellen's nutritional status. She had a serious mineral imbalance that manifested in several forms, including a craving for sweets, and this seriously affected her immune system; she had musculoskeletal and joint problems mostly from her weight and physical inactivity. In Ellen's case, skin disorders and digestive symptoms indicated a mineral imbalance, Dr. Labriola explains. To help restore balance, he gave Ellen amino acids, vitamin B complex, antioxidants, essential oils, vitamins, and specific herbs.

***"Compliance is the biggest challenge every physician has," Dr. Labriola says. "If we could all get compliance, our success rates would double, or more. I spend a lot of time trying to make it possible for my patients to comply with the program we develop."***

"She needed nearly *everything*, so she was on a careful cycle of nutrition," says Dr. Labriola. In addition, he advised Ellen to practice basic light exercises to help prevent further weight gain. The nutritional supplements helped her reduce her sweets cravings and to lose a small amount of weight. "She was feeling better and had more energy. We built her up to the extent that she was in good shape and ready for the treatment. We did a great deal to balance Ellen's immune system."

During the chemotherapy, Dr. Labriola's efforts were aimed at "keeping her comfortable and alive, literally." The procedure involved removing a certain amount of healthy stem cells, then administering highly toxic, high-dose chemotherapy; meanwhile, the stem cells are cleansed of all diseases, impurities, and traces of cancer, and stored; when the chemotherapy is finished, leaving the immune system nearly destroyed, the stem cells are reinfused into the body. Ellen received some nutritional supplements by intravenous infusion in a program Dr. Labriola worked out with her oncologist. "We played it carefully because we were afraid if this patient did badly with side effects she would probably abandon everything, including her life," says Dr. Labriola.

Dr. Labriola was fortunate in finding a relatively enlightened oncologist with whom to collaborate. "He was an oncologist who knew how to ask the right questions, which is important. He and I had seen other patients who had used alternative methods incorrectly, so he knew where the risk areas are." In fact, this oncologist had attended one of Dr. Labriola's professional seminars for physicians. "He ended up asking me all the questions I had taught him he needed to be asking when he was dealing with anybody working with alternatives. He got to see the system work and he was happy with that. His whole attitude toward alternative medicine in cancer treatment changed."

***"The key to long-range survival is to not march down the same road you marched down to get this tumor in the first place," Dr. Labriola says.***

During the complicated procedure of stem cell replacement and transplantation, Dr. Labriola was careful not to do anything that would interfere with the process. "As a result, Ellen was relatively symptom free through this procedure. She gradually lost her hair, but not for long; it grew back quickly. She hardly had any mouth sores which are highly common with this treatment, which, incidentally, was at a higher dosage than her earlier chemotherapy. Ellen's treatment was more intensive this time yet she had far fewer side effects. The nurses were amazed."

Even more impressive was the fact that during her earlier series of chemotherapy, Ellen had been out of work for 4-5 months, but in this round, with naturopathic support, she missed only 1 week in all. Following the naturopathically supported chemotherapy, Ellen began to improve. She lost weight and her joint problems disappeared. She eliminated much of the excessive fats from her diet which, in turn, greatly reduced the powerful mood swings and sweets cravings she had been subject to formerly. Ellen also began regular therapy sessions with a counselor and was able to discharge many of the emotional issues attending her condition, Dr. Labriola says. "After 18 months, all her cancer markers are down and she has had no recurrence. She's doing very well. Her life is good."

## SUCCESS STORY

### Naturopathic Support during the Conventional Treatment of Leukemia

Tommy, aged 11, suffered from an early form of leukemia. His parents had been advised to enroll him in a bone marrow transplant program and that his chances for survival were slim without it. His immune system was highly dysfunctional, providing little "raw material" capable of responding to natural support, says Dr. Labriola.

> ***Following the naturopathically supported chemotherapy, Ellen began to improve. Ellen also began regular therapy sessions with a counselor and was able to discharge many of the emotional issues attending her condition, Dr. Labriola says. "After 18 months, all her cancer markers are down and she has had no recurrence. She's doing very well. Her life is good."***

In addition, Tommy had multiple risk factors. He had a high degree of toxicity as he had been around motors, automotive chemicals, and solvents for years, and had lived close to a garbage dump where he inadvertently inhaled the toxic fumes when the garbage was burned. Industrial toxins from these sources had compromised his immune system, says Dr. Labriola. A bone marrow transplant was decided upon and Dr. Labriola agreed to provide naturopathic support. In this medical procedure, bone marrow is harvested from the patient and set aside; then high-dose chemotherapy and, in Tommy's case, total body irradiation, are administered; then the bone marrow is returned to the patient. In Tommy's case, his bone marrow was not good enough for the procedure, so his doctors used bone marrow from his sister.

In the time before the combined chemotherapy and radiation, Dr. Labriola built up Tommy's immune system and general health, using nutritional and botanical supplements. Dr. Labriola worked in collaboration with Tommy's attending physician; the hospital eventually gave Dr. Labriola attending status and was highly cooperative with his program, he says. "I was there every day for months," says Dr. Labriola. Using a classical naturopathic technique, he gave Tommy hot and cold packs (hydrotherapy) and mild electrical stimulation to get the immune system "up and kicking." During the recovery stage, Dr. Labriola repeated the hydrotherapy to reduce the side effects of the treatment.

Tommy not only survived the treatment and the cancer, but 10 years later, was "an adult and doing wonderfully." There had been some fear that the toxic treatments might stunt his growth (at the time he was 5'5"), but the naturopathic immune system support avoided this and Tommy eventually grew to be 6' tall.

***"The bone marrow graft went well and he had an absolutely spectacular recovery," comments Dr. Labriola. "This is in part because Tommy received considerable nutritional care and because the hospital was skilled in providing their care. Choosing your hospital and oncologist carefully has a great deal to do with your survival."***

"The bone marrow graft went well and he had an absolutely spectacular recovery," comments Dr. Labriola. "He had some mouth sores and hair loss but he fared not nearly as badly as other patients receiving similar treatments without the naturopathic support. This is in part because Tommy received considerable nutritional care and because the hospital was skilled in providing their care. Choosing your hospital and oncologist *carefully* has a great deal to do with your survival."

For information on **low-dose chemotherapy**, see Chapter 30: The New Pharmacology for Treating Cancer. pp. 849-850.

For a health maintenance plan, Dr. Labriola advised Tommy to stay away from petrochemicals whenever possible and to wear a respiratory mask and gloves when he worked around gasoline engines. Eventually he abandoned this work in favor of his health.

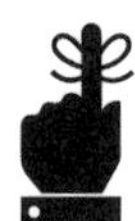

According to Dr. Labriola, some alternative and conventional treatments work better in combination than in isolation, working with each other rather than against each other.

## Certain Alternative and Conventional Methods Work Better Together

A shift in treatment emphasis to combine naturopathic and conventional oncological methods makes sense on the biological level, at least for certain advanced cases. It serves as the functional basis for much of Dr. Labriola's approach to cancer. "All of the positive health-promoting and sometimes curative substances and procedures we have available in alternative care are of tremendous value. But like it or not, there are many good acute-care procedures and medicines in conventional oncology that work," he contends. "In some cases, if you're going to be 100% effective, you need to have the flexibility to provide conventional services as well."

According to Dr. Labriola, some alternative and conventional treatments work better in combination than in isolation, working *with* each other rather than *against* each other. "There is definitely a synergy between the two sides when they are carefully combined. The patient can receive the best of both worlds." Physicians cannot afford to be biased in either direction, conventional or alternative, and must be more rigorously objective in their entire approach to cancer, Dr. Labriola says.

From the biological perspective, using conventional treatment immediately removes the "tumor burden" (the total cost of the tumor's presence) on the body through surgery and/or cell-killing (cytotoxic) methods. Here it is helpful to understand that the tumor is "probably the weakest, most vulnerable tissue in the body," Dr. Labriola explains. "People have a tendency to think the cancer tissue is the toughest tissue, but it isn't. It's not strong. It's not flourishing. It struggles to get blood supply. It is not well organized. The problem is that it grows in places where it interferes with body function. That is why cancer tumors can be as devastating as they are. Chemotherapy drugs were developed to prioritize their action against tumor tissue."

Eliminating the most overt and objective signs of the cancer is the most significant thing that happens with traditional oncology, says Dr. Labriola. "In some cases conventional oncologists are good at doing that. There are some exceptions and this is where naturopathic or alternative treatments alone will often suffice."

Dr. Labriola's specific advice to cancer patients concerning the application of a complementary approach is as follows:

1) If you have a tumor with good margins—that is, it is well-defined or well-differentiated, or has all the characteristics of a tumor that can be removed surgically without concern for metastasis—then surgery might be a good idea. Dr. Labriola notes that chemotherapy and radiation may be unnecessary in some of these cases and may even result in an increased risk for future cancer; nutrition, botanicals, and other alternative treatments should be used instead.
2) If the tumor's margins are not clear or well-differentiated, then other conventional cancer treatments may be helpful, such as low-dose ("fractionated") chemotherapy. "Certain leukemias and lymphomas

actually respond well, often permanently, to chemotherapy," says Dr. Labriola. "It always gives me a little indigestion to tell anyone that there is something good about chemotherapy. But there are some occasions for which chemotherapy is the best shot we know of for certain cancers." Depending on the disease, its staging and the drugs used, often there is a lifetime remission, he adds, though this depends almost entirely on the use of nutritional and botanical support.

3) The next priority is to take all the steps needed to safeguard against a recurrence. Such "secondary prevention" is an essential part of cancer treatment and should be emphasized as strongly as the so-called curative phase. "The key to long-range survival is to not march down the same road you marched down to get this tumor in the first place," Dr. Labriola says. "Naturopathic medicine was doing this years before prevention became a buzzword." When patients go into remission or are declared medically stable (no further tumor to be removed), naturopathic protocols can help prevent future recurrence.

***"The language a doctor uses with the cancer patient must be carefully chosen at times," says Dr. Labriola. "But most importantly, we discuss life, success, and happiness. We must always be clear and truthful with patients, but hope never hurt anyone and no physician has the right to take it away."***

A key factor in the success of any outcome, but particularly one blending conventional and alternative approaches, is patient compliance, says Dr. Labriola. "One of the things I do is to make certain that patients are doing something with which they can comply. On the other hand, my patients do not get away without some lifestyle changes. Compliance is the biggest challenge every physician has. If we could all get compliance, our success rates would double, or more. I spend a lot of time trying to make it possible for my patients to comply with the program we develop. I tailor each program to what the patient is likely to do without feeling as though they're being punished or undertaking something that significantly reduces their quality of life."

## Nutritional Support Is Crucial after Chemotherapy

Preventing recurrences makes the critical difference if someone has chosen to undergo low-dose chemotherapy or localized radiation. "The amount of support *after* the chemotherapy or whatever treatment they've had is the crucial factor. You can read about studies showing high rates of leukemia among people who received chemotherapy for Hodgkin's lymphoma and perhaps other cancers, but you have to remember that all those statistics are based on conventional treatment without any follow-up alternative therapies, which greatly enhance the person's resistance to cancer."

The five keys to support are (1) balanced nutrition, (2) optimal botanical support, (3) lifestyle adjustments (e.g., exercise and relaxation techniques), (4) environmental considerations (avoiding toxins), and (5) psychological support. "When you try to fully inform patients and give them the sense that they're in control, their stress level drops dramatically. This moves them out of the victim phase and into the empowered phase where they need to be."

Dr. Labriola tells his patients at every juncture in their treatment program that they will be making tough decisions at times, and that his role is to provide them with enough information so that they can choose their strategies appropriately. He tells his patients: "You must make these decisions based on what's inside you, tempered by what we, the physicians, determine to be appropriate based on our measurements and evaluations."

The language a doctor uses with the cancer patient must be carefully chosen at times. "I don't like the words 'terminal,' 'hopeless,' or 'incurable.' We do discuss death and dying, because that is an issue that exists in all of our lives. But most importantly, we discuss life, success, and happiness. We must always be clear and truthful with patients, but hope never hurt anyone and no physician has the right to take it away."

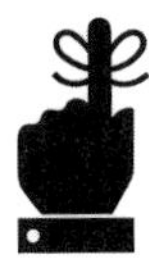

*The successful approach*

*to reversing cancer and preventing*

*its future recurrence*

*is always multimodal. No single*

*therapy, technique, or*

*substance can prevail against the*

*complexity of this disease.*

## CURRICULUM VITAE

# Victor A. Marcial-Vega, M.D.

4037 Poinciana Avenue, Coconut Grove, FL 33133;
tel: 305-442-1233; fax: 305-445-4504.

Dr. Marcial Vega received his M.D. from the University of Puerto Rico School of Medicine in San Juan, Puerto Rico, and completed a 4-year internship and residency in radiation oncology at Johns Hopkins Hospital in Baltimore, Maryland. From 1988-1990, Dr. Marcial-Vega was chief of Head and Neck Cancer Service at Mallinckrodt Institute of Radiology, Washington University School of Medicine in St. Louis, Missouri; from 1990-1994, he was clinical assistant professor in the Department of Radiation Oncology at the University of Miami School of Medicine; and from 1990-1993, he was in practice as a radiation oncologist at Baptist Hospital in Miami, Florida. Dr. Marcial-Vega has contributed articles to the *International Journal of Radiation Oncology* and *Biological Physics* and written chapters for various medical texts on cancer treatment.

***"At least 95% of all of cancer patients are immunosuppressed due to physical, chemical, mental, and/or environmental causes," Dr. Marcial-Vega says. "When someone's immune system becomes suppressed, then they are more susceptible to cancer. If you don't address the immune system, you're treating the cancer without really treating the cause of the cancer."***

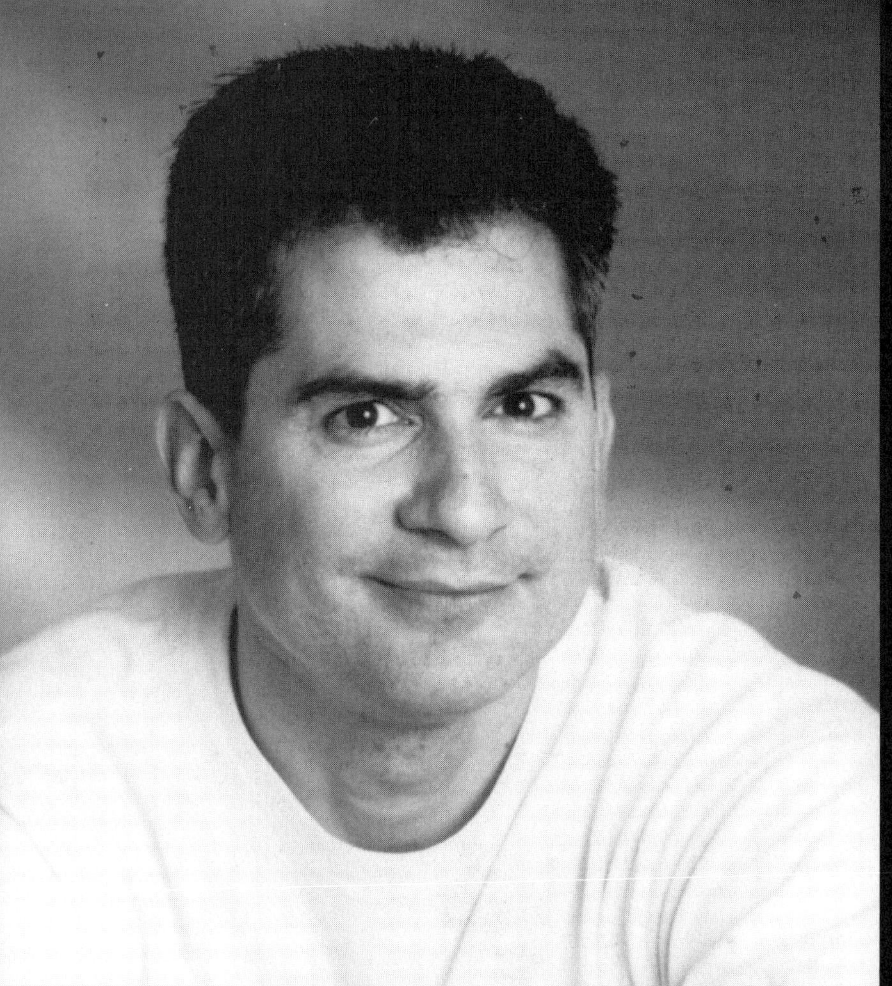

# *Victor A. Marcial-Vega, M.D.*

**THE SUCCESS OF A CANCER** treatment program, and perhaps the avoidance of cancer itself, depends on the health and function of the immune system, says Dr. Marcial-Vega, whose multifaceted nutritional and herbal supplementation program supports and strengthens a patient's own inner defenses.

Dr. Marcial-Vega's basic philosophy of cancer treatment is that the laws of health are inseparable from the laws of Nature. "Once we live according to the laws of Nature, we are never sick and healing occurs effortlessly, in an orderly way. Our main source of nourishment, the basis of our health, is air, water, and food. It has nothing to do with medications or high-tech gadgetry." The body and mind are nourished by such "natural" elements as silence, music, and relationships.

"The less solid or tangible a nourishment, the more powerful its impact can be on health. We can survive longer without food than without water and longer without water than without air. It logically follows that what our senses take in is even more powerful in sustaining us."

For Dr. Marcial-Vega, the key to successful cancer therapy is strengthening the immune system. "At least 95% of all cancer patients are immunosuppressed due to physical, chemical, mental, and/or environmental causes," Dr. Marcial-Vega says. "When someone's immune system becomes suppressed, then they are more susceptible to cancer. If you don't address the immune system, you're treating the cancer without really treating the cause of the cancer."

By "immunosuppression" Marcial-Vega means that his patients have a total lymphocyte count of less than 1200 cells/mm$^3$. The low lymphocyte number can be detected by a Complete Blood Count (CBC), a rou-

# Dr. Marcial-Vega's Generalized Model for Cancer Treatment

| STRATEGY | DOSAGE/ KEY COMPONENTS | FOR MORE INFORMATION see page # |
|---|---|---|
| **Nutritional Plan** | | |
| Mainly vegetarian, with occasional use of fish | steamed and raw vegetables, whole grains; beans, nuts, seeds; raw fruit and fresh juices | 749 |
| Vitamin C | 10-12 grams, divided into 4 doses and taken orally | 786 |
| Niacinamide | 300-1500 mg daily (start at the lowest dose) | 785 |
| B complex | 1 tablet, 3X/day | 784 |
| Vitamin E | 400 IU, 2X/day | 790 |
| Selenium | 400-600 mcg, 2X/day | 783 |
| Coenzyme Q10 | 250-300 mg/day | 766 |
| Beta carotene | 20,000-25,000 units IU, 4X/day | 764 |
| Green concentrates (blue-green algae, spirulina, etc.) | 1 serving, 4X/day | 809 |
| Multivitamins | 1 tablet with each meal | — |
| Herbal remedies<br>1) *Tristerix tetrandus chilensis*<br>2) *Urtica urens*<br>3) *Taraxacum officin*<br>4) *Plantago mayor*<br>5) *Quinchamalium majus* | amounts and combinations vary depending on patient condition | 273 |
| Willard's Water | 1 oz stirred in a gallon of spring water; 1 gallon daily | 274 |
| **Natural Cancer Complements** | | |
| Essiac | 3 ounces of Essiac, 3X/day prepared as directed | 815 |
| Bovine cartilage | 9 g per day, or 3 grams 3X/day | 861 |
| Enzymes (Intenzyme) | dosage varies depending on patient condition | 928 |
| Vitamin C | 50-150 g given intravenously 3X/week | 786 |
| VMV Product: Natural clay/ 18 Herbs | 1/2 tsp. orally 1-2X/day, 30 minutes before meals; also topical application near tumor site | 276 |

*Continued*

## Dr. Marcial-Vega's Generalized Model for Cancer Treatment (cont.)

| STRATEGY | DOSAGE/ KEY COMPONENTS | FOR MORE INFORMATION see page # |
|---|---|---|
| Aromatherapy essential oils | orange, lavender, peppermint: 1-2 drops, rubbed on hands, inhaled 4X daily; 2 drops lavender oil taken orally with food 4X daily; lavender and orange oil: applied topically 4X daily to skin over tumor site; added to bath water: 5 drops of ylang-ylang, orange, patchouli, or cedarwood | 275 |
| **Psychospiritual Strategies** | | |
| Psychospirtual counseling | tailored to individual needs | 277 |
| Meditation and/or prayer | tailored to individual needs | |
| Visualization, imagery | tailored to individual needs | |
| Neurolinguistic programming | tailored to individual needs | |

For more information on **lymphocytes** and a summary of key immune system components, see Chapter 25: What Causes Cancer?

tine and inexpensive medical test. The total lymphocyte count, however, is not always a reliable measure of immunosuppression. Some cancer patients have a normal lymphocyte count, but they are exceptions to the rule. In many of these unusual cases, the person's natural killer (NK) cell activity is low. When NK cell activity is depressed, the body's ability to fight cancer is diminished. Other components of the immune system that may be compromised include the T4 lymphocytes (T helper cells), macrophages, and antibody production. Dr. Marcial-Vega points out that the majority of cancer cases can be determined based on lymphocyte count.

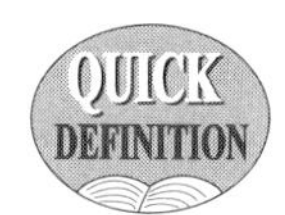


A **lymphocyte** is a form of white blood cell, representing 25-33% of the total count, whose numbers increase during infection. Lymphocytes, produced in the bone marrow, come in two forms: T cells, which are matured in the thymus gland (behind the breastbone) and have many functions in the body's immune response; and B cells, which produce antibodies to neutralize an antigen—foreign and potentially dangerous matter in the blood. Each lymphocyte produces a single and specific antibody.

Before a person receives any form of treatment, Dr. Marcial-Vega employs 2 other tests to assess a patient's systemic ability to fight cancer. A Pantox lab test allows him to assess the balance and availability of key antioxidants in the cancer patient's body. Specifically, this test compares the patient's levels of vitamins A, E, coenzyme Q10, C, beta carotene, and ferritin to the percentile scores for a normal population.

A score of 100% is optimal; 1% to 5% is extremely low.[1] A relatively high antioxidant index correlates with a higher survival rate in cancer patients, Dr. Marcial-Vega notes.

Also helpful are measurements of 2 antioxidant enzyme systems, adds Dr. Marcial-Vega. One is the individual's glutathione blood level, which indicates how depleted antioxidants are in the liver. Another measures the levels of lipid peroxidase, which in turn reflects the toxic load on the body and consequently the patient's antioxidant status.

For more information about the **Pantox** test for antioxidants, see Chapter 27: Early Detection and Prevention of Cancer, p. 742.

## SUCCESS STORY

### Reversing Uterine Cancer

Janet, aged 47, was a hardworking housewife who had always considered herself to be in good health. One winter, she began to experience severe abdominal pains and shortly afterward she was diagnosed with endometrial carcinoma; the following spring she underwent surgery to have her uterus removed by total abdominal hysterectomy.

CAUTION

This chapter includes information regarding actual treatments used by Dr. Marcial-Vega only after his careful diagnosis of each patient. All cancer patients are unique. **Do not administer these treatments to yourself or others.** Discuss these treatments with your physician or other qualified health-care professional. Readers should not interpret this material as therapeutic advice, but should see a physician in all cases.

About 2 years later, Janet experienced severe vaginal bleeding and, once again, abdominal discomfort. Her cancer had returned. Located in her abdominal cavity was a palpable mass in the left pelvis; a CT scan showed that peritoneal spreading was under way. By conventional standards, Janet's condition was expected to worsen, with death likely in less than a year. Her medical prognosis, according to her oncologist, was "terminal."

At this point, Janet consulted Dr. Marcial-Vega who placed her on an intensive program of Essiac, shark cartilage, vitamins C, E, B complex, selenium, and coenzyme Q10. During this time, Janet received no chemotherapy or radiation. Within 2 weeks of beginning this program, Janet began to experience "a renewed sense of vitality and well-being," states Dr. Marcial-Vega. Two years after the cancer recurrence, she showed no evidence of cancer based on CT scans and other medical tests. Her overall health was much better than it had been prior to her diagnosis of cancer. "Today, Janet's overall health is excellent," says Dr. Marcial-Vega.

## Marshaling a Complementary Response to Cancer

Dr. Marcial-Vega has developed a 3-pronged strategy for treating cancer.

The first component is primarily aggressive: overpower the cancer before it takes a person's life. The second component involves botanical support and detoxification. The third component addresses the psychological aspects of healing. Regarding the first component, Dr. Marcial-Vega says, "The more advanced or aggressive forms of cancer can kill a person within a week or month, so quick and decisive action is warranted. The most powerful form of counterattack can entail a combination of conventional and alternative therapies."

In his view, while some patients may need chemotherapy, radiation, or surgery to overpower the cancer, most do not. "I use it as a tool where appropriate because it has its place in modern medicine." Dr. Marcial-Vega contends that these methods are often overutilized or abused by oncologists. "This is especially the case in advanced or metastatic cancers where chemotherapy or radiation have no benefit. Even so, these patients get the most of both of these therapies and often succumb from the treatment rather than the cancer."

***While some patients may need chemotherapy, radiation, or surgery to overpower the cancer, most do not. Dr. Marcial-Vega contends that these methods are often overutilized or abused by cancer doctors.***

If people would use natural treatments in the *early* stages of their cancer, they might not have to endure the harsh conventional methods later, says Dr. Marcial-Vega. Unfortunately, many people wait until they have exhausted all those possibilities and are in the advanced stages of cancer before turning to the gentler medical alternatives. "The medicine of the future will strengthen the human body, mind, and spirit to such a degree that we will not need any artificial tools, such as radiation, drugs, or chemotherapy. That medicine of the future is already here today."

Most of Dr. Marcial-Vega's patients are in the advanced stages of cancer. "But even with that dismal prognosis, I have patients who have been cured by the natural treatments only." He estimates that 5-10% of those who come to him when the cancer is in the advanced stage have their tumors reversed by his treatments and that 90% are helped to varying degrees. "Imagine the results if people with cancer would start this alternative approach immediately upon learning the diagnosis," he observes.

**Essiac**—Dr. Marcial-Vega has observed that Essiac tea placed on top of cancer cells on the skin will dissolve the cells. "In addition to helping bolster the immune system, Essiac acts directly on the cancer cells," he notes. He generally recommends taking 3 ounces of Essiac 3 times a day, prepared as directed and consumed on an empty stomach, between meals.

**Cartilage—**Dr. Marcial-Vega has recommended shark cartilage, but he says bovine cartilage is easier to take because it is required in a much smaller quantity and lacks the fishy taste; either can work depending on the individual. His recommended amount of bovine cartilage is generally about 9 g per day, or 3 g 3 times per day, taken on an empty stomach between meals.

**Enzymes—**Enzymes not only digest food, but also help the immune system eliminate cancer cells. "When we're healthy, we produce numerous enzymes that help dismantle cancer cells. If you don't have sufficient enzyme production in the digestive tract, you also tend to lack the ability to enzymatically break down cancer cells elsewhere in the body." His recommended brand of enzyme is called Intenzyme; Dr. Marcial-Vega's typical recommended dosage for Intenzyme is variable, from 10-30 capsules 3 times a day with the dosage slowly increased. It is vital to take the enzymes between meals, on an empty stomach, and preferably not at the same time as Essiac or cartilage, stresses Dr. Marcial-Vega.

**Intravenous Vitamin C—**Dr. Marcial-Vega regards vitamin C as a versatile form of "natural chemotherapy." Research shows that vitamin C boosts natural killer cell activity against cancer cells, and that this increased activity is greatest between 8 and 24 hours after ingesting the vitamin.[2] Dr. Marcial-Vega often gives his patients between 50 g and 150 g of vitamin C intravenously 3 times a week, usually on Monday, Wednesday, and Friday. "This can be done for as many weeks as seems necessary, but it must be a *slow* infusion, over a period of about 4-5 hours. The individual who receives this megadose of vitamin C should be taken off of it only very gradually and should be supplemented throughout with oral vitamin C."

These 4 therapies—Essiac, cartilage, enzymes, and vitamin C—may be offered to everyone with cancer, says Dr. Marcial-Vega. "Not only do they increase the cure rate, but they also dramatically decrease the side effects of chemotherapy and radiation. We now have evidence that chemotherapy, radiation, and surgery flush out vitamins and minerals from the body from day one. Without nutritional supplements, the patient will most likely get sicker, and it's not from the chemotherapy and radiation *per se*, but from the lack of nutrition to protect them from the conventional treatments."

Another reason a patient under conventional treatment feels sick is the accumulation of cellular debris from the killing of cancer cells; the technical name for this is cancer necrosis. If the body does not eliminate these toxins, the person feels sick, experiencing nausea, flu-like symptoms, achy joints, and headaches. The connection is simple: a lack of adequate nutrition and proper elimination of toxins are major reasons why cancer patients receiving conventional treatment become sicker, says Dr. Marcial-Vega. Simple ways to increase toxin elimination are increasing water intake and having enemas.

***"Chemotherapy, radiation, and surgery flush out vitamins and minerals from the body from day one," says Dr. Marcial-Vega. "Without nutritional supplements, the patient will most likely get sicker, from the lack of nutrition to protect them from the conventional treatments."***

## Nutrition, Botanicals, and Detoxification Strategies

The second component of Dr. Marcial-Vega's treatment approach, herbal and nutritional supplements, supports numerous aspects of the body's self-healing ability. Some of these relate to immune and hormonal mechanisms while others involve detoxification mechanisms and the removal of toxic substances from the cells. "Sometimes, the cancer is eliminated through the skin," says Dr. Marcial-Vega. "Other times, it's eliminated through the stool and urine. In any case, when the body is functioning optimally, cancer is quickly disposed of because the healthy body expels anything that doesn't belong in it. Then the internal environment no longer supports the existence of cancer cells."

**Vitamin C (Oral)—**Oral supplements need to be taken during the administration of intravenous vitamin C to maintain a stable, continuous supply of nutrients, says Dr. Marcial-Vega. He prefers the ascorbate type of oral vitamin C, which can be prepared by mixing 3 g of vitamin C powder and 1.5 g of baking soda (sodium bicarbonate, without aluminum) in a glass of distilled water. This mixture equals 3 g of vitamin C ascorbate. The recommended dose is 10-12 g a day, in 4 divided doses (2.5 to 3 g for each dose). If loose stools, diarrhea, or stomach pains develop, decrease the dose.

**Niacinamide**—Dr. Marcial-Vega recommends working within a range of 300-1500 mg a day. Start with 300 mg and increase it every few days until you reach 1500 mg daily, he advises.

**Vitamin E**—Dr. Marcial-Vega recommends the succinate form of vitamin E, 400 IU twice a day.

**Selenium**—Dr. Marcial-Vega's preferred dosage range is 400 to 600 mcg a day, with close monitoring of blood levels to avoid toxicity.

**Beta Carotene**—Dr. Marcial-Vega recommends taking 20,000-25,000 IU of beta carotene 4 times a day (a total daily intake of 80,000-100,000 IU). One of his patients with chronic lymphatic leukemia achieved a normal blood count through taking this amount.

**Green Concentrates**—These vegetable concentrates contain a wide variety of vitamins and minerals, as well as various "probiotics," substances that aid in digestion, detoxification, and other key functions. Dr. Marcial-Vega prescribes a serving of any 1 or combination of the following green concentrates 4 times day: blue-green algae, spirulina, wheat grass, watercress, or Green Magma. If the stool turns loose or gas develops, decrease the frequency then slowly increase it again.

**Multivitamin**—This all-purpose supplement (1 tablet with each meal) is designed to ensure that nutritional deficiencies do not take place during cancer treatment and recovery from the disease. Dr. Marcial-Vega says it is important to pay attention to how you *feel* as you take these supplements. "If any changes occur, contact your physician immediately. Monitoring your own body is essential for determining your optimal dosage. Be sure to drink plenty of water, either pure spring water or water purified by reverse osmosis, at the rate of about 6-10 glasses (8 ounces each) a day."

**Herbal Medicines**—In addition to Essiac, Dr. Marcial-Vega recommends

***"Clinical data show that Willard's Water helps patients to eliminate toxic chemicals and heavy metals from their bodies," says Dr. Marcial-Vega.***

various herbs to bolster immunity and assist in other bodily processes involved in one's ability to fight cancer. Herbs tend to improve overall health because "they improve the body's ability to fight disease and act non-specifically, in support of many body systems simultaneously." Among the herbs he uses: stinging nettle (*Urtica urens*); dandelion (*Taraxacum officin*); plantain (*Plantago mayor*); and South American rain forest herbs such as *Quinchamalium majus* and *Tristerix tetrandus chilensis.* Since the amounts and combinations of these herbs will vary depending on one's condition, be sure to consult a doctor well-versed in the use of botanical medicines.

QUICK DEFINITION

**Willard's Water**, which claims 21 U.S. patents, is water into which a catalyst has been introduced, changing the water's molecular structure and its properties, according to its manufacturer. Its makers refer to it as "catalyst-altered water," based on a catalyst (called a "micelle," comprising tiny electrically charged particles) discovered by John W. Willard, Ph.D., Professor Emeritus at South Dakota School of Mines and Technology, in Rapid City.

**Willard's Water**—To facilitate the removal of toxins, Dr. Marcial-Vega recommends the use of Willard's Water, a special, mineral-rich prepared water that can be obtained from most health food stores. An ounce of this water is placed in a gallon of spring water, then stirred; the cancer patient drinks a gallon of this water daily. "Clinical data show that people drinking the dilute Willard's Water have increased levels of toxic metals in the urine," says Dr. Marcial-Vega, "meaning it helps patients to eliminate toxic chemicals and heavy metals from their bodies."

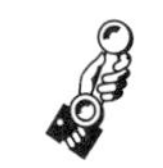

For **Willard's Water,** contact Dakota Providers, P.O. Box 8023, Fargo, ND 58109; tel: 701-235-4064 or 800-447-4793; fax: 701-235-3432. For information on the **Intenzyme Forte** and **Retenzyme Forte** brand of enzymes used by Dr. Marcial-Vega, contact Biotics Research Corp., P.O. Box 36888, Houston, TX 77236; tel: 713-240-8010; fax: 713-240-2304. For information on the **Essiac** formulation Dr. Marcial-Vega uses, contact: Essiac USA, Inc., 26 Union Street, Newburyport, MA

**Coffee Enema**—When the cancer patient has cold or flu-like symptoms, such as from a rapid death of cancer cells and the subsequent release of toxins into the blood circulation, Dr. Marcial-Vega may recommend the temporary use of coffee enemas to stimulate excretion and elimination of toxins. The coffee enema is among the only pharmaceutically effective choleretics (which increase the flow of toxin-rich bile) noted in the medical literature that can be safely used many times daily without toxic effects.[3]

Dr. Marcial-Vega is not in favor of the regular use of enemas, however, because they can be uncomfortable and he contends they tend to upset the balance of intestinal flora, which have important immune and detoxification functions. If his patients do use a coffee enema, Dr. Marcial-Vega recommends taking a supplemental *Lactobacillus* supplement 3 times a day.

**Aromatherapy Essential Oils**—Essential plant oils have become an integral part of Dr. Marcial-Vega's anticancer approach. "They are very important in any case where herbs are prepared in their dry form, which is the case in more than 99% of the herbal preparations used in the U.S. as the USDA allows only dry herbs to enter the country," he comments.

"This renders a product that has lost most of its healing qualities because of the lack of essential oils." Essential oils, prepared by distillation or extraction, have several key properties of interest to the cancer physician, including antibacterial, antifungal, antiviral, antiparasitic, and anticancer, Dr. Marcial-Vega says. As part of a treatment program prescribed by a physician, they may be inhaled, applied topically, or taken orally.

For more information about **coffee enemas,** see Chapter 4: Etienne Callebout, M.D., pp. 101-103.

***"At least 95% of all of my cancer patients are immunosuppressed due to physical, chemical, mental, and/or environmental causes," Dr. Marcial-Vega says.***

Dr. Marcial-Vega has found that lavender and orange essential oils are powerful anticancer oils when used both orally and topically on the skin. Regarding lavender, 1-2 drops can be rubbed on the palms of the hands, cupped over the nose, and inhaled until the aroma is gone; this can be repeated 4 times daily. Dr. Marcial-Vega says that lavender oil may also be taken orally at the dosage of 2 drops with food, 4 times daily. "Attention must be paid to any gastrointestinal symptoms arising because the oils may be irritating to the mucosa. In such a case, start slowly and increase the dose over a 2-week period." Orange essential oil may be taken according to this same procedure, he adds.

Another advantage to taking essential plant oils orally is that parasites can be eliminated, says Dr. Marcial-Vega. Peppermint is a powerful antiparasitic oil and can be taken 1 drop with every meal, sprinkled over the food. In addition, lavender and orange may be applied topically 4 times daily over the skin areas overlying the tumor. "Essential oils will penetrate the skin and go inside the body," says Dr. Marcial-Vega. "They can also be used for relaxation and stress reduction." Here he generally recommends

5 drops of any of the oils mentioned above in either a whole-body bath or a foot bath. Remain immersed in the water for at least 20 minutes. "Let the oils permeate the air in the room so you can also inhale them as well as absorb them through the skin." He generally recommends ylang-ylang, orange, patchouli, and cedarwood.

Not all commercial essential plant oils are of the highest quality, Dr. Marcial-Vega cautions. "I have found very few oils that meet the criteria I require for the above-mentioned regimen, which is why I helped to formulate a special line for clinical use."

***"The only way to fully recover from cancer is to identify and connect with those parts within oneself that are wounded, repressed, or in need of healing attention," says Dr. Marcial-Vega.***

**VMV Product: Natural Clay/18 Herbs**—Dr. Marcial-Vega has also devised and is experimenting with a preparation that includes natural clay from volcanic areas around the world combined with extracts of 18 herbal roots from the rain forest. Dr. Marcial-Vega gathered these materials personally during several trips to rain forest areas. "This was originally prepared with the intention of offering all the essential minerals and most of the water-soluble vitamins in a natural form," he explains. "In the initial months in which I have explored it, I have found this to be anticancerous as well as highly nutritious, as noted by the decrease in tumors as well as the increase in patient well-being and energy."

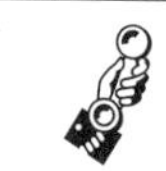

For information about **aromatherapy oils** and **volcanic clay**, contact: Phyto Medicine Company, 6701 Sunset Drive, Suite 100, Miami, FL 33143; tel: 305-662-6396; fax: 305-667-5619.

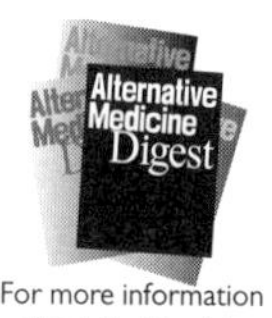


For more information about Dr. Marcial-Vega's use of **VMV Product** and **aromatherapy essential oils**, see "Aromatherapy Oils as Oral Remedies," #16, pp. 30-35.

Dr. Marcial-Vega's patients take 1/2 level teaspoon of the mixture (orally) 1-2 times daily 30 minutes before meals. It is mixed well with saliva until it is liquified in the mouth, then swallowed. The mixture can also be applied over body areas where tumors are located as well as in an intrarectal form for prostate cancer, colitis, prostatitis, and rectal cancer, he notes. "One patient with anal cancer has had a remission documented by CT scan of the pelvis, and another is experiencing a decrease in his prostate specific antigen (PSA) count. Still another is applying this mixture topically for a breast cancer and the tumor is now half the size after 5 weeks of application." The topical applications are performed at night, the clay is allowed to dry, and the patient then goes to sleep.

## Psychological Strategies for Healing

The third area of Dr. Marcial-Vega's approach is addressing the psychological and spiritual dimensions of the cancer patient. "The best approach to cancer is one that combines interventions for the mind, body, soul, and current emotional state. The only way to fully recover from cancer is to identify and connect with those parts within oneself that are wounded, repressed, or in need of healing attention."

A willingness to pay attention to inner signals is the first step toward greater self-awareness and a clearer, more expansive sense of self. "True healing is largely a process of getting to know oneself," Dr. Marcial-Vega says. "It's about learning to listen to your body. Any time there's something painful or uncomfortable, the healing mind pays attention to what's going on inside the body. It doesn't try to lay blame on people or things outside of oneself." To instruct people in this "inner listening," Dr. Marcial-Vega offers his patients tapes and books to help them find a self-help approach that feels comfortable.

> ***"True healing is largely a process of getting to know oneself," Dr. Marcial-Vega says. "It's about learning to listen to your body. Like any other illness, cancer is a sign that one's life is out of balance. The trouble is, many of us are actually in disease, eating poorly, getting stressed-out on the job, or not choosing mutually enhancing relationships."***

Basic to the therapeutic process is helping cancer patients learn to see their condition as a signal to reorient their inner and outer lives. "Like any other illness, cancer is a *sign* that one's life is out of balance. If we're at ease with life, enjoying our quality of life and doing exactly what we want to, we're not going to be sick. The trouble is, many of us are actually in *dis*ease, eating poorly, getting stressed-out on the job, or not choosing mutually enhancing relationships." When the human body is free from chronic distress, it is far more resistant to toxic insults from the environment that can trigger the onset of cancer.

To get a picture of this cancer-creating context, Dr. Marcial-Vega compares it to the ulcer-prone work pattern. "Let's say I'm feeling depressed at my job because I don't like what I'm doing. Every morning I have a stomachache, but instead of *listening* to this signal, I take antacid medications to make the ulcer go away. As a result, the cause of my ulcer, which is my per-

***It is a grave error, says Dr. Marcial-Vega, for doctors to prescribe supplements and other nontoxic strategies without paying attention to the person's areas of denial or repression.***

ception of the world around me, is never dealt with." The body eventually succumbs to either an ulcer or some form of serious, stress-related illness. Similarly, many potential sources of emotional or psychosocial stress can depress the immune system and contribute to one's susceptibility to cancer.

In probably 9 out of 10 cases, this stress involves some form of denial or emotional repression, shutting down of one's feelings or not paying attention, says Dr. Marcial-Vega. Most Americans pay attention to their thoughts while ignoring body signals. "We get locked into intellectual fixations and block out what our bodies are telling us. We tune out our inner sensations and feelings, and when the tuning-out becomes habitual, it can promote all kinds of illness, including cancer." Symptoms of illness can be triggered as much by emotional and psychosocial stress—a tense relationship with one's employer, inadequate communication with a spouse—as they can by poor diet or erratic exercise.

For more information about **emotions** and **psychological conditions** as contributing causes to cancer, see Chapter 25: What Causes Cancer? pp. 615-619.

It is a grave error, says Dr. Marcial-Vega, for doctors to prescribe supplements and other nontoxic strategies without paying attention to the person's areas of denial or repression. "If I say that just taking this herb, vitamin, or diet will cure your cancer, I'd be guilty of the same irresponsible medicine that prescribes drugs in an unprincipled way. The philosophy behind this mode of medical action is wrong because it's symptomatic and doesn't deal with root cause."

## REINFORCING THE PATIENT'S WILL TO HEAL

Everything is individualized: for 2 people with the same type and stage of cancer, what constitutes a cure for one person can be poison for the other. Dr. Marcial-Vega's emphasis on the individuality of each patient extends from diet and exercise to addressing all aspects of the individual's psyche and social sphere. "If some doctor was to get hold of my nutritional guidelines and simply start prescribing, he could end up damaging people. Everyone's needs are unique and each person must pay attention to the needs of their body."

Before Dr. Marcial-Vega recommends the use of any therapy, including conventional treatment, he assesses the individual's frame of reference regarding each option. "Some people benefit from chemotherapy and radiation while others become poisoned and die. The conventional treatments are particularly helpful for people who are not as able to dig inside themselves to find the underlying causes, those factors that are promoting and reinforcing the disease process." Accordingly, the doctor must discern the individual's beliefs regarding therapeutic strategies and how trustful they are of a particular approach.

Dr. Marcial-Vega says that he can usually tell how well an individual will respond to an approach by talking with them for a while. "By listening carefully and impartially to what they're saying, I'll know if they are able to do this or not." In general, people who tend to ask many intellectual or skeptical questions about alternative medicine tend to fare poorly with the nontoxic therapies alone. Those who feel more aligned with the principles behind radiation and chemotherapy, or believe more strongly in these conventional treatments, will tend to benefit more from those strategies.

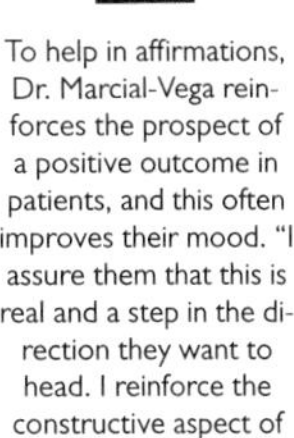

To help in affirmations, Dr. Marcial-Vega reinforces the prospect of a positive outcome in patients, and this often improves their mood. "I assure them that this is real and a step in the direction they want to head. I reinforce the constructive aspect of themselves and make them aware of the destructive aspects as well, so they do not fall back into *dis*ease."

If a person comes to Dr. Marcial-Vega with incessant questioning and skepticism, rather than showing an impartial willingness to experience the benefits of his therapies, then he often will give them information to the point of overload. Once they have become overfilled with facts, they tend to let go of rigid or close-minded attitudes and begin sensing their own needs and desires.

"I tell my patients to work on 2 areas," Dr. Marcial-Vega explains. "One is how to get out of disease and the other is to understand how they got into it. If I do not assist patients in both areas, they can fall into disease again. To get out, one simply has to stop and say, 'I want to head in this other direction,' and it will eventually happen, if they repeat it enough. I believe that a force—call it God, Universe, Mother Earth, or whatever—is waiting for all of us to ask. When we ask, we always receive."

To help this affirmation, Dr. Marcial-Vega reinforces the prospect of a positive outcome in patients, and this often improves their mood. "I assure them that this is real and a step in the direction they want to head. I reinforce the constructive aspect of themselves and make them aware of the destructive aspects as well, so they do not fall back into *dis*ease."

Not only does Dr. Marcial-Vega work closely with his patients, but he helps other physicians who want to master the alternative approaches, often by way of training seminars. "Training physicians is an integral part of my practice," he says. "I assist them to reach a state where they can diagnose and treat disease with a high degree of accuracy and results. I also help them make the transition from their previous practice to a holistic approach, ensuring them success."

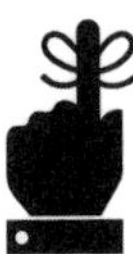

*Even if a tumor is not yet visible by conventional means, it is still active as cancer and a serious health threat waiting to announce itself. Knowing that early detection of the growing tumor allows for early treatment and better chances of survival, holistically minded physicians have begun seeking ways to diagnose precancerous conditions—those that precede the actual appearance of the cancer.*

## CURRICULUM VITAE

# Martin Milner, N.D.

Center for Natural Medicine, Inc.,
1330 SE 39th Avenue, Portland OR 97214;
tel: 503-232-1100; fax: 503-232-7751;
e-mail: martinm@teleport.com

Dr. Milner received his N.D. from the National College of Naturopathic Medicine in Portland, Oregon, where he is associate professor of cardiovascular and pulmonary medicine. Dr. Milner is co-founder (with Mary Milner) and medical director of the Center for Natural Medicine (established in 1991) and, before this, was in practice at the Center for Holistic Medicine, in Portland, Oregon. He has been treating cancer patients since 1982. His articles have appeared in *The Naturopathic Physician*, *Townsend Letter for Doctors and Patients*, and *Alternative & Complementary Therapies*. Other physicians at Dr. Milner's center include 2 M.D.s, a nurse practitioner, 3 chiropractors, an acupuncturist, 9 licensed massage therapists, and a colon hydrotherapist. A wide range of health-enhancement and lifestyle adjustment classes are integrated into the delivery of health care and illness management at Dr. Milner's clinic.

***"The increased incidence of cancer requires both physicians and the public to carefully scrutinize natural cancer treatment options," Dr. Milner says. "Even so, getting rid of the tumor is only the beginning of comprehensive treatment. The real battle is in making sure the cancer never has a chance to come back."***

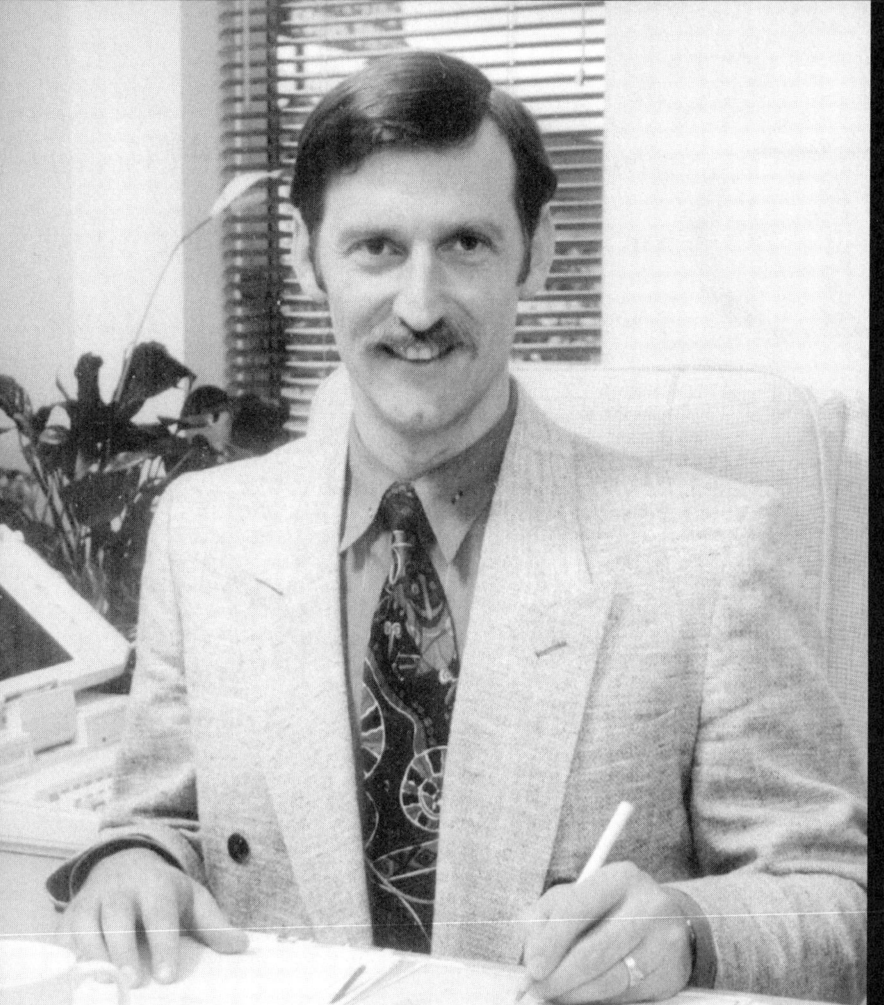

Chapter 14

# *Martin Milner, N.D.*

**THE NATUROPATHIC APPROACH** to cancer treatment calls for collaboration among many medical specialties, in addition to a firm foundation of nutritional and herbal supplementation, exercise, stress reduction, and dietary change, says Dr. Milner.

Dr. Milner and his colleagues at the Center for Natural Medicine have identified a wide range of natural, nontoxic medications and therapies that have shown effectiveness against various types of cancers. Dr. Milner provides medical information to his patients regarding these modalities so that they can select a plan of action that makes sense to them. But he adamantly discourages patients from constructing their own cancer treatment program without consulting him or other physicians well trained in natural therapeutics.

To the cancer patient, Dr. Milner recommends: "Please contact your conventional physician and inform him about your decision to augment your conventional treatment with natural therapies," says Dr. Milner. "No patient should self-prescribe and no patient should use all of the therapies listed," Dr. Milner says.

"Certain therapies are contraindicated and cannot be used in combination with other therapies; further, some absolutely require supervision and close monitoring by the physician. No one should assume that these therapies offer definitive treatment or a *cure* for cancer. The increased incidence of cancer requires both physicians and the public to carefully scrutinize natural cancer treatment options. Practitioners and patients alike have the opportunity to share information and resources in the challenge

# Dr. Milner's Generalized Model for Cancer Treatment

| STRATEGY | DOSAGE/ KEY COMPONENTS | FOR MORE INFORMATION see page # |
|---|---|---|
| **Dietary Intervention** | | |
| **Consume a low-fat, high-fiber diet: organic whole grains, fresh organic fruits and vegetables. No red meat, refined carbohydrates, alcohol, or caffeine. Test for IgG4/IgE food allergens. Ensure optimal caloric and adequate protein intake if patient with weight loss. Low acid diet, especially with Alavazatos and chronic pain patients. | optimal total nutrition; increase transit time; reduce oxidative stress; reduce toxic and carcinogenic load; fruits minimize dietary antigens/ allergens to enhance immunity | 749 |
| **Enzyme and Digestive Support** | | |
| **Acidophilus, high potency, refrigerated, assayed, 1/4-1 tsp, 2 times a day | reduces carcinogenic intestinal bacteria and optimizes biological terrain/intestinal flora | 762 |
| **Coenzyme Q10, 50-100 mg tablets, total of 300-600 mg daily | immune stimulation, antioxidant, antitumor | 766 |
| **Enterically coated digestive enzymes (only available by prescription), potencies vary, 3-10 pills, 3 times a day between meals | break fibrin coat of cancer cells, especially indicated in pancreatic and liver involvement or GI tract cancers; contraindicated with certain other therapies, consult your physician | 928 |
| **High-potency digestive enzymes with plant- and/or animal-based protease, amylase, and lipase; potencies vary, 1-3 pills, 3 times daily with meals | optimize digestion, energy, and metabolism; especially indicated in pancreatic and liver involvement or GI tract cancers | 928 |
| **Food Concentrates** | | |
| **Food concentrates with cancer protective qualities (broccoli, soybean, carrots, thick-skinned berries, legumes, figs, vegetables in the mustard family) | antitumor | — |
| **Liver concentrates or extracts; doses vary with manufacturer | source of small amounts of iron; important in advanced cancer and with anemic patients | — |
| **Protein powder with free-formed amino acids and other nutrients; 1-2 scoops twice a day | source of free amino acids, easily digested with minimal strain on liver and GI tract; especially important for patients with wasting | 762 |

*Continued*

# Dr. Milner's Generalized Model for Cancer Treatment (cont.)

| STRATEGY | DOSAGE/ KEY COMPONENTS | FOR MORE INFORMATION see page # |
|---|---|---|
| **Maitake mushroom extract "D" fraction, beta 1,3 glucans | active constituent in maitake mushrooms; immune function enhancer; dosage variable | 833 |
| *Beta 1,3 glucans, 2.5 mg, derived from the cell wall of baker's yeast: take 1 tablet, 3X daily with meals | enhances immune response and macrophage activity, protects against radiation, works as antioxidant, aids tissue repair | — |
| *Lactoferrin: 350 mg, 2-4 daily, before bedtime | binds iron (a strong free radical), absorbs excess iron, deprives bacteria of iron, improves intestinal bacterial flora, helps regulate immune system, improves CD4 cell counts | — |
| *Modified citrus pectin: 10-15 g daily, or 1 tsp (4 g), 3X daily | inhibits cancer (prostate, melanoma) by reducing the tumor cells' adhesion to target organ vascular endothelium | 834 |

## Herb and Plant Extracts

| STRATEGY | DOSAGE/ KEY COMPONENTS | FOR MORE INFORMATION see page # |
|---|---|---|
| ***Antiparasitic herbs (clove, green walnut hulls, wormwood) 1-2 tsp as tea 3 times a day | kills parasites | — |
| **Astragalus, 500 mg, 2-3, 3 times a day between meals | immune enhancement | 813 |
| ***Bromelain, 1000-3200 units, 2-3 with meals, especially if using shark cartilage | breaks cancer coat, anti-inflammatory | — |
| **Cat's claw, 1000 mg, 3 times a day between meals | immune enhancement | 814 |
| **Green concentrates including wheat grass, chlorella, other green plants, with herbs, bulk fiber, and anticancer food concentrates, 9 g daily | immune enhancement, detoxification and toxin neutralization, adaptogenic and antitumor effects | 809 |
| ****Echinacea*, 500 mg, 3 times a day, alternate weeks or avoid completely | immune enhancement, some controversy of efficacy with cancer and AIDS | 815 |
| **Flaxseed oil (organic), 1-2 tbsp daily | prostaglandin and immune modulation | 768 |
| **Genistein, 1000 mg, 2-3 times a day | anticancer agent in soybean; you can get the same by eating large amounts of tofu and soy products daily | 824 |

| STRATEGY | DOSAGE/ KEY COMPONENTS | FOR MORE INFORMATION see page # |
|---|---|---|
| **Grape seed extract, 50 mg, 1-3 daily | potent antioxidant; do not use this as an alternative to other proven antioxidants (selenium and vitamins A, C, and E) | 822 |
| *Hoxsey-like formula (red clover, stillingia, potassium iodide, phytolacca, et al) 1 tsp in hot water 3-4X daily | shifts sodium/potassium ratio; antitumor effects; blood and lymphatic purification | 827 |
| **Silymarin (in liver cancer), 200 mg 3X daily, between meals | liver support and potent liver antioxidant and detoxifier | 835 |
| ***Taheebo tea, 1 tsp as tea, 3X daily | immune enhancement | — |

## Homeopathy

| | | |
|---|---|---|
| *Commonly indicated homeopathic medications | Arsenicum, Carcinocin, Conium, Lachesis, Phytolacca, Viscum Album, for organ drainage; mixed low-potency formulas, or remedies treating any inherited or acquired miasms. Treat cancer by stimulating the patient's immune response to destroy cancer cells. Especially effective at the lower potencies of 3C to 9C | — |

## Hormones

| | | |
|---|---|---|
| *Adrenal optimization with DHEA, if needed, 5-25 mg daily | most studies show DHEA to be cancer-protective; doses higher than 25 mg may cause acne or irreversible hair growth and liver tumors | 939 |
| ***Melatonin optimization, if needed, 0.5-6 mg daily | bolsters antioxidant and immune responses, anticancer effects | 941 |
| *Thyroid extract, if needed, with glandular T3/T4, synthetic T4 or natural time-released T3; dosage variable | optimal thyroid function essential in battling cancer; a low metabolic rate slows the immune response | 944 |
| Thymus extract, variable dosage, but 1-3 doses, 3X daily is typical | stimulates immune function | 944 |

## Hyperthermia

| | | |
|---|---|---|
| ***Raising core body temperature | patients must be strong in their stage of disease to tolerate this therapy; raising the core temperature enhances the immune response if done safely and under proper supervision | 998 |

*Continued*

# Dr. Milner's Generalized Model for Cancer Treatment (cont.)

| STRATEGY | DOSAGE/ KEY COMPONENTS | FOR MORE INFORMATION see page # |
|---|---|---|
| **Colon Hygiene** | | |
| *Colonics, enemas (coffee, shark cartilage, or *acidophilus*), wheat-grass implants | cleansing and detoxification; dilation of common bile duct | 949 |
| **Intravenous/Injectable Formulas** | | |
| ***Alavazatos (Metbal) formula | disrupts cancer cell coat/membrane | — |
| ***Glyoxylide (Koch treatment) | oxygenation, tumor-killing activity | 922 |
| ***Iscador | tumor-killing activity | 830 |
| ***Rodaquin | tumor-killing activity | — |
| ***Vitamin B complex, folic acid, B12 | energy for patients with wasting and/or anemia | 784 |
| ***Vitamin C with other vitamins and minerals | antioxidant, detoxifier, antitumor | 786 |
| **Misc. Agents** | | |
| ***Hydrazine sulfate, 60 mg daily from 4 days to 2 weeks | Cancer inhibition; reduces toxic side effects of chemotherapy | 868 |
| ***Amygdalin (laetrile; B17), 500-1500 mg daily orally, or 1-2 vials, 1-4 times daily, gradually increased, intravenously | anticancer; thiocyanate toxicity can result; patient must be under a doctor's supervision for the monitoring of blood levels | 812 |
| **Mind/Body Therapies** | | |
| *Key Modalities | affirmations, counseling, emotional mind/body release, life purpose, meditation, mental attitude adjustments when appropriate, prayer, guided visualizations, breathing exercises, family support, support group work | — |
| **Shark Products** | | |
| **Shark Cartilage (Benefin, Lane Labs) 6 g per scoop, 2-4 scoops 4X daily on an empty stomach in water, V-8 juice with lemon, or non-citrus fruit juice; avoid cranberry juice | angiogenic inhibition; immune modulation | 863 |

| STRATEGY | DOSAGE/ KEY COMPONENTS | FOR MORE INFORMATION see page # |
|---|---|---|
| **Shark Liver Oil (Immunofin, Lane Labs) 250 mg containing 20% GE lipids, 2-4 capsules, 3X daily with meals | antitumor; reduces harmful effects of radiation; especially indicated for leukemic and lymphatic patients | — |

## Topical Agents

| STRATEGY | DOSAGE/ KEY COMPONENTS | FOR MORE INFORMATION see page # |
|---|---|---|
| ***Black salve, phytolacca oil (pokeroot oil), sanguinaria, shark cartilage, shark liver oil, thuja oil, zinc chloride | works mostly by sclerosing/ hardening/ulcerating or through angiogenic inhibition | — |

## Vitamin and Mineral Supplementation

| STRATEGY | DOSAGE/ KEY COMPONENTS | FOR MORE INFORMATION see page # |
|---|---|---|
| *Potassium (if not taking Hoxsey, with sodium limitation) | increase potassium/sodium ratio | 783 |
| *Vitamin A (fish oil) 25,000 IU, without vitamin D, 1-2 daily, monitored carefully and reduced after 2-4 weeks | antioxidant | 784 |
| *Vitamin A (beta carotene) 20,000-25,000 IU, 1-4 daily, monitored carefully and reduced after 2-4 weeks | antioxidant | 764 |
| *Vitamin and mineral, multiple, high potency, 6-8 daily | protects against deficiencies, especially minerals with antioxidant support in a balanced formula | — |
| **Vitamin antioxidant formula (vitamins A, C, and E, selenium, zinc, silymarin, glutatathione); take 1-4 tablets 3X daily with meals; dosage varies with manufacturer | antioxidant protection | 784, 786, 790, 783, 793, 835, 868 |
| **Vitamin C, 1-5 g, 4 times daily, or to bowel tolerance, with meals | antioxidant | 786 |
| *Vitamin E, 400 IU, 2X/day | antioxidant | 790 |
| **Lipotropic Complex (factors with herbs), take 1-2, capsules 3X daily | liver support, detoxifier | — |
| ***Carotenoids, mixed, dosage varies depending on manufacturer blend | antioxidant with skin and mucous membrane specificity | 764 |

*Continued*

## Dr. Milner's Generalized Model for Cancer Treatment (cont.)

| STRATEGY | DOSAGE/ KEY COMPONENTS | FOR MORE INFORMATION see page # |
|---|---|---|
| ***Calcium D-glucarate; dosage remains experimental | potent carcinogenic detoxifier, lowers extrogen levels | — |
| *Reduced glutathione: 300-700 mg, 3X daily (800-2000 mg daily), on an empty stomach at least 1/2 hour before or 2 hours after food or medication | the primary intracellular defense against oxidative stress and free radicals; chemical detoxification; aids in DNA synthesis and repair. | 868 |

*Therapies designated with * are those used regularly by Dr. Milner, those designated with ** are a protocol shared by Dr. Milner and naturopathic doctor consultant, Dante Ruccio, N.D.C., of Newark, New Jersey (675 North 5th Street, Newark, NJ 07107; tel: 201-485-7656), and those designated with *** are well researched yet not often used by Dr. Milner.

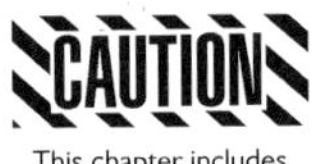



This chapter includes information regarding actual treatments used by Dr. Milner only after his careful diagnosis of each patient. All cancer patients are unique. **Do not administer these treatments to yourself or others.** Discuss these treatments with your physician or other qualified health-care professional. Readers should not interpret this material as therapeutic advice, but should see a physician in all cases.

to find mixtures of natural therapies that reverse disease when possible and optimize each patient's quality of life."

SUCCESS STORY

### Reversing Prostate Cancer

After Bob, aged 67, was diagnosed with prostate cancer (clinical name: prostatic adenocarcinoma), he underwent surgical removal of his prostate, a procedure called radical prostatectomy. For the next decade, Bob lived with the hope that the oncologists had removed all the malignant prostate cells and that his life could return to normal. But in the tenth year after the operation, Bob began to experience severe bone pain.

Laboratory tests revealed high levels of prostate specific antigen (PSA, a cancer marker), indicating the presence of a prostatic tumor. Four months later, bone scans revealed that the prostate cancer had metastasized to the bone; 6 months later, Bob underwent surgical removal of his testes (bilateral orchiectomy) in an effort to halt hormonal stimulation of the cancer. But one week before the surgery, Bob started taking shark cartilage at the rate of 5 g daily.

By the time of the surgery, the excruciating pain in his bones had disappeared. However, the cancer had spread to his shoulders, sacrum (tailbone), left thigh bone and right hip bone. With the cancer spreading so rapidly through his bones, Bob's doctors did not expect him to live more than a few months.

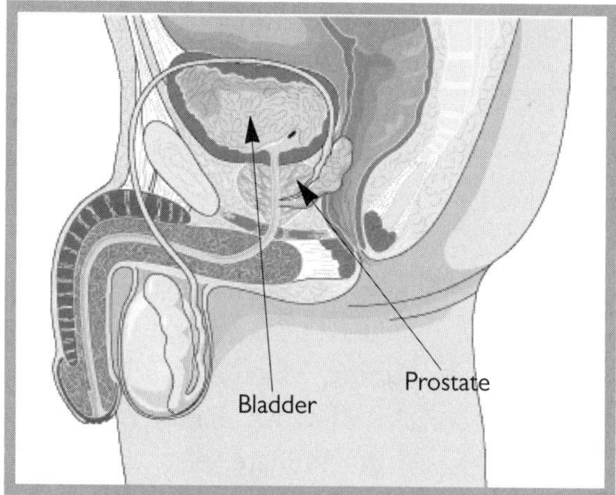

**Figure 14.1—The prostate gland**

After the surgery, Bob increased his shark cartilage intake gradually from 5 g to 60 g. Two months later, he doubled this dosage, and after another 5 months, it was up to 150 g per day. Bob was also taking 250 mg of grape seed extract, twice daily. Within 3 months of beginning this program of intensive supplementation, bone scans revealed that the metastasis had stopped and was beginning to reverse itself.

> ***"It is unfair and wholly unethical to deny a well-informed patient the right to choose a safe combination of natural therapies that may have a beneficial effect on improving quality of life or health outcomes," says Dr. Milner.***

About 9 months later, Bob's oncologist noted that the previously identified sites of metastasis were less diseased or active and that no new lesions were present. All the bone scans indicated general improvement and his PSA levels were 17 times lower than before, a highly encouraging sign.

"By this time, Bob's metastatic prostate cancer had clearly improved according to standard medical tests," says Dr. Milner. "In addition, he was now pain free. We attribute this success to the combination of shark cartilage and orchiectomy, since such results are virtually unheard of with orchiectomy alone." Today more than 3½ years since the metastasis was diagnosed, Bob has survived well beyond what his conventional doctors "expected."

## SUCCESS STORY
### Reversing Soft Tissue Sarcoma

Paul, aged 63, was diagnosed with an aggressive soft tissue sarcoma in his

**Naturopathy** is an umbrella term to describe the original basis of natural, holistic, and alternative medicine, as first formulated by 19th-century European physicians. In essence, it understands that Nature heals, that the body is inherently self-healing, given the appropriate support therapies, such as diet, herbs, nutritional supplementation, exercise, heat and water therapy, massage, bodywork, counseling, and relaxation. Naturopathic medicine emphasizes disease prevention and health promotion. It is currently licensed as a medical profession in 11 states. In a few states naturopaths function as primary care physicians, and insurance companies cover their services.

right leg. This is a type of cancer that affects the tissues, muscles, or connective tissue and is clinically known as a malignant fibrous histiocytoma. Paul underwent chemotherapy and amputation of the right leg and part of his pelvis. Soon after, he developed 2 pelvic tumors against which extensive chemotherapy treatment had no effect.

Four months later, Paul started shark cartilage and a range of nontoxic therapies. After 4 months on this program, Paul's CT scans confirmed a dramatic reduction in his pelvic tumors, which had shrunk from "lemons to walnuts," notes Dr. Milner. Radiation treatment was given a few months later to eliminate these "walnuts."

For the next year, Paul's CT scans were negative and he appeared to be in clinical remission with no sign of cancer. He continued to receive shark cartilage, 60-70 g per day, for 9 months, when his dosage was shifted to 7.5 g per day, mainly for maintenance; Paul also took various supplements, including vitamins C and E, a multivitamin, acidophilus, garlic, cod liver oil, and zinc.

A biopsy late in the following year indicated residual cancer, though many areas of previously cancerous tissue were now clear. During the most aggravated stage of his illness, he was sleeping 20 hours a day. But today, Paul is in fine shape, walking, doing yard work, and playing golf on a regular basis, says Dr. Milner.

"Paul's treatment resulted in a clear reduction in the cancer mass as well as a marked reduction in the normal rate of metastasis," he adds. "With this integrated approach, his life span has already increased by more than 2 years beyond what is 'expected' for this type of cancer, and he remains remarkably healthy today."

## SUCCESS STORY

### Reversing Lymphocytic Lymphoma

Joan, aged 72, was diagnosed with an aggressive form of lymphoma called "B-cell malignant, poorly differentiated, lymphocytic lymphoma." She received no radiation, chemotherapy, or surgery. Instead, Joan chose intravenous infusions—52 in all—of various vitamins and other alternative medications. About 9 months later, Joan started taking shark cartilage at the rate of 120 g daily.

Joan's mood and energy levels soon began to improve. She continued to take the high doses of shark cartilage for another 4 months, after which CT scans confirmed that the lymphoma had disappeared. "By all indications, Joan's energy levels are good and gradually improving," says Dr. Milner.

"Conventional medicine would call this a spontaneous remission, since no 'conventional' treatment was used. We call it a complete remission of lymphoma using shark cartilage and intravenous nutritional therapy and no conventional treatment," adds Dr. Milner.

## Collaboration and Communication among the Medical Specialties

According to Dr. Milner, many of the naturopathic therapies can greatly enhance the action of conventional anticancer treatments while simultaneously minimizing their toxic side effects such as nausea, hair loss, chronic fatigue, and immunosuppression. Dr. Milner tends to view naturopathic medicine and conventional medicine as potentially complementary in treating cancer and his Center for Natural Medicine encourages collaboration and communication among various types of medical professionals.

***According to Dr. Milner, many of the naturopathic therapies can greatly enhance the action of conventional anticancer treatments while simultaneously minimizing their toxic side effects such as nausea, hair loss, chronic fatigue, and immunosuppression.***

"I'm committed to conducting research into health outcomes for cancer patients using natural therapies either alone or in combination with conventional surgery, chemotherapy, and radiation," Dr. Milner notes. "In the cancer treatment field, we are beginning to realize that often you can't stop advanced or aggressive cancers without some strong cell-killing measures. Sometimes that means using tools of conventional medicine, but with the essential *support* of naturopathic medicine."

In the initial consultation, Dr. Milner makes a comprehensive inquiry into the patient's medical history, and examines pathology laboratory and medical records in conjunction with a physical examination. Dr. Milner and his team identify factors that have contributed to the onset of the cancer, such as exposure to toxic substances in the home or work environment.

Next, they search for biological stressors that impair an optimal immune response. Such stressors typically include dietary imbalances, food allergies, exposure to heavy metals (lead, mercury, arsenic, cadmium), depressed hormone function (thyroid, adrenal), and other factors or influences that suppress immune function. "Getting rid of the tumor is only the beginning of comprehensive treatment," Dr. Milner says. "The healing process continues in making sure the cancer never has a chance to come back."

Dr. Milner commonly makes recommendations that incorporate natural therapies, sometimes accompanied by advice to consider surgery, chemotherapy, or radiation. While surgery, radiation, and chemotherapy may have their place in the management of certain types of cancer at certain stages, says Dr. Milner, their potential benefits should be carefully weighed against the harm they usually cause.

When these conventional interventions are known to be ineffective against certain types of cancer or to have no beneficial effect on the quality of life, the risk of side effects and the high cost of therapy make them poor treatment choices, he advises. Dr. Milner urges anyone facing these types of cancer to possibly avoid conventional therapy altogether and to seriously consider natural treatment options, including dietary recommendations, lifestyle changes, supplementation, and specific nontoxic therapies.

"While acknowledging that it is unfair to offer idle hope that an unproven conventional or natural therapy will reverse 'terminal' cancer, patients deserve the right to seek out viable therapies as long as they are fully informed about their strengths and weaknesses as reported in scientific studies," says Dr. Milner. He adds that every cancer patient should have the right to choose something they firmly believe in, particularly when the treatment is nontoxic. "It is unfair and wholly unethical to deny a well-informed patient the right to choose a safe combination of natural therapies that may have a beneficial effect on improving quality of life or health outcomes."

Dr. Milner's experience in working with hundreds of patients fighting cancer has indicated that a patient's *will to live*—a powerful healing force in its own right—is closely tied to their beliefs in the usefulness of the therapies they choose. He finds that when people feel confident about the therapies they choose, they are more likely to obtain significant benefits.

## Nutritional Oncology: A Clean and Vital Diet

Dr. Milner begins his naturopathic anticancer program by having all his patients make changes in their diet. This includes buying organically-grown foods. Our modern food supply is a significant source of exposure to carcinogenic pesticide and insecticide residues in fruits, vegetables, and grains. In addition to being free of pesticides, the nutritional content of organic produce can be substantially higher, containing, for example, more protein[1] and vitamin C[2] than conventionally-grown crops. The mineral content of organically-grown foods is 2-4 times higher, including more boron, copper, chromium, calcium, magnesium, manganese, molybdenum, selenium, and zinc.[3]

Next, Dr. Milner analyzes the patient's diet for total calories, protein, fat, carbohydrate, vitamin, and mineral content and prescribes appropriate supplementation whenever deficiencies or imbalances are indicated. The scientific literature on dietary recommendations for many cancers, especially breast and colon cancer, strongly points to the protective value of a low-fat, high-fiber diet—primarily vegetarian—with no refined sugars or carbohydrates, and with limited salt and avoidance of red meat.

"If the research is correct, then there may be a viral carcinogen in chicken," Dr. Milner says. "Many commercially available animal products are contaminated with hormones, chemical residues, or heavy metals, and these factors tend to compromise our cancer resistance." Dr. Milner is a proponent of a modified vegetarian diet consisting of whole grains, legumes, a wide variety of vegetables, fruits, nuts, seeds, and occasional servings of fish.

***"Many commercially available animal products are contaminated with hormones, chemical residues, or heavy metals," says Dr. Milner, "and these factors tend to compromise our cancer resistance."***

For information on **carcinogens** in foods, see Chapter 25: What Causes Cancer?, pp. 568-574; for more on **exercise benefits**, see Chapter 33: Physical Support Therapies, pp. 1003-1005; for more on **oxygen** and the cancer process, see Chapter 32: Enhancing Whole-Body Metabolism, pp. 915-927; for psychological factors and **stress**, see Chapter 25: What Causes Cancer?, pp. 613-615.

## Moderate, Regular Exercise Aids Cancer Recovery

Dr. Milner advocates regular exercise for cancer patients, encouraging them to move as much as possible, short of excessive strain or energy depletion. Physical activity helps move the lymph through its channels and thus aid detoxification. In general, when a person participates in a regular form of movement such as walking or calisthenics, their system is more capable of neutralizing poisons and eliminating toxins from the fatty tissues, explains Dr. Milner.

Lower rates of cancers have been observed among people who engage in regular physical exercise.[4] For example, former college athletes have lower rates of cancers of the breast and reproductive system,[5] people engaged in a regular walking program have increased natural killer (NK) cell activity;[6] and cyclists have significantly increased NK activity when compared to less active people.[7]

Similar results have been observed in elderly women who followed regular exercise routines: the tumor-cell-killing activity in these women is significantly higher compared to their more sedentary counterparts.[8] Vigorous exercise raises the body temperature and increases the production of pyrogen, a special substance that enhances the function of white blood cells.[9]

***"By increasing the oxygen supply to body tissues, you are more likely to repel cancer cells, which tend to proliferate in a low-oxygen environment," says Dr. Milner.***

If the cancer patient is able to exercise, Dr. Milner recommends a program of moderate walking or aerobics with the level of exercise intensity set slightly below the target aerobic heart rate for 20-30 minutes every other day. If the individual is able to do aerobic exercise, then Dr. Milner recommends Oxygen Multistep therapy developed by Dr. von Arden of Germany; this program "seems to permanently improve oxygen uptake and utilization at a cellular level," Dr. Milner says. "By increasing the oxygen supply to body tissues, you are more likely to repel cancer cells, which tend to proliferate in a low-oxygen environment."

Dr. Milner explains that Oxygen Multistep therapy involves taking a packet of nutrients that increases cellular uptake and utilization of oxygen before exercise. The patient, under physician supervision, then exercises at varying rates depending upon the condition and health status. While exercising, the patient receives high flow rates of oxygen orally delivered through a bag-mask device. Dr. Milner monitors the patient's heart rate and function on an electrocardiogram screen; the exercise period typically lasts 10-20 minutes and is repeated afterwards as needed.

If the individual's condition is too weak, aerobic exercise is inadvisable, says Dr. Milner, but substitutions can be made, such as: (1) deep breathing; (2) stationary range of movement and resistance exercises (weights, pull-ups); and (3) relaxation/stretching movements, such as yoga postures or tai chi. "I tell all my patients to schedule exercise, relaxation, or meditation in their daily routines because it's just as important as every other aspect of therapy."

## The Importance of Reducing Stress as a Cancer-Fighting Approach

Exercise is important to the cancer patient's ability to handle stress, comments Dr. Milner. Aerobic exercise on a regular basis can reduce both anxiety and depression, probably by releasing endorphins, the natural opiate-like compounds, into the bloodstream.[10,11] Animals exposed to uncontrollable stress show low NK activity and increased susceptibility to tumors.[12]

"People who exercise are frequently amazed by how much more relaxed they feel afterward," says Dr. Milner. "This is an effective way to let off tension and directly promote your cancer-fighting ability at the same time. The development of life-threatening illness is a major stressor all on its own, so people diagnosed with cancer need to cultivate their own regular program of therapeutic relaxation." For example, a hot bath by candlelight or a walk in the park or woods can provide comfort and relaxation at the end of a pressure-filled day.

> ***"The development of life-threatening illness is a major stressor all on its own, so people diagnosed with cancer need to cultivate their own regular program of therapeutic relaxation," says Dr. Milner.***

One's emotional attitude and psychological stance are important, too, says Dr. Milner. People who feel helpless in the face of cancer, who engage in passive ways of coping, are more likely to produce *excessive* amounts of the brain's natural painkiller chemicals, the endorphins.[13] The danger here is that research shows that this oversecretion of endorphins suppresses the cancer-fighting activity of NK cells and increases the likelihood of tumor growth.[14] The more positive your mental attitude, the better your immune system fights cancer, yet this does not mean that one should deny emotions such as sadness or anger. "The key to emotional healing involves a balance of expressing one's feelings, getting them out in the open, as it were, and cultivating a positive, enthusiastic view of life," says Dr. Milner. He encourages his patients to adopt an assertive attitude

## The Importance of a Fighting Spirit

A 15-year study of breast cancer patients concluded that those who showed a fighting spirit and a healthy sense of denial (e.g., downplaying the gravity of the situation) had significantly better survival rates than those who held on to a helpless-hopeless attitude or one of stoic acceptance.[16] Dr. Milner adds that it is crucial that the patient have a loving, supportive home life and participate in some form of counseling with a cancer support group. "Any issues standing in the way of the patient's healing must be addressed and processed until they are resolved," Dr. Milner says.

or "fighting spirit" toward their condition, even when faced with daunting odds. Studies found a significant association between passive or helpless coping styles and poor survival rates among cancer patients.[15]

### Dr. Milner's Nutritional and Botanical Program to Reverse Cancer

**Cat's Claw**—Recent studies indicate that this plant contains substances that have immune- and digestion-enhancing properties including several types of antioxidant compounds.[17] Dr. Milner often advises his cancer patients to take between 3-6 g of cat's claw per day, but, for more advanced cases of cancer, he may substantially increase the dosage.

QUICK DEFINITION

The **thyroid** gland (located near the trachea in the throat) is the body's metabolic thermostat, controlling body temperature, energy use, and, for children, the body's growth rate. The thyroid hormones T3 (triiodothyronine) and T4 (thyroxine, accounting for almost 93% of the thyroid's hormones which are active throughout the body) are regulated by thyroid-stimulating hormone, or TSH, secreted by the pituitary gland in the brain. Thyroid-related health problems include chronic fatigue, an inability to lose weight, anemia unrelieved by iron supplementation, feeling cold in the extremities even in warm climates, lethargy, concentration and memory problems, depression, skin problems, swelling and fluid retention, and chronic muscle pain and weakness, among others.

**Flaxseed Oil**—This is a highly unusual plant oil because it contains a high concentration of the "good fats" known as the omega-3 fatty acids: close to 60% of flaxseed oil is alpha-linolenic acid (ALA), an omega-3 which helps us maintain the levels of health-promoting eicosanoids and inhibits the production of tumor-promoting eicosanoids. Dr. Milner's typical dosage is 1-2 tablespoons of flaxseed oil mixed in ¼ cup of fat-free cottage cheese.

CAUTION

Because flaxseed oil is highly unsaturated, it readily oxidizes when exposed to the open air. For this reason, it has a short shelf life. It must be bought as fresh as possible and kept tightly sealed in a 500-ml bottle in the refrigerator. Never heat or cook the oil. If these guidelines are not followed, the resulting rancidity makes this oil unfit for human consumption. If the oil becomes highly oxidized, it can be dangerous for cancer patients.

**Thyroid Extract**—Dr. Milner generally recommends using time-released thyroid extracts on a regular basis for his cancer patients who show consistent midday oral temperatures less than 98.6° F. This lowered metabolic rate compromises the body's immune regulating mechanisms. Dr. Milner's typical prescription is glandular thyroid (1/4-2 grains), or L-thyroxin (0.125-0.2 mg), or natural time-released T3 (7.5 mcg or more, every 12 hours). This third therapy is dosed cyclically; the dose is increased by 7.5 mcg every 2 days until the patient's temperature is 98.6° F. Then the medicine is gradually reduced as the new 98.6° F temperature is maintained, Dr. Milner explains.

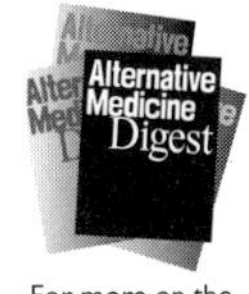


For more on the thyroid, see "The Hidden Reason," #16, pp. 52-56.

**Thymus Extracts—**Thymosin and other thymus extracts stimulate immune function and are best combined with enzyme treatment. The dosage varies depending upon the manufacturer, but generally 1-3 doses, taken 3 times daily, is advisable, says Dr. Milner. Certain extracts have been researched and proven to be more effective than others, he adds.

**Hydrazine Sulfate—**This is an experimental therapeutic agent which seems to retard or inhibit the loss of protein or body mass caused by cancer, while at the same time exerting indirect antitumor effects. Most of the research on hydrazine sulfate shows that the substance leads to significant subjective improvements (notably in controlling pain and nausea) as well as favorable clinical outcomes for many types of cancer.[18] Use cautiously. Dr. Milner generally advises using it for short periods of about 2 days to 2 weeks only at a time, then at 60 mg once daily from 1-2 weeks.

**Green Concentrates—**Dr. Milner typically advises patients to have 3 servings daily (or 1 large dose of 9 g) of 1 or a combination of the following green "superfood" concentrates (or phytogreens): blue-green algae, spirulina, wheat grass, watercress, or Green Magma. If the stool turns green or diarrhea develops, decrease the intake frequency.

**Castor Oil—**Tumors and cysts of all sizes may be reduced in size or eliminated with castor oil packs. In a study of the immune-stimulating properties of castor oil packs conducted on 36 people, those treated with castor oil packs showed significant improvement in the total production of lymphocytes and other immune cells.[19] Dr. Milner cautions that local warm applications increase circulation and may stimulate tumor growth.

**Amygdalin (Laetrile)—**"Amygdalin, although not licensed by the FDA for sale in the U.S., deserves to have a regular place in cancer therapy," says Dr. Milner. "Amygdalin converts into thyiocyanate and blood levels need to be monitored regularly to avoid toxicity. Optimal blood serum thyiocyanate levels should be 3-7%."

**Vitamin C**—Dr. Milner usually starts patients on vitamin C at between 5 g and 10 g per day, then increases it until bowel tolerance is attained. The dosage is then reduced to just below that level and maintained for several months or more. Intravenous vitamin C is also used as part of Dr. Milner's aggressive naturopathic strategy when cancers are unresponsive to other therapeutic combinations.

**Vitamin E**—This fat-soluble vitamin, one of the body's primary agents for protecting cell membranes, is also among the major nutrients required for a strong immune response.[20] Dr. Milner generally recommends the succinate form of vitamin E at 400 IU taken twice a day.

**Beta Carotene**—Beta carotene, a key antioxidant and precursor to vitamin A, has repeatedly been shown to enhance the activity of natural killer cells and other immune cells against tumors.[21,22,23] Dr. Milner often recommends cancer patients take 20,000-25,000 units of beta carotene 4 times a day, for a total daily intake of 80,000-100,000 units, reducing the dose after 2-4 weeks. He advises medical monitoring for carotenemia (excess carotene accumulation that may cause the skin to turn yellow) based on blood work and physical examination.

**B Complex**—Deficiencies of any one or more of the B vitamins inhibit the immune system's ability to fight cancer.[24,25] Cancer patients are frequently deficient in folic acid, which has been shown to inhibit the growth of chemically induced tumors.[26] Dr. Milner often uses B complex for maintaining optimal functioning of the immune and nervous systems and to reinforce the effects of vitamin B1 and B3.

**Zinc**—Dr. Milner will occasionally recommend zinc as a temporary supplement (30-60 mg per day), but only if the person shows definite signs of a zinc deficiency. The reason is that excessive zinc can induce a copper deficiency and copper is essential to proper functioning of a wide range of immune cell types, including antibody-forming cells, T helper cells, and macrophages, all of which may help the body defend against cancer.[27] Like selenium, zinc supports many aspects of the immune system, and its deficiency can potentially make us more vulnerable to certain cancers.[28]

## A Special Focus on Shark Cartilage's Therapeutic Benefits

Since 1991, Dr. Milner has investigated the therapeutic potential of shark cartilage and has advised numerous cancer patients concerning its use. Tumors must be supported by nutrients, hormones, and other factors provided through the bloodstream. With these nutrients, they are able to form new blood vessels a (process called angiogenesis), which is essential to the spread of cancer cells. Shark cartilage has been shown to inhibit angiogenesis both in test-tube conditions and in living organisms.[29] Consequently, many investigators agree that anti-angiogenic agents are promising anticancer therapies.[30]

In 1996, Dr. Milner reported on the results of 21 cancer patients using shark cartilage in combination with other natural therapies. Cancers included prostate (7), breast (5), brain (4), and 5 other cancer types. All patients reported beneficial effects of shark cartilage; 5 used shark cartilage and other natural therapies without any other conventional treatment while the rest combined conventional treatment either with shark cartilage alone, or with a blend of shark cartilage and other alternative therapies.

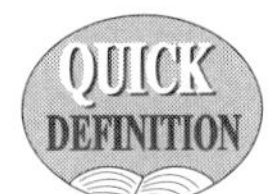


**Prostate specific antigen** (PSA) is a cancer marker, or blood test, for the detection of prostate cancer. A normal reading is 0-4; an elevated reading is anything over 4, with the higher the number the greater the presence of cancer. Ideally, after cancer treatment, the elevated numbers drop (e.g., from 25 to 0.4), indicating that the cancer has been eliminated. If a man is retested some time later and the numbers are again elevated (e.g. to 40), this may indicate that the cancer has recurred in the prostate or spread to the lymph nodes or bone, which are the most common areas of metastasis in prostate cancer.

All the prostate cancer patients in this study showed significant reduction in their prostate specific antigen (PSA) counts. Eleven of 18 patients (61%) with tumors showed a reduction or remission of their tumors. Most of the cancer patients (87%) reported that their quality of life, as measured by energy levels, pain reduction, and mood changes, had improved significantly since beginning the shark cartilage and integrated naturopathic protocols.[31]

Dr. Milner is careful to point out that this study is not formal proof that shark cartilage can reverse cancer. "This is a retrospective, non-randomized pilot study to see what kinds of responses patients were reporting after receiving shark cartilage," he notes. "Our objective was not to see if shark cartilage is inherently valid, but to see if there is some indication of a response. Since there was, we have begun to track patients who are being treated successfully with shark cartilage alone or in combination with other natural therapeutics to determine if there's a consistent pattern of response."

Much of the controversy surrounding the potential clinical benefits of shark cartilage has centered around the question of whether or not anti-angiogenic compounds are absorbed in an intact form via the intestinal tract. "Anti-angiogenic compounds are typically large protein structures," says Dr. Milner. "Conventional theory holds that the size of these proteins makes them too large to be absorbed intact through the gastrointestinal tract. We now have definitive evidence that many large molecules are absorbed intact from the human intestine into the bloodstream under normal conditions."[32]

***"I invite all physicians and their patients to share their successful case stories, as well as their treatment protocols, in order to help us expand our database," says Dr. Milner.***

No research as yet has been conducted on any of the phenolic compounds or other chemical constituents in shark cartilage such as its high concentrations of calcium. "These substances may play a role in angiogenesis inhibition or tumor reduction by other currently unidentified mechanisms," Dr. Milner says. "Additionally, we now know that the mucopolysaccharide content in shark cartilage is a potent immune modulator. "Further study and clinical trials using shark cartilage are warranted as a single therapeutic intervention in the treatment of certain cancers."

## Compiling a Database of Successful Outcomes

"The challenge of evaluating mixed natural therapies in medicine is immense," Dr. Milner says. "No one has made the effort to track those people who decide to use alternative therapies, so that's what we're trying to do." Under Dr. Milner's supervision, a comprehensive "health outcomes" database of patients using natural therapies is updated regularly, and individual cancer treatment protocols are being revised as new research data is accumulated. "If physicians adhere to implemented standardized protocols, health outcomes can be scientifically tracked," he says.

The protocols Dr. Milner is developing will be shared with physicians who agree to use them unaltered in exchange for sharing their patient outcomes data with Milner and his colleagues for further study. "This is a practical and effective way of making significant and cost-effective progress in natural medicine cancer research," he says. "I invite all physicians and their patients to share their successful case stories, as well as their treatment protocols, in order to help us expand our database. As data is accumulated, the protocols will be carefully scrutinized and modified." Finally, Dr. Milner notes that if these protocols are standardized and implemented, this could "pave the way to furthering the scientific search for effective natural therapeutics in cancer management."

## CURRICULUM VITAE

# Emanuel Revici, M.D.

Emanuel Revici, M.D., The Revici Life Science Center, Inc.,
200 West 57th Street, Suite 402, New York, NY 10019;
tel: 212-246-5122; fax: 212-246-5711.
Kenneth Korins, M.D., is handling new cases using
Revici therapy at The Revici Life Science Center.

Dr. Revici was first licensed to practice medicine and surgery in Romania in 1921 when he joined the faculty of medicine at the University of Bucharest. From 1937-38, he was sub-director of the Pasteur Institute in Paris, France, where he published 5 articles on lipids in cancer care and the management of pathological pain through the National Academy of Science in France. In 1942, Dr. Revici founded the Institute of Applied Biology in Mexico City, Mexico, then in 1946, the University of Chicago sponsored him to continue his cancer research in the U.S.

**"There are simply no 2 cancers which are alike, just as no 2 individuals are alike," says Dr. Revici. "We are fully entitled to consider my approach not only a highly beneficial treatment which can be offered now for this disease, but even a major step nearer to the solution of the problem of the therapy of cancer."**

In 1947, Dr. Revici founded the Institute of Applied Biology in New York City and obtained a New York State medical license. In 1955, he purchased Trafalgar Hospital in New York City and became chief of the department of oncology; this closed in 1978. In 1961, with the publication of *Research in Physiopathology as Basis of Guided Chemotherapy with Special Application to Cancer*, the American Cancer Society put Dr. Revici's therapy on its infamous list of "unproven methods" and officially blacklisted him. In 1990, the Office of Technology Assessment of the U.S. Congress issued a report on "unconventional" cancer treatments and covered Revici therapy accurately. In addition to his book, Dr. Revici has published at least 30 scientific articles on his approach to cancer.

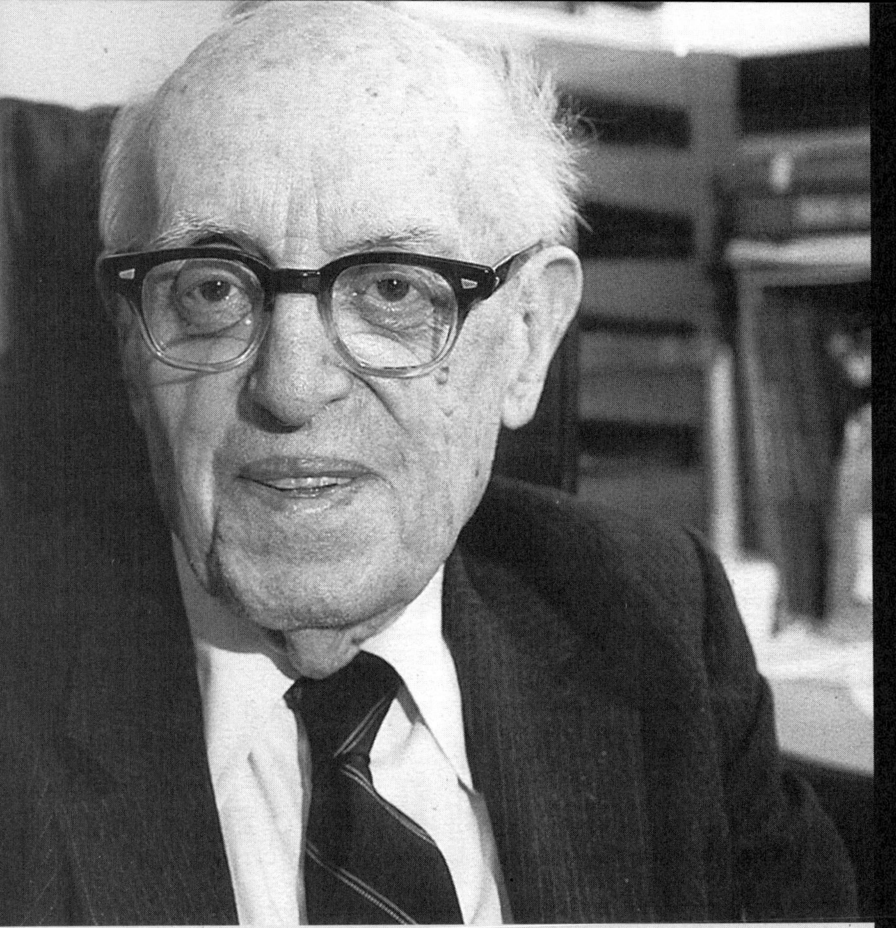

Chapter 15

# *Emanuel Revici, M.D.*

**AN EFFECTIVE APPROACH TO** cancer treatment can be based on a deep knowledge of the body's metabolic processes and which nutrients can most effectively rebalance it, says cancer pioneer Dr. Revici, who uses fatty acids and sterols, enzymes, high-dose selenium, dietary changes, and "biologically guided, nontoxic, true chemotherapy" in its original sense.

Emanuel Revici, M.D., still alive and practicing medicine at age 100 and widely regarded as a major cancer treatment pioneer, summarized his scientific and clinical findings about cancer in 1961 in his *Research in Physiopathology as Basis for Guided Chemotherapy with Special Application to Cancer.* His treatment, he claimed, "when correctly applied, can, in many cases, bring under control even far-advanced malignancies." To support this claim, he presented many cases histories of cancer patients who underwent partial or complete remissions following his therapy.

Dr. Revici concluded: "The results obtained and especially their high proportion, even in far advanced cases, permits a fair judgment of the place of the present form of application of this method in the fight against cancer. Based on these results, we are fully entitled to consider it not only a highly beneficial treatment which can be offered now for this disease, but even a major step nearer to the solution of the problem of the therapy of cancer."[1]

## "A Highly Beneficial Treatment"— The Emanuel Revici Story

Emanuel Revici was born in 1896 in Bucharest, Romania. He graduated at the top of his class from the University of Bucharest Medical School in 1920. Dr. Revici ran a private practice until 1936, at which time he became subdirector of the Pasteur Institute in Paris, France. In 1941, Dr. Revici fled

## Dr. Revici's Biologically Guided Chemotherapy[2]

### For patients with ANABOLIC (STEROL) predominance:

- lipid-bound selenium
- fatty acids (including some obtained from human and animal sources)
- aldehydes
- hydrines (e.g., epichlorohydrin)
- sulfur compounds (e.g., sodium thiosulfate and colloidal sulfur)
- male hormones (testosterone)
- mustard compounds

### For patients with CATABOLIC (FATTY ACID) predominance:

- sterols (e.g., cholesterol)
- alcohols (e.g., butanol)
- female hormones (estrogens)
- amines (e.g. aminobutanol)
- halogens (e.g., iodine)
- metals (iron, mercury, bismuth)

from Nazi-occupied Paris to southern France, lending medical aid to the French Resistance while continuing his research. He relocated that same year to Mexico City, where he set up a free clinic and spent 5 years treating many cancer patients.

During his stay in Mexico City, Dr. Revici attracted the attention of prominent U.S. physicians and medical institutions. In 1946, he was invited to share his research findings at the University of Chicago School of Medicine. The following year, he moved to New York City, where he founded the Institute of Applied Biology, whose primary function was to apply laboratory breakthroughs to patient care as swiftly as possible.

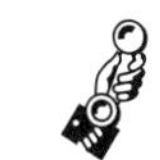

For more information about **Dr. Revici's protocols** for cancer and other diseases, see: *The Man Who Cures Cancer*, William Kelley Eidem (1996), Be Well Books, c/o American Educational Systems, 173 West 81st Street, Lower Level, New York, NY 10024: tel: 212-501-8181; fax: 212-501-8926. His classic work, *Research in Physiopathology as Basis of Guided Chemotherapy with Special Application to Cancer* (1961) is available from the Revici Life Science Center.

## SUCCESS STORY
### Reversing Colon Cancer

Mark, aged 48, had been diagnosed with advanced-stage colon cancer. The cancer spread to the lymph and tissue around the colon and exploratory surgery confirmed the presence of metastatic cancer around the colon. Mark received no chemotherapy or radiation for his condition. Instead, he traveled to New York City to undergo Revici therapy. Within a few weeks of treatment, Mark's energy levels rose, his weight increased, and all signs of poor health disappeared. Some 3 years later, a colonoscopic examination revealed a healthy, normal colon, and CAT scans of the pelvis showed no signs of cancer.

***Dr. Revici found that catabolic agents dramatically reduce the percentage of spontaneous tumors in laboratory animals, while anabolic agents increase the number of animals that develop such tumors.***

## SUCCESS STORY
### Reversing Bone Cancer

At age 34, Tony had undergone above-the-knee amputation of his left leg because of bone cancer. Subsequently, the cancer spread to both lungs and kidneys. With the cancer's progression showing no sign of slowing down, his prognosis was "terminal." Despite this pronouncement, or because of it, Tony decided to undergo Revici therapy. Within a few months, he gained back 20 pounds, always a sign of returning health for a cancer patient. An X ray of Tony's chest showed that the tumors were stabilized in his lungs, while other tests showed that the tumor in his left kidney was decreased in size. Tony also had increased energy and a more positive outlook on life. Seven years later, Tony was reported to be well and without any signs of cancer.

## SUCCESS STORY
### Reversing Lung Cancer

Nancy, aged 62, was diagnosed with adenocarcinoma of the lung. Her cancer was considered inoperable because it had spread to the lymph nodes and was hard to reach surgically. Nancy received 2 courses of radiation therapy then began Revici therapy; she continued it for 5 years with considerable success. Some 6 years after finishing therapy, Nancy continues to do well and has no signs of lung cancer.

## SUCCESS STORY

### Reversing Brain Cancer

After Jane, aged 39, was diagnosed with brain cancer, she underwent surgery to have the tumor removed, but the doctors could not remove all the cancerous tissue. After leaving the hospital, she received a course of 28 radiation treatments that left her unable to move her arms or legs, effectively making her a quadriplegic. In addition, she could not talk or breathe normally, swallow or feed herself. An MRI scan 6 years later revealed a small tumor at the base of her brain.

At this point, Jane underwent Revici therapy and quickly regained her ability to talk. In a few months, she was able to move her arms and legs again. She now feeds herself and has regained normal functioning. By all indications, her brain cancer is in remission.

***Cancer results when the body's defense system is arrested in the lipidic phase, Dr. Revici claims. When this occurs, either fatty acids or sterols are produced in excessive quantities and this, in turn, promotes the development of cancer.***

## TRUE NONTOXIC "CHEMOTHERAPY": BASED ON THE BODY'S METABOLISM

"There are simply no 2 cancers which are alike, just as no 2 individuals are alike," says Dr. Revici. Dr. Revici's primary contribution to oncology has been the development of a nontoxic form of chemotherapy that uses specific preparations of lipids—that is, organic compounds such as fatty acids and sterols—to strengthen and fine-tune the body's cancer-fighting ability. Dr. Revici's approach is founded on a profound knowledge of the body's metabolism.

For more information about **metabolism** and metabolic therapies, see Chapter 32: Enhancing Whole-Body Metabolism for Treating Cancer.

Metabolism is the sum total of all the biochemical processes going on inside the body, and metabolic therapies focus on ways to balance these chemical processes—enabling normal cells to thrive and cancer cells to become depleted and die, or revert back to normal. The therapeutic goal of metabolic therapies is to rebuild and revitalize all of the body's life-sustaining functions, thereby helping to stop and reverse cancer, or to prevent a recurrence.

Metabolism consists of 2 fundamental phases, says Dr. Revici.

**Lipid** is a biochemist's term for a fat, which is one of the 6 basic food groups. Fats and oils are made of building blocks called fatty acids. Of these long-chain molecules (comprising atoms of carbon, hydrogen, and oxygen) the "fatty" end does not dissolve in water, whereas the "acid" end does. Fats are also called triglycerides as they consist of 3 (tri) fatty acid molecules joined to one molecule of glycerol, a kind of sugar. Unsaturated fats required in the diet are called **essential fatty acids**, and include linoleic acid (an omega-6 oil), found in corn and beans, and alpha linolenic acid (an omega-3 oil), found in fish, flaxseeds, and walnuts.

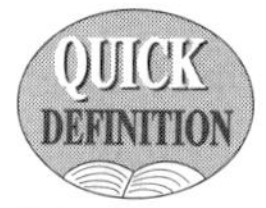


A **steroid** is a large family of similarly configured chemical substances that make up many hormones, body constituents, and, in synthetic form, conventional drugs. Natural steroid hormones are mainly produced in the adrenal gland and gonads and include androgens, progesterones, estrogens, and corticosteroids from the adrenal cortex. Steroids comprise at least 8 different subgroups (such as gonanes, estranes, and androstanes) based on small differences in their chemical structure. Sterols are a type of steroid, and include cholesterol, ergosterol, and sitosterol, among others.

Anabolism is the constructive, building-up phase, fostering growth and order, storage of energy, and production of organic substances such as enzymes, hormones, antibodies, and cell membrane receptors. Catabolism is the destructive phase, in which matter is broken down and energy is used.[3]

All fundamental biochemical processes are either anabolic or catabolic in nature and Dr. Revici regards health as a dynamic balance between these 2 opposing metabolic phases.[4] Certain organic compounds (such as positively charged alcohols, amines and amides) have an anabolic character in the body, while others (negatively charged acids, aldehydes, and ketones) have a catabolic character.[5] Practically any therapeutic agent can be classified according to its anabolic or catabolic character. Vitamins showing catabolic activity are A, D, B6, and B12, whereas vitamins B1, B2, K, E, pantothenic acid, niacin, and nicotinamide have anabolic properties. The ascorbic acid form of vitamin C is neutral.

Ordinarily, the body cycles between anabolic and catabolic phases, but when health begins to decline, this alternating rhythm becomes altered. According to Dr. Revici, it is the sustained predominance of either phase that leads to the onset of illness.

There is one more element central to his thinking. Dr. Revici described the body's defense system in terms of 4 successive phases: (1) enzyme phase, or the breaking down of foreign substances (antigens) by enzymes; (2) the lipidic phase, in which either fatty acids or sterols are produced; (3) the coagulant antibody phase, in which antibodies gather at the site of the foreign substance; and (4) the globulinic antibody phase, in which the foreign substance is fully neutralized and rendered harmless. Cancer results when the body's defense system is arrested in the lipidic phase, Dr. Revici claims. When this occurs, either fatty acids or sterols are produced in excessive quantities and this, in turn, promotes the development of cancer.

If every cancer has either an anabolic or a catabolic character, then the therapeutic strategy is to use substances that counterbalance one or the other. For example, in rats, sodium chloride enhances the growth in transplanted tumors having an anabolic character because of the anabolic activity of both sodium and chloride. However, when 2 catabolic agents, either magnesium or bivalent negative sulfur, are administered to these rats, the noxious action of sodium chloride is completely prevented.[6]

Dr. Revici found that catabolic agents dramatically reduce the percentage of spontaneous tumors in laboratory animals, while anabolic agents increase the number of animals who develop such tumors. Alternating the administration of sulfur and selenium produces the best results for cancer prevention, according to Dr. Revici.

Dr. Revici is among the first research clinicians—if not the first—to discover effective chemotherapy agents that can work and produce only negligible toxicity. In fact, over the years he produced some 100 of his own medicines (and patented many of them) based on isolating and concentrating key catabolic or anabolic components in foods. Dr. Revici has developed medicines from special formulations of selenium, copper, sulfur, zinc, calcium, nickel, beryllium, mercury, lead, and other elements with a general toxicity level less than 1/1000 of these substances in their ordinary form.

His selenium preparation, for example, in which he incorporated a molecule of fatty acid into a bivalent negative selenium molecule, enables him to administer 1 g (1 million mcg) of selenium by injection daily, reportedly with no side effects that would otherwise be expected for so high a dose of selenium. In contrast, selenite (hexavalent-positive selenium) usually is limited to about 100-150 mcg daily when taken orally. These agents

## Anabolic and Catabolic Qualities of Foods and Substances

CATABOLIC (breaking down, digestion): meats, breads, nuts, grain, fried eggs, anything fried, fermented cheese, cherries, cranberries, pasta, tuna fish, fish oils; vitamins A, D, B6, and B12, folic acid, selenium, magnesium, calcium, silver, silicon, lead; testosterone, progesterone, epinephrine; surgery, radiation, chemotherapy (depending on type)

ANABOLIC (building up, cell growth): dairy, fruits, sugar, green leafy vegetables, poached/boiled eggs, soy sauce, fresh cheese, chocolate, alcohol, coffee, black tea, butter, honey, fresh fish, olive, safflower, or corn oil; vitamins B1, B2, B3, B5, E, K, and zinc, rutin, sodium, potassium, chromium, iron, mercury, bismuth, iodine, fluorine, chlorine, cortisone, insulin, estrogen, codeine, cocaine, morphine, aspirin, caffeine, chemotherapy (depending on type).

are lipids or lipid-based compounds, not dissolvable in the blood, that can travel in the bloodstream to cancerous lesions or sites showing a tendency to develop cancers; there they form chemical bonds with lipids, as the lesions are rich in lipids.

In this way, Dr. Revici's anticancer agents show a high degree of "tumor specificity" and are less likely to become concentrated in normal cells or healthy tissues. Lipid-based agents are even capable of penetrating the blood-brain barrier, thus acting against brain tumors; further, the lipids help reduce harmful oxidative processes in normal cells.

Specific kinds of lipid imbalances are the underlying basis for most if not all cancers, explains Dr. Revici. This is not to say they are the primary cause.[7] Instead, the imbalances result in poor internal regulation such that the body's defense system can no longer keep cancer cell growth and multiplication in check. This information enables Dr. Revici to classify cancers into types. The catabolic cancer has a predominance of fatty acids (relative to sterols) and other related factors;[8] the anabolic cancer has a predominance of sterols, resulting in marked cellular changes.[9]

***Dr. Revici is among the first research clinicians—if not the first—to discover effective chemotherapy agents that can work and produce only negligible toxicity.***

Dr. Revici isolated (fractionated) certain active and powerful components in lipids and prepared them as non-water-soluble therapeutic agents. For a catabolic cancer, sterols and other agents with a positive electrical charge (to counteract the negatively charged fatty acids) are used; anabolic tumors can be treated with fatty acids and other agents that raise the metabolic activity of fatty acids.[10] These agents are given either orally or by injection and all are prepared according to Dr. Revici's instructions.

## Intravenously Administered Minerals Penetrate the Cell Membranes

Among the more powerful components of Revici therapy is the use of an organic selenium compound, as well as other mineral-containing compounds that help rebalance the body's chemistry. These mineral elements are administered intravenously in a lipid form to allow for greater penetration of the cell membranes, more efficient transportation in the circulatory system, greater concentration in the tumor, and a slow but sustained therapeutic reaction.

This approach not only allows for megadoses of these compounds to be taken without causing any toxicity, it enables them to serve as tumor-targeting and antiviral agents as well. Dr. Revici's lipid-incorporated selenium is the only form of this mineral that can be taken at the high doses required to maintain adequate cellular levels of selenium without adverse reaction.

Selenium can be toxic when taken in doses greater than 150-200 mcg per day, according to the National Research Council, a division of the National Academy of Sciences. Dr. Revici's form of selenium (he calls it "bivalent negative selenium") is reportedly nontoxic even in huge quantities—up to 1 million mcg, in fact, have been injected without ill effects.[11] This organic selenium complex is usually a combination of the mineral with various lipid compounds, such as the fatty acids of sesame oil. The 1 million mcg level has been used for treating drug addiction; much lower doses, approximately 10,000 mcg, are typically used for treating cancer.

A slightly different selenium compound devised by Dr. Revici was tested by the Imperial Cancer Research Fund and Westminster Hospital in London, England, against various tumors in animals. This selenium compound was shown to be active against early tumor growth, leukemia, and lung and liver metastases; when the compound was studied for potential toxicity (both acute and chronic), the dosage range within which antitumor activity was present was still below the toxic dose.[12]

***While Revici therapy may be given to destroy or reduce tumors, its fundamental use is to fine-tune metabolic processes that have allowed the growth of tumors.***

While Revici therapy may be given to destroy or reduce tumors, its fundamental use is to fine-tune metabolic processes that have allowed the growth of tumors. It's important to remember that chemotherapy often fails to kill *all* the cancer cells, rendering those that survive highly resistant to further treatment. Dr. Revici discourages talk of a "cure" for cancer, particularly as current diagnostic techniques are too gross for detection of micrometastases (microscopic masses of cancer cells that have spread from their original site) that may remain after treatment.

## Know Your Metabolic Cycles Via a Urine Test

The cancer patient typically shows a predominance of either the anabolic or catabolic phases in their metabolic cycle. This pattern is reflected in the regular alternation between alkalinity (anabolic tendency) and acidity (catabolic tendency) in the body fluids, most notably, in the urine. To map out these characteristic cycling patterns and detect changes resulting from therapy, Dr. Revici relies on a urine pH test. Dr. Revici favors the urine over the blood test because it is quick, easy, and accommodates a wider range of pH values.

To test the pH of the urine, one puts a few drops of the test solution in a sample of urine which then changes the color of the urine. Placing the colored urine inside a device called a colorimeter can measure the exact wavelength of light coming from the color and correlate that to an exact pH. In this case, red indicates catabolic, green indicates anabolic.

Normally, the anabolic phase predominates at night, which is why most people show a green urine test in the morning; during the day, as metabolic processes accelerate and shift toward a catabolic phase, the urine turns more acidic, showing a red test result. Dr. Revici's cancer patients are instructed to take their own urine samples at home and to keep a record of results. If the patient is not cycling from acid to alkaline, then a problem exists; improper cycling calls for adjusting or supplementing the medication.

## A Progressive Approach Validated by His Medical Peers

Several independent studies have validated Dr. Revici's conclusions. In 1984, Eduoardo Pacelli, M.D., a physician practicing in Naples, Italy, presented his findings on the use of Revici therapy with 372 cancer patients representing 6 different types of cancers. None of the patients studied were considered curable at the start of treatment. Of these patients, 186 had lung cancer. Revici therapy produced a cesssation in the coughing up of blood for 75% of the lung cancer patients, a pain reduction or elimination for 80%, and a regaining of proper body weight after 3 months for 75%.

While the lung cancer patients had been expected to survive for only 80 days, their average survival under Revici therapy was doubled to 172 days; however, 45% survived well beyond the date Dr. Pacelli's report was filed.

Of stage IV breast cancer patients (53), 80% received either pain reduction or elimination with a doubling of survival time to 180 days. For patients with intestinal cancers (57), life expectancy jumped from an average of 60 days to 245 days, with 21 patients outlasting the study. About 66% experienced major pain reduction, 85% found their persistent fevers went away, and 70% saw their excess abdominal fluid clear up.

Uterine cancer accounted for 27

patients. Their life expectancy had been estimated at 90 days, but under Revici therapy, this extended to 270 days, with some outlasting the study. In addition, 71% experienced a significant pain reduction and a doubling in their quality-of-life index from 35 to 70 (out of 100). Results of an equivalent nature were obtained for patients with liver and stomach cancers.

These were impressive results considering that normally Dr. Revici prefers the administration of his multifaceted therapy much earlier in the development of cancer, as he explained in a 1955 monograph, *The Control of Cancer with Lipids:* "It is our feeling that the method of cancer chemotherapy that we are utilizing ought to be applied in cases of cancer as soon as possible after the diagnosis has been determined. Generally, we believe that it is preferable to apply the method before, rather than after the disease has reached the systemic phase."[13]

Another clinical trial of his methods was conducted in Belgium by Professor Joseph Maisin, director of the Cancer Institute of the University of Louvain and president of the International Union against Cancer, on 12 advanced cancer patients. Dr. Maisin reported dramatic improvements in 9 of the 12 (75%), including the regression of tumors and metastases.[14]

Seymour Brenner, M.D., a board-certified radiation oncologist practicing in New York City, examined the medical records of 10 patients treated by Dr. Revici. In presenting these cases at the March 1990 meeting of the Advisory Panel for the U.S. Office of Technology Assessment, Dr. Brenner publicly stated that he believed these 10 patients to be examples of successful treatment with Revici therapy, citing evidence of tumor regression, survival greater than expected, and enhanced quality of life.[15] In 1996, Dr. Brenner declared: "Dr. Revici has cured many people who were otherwise considered incurable. It is my professional opinion that his medicines have worked for many of the patients whose records I have examined."

Even more convincing is the fact that Dr. Brenner allowed Dr. Revici to treat him for elevated prostate specific antigen (PSA), a precursor of prostate cancer. Dr. Brenner's PSA at the time was 6.2 (less than 4 is normal); after taking Dr. Revici's medications for one year, his PSA dropped to 1.6 with "no apparent ill effects." After being off the medicines for sev-

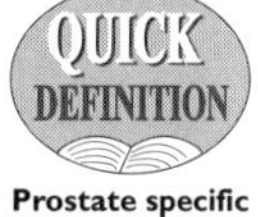


**Prostate specific antigen** (PSA) is a cancer marker, or blood test, for the detection of prostate cancer. A normal reading is 0-4; an elevated reading is anything over 4, with the higher the number the greater the presence of cancer. Ideally, after cancer treatment, the elevated numbers drop (e.g., from 25 to 0.4), indicating that the cancer has been eliminated. If a man is retested some time later and the numbers are again elevated (e.g. to 40), this may indicate that the cancer has recurred in the prostate or spread to the lymph nodes or bone, which are the most common areas of metastasis in prostate cancer.

eral years, Dr. Brenner's PSA remained low and healthy at 2.5.[16]

The largest study of Dr. Revici's work to date was conducted by Robert Ravich, M.D., who worked with Revici at his Institute of Applied Biology. Dr. Ravich's study focused on 1,047 cancer patients who were treated at the Institute between 1946 and 1955. Most were either "far advanced" or "terminal" cases and had already been treated by conventional means, but without success. Accordingly, the majority in this study population were expected to die. When they were treated with Revici therapy, 206 responded well to the treatment, and of these, 100 had both favorable objective and subjective responses.[17]

Biochemist Gerhard Schrauzer, Ph.D., in a letter to the State of New York defending Dr. Revici's reputation, noted that he is an "innovative medical genius, outstanding chemist and a highly creative thinking [person] ... Dr. Revici deserves credit for having discovered pharmacologically active selenium compounds of very low toxicity ... The National Cancer Institute has recognized the importance of selenium only within the past few years. Would one thus not have to conclude that Dr. Revici, in this one instance, was 40 years ahead of his time?"[18]

## Timing the Intake of Supplements in Revici Therapy

Medications and supplements work better at certain times of the day than others because of the body's metabolic cycles. If a person's biological rhythms are found to be cycling improperly, the Revici practitioner adjusts the dose of the medications to shift them appropriately. Normally, one goes through an anabolic and a catabolic phase each day. Therapeutic agents classified as catabolic should be taken during a person's catabolic phase, usually in the daytime. Similarly, anabolic substances should be taken during a person's anabolic phase, usually at night. If the urine test results indicate inappropriate pH changes, the supplementation pattern should be changed accordingly.

The term **pH,** which means "potential hydrogen," represents a scale for the relative acidity or alkalinity of a solution. Acidity is measured as a pH of 0.1 to 6.9, alkalinity is 7.1 to 14, and neutral pH is 7.0. The numbers refer to how many hydrogen atoms are present compared to an ideal or standard solution. Normally, blood is slightly alkaline, at 7.35 to 7.45; urine pH can range from 4.8 to 7.5, although normal is closer to 7.0.

Dr. Revici advises most patients to stop their former supplementation programs so that their bodies can begin cycling properly. The use of high-dose vitamins—except for those prescribed by Dr. Revici—is generally discouraged because high-dose nutrients can shift the metabolic phase and stop the action of the therapy by biochemically overwhelming the cells. If supplements are used in a kind of "shotgun" fashion, i.e., not specifically tailored to the individual's needs, the resulting interactions may cancel their effectiveness.

## CURRICULUM VITAE

# Robert C. Rountree, M.D.

Bob Rountree, M.D., Helios Health Center, 4150 Darley Avenue, Suite 1, Boulder, CO 80303; tel: 303-499-9224; fax: 303-499-9593.

Dr. Rountree received his M.D. from the University of North Carolina School of Medicine at Chapel Hill in 1980. He subsequently completed a 3-year residency in family and community medicine at the Milton S. Hershey Medical Center in Hershey, Pennsylvania, after which he was certified by the American Board of Family Practice. He augmented his medical training with extensive postgraduate studies in nutritional and herbal pharmacology and neurolinguistic programming. In private practice since 1983, Dr. Rountree co-founded the multidisciplinary Helios Health Center in 1993. Dr. Rountree is the coauthor of *Smart Medicine for a Healthier Child* (Avery, 1994); he hosts "HealthSmart" on the Colorado radio station, KHOW; and he serves as assistant clinical professor in the department of family medicine at the University of Colorado School of Medicine.

***"Most of my patients have already received chemotherapy and radiation, so I must not only treat the cancer, but also the side effects of those orthodox treatments," says Dr. Rountree. "Many people who have had chemotherapy suffer from nutritional deficiencies, since their oncologists do not pay close attention to this issue. One of the greatest virtues of alternative medicine is its ability to greatly diminish, if not eliminate, these side effects and thereby improve the chances for a full and enduring recovery."***

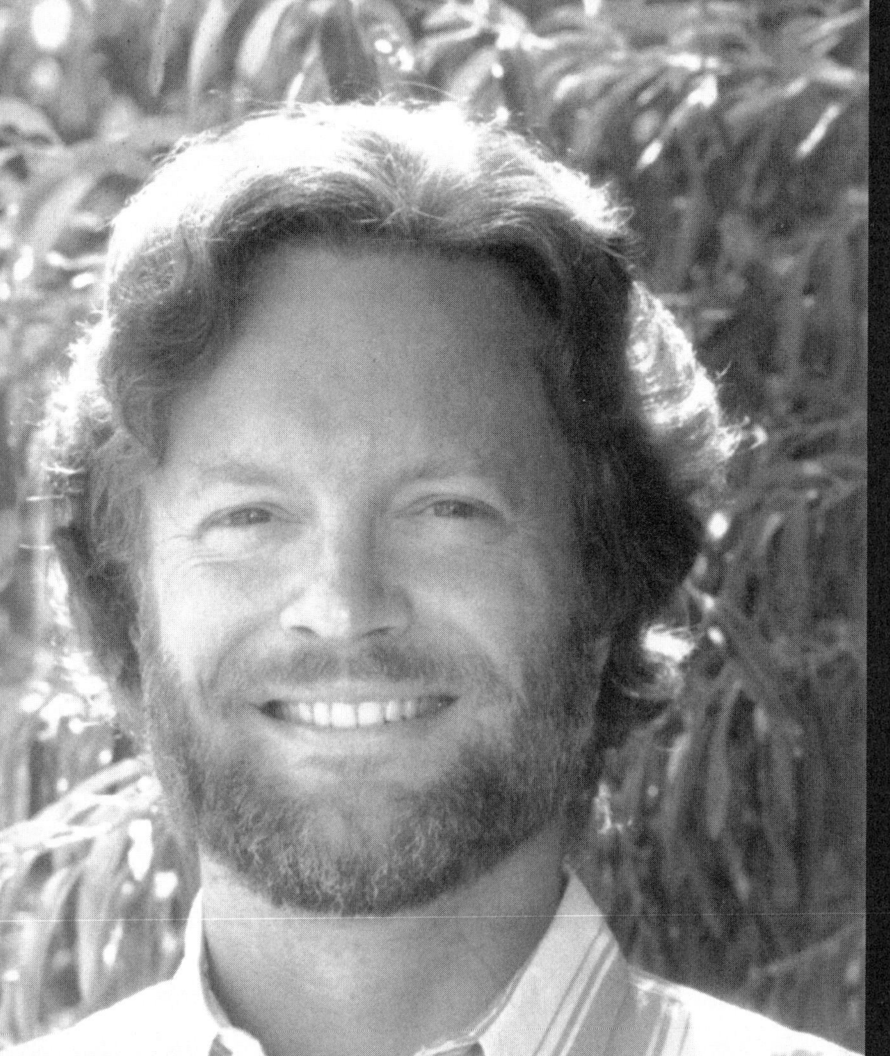

Chapter 16

# *Robert C. Rountree, M.D.*

**FOR CANCER PATIENTS WHO** feel they must undergo conventional treatment, the precise adjunctive use of nutritional and herbal supplements can reverse much of the damage and support the immune system in its struggle to recover, says Dr. Rountree.

Early on in his medical studies, Dr. Rountree became deeply interested in a patient-centered holistic approach to health and healing. Over the years, he has found that this approach allows him to use a wide range of therapies based on their effectiveness for a *specific individual* instead of following rigid protocols for a specific disease. In addition, his certification as a master practitioner of neurolinguistic programming (NLP), which is a psychological modality, has helped him understand his patients' information-processing styles and thus enabled him to communicate more effectively with them. The result is a successful integration of traditional family medicine, nutrition, botanicals, and mind/body medicine.

In general, Dr. Rountree sees 3 kinds of patients at his Helios Health Center. First, there is the patient who has been attending his family practice for regular checkups and comes in with a suspicious finding, such as a lump or skin lesion, suggesting the presence of a tumor. "If they have a large lymph node in the neck, I send them to a surgeon to have it biopsied," says Dr. Rountree. "They then undergo a thorough investigation so we know what kind of tumor it is, whether there is metastasis, and what

# Dr. Rountree's Generalized Model for Cancer Treatment

| STRATEGY | DOSAGE/ KEY COMPONENTS | FOR MORE INFORMATION see page # |
|---|---|---|
| **Dietary Plan** | | |
| Low-fat, high-fiber diet as starting point; move into macrobiotic diet | fat intake no more than 20% of total daily caloric intake, lower if possible; plenty of organically grown grains, legumes, and vegetables | 749 |
| **Supplements** | | |
| Vitamin A | in mycellized form; 5000 IUs in a single drop, 1-4 drops daily, depending on one's clinical status | 784 |
| Vitamin E | in mycellized form; 150 IUs per drop, 150 IUs daily | 790 |
| Vitamin C | 10-12 g/day | 786 |
| Methoxyflavone C | contains 500 mg vitamin C and 500 mg bioflavonoid complex; 2 tablets/day | 324 |
| Basic Preventive™ | 3 tablets, 2X daily | 332 |
| Basic Antiox™ | 4 capsules/day | 332 |
| Maitake mushroom (*Grifola frondosa*) "D Fraction" | 6-9 caplets (500 mg each) and 2 droppersful of liquid D-fraction daily | 833 |
| Green drinks ("supergreen concentrates") | 2-3 tbsp/day, Green Vibrance brand | 809 |
| Bovine cartilage | 12 capsules/day, 750 mg/capsule, Vita-Carte brand | 861 |
| Shark liver oil extract (Alkyrol) | 3 capsules/day, 500 mg/capsule | 333 |
| Modified citrus pectin | 5-15 g/day (15 g= 3 tsp), to stop cancer spread and to stimulate natural killer cells | 834 |
| Soy protein isolate | Genista brand, 30-60 g/day (containing 20 mg genistein/g); or Haelan 851 Platinum formula (fermented soy protein beverage), 8 oz daily | 824 |
| Aloe vera juice | 4-8 oz/day | 812 |
| Coenzyme Q10 | 300-400 mg/day | 766 |
| Flaxseed oil | 1 tbsp/day | 768 |
| Garlic extract | Garlicin brand, 3-6 capsules/day | 818 |

*Continued*

# Dr. Rountree's Generalized Model for Cancer Treatment (cont.)

| STRATEGY | DOSAGE/ KEY COMPONENTS | FOR MORE INFORMATION see page # |
|---|---|---|

## Counterbalancing Toxic Effects of Conventional Treatment and Immune Support

| | | |
|---|---|---|
| Astragalus | 1 dose of 250-500 mg powder, 2-3X/day; as tincture, 1-5 ml/day | 813 |
| Ginger or peppermint tea | relieves nausea; 1 cup as needed | 334 |
| Siberian ginseng | 100-400 mg standardized powder or 1-5 ml of fluid extract, once daily | 821 |
| Shiitake mushroom | 2-3 whole mushrooms in the diet per day or dosage of supplement product | 335 |
| Homeopathic *Arnica Montana* (Leopard's Bane) | 1 dose of 30C after conventional treatment | 335 |
| Homeopathic *Nux Vomica* (Poison Nut) | 1 dose of 6C as needed, after conventional treatment | 335 |
| Homeopathic *Aconite* (Monkshood) | 1 dose 6C-30C, after conventional treatment | 335 |
| Tri-Butyrate | 20-40 g daily, based on 0.5-0.6 g/kg body weight, for severe cases only; the substance, which must be ordered from Sweden under "compassionate use" protocol, starves cancer cells by depleting supplies of glutamine (from Triple Crown America, tel: 215-453-2500) | — |

## Prevention of Childhood Cancers

| | | |
|---|---|---|
| Diet above | | |
| Eliminate tobacco smoke | | 329 |
| Test your house for radon | radon test kit available at hardware stores | 329 |
| Limit exposure to chemical fumes | including fumes from paints, solvents, gasoline, pesticides, glues, oven cleaner, nail polish remover, among other household chemicals | 330 |
| Don't sunburn | use sunscreen that screens both UVA and UVB rays, SPF of 10 or higher; have child wear sunglasses and hat; limit outdoor play in middle of day; supplement with carotene complex | 330 |

implications this has for the rest of the body."

**CAUTION**

This chapter includes information regarding actual treatments used by Dr. Rountree only after his careful diagnosis of each patient. All cancer patients are unique. **Do not administer these treatments to yourself or others.** Discuss these treatments with your physician or other qualified health-care professional. Readers should not interpret this material as therapeutic advice, but should see a physician in all cases.

Second, there is the patient who has come referred by another practitioner. Dr. Rountree not only receives referrals from chiropractors, acupuncturists, and herbalists, but also from local oncologists who regard him as a professional who will cooperate with them. They consult over patients and Dr. Rountree then provides therapies that reduce and even eliminate the toxic side effects of conventional treatments those referred patients have received.

Third, Dr. Rountree sees the patient with advanced cancer who arrives having already fruitlessly explored many options. Perhaps this patient heard him speak on the radio, read about his approach, or heard favorably about him from a friend. "I try to understand where the person is, both objectively and subjectively," Dr. Rountree says. "Is their condition life-threatening? Should I be aggressive in my treatment or should I suggest that they let go?"

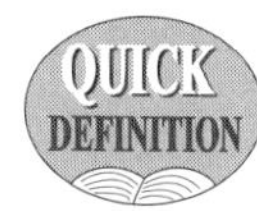


**Staging** in cancer terminology is a relative index of how much cancer exists in the body, its size, location, and containment or metastasis. *Stage I*, the earliest, most curable stage, shows local tumor involvement. *Stage II* indicates some spreading of cancer to the surrounding tissues and perhaps to nearby lymph nodes. *Stage III* involves metastasis to distant lymph nodes. *Stage IV*, the most advanced and least easily cured, means the cancer has spread to distant organs.

Dr. Rountree generally advises his patients to consult with an oncologist to ensure that the cancer is adequately staged—a term that refers to the process by which doctors determine how much cancer there is in the body and where it is located. Staging helps doctors make decisions about treatment and it helps them communicate with each other about specific cases. When an advanced cancer stage has been reached, Dr. Rountree will often propose an aggressive combination of alternative and conventional therapies. "My patients are presented with information on both conventional and alternative therapies. They then make the decision on whether they want to take this or that route. It's not up to me to tell them which way to go—I'm just one player in a bigger game."

## SUCCESS STORY

### Reversing Breast Cancer

Sarah, aged 50, was diagnosed with metastatic breast cancer. Technically, the clinical name for her condition was "infiltrative ductal carcinoma, aggressive cell type." She received conventional treatment that involved a mastectomy, extensive lymph node resection, local radiation therapy, and chemotherapy. By the time she came to Dr. Rountree, Sarah had completed about two-thirds of the chemotherapy and one-sixth of the scheduled radiation treatments.

She reported feeling fatigue, nausea, and painful swallowing from a tongue swollen with canker sores. Sarah's intention was to receive nutritional counseling from Dr. Rountree so she could enhance her immune system function, gain energy, and minimize the harmful effects of her conventional treatments.

Dr. Rountree's treatment approach had 3 components. First, for the oral lesions, he gave her an herbal tincture of *Echinacea*, red root, bee propolis, and the herb usnea (an extract from moss), taken 4 times daily, and zinc lozenges, also taken 4 times daily. Second, for the chemotherapy-induced nausea, Dr. Rountree prescribed a drink made from Japanese salt plum paste (*umeboshi*), kuzu root, and grated ginger, to be taken as needed.

Third, to support Sarah's immune function, Dr. Rountree gave her a series of prepared supplements: Basic Preventive™ (a multiple vitamin/mineral trace element supplement), 3 tablets, twice daily; Methoxyflavone-C (bioflavonoid complex with vitamin C), 1500 mg daily; Green Vibrance, 1 tablespoon daily; reishi/shiitake mushroom standardized solid extract, at the rate of 1 capsule 3 times daily; Betaplex (a carotenoid complex), taken as 1 drop daily; and flaxseed oil, 1 tablespoon daily.

Several months later, Dr. Rountree modified Sarah's program to include shark liver oil (Alkyrol) at the rate of 500 mg, 3 times daily. Maitake mushroom "D fraction," 1 dropperful twice daily, was substituted for the reishi/shiitake mixture.

While Sarah remained on this program, she was able to tolerate the chemotherapy much better, says Dr. Rountree. "Her mouth ulcers resolved, and the nausea responded well to the *umeboshi* drink. Her energy increased, her appetite improved, and she began to gain weight." On her last follow-up visit, Sarah was "doing very well, with good mood and energy," adds Dr. Rountree. Her white blood cell count, which had been low after chemotherapy, was gradually returning to normal.

Her only complaint was a persistent swelling of the lymph nodes of her right arm, a condition that developed after her surgery. To remedy this, Dr. Rountree prescribed 1 dropperful twice daily of horse chestnut seed extract. In addition to the nutritional supplements, Sarah also took tamoxifen. At this point, a blood test for CA 27.29, an antigen associated with breast cancer, was less than 25; normal is anything under 38.

Her natural killer cell activity level, which correlates closely with overall immune system function because it relates to the body's ability to fight off cancer, was a little under normal at 19.02 LUs (lytic units) compared to the reference range of 20-50 LUs, says Dr. Rountree. "As a consequence I recommended she continue with the supplement program adding Genista, a soy protein isolate standardized for genistein content [from Natus Global, Inc.], at the rate of 2-4 scoops daily."

***"My patients are presented with information on both conventional and alternative therapies. They then make the decision on whether they want to take this or that route," says Dr. Rountree.***

## Developing a Full Picture of the Patient's Condition

Nutritional assessments are a key part of Dr. Rountree's initial evaluation of cancer patients. Dr. Rountree examines the skin for evidence of an essential fatty acid deficiency and other signs of malnourishment. The results of blood tests, tissue samples, and dietary questionnaires give him a better picture of what specific types of nutritional and botanical aids will best support the patient.

"Most of my patients have already received chemotherapy and radiation, so I must not only treat the cancer, but also the side effects of those orthodox treatments. Many people who have had chemotherapy suffer from nutritional deficiencies, since their oncologists do not pay close attention to this issue. One of the greatest virtues of alternative medicine is its ability to greatly diminish, if not eliminate, these side effects and thereby improve the chances for a full and enduring recovery."

Patients who have undergone chemotherapy and radiation may also be anemic and require a blood transfusion. If they have lost a substantial amount of muscle mass, they may need a protein supplement along with a gentle exercise routine. Liver damage or damage to the colon after surgery might also be interfering with nutrient absorption."

After Dr. Rountree looks at his patients in this more general way, he then starts zeroing in on more specific needs. If someone comes to him af-

## What Causes Childhood Cancer?

Several factors have been identified as contributing to childhood cancers. These include exposure to: (1) electromagnetic radiation, especially through nearby power lines and transformers, (2) radioactivity or low-level ionizing radiation, such as from contamination of the food supply ; (3) certain medications, particularly chemotherapy drugs and diethystilbestrol, or DES; (4) food additives and pesticides; and (5) cigarette smoke, which most children are exposed to indirectly as "secondhand" smoke.

ter extensive radiation treatment, they may have chronic diarrhea. In this case, he would do a stool analysis for parasites or yeast infections, both of which interfere with recovery. He would ask a series of questions related to the problem, such as: If one is short of breath, is it anemia? If one has developed anemia, did it result from the chemotherapy or from a specific nutrient deficiency? If it is a nutrient deficiency, was it something lacking in the diet or something that interfered with the nutrient's absorption?

The prognosis depends on the type of cancer found, its location, the patient's response to treatment, and overall state of health at the time of diagnosis. Because each person is biochemically unique, the response to the disease and treatment will also be unique. It is vitally important, says Dr. Rountree, to ask the person questions regularly regarding energy levels, nausea, appetite, and general feelings of well-being. He advises all cancer patients: "Relay whatever you find out to the health-care practitioners you have chosen to work with, and make sure each of these professionals knows what the other is doing. The interventions of one can affect those prescribed by the other." This is particularly so in the case of childhood cancers.

Although treating childhood cancer is not Dr. Rountree's prime focus, his experience here has yielded crucial insights into the kinds of treatments appropriate for this age group. In the 1930s, cancer ranked tenth as a killer of children, but today, cancer ranks second only to accidents as a killer of children 14 years and younger; leukemia and cancers of the lymphatic and nervous systems are now the most common childhood cancers.

In light of this, if you have a child who is diagnosed with cancer, you may tend to experience overwhelming feelings of guilt and responsibility, says Dr. Rountree. "Many parents think they probably did something to cause the cancer. They blame themselves endlessly for not seeing it sooner or for not taking adequate steps to educate themselves in cancer prevention. The fact is many cases of childhood cancer cannot be ascribed to any one cause, so blaming yourself is a futile gesture."

Fortunately, much can be done to help children become cancer free and stay that way for a lifetime. It is important, in Dr. Rountree's view, not to assume that once the cancer is gone, the battle is over. Later in this chapter, Dr. Rountree describes his recommendations of nontoxic measures to detoxify the child's body and strengthen the immune system along with suggestions for lifestyle adjustments to keep the child strong into adulthood.

Dr. Rountree urges parents to initially seek out a pediatric oncologist—a medical doctor specializing in childhood cancer—as well as an alternative medical practitioner, to bring out the child's healing potential. The treatment of all cancers is a complex and long-range process. "To help keep your child in remission, carry out frequent follow-up appointments with your doctor, for as long as your doctor suggests," he says. "Cancer can reappear at any time, particularly if the child is stressed-out or depressed, so treatment may need to be reinitiated."

According to Dr. Rountree "herbs, homeopathy, acupressure, diet, and nutritional supplements—all these can be used to enhance your child's immune system and ease the discomforts of conventional cancer therapies, if they are used." One of the greatest virtues of alternative medicine is its ability to greatly diminish, if not eliminate, side effects and thereby improve the chances for a full and enduring recovery."

## Prevention of Childhood and Adult Cancers

The processes that encourage the development of childhood cancer are not well understood, although diet and environmental factors probably play a primary role. Childhood cancers appear to be especially difficult to prevent, says Dr. Rountree, in part because they develop so quickly compared to adult cancers. Children who inherit "immunodeficiency diseases" (such as agammaglobulinemia, or lack of antibodies) are more susceptible to certain cancers; and young children are also particularly vulnerable to the effects of ionizing radiation. For example, infants treated with X rays to reduce an enlarged thymus gland sustain an 83-fold greater rate of thyroid cancer later in life.[1]

If your child is treated with chemotherapy and radiation, the importance of preventing a recurrence becomes greatly magnified, says Dr. Rountree. That is, the child so treated may be at an *increased* risk that cancer will eventually reappear. Consider Hodgkin's lymphoma, often found in older children; this cancer has long been cited as an example of chemotherapy's effectiveness. Yet according to a recent study, Hodgkin's patients receiving the standard chemotherapy treatment were 14 times more likely to develop cancer later on than Hodgkin's patients who did not receive chemotherapy.[2] Had these patients received the chemotherapy *along with* nutritional, botanical and homeopathic supports, such risks might have been greatly reduced, says Dr. Rountree.

Dr. Rountree recommends the following measures for adults and to help safeguard children from known risks that might encourage the onset of cancer.

**Eat a Healthy Diet—**As a starting point, follow a low-fat, high-fiber diet, plenty of grains, legumes and vegetables. Limit the amount of dietary fat to no more than 20% of calories consumed, and even lower if possible. "Eating too much fat and too little fiber contributes to the development of colorectal and other cancers. While these conditions may not develop for many years, it's best to start your child off eating well now." Children seem to recover faster from the negative effects of conventional cancer treatments when they are placed on a diet of this type, Dr. Rountree adds. If a child is placed on a dairy-free vegetarian or vegan diet, Dr. Rountree advises parents to make sure that adequate sources of dietary calcium are included, possibly through using a calcium supplement.

**Macrobiotics** is a specialized diet and food philosophy roughly based on Chinese medicine and filtered through contemporary Japanese culture and American representatives such as Georges Ohsawa and Michio Kushi. The diet emphasizes balancing the energy qualities of fresh, whole foods to maximize their delivery of *Qi*, or vital life force, to the body. The diet comprises cooked whole grains, beans and bean products, vegetables, fruits, nuts, seeds, small amounts of saltwater fish (salmon), fermented soybean products (miso), seaweeds, shiitake mushrooms, and special pickles and condiments. Macrobiotics has been used successfully when clinically prescribed as a curative and restorative diet in treating chronic and serious illness, including cancer; as a health-maintenance diet, it has produced excellent results for many people.

Patients who are malnourished may initially need to consume extra fat, such as from the omega-3 sources (fish and flax oil) or omega-9 sources (olive oil). "Instead of putting people immediately on a vegetarian diet, which I consider optimal, I have them cut down on the most obvious problem foods—fried foods, 'junk' foods, dairy products and red meat. Then I gradually phase them into a stricter, vegetarian or macrobiotic type of diet." Dr. Rountree often advocates the macrobiotic diet as a "good, comprehensive approach to healing with foods;" in such cases, Dr. Rountree urges his adult patient to take macrobiotic cooking classes as a way of becoming familiar with the approach.

For any cancer patient wishing to prevent a recurrence, this type of diet can be helpful. However, it is less helpful for patients who need immediate, aggressive, and, most often, conventional therapy.

**Eat Organic Foods**—It's important to serve organically-grown foods whenever available. Children may be particularly susceptible to the toxic effects of pesticides, herbicides, and other contaminants in the food supply, many of which are carcinogenic. "If you can't buy organic produce, consider growing your own. If you do use conventionally-grown produce, make sure you wash it thoroughly before preparing to eat it."

**Eliminate Tobacco Smoke**—Parents are advised to refrain from smoking tobacco products around their children. Better yet, quit smoking altogether, says Dr. Rountree. Over 2,000 compounds are generated by tobacco smoke and many of these are poisonous.[3] "Secondhand smoke may be even more dangerous than the smoke the smoker inhales. People who smoke may erroneously believe they can have their children out of a smoke-filled room one moment, and in the room the next, but it doesn't work that way." Secondhand smoke causes 1 in every 5 lung cancers in the U.S. not attributed directly to smoking, accounting for about 3000 lung cancer deaths each year among nonsmokers.[4]

**Test Your House for Radon**—Radon is a naturally-occurring radioactive gas

## Nutrients in BASIC PREVENTIVE™

- vitamin A (fish liver oil), 10,000 IU
- beta carotene, 15,000 IU
- vitamin D (fish liver oil), 100 IU
- vitamin E (d-alpha tocopheryl succinate), 400 IU
- vitamin K, 60 mcg
- vitamin C, 1200 mg
- vitamin B1, 100 mg
- vitamin B2, 50 mg
- niacin, 50 mg
- niacinamide, 150 mg
- pantothenic acid, 400 mg
- vitamin B6, 50 mg
- folic acid, 800 mcg
- vitamin B12, 100 mcg
- biotin, 300 mcg
- choline, 150 mg
- calcium (citrate, ascorbate), 500 mg
- magnesium (aspartate-ascorbate complex, amino acid chelate), 500 mg
- potassium (aspartate-ascorbate complex), 99 mg
- copper (amino acid chelate), 2 mg
- manganese (amino acid chelate), 20 mg
- zinc, (amino acid chelate), 20 mg
- iodine (kelp), 150 mcg
- chromium GTF (ChromeMate), 200 mcg
- selenium (amino acid complex), 200 mcg
- molybdenum, (amino acid chelate), vanadyl sulfate, 200 mcg
- boron (aspartate-citrate), 2 mg
- PABA, 50 mg
- inositol, 50 mg
- citrus bioflavonoids, 100 mg.

For more information about how to **remove toxins** from your food, see Chapter 33: Physical Support Therapies, p. 962. For more information about the health hazards of **tobacco smoke** (pp. 582-586), **sunlight** (pp. 551-552), and **radon** and **household carcinogens** (pp. 559-561), see Chapter 25: What Causes Cancer?

that seeps from granite-containing soils and rocks. If your house is not properly ventilated, radon gas can become concentrated, possibly paving the way for lung cancer, stomach cancer, and leukemia. "If you live in Colorado, Pennsylvania, or other parts of the country where radon can be a problem, you should have your house and water tested for the presence of the gas," Dr. Rountree says.

Since the gas is invisible and odorless, the only way to know whether it is present is to use a radon test kit. These can be found at many hardware stores. If you find that there is radon in your home, you can usually correct the problem by sealing cracks in the basement and improving ventilation throughout the house.

***Infants treated with X rays to reduce an enlarged thymus gland sustain an 83-fold greater rate of thyroid cancer later in life.***

**Limit Exposure to Chemical Fumes—**Researchers have identified a wide range of chemicals in the modern environment that may be carcinogenic.[5] These include fumes from paints, solvents, gasoline, pesticides, herbicides, and even such items as glues, oven cleaners, nail polish remover, and other common household chemicals. Many of these substances are known to either cause or contribute to the development of cancer. The fumes emitted by these products can be inhaled directly, so children must be protected from all unnecessary exposures.

**Don't Sunburn—**Frequent intense exposure to sunlight raises the risk of developing malignant melanoma, a potentially deadly form of skin cancer. Fair-skinned people who burn easily are at greater risk as are people with a history of multiple sunburns. "Your child's delicate skin should be sheltered from the sun. Even a single severe sunburn in childhood increases the risk of developing skin cancer later on."

In addition, Dr. Rountree adds, if your child's diet is nutritionally inadequate or imbalanced, the risk may be amplified. Dietary antioxidants such as vitamin E and zinc may protect against sun-induced damage resulting in melanoma. One study found that people whose diets contained high levels of vitamin E were 3 times less likely to develop melanoma, while those with high zinc intakes (from both food and supplements) were half as likely to develop melanoma, compared to people with low consumption of these nutrients.[6]

To prevent sunburn, you must, Dr. Rountree insists, apply a sunscreen to your child's skin before the child goes outside on a sunny day. Select a formula that screens out both UVA and UVB rays, that has a "Sun Protection Factor" (SPF) of 10 or higher and that is specifically designed for your child's skin, says Dr. Rountree. An SPF of 10 implies that one can endure 10 times more sunlight exposure than the current exposure level before developing a burn, Dr. Rountree explains. In general, children need a higher SPF than adults, to 15 or higher, says Dr. Rountree; children with especially light skin (such as an "Irish" complexion, need an even higher SPF, approaching 40.

"Make sure your child wears sunglasses and a hat if possible, and limit outdoor play in bright sunlight during the middle of the day when sunlight is strongest. Your child can start off with short exposures and gradually work up to longer periods of exposure by the end of the season." Finally, supplementing the diet with carotene complex containing all the carotenes may help protect against burns, notes Dr. Rountree.

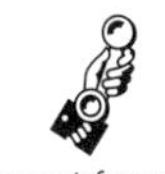

For more information about **Betaplex**, contact: Spectrum Naturals, 133 Copeland Street, Petaluma, CA 94952; tel: 707-778-8900; fax: 707-765-1026. For more information about **Basic Preventive**™, contact: Amni, Advanced Medical Nutrition, Inc., 2247 National Avenue, P.O. Box 5012, Hayward, CA 94550; tel: 800-437-8888; fax: 510-783-8196. For **Basic Antiox**™, contact: Allergy Research Group, 400 Preda Street, San Leandro, CA 94577; tel: 800-545-9960) For information about **mycellized vitamins A, E,** and **Metho-yflavone C,** contact: Metagenics, 971 Calle Negocio, San Clemente, CA 92672; tel: 800-692-9400. For **Genista**, contact: Cartilage Technologies, 200 Clearbrook Road, Elmsford, NY 10523; tel: 800-700-6300; tel: 914-345-6300; fax: 914-592-7166.

## A Specially Designed Nutrient Supplementation Program

The careful use of supplements can aid both the treatment and prevention of cancer, as well as counteract the harmful effects of environmental pollution and conventional treatments, says Dr. Rountree. Many supplements help reduce the burden of free radicals that further weaken the cancer-afflicted body.

"Our body cells and tissues are constantly being damaged by toxic free radicals which are produced during normal metabolism, by chemical reactions, and by toxic agents in the environment." A key focus of his approach is to stop the *uncontrolled* production of free radicals, which, as so many have testified, are a major contributing factor in immune-system breakdown and disease progression.

Dr. Rountree generally relies on a standardized list of supplements, knowing that individual cases require precise modification. For example, for women diagnosed with early cervical dysplasia, he may paint the cervix with a micellized form of vitamin A which delivers the vitamin right into the tip of the cervix, and also advise oral folic acid at 10 mg daily. For people with prostate cancer, he recommends saw palmetto (160-mg tablet, 3 times a day) and flax oil (3 tbsp per day), along with the supplements listed below. Dr. Rountree starts patients off with an antioxidant or multivitamin preparation, then draws upon either the Basic Preventive or Basic Antiox systems (using one or the other, but not both).

A **free radical** is an unstable molecule with an unpaired electron that steals an electron from another molecule and produces harmful effects. Free radicals are formed when molecules within cells react with oxygen (oxidize) as part of normal metabolic processes. Free radicals then begin to break down cells, especially if there are not enough free radical quenching nutrients, such as vitamins C and E, in the cell. While free radicals are normal products of metabolism, uncontrolled free radical production plays a major role in the development of degenerative disease, including cancer, heart disease, and aging. Free radicals harmfully alter important molecules, such as proteins, enzymes, fats, even DNA. Other sources of free radicals include pesticides, industrial pollutants, smoking, alcohol, viruses, most infections, allergies, stress, even certain foods and excessive exercise.

**Basic Preventive™**—This adult supplement, an AMNI (Advanced Medical Nutrition, Inc.) product, contains 30 essential nutrients and cofactors. "This is a potent antioxidant formula that has provided superb nutritional support for my patients," says Dr. Rountree. "It is the first supplement I will recommend to help people reverse cancer and improve their health."

Basic Preventive™ contains natural beta carotene, and vitamin E, a full-spectrum trace element supplement, a significant source of bioavailable calcium and magnesium, and a high-potency B-complex supplement. One important feature of this supplement is that it is iron free, which is significant because iron promotes free radical damage when taken in excess. According to Dr. Rountree, "About 80% of the U.S. population gets too much iron in their diet, mostly from red meat, which just adds to the biological burden and lowers the threshold of cancer resistance." His recommendation for cancer patients is 6 capsules daily.

A **micellized** vitamin (from micelle, which means "a colloid particle") is formulated to resemble a small, highly absorbable fat droplet, ready to be absorbed by the mucosa under the tongue. The result is that you need less. For example, you need only 1 drop of micellized vitamin A per day to meet recommended daily requirements.

**Basic Antiox™**—This multinutrient package is formulated to supply significant amounts of key antioxidants, including vitamin E (1200 IU per day), vitamin C (3200 mg per day), and other antioxidants necessary to eliminate free radicals in the body. Cancer patients generally take 4 capsules per day.

**Maitake Mushroom Extract**—Other extracts can be effective, but they are less effective when taken orally, Dr. Rountree notes, adding that most published studies on the use of shiitake mushrooms for cancer involve dosages given intravenously. Unlike other mushroom extracts, maitake's D-fraction shows potent anticancer activity even when ingested orally. "There appears to be a synergistic action between the caplets and the liquid D-fraction," Dr. Rountree says, who generally recommends about 6 caplets ( 500 mg each), and 2 droppersful of the liquid D-fraction daily.

**Green Drinks**—These "supergreen" food concentrates contain vitamins, minerals, phytochemicals, and probiotics drawn from sea vegetables, barley greens, blue-green algae, spirulina, chlorella, *Echinacea*, *Gingko*, and astragalus. Dr. Rountree generally recommends 2-3 tablespoons per day.

**Bovine Cartilage**—"In recent years, I have been using more bovine than shark cartilage, because it's less expensive and seems to be more potent," says Dr. Rountree. "The greatest advantage is that its taste is tolerable, whereas shark cartilage is far less palatable."

***"The toxic side effects of chemotherapy can greatly diminish the child's sense of well-being and overall quality of life," says Dr. Rountree.***

**Shark Liver Oil Extract (Alkyrol)**—This product may be valuable in helping people tolerate both chemotherapy and radiation. "[It] has been mostly promoted as a way to help mitigate the toxic effects of radiation, surgery, and chemotherapy," says Dr. Rountree, "but if you look at the research, you find that it seems to have antitumor effects all on its own." Shark liver oil is also useful for raising a low white blood cell count, Dr. Rountree adds.

## Counterbalancing the Toxic Effects of Conventional Treatment

Chemotherapy is commonly used to treat leukemia and other childhood cancers, and this treatment is among the only ones in which modern medicine has been able to claim any success in the "war on cancer." For those receiving such drastic treatment, however, the term "success" is highly relative. Toxic side effects of chemotherapy can greatly diminish a person's sense of well-being and overall quality of life.

In addition, many who manage to recover after such treatments run a high risk of developing "secondary" cancers later on. The reason is that chemotherapy not only suppresses the immune system, but it can actually trigger the eventual development of cancer itself. Recurrences usually mean having to undergo even more intensive forms of conventional treatment, resulting in more serious side effects and a reduced likelihood of success each time around.

It is for this reason that, in addition to the supplements listed above, Dr. Rountree recommends a combination of botanical and homeopathic medicines to help his patients successfully undergo conventional treatment and to further improve their chances of long-term survival.

**Astragalus**—(*Astragalus membranaceous*). This herb can support the immune system while a child or adult is undergoing chemotherapy. "It seems to substantially diminish some of the side effects of chemotherapy, including poor appetite, hair loss, and depression," says Dr. Rountree. Generally, he suggests one dose, taken 2-3 times daily.

**Ginger or Peppermint Tea**—These teas can be taken on their own or together. They are helpful in reducing the nausea produced by chemotherapy or radiation treatment. One cup of these herbs as tea can be taken as a palliative or on an as-needed basis. "If you are drinking it yourself or giving your child a tea containing peppermint as well as a homeopathic preparation, be sure to allow one hour between the two," he says. "Otherwise, the strong smell of the mint may interfere with the action of the homeopathic remedy."

Many classical homeopaths maintain that aromatics can interfere with the action of many (but not all) homeopathic remedies for as long as up to several weeks, and for this reason, aromatic substances should be avoided while on a homeopathic remedy. "There is a lot of debate on this matter, but as far as I know, no controlled studies show how, specifically, the aromatic substances interfere and for how long," says Dr. Rountree.

**Siberian Ginseng**—Ginseng is effective in enhancing energy levels and is useful for a child experiencing fatigue or exhaustion. "Siberian ginseng has long been known to help protect the liver from damage by chemotherapy and radiation treatments," says Dr. Rountree. "There is no reason that oncologists all around the world should not be using this one botanical as an adjunctive treatment on a regular basis."

**Shiitake Mushroom**—This mushroom is best added to soups in its whole form but it is also available in capsule form. Dr. Rountree suggests including 2-3 whole shiitake mushrooms in the daily diet or following the dosage directions on the supplement product label.

**Homeopathic Remedies**—Even though homeopathics must be specifically matched to a client's unique conditions, there are some generic formulas believed to be of benefit as an adjunct in a cancer treatment program. The following low-potency homeopathic remedies are available over the counter without prescription.

- **Aconite (Monkshood):** This remedy is used to help counteract the physical and mental shock that typically accompanies the first chemotherapy treatment. "It is helpful for both the child and parents following the treatment," Dr. Rountree says. Take one dose of low-potency Aconite (6C-30C) after the treatment.
- **Arnica Montana (Leopard's Bane):** This remedy can help reduce the dull pain or achiness associated with chemotherapy treatment. Dr. Rountree generally recommends giving your child one dose of Arnica at a strength of 30C after each treatment.
- **Nux Vomica (Poison Nut):** This remedy is helpful in lessening the nausea associated with chemotherapy. Dr. Rountree often advises parents to give their child one dose of Nux vomica at a strength of 6C as needed.

## CURRICULUM VITAE

# Geronimo Rubio, M.D.

American Metabolic Institute
555 Saturn Blvd., Building B, M/S 432
San Diego, CA 92154
tel: 619 267-1107, 619-229-3003,
or 800-388-1083; fax: 619-267-1109
In Mexico, tel: 52-6621-7602 or 52-6621-7603.

Dr. Rubio received his M.D. from the University of Autonoma de Baja California Medical School in Mexico and has conducted research in physiology, biochemistry, bacteriology, and parasitology. Some of this research resulted in his discovery that flowers brought into hospital rooms were infecting patients with bacteria. In 1987, Dr. Rubio began researching RNA transference in immune system cells which led to the development of a process to prepare immune-boosting vaccines from an individual's own blood and cancer cells.

Dr. Rubio is currently the medical director of American Metabolic Institute in La Mesa, Mexico, where his vaccines are combined with Rife technology, herbal medicines, and other therapies to reverse cancer.

***The success rate of Dr. Rubio and the American Metabolic Institute in reversing Stage III and IV cancers is 65 to 75%, but when they are able to work with cancers at an earlier phase of development, such as Stages I and II, their reversal rate is about 80% "If the patient follows the program, the patient's system will respond favorably to treatment," says Dr. Rubio.***

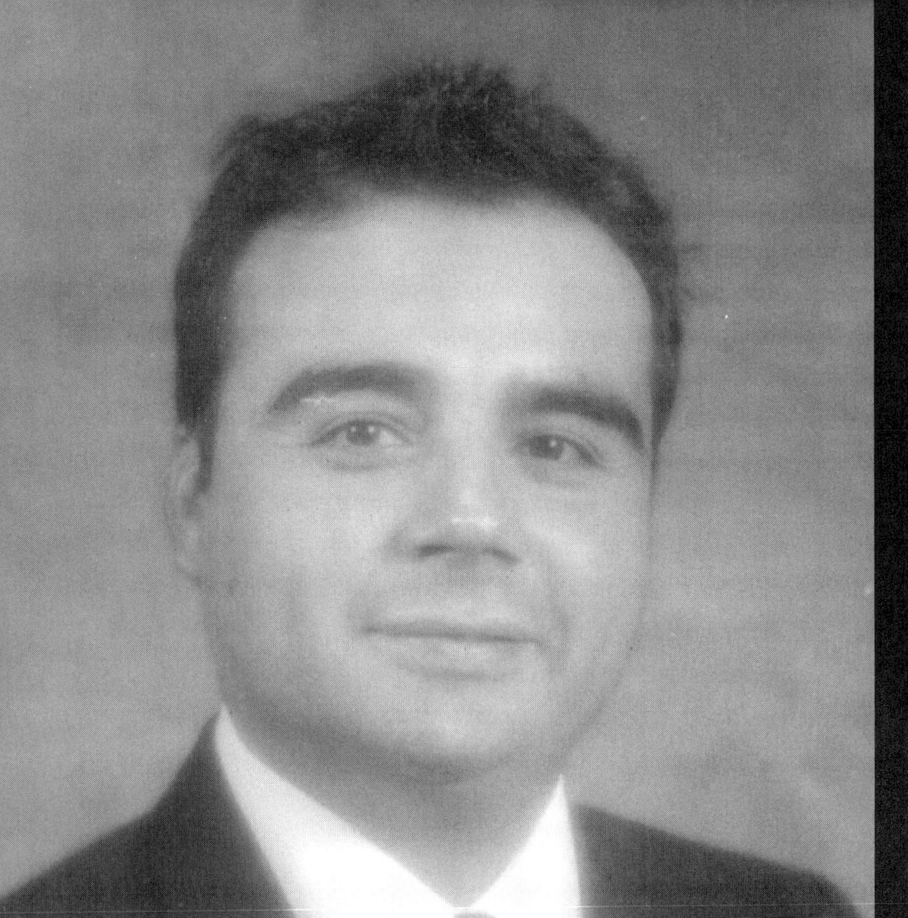

Chapter 17

# *Geronimo Rubio, M.D.*

**TO SUCCESSFULLY REVERSE CANCER** you must teach the patient's immune system how to respond effectively to the cancerous cells, says Dr. Rubio. He uses up to 150 different nontoxic medications and therapies to train the immune system to eliminate cancer.

To successfully reverse cancer, you must teach the patient's immune system how to respond effectively to the cancerous cells, says Geronimo Rubio, M.D., medical director of the American Metabolic Institute. This may sound obvious but when the body has a cancer process under way, clearly the immune system has become dysfunctional and is either unable or has forgotten how to eliminate the foreign cells.

## Developing Individual Treatment Plans

Dr. Rubio administers a 16-bed facility for treating cancer in La Mesa, Mexico, a few miles south of San Diego, California. Typically, patients stay for 3 to 5 weeks while they receive treatments from a diverse roster of alternative modalities, from enzymes to special vaccines, oxygen therapy to visualizations, physiotherapy to energy frequencies. Dr. Rubio draws upon 150 different medications in developing his individual treatment plans. American Metabolic's small in-patient population enables Dr. Rubio's staff to concentrate their medical attention on patients virtually around the clock.

According to statistics developed by American Metabolic Institute, based on their clinical work since their founding in 1983, their success rate in reversing Stage III and IV cancers is 65 to 75%, but when they are able to work with cancers at an earlier phase of development, such as Stages I and II, their reversal rate is about 80%, says Dr. Rubio. "If the patient follows the program, the patient's system will respond favorably to treatment," he says.

**Staging** in cancer terminology is a relative index of how much cancer exists in the body, its size, location, and containment or metastasis. *Stage I*, the earliest, most curable stage, shows only local tumor involvement. *Stage II* indicates some spreading of cancer to the surrounding tissues and perhaps to nearby lymph nodes. *Stage III* involves metastasis to distant lymph nodes. *Stage IV*, the most advanced and least easily cured, means the cancer has spread to distant organs.

# Dr. Rubio's Generalized Model for Cancer Treatment

| STRATEGY | DOSAGE/ KEY COMPONENTS | FOR MORE INFORMATION see page # |
|---|---|---|
| Dietary plan | individualized and by blood type: type O, organically raised chicken or shark at least 3 times weekly; type A or B blood, protein from vegetable sources such as grains and soybeans | 749 |
| Fasting | 3-day limited fast, fresh vegetable juices only; day 4, vegetable broth; day 5, start blood type-specific diet | 341 |
| Detoxification | organ cleansers (Kdne-Rinse, Colon Rinse, Liv-Rinse; *acidophilus*, 3 capsules/day; shark, bovine, chicken, and/or snake cartilage enemas (15 g per enema); maitake and shiitake mushroom enemas, coffee enemas | 949 |

## Supplements

| | | |
|---|---|---|
| Botanicals | cascara sagrada for intestinal cleansing; licorice root, lemon, and cornsilk for the kidneys; pau d'arco for the immune system; fresh celery, lettuce, green pepper, carrot, cactus, pineapple, or beet juice taken daily, sometimes hourly; Mexican herbs, cuachalalate and candurango | 343, 834 |
| Digestive enzymes | Wobenzym N, 2 tablets before each meal | 928 |
| Intravenous infusions | selenium, zinc, chromium, copper, magnesium, vitamins A (100,000 IU), B, C (150 g), D, E, and K, pycnogenol (1500 mg) | 749, 822 |

## Other Therapies

| | | |
|---|---|---|
| Oxygen therapy | oxygen mixed with germanium through the patient's nose (3 times daily, 10 minutes per session); ozone, rectally or in an ozone chamber, 3 times/day, up to 20 minutes/session | 915, 771 |
| Vaccines cultured from patient's blood and tumor cells | injection once weekly for 3-5 weeks; follow-up injection once every 3 months for next 2 years, then twice yearly for another 3 years | 344 |

*Continued*

## Dr. Rubio's Generalized Model for Cancer Treatment (cont.)

| STRATEGY | DOSAGE/ KEY COMPONENTS | FOR MORE INFORMATION see page # |
|---|---|---|
| Anticancer agents | over 150, including concentrated shark liver oil, Clodronate, intravenously delivered laetrile (amygdalin) | 837 |
| Rife frequency generator | individually determined | 345 |
| Visualizations | individually determined | 345 |
| Low-dose radiation | 1000 rads followed by steps to minimize immune system damage: fresh raw cabbage poultice on external site of radiation, then whole-body bath with baking soda, sea salt, and ginger | 849 |

**CAUTION**

This chapter includes information regarding actual treatments used by Dr. Rubio only after his careful diagnosis of each patient. All cancer patients are unique. **Do not administer these treatments to yourself or others.** Discuss these treatments with your physician or other qualified health-care professional. Readers should not interpret this material as therapeutic advice, but should see a physician in all cases.

### SUCCESS STORY

### Reversing a 3-Year Lymphoma

Claudette, aged 55, had suffered from non-Hodgkin's lymphoma for 3 years before seeing Dr. Rubio. The lymph glands in Claudette's abdomen and pelvis were cancerous, and her left leg was seriously swollen and painful (from bone metastases) preventing her from walking. She had received chemotherapy, but this had failed to reverse the lymphoma. Dr. Rubio administered his program including detoxification, diet, supplements, herbs, and vaccine. For example, Claudette took Liver, Kidney, and Colon Rinse formulas twice daily, Acidophilus (3 times daily), oxygen with germanium, shark liver oil, Clodronate, laetrile, enzymes, another nontoxic formula called Oncotax, and a preparation devised by Dr. Rubio to block the flow of hormones that otherwise support the cancer.

In addition, Dr. Rubio gave Claudette 10 treatments of low-dose radiation (3000 rads) to address the cancers that had spread to her bones.

"We started seeing her respond within the first week and the pain and pressure in her leg started to diminish," says Dr. Rubio. He estimates that Claudette experienced a 40% reduction in her pain in this first week; after 10 days, all the leg pain was gone. After 3 weeks of this combined treatment, Claudette's leg was healed and returned to normal, allowing her to walk comfortably.

During this time, her tumors shrunk noticeably, says Dr. Rubio. A CAT scan after 5 months on the program showed that the tumors had disappeared and that Claudette's cancer had been reversed. A year after the treatment began, Claudette was "still doing excellently," says Dr. Rubio.

## Blood Tests to Provide a Complete Health Picture

American Metabolic performs standard blood tests (including identifying blood type) along with CAT scan, MRI, and ultrasound evaluations of each patient as needed. Using a darkfield microscope, Dr. Rubio can examine a sample of the patient's live blood for signs of toxicity and immune dysfunction. A toxic liver, for example, will be indicated by dark specks amidst the living red blood cells under the microscope. With the information from these tests, Dr. Rubio can proceed in developing the patient's treatment plan.

## Components of the Individualized Treatment Plan

### DIETARY PLAN

Physicians at American Metabolic coordinate a dietary program with a patient's blood type. For example, a patient with type O blood needs to eat some meat regularly to build strong blood and may become anemic on a vegetarian diet, says Dr. Rubio. These patients are advised to eat organically raised chicken or shark at least 3 times weekly. A patient with type A or B blood does not require animal protein and may draw their protein from vegetable sources instead, such as grains and soybeans. "This is a more specific way of prescribing a diet and does not distress the patient with an inappropriate eating plan," Dr. Rubio explains.

QUICK DEFINITION

Blood is classified into 4 **blood types** or groups according to the presence of type A and type B antigens on the surface of red blood cells. These antigens are also called agglutinogens and pertain to the blood cells' ability to agglutinate, or clump together. Type O blood (containing neither type) is found in 47% of the Caucasian population; type A, 41%; type B, 9%; type AB, 3%. Another form of blood grouping is according to Rh positive and Rh negative types, based on the distribution of 6 different Rh antigens. About 85% of all white people and 95% of American blacks have Rh positive blood.

### FASTING

If the patient has enough energy reserves, they undergo a 3-day limited fast, consuming only fresh vegetable juices, in order to cleanse the body. On day 4, the patient has vegetable broth; on day 5, they start their blood type-specific diet. For patients who have lost too much weight already and must receive some nourishment, nutrients are provided through intravenous infusion during the 3-day fast, explains Dr. Rubio.

## DETOXIFICATION

Every cancer patient has a body overloaded with toxins, derived from foods, previous conventional medical procedures, and the environment, says Dr. Rubio. Hence, American Metabolic places a strong emphasis on detoxifying each patient. In addition, once the immune system is stimulated to start destroying the cancer, the dead cancer cells must be safely removed from the body.

Sources of toxicity often include mercury amalgam dental fillings, says Dr. Rubio. "We find these can leak mercury and diminish the immune system. A patient who has measurable mercury levels in the body must have it removed for the immune system to respond properly." Almost always, this involves the careful removal of all mercury fillings, which American Metabolic handles on site.

**Organ Cleansers**—Dr. Rubio relies on a series of prepared oral formulas for cleansing different organs. For example, Kidney Rinse combines comfrey, kidney beans, cranberry powder, kelp, and other natural substances to help flush toxins out of the kidneys. There is also a Colonic Rinse (with bentonite powder, psyllium husk, citrus pectin, diatomaceous earth, and various herbs) and a Liver Rinse.

Patients take Acidophilus (3 capsules daily) to recolonize the intestines with "friendly" bacteria. Dr. Rubio also dispenses a preparation called Perfect 7 (an herbal laxative containing plantago and psyllium) to heighten intestinal waste elimination.

**Enemas**—American Metabolic administers enemas using shark, bovine, chicken, or snake cartilage, often in combination and up to a total of 15 g per enema. When these substances are introduced intravenously, the body can handle a dosage of up to 150 g, says Dr. Rubio.

Biochemically speaking, a cartilage component called mucopolysaccharide helps block the tumor from growing and spreading. Dr. Rubio prefers the snake cartilage for patients with lymphomas, or cancers of the lymph system. For patients with cancers in their digestive system, such as stomach, pancreas, or colon, Dr. Rubio adds colostrum (mother's milk produced immediately after an infant's birth—in this case, from cows) to the cartilage enema. Enemas containing medicinal extracts of maitake and shiitake mushrooms as well as the more standard coffee enema are also used.

## SUPPLEMENTS

**Herbs**—Various botanical supplements are given to help cleanse the patient's liver, lungs, skin, and intestines, says Dr. Rubio. For example, Cascara sagrada is given for the intestines, while licorice root, lemon, and cornsilk are for the kidneys, and pau d'arco helps the immune system. Juices freshly made from celery, lettuce, green pepper, carrot, cactus, pineapple, or beet are taken daily, sometimes hourly. Dr. Rubio also relies on herbs native to Mexico such as cuachalalate and candurango.

***Every cancer patient has a body overloaded with toxins, derived from foods, previous conventional medical procedures, and the environment, says Dr. Rubio. Hence, he places a strong emphasis on detoxifying each patient.***

**Enzymes**—Dr. Rubio frequently prescribes digestive enzymes to help remove the protective coating around cancer cells that otherwise enables them to avoid being destroyed by the immune system. In most cancer patients, enzymes required for food digestion are usually deficient, leading both to nutritional shortfalls and intestinal toxicity. Dr. Rubio generally recommends German-made Wobenzym N which contains pancreatin, trypsin, papain, and other key enzymes. A typical dose is 2 tablets before each meal.

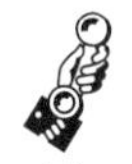

For more information about **Wobenzym N enzymes**, contact: Bio-Future, 1223 Wilshire Blvd., Box 315, Santa Monica, CA 90403; tel: 800-759-0331. For **Colonic Rinse** ™, **Liv-Rinse**™ (Liver Rinse), and **Kdne-Rinse**™ (Kidney Rinse), contact: Vitality Unique Products, Inc., P.O. Box 1003, Agoura Hills, CA 91376; tel: 818-889-7739; fax: 818-889-4895. For **Perfect 7**, contact: Agape Health Products, P.O. Box 2277, Seal Beach, CA 90740; tel: 800-767-4776 OR 714-229-8866; fax: 714-229-8866.

**Intravenous Nutrients**—Dr. Rubio administers a range of high-dose nutritional supplements and antioxidants such as selenium, zinc, chromium, copper, magnesium, and vitamins A, B, C, D, E, and K, usually by intravenous infusion. Among these daily nutrients, vitamin A is given at a dosage of 100,000 IU, vitamin C at 150 g, and pycnogenol (an antioxidant from Maritime pine bark or grape seed) at 1500 mg.

## OXYGEN THERAPY

Research has proven that cancer cells grow best in the absence of oxygen and that oxygen, therefore, is deadly for tumors. Dr.

Rubio administers oxygen mixed with germanium (a natural element believed to enhance oxygen supplies) through the patient's nose (3 times daily, 10 minutes per session) to raise body oxygen levels. Patients receive ozone (a variant of oxygen) through a self-contained ozone chamber or rectally, often 3 times daily for up to 20 minutes per session.

## VACCINES

A central feature of Dr. Rubio's cancer approach is to culture a special immune-boosting vaccine from the patient's own blood and cancer cells. "All cancer patients need this cancer vaccine because it teaches their immune system to recognize the tumor." The nontoxic medications, including herbs, minerals, vitamins, oxygen therapies, and detoxification, all prepare the cancer patient's system for handling the vaccine, Dr. Rubio explains.

First, he extracts a small cell sample of the cancer by needle biopsy and removes the cancer cell coating that blocks recognition by the immune system. Second, Dr. Rubio allows the tumor to grow outside the patient in a laboratory container; then he introduces living white blood cells from the patient into the tumor culture where they coexist for 14-21 days. In the case where a cancer tissue sample cannot be extricated, such as in the brain, Dr. Rubio collects tumor antigens (protein samples of the cancer) from the blood and uses them instead.

> "I am the happiest woman that I know today. On April 10, 1996, the doctors in Detroit, Michigan, gave me two months to live because I had uterine cancer and intestinal cancer. It is August 23, 1996, and I am cancer free.
>
> I have no cancer because of Dr. Rubio, his program, and his staff. His conviction that people who have cancer can live and heal rather than viewing cancer as a death warrant has saved many lives including mine. The vaccines he has developed combined with the medications, diet, food supplements, physical and emotional therapies as well as the home program saved my life and many others, I am sure."
>
> —Maureen Woods, Southfield, Michigan

The goal is to use this small-scale setting to "train" the patient's immune cells to recognize the cancer cells and "learn" how to destroy them. After the culturing process, the white blood cells are extracted and injected back into the patient's body as an immune-building vaccine. As Dr. Rubio explains, "These white blood cells send biochemical 'messages' to the patient's bone marrow (where such cells are made) to stimulate it to produce the same type of immune cells capable of recognizing cancer."

The patient receives the vaccine by injection once weekly for the 3-5 weeks they reside at the hospital. Afterwards, they must return once every 3 months for a follow-up injection for the next 2 years, then twice yearly for another 3 years.

## NATURAL ANTICANCER AGENTS

Among the 150 anticancer medications Dr. Rubio has at his disposal, there are concentrated shark liver oil and intravenously delivered laetrile (amygdalin, from apricot kernels). Both have clinically and scientifically proven anticancer effects. Dr. Rubio also uses several innovative medicines including Clodronate (dichloromethylene bisphosphonate) which is especially effective against bone cancer.

## RIFE FREQUENCY GENERATOR

In the 1930s, American medical inventor Raymond Royal Rife developed a device that could transmit specific electronic signals to deactivate or destroy living organisms such as pathogens, bacteria, and cancers. Rife's concept was that if you match the energy signal (frequency or rate of vibration) of a cancer cell, for example, with an electronically transmitted frequency, it would cause the cancer cell to explode from an excess of energy. Dr. Rubio's staff regularly use the Rife generator with their cancer patients.

## VISUALIZATIONS

It is vital to attend to the thoughts and emotions of the cancer patient and to encourage them to develop a strong positive attitude about their eventual success in reversing cancer, says Dr. Rubio. A staff psychologist works daily with patients in putting their minds creatively to work in dissolving their tumors through guided mental imagery in which they visualize their immune system destroying cancer cells.

"This is an important technique and patients who use it respond better to all the other therapies we provide," says Dr. Rubio. Other related approaches used at American Metabolic include color, art, and music therapy.

## LOW-DOSE RADIATION

"Radiation therapy will not cure the cancer but it will sometimes slow down the process to give us time for the alternative therapies to work," says Dr. Rubio.

Here, a very low dose of radiation—typically, 1000 rads compared to a normal protocol of 5000 rads—will encapsulate the tumor. This can be strategically valuable if the tumor is located on a bone and is progressively weakening the bone structure, leaving it prone to fracture, or if it is located in the chest wall or lungs and is putting a life-threatening amount of pressure on vital blood vessels.

Immediately following the low-dose radiation therapy, Dr. Rubio employs several procedures to minimize the otherwise inevitable damage to the immune system. First, a poultice made of fresh raw cabbage is placed at the external site of radiation to draw out the toxins. Second, the patient is immersed in a whole-body bath containing baking soda, sea salt, and ginger to remove radiation from the body.

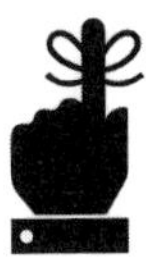

*An important goal of this book is to illuminate the dark fact that most of what you have heard over your lifetime about cancer treatments is not the truth. At the very least, you have received an incomplete picture. If you believe the propaganda you have been fed and you develop cancer, it can cost you your life.*

## CURRICULUM VITAE

# Michael B. Schachter, M.D.

Michael B. Schachter, M.D., Schachter Center for Complementary Medicine, Two Executive Boulevard, Suite 202, Suffern, NY 10901; tel: 914-368-4700; fax: 914-368-4727.

Dr. Schachter received his M.D. from Columbia College of Physicians and Surgeons, in New York City, New York, and he completed a 3-year residency in psychiatry at Kings County Hospital in Brooklyn, New York. He is licensed to practice medicine in New York, California, Mississippi, and New Jersey, and licensed to practice homeopathy in Arizona and Connecticut. In addition, he is certified by the American Board of Chelation Therapy and certified in psychiatry by the American Board of Psychiatry and Neurology. He belongs to 12 medical professional societies.

Dr. Schachter is a past president of the American College for Advancement in Medicine (ACAM) and current president of the Foundation for the Advancement of Innovative Medicine (FAIM); from 1983 to 1996, he was the recipient of the American Medical Association's Physician's Recognition Award in Continuing Medical Education. Dr. Schachter is the author of *The Natural Way to a Healthy Prostate* (Keats, 1995), *Food, Mind, and Mood* (with D. Sheinkin and R. Hutton, Warner Books, 1980), and he has published articles in *Townsend Letter for Doctors*, *Journal of Advancement in Medicine*, *Innovation*, *Annals of Emergency Medicine*, and others.

***"My goal is to help my cancer patients choose a treatment path that makes sense to them, that they can follow with conviction and enthusiasm," says Dr. Schachter. "This may include some conventional treatment modalities as well as alternative treatments. However, I believe that in many cases, patients who select only the alternative program and leave out the more destructive elements of conventional treatment will do better."***

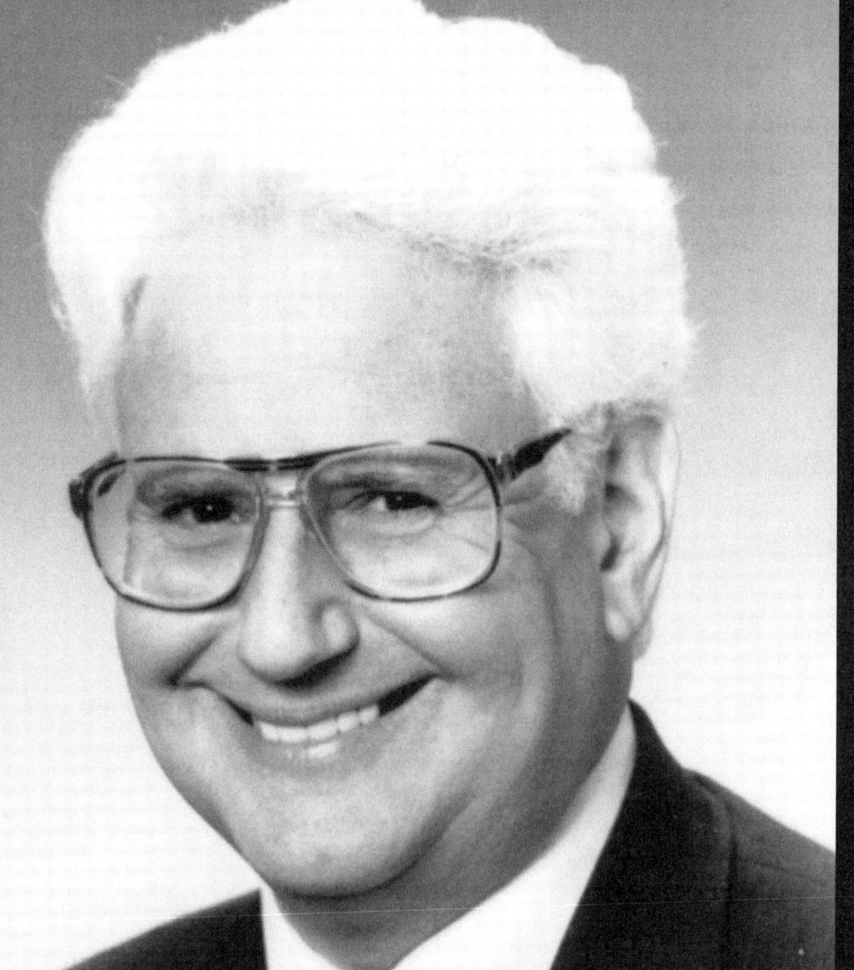

# *Michael B. Schachter, M.D.*

**"PERSONALLY, I BELIEVE** that in many cases, patients who select only the alternative program and leave out the more destructive conventional treatment will do better," Dr. Schachter says.

The multifaceted cancer treatment approach of the Schachter Center for Complementary Medicine is founded on this key idea: "You should try a *variety* of alternative treatments against cancer, either with, or sometimes instead of, the conventional treatments—surgery, radiation, and chemotherapy."

The Center's comprehensive approach emphasizes a health-promoting diet and lifestyle in which toxins from foods and the environment are avoided as much as possible and an array of natural substances are administered both orally and in injectable form. Over the years, these methods have demonstrated effectiveness against cancers of the ovary, lung, pancreas, lymphatic system, brain, prostate, and breast, including some advanced metastatic cancers.

In many of these cases, the patients' previous doctors had told them to go home and take care of their final affairs as nothing else could be done for them with conventional medicine. Even when a patient is given a poor prognosis, Dr. Schachter believes that a trial of alternative treatment is worthwhile because, for some, it produces results.

Dr. Schachter's thriving practice occupies almost 10,000 square feet in a spacious office building in Suffern, New York, about 30 miles north of New York City. His practice is versatile and diverse, incorporating a range of disciplines including nutritional therapy (involving extensive use of supplements and biological response modifiers), oxygen therapy, herbal medicine, chelation therapy, acupuncture, homeopathy, and mind/body/spiritual counseling.

In addition to Dr. Schachter, the Center's medical staff includes 2 other physicians (one an osteopath) with experience in alternative medicine, an acupuncturist, a chiropractor, a classical homeopath, 2 physician assistants,

# The Schachter Center's Generalized Model for Cancer Treatment

Although certain elements of the program apply to most or even all cancer patients, the Center tailors each treatment plan to the individual.

| STRATEGY | DOSAGE/ KEY COMPONENTS | FOR MORE INFORMATION see page # |
|---|---|---|
| **Nutritional/Pharmacologic Support** | | |
| Low- to moderate-fat, high-fiber diet of whole grains, fruits and vegetables, with modest amounts of nuts, seeds, fish, and organic chicken. Restricted use of eggs and dairy products. | flexible portions, based on individual need and cravings; if tolerated, 50% of diet should be raw foods, such as fresh juices; eggs used sparingly, dairy infrequently | 749 |
| **Avoid:** | tobacco smoke, alcohol, sugar, white flour, "junk food," caffeine, artificial sweeteners, preservatives, food additives, pesticides, fluoridated and chlorinated water, fluoride in all forms including toothpaste, margarine, aluminum cookware | ↓ |
| Vitamins: A, C, E, D, B complex (including folic acid and B12) | daily: vitamin A, 10,000-100,000 IU, and 50,000 IU of beta carotene; vitamin C, 10-12 g; vitamin E, at least 400 IU; vitamin D, 400-1000 IU; most B complex, 10-100 mg; B3, 100-3000 mg; folic acid, 1-10 mg; biotin, 600 mcg to 5 mg; B12 as needed, 250-3000 mcg | ↓ |
| Minerals/trace elements: magnesium, calcium, iron, selenium, zinc, copper, molybdenum, manganese, chromium, iodine, germanium sesquioxide | daily: magnesium, 400-800 mg; calcium, 800-1000 mg; iron (depends on serum ferritin level); selenium, 200-1000 mcg; zinc, 15-30 mg; copper, 2-4 mg; molybdenum, 100-1000 mcg; manganese, 5-20 mg; chromium, 200-600 mcg; iodine, varies; germanium sesquioxide, 200-1000 mg | ↓ |
| Amino acids: L-methionine, L-cysteine, L-lysine, L-arginine, L-glutamine | L-methionine, 500 mg, 2-3x/day; L-cysteine, 500 mg, 2-3x/day; L-lysine, 500 mg, 2-6x/day; L-arginine, 500 mg, 2-6x/day; L-glutamine, 2-40 g daily | 762 |
| Essential fatty acids: evening primrose oil, flaxseed oil, cod liver oil | evening primrose oil, 2-3 capsules, 500 mg each, 3X/day; flaxseed oil, 1-3 tbsp daily; cod liver oil, 1/2 to 1 tbsp daily | 768 |
| Enzymes: pancreatic enzymes plus bromelain and papaya for an enzyme mix | individually determined amounts | 928 |

*Continued*

# The Schachter Center's Generalized Model for Cancer Treatment (cont.)

| STRATEGY | DOSAGE/ KEY COMPONENTS | FOR MORE INFORMATION see page # |
|---|---|---|
| Botanicals: FlorEssence, Vitae Elixxir | FlorEssence, 2 oz mixed with 2 oz boiled water, 2x/day; Vitae Elixxir, max dosage is 6 drops, 3x/day, or 18 drops daily | 382 |
| Accessory food factors (AFFs): choline, inositol, bioflavonoids, carotenoids, modified citrus pectin, pycnogenol, lycopene, other phytonutrients | individually determined amounts | 809 |
| Therapeutic foods: garlic, chlorella, spirulina, barley greens, wheat grass, green kamut, maitake mushrooms, amygdalin (laetrile), shark cartilage, bovine tracheal cartilage (BTC) | shark cartilage, 1-3 heaping tbsp in 6 oz of fluid, 2-4x/day, orally in tomato or other juice, or in water as a rectal retention enema; BTC, 4 capsules of 750 mg each, 3x/day; amygdalin, 500 mg tablet, 1-3X/day | 809, 863, 861 |
| Additional antioxidant supplements: coenzyme Q10, N-acetyl cysteine, thioctic (alpha lipoic) acid | coenzyme Q10, 100-1000 mg/day; N-acetyl cysteine, 500 mg, 2-3x/day; thioctic acid, 100-1200 mg/day | 766, 868 |
| Intravenous infusions: vitamin C and amygdalin most commonly used; also, calcium, magnesium, potassium, zinc, selenium, manganese, chromium, glutathione, heparin. On occasion, vitamin B6 and pantothenic acid; B complex injected intramuscularly; staphage lysate (when available) | vitamin C, 7.5-10 g as intravenous push or 25 g as intravenous infusion; amygdalin, 3-9 g. amounts and proportions for the remainder of these substances will vary depending on the patient's specific needs. | 379 |

## Detoxification Methods

| STRATEGY | DOSAGE/ KEY COMPONENTS | FOR MORE INFORMATION see page # |
|---|---|---|
| The 4 Rs to improving GI function: (1) Remove abnormal microorganisms (2) Replace digestive acid and enzymes (3) Reinoculate with friendly bacteria (4) Repair lining with nutrients | determined by testing | 370 |
| Cleansing enema and colonics, followed by *L. acidophilus, bifidus,* and other friendly bacteria | individually determined | 949 |
| Removing heavy metals: chelation with DTA or DMPS; biological dentistry | individually determined | 973, 980 |
| Sweating via saunas & exercise | individually tailored exercise program; exercise for at least 25 min a session, 3-4X/weekly, as tolerated | 996, 1003 |

| STRATEGY | DOSAGE/ KEY COMPONENTS | FOR MORE INFORMATION see page # |
|---|---|---|
| Liver detoxification via botanicals such as silymarin (milk thistle) and thioctic acid, nutritional supplements, dietary changes, coffee enemas, and accessory food factors (choline and inositol) | silymarin, 2-6 capsules daily; thioctic acid, 1-4,3X/day; choline and inositol, 500 mg 1-6X/day of each; others individually determined | 835, 776 |

## Oxygen (bio-oxidative) Therapies

| | | |
|---|---|---|
| Intravenous hydrogen peroxide, intravenous ultraviolet blood irradiation, and/or ozone therapy | individually determined, from 1X/week to daily | 915 |

## Hormonal Balancing

| | | |
|---|---|---|
| DHEA (oral) | 5-15 mg daily, occasionally increasing to 25-100 mg, depending on DHEA sulfate levels | 939 |
| Thyroid (oral, desiccated thyroid extract) | usually 1/4 to 2 grains daily | 944 |
| Thymus extract | individually determined | 944 |
| Melatonin (oral) | less than 1 mg to 10 mg daily | 941 |
| Natural progesterone (topical) | usually 1/4 tsp, 1-2X/day | 383 |

## Other Adjunctive Methods

| | | |
|---|---|---|
| Hydrazine sulfate | 30 mg or 60 mg depending on weight, 2-3x/day | 868 |
| Pamidronate (Aredia) for bone metastases | 90 mg in 250 ml saline or dextrose and water given intraveneously over 3-4 hours every 3-4 weeks for 6-8 (or more) treatments | 387 |
| Urea and creatine monohydrate | 15-30 g urea and 25 g creatine monohydrate dissolved in qt of water or juice/daily, divided in 4-8 doses; BUN test to monitor urea dosage | 874 |
| Homeopathic remedies | individually determined | 384 |
| Magnetic therapy | individually determined | 1032 |
| Acupuncture | individually determined | 385 |
| Acupressure | individually determined | 385 |

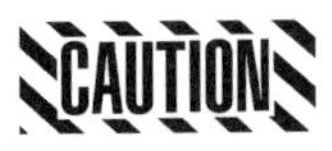

This chapter includes information regarding actual treatments used by Dr. Schachter only after his careful diagnosis of each patient. All cancer patients are unique. **Do not administer these treatments to yourself or others.** Discuss these treatments with your physician or other qualified health-care professional. Readers should not interpret this material as therapeutic advice, but should see a physician in all cases.

For more information on laboratory tests for **heavy metal toxicity** levels, see Chapter 27: Early Detection and Prevention of Cancer, pp. 738-740.

a nurse practitioner, 5 registered nurses, 5 laboratory technicians, a stress management counselor, and 3 lifestyle counselors. Dr. Schachter refers some of his patients to a holistic dentist next door when it's necessary to have their mercury dental amalgams removed as part of an overall detoxification program.

## Comprehensive Tests Help Chart the Course of Individual Treatment

Each patient entering the Center is carefully evaluated so that a practical, mutually agreed upon therapeutic program can be designed and implemented. Diagnostic testing is individualized and based in part on what tests and procedures have been done prior to the initial visit. Tests that are considered include not only the usual X rays, scans, sonograms, and blood and urine chemistries, but also an assessment of hormonal balance (notably thyroid and adrenal hormones), nutrition parameters (with careful attention given to screening for trace element deficiencies, such as selenium, zinc, copper, and molybdenum), blood cancer markers (which give a rough indication of the progress of a cancer), and an immune system profile.

Other tests can provide directions for detoxification protocols. First, it helps to know what kinds and quantities of toxic substances are present in the body. For example, a mineral analysis of hair or a urine sample may be used to screen for heavy metal toxicity—lead, cadmium, aluminum, mercury, arsenic, and others. An even more precise way of screening for heavy metal toxicity is to administer a chelating agent, which is a substance capable of tightly binding to minerals; both then pass from the body in the urine. Urine samples are collected, usually over 24 hours, and tested for heavy metal content. If a cancer patient has a history of exposure to heavy metals (at work, for example) or heavy metal toxicity shows up in a physical examination or in blood, urine, or hair samples, Dr. Schachter is likely to recommend this test.

Different chelating agents may be needed to check for different minerals. For example, the chelating agent EDTA (ethylene-diamine-tetraacetic acid) is excellent for lead and cadmium, but poor for mercury, while the chelating agent DMPS is excellent for mercury.

If heavy metal toxicity is found, the source of contamination must be eliminated. For example, mercury toxicity is frequently caused by silver amalgam fillings in the teeth, which are 50% mercury. In such a case, Dr. Schachter may recommend evaluation for removal of these fillings by a biological dentist. Additionally, an appropriate chelating agent may be given to remove the accumulated heavy metal from the tissues of the body.

Aside from heavy metals, other toxins may be present in the body as a result of environmental exposure via air, water, or food. Blood and urine screens can also be carried out for toxic organic compounds, such as pesticides, which are known to be carcinogenic.

Allergies, which are reactions to substances that are toxic to some people but not to others, need to be evaluated in some patients, as allergic reactions may tend to occupy the immune system, thus preventing it from properly dealing with cancer growth. Allergies may be determined by many methods including various blood tests, skin tests, electrodermal testing, and food elimination and challenges. At the Schachter Center, several of these methods are used: checking the blood for IgE antibodies to allergens; viewing through a microscope the responses of blood cells to allergens; and electrodermal testing. Once the presence of allergies is established, therapeutic measures may be taken.

Toxicity may also be caused by the presence in the gastrointestinal system of microorganisms that do not belong there or are there in excessive amounts. These may include *Helicobacter pylori* in the stomach, an overgrowth of anaerobic (not needing oxygen) bacteria in the small intestine, the presence of parasites (such as *Giardia* or *Entamoeba histolytica*) anywhere in the gastrointestinal tract, or *Candida* or other yeast or fungal overgrowth, usually in the colon. These abnormalities may be diagnosed with stool analysis and cultures and antibody tests of blood or saliva.

The second aspect of laboratory testing related to detoxification protocols has to do not with measuring toxic substances in the body but with determining how the organs of detoxification in the body are functioning. These tests focus on the gastrointestinal system and the liver. For example, a Heidelberg capsule test may be used to determine if the stomach lacks the ability or has a reduced capacity for forming hydrochloric acid, which is necessary for both digestion and for killing bacteria, parasites, and fungi that enter the stomach with food (see page 375). A Chymex test may be used to determine the ability of the pancreas to produce enzymes for digestion.

Another simple test can be done to determine if the intestines have a problem with malabsorption or a so-called leaky gut. With malabsorption, proper absorption of nutritive food substances from the intestine into the bloodstream does not occur. With leaky gut syndrome, substances entering the intestine that are supposed to be kept out of the bloodstream find their way into it, causing toxicity or inducing allergic reactions.

To check for these conditions, the patient drinks a solution containing the sugars mannitol and lactulose. Urine is then collected over the next several hours and brought to the laboratory for analysis. Mannitol is generally better absorbed than lactulose. By determining the absolute amounts of each of these sugars in the urine and also looking at the ratio between them, the physician can determine if either malabsorption or a leaky gut is present. If either one or both is present, therapeutic measures may be taken to correct the problem.

Along with evaluating intestinal function, tests for how the liver is functioning are extremely important. The usual "liver function tests" that are included in a blood chemistry screen (e.g., SGOT, SGPT, alkaline phosphatase, LDH) generally reflect damage to liver cells and do not indicate how well the liver is functioning with respect to detoxifying substances that need to be removed from the body.

There are 2 phases in the liver's detoxification process. In Phase I, substances are oxidized or chemically changed to make them ready for Phase II. In Phase II, the oxidized substance is combined with one of many substances in the liver, such as glycine, glucuronic acid, or sulfate to make the substance more soluble, so that it may be eliminated in the bile from the liver or in the urine from the kidneys after being brought to the kidneys via the bloodstream.

When either Phase I or Phase II are impaired or out of balance with each other, the patient will accumulate toxic substances, develop symptoms, and have difficulty recovering from a chronic disease, such as cancer.

A simple test involving the one-time administration of caffeine, acetaminophen (Tylenol), and aspirin, followed by collecting saliva and urine samples, can clarify how Phase I and Phase II liver detoxification are working. Measures can then be taken to correct any abnormality. This diagnostic procedure is particularly important for patients who undergo chemotherapy, which involves the administration of poisons. Those patients with abnormal liver detoxification profiles are probably the ones who will have the most severe adverse reactions to chemotherapy.

During a patient's first visit to the Schachter Center, tests are ordered and a tentative treatment program outlined. Treatment may then be modified, depending on the results of the laboratory tests.

"My goal is to help my cancer patients choose a treatment path that makes sense to them, that they can follow with conviction and enthusiasm," says Dr. Schachter. "This may include some conventional treatment modalities as well as alternative treatments. However, I believe that in many cases, patients who select only the alternative program and leave out the more destructive elements of conventional treatment will do better."

## SUCCESS STORY

### Reversing Lung Cancer

When she was 61, a routine X ray of Michelle's chest revealed a dark mass in the upper lobe of her left lung. A biopsy confirmed her worst fear: lung cancer. One month later, believing that the tumor was operable and that adjacent lymph nodes were not involved, her surgeon removed the left lobe of the lung. However, during the operation, the surgeon found, much to his dismay, that some lymph nodes in the tissue structure between the 2 lungs (the mediastinum) were involved, which meant a poor prognosis.

Michelle relates that the surgeon told her she had only a few months to live. The radiation oncologist recommended "palliative radiation" (aimed at reducing intensity of symptoms, but not producing a cure), but said it would improve the prognosis only slightly.

Michelle was determined to defy the medical odds. She sought the guidance of Dr. Schachter, whom she had previously consulted for headaches and nasal allergies (allergic rhinitis). Dr. Schachter immediately placed her on extensive oral supplements and an injectable program consisting of intramuscular injections of crude liver extracts and intravenous infusions of vitamin C, hydrogen peroxide, and amygdalin (both orally and intravenously), along with other therapeutic substances.

Dr. Schachter designed the regimen not only to help Michelle's body ward off the cancer, but also to help her cope with the adverse aftereffects of surgery and the radiation she chose to undergo in combination with the alternative treatment. She received the "palliative radiation" 5 days a week for 5 weeks. Since radiation disables the immune system for weeks, or even months, at a time, a key part of Dr. Schachter's strategy was to get Michelle's immune system functioning as quickly as possible to help her own body fight and eliminate cancer cells.

The strategy paid off, because a little less than a year later, Michelle's pulmonary specialist at New York Hospital remarked that she looked "more robust and energetic" than all his other radiation patients. Along with a maintenance intravenous program which Dr. Schachter gradually tapered off in the years to follow, he placed her on a primarily vegetarian diet and had her take various supplements common to his program.

Since then, Michelle has enjoyed more than 11 years of good health. Every few months, she comes to the Schachter Center for a follow-up evaluation. "At this point, it's unclear whether or not she has any cancer in her body," Dr. Schachter says. "Even though the lymph nodes, according to her chest X ray, are still enlarged, we do not recommend chemotherapy to reduce the size of these nodes." Instead, Dr. Schachter advises Michelle to stay on her anticancer supplement program.

## SUCCESS STORY

### Controlling Pancreatic Cancer

Ron, aged 71, had experienced severe abdominal pain, nausea, vomiting, and a 40-pound weight loss over 6 months. A CT scan of the abdomen showed an enlargement of the tail of the pancreas and lesions in the liver, suggesting liver metastases. A biopsy of the pancreas revealed pancreatic cancer. The conventional medical prognosis in such a case is death within a few months.

Ron received 5 rounds of chemotherapy (5FU and leukovorin), but had such a severe reaction that he stopped the treatments. When he came to the Schachter Center, he weighed 129 pounds (5' 2" height). Dr. Schachter put him on a program of oral Vitae Elixxir (6 drops, 3 times a day) as well as foot soaks, shark cartilage enemas (up to 5 daily, 1 heaping tbsp each), vitamin C (3 g daily), hydrazine sulfate (60 mg twice a day), and low doses of pancreatic enzymes.

Within 3 months, Ron had improved significantly; his energy and appetite were better, he had gained 15 pounds, and his abdominal pain has lessened considerably. At this point, he was on the same dosage of Vitae Elixxir and hydrazine sulfate, still doing the shark cartilage enemas and

Vitae foot soaks (with DMSO as well), and also taking amygdalin (500 mg, 3 times a day). Six months later, a repeat CT scan showed evidence of some progression of the liver metastases, but no change in the pancreas.

Over the next several months, Ron continued to do reasonably well despite multiple complications in his condition, including angina, cramp-like pains in the calves when walking (called intermittent claudication, associated with atherosclerosis), gastric and duodenal ulcers, abdominal hernias, 2 surgeries to repair the hernias, constant pain medication for the abdominal pain, other medication administered to him by his conventional doctors, and severe anxiety and depression, which may have been caused in part by interactions of his medications and/or overdosage of pain pills. The fact that Ron was being treated by 2 medical teams with conflicting philosophies created a further complication.

For example, he frequently was given morphine for abdominal pain because his physicians believed that the pain was due to the pancreatic cancer. It was actually being caused by the ulcers which should have been treated with other, more appropriate medications. The morphine and other drugs given for anxiety and depression actually caused Ron to become confused and more agitated and depressed. This was especially true because some of these drugs were contraindicated by the hydrazine sulfate he was taking. Ron was on these conflicting drugs for a while before Dr. Schachter became aware of it and asked him to discontinue the hydrazine sulfate.

Ron faithfully followed the Schachter Center program and for 18 months did well. Nine months after the second CT scan, however, he began experiencing severe pain again, his morphine dosage was increased, and he was soon hospitalized. Another CT scan showed no progression of the cancer, but Ron never left the hospital. Increasingly agitated and confused by large doses of pain and psychotropic medications, he died 23 months after the original diagnosis of pancreatic cancer and liver metastases. The cause of death was listed as congestive heart failure.

"I don't think cancer was in any way associated with Ron's death," says Dr. Schachter. "Rather, this appears to be a clear example of how inappropriate use of drugs in the course of therapy can lead to complications which end up killing the patient."

# SUCCESS STORY

## Controlling Prostate Cancer

At age 60, Lou received a diagnosis of prostate cancer, based on a biopsy which revealed a Gleason 7 (moderately malignant) adenocarcinoma. The urologist advised surgical removal of the prostate. A second biopsy, conducted at another institution, came back with a Gleason score of 8, indicating severe malignancy.

For information on prostate cancer and the negative effects of radiation therapy, see Chapter 30: The New Pharmacology for Treating Cancer, p. 846.

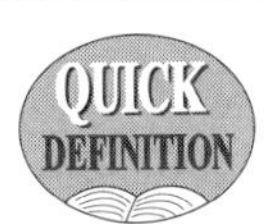


The **Gleason score** is a way of grading the microscopic appearance of prostate cancer. First, different areas of the slide are rated from 1 to 5 with 1 appearing most benign and 5 appearing most malignant. Then the 2 most predominant patterns are added together for a Gleason score, with 2-4 being mildly malignant, 5-7 moderately malignant, and 8-10 severely malignant. The higher the score the worse the prognosis.

**Prostate specific antigen** (PSA) is a cancer marker, or blood test, for the detection of prostate cancer. A normal reading is 0-4; an elevated reading is anything over 4, with the higher the number the greater the presence of cancer. Ideally, after cancer treatment, the elevated numbers drop (e.g., from 25 to 0.4), indicating that the cancer has been eliminated. If a man is retested some time later and the numbers are again elevated (e.g. to 40), this may indicate that the cancer has recurred in the prostate or spread to the lymph nodes or bone, which are the most common areas of metastasis in prostate cancer.

His urologist recommended either surgery or radiation for his condition. One radiation oncologist recommended placement of radioactive needles in Lou's prostate. Another thought the cancer was too advanced and that external beam radiation therapy was the appropriate treatment. In this, the prostate is radiated from an external source, as opposed to brachytherapy, in which radioactive rods are inserted into the prostate and radiate the gland from within. Radiation oncologists regard brachytherapy as an accurate way of irradiating an organ and not the surrounding vital structures, but it may be used only when the cancer is clearly confined to the organ being irradiated. External beam radiation may be used when the cancer is too large for brachytherapy or is located beyond the bounds of the organ.

When Lou decided to undergo Dr. Schachter's treatments instead of the conventional approach, his urologist wrote a formal letter to Lou strongly criticizing this decision and repeating his recommendation to have either a radical prostatectomy or radiation treatment.

Unfortunately, Lou's insurance would not cover Dr. Schachter's injectable program (although they would pay for prostate surgery or radiation), so Lou had to forgo injections. Instead, he began an intensive program of oral supplements along with proteolytic enzyme and shark cartilage rectal retention enemas. The oral supplements included vitamin C, beta carotene, shark cartilage, amygdalin, sodium selenite, flaxseed oil, Vitae Elixxir, cod liver oil, maitake mushrooms, FlorEssence (a form of Essiac herbs), coenzyme Q10, pycnogenol, apricot kernels, hydrazine sulfate, and a multivitamin/mineral formula. The modalities were introduced over a 6-week period.

Within a month, Lou's energy levels improved and he reported feeling well. His prostate symptoms, which included occasional bedwetting, were much reduced. Over the next year, Lou's prostate specific antigen (PSA) counts fluctuated considerably, but eventually showed a continual downward trend, dropping from a high of 17.8 to stabilize at 8.23, which is a moderate count (normal being 0 to 4).

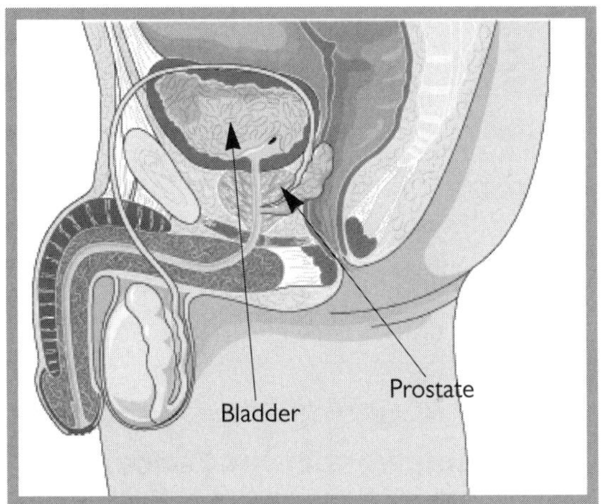

Figure 18.1—The prostate gland

According to Dr. Schachter, Lou continues to feel well and remains physically active. His only symptoms are waking once nightly for urination and occasional bed-wetting, which had begun prior to his first consultation. Some 28 months after his diagnosis, Lou's PSA was 9.79, still within the moderate range, his prostatic acid phosphatase was 1.4, which is normal. (This blood test, known as the male PAP, is less sensitive than the PSA in monitoring prostate cancer. Usually when it is elevated, there are metastases to the bones.) Lou continues to feel well, working full time and playing racketball for 3 hours at a stretch several days each week, reports Dr. Schachter.

## SUCCESS STORY

### Preventing a Recurrence of Breast Cancer

When Lisa, aged 56, came to Dr. Schachter, she had been diagnosed with metastatic breast cancer. After experiencing stabbing pains in her right breast for several months, Lisa had a mammogram and it suggested cancer. A subsequent hospital consultation led to a lumpectomy, in which surgeons removed a tumor 1.5 cm in diameter along with 17 lymph nodes, 4 of which tested positive for cancer. Radiation and chemotherapy were recommended, but after the first chemotherapy treatment, Lisa felt extremely weak and shaky.

Lisa decided to forgo any further chemotherapy and radiation. Instead, she elected to follow Dr. Schachter's program. More than 6 years later, there is no evidence of cancer, reports Dr. Schachter.

Lisa continues to receive intravenous infusions about once a month and to promote her health in other ways to prevent a recurrence of cancer. "This is a fine example of active preventive medicine," says Dr. Schachter. Lisa is one of many of the Schachter Center's breast cancer patients who forgo radiation and chemotherapy after surgery and opt for the intensive, nontoxic, noninvasive alternative program instead.

## SUCCESS STORY
### Reversing Testicular Cancer

Paul, aged 27, had undergone surgery and chemotherapy for testicular cancer, which had begun spreading to the lymph nodes. He was told that this course of treatment had a 95% chance of cure. Some 3-4 months after he finished conventional treatment, however, a blood cancer marker associated with testicular cancer started to increase, indicating that the chemotherapy had failed.

**Alpha fetoprotein** (AFP) is a protein normally made by the human fetus. A high AFP level can indicate the presence of neural tube defects such as *spina bifida* (a defect in the vertebral column) and anencephaly (defects in brain hemisphere development) in a fetus. In adults, high serum levels of AFP may indicate the presence of certain cancers, such as liver (hepatocellular carcinoma), testicular, and ovarian, and to a lesser extent, carcinomas of the pancreas, stomach, colon, or lung. As such, elevated AFP levels are interpreted as a cancer tumor marker.

Paul's doctors told him he needed a formidable series of chemotherapy treatments, followed by a bone marrow transplant, which alone would cost $150,000. In addition, he would require 3 months of isolation after chemotherapy because his immune system would be severely weakened by that treatment, leaving him highly susceptible to developing a life-threatening infection.

None of this appealed to Paul. Instead, he went on Dr. Schachter's intensive metabolic program. Within 6 weeks, Paul's alpha fetoprotein (AFP) levels, the cancer marker which had been elevated to 25, dropped down to the normal value of 2.5. Paul continued intensively on Dr. Schachter's program for about a year. Now, more than 5 years since his original diagnosis, Paul works full time and has no evidence of cancer, says Dr. Schachter.

## SUCCESS STORY

### Stabilizing Kidney Cancer with Lung Metastases

Caleb, 63, was diagnosed with kidney (renal) cancer with widespread metastases involving both lungs. His left kidney had been removed because of kidney cancer 6 years earlier. The usual life expectancy for this condition of metastatic cancer to both lungs from the kidney is less than a year. He came to the Schachter Center to see if he could avoid the chemotherapy his conventional doctors recommended. He was already on an extensive daily supplement program which he had designed himself. It included a B-complex vitamin, vitamin C (3 g), vitamin E (400 IU), vitamin A (10,000 IU), beta carotene (25,000 IU), fish oil, garlic, selenium (150 mcg), chromium, zinc, coenzyme Q10 (90 mg), magnesium, and calcium.

To this daily program, the Center added powdered shark cartilage (3 heaping tbsp), hydrazine sulfate (60 mg, 3 times daily) for 6 weeks on and 2 weeks off during the first year, amygdalin, apricot kernels, proteolytic enzymes, and intravenous vitamin C infusions followed by intravenous amygdalin about once a week. When a CT scan revealed a new lesion in his lungs and an adrenal tumor 5 months later, the Center doctors added the herbal product, Vitae Elixxir (18-21 drops daily).

Caleb has remained on this program, with some reductions in the frequency of intravenous treatments after a few years. As he hoped, he has been able to avoid chemotherapy. A recent CT scan showed slight worsening, but 3½ years after his diagnosis, Caleb is doing well and even works part time.

## SUCCESS STORY

### Non-Hodgkin's Lymphoma in Remission without Conventional Treatment

Ahmed, 47, discovered a lump in the area of his left elbow which turned out to be an enlarged lymph node. Six months later, a second enlarged lymph node appeared on his right upper thigh. After multiple bone marrow biopsies a year after that, he was diagnosed with stage IV non-Hodgkin's lymphoma, involving the bone marrow. The 5-year survival with conventional treatment is 46% or less, as determined by the Ann Arbor and Working classifications (a predictive scale for the prognosis of different stages of non-Hodgkin's lymphoma).

CT scans of Ahmed's chest, abdomen, and pelvis failed to identify any major organ involvement besides the bone marrow. However, the scans revealed additional enlarged lymph nodes in the left groin region. Ahmed was not experiencing significant symptoms at that time. Although most oncologists would have recommended chemotherapy, his hematologist-oncologist took a conservative approach, suggesting that early chemotherapy was ill-advised at that point; he offered no other treatment.

Ahmed's medical history included a herniated disk and spastic colon (irritable bowel syndrome). A long-term smoker and moderate drinker, he also had poor dietary habits. Running was his primary mode of exercise, but was often restricted due to his disk herniation.

Six months prior to visiting the Schachter Center, Ahmed had sought the assistance of alternative medicine and was started on a program of lifestyle modification, nutritional supplementation, and intravenous vitamin C and other immune-enhancing factors. Being overweight at the time, he was happy to lose a total of 25 pounds and felt that his energy level had greatly improved on this program. Ahmed came to the Schachter Center seeking additional complementary treatments to the ones he was already using.

***Dr. Schachter presents dietary information in a gentle, sensitive way, emphasizing that the proposed changes are goals to strive for at a pace comfortable for the cancer patient.***

After laboratory testing for indicators of immune system competence, vitamin and mineral deficiencies, hormonal balance, and toxic metabolites, the Center continued Ahmed's intravenous infusions of vitamin C with calcium, adding amygdalin, and alternating days with hydrogen peroxide infusions. Hydrazine sulfate was added to his oral supplementation program, which included a diverse regimen of vitamins, minerals, and herbs designed for detoxification and immune system enhancement in order to combat the malignancy. Ahmed met with lifestyle counselors who recommended diet modifications and exercise options.

Every few months, Ahmed was examined by his hematologist-oncologist. After the lymph node enlargements disappeared, Ahmed's oncologist declared him "in remission." Today, more than 5 years after the original diagnosis, Ahmed is active, works full time, and continues to conduct a normal life with his family. He remains on a heavy oral supplementation program and still receives intravenous infusions every 2 weeks.

## Achieving Dietary Goals at a Comfortable Pace

Over the years, Dr. Schachter has learned to present dietary information in a gentle, sensitive way, emphasizing that the proposed changes are goals to strive for at a pace comfortable for the cancer patient. "If we tell people whose appetites are already reduced to radically change their diet overnight, we generally will not achieve positive results," says Dr. Schachter. "Therefore, we begin the dietary program at whatever level the patient can handle."

Dr. Schachter divides his dietary guidelines into 2 categories: what to avoid and what to eat. The avoidance list includes alcohol, white sugar, white flour, caffeine, artificial sweeteners, preservatives and other food additives, pesticides, fluoridated water and all fluoride-containing products (such as toothpaste), chlorinated water, hydrogenated fats (i.e., margarine), and foods with added aluminum products, such as those containing aluminum-based baking powder.

Aluminum cookware and antiperspirant deodorants containing aluminum are also on the avoid list. The goal is to remove these substances from one's diet and water supply. Although not a dietary guideline, but related in its impact on the body, exposure to tobacco and tobacco smoke is also to be avoided.

On the good-to-eat side of dietary matters, Dr. Schachter recommends a low- to moderate-fat, high-fiber, moderate- to high-complex-carbohydrate, moderate protein diet centered around whole grains, fresh fruits and vegetables, and modest amounts of nuts, seeds, fish, and organically raised poultry. If tolerated, Dr. Schachter recommends consuming approximately 50% of the diet as raw food, mainly in the form of fresh raw vegetable juices. For most people, he allows 6-8 soft-boiled organic eggs per week and some organic dairy products, preferably yogurt, 2-3 times a week. Depending on the patient's "metabolic type," Dr. Schachter may allow organic red meat on an occasional basis.

***Dr. Schachter recommends a low- to moderate-fat, high-fiber, moderate- to high-complex-carbohydrate, moderate protein diet centered around whole grains, fresh fruits and vegetables, and modest amounts of nuts, seeds, fish, and organically raised poultry.***

In every case, Dr. Schachter's guiding dietary principle is flexibility. "We will follow these patients and try to help them with their programs as long as they seem to be doing well. If they begin to decline, we will suggest dietary modifications which, based on our own clinical experience, may be of value."

## Employing Supplements to Reverse Cancer

**Vitamin A**—Many studies have shown vitamin A in its various forms to have anticancer and immune-enhancing properties. This supplement is usually used in the form of either fish oil or oil-based vitamin A capsules, with a typical starting dosage between 10,000 and 100,000 IU daily, says Dr. Schachter. For patients having problems with absorption of fat-soluble vitamins, a water-soluble form may be used.

To prevent vitamin A toxicity, Dr. Schachter periodically checks the patient's vitamin A blood levels. Evidence of vitamin A toxicity may also show up as an elevation of certain liver enzymes that are checked in routine blood chemistry tests. Symptoms such as dry lips and skin, headaches, and joint pains may also indicate vitamin A toxicity. Evidence of any vitamin A toxicity requires either lowering the dose or temporarily discontinuing it.

**Vitamin C**—This antioxidant has proven anticancer ability and is usually taken orally in high doses of 10 to 12 g or more, divided over a day. However, some patients develop diarrhea at these high levels and the dose needs to be reduced to 3 to 5 g or less daily. In general, the idea is to increase the vitamin C dosage to bowel tolerance (development of diarrhea) and then reduce the dosage to the point that the patient no longer experiences diarrhea or uncomfortable gas and bloating, says Dr. Schachter.

**Vitamin E**—Dr. Schachter often prescribes 800 IU or more daily. Vitamin E increases the effectiveness and specific toxicity of chemotherapy agents on tumors[1] and helps protect against the toxic effects of radiation treatments.[2] This can prove extremely useful to those patients of Dr. Schachter's who are also receiving conventional treatments.

**Vitamin D**—The vitamin D supplement may be given in the range of 400 units to 1000 units daily, says Dr. Schachter. Many recent studies show evidence for anticancer activity of vitamin D in prostate cancer and other cancers.

**B-Complex Vitamins**—The B-complex vitamins have numerous metabolic functions, such as aiding in the production of energy in all cells of the body. A deficiency of any one of them can result in impaired brain and immune functions. Although a balanced diet will tend to supply enough B vitamins to the healthy individual, a person with cancer may require higher doses for optimal functioning.

Thus, Dr. Schachter usually recommends oral supplements containing B vitamins, either as the B complex or in the form of a multivitamin and mineral formula. The dosage for vitamins B1 (thiamine), B2 (riboflavin), B3 (niacin or niacinamide), B5 (pantothenic acid), and B6 (pyridoxine) is usually 10 to 100 mg daily in divided dosages.

There is evidence that higher doses of vitamin B3 (from 500 to 3000 mg daily) and vitamin B5 (100 mg to 1500 mg) may be helpful to some cancer patients. Dosages of other B-complex vitamins are as follows: biotin, 600 mcg to 5 mg; folic acid, 1 to 10 mg; and B12, 250 to 3000 mcg. Vitamin B12 is extremely important for the nervous system, to prevent anemia, and for immune function. "Cancer patients are frequently deficient in B12 because of absorption problems associated with inadequate hydrochloric acid in the stomach, surgical removal of part of the stomach or intestine, or inadequate intake, especially in vegetarians," says Dr. Schachter.

***"Cancer patients are frequently deficient in B12 because of absorption problems associated with inadequate hydrochloric acid in the stomach, surgical removal of part of the stomach or intestine, or inadequate intake, especially in vegetarians," says Dr. Schachter.***

B12 may be given as a sublingual preparation to be dissolved under the tongue or as an injection if there are absorption problems or if B12 needs to be replaced quickly. The injectable mode of administration is more effective than the sublingual route, although the latter is better than simply taking B12 oral supplements. Since there is evidence that, along with stimulating immune function, B12 may stimulate cancer growth, it is wise not to give high doses of it (more than 1000 mcg by intramuscular injection twice a week or more than 3000 mcg orally or sublingually per day). Certain functional vitamin tests, such as the measurement of plasma homocysteine and/or methylmalonic acid can help determine if B12 is needed.

CAUTION

To avoid overloading the body with iron, you should have your iron levels tested before beginning iron supplementation. The best test for doing this is the measurement of serum ferritin, a protein that bonds iron stores in the body. The test can be done in any commercial laboratory. Dr. Schachter recommends that an iron supplement be used only when the level of serum ferritin is below 20 or 30 mcg per liter of blood. Sometimes, as a result of inflammation associated with the cancer, there may be an elevation of serum ferritin in the presence of anemia and inadequate iron stores. In such a case, a therapeutic trial of iron supplementation may be warranted.

## MINERALS

Dr. Schachter generally prescribes a multivitamin-mineral formula with the full range of known essential minerals (calcium, magnesium, zinc, copper, manganese, chromium, molybdenum, iodine, and selenium) except perhaps for iron, with additional individual minerals being added either because larger amounts of that mineral are necessary for cancer patients or because the patient shows evidence of a specific mineral deficiency.

His patients have done well using mineral solutions, especially when in colloidal form. "Some patients respond positively to a colloidal mineral formula in a way that never occurred when they took only the known essential minerals in pill form," reports Dr. Schachter. "This may be because they are able to absorb them better." In addition, colloidal mineral formulas contain as many as 70 or more trace minerals in minute quantities, which probably yield therapeutic benefits. For example, minute quantities of both arsenic and aluminum have recently been shown to be essential for general health.

**Selenium—**All Schachter Center cancer patients receive relatively high doses of selenium (400 to 1,000 mcg daily, in divided doses), as research has shown that this mineral clearly is involved in cancer prevention and treatment. According to Dr. Schachter, "Selenium is the single most important mineral for fighting cancer."

**Zinc and Copper—**Dr. Schachter often prescribes zinc at 15 to 30 mg daily and copper at 2 to 4 mg daily. Zinc is intimately involved in immune system functioning, and its deficiency may readily increase one's susceptibility to cancer.[3] Copper is essential to proper functioning of a wide range of immune cell types, including antibody-forming cells, T helper cells, and macrophages, all of which may help the body defend against cancer.[4] Since excessive amounts of either copper or zinc may deplete the other, Dr. Schachter advises that their intake be carefully controlled under medical supervision. The usual safe ratio of zinc to copper is 7-14 to 1.

**Iron—**"Iron supplements are generally unwarranted unless there is evidence of iron deficiency, which tends to depress the immune system and cause anemia," says Dr. Schachter. However, anemia is not always caused by iron deficiency. It may occur as a result of the body's inability to utilize iron to make hemoglobin even though adequate iron stores are present. This can be as a consequence of the cancer disease process itself or the administration of chemotherapy. In such a case, it is unwise to supplement with iron because iron may increase free radical formation, which may, in turn, promote the growth of tumors.[5]

**Manganese**—Dr. Schachter recommends a manganese supplement (5 to 20 mg daily) because this trace element bolsters immunity and assists the body in utilizing amygdalin properly.

**Molybdenum**—According to Dr. Schachter, molybdenum (100 to 1,000 mcg daily) is useful in phase 1 liver detoxification to help oxidize sulfites (found in many preservatives), alcohol (in beverages and medications), aldehydes (a toxic by-product of metabolizing various chemicals), and other toxic substances. A low molybdenum level can be detected by a urine or blood test for this mineral.

***"The cancer patient may have increased production of internal toxins as a result of the cancer itself and metabolic products that are formed as a result of cancer breakdown," says Dr. Schachter.***

## The Importance of Detoxification in Reversing Cancer

"External toxins, including petrochemicals such as pesticides and heavy metals such as mercury, play a major role in the development and growth of cancer," says Dr. Schachter. He stresses that it is important to remove them as much as possible to both prevent and treat cancer.

Toxins may originate from inside the body as well. "The cancer patient may have increased production of internal toxins as a result of the cancer itself and metabolic products that are formed as a result of cancer breakdown." The body uses the skin, lungs, kidneys, liver, and colon to remove the toxins. "Our job in the course of healing is to *support* those organs through a variety of detoxification methods," Dr. Schachter explains. His basic approach to detoxifying involves stimulating and nourishing the organ systems to rid the body of toxins as quickly and as painlessly as possible.

***The body uses the skin, lungs, kidneys, liver, and colon to remove the toxins. "Our job in the course of healing is to support those organs through a variety of detoxification methods," Dr. Schachter explains.***

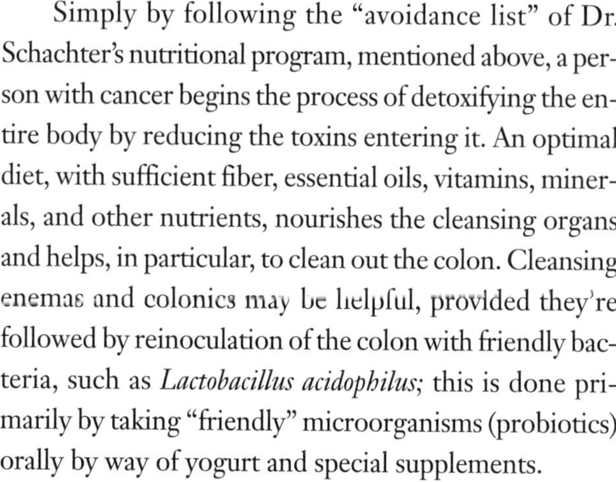

Simply by following the "avoidance list" of Dr. Schachter's nutritional program, mentioned above, a person with cancer begins the process of detoxifying the entire body by reducing the toxins entering it. An optimal diet, with sufficient fiber, essential oils, vitamins, minerals, and other nutrients, nourishes the cleansing organs and helps, in particular, to clean out the colon. Cleansing enemas and colonics may be helpful, provided they're followed by reinoculation of the colon with friendly bacteria, such as *Lactobacillus acidophilus;* this is done primarily by taking "friendly" microorganisms (probiotics) orally by way of yogurt and special supplements.

**Improving Gastrointestinal Function—**Generally, any detoxification program needs to begin with an avoidance of external toxins in air, water, and food as much as possible, along with attention to overall gastrointestinal function, according to Dr. Schachter.

For more information on **detoxification** (pp. 949-980) and protocols for **detoxifying mercury** (pp. 984-989), see Chapter 33: Physical Support Therapies. For more information on the health hazards of **mercury** fillings, see Chapter 25: What Causes Cancer?, pp. 594-600.

His approach to gastrointestinal function can be summarized by the four Rs: (1) **R**emove; (2) **R**eplace; (3) **R**einoculate; and (4) **R**epair. Through laboratory testing of stool, blood, or saliva, the diagnosis of one or more parasites, small intestine overgrowth of bacteria, or *Candida* overgrowth may be established. The first step then in restoring proper gastrointestinal function is to **remove**, as much as possible, any abnormal microorganisms. This may be done with natural substances, such as herbs (e.g., *Artemisia annua*) or grapefruit seed extract, medications, or both.

If the patient lacks hydrochloric acid in the stomach or pancreatic enzymes, these may be **replaced** with the administration of betaine hydrochloride or glutamic acid for the stomach acid and enzyme supplements for the pancreatic deficiency. The bowel then should be **reinoculated** with friendly bacteria by oral administration of yogurt, friendly bacteria supplements (*Lactobacillus acidophilus*, *bifidus*, and others), and fructooligosaccharides (FOS, special sugars that are not absorbed, but promote the growth of friendly bacteria in the colon).

Finally, any damage to the lining of the gastrointestinal system should be **repaired** by supplying the necessary nutrients for repair, such as zinc, vitamin A, vitamin C, glutamine, and others.

**Liver Detoxification**—Based on the results of testing phase 1 and phase 2 liver detoxification as discussed earlier, the appropriate steps are then taken to improve and balance the 2 phases. These may include (1) reducing external toxin intake; (2) nutrient supplements to support phase 2; (3) herbs such as silymarin (more commonly known as milk thistle); (4) nutrients such as choline and inositol (both needed for proper cell membrane functioning); (5) special therapeutic foods such as garlic, barley grass, and chlorella; and (6) coffee retention enemas, which stimulate bile release from the liver and often leave the patient feeling invigorated.

***Dr. Schachter refers many of his patients to a biological dentist for the careful removal of their mercury amalgams and replacement with a composite resin material.***

**Chelation**—After testing for the levels and types of heavy metal toxicity as discussed earlier, the appropriate chelating agent can be administered to eliminate them from the body. Chelation refers to a method of binding ("chelating") a chelating agent to a metallic ion with a positive electric charge (e.g., a heavy metal) and removing it from the body. Chelation has proven particularly effective in removing high levels of cadmium, copper, lead, and mercury.[6]

One type of chelation therapy involves the chelating agent disodium EDTA mixed with magnesium, vitamin C, and a few other substances in a 500-ml solution and given as an intravenous infusion over a 3½ hour period. Usually 20 to 30 treatments are administered at the rate of 1 to 3 sessions per week. This treatment improves circulation throughout the body, reduces misplaced soft-tissue calcification, reduces free-radical pathology, and increases oxygen to the cells.

Chelation therapy is extremely beneficial for all forms of atherosclerotic cardiovascular disease including angina pectoris and coronary artery disease, intermittent claudication and gangrene in atherosclerotic cardiovascular disease of the legs and feet, and strokes and transient ischemic attacks in atherosclerotic cardiovascular disease of the neck and brain arteries.

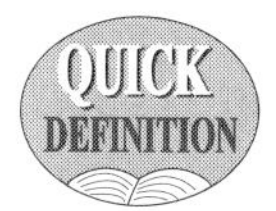

**Biological dentistry** stresses the use of nontoxic restoration materials for dental work and focuses on the unrecognized impact that dental toxins and hidden dental infections can have on overall health. Typically, a biological dentist will emphasize: the safe removal of mercury amalgams; in many cases, either the avoidance or removal of root canals; the investigation of possible jawbone infections (cavitations) as a "dental focus" or source of bodywide illness centered in the teeth; and the health-injuring role of misalignment of teeth and jaw structures.

**DMPS** (2,3-dimercaptopropane-1-sulfonate) is the chelating (binding-up) agent of choice for the removal of elemental mercury from the human body. It can be given orally, intravenously, or intramuscularly and is useful for people who have had exposure to mercury amalgam through their dental fillings or those who show evidence or suspicion of heavy metal toxicity from other sources.

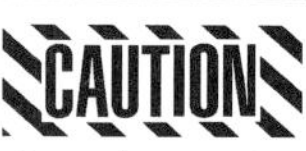

To avoid exposing the patient to toxicity caused by mercury vapors, amalgam removal should only be performed by dentists trained in the procedure; a detoxification program involving nutrient supplementation should also be undertaken at the same time.

**Biological Dentistry—**The mercury contained in dental amalgams has been proven to leach out of the amalgam and infiltrate various bodily tissues, paving the way for cancer, immune system breakdown, and other conditions. Many studies have shown, for example,that mercury from silver amalgams promotes free radical damage[7] as well as immune system suppression.[8] Dr. Schachter refers many of his patients to a biological dentist next door to his office for careful removal and replacement of the mercury amalgams in the teeth. They are usually replaced with a composite resin material.

A chelating agent known as DMPS is also effective in removing some heavy metals from the body, says Dr. Schachter. DMPS (2,3-dimercaptopropane-1-sulfonate), is the chelating (binding-up) agent of choice for the removal of elemental mercury from the human body. DMPS can be given orally, intravenously, or intramuscularly with a maximum dose of 3 mg/2.2 pounds of body weight, with 250 mg being the typical dose.

People who have had exposure to mercury through their fillings commonly require 3-5 injections, but sometimes more. Those who have never had amalgam fillings, but show evidence or suspicion of heavy metal toxicity through other sources, may require only 1-2 injections. An injection every 4-6 months thereafter may be recommended for patient maintenance. Usually, the patient will begin to notice improvement within 3-4 weeks following the DMPS injections.[9]

**Saunas and Moderate Aerobics—**To help rid the body of fat-soluble toxins, saunas may be helpful, but only if the person can tolerate the heat, says Dr. Schachter. Sweating from aerobic exercise causes an increased discharge of toxins through the skin, while exercise in general, with or without sweating, reinforces the detoxification process. Bouncing on a rebounder or doing yoga or other muscle stretching exercises stimulates the lymphatic system, aiding in detoxification.

## Amino Acids and Essential Fatty Acids to Reinforce Cancer Resistance

For Dr. Schachter, vitamins and minerals are only the tip of the therapeutic iceberg of potential supplements that may be helpful for cancer patients. Also important are anticancer factors found in the fats (lipids) and proteins in our food. Certain fatty acids found in fats and amino acids found in proteins may be given as supplements.

### AMINO ACIDS

Amino acids are the building blocks of protein, the main structural material of all living things. Although cancer patients should be careful not to get too much protein, they still need enough to supply the amino acids which in turn help the body maintain its cancer defense systems. For example, antibodies are made of proteins; the cell membrane surrounding the immune cells (lymphocytes), as well as other body cells, consists of various specialized proteins embedded in a double layer of fat.

**L-Methionine and L-Cysteine**—Dr. Schachter sometimes recommends one or more individual amino acids for his patients, depending on their treatment and condition. Two amino acids which are sometimes deficient in a vegetarian diet are the sulphur-containing essential amino acid L-methionine and its derivative L-cysteine. These amino acids fill numerous important functions, including helping the liver to detoxify, but they are particularly important for cancer patients receiving amygdalin. Cancer patients receiving amygdalin require at least one of these amino acids in the diet or as a supplement to supply sulfur, which is necessary to convert cyanide (in amygdalin) into a harmless compound called thiocyanate.

Amygdalin is generally safe, but cancer patients on a sulfur-deficient diet may experience some discomfort or a lack of benefit from taking amygdalin, unless methionine or cysteine are added to the program, says Dr. Schachter. Cysteine, which may be converted into glutathione (part of a major antioxidant system, glutathione peroxidase), may greatly reduce the toxic side effects from both chemotherapy and radiation treatments.[10] Methionine supplements may reduce the body's uptake of mercury, thereby freeing up the immune cells to more actively ward off cancer.[11]

L-methionine or L-cysteine may be taken as individual amino acid supplements at 500 mg, 2-3 times a day. Cysteine may be better absorbed in the form of N-acetyl cysteine at the same dosage.

**L-Glutamine**—In relatively high doses (8 to 40 g daily), this amino acid prevents muscle breakdown, supports the liver, aids acid-base balance, stimulates the immune system, helps in glutathione formation, and repairs the lining of the digestive tract, says Dr. Schachter.

There is some controversy about taking glutamine in high doses because theoretically it may stimulate the growth of cancer. However, recent studies in animals and humans indicate that, overall, glutamine is extremely helpful to cancer patients and does not stimulate cancer growth.

## ESSENTIAL FATTY ACIDS

**Omega-3 Fatty Acids**—Dr. Schachter includes an omega-3 source for most of his cancer patients. Omega-3 fatty acids come primarily from the following sources listed in order from highest to lowest concentrations: flaxseed oil (50%), fish oils, including cod liver oil (20%), walnut oil (13%), canola oil (11%), and soy oil (5%). He most often recommends 1 to 3 tablespoons of flaxseed oil daily and 1/2 to 1 tablespoon of cod liver oil daily. Both for taste and for increased therapeutic value, the flaxseed oil may be mixed with cottage cheese in the ratio of 1 tablespoon of flaxseed oil to 2 tablespoons of cottage cheese.

**Lipid** is a biochemist's term for a fat or oil, which is one of the 6 basic food groups. Fats and oils are made of building blocks called fatty acids. Of these long-chain molecules (comprising atoms of carbon, hydrogen, and oxygen) the "fatty" end does not dissolve in water, while the "acid" end does. Fats are also called triglycerides as they consist of 3 (tri) fatty acid molecules joined to one molecule of glycerol, a kind of sugar. Unsaturated fats required in the diet are called essential fatty acids, and include linoleic acid (an omega-6 oil), found in corn, beans, and some nuts and seeds, and alpha linolenic acid (an omega-3 oil), found in fish, flaxseed, and walnuts.

**Omega-6 Fatty Acids**—Examples of omega-6 fatty acids include linoleic acid, arachidonic acid, and gamma linolenic acid. Linoleic acid is found in most vegetable oils, such as corn, safflower, and sunflower. Arachidonic acid, found in red meat and dairy products, is a precursor of certain local hormones that tend to be carcinogenic. Dr. Schachter recommends that his patients limit these classes of foods.

One hormone that appears to have anticancer properties is prostaglandin E1. Its precursor is gamma linolenic acid, which is normally formed from linoleic acid. However, for a variety of reasons, especially in cancer patients, this conversion is not made easily. Consequently, a natural source of gamma linolenic acid is necessary to help produce therapeutic levels of prostaglandin E1 to aid the cancer patient.

The major sources of gamma linolenic acid are primrose, borage, and black currant oils. Dr. Schachter frequently includes one of these in his therapeutic program. He prefers primrose oil (500 mg capsules, 2-3 capsules 3 times per day) as most of the research in this area has been done with that oil.

## Prescribing Enzymes That "Eat" Cancer

According to Dr. Schachter, most cancer patients are deficient in protein-degrading (proteolytic) enzymes. These are natural compounds that help the body digest food. In a healthy, cancer-free person, this class of enzymes is produced in adequate amounts by the pancreas. However, a person who lacks these enzymes has difficulty breaking down, absorbing, and utilizing the nutrients in food.

For this reason, Dr. Schachter often prescribes oral pancreatic enzymes to be taken with meals to help break down proteins, fats, and carbohydrates. Hydrochloric acid, the major digestive stomach acid, is occasionally added to the mix in the form of betaine or glutamic acid if there is evidence of low stomach acid, as determined by the Heidelberg capsule. This is a capsule, the size of a B-complex capsule, that has a pH meter and a radiotransmitter inside. The patient swallows it and a radio receiver over the patient's stomach picks up and records the pH of the stomach. The capsule can pass through the GI tract into the stool or a string can be attached so that the capsule can be pulled out after the test. When a string is used, while the capsule is in the stomach, small samples of bicarbonate of soda solution (high pH) can be given and the physician can observe if and how long it takes for the stomach acid to neutralize the bicarbonate. This measures the acid reserve of the stomach.

Pancreatic enzymes also serve a more cancer-specific function. When taken between meals, some of these enzymes are absorbed intact and can have systemic effects that are beneficial to the cancer patient. These actions include an anti-inflammatory effect and a tendency to dissolve the protective coating around cancer cells.

For more information on **enzymes**, see Chapter 32: Enhancing Whole-Body Metabolism for Treating Cancer, pp. 928-934; for more on **therapeutic foods**, see Chapter 29: Botanicals as Cancer Medicine.

**Enzymes** are specialized living proteins fundamental to all living processes in the body, necessary for every chemical reaction and the normal activity of our organs, tissues, fluids, and cells. There are hundreds of thousands of these Nature's "workers." Enzymes enable your body to digest and assimilate food. There are special enzymes for digesting proteins, carbohydrates, fats, and plant fibers. Specifically, protease digests proteins, amylase digests carbohydrates, lipase digests fats, cellulase digests fiber, and disaccharidases digest sugars.

Dr. Schachter uses pancreatic enzyme tablets, bromelain, papaya, and combinations of these and other enzymes.[12] The amounts of these enzymes vary considerably, according to how they're administered (i.e., orally or as a rectal enema, which allows for more rapid entry of the enzymes into the blood circulation.)

## Therapeutic Foods and Accessory Food Factors (AFFs)

Substances found in food that appear to be useful for health, but do not fall into the old nutritional categories of macronutrients (proteins, fats, and carbohydrates), vitamins, or minerals are termed accessory food factors (AFFs). Many of these are available as oral nutritional supplements and Dr. Schachter sometimes adds these to his program. For liver support, choline and inositol (500-1500 mg of each daily) may be helpful. Mixed carotenoids, including beta carotene, pycnogenol, and other bioflavonoids may be added for their varied effects.

***"As part of a comprehensive health-enhancing program, amygdalin is a useful natural substance for fighting cancer," Dr. Schachter says.***

Therapeutic foods include garlic, barley greens, wheat grass, spirulina, chlorella, various mushrooms (such as maitake), soy compounds or extracts containing large doses of isoflavones, amygdalin (laetrile), bovine tracheal cartilage and/or shark cartilage, and many others. Many of these foods contain compounds which do not directly kill cancer cells, but do so through stimulation of elements within the body's immune system.

**Amygdalin (Laetrile)**—Amygdalin is a natural cyanide-containing substance, present in numerous foods, which has been used to prevent and treat cancer for many years. Dr. Schachter, who has used it for more than 20 years with cancer patients, remarks, "As part of a comprehensive health-enhancing program, amygdalin is a useful natural substance for fighting cancer."

Amygdalin may be given as an oral supplement (a 500-mg tablet, 1 to 3 times daily). It may also be administered intravenously. By eating amygdalin-rich foods, patients may get substantial amounts in their diet. One source is bitter apricot kernels which are safe at the rate of 3-5 apricot kernels 3 times daily.

**Cartilage**—The use of cartilage for cancer patients has become an increasingly important tool at the Schachter Center. The dosage of shark cartilage for patients with advanced cancer is from 1/2 to 1 g per pound of body weight (roughly 60 to 200 g) daily in divided doses. The dosage should be started low and gradually increased. Since shark cartilage capsules are usually 750 mg (or 3/4 of a gram), the number of capsules required per day would obviously be prohibitive for most patients, says Dr. Schachter.

For this reason, it is usually administered in powdered form, mixed in tomato juice (or some other form of juice), and preferably taken on an empty stomach 2 to 4 times daily. A rounded tablespoon is about 15 g of shark cartilage, so a patient could be taking 4 to 12 tablespoons daily. The high dosages of cartilage may be slowly reduced as the patient responds to the program. For less advanced cancers or for prevention, much lower doses of shark cartilage may be used. The dosage is determined by the weight of the patient, the severity of the condition, and response to treatment.

For patients who cannot tolerate taking shark cartilage orally or whose appetite is suppressed by doing so, an alternative is a rectal retention enema, explains Dr.

## Shark Cartilage Made the Difference in Colon Cancer

A 43 year-old fireman, Jared was suffering from jaundice and had lost 20 lbs of body weight, but gained 35 lbs of fluid in his abdominal cavity. Testing revealed widespread cancer in the abdominal cavity from a primary cancer in the colon. Prior to his visit to the Schachter Center, Jared had received 5 chemotherapy treatments without an apparent response.

Dr. Schachter put him on shark cartilage (40 g administered as a rectal retention enema twice a day for a total of 80 grams), herbs, and vitamins. Jared continued to receive chemotherapy with the Schachter program. Within 3 weeks, he lost 17 lbs of fluid, his weight falling from 186 to 169 lbs. At 8 weeks, he had lost another 18 lbs of fluid and was down to 151. At 16 weeks, he was back to his normal weight of 175 lbs without any evidence of fluid. In 6 months, his cancer marker CEA (carcinoembryonic antigen, used especially for colon cancer; normal is less than 2.5) dropped from 100 to 2.4. At that time, he was fully active and felt great, continuing on his conventional program, along with the shark cartilage, vitamins, and herbs. His oncologists expressed amazement, reporting that they had never seen such a response from chemotherapy alone.

During Jared's visit to his oncologist a month later, however, his CEA had gone up slightly. The oncologist told Jared the shark cartilage might be interfering with the chemotherapy and advised him to stop it, which he did. He went downhill quickly after that and was bedbound within a few weeks. Two months after discontinuing the shark cartilage, he died.

"This is pretty strong evidence that the shark cartilage was responsible for his dramatic positive improvement and the removal of it was the cause of his precipitous decline and demise,"states Dr. Schachter.

Schachter. To do this, the patient empties a Fleets enema bag and fills it with a suspension of 1 to 3 heaping tablespoons (20 to 60 grams) of shark cartilage powder mixed in 6 ounces of pure water. All of the contents are inserted into the rectum and retained for at least 30 minutes. This may be repeated 2 or 3 times daily. Some patients will take 1 or 2 dosages orally and 1 or 2 doses by rectum.

Generally, shark cartilage should be used for 2 to 4 months before assuming that it isn't working. If it is effective, it probably needs to be continued indefinitely with the dosage being adjusted up or down, depending on the patient's response.

A form that is much easier to take is frozen shark cartilage extract which contains the protein in the cartilage that appears to be responsible for some or all of the antiangiogenesis (blocking blood vessel formation in tumors which they need in order to grow) activity. It is available as a nutritional supplement. To retain the antiangiogenic function, the protein solution must be kept frozen until used by the patient. It is shipped in dry ice and must be stored in a freezer. It comes in 7-cc vials and the usual dosage is 1 vial daily. When ready to take the solution, warm the vial in your hand until the frozen preparation melts. Half of the solution is placed under the tongue, kept there for 5 minutes, and then swallowed. This is repeated with the second half of the solution.

***"Maitake mushroom does not kill cancer cells directly, but stimulates the immune-competent cells to destroy the cancer cells," Dr. Schachter says.***

Frozen shark cartilage extract may be used instead of powder in some cases or in addition to it in patients with more advanced disease. For the latter, the Schachter Center may also utilize bovine tracheal cartilage and one or more forms of shark cartilage. The decision as to which type of cartilage or which form should be used for a particular patient is determined by factors such as the severity of the disease, the patient's willingness and ability to do the treatments, and the cost, among other factors.

"Although there is insufficient formal research to state that cartilage is of proven benefit in treating cancer patients, like many other nontoxic substances, there is enough theoretical evidence and there are enough clinical reports to justify its use in willing patients," says Dr. Schachter.

**Matiake Mushroom (*Grifola*) Extract**—This mushroom has powerful immune-enhancing potential and cancer-fighting ability. "Maitake does not kill cancer cells directly, but stimulates the immune-competent cells to destroy the cancer cells," Dr. Schachter says. It shows strong anticancer activity even when it is administered orally.

## Dr. Schachter's Injectable Program for Reversing Cancer

Another key component in Dr. Schachter's approach is nutrients and other medicinal substances given by injection because this method delivers them directly to the bloodstream. If the cancer patient has intestinal absorption problems, the injections ensure that the patient will receive optimal levels of certain key nutrients and biologically-active substances. As Dr. Schachter notes, "The blood and tissue levels can be much higher with the injectable method than with oral administration. This high concentration may be necessary to turn on certain enzyme systems as well as achieve other therapeutic effects."

Patients usually come to Dr. Schachter's office 1-3 times per week for the first 1-2 months to receive either brief injections, called "pushes," or prolonged IV infusions. The shorter IV pushes take 10-20 minutes and usually consist of 7.5-10 g of vitamin C, with calcium, magnesium, and trace minerals. The longer infusions normally consist of 25 g of vitamin C, calcium, magnesium, potassium, zinc, selenium, manganese, chromium, glutathione, and a small amount of heparin (naturally produced by the body; also a conventional drug for thinning the blood and, in this case, preventing irritation to the vein from repeated infusions), combined in 500 ml of sterile water and dripped in over a period of 1-3 hours. (In comparison, EDTA chelation infusions usually last 3-4 hours.)

On some occasions, Dr. Schachter adds vitamin B6 and pantothenic acid to the IV infusion mixture. Toward the end of the infusion, amygdalin (3-9 g) is added to the IV or given a separately after the vitamin C infusion has finished. Under certain medical circumstances, such as fluid retention, an injection of 7.5-10 g of vitamin C and smaller amounts of the minerals mentioned above are given as a 60-cc sterile-water infusion instead of the larger infusion. Again, this may be followed by an injection of amygdalin at the dosage of 3-9 g. Vitamin C in high concentrations can actually kill cancer cells and leave normal cells alone, but this cancer cell-killing effect may be obtained *only* with intravenous infusions of vitamin C, says Dr. Schachter.

There is a possible problem here, says Dr. Schachter, in that the benefit of the vitamin C cytotoxic mechanism may require that high levels of vitamin C be in contact with the cancer for many hours. The usual office infusion of vitamin C given over 1-3 hours may not be sufficient. Consequently, Dr. Schachter sometimes recommends a home infusion program for cancer patients; here they can receive intravenous infusions of 25-50 g or more of vitamin C over an 8-12 hour period, anywhere from 1-7 times weekly. Dr. Schachter is in the process of evaluating whether this approach in the delivery of vitamin C to cancer patients will result in a significant improvement in therapeutic results.

**Intramuscular Vitamin B Complex**—For patients who show low energy levels, Dr. Schachter sometimes uses intramuscular injections of vitamins and minerals, especially vitamin B12 and magnesium, along with calcium, which reduces the pain of the injection. These injections not only enhance immunity and improve energy levels, but tend to stimulate one's appetite as well, according to Dr. Schachter.

**Staphage Lysate (SPL)**—Since 1981, Dr. Schachter has stimulated the immune systems of his cancer patients by giving injections of staphage lysate. This consists of remnants of a common bacterium called *Staphylococcus aureus*, as well as viruses (phages) which attack the bacterium.

The basic principle is that the immune system is "tricked" into producing cells that would target and eliminate not only these foreign entities, but also any cancer cells in the system. Recent research found that staphage lysate increases delayed cellular immunity and other immune functions that play a role in cancer resistance.[13,14] Unfortunately, the FDA "temporarily" removed SPL from the market a few years ago, allegedly because of labeling problems. As of this writing, it is still not available.

## Oxygen and Bio-oxidative Therapies

Cancer cells do not survive well in an oxygen-rich (aerobic) environment; hence "bio-oxidative" therapies hold promise for cancer patients. Bio-oxidative therapies have profound immune-enhancing effects on the body, as demonstrated by numerous studies in animals and humans, and have been in continuous use for more than 100 years in many countries, including the United States. The oxidative modalities currently used at the Schachter Center include intravenous hydrogen peroxide infusions, ultraviolet irradiation of blood, and ozone therapy.

**Hydrogen Peroxide ($H_2O_2$)—**This is a natural substance made by normal healthy human cells in the body to regulate metabolism and act as a poison to destroy invaders. The procedure used at the Schachter Center for cancer patients consists of adding pure hydrogen peroxide to a 250-ml sugar-water solution (5% dextrose in water to form a weak solution of 0.03% hydrogen peroxide) and infusing it slowly into a vein over a period of 1 to 1 ½ hours.

This treatment is quite safe, Dr. Schachter says hundreds of patients have received it at the Schachter Center since 1986. Often, the hydrogen peroxide infusion is alternated with intravenous vitamin C drips, with the 2 being given on different days, usually at least 24 hours apart.

**Ultraviolet Blood Irradiation—**Another bio-oxidative modality recently introduced at the Schachter Center is ultraviolet blood irradiation, which has been in medical use since the 1930s. This technique was used to combat the polio virus. It involves removing approximately 250 ml of blood, passing it through a chamber where it is exposed to ultraviolet light at therapeutic wavelengths, and reinfusing it into the patient. These blood cells, once returned to the body, transfer their radiant energy to neighboring cells until most of the cells in the body have the benefit of this energy. The entire procedure takes about an hour.

Also called photo-oxidation or photo-luminescence, ultraviolet blood irradiation has been shown to inactivate toxins, destroy and inhibit bacteria and viruses, increase the oxygen in the blood, cause the blood vessels to widen (vasodilation), activate white blood cells, stimulate cellular and humoral immunity, increase destruction of clots (fibrinolysis), decrease blood thickness (viscosity), improve microcirculation, and decrease platelet aggregation. The procedure is done from once, in the case of acute viral infection, to as often as daily for a short period in treating cancer and other immune system disorders.

**Ozone Therapy**—Several different methods are used in the application of ozone. Intravenous application, colonic irrigation (with ozonated water), rectal insufflation (ozone gas administered through a tube into the rectum), bagging (a noninvasive topical application to wounds, burns, and gangrene), and autohemotherapy are just a few of the techniques used worldwide.

The Schachter Center practices the technique known as major autohemotherapy, which involves removing approximately 100 to 250 ml of the patient's blood. Ozone and oxygen are mixed with the blood for several minutes and then reinfused into the patient's bloodstream. The entire procedure takes about 45 minutes. It is probably the most common ozone therapy used today. Side effects are usually minimal to nil.

## Special Botanical Formulas May Help in Cancer Reversal

Botanical medicine plays an increasingly vital role in Dr. Schachter's treatment of cancer patients. In some cases, he uses single herbs for specific purposes, such as to improve digestion or speed up detoxification. In most cases, however, he uses combinations of herbs which appear to have a reasonable track record.

**FlorEssence**—Thousands of cancer patients have been treated with this herbal tea (a variant of Essiac), and many have claimed that it has merit in treating cancer. The tea can be made at home following the precise insructions that come with the tea. Although research in this area is limited, Dr. Schachter believes there is enough anecdotal evidence to support its use, especially since it is nontoxic. For cancer patients, Dr. Schachter generally advises taking FlorEssence twice daily; mix 2 ounces of it with 2 ounces of boiled, purified water, sip slowly for 4-5 minutes on an empty stomach an hour before breakfast and at bedtime.

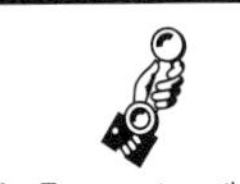

**FlorEssence** is available in health food stores, or contact: Flora, Inc., P.O. Box 950, Lynden, WA 98264; tel: 800-446-2110. For information on Vitae Elixxir, call 307-266-5710.

**Vitae Elixxir**—Dr. Schachter often uses FlorEssence in combination with another herbal-mineral mixture called Vitae Elixxir. This mixture can be taken orally as drops mixed with food or drink, gradually increasing the dosage over several days. Generally, the maximum dosage of Vitae Elixxir is 6 drops taken 3 times a day, for a daily total of 18 drops.

Alternatively, Vitae Elixxir can be used as a foot bath when mixed with

DMSO (dimethyl sulfoxide). This method works well in the case of extremely ill patients or those unable to tolerate taking Vitae Elixxir orally due to digestive problems or to severely impaired appetites. Although a number of his patients have used this combination with apparent benefit, Dr. Schachter cautions that his own experience is still too limited for him to make any compelling statements about the efficacy of using either Essiac or Vitae Elixxir for the treatment of cancer. He also cautions that it is best to use both FlorEssence and Vitae Elixxir under medical supervision, so that responses to treatment can be monitored.

CAUTION

Dr. Schachter warns patients against using DHEA on a casual, nonprescriptive basis as the substance may promote hormone-sensitive cancers like breast cancer and prostate cancer; this is possible because DHEA is a precursor for both testosterone and estrogen.

For more informaiton on **thyroid hormone** and other glandular extracts, see Chapter 32: Enhancing Whole-Body Metabolism for Treating Cancer, pp. 935-945.

## The Benefits of Balancing the Hormones

Many cancer patients have hormonal imbalances, notably those hormones produced by the thyroid and adrenal glands. After screening for gross thyroid dysfunction with routine thyroid blood tests, Dr. Schachter often asks patients with suspected low thyroid function to check their basal body temperature over several days. Low temperatures may indicate poor or marginal thyroid functioning—even when thyroid hormone levels appear to be normal in the blood—and this reduces the body's cancer-resisting ability. If low, thyroid hormones can be given.

**DHEA**—Another hormone important to the cancer process is DHEA, an adrenal secretion with many functions. When adrenal function is overly stressed or weak, perhaps due to stressful lifestyle, the blood levels of DHEA tend to be low. In these cases, Dr. Schachter may recommend 5-15 mg of oral DHEA daily, only rarely increasing this to 25-100 mg; the dosage is adjusted according to the actual DHEA sulfate levels measured in the patient's blood.

Recently, the Schachter Center has begun to do a more complete assessment of adrenal function by checking saliva levels of DHEA and cortisol several times over a 24-hour period, thus determining accurately the overall state of the adrenals. To correct problems, glandulars, nutrients, herbs, or physiologic (equal to what the body would naturally produce) doses of natural hormones may be used.

**Progesterone and Estriol**—These natural female hormones may play a

***"Homeopathic remedies can help improve mood and outlook, reduce pain, and enhance the immune system; they are nontoxic and will probably play a major role in managing cancer patients in the future," Dr. Schachter says.***

role in cancer prevention in women who are deficient in them. Some evidence indicates that they have anticancer properties. However, their role in actually treating cancer is not clear at this time. Natural progesterone, taken either orally or used as a skin cream, is well absorbed and helps to overcome the condition of estrogen dominance, which predisposes a woman to the development of breast and probably ovarian cancer.

Estriol, a form of estrogen, has weak estrogenic effects and seems to have anticancer activity, in contrast to the other forms of estrogen (estradiol and estrone). So when Dr. Schachter prescribes estrogen replacement therapy for postmenopausal women, most of the estrogen prescribed will be estriol. Any patient receiving hormonal therapy should be under medical supervision with monitoring of hormone levels through saliva or blood tests.

QUICK DEFINITION

**Homeopathy is** now practiced according to two differing concepts. In classical homeopathy, only one single-component remedy is prescribed at a time in a potency specifically adjusted to the patient; the physician waits to see the results before prescribing anything further. In complex homeopathy, typified by *Hepar compositum*, a prescription involves multiple substances given at the same time usually in low potencies.

**Melatonin—**Regarding the hormone melatonin, Dr. Schachter recommends that it be taken only at night, since it promotes sleep; he recommends it in dosages from less than 1 mg to 10 mg daily, as a sleep aid. Recent research on melatonin suggests it is a strong, nontoxic antioxidant that is available to every cell of the body. It appears to protect against the toxic effects of radiation. Some research protocols for cancer patients call for 40 mg daily of melatonin. Dr. Schachter is considering trying higher doses with some of his cancer patients.

## Energy Therapies Are Key Adjuncts in the Program

Energy-based therapies, such as homeopathy, spinal adjustments (both chiropractic and osteopathy), acupuncture, and magnetic therapy, are useful in the treatment of cancer, says Dr. Schachter. The combination of approaches depends on the individual patient's needs and desires.

**Homeopathy—**Dr. Schachter believes that homeopathy is useful for some of his cancer patients to help with pain control and psychological disturbances associated with the cancer, and to strengthen the body's defenses against the cancer. He refers these patients to a classical homeopath on his staff who is familiar with the work of A.H. Grimmer, a classical homeopath who worked extensively with cancer patients in the early 1900s.

Generally, it is not a matter of simply matching a homeopathic remedy with a particular type of cancer, but matching the remedy to the individual person, whose total picture includes the cancer. Nevertheless, certain classical homeopathic remedies frequently apply to states found in cancer patients or in certain types of cancer, says Dr. Schachter.

For example, patients with "wasting" (loss of lean body mass as a result of cancer growth) who are in a state of agitated restlessness and fearful of death will often benefit from the remedy *Arsenicum album.* Prostate cancer patients often are helped by *Conium* or *Lycopodium,* while breast cancer patients often respond to *Conium, Phytolacca,* or *Silica.* These are only possibilities—each case must be completely individualized. "Homeopathic remedies can help improve mood and outlook, reduce pain, and enhance the immune system," Dr. Schachter says. "They are nontoxic and will probably play a major role in managing cancer patients in the future."

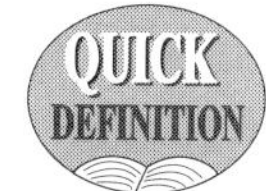


**Electrodermal screening** is a form of computerized information gathering, based on physics, not chemistry. A noninvasive electric probe is placed at specific points on the patient's hands, face, or feet, corresponding to acupuncture meridian points at the beginning or end of energy meridians. Minute electrical discharges from these points serve as information signals about the condition of the body's organs and systems, useful for a physician in evaluation and developing a treatment plan.

For more information on **electrodermal screening** and **magnetic therapy**, see Chapter 34: Energy Support Therapies, pp. 1021-1045; Chapter 20: Vincent Speckhart, M.D., pp. 422-431.

**Electrodermal Screening**—The Schachter Center uses electrodermal screening (EDS) to measure imbalances in acupuncture meridians[15] and determine with some degree of success which homeopathic remedies will work best for individual cancer patients. EDS can also measure the positive or negative effects on the patient's body of foods, nutritional supplements, and other substances.

By measuring the electric skin resistance at acupuncture points and placing one or more of the substances to be tested in linkage with the instrument and the patient's acupuncture points, a reasonable assessment may be made as to whether or not the substance is helpful to the body and whether or not it will be tolerated.

**Acupuncture, Acupressure, and Massage**—Dr. Schachter also recommends the use of acupuncture and acupressure to stimulate the body's internal energy which runs along energy pathways known as meridians. In most cases, both therapies are used to reduce pain and stimulate the body's immune defenses. Therapeutic massage can also enhance the patient's sense of well-being and induce deep relaxation.

For more detail on **hydrazine sulfate**, see Chapter 26: How Cancer Politics Have Kept You in the Dark, pp. 668-674; and Chapter 30: The New Pharmacology for Treating Cancer, pp. 868-869.

The application of hydrazine sulfate to cancer therapies warrants further research in which appropriate protocols are used.

**Magnetic Therapy**—Another useful adjunctive approach is magnetic therapy, which is the clinical application of permanent magnets (and their magnetic fields) to tumors and areas of pain. "I have seen dramatic results when the north magnetic pole (also known as the negative magnetic energy pole or south-seeking magnetic pole) is applied to a cancer or an area of inflammation," Dr. Schachter says. "The north pole tends to inhibit inflammation and inhibit cancer growth, whereas the south pole tends to stimulate it." One patient with an inflamed breast and another with brain cancer both showed clear-cut benefits with magnetic therapy. Others have also reported benefits.

## Additional Potentially Beneficial Substances for Cancer Treatments

Occasionally, Dr. Schachter finds it appropriate to prescribe conventional drugs of proven low toxicity.

**Hydrazine Sulfate**—This substance seems to retard or inhibit the loss of protein or body mass caused by cancer while at the same time exerting indirect antitumor effects. According to Dr. Schachter, "Hydrazine sulfate seems to starve out cancer cells while leaving normal cells alone." Hydrazine sulfate is a relatively inexpensive medication and appears to be nontoxic when administered properly.

Hydrazine sulfate must not be used by patients who are taking certain drugs, such as alcohol, barbiturates, antidepressants, and antipsychotics, cautions Dr. Schachter. Pain medications may be safely used without interfering with hydrazine sulfate, but dosages of more than 25 mg of vitamin B6 and more than 3 g of vitamin C may interfere with hydrazine sulfate's activity.

A number of clinical studies throughout the world have shown the benefits of hydrazine sulfate in treating cancer. However, it is an extremely controversial product; it was on the American Cancer Society's "Unproven Cancer Cures" list for years, until its removal in 1982. The FDA has not approved it as a cancer treatment, based on the results of FDA-approved clinical trials.

According to Joseph Gold, M.D., who developed the treatment, these FDA-approved clinical trials were flawed, using the wrong dosage or using incompatible drugs at the same time. Nevertheless, because of the FDA's "compassionate use" provisions, cancer patients are usually able to obtain the drug for their own use from sources outside of the United States or sometimes from compounding pharmacies within the United States when it is prescribed by a physician.

**Urea and Creatine Monohydrate**—A natural chemical produced by the liver, synthesized urea, given orally, increases urea concentrations in the bloodstream sufficient to inhibit cancer growth in the liver, says Dr. Schachter. Observations made over an 11-year period indicate substantial clinical benefits of using urea to treat primary or secondary (metastatic) liver cancer.[16] A typical dosage for urea is 15-30 g in powder form, dissolved in a quart of water or juice, and imbibed over the course of the day, in at least 4 (preferably 8) divided doses.

Recent evidence indicates that the results of this treatment may be improved by adding creatine monohydrate to the urea. This substance, also natural to the body, is associated with muscle activity. The dosage of creatine monohydrate in the mixture remains constant at 25 g added to the quart. The mixture must be shaken vigorously immediately prior to each ingestion because the creatine monohydrate is not completely soluble.

## Pain Relief for Bone Cancer

Dr. Schachter sometimes uses another drug called pamidronate (brand name, Aredia) as an intravenous transfusion to treat bone metastases. This treatment appears to reduce pain and slow up the progression of the disease. It sometimes even reverses, at least temporarily, the size of the bone metastases. Pamidronate has been approved by the FDA for the treatment of elevated blood calcium (hypercalcemia, which can cause cardiac arrest) often due to cancer in the bone, and cancerous bone lesions associated with 2 cancers—multiple myeloma and breast cancer—even if hypercalcemia is not present.

The dosage of pamidronate generally used by Dr. Schachter is 90 mg dissolved in 250 ml of saline or dextrose and water, given intravenously over a 3-4 hour period, every 3-4 weeks for 6-8 or more treatments; the patient is then reevaluated for further treatment. Since pamidronate is FDA-approved, it is available by prescription.

***"Even if a person with cancer gets in only 2-5 minutes of walking outdoors, that's a good start because every little bit helps," says Dr. Schachter.***

The dosage of urea varies, depending upon the results of a monitored blood test. After 2 weeks of 15 g of urea, a blood test measuring blood urea nitrogen (BUN) is taken towards the end of the day after the patient has ingested several dosages. The desired BUN level, assuming normally functioning kidneys, is between 35 and 40 mg/100 ml of serum. If the BUN is below this level, the dosage of urea added to the mixture should be increased to 20 g and the BUN should be rechecked in 2 more weeks. The dosage of urea may sometimes go as high as 25 or 30 g added to the mixture. Once the dosage is found, it should be maintained with periodic checks on the BUN.

For more information on **exercise** benefits, see Chapter 33: Physical Support Therapies for Reversing Cancer, pp. 1003-1005; for more on **psychological factors**, see Chapter 25: What Causes Cancer?, pp. 613-615.

Urea and creatine monohydrate are both available over the counter in selected pharmacies and health food stores.

## Making Environmental and Lifestyle Adjustments

Environmental factors can also support the process of recovering from cancer. Primary among Dr. Schachter's recommendations is getting ample exposure to sunlight and fresh air. The reason is that both support optimal immune functioning and enhance the results of other alternative cancer treatments. A landmark study showed that cancer patients who spent 2 or more hours each day outdoors had greater longevity compared to cancer patients who stayed indoors.[17]

Dr. Schachter advises his patients to avoid exposure to electric blankets, high-voltage electric fields, and fluorescent lighting (unless it is full-spectrum fluorescent lighting) because these energies appear to be harmful to the delicate electromagnetic energy systems of the body.

Starting a program of aerobic exercise is another important lifestyle adjustment. "Ideally, cancer patients who are strong enough should seek out an exercise program in which the amount of oxygen taken in is equal to the amount being used," says Dr. Schachter. "This is accomplished through the action of the body's large muscles in activities such as rapid walking, bike riding, or swimming."

Dr. Schachter generally recommends that people exercise for a minimum of 25-30 minutes, 3-4 times weekly. Though many cancer patients have trouble reaching this goal at first, they can gradually work up to it. "Even if a person with cancer gets in only 2-5 minutes of walking outdoors, that's a good start because every little bit helps." Stretching exercises may complement any other exercise program because they help relax the muscles and prepare them for activity.

However, if a patient feels exhausted or distressed after exercise, one needs to tone down the efforts or even stop temporarily, Dr. Schachter cautions. Excessive exercise can actually cause toxicity through the creation of free radicals, so overexertion is not recommended. The dietary and supplement program must be maintained at all times to maintain an ample supply of antioxidants, minerals and other nutrients which will reinforce the benefits of exercise.

***"It is important to help the patient reframe the cancer experience as a message that one's life is not in harmony or balance and that changes in lifestyle would be helpful," Dr. Schachter says.***

## Education and Counseling That Support Healing

Patient education forms an invaluable part of Dr. Schachter's approach. Adjoining his waiting room is a small store offering books, audio and video cassettes relating to health, mind/body interactions, and alternative cancer treatments. "The videotapes in particular are great motivators. They've inspired many of my patients to take a more active role in their treatment by educating themselves and discussing any questions or issues with me and my staff." After all, "it is difficult to imagine a more stressful circumstance than being told that you have cancer and then have to deal with it."

Intense stress and anxiety such as this can directly impair the immune system, reducing one's chances of recovery. This is why Dr. Schachter's staff includes therapists who work with cancer patients both individually and in groups using mind/body treatment modalities of Carl Simonton, M.D., Bernie Siegel, M.D., and Lawrence LeShan. Each of these authorities is renowned for his insight into the psychological, emotional, and spiritual factors involved in cancer and the need to resolve these factors as part of the cancer treatment. "It is important to help the patient reframe the cancer experience as a message that one's life is not in harmony or balance and that changes in lifestyle would be helpful," Dr. Schachter says.

Dr. Schachter's training in psychiatry deepened his ability to understand people and emphathize with the psychological dynamics of the doctor-patient relationship. Among the pivotal insights gained from his work with cancer patients over the years is recognizing the need to meet them at their own level. "Sometimes people aren't ready to do meditation, guided imagery, or other kinds of mind/body work," Dr. Schachter says. "Doctors must be able to recognize the defense mechanisms of their patients and to respect where they're at psychologically at the time, not just go in like a bull in a china shop and try to adjust their whole world view."

Understanding how the patients see their world, themselves, and their illness is a first step toward forging a successful alliance with the patient, one more likely to result in a solid commitment to healing and to long-term survival, says Dr. Schachter. The potential success of a treatment often can be gauged during the first visit. "Consider the cancer patient who is dragged in by his family and doesn't really want to be there. His outcome will likely be far worse than that of the patient who does his homework and knows firmly what he wants to do—that he wants to do *whatever* needs to be done to survive."

At the same time, Dr. Schachter doesn't turn away patients who seem to lack either the motivation or the support to fully engage in his comprehensive program. "I try to work with whoever comes through the door. My goal is not to try to change them in any fundamental way, but to help them choose a path that makes sense to them, a path they will follow with conviction and enthusiasm."

With so many alternative cancer therapy options, it is literally impossible to do "everything." This is where the *art* of medicine comes in. To understand patients and their total situation, as well as the current available information on alternative therapies, which literally changes every day, the physician must integrate all of the information and, together with the patient and patient's family, choose the elements of the program that will most likely work for that particular person. Then a reasonable trial should be given with careful observation. A willingness to shift gears and either remove or add elements of the program should be maintained in order to increase the chance of a successful result.

Many of Dr. Schachter's patients are exposed to conventional therapies before receiving his treatment. He believes that patients receiving conventional cancer therapy while also on his metabolically supportive regimen do better than those who undergo conventional therapy without receiving such support.

Dr. Schachter is in the process of conducting retrospective studies with certain types of cancer patients to compare the efficacy of his program alone with that of patients receiving his program along with conventional treatment of chemotherapy and radiation. He expresses his present position as follows: "Personally, I believe that in many cases, patients who select only the alternative program and leave out the more destructive conventional treatment will do better."

## CURRICULUM VITAE

# Charles B. Simone, M.MS., M.D.

Simone Protective Cancer Center, 123 Franklin Corner Road, Lawrenceville, NJ 08648; tel: 609-896-2646

Dr. Simone received his Master's of Medical Science and M.D. from Rutgers College of Medicine in Piscataway, New Jersey. While there, he investigated the cancer-killing properties of plant extracts called lectins. Between 1977 and 1982, Dr. Simone worked at the National Cancer Institute (NCI) as a clinical associate in the immunology branch, then as investigator in the pharmacology branch; while at NCI, he trained in medical oncology and clinical immunology. Between 1982 and 1985, Dr. Simone trained in radiation oncology at the University of Pennsylvania and then became associate professor in radiation oncology and nuclear medicine at Thomas Jefferson University (1985-1988), both in Philadelphia. In 1988, he founded the Simone Protective Cancer Center.

Dr. Simone is the author of 25 peer-reviewed medical articles, and 350 consumer articles; he has appeared on 400 television shows (including *60 Minutes*, *Prime Time*, *The Today Show*) and 1500 radio shows. In addition, he is the author of *Cancer and Nutrition: A Ten-Point Plan to Reduce Your Chances of Getting Cancer* (McGraw Hill, 1982; revised, 1994, Avery Publishing Group), *Breast Health* (Avery, 1995), *Shark Cartilage and Cancer* (Paradigm Press, 1995), and *Prostate Health* (forthcoming).

***Lifestyle modifications according to Dr. Simone's Ten-Point Plan can decrease cancer-initiating and promoting factors while enhancing the immune system. With a focus on diet, nutrition, and other controllable factors, the Ten-Point Plan is designed to reduce the risk of developing cancer, to halt the progress of an existing tumor, and to decrease the rate of recurrence.***

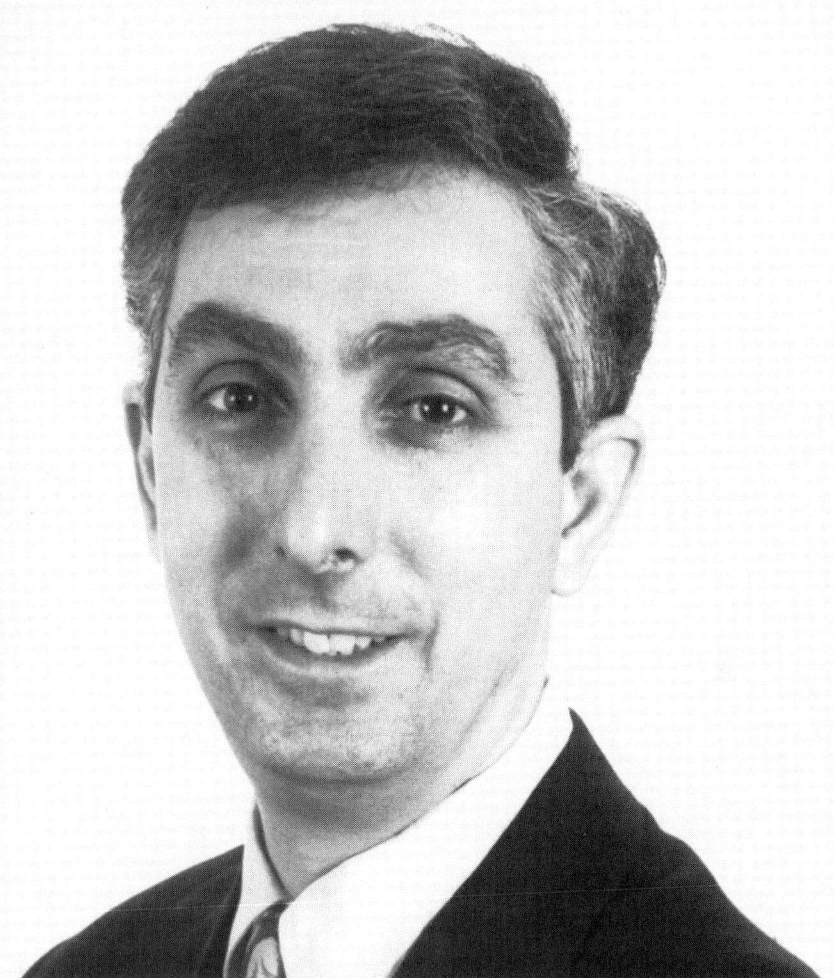

# *Charles B. Simone*, *M.MS.*, *M.D.*

**"THE RISING INCIDENCE OF** cancer compelled me to begin investigating the effects of nutrition on cancer and the possibilities of cancer prevention," says Dr. Simone. "If more people are made aware of risk factors and implement their modification, the incidence of cancer will decrease."

Dr. Simone is convinced that proper nutrition, nutrient supplementation, and lifestyle modification help protect a person from developing cancer and can be used as an adjunct to conventional therapies. The majority of his practice since 1982 has been with patients who have breast cancer or benign breast disease, and those who want to prevent both. The ultimate goal of Dr. Simone's approach is to win the war on cancer through prevention, early detection, and treatment "in which all options are fully explored," says Dr. Simone.

His thoughts are clear regarding what is needed in cancer care. "What is needed is some person, some institution, some inescapable 'force' that captures the imagination of our citizens and demonstrates that cancer will be eliminated only when each of us comes to understand that its elimination can only occur as part of a lifelong process of sanity, balance, moderation, and self-respect."

One of the first cancer patients Charles B. Simone, M.D. treated was former Vice President Hubert Humphrey, who in the 1970s was dying of malnutrition related to his cancer. Later, a man diagnosed with a rare cancer, who was Dr. Simone's own age, came to him and asked to be kept alive for the birth of his child. Though chemotherapy eradicated the cancer, the man did not improve. "As a last resort, I gave him high doses of vitamins and minerals, and these quickly produced a seemingly miraculous recovery," Dr. Simone says. The man lived long enough to see the birth of his son.

These incidents sparked Dr. Simone's interest in nutrition. "At this

# Dr. Simone's Generalized Model for Adjunctive Cancer Care

| STRATEGY | DOSAGE/ KEY COMPONENTS | FOR MORE INFORMATION see page # |
|---|---|---|
| **Dietary Plan** | | |
| Low-fat, high-fiber diet | 1) fat intake no more than 20% of total daily caloric intake; 2) 25-30 g of dietary fiber daily; best sources are whole grains (especially rice, barley, and buckwheat), legumes, vegetables (especially of the cabbage family); 3) fresh fruit preferable, but unsweetened juices and unsweetened cooked, canned, or frozen fruit allowable | 749 |
| Avoid most animal products | 1) exceptions are 2-4 servings per week of free-range poultry (cooked without skin) or any fish except shellfish, mackerel, sardines, or fish canned in oil or high in fat; 2) avoid most dairy products except occasional use of nonfat milk products or yogurt; 3) avoid smoked, salt-cured, barbequed, and charcoal-broiled foods. | 401 |
| Avoid products that contain added sugar and refined flour | avoid added sugar, bleached white flour, grain products made with fats, oils, or egg yolks; commercial biscuits, muffins, doughnuts, butter rolls, sweet rolls, egg bread, cheese bread, and commercial mixes containing dried eggs and whole milk. | 403 |
| Avoid all alcohol and caffeine | | 404 |
| **Supplement called Onccor™ developed by Dr. Simone includes:** | | |
| Carotenoids | | |
| beta carotene | 30 mg daily | 764 |
| lycopene | 10 mcg daily | — |
| lutein | 10 mcg daily | — |
| Vitamin A | 5000 IU daily | 784 |
| B Vitamins | daily dosages: B1, 10 mg; B2, 10 mg; niacinamide, 40 mg; B5 (pantothenic acid), 20 mg; B6, 10 mg; B12, 18 mcg; biotin, 150 mcg | 784-786 |
| Folic acid | 400 mcg daily | 784 |
| Vitamin C | 350 mg daily | 786 |
| Vitamin D | 400 IU daily | 789 |
| Vitamin E | 400 IU daily | 790 |

*Continued*

# Dr. Simone's Generalized Model for Adjunctive Cancer Care (cont.)

| STRATEGY | DOSAGE/ KEY COMPONENTS | FOR MORE INFORMATION see page # |
|---|---|---|
| Chromium (organic) | 125 mcg daily | 766 |
| Copper | 3 mg daily | 767 |
| Iodine | 150 mcg daily | 776 |
| Manganese | 2.5 mg daily | 780 |
| Molybdenum | 50 mcg daily | 780 |
| Potassium | 30 mg daily | 783 |
| Selenium (organic) | 200 mcg daily | 783 |
| Zinc | 25 mg daily | 793 |
| Inositol | 10 mg daily | 776 |
| Amino acid L-cysteine | 20 mg daily | 762 |

## Lifestyle Modifications

| | | |
|---|---|---|
| Avoid tobacco | don't smoke or chew tobacco, use snuff, or inhale your own or other people's tobacco smoke | 403 |
| Avoid unnecessary drugs | birth control pills, body-building steroids, any other nonessential drugs | 409 |
| Clean up your home and work environments | 1) get rid of indoor pollution—chemical fumes from furnishings, cleaning products, air fresheners, paints, glues, solvents, varnishes; improper ventilation, dirty filters in air systems<br>2) avoid use of pesticides, fungicides, and other gardening chemicals<br>3) use reverse osmosis water, install a water filtration system, buy spring or filtered water; best, use distilled water<br>4) demand that your elected officials keep your community's air and water clean | 408 |
| Avoid radiation exposure | 1) ionizing (X rays, mammograms, and other medical technologies, and industrial emissions, as from nuclear power plants);<br>2) non-ionizing (electromagnetic fields generated by power lines, computer monitors, copy machines, dimmer switches, poorly insulated electric wiring, waterbed heaters, electric blankets) | 406 |
| Exercise | supports anticancer defenses | 411 |
| Stress reduction | immune-strengthening psychotherapy, support group, relaxation techniques, guided imagery, biofeedback, hypnosis | 411 |

point I realized that, despite all the existing cancer treatments, the results were limited," Dr. Simone says. "The rising incidence of cancer compelled me to begin investigating the effects of nutrition on cancer and the possibilities of cancer prevention." He went on to carry out extensive research on health-related lifestyle changes, with a primary focus on "adjuvant nutrition for cancer treatment"—that is, dietary and supplementation strategies that support the successful treatment of cancer. "International studies indicate that people with diets rich in beta carotene have a lower incidence of cancer. If more people are made aware of risk factors and implement their modification, the incidence of cancer will decrease."

**CAUTION**

This chapter includes information regarding actual treatments used by Dr. Simone only after his careful diagnosis of each patient. All cancer patients are unique. **Do not administer these treatments to yourself or others.** Discuss these treatments with your physician or other qualified health-care professional. Readers should not interpret this material as therapeutic advice, but should see a physician in all cases.

In July 1996, the *Journal of the National Cancer Institute* recognized Dr. Simone's contribution to cancer treatment and research. "In 1981, Dr. Simone was the first to recognize the need and then develop a single supplement having multiple chemopreventive agents."[1]

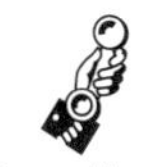

**Onccor**™ and **Calcor**™ are available from Simone Protective Pharmaceuticals, Inc., 123 Franklin Corner Road, Lawrenceville, NJ 08648; tel: 609-896-2646.

## SUCCESS STORY

### Metastatic Breast Cancer

Laura, aged 37, was a songwriter who developed breast cancer for which she received conventional treatment. The doctors told her after treatment that there was no detectable sign of cancer. But the cancer returned and in a far more deadly form, metastasizing to her bones. Laura underwent an extensive series of radiation and chemotherapy treatments to fight the metastases, but these failed. The bone cancer became extremely painful. Owing to the extensive nature of her metastases, she was told she probably had only a few months to live.

When Dr. Simone consulted with Laura on her first visit, she agreed to follow the Simone Ten-Point Plan. In addition she took the nutrient supplements called Onccor™ and Calcor™, developed by Simone Protective Pharmaceuticals. At first, she had difficulty adhering to all the guidelines because of her attachment to certain lifestyle habits. "These same unhealthy habits probably initiated the cancer," said Dr. Simone. "Even with a life-threatening diagnosis like cancer, many people still find that changing their lifestyle habits is a big challenge, especially after so many years of living life a certain way."

After several weeks, Laura began feeling stronger and had less bone pain. She stayed with the Simone Ten-Point Plan (including Onccor™ and Calcor™) and began telling other people about her recovery and the importance of adopting a health-promoting lifestyle. Her bone pain continued to decrease, and eventually she became pain free. She resumed writing songs. Laura lived 15 more years and kept highly active in her songwriting and other creative pursuits. She wrote her most famous song during this time.

Looking back on Laura's case, Dr. Simone recalls how happy she was to have a chance to reclaim her life with a heightened sense of balance and personal fulfillment. "Laura's healing was in being able to live more fully, which she did for another 15 years," says Dr. Simone.

## SUCCESS STORY
### Reversing Prostate Cancer

John, aged 53, had prostate cancer that spread to his bladder and certain bones. According to conventional oncology, with metastatic cancer of this degree, John's life expectancy should have been 12-14 months. However, he agreed to radically change his lifestyle and to adopt all the recommendations in Dr. Simone's Ten-Point Plan.

He was an avid lover of ice cream and all the other fatty foods yet he gave these up for his recovery. During the first 12 months, John was allowed only minimal amounts of fatty foods but, in the next 6 months, his fat consumption was cut back to nothing. In addition to the Plan, Dr. Simone put John on male hormone therapy (Lupron, an antitestosterone hormone) as a once-monthly injection; he remained on this for 18 months. He received no other form of conventional therapy during this 18-month period nor did he deviate from Dr. Simone's program.

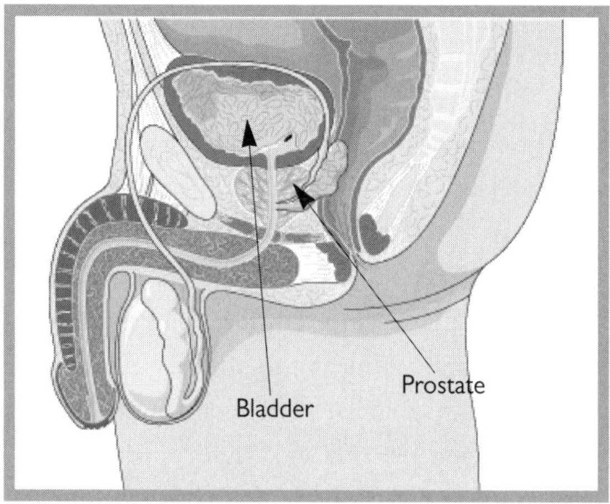

**Figure 19.1—The prostate gland**

Within the first year, John's prostate specific antigen (PSA, a cancer marker) dropped to zero. Six years later he was still alive and doing well, some 60 months beyond his supposed life expectancy. "This example points out the fact that if you change your lifestyle, especially with a diet-sensitive tumor (such as prostate, breast, endometrial, or rectal), you can improve your survival. This is the only approach that's been shown to do this—not chemotherapy, radiation, or surgery—but lifestyle changes. If you change your lifestyle, you *will* live longer."

## Modifying Cancer's Risk Factors—The Ten-Point Plan

*"In theory, most cancers can be entirely prevented if the factors that cause them are controlled and eliminated," says Dr. Simone.*

Between 80 and 90% of all cancers, Dr. Simone asserts, are related to 3 major groups of risk factors: (1) nutrition, specifically a high-fat, high-cholesterol, low-fiber diet (60% of women's and 40% of men's cancers are related to nutritional factors alone, he says); (2) lifestyle, including tobacco smoking, alcohol consumption, stress, illegal drug use, and sedentary living; and (3) environment (industrial toxins, electromagnetic radiation, chemical carcinogens, and air and water pollution).

For more information on the 33 **contributing factors** to cancer, see Chapter 25: What Causes Cancer?

"In theory, most cancers can be entirely prevented if the factors that cause them are controlled and eliminated," says Dr. Simone. "Some exposures, though, are difficult to control. Many people are exposed to chemicals without knowing that cancers are associated with these exposures." Many chemicals that may initiate cancer, he notes, are present in small amounts and exert their harmful effects in combination with other chemicals. Such combinations are unique to a person's culture and environment.

Of all the factors affecting the development of cancer, nutrition is the most controllable and exerts the most profound effects on a day-to-day basis. "Improper nutrition and smoking are the main risk factors for the development of cancer," Dr. Simone says. "If you eat a poor diet and/or smoke regularly, you considerably raise your risk of developing cancer. Probably the majority of smokers also have poor diets, which only amplifies their susceptibility to cancer."

Though Dr. Simone's approach to cancer is primarily oriented toward prevention, he acknowledges that many of the same factors that de-

## Dr. Simone's Ten-Point Plan to Prevent Cancer and Cancer Recurrence

1. Adopt a healthy nutritional strategy
2. Avoid tobacco products and tobacco smoke
3. Avoid alcohol and caffeine
4. Minimize radiation exposure
5. Keep your environment clean
6. Modify hormone-related and sexual-social factors
7. Learn the 7 cancer warning signs
8. Exercise to support your anticancer defenses
9. Modify your stress level
10. Get a physical exam and assess your risk profile

termine the risk of cancer also affect its progression. "In general, the same dietary factors that act as promoters of carcinogenesis may influence the growth of tumors," he says. "Fat is a good example of a dietary factor that contributes to both the onset and progression of cancer. Cancer patients can greatly benefit by lowering their fat intake."

Thus, the same overall dietary approach used in cancer prevention can be applied to cancer treatment as well. To bolster your body's cancer resistance, Dr. Simone recommends modifying the main risk factors for cancer and adhering to his Ten-Point Plan.

Dr. Simone's approach aims at decreasing the risk of developing cancer and also decreasing the risk of its progression if a tumor has been created. "The scientific data is very clear," he says. "Lifestyle modifications according to my Ten-Point Plan can decrease cancer-initiating and promoting factors while enhancing the immune system." All of Dr. Simone's guidelines for prevention also apply to decreasing the recurrence rate of cancer—a concern for many people, especially since cancer, when it recurs, typically does so in a more aggressive, life-threatening form.

***"Lifestyle modifications according to my Ten-Point Plan can decrease cancer-initiating and promoting factors while enhancing the immune system," Dr. Simone states.***

### POINT 1: ADOPT A HEALTHY NUTRITION STRATEGY

"The first step is to change one's diet to a low-fat, high-fiber diet, supplemented with certain vitamins and minerals," Dr. Simone says. "If more people are made aware of risk factors and how to modify them, the incidence of cancer will decrease, and long-range survival odds will improve as well." This translates into a diet that contains few animal products, since cholesterol is a fatty substance that comes only from animal sources. A total of 2-4 servings of fish and/or free-range poultry (cooked without the skin) per week is advisable. The foods Dr. Simone recommends provide more than enough fats necessary for all bodily functions, and, at the same time, modify one's cancer risk.

One basic principle of the nutrition program is to maintain an ideal weight, even losing 5-10 pounds if necessary. This tends to occur automatically as one follows Dr. Simone's dietary plan, particularly when complemented by a moderate exercise routine.

**20% Total Caloric Fat Intake**—A person's daily fat intake should not exceed 20% of the diet's total caloric value. According to Dr. Simone, this calls for avoidance of most animal products, with the exception of lean white meats such as low-fat game birds (always remove the skin before cooking). All fish are fine except shellfish, mackerel, sardines and any other fish canned in oil or any fish high in fat or cholesterol.

Dr. Simone also recommends avoiding all red meats like beef, bacon, hamburger, spareribs, sausage, luncheon meats, sweetbreads, hot dogs, kidney, brains, liver, etc., because they are high in fats. Smoked, salt-cured, barbecued, and charcoal-broiled foods should be strictly avoided. Avoid most dairy products, with the exception of occasional use of nonfat milk or yogurt.

For more information on **pesticides** and cancer, see Chapter 25: What Causes Cancer? pp. 568-574.

One of the many ways that fat increases the risk of cancer is that fat tends to concentrate certain chemicals, such as pesticides, another potential risk factor for cancer. Low-fat foods typically have a low-pesticide content. "Pesticide use in food production is widespread and often excessive," says Dr. Simone.

"The link between pesticides and cancer is not direct, but the findings of many studies are substantial enough to dictate the reduction in pesticide use from a public health standpoint." In studies comparing cancerous breast tissue with healthy breast tissue from the same woman, the concentration of toxic chemicals such as DDT (a pesticide) and PCB (an industrial chemical) was "much increased in the malignant tissue compared to the normal breast and adjacent adipose tissue."[2] In other words, while studies have identified that the fats in breast tissue were laden with pesticides, in Dr. Simone's view, you cannot say definitively that these pesticides causes the breast cancer.

SHARK CARTILAGE

## An Investigational Protocol of Merit

In 1994, the FDA granted Dr. Simone an Investigational New Drug (IND) approval for his protocols describing the treatment of advanced cancers using shark cartilage.

Tumors grow, in part, because they develop their own blood supply. Most tissues and organs also do this in a process known as angiogenesis, Dr. Simone explains. If you want to kill a tumor or stop its growth, cutting off the blood supply can be an effective strategy. Shark cartilage contains substances, called angiogenesis inhibitors, that appear to be capable of doing this. According to Dr. Simone, shark cartilage also appears to suppress inflammation and slightly enhance immune system function. Shark cartilage contains an abundance of "antiangiogenic factors" that effectively interrupt the formation of new blood vessels needed to sustain tumor growth.

After reviewing the favorable results of his clinical trial involving shark cartilage, and with prompting from the National Institutes of Health's Office of Alternative Medicine, Dr. Simone decided to conduct his own investigations by way of a clinical trial in Cuba in 1993. The trial included collecting approximately 100 patients who were diagnosed with various advanced cancers—all involving metastases, and most considered to be "terminal" cases by conventional oncologists. These patients had taken shark cartilage as a supplement in some form prior to coming to see Dr. Simone, so they were open to the therapy.

Thirty-five patients who failed all conventional treatments requested to go on Dr. Simone's intensive shark cartilage program while following the Ten-Point Plan and no other treatment (group A). Another group of patients asked to enter Dr. Simone's cartilage program but continue with their chemotherapy (group B).

Overall, 34% of the group A patients (12 out of 35), showed some improvement in response to the shark cartilage regimen combined with the Simone Ten-Point Plan.

Complete remissions occurred in 3 patients, including a case of gallbladder cancer with metastasis to the liver, breast cancer with metastasis to the liver, and lung cancer with metastasis to the liver. Partial responses (greater than 50% reduction in cancer) were seen in 9 patients, all of whom had metastatic disease.

Dr. Simone notes that all 30 patients in group A and half of those in group B reported an improved quality of life. The improvements included better energy levels, less pain, enhanced appetite, and more positive moods. "Perhaps the most notable change in most patients with bone metastases was that the pain from bone metastasis resolved within 3-4 weeks," Dr. Simone says. "That kind of intense pain usually doesn't resolve so quickly."

**5-30 Grams of Dietary Fiber—**This level of intake requires regular daily consumption of whole grains, legumes, and vegetables. "It is easy to attain this level of fiber consumption every day," says Dr. Simone. "High-fiber cereals, including whole or slightly milled grains such as rice, barley, and buckwheat, are the highest sources, but whole-grain breads and vegetables of the cabbage (*Brassicaceae*) family are excellent sources as well." Dr. Simone adds that whole wheat bread and whole wheat pasta, cereals, and other grain products are good fiber sources on a daily basis. Though fresh fruit is preferable, Dr. Simone says unsweetened fruit juices and unsweetened cooked, canned or frozen fruit can also be eaten.

At the same time, avoid any products that contain added sugar, bleached white flour, and grain products made with fats, oils or egg yolks; also avoid commercial biscuits, cakes, muffins, doughnuts, butter rolls, sweet rolls, egg bread, cheese bread, and commercial mixes containing dried eggs and whole milk.

## POINT 2: AVOID TOBACCO

Dr. Simone advises people not to smoke or chew tobacco, use snuff, or inhale tobacco smoke, their own or that of other smokers. Exposure to tobacco particles is considered to be the second major cause of cancer and the number one cause of cancer-related death, mainly due to lung cancer. Smoking has been linked to cancers of the head and neck, mouth, throat, vocal cords, bladder, kidney, stomach, cervix, and pancreas, as well as to some leukemia; additionally, smokeless tobacco has been linked to cancers of the lip and tongue.[3] Involuntary inhalation of tobacco smoke causes about 17% of lung cancers, particularly for those who inhale between ages 3 and 15, says Dr. Simone.

For more information on the cancer-causing role of **poor nutrition,** (pp. 604-613) **smoking** (pp. 582-586), **alcohol** (pp. 612-613), and **household pollution and carcinogens** (pp. 559-561), see Chapter 25: What Causes Cancer?

Smoking leads to 2 primary health-related problems, according to Dr. Simone: (1) production of harmful free radicals and (2) adverse effects on the human immune system. "People who smoke tend to have an extraordinary amount of free radical activity in their bodies, which can damage their DNA and set the stage for cancer," he says. "At the same time, the smoke alters the balance of key immune cells and suppresses the natural killer (NK) cells and IgA antibodies, which is a first line of defense against viruses and bacteria." Since NK cells ordinarily would destroy cancer cells in the bloodstream, the suppressive effect on this cell population could explain why smokers are more vulnerable not only to lung cancer, but to other cancers as well.[4]

To make matters worse, smokers tend to have lower blood levels of vitamin C and several other antioxidants that would otherwise scavenge or neutralize the free radicals. As a result, tobacco smoke offers the perfect formula for initiating and promoting cancer: carcinogens, toxins, free radicals, antioxidant deficiencies, and immune suppression.

## POINT 3: AVOID ALCOHOL AND CAFFEINE

"What few people realize is that alcohol is not merely a risk on the road but also at home [leading to accidents, abuse, and divorce]," says Dr. Simone. "An alcohol habit can greatly increase the risk for cancers of the breast, mouth, throat (pharynx, larynx and esophagus), pancreas, liver, and head and neck."

Alcohol interacts with tobacco smoke to heighten the risk of developing cancers of the digestive and urinary tracts.[5] It is estimated that this toxic combination accounts for 75% of all oral cancers in the U.S. Mounting evidence has shown that alcoholism significantly raises the risk of smoking-related cancers as well, according to Dr. Simone.

***If you intend to drink coffee, drink no more than 2 cups of decaffeinated coffee a day, and select only the organically grown coffees sold at health food stores, says Dr. Simone.***

Alcoholics, like smokers, are prone to develop nutritional problems. "Alcoholics have more nutritional deficiencies than all other groups of people, mainly because alcoholics consume most of their daily caloric intake as alcohol," says Dr. Simone. "As a result, they tend to develop deficiencies of vitamin C, various B vitamins, calcium, zinc, and magnesium. Not surprisingly, then, alcoholics are more likely to have depressed immune systems that leave them vulnerable to cancer and infection." Dr. Simone proposes that alcohol be classified as an immune-suppressive drug with far-reaching effects.

If you already have cancer, alcohol can greatly speed up the disease, especially in the case of breast cancer. Dr. Simone cites a study in which animals were injected with breast cancer cells, which always spread (metastasize) to the lungs; at the time of injection, the animals were allowed to consume alcohol. "Those with a blood alcohol content of 0.15 percent, which represents about 4-5 drinks an hour, later developed more than twice the number of new lung metastases compared to the animals that did not drink," Dr. Simone reports. "Those with a blood level of 0.25 percent had 8 times more tumors in their lungs." For comparison, these same levels of alcohol are seen in humans who drink excessively for one hour. He notes that women who drink this amount are at an increased risk for developing tumors as well as metastatic breast cancer.

Other research has found that women who consume 2-3 alcoholic drinks per week—not per day—have a 2-3 times higher risk for developing breast cancer, and this added risk is independent of other breast cancer risk factors.[6] Dr. Simone reminds us that each alcoholic drink is the equivalent of either 12 ounces of beer or 4 ounces of wine, or 1½ ounces of whiskey. "It comes as a bit of shock to most people that a seemingly small amount of alcohol is a very potent carcinogen," Dr. Simone says.

Alcohol may accelerate the growth of an existing cancer by suppressing NK cells, immune cells which would otherwise help repel cancer.[7] Heavy alcohol consumption, over time, can also damage the liver, limiting its ability to detoxify pollutants that enter the bloodstream. These effects, taken together, would seem to make alcohol a poor choice for a beverage if you have been diagnosed with cancer.

***Women who consume 2-3 alcoholic drinks per week—not per day—have a 2-3 times higher risk for developing breast cancer, and this added risk is independent of other breast cancer risk factors, says Dr. Simone.***

Caffeine, the most popular drug in North America, is found in coffee, tea, cola beverages, and chocolate. Coffee drinking has been linked to cancer of the lower urinary tract, including the bladder;[8] the risk is greatest in people who drink more than 3 cups of coffee a day. Caffeine can cause damage to genetic material, and any change in the DNA could potentially lead to the development of cancer.[9]

"Although there is no direct link of caffeine to cancer, caffeine does increase the risk and progression of benign lumps on the breast, which are a risk for breast cancer," says Dr. Simone. In all likelihood, substances in coffee other than caffeine compound the risk. For this reason, says Dr. Simone, if you intend to drink coffee, drink no more than 2 cups of decaffeinated coffee a day, and select only the organically grown coffees sold at health food stores.

Dr. Simone asserts that there are several other important reasons for avoiding coffee or other caffeinated beverages. "Excessive coffee consumption has been associated with heart disease, osteoporosis, malformed fetuses, and low-birth-weight infants," he says. "Of course, the decision to consume it, as well as alcoholic beverages, is yours. You are the only one who can decide the status of your health."

***"Now mammograms can detect the cancer earlier, at about year 7 or 8, versus year 11 or 12, so the patient appears to live longer, but actually does not," says Dr. Simone.***

## POINT 4: MINIMIZE RADIATION EXPOSURE

As a basic guideline, Dr. Simone advises people to avoid or minimize exposures to both ionizing and non-ionizing forms of radiation. Evidence exists for a connection between cancer and the most common source of ionizing radiation: the medical technologies used for diagnosis and treatment.

For more information about the **disadvantages of mammography,** see Chapter 27: Early Detection and Prevention of Cancer, pp. 716-725; for more information about **electromagnetic field exposures,** see Chapter 25: What Causes Cancer?, pp. 552-556.

**Ionizing Radiation—**For the general population, exposure to ionizing radiation could be greatly reduced if health-care practitioners made more judicious use of X rays and other medical technologies that emit such radiation. For example, doctors could probably halve the dose of X rays to the population without sacrificing the accuracy of their diagnoses.[10] The most common X rays are of the chest and teeth; they account for almost half the total.

Screening for breast cancer is important, Dr. Simone says, but in many cases screening relies too much on mammography. Instead, he proposes that physician breast examination always precede or take precedence over the mammogram. "The physician breast examination is as effective or more effective than mammograms," Dr. Simone says. "Physicians who spend 10 to 15 minutes doing the exam have a higher likelihood of identifying problems. Also, there is no survival benefit in mammography screening for women aged 40-49 or those older than 65—absolutely none."

Dr. Simone concludes that only women between the ages of 50 and 65 should receive screening mammograms, every 1-2 years. This should only occur after a *thorough* breast examination by a physician. Mammograms tend to cause women a great deal of stress, mainly because of a high rate of "false positives," tests that indicate the presence of cancer when no such cancer exists.

"About 5% of screening mammograms are positive," Dr. Simone says. "Of these, however, about 80% to 90% are *false* positives that require excessive workups such as surgery. This translates into a great deal of undue emotional distress." Negative mammography readings provide false assurances in 10% to 15% of women. Dr. Simone says the annual cost per "life saved" is about $1.3 million.[11]

He also expresses concern regarding the cumulative radiation hazard of annual mammograms. "Until recently, mammography screening had been promoted as safe and reliable for early detection of breast cancer," Dr. Simone says. "But the radiation dose from current mammographic examination techniques is extremely damaging to the glandular tissue of the breast." Prevention should take precedence over the business of detecting and treating breast cancer, he adds.

The irony is that women screened by this procedure are unwittingly subjecting themselves to a source of radiation that *causes* breast cancer. "Mammograms increase the risk for developing breast cancer and raise the risk of spreading or metastasizing an existing growth," says Dr. Simone. "By some estimates, one per 10,000 women screened get breast cancer as a result of mammography."

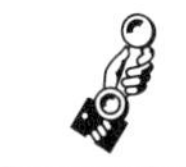

To measure **low-frequency EMFs** in your home, order a Safe ELF Gauss Meter, which measures field strength in milligauss units. For information, contact: Safe Technologies Corporation, 145 Rosemary Street, Needham, MA, 02194; tel: 617-444-7778.

Even the National Cancer Institute and National Academy of Sciences admit that mammography promotes cancer.[12] Their justification for endorsing the technology as a regular screening method is that for all the cancers detected early on, the relatively small number of cancers caused by this procedure make it worthwhile. "Remember," says Dr. Simone, "mammograms can detect a cancer earlier, but earlier detection has not translated to a longer life. If breast cancer is a 15-year disease, the mammograms of the older technology were able to detect the cancer at about year 11 or 12, so the patient lived 3-4 more years. Now mammograms can detect the cancer earlier, at about year 7 or 8, so the patient *appears* to live longer, but actually does not."

There are cancer risks associated with living near nuclear power plants or eating food tainted by the radioactive releases from such plants. Among the main hazards are the small amounts of radioactive gases released daily from nuclear reactors at levels deemed "permissible" by the U.S. Department of Energy. This low-level radioactive pollution enters rain that falls and then accumulates in the soil and the food chain.

**Non-Ionizing Radiation (EMFs)**—Dr. Simone recommends minimizing exposures to electromagnetic fields, or EMFs, which are generated by electrical currents. Studies have consistently found associations between residential EMF exposure and cancer, particularly in the case of childhood leukemia.[13] Among adults, there seems to be a stronger association between EMF exposure and brain cancer[14] and, to a lesser extent, breast cancer.[15]

Dr. Simone says the priority is to avoid chronic exposure to EMFs in the home environment. Among more hazardous sources is the electric blanket, which has been linked with childhood cancers.[16] Other chronic EMF sources are computer monitors, copiers, dimmer switches, waterbed heaters, poorly insulated electric wiring, power lines, and the grounding of the electrical system to the plumbing system, which effectively produces 2 powerful, unhealthy EMF sources in the home.

For more information about **indoor pollutants** and the **sick building syndrome** (pp. 559-561) and **radiation exposure** (pp. 561-568), see Chapter 25: What Causes Cancer?

## POINT 5: KEEP YOUR ENVIRONMENT CLEAN

As part of his cancer-fighting strategy, Dr. Simone recommends carefully upholding high standards for environmental quality at home and at work. Examples of contaminants commonly found in homes and offices include formaldehyde fumes from pressed-wood furniture and cabinets; fumes and vapors produced by cleaning products, air fresheners, paints, hobby supplies (glues, varnishes, etc.), and improperly vented gas stoves and dryers; lead and other chemicals found in drinking water; office or home air systems that can fill the air with bacteria, mildew, and viruses; and radon gas infiltration.

"Avoid prolonged exposure to household cleaning fluids, solvents, and paint thinners," Dr. Simone says. "Some may be hazardous if inhaled in high concentrations. Pesticides, fungicides, and other home garden and lawn chemicals are also potentially dangerous."

Occupational exposures to chemicals may, in some cases, carry serious cancer risks. "Several specific industries, such as the manufacture of boots, shoes, furniture, and cabinets, are risk factors for the development of cancer of the nasal sinuses," says Dr. Simone.

Polluted air and water also contribute to the risk of breast cancer, but to a moderate degree, says Dr. Simone. Air pollution includes smog, automobile exhaust, acid rain (which leaches heavy metals into the food chain), excessive exposure to UV light (from destruction of the ozone layer), and polluted indoor air not vented to the outside. Water pollution includes harmful organic and inorganic chemicals, chlorination by-products, carcinogens, fluoride, radioactive materials, living organisms, and solid particulates like asbestos.

## POINT 6: MODIFY HORMONE-RELATED AND SEXUAL-SOCIAL FACTORS

Hormonal factors and sexual-social behavior have become increasingly important in the creation of cancers. Cancers of the breast, ovary and prostate, are considered "hormone-sensitive" because sex hormones (estrogen in the case of breast and ovary, testosterone in the case of prostate cancer) can accelerate their growth.

Dr. Simone says that the risk for developing breast cancer is greatly increased if the woman began menstruating early at age (10 or 11), experienced a late pregnancy (35 or older), or had a late menopause. Other risks include never breastfeeding, never getting pregnant, and having a first pregnancy termination (from miscarriage or abortion) in the first trimester. If your mother used estrogen during pregnancy with you, this increases your risk of developing cancer later on. Breast cancer risks also increase with the use of oral contraceptives as well as estrogens for postmenopausal symptoms.

Other sexual-social factors that may promote cancers in either men or women are as follows:

- Female promiscuity: According to Dr. Simone, the earlier the age of starting sexual intercourse and the more male sexual partners a female has, the greater her risk of developing cervical cancer. The risk increases with uncircumcised male partners who practice poor hygiene.
- Male promiscuity: "Practice safe sex," says Dr. Simone. This means wearing condoms and abstaining from anal intercourse or other practices that suppress the immune system.
- Poor hygiene in uncircumcised males: Dr. Simone says uncircumcised men need to bathe thoroughly, as poor hygiene may lead to cancer of the penis.
- Birth control pills: Oral contraceptives should be avoided, Dr. Simone suggests, as should the use of estrogens to treat other conditions. "Other means of birth control should be consistently used."
- DES exposure: Dr. Simone recommends reporting to a physician if you were exposed to DES (diethylstilbestrol), or if you are the daughter or son of a DES-exposed mother.
- Androgens: More commonly known as sex steroids, androgens

should not be used for body-building or any other purpose. "Build your body by working out," says Simone. "In every way, it's the healthier path to take."

- Drugs: Dr. Simone recommends avoiding all unnecessary drugs. "Take drugs only when they are prescribed by your physician, and check to see if the drug interferes with vitamin function."

## POINT 7: LEARN THE SEVEN WARNING SIGNS OF CANCER

Early detection is imperative for the most effective treatment of cancer. If any of these signs appear, Dr. Simone recommends that you contact your physician immediately.

***Dr. Simone notes that exercise raises the body temperature and increases the production of pyrogen, a special substance (lymphokine) that enhances the function of white blood cells (lymphocytes).***

- A lump or thickening in the breast or testicles.
- A change in a wart or mole may be indicative of melanoma. Skin cancers may appear as dry, scaly patches, as pimples which never go away, or as inflamed or ulcerated areas. Warts or moles which grow or bleed should be checked, says Dr. Simone, as should sores in the mouth that persist.
- A skin sore or a sore throat that does not heal may also be indicative of melanoma. A sore throat that does not go away, hoarseness, a persistent lump in the throat, and difficulty swallowing may indicate cancer of the larynx.
- A change in bowel or bladder habits. Continuing urinary difficulties, constipation, diarrhea, gas pains, rectal bleeding, or blood in the stool should not be ignored.
- A persistent cough or hoarseness.
- Constant indigestion or trouble swallowing. Difficulties in swallowing, continued indigestion, nausea, heartburn, bloating, and loss of appetite may all be symptoms of cancer of the upper gastrointestinal tract, such as esophagus or stomach.
- Unusual bleeding or discharge from the vagina can indicate early stages of uterine cancer and later stages of cervical cancer.

## POINT 8: EXERCISE TO SUPPORT THE ANTICANCER DEFENSES

Dr. Simone encourages his patients to start a program of regular exercise after seeing a physician to check for risk factors of cardiovascular disease. He suggests starting out slowly, then increasing the exercise to a comfortable level. Fast walking several times a week is a good form of exercise and 2 miles is a satisfactory distance for brisk walking 4 days a week. "I stress fast walking because it is easier to do than other forms of exercise—no equipment to buy, no change of clothing, no one to rely on except yourself," Dr. Simone says.

Calisthenics, such as 5-10 sit-ups with knees bent, help to firm up abdominal-wall muscles. Any form of vigorous movement helps move the lymphatic system; exercise also speeds up detoxification and stimulates the activity of natural killer cells and other components of the body's anticancer defenses.[17]

Dr. Simone notes that exercise raises the body temperature and increases the production of pyrogen, a special substance (lymphokine) that enhances the function of white blood cells (lymphocytes).[18] Another major benefit of exercise is that it increases the oxygen supply to body tissues. Since cancer operates in an oxygen-poor environment, the well-exercised body is far more likely to repel cancer cells or keep them from propagating.

The bottom line in beginning an exercise program is to avoid excessive strain of any kind and maintain some level of consistency with the practice. "Some amount of exercise is always better than none," says Dr. Simone. "A little every day will benefit you enormously. Choose an exercise program that you are likely to follow, and then stick with it." Set realistic goals for yourself, he adds. "Only gradually work up to a more vigorous level of walking or other exercise." Dr. Simone agrees with those who say that the best exercise program—the one people are most likely to continue on a regular basis—involves an activity they enjoy.

## POINT 9: MODIFY YOUR STRESS

Stress suppresses the immune system, thereby increasing one's susceptibility to cancer and infectious diseases. Among the stress-related factors now thought to play a role in increasing cancer risk are repressed anger, hopelessness, helplessness, and a high degree of passivity or social conformity.[19]

## Stress-Handling Exercise

As a practical way of handling stress, Dr. Simone offers this exercise to his patients:

Get into a comfortable lounging position. Concentrate on feeling every part of your body with your mind. Think about your right foot, then your right ankle, right leg, right thigh, then left foot, etc. Then move from your hands up to your shoulders and neck, and so on. Now, start to tense specific muscle groups as hard as you can; hold them tense for 20-30 seconds, then relax them. Again, start with your foot muscles (tense, relax), the leg muscles (tense, relax), and so on. Repeat the entire sequence through your whole body once or twice.

While you are doing this, tell yourself that you are tightening your muscles each time you do so, and, provided that your effort is strenuous, you will look forward to relaxing each muscle group. While relaxing, think of a pleasant place that evokes fond memories.

This sequence should produce relief and relaxation, and decrease your anxiety levels. Stress is another risk factor over which you have a great deal of control.[20]

"Emotional suppression or being overly accommodating is a real risk factor for cancer, not simply a reaction to a cancer diagnosis," says Dr. Simone. "It's also quite clear that emotional suppression is linked to symptoms of depression and anxiety among many cancer patients." Through psychotherapy and other techniques, he suggests that a person can learn to better express his or her emotions, thereby removing this mind-body onus from the immune system.

Methods such as guided imagery, biofeedback, hypnosis, and relaxation training have helped cancer patients better cope with the unpleasant effects of cancer and may bolster the body's cancer-fighting ability.[21] Relaxation training can significantly reduce the severity of side effects—nausea, vomiting, distress, and other undesirable symptoms—caused by chemotherapy and radiation.[22] Whether or not life is actually extended by mind-body techniques, the quality of life definitely improves, and that alone is of value to the person with cancer, says Dr. Simone. Four more common ways of reducing stress include hot water baths, listening to music, prayer, and sexual intimacy, says Dr. Simone.

Social support may be of great benefit to cancer patients. In a study of breast cancer patients, a treatment group met weekly for a supportive group therapy session, with training in self-hypnosis for pain management; the control group did not have any such psychosocial support. After 10 years of follow-up, survival in the treatment group was almost double the time (36.6 months) compared to the control group (18.9 months).[23] "If you have cancer, it helps to feel supported," says Dr. Simone. "Don't just settle for relaxation techniques—get involved in support groups, or start one yourself."

## POINT 10: GET A PHYSICAL EXAM AND ASSESS YOUR RISK PROFILE

People who are diagnosed with localized cancer will live longer than those who present with widespread (disseminated or metastatic) cancer. For this reason, Dr. Simone urges everyone, age 35 and older, to have an annual comprehensive medical history and physical examination with appropriate laboratory studies in order to prevent or detect early cancer. "Early detection means early treatment."

Dr. Simone offers the following suggestions for undergoing a successful physical examination to detect early cancers:

- As part of a thorough physical checkup, laboratory tests should be done and blood and urine taken and assayed.
- Testing of stools is important: the presence of blood may indicate digestive tract cancers. "It is important to completely avoid all red meat for 3 entire days prior to and during the stool sampling period," says Dr. Simone. "That's because red meat contains animal blood, which will produce a [false] positive result in the test."
- A fiberoptic laryngoscope may be used to detect nose and throat lesions (in the nasopharynx and larynx), important when examining patients who have involuntarily inhaled tobacco smoke.
- A fiberoptic colonoscope can be used to examine the colon and survey for colon cancer, polyps, and chronic inflammatory bowel disease, which places undue stress on the immune system. The colonoscopy is also indicated in the case of unexplained iron deficiency anemia and when an abnormality is found with a barium enema.
- An annual chest X ray should be reserved *only* for high-risk patients who smoke, drink, and generally abuse their health.
- Self-examination of the breasts should be carried out once a month by all women, regardless of age. "Because men, too, can get breast cancer, they should examine their breasts as well," says Dr. Simone. "Self-examinations of the testicles should also be performed by men, especially between the ages of 20 and 40."

## Achieving a Better Quality of Life for Breast Cancer Patients

Nutrition can profoundly reduce toxic side effects and improve the results of conventional treatments, says Dr. Simone. Dr. Simone cites 50 peer-reviewed studies, both human and animal, in which the tumor-killing effects of radiation and chemotherapy were enhanced by nutritional strategies involving antioxidant supplements.

In a recent study of 50 patients with early-stage breast cancer, Dr. Simone evaluated side effects of treatment with radiation alone or radiation combined with chemotherapy in women taking therapeutic doses of nutrients according to his ten-point program. Patients were asked to evaluate the impact of their treatment on "quality-of-life" measures, such as: physical symptoms, performance, general well-being, cognitive abilities, sexual dysfunction, and life satisfaction.

***A major rationale behind Dr. Simone's nutritional plan is that it contains a well-rounded supply of free-radical scavengers and immune-strengthening nutrients.***

In addition to following the Simone Ten-Point Plan and taking the recommended supplements called Onccor™, the women took Calcor™, which includes calcium carbonate (1000 mg), magnesium (280 mg), boron (2 mg), L-lysine (2 mg), L-threonine (2 mg), and silicon (2 mg). Each decided whether the nutrients used during conventional treatments had improved, worsened, or made no change in her life during the treatment period.

A major rationale behind Dr. Simone's nutritional plan is that it contains a well-rounded supply of free-radical scavengers and immune-strengthening nutrients. "This regimen is designed to protect the body against the harm generated by radiation and chemotherapeutic agents without diminishing the effect of those treatments on the cancer cells," says Dr. Simone. "The cell-killing effect of chemotherapy and radiation produces free radicals as well. The nutrients make conventional treatment far more selective for the cancer while protecting the rest of the body."

The results of this study were supportive of Dr. Simone's claims:

- 49 out of 50 (98%) breast cancer patients reported improvements in their physical symptoms, one indicated no change at all
- 47 out of 50 (94%) patients observed improvement in their cognitive ability, the other 3 noted no change

- 46 out of 50 (92%) patients noted improvement in their performance (energy levels, coordination, physical function); the remaining 4 reported no change
- 40 out of 50 (80%) patients observed improvements in sexual function; the other 10 noted no change
- For the 2 other quality-of-life measures—general well-being and life-satisfaction—the entire group reported improvement

Not one subject in the entire group reported a worsening of symptoms. "Our study clearly shows that breast cancer patients who followed the Ten-Point Plan and used certain supplements had very few side effects from conventional treatments, and most actually got better," says Simone, adding, "The ability to kill the tumor while at the same time protecting normal cells should be a priority of every aggressive treatment program."

In summary, Dr. Simone states: "The Ten-Point Plan will decrease your risk of developing cancer and decrease the risk of promoting an existing cancer. Lifestyle modification is *your responsibility*."

***Overall, 34% of the patients (12 out of 35), showed some improvement in response to the shark cartilage regimen combined with the Simone Ten-Point Plan.***

## CURRICULUM VITAE

# Vincent Speckhart, M.D., M.D.H.

902 Graydon Avenue, No. 2, Norfolk, VA 23507;
tel: 804-622-0014; fax: 804-622-9808.

Dr. Speckhart received his M.D. from New York Medical College in New York City and completed a postdoctoral fellowship in Medical Oncology at the Medical College of Virginia. From 1970-1992, Dr. Speckhart was in private practice as an oncologist and since 1989 has practiced homeopathy as part of his overall medical program. From 1970-1990, he was director of the Tumor Clinic at DePaul Medical Center in Norfolk, Virginia; from 1974-1991, he was assistant clinical professor of medicine at Eastern Virginia Medical College. Dr. Speckhart is board certified in chelation therapy by the American Board of Chelation Therapy and is a licensed homeopathic physician (M.D.H.).

In 1994, he was appointed by the governor of Virginia to the Joint Subcommittee to study the commonwealth's Current Laws and Policies related to Acute and Cancer Pain Management. Dr. Speckhart has been appointed to the faculty of the Medical College of Virginia to teach electrodermal screening to 4th-year medical students who choose alternative medicine as part of their curriculum electives.

***"Electrodermal screening (EDS) provides the attentive physician with valuable insights into the nature and origin of cancer," says Dr. Speckhart. "We're finding that energy dysfunction always precedes the physical changes. By enabling doctors to identify the dysfunction before cancer develops, EDS helps doctors prescribe effective, individualized preventive measures."***

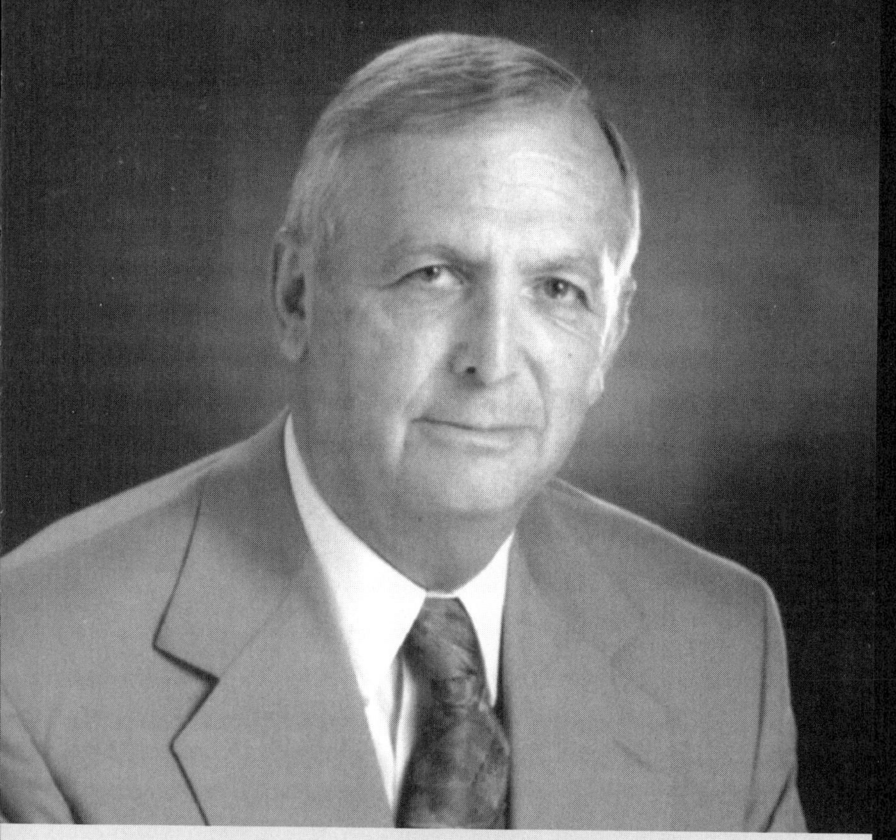

Chapter 20

# *Vincent Speckhart, M.D., M.D.H.*

**FOR DR. SPECKHART,** the skillful use of electrodermal screening can help identify the multiple sources of toxicity characteristic of cancer patients, while the precise use of homeopathic remedies, herbs, and nutritional supplements can often complete the cancer reversal process by removing toxins from the system and repairing the immune system.

According to Vincent Speckhart, M.D., who practiced as an oncologist for 22 years before turning to homeopathic medicine, cancer is the *result* of ill health, not its *cause*. "In cancer therapy, the generally accepted treatments are directed toward destroying the cancer lumps. With surgery, radiation, chemotherapy, and, more recently, with biological response modifiers, the cancerous growth is looked upon as the problem, when in fact it is the result of a failure of the host in which it is growing to maintain a healed state."

One of the frustrations in cancer management has been the inability to identify the cause of cancer development, Dr. Speckhart notes. But new developments in diagnostic methods have changed this. Foremost among new tools being used is an energy-information-gathering device called electrodermal screening (EDS).

***"Electrodermal screening gives us powerful clues about the multiple factors associated with malignancy," says Dr. Speckhart.***

"Electrodermal screening gives us powerful clues about the multiple factors associated with malignancy." In addition to his training in standard cancer oncology, Dr. Speckhart is accomplished in the use of EDS to understand the cancer process in individual patients, has a strong background in anticancer vaccines and oxygen therapy, and is recognized as a highly experienced practitioner of homeopathy as applied to cancer treatment.

# Dr. Speckhart's Generalized Model for Cancer Treatment

| STRATEGY | DOSAGE/ KEY COMPONENTS | FOR MORE INFORMATION see page # |
|---|---|---|
| **Dietary Plan** | | |
| Depending on individual | some thrive on vegetarian diet; others do better on a more omnivorous diet, including lean-meat animal products such as fish or poultry | 749 |
| **Alternative Cancer Therapies** | | |
| EDTA chelation | per standard protocols; not a cancer therapy per se, but is of main benefit for heart and circulation and removal of heavy metals (a possible cancer precursor) | 973 |
| Electrodermal screening | provides precise information about individual's cancer and most appropriate homeopathic remedies | 1021 |
| Homeopathic remedies | individually determined | 422 |
| Urea therapy | oral dosage, depending on individual | 874 |
| **Supplements** | | |
| Vitamin A | 5000 IU daily | 784 |
| Beta carotene | 25,000 IU daily | 764 |
| Vitamin B6 (pyridoxine) | 100-300 mg daily | 786 |
| Vitamin C | dosage to tolerance, 5,000-10,000 mg daily | 786 |
| Vitamin E | 400-800 IU daily | 790 |
| Selenium | 600 mcg daily | 783 |

## SUCCESS STORY
### Reversing Hodgkin's Lymphoma

Paula, aged 35, experienced a recurrence of her Hodgkin's lymphoma after completing a full course of chemotherapy and radiation therapy. When Dr. Speckhart first saw her, he used electrodermal screening (EDS) to develop his diagnosis. He discovered that she was highly toxic from the chemotherapy. Specifically, Adriamycin, the chemotherapeutic agent used, was imparting toxicity to her heart, and another chemotherapeutic agent, vincristine, was acting as a toxic factor for her stomach.

Technically, these chemical residues were affecting Paula's system negatively through specific acupuncture points on her body, the endocardium (Heart 8B) and parasympathetic (Stomach 10A points), respectively. The EDS diagnosis was able to pinpoint which energy points in Paula's body were being adversely affected; once the energy points were known, Dr. Speckhart could further identify which organs and organ systems were involved. EDS practitioners have extended the inventory of classically defined acupuncture meridians and points by developing empirically founded additional pathways and access points. With this expanded inventory, Dr. Speckhart also determined that silicone breast implant toxicity was registering in certain points in Paula's system.

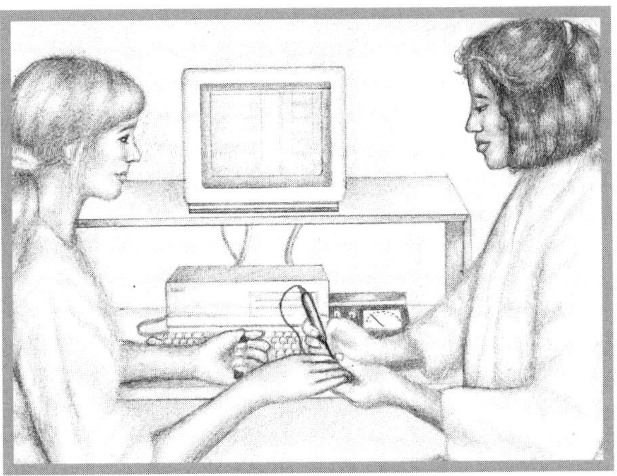

**Figure 20.1—Electrodermal Screening**

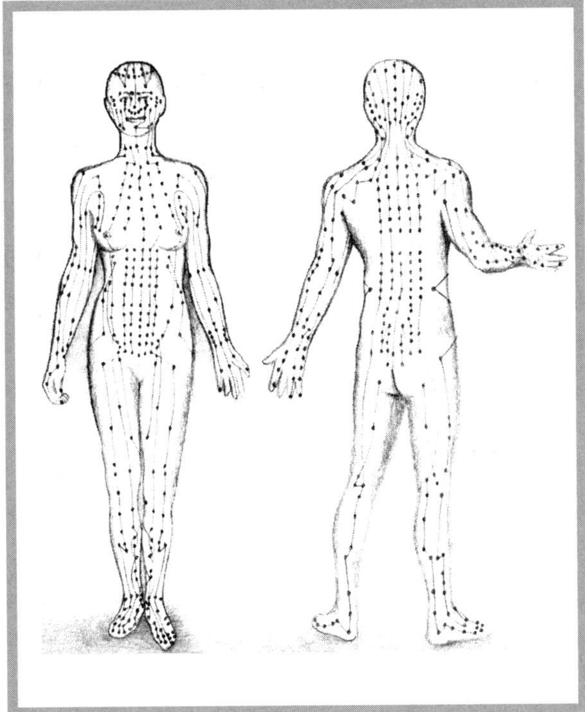

**Figure 20.2—Acupuncture points, front and back views**

Over the next few visits, Dr. Speckhart identified more points of toxicity involving bacteria, virus-

CAUTION

This chapter includes information regarding actual treatments used by Dr. Speckhart only after his careful diagnosis of each patient. All cancer patients are unique. **Do not administer these treatments to yourself or others.** Discuss these treatments with your physician or other qualified health-care professional. Readers should not interpret this material as therapeutic advice, but should see a physician in all cases.

es, fungi, toxic metals, and numerous chemicals. Once these "signals" were registered by the EDS device, Dr. Speckhart was able to deactivate them and cancel out their influence in Paula's body using homeopathic remedies. He also found evidence of Hodgkin's lymphoma in various acupuncture testing points on her body—those corresponding to the liver, spleen, and bone marrow.

On Dr. Speckhart's recommendation, Paula had her mercury amalgams and silicone breast implants removed to reduce the toxic load on her system. Within 2 years, EDS no longer picked up any signals indicating Hodgkin's lymphoma; a standard chest X ray also showed no evidence of disease.

QUICK DEFINITION

**Silicone implant disease** (also called human adjuvant disease or silicone-induced illness) is a new illness category developed by physicians now treating women with implants. Typically the disease produces a cluster of symptoms including any of the following: severe weight loss, hair loss, liver dysfunction, lymph node swelling, fatigue, weakness, granulomas, breast and nipple inflammation, skin shedding, circulation problems, arthritic pain, autoimmune symptoms, and chronic muscle pain and stiffness.

A homeopathic **nosode** is a super-diluted remedy made as an energy imprint from a disease product, such as bacteria, tuberculosis, measles, bowel infection, influenza, and about 200 others. The nosode, which contains no physical trace of the disease, stimulates the body to remove all "taints" or residues it holds of a particular disease, whether it was inherited or contracted. Only qualified homeopaths may administer a nosode.

## SUCCESS STORY

### Reversing Testicular Cancer

Keith, aged 37, suffered from cancer of the testes that failed to go away after a full course of chemotherapy. When he first consulted Dr. Speckhart, Keith had a 10-centimeter wide tumor in the right side of his abdomen. Understandably, Keith was depressed.

Using EDS, Dr. Speckhart was able to pinpoint specific energy points that were affected by the cancer or whose imbalance may have contributed to the cancer. Then Dr. Speckhart used EDS to identify which substances could correct these and other energy imbalances registered at key acupuncture testing points. Keith tested positive for *Natrum* and *Muriaticum Mandragora*, homeopathic remedies often prescribed to help relieve depression.

Further EDS investigation identified energy signals of cisplatinum (a chemotherapy drug), toluene, and xylol (toxic chemicals) in his system. These influences were neutralized by specific homeopathic remedies. Soon after, the mass in Keith's abdomen had decreased in size and he felt much better; he was no longer depressed and EDS no longer registered a signal indicating the need for *Natrum Muriaticum.* During the next 2 visits, signals for lymphogranuloma (an infectious disease

A homeopathic **miasm,** as originally described by Samuel Hahnemann, the 19th-century German founder of homeopathy, is a subtle taint or energy residue of previous illness, even across the generations. As an inherited predisposition for chronic disease that is far more subtle than anything genetic, miasms are broad-focused, predisposing individuals and families to specific illnesses, such as tuberculosis or cancer. According to Hahnemann, 3 miasms underlie all chronic illness and parallel broad stages in the history of human experience with primary disease states. They are the *Psoric* miasm (from psora, meaning "itch"), the *Syphilitic* miasm (deriving from syphilis), and the *Sycotic* miasm (arising as a residue of gonorrhea). Some homeopaths add a fourth Cancer miasm, and a fifth Petroleum miasm.

of the lymph glands) and the need for the homeopathic remedy *Psorinum* became prominent. Keith received homeopathic potencies of these energies, including *Psorinum*, which is a nosode (from scabies-infected tissue) for the *Psoric* miasm, as defined by homeopathy. "Cancer patients are twice as likely as a control group to have a *Psorinum* miasmic signal," says Dr. Speckhart.

By his eighth visit, 14 months after Dr. Speckhart initially balanced his acupuncture points, there was no physical or electrodermal evidence of cancer, and his cancer markers were normal. In other words, according to both conventional and energy indexes, Keith was cancer free.

Subsequent testing with ultrasound of Keith's abdomen failed to identify any tumor. "His body energy is currently focusing on his dental problems, specifically, for mercury amalgams and methylmercury, its by-product," Dr. Speckhart says. This means that among the energy signals in Keith's system, those related to dental products and their toxins were the "loudest" and most significant. "He is in the process of having his mercury amalgams replaced with a non-metal-containing composite, and he's taking garlic and chlorella for mercury detoxification."

## Interpreting the Multiple Energy Signals of Disease

As early as 1971, Dr. Speckhart began working with chemotherapy as a primary treatment for cancer. Although chemotherapeutic drugs were then hailed as the oncologist's prime tool, Dr. Speckhart's initial impressions of this modality were less enthusiastic. "After a while it became fairly evident that we were not getting the results we wanted with solid tumors," he recalls. "People often seemed to be getting worse instead of better. Chemotherapy is like trying to remove a fungus growing on a tree by spraying toxic chemicals on it. This approach doesn't eliminate the underlying conditions of the soil and tree that feed the fungus or disease."

The central focus of Dr. Speckhart's approach to cancer today is a combination of electrodermal screening (EDS) and homeopathy. EDS provides valuable clinical information about a person's energy state and suggests possible imbalances and toxic interferences; homeopathy provides subtle, highly potentized remedies to correct these disturbances.

EDS is based on the concept that a person's energy field influences the development and progression of disease and registers its progress, but it is also the means by which the practitioner can usefully interact within the patient's energy and biochemical domains and suggest therapeutic substances for healing. The EDS practitioner gathers information about the entire body by probing certain key points on the patient's hands and feet; these points are fully described by traditional Chinese medicine (TCM) in its classical model of energy pathways (meridians) and treatment points (acupoints).

***EDS enables the practitioner to detect early cancer-like signals from the patient's energy field, and provides highly specific information that assists the physician in selecting the therapies most appropriate for* that *patient.***

In this model, basic life force or vital energy, known as Qi (pronounced CHEE), circulates continuously, much like a river and its tributaries, passing through about 22 primary energy pathways. The presence of more than 1000 treatment points (acupoints, or places where the Qi is stronger and more easily accessed) enable the practitioner to influence, in various ways depending on the practice modality, the quality of the energy on that pathway. They also enable the skilled EDS practitioner to "listen" to the variations and nuances of the patient's energy flow and gather evidence of imbalances.

In fact, so finely tuned is EDS to the flow of Qi that it can differentiate specific factors believed to obstruct, block, or stagnate this energy. Such factors include toxins such as heavy metals, pesticides, parasites, allergens, "unfriendly" microorganisms, dental mercury, and many others. The more sophisticated EDS computer program may contain up to 3000 different energy "signals" corresponding to beneficial and harmful substances; this inventory (called the Product Library) also includes a database of remedies and therapeutic substances.

When the practitioner probes the patient's system for evidence of specific imbalances, the computer is able to compare its inventory of 3000+ signals with the energy information it is receiving electrodermally (through the skin by electronic sensors); the practitioner then correlates this information, interprets its significance, and weaves the information into the overall diagnosis.

## Modifying the Therapy to Fit the Individual's Unique Needs

EDS enables the practitioner to detect early cancer-like signals from the patient's energy field, and, further, provides highly specific information that assists the physician in selecting the therapies most appropriate for that patient. In effect, it often enables the physician to see disease before it manifests as pathology or to detect it at its earliest stage of manifestation. Even better, the specificity of EDS allows the physician to select the appropriate dose and strength, enabling the adjustment and calibration of the dose *precisely* to the unique energy and biochemical parameters of the individual patient.

This is so unlike conventional drug-based chemotherapy as to seem futuristic, yet *specificity* is the hallmark of alternative medicine, and most keenly, of homeopathy. Here, a one-strength dose does not fit all patients; instead, each patient requires different remedies at different strengths. The value of EDS, Dr. Speckhart explains, is that it can help the physician achieve this degree of *necessary* specificity.

Furthermore, EDS is highly empirical, based on observed results and clinical outcomes, the gold standard of true science and medical practice. The computer stores the energy signals of thousands of different substances, toxins, and remedies. Physicians can work with an energy biofeedback loop between patient, EDS device, and their own understanding. The EDS device is finely calibrated and registers changes in the patient's energy state, recording the actual response to the introduction or removal of these signals. "With EDS, you can find where tumor signals are located in the body," Dr. Speckhart says.

In EDS language, the acupuncture points that correspond to specific organs and tissues are known as control measurement points (CMP). Also known as "summation measurement points," these act as an information window, providing a general indication of the health of a particular meridian. If the CMP for a particular organ gives a poor reading, indicating what Dr. Speckhart calls an "energy disturbance," the CMPs for the various parts of that organ can then be checked. The physician can then assume that whichever part of the organ shows an imbalance is the site of the dysfunction.

If a patient has a lesion in the lung, for example, an EDS signal picked up on the Lung-11 point on the right side of the body may be consistent with an adenocarcinoma of the lung, even if it is at its earliest stage of manifestation, or even before it has become clinically evident. "You would then order other diagnostic tests to confirm your EDS impression," says Dr. Speckhart. If a particular meridian is not conducting energy well, this is called an indicator drop; the primary goal of treatment is to restore conductivity to those points.

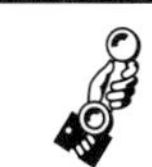

For information about the **political aspects of breast implants**, see *Informed Consent*, John A. Byrne, New York: McGraw Hill, 1996; *Silicone-Gate: Exposing the Breast Implant Scandal*, Henry Jenny, M.D., 1994 (self-published); and "Silicone Implants: How to Get Well Again After the Implants Come Out," *Alternative Medicine Digest* 10 (1996), 38-41.

EDS can indicate not only what area of the body is being affected, but the exact source of the problem as well. The screening is done by having the patient hold, one at a time, sample homeopathic dilutions of known disease substances, such as bacteria, viruses, or diseased tissue. When the patient is holding the one directly related to the cause of the problem, the EDS reading will return to normal. This means that particular homeopathic preparation will have a restorative or rebalancing effect on the immediate energy disturbance. In effect, the patient's body responds positively to what it perceives as "good medicine."

For more information about homeopathic **miasms**, see Chapter 25: What Causes Cancer?, pp. 640-642.

In the case of cancer, the tumor itself is less important than the kinds of signals that arise corresponding to that particular area of the body, says Dr. Speckhart. Correcting these signals with homeopathic remedies and detoxification strategies helps stimulate the body to react favorably against the cancer. Later on, Dr. Speckhart will check the point again to see how that particular meridian was modified; in other words, the EDS process is one of constant evaluation, followed by treatment and more evaluation. Over time, a skilled and attentive EDS practitioner such as Dr. Speckhart is able to build an empirical database of probable correlations between energy signals and pathologies or imbalances. "That's what we're trying to establish—the subtle energy characteristics of each type of cancer."

Energy flow can be disrupted by toxic insults to the tissues from heavy metals, ionizing radiation, or other sources of free radicals. "Heavy metals like cadmium or mercury may affect the Lung meridian in a case of lung cancer, or you could have a DDT signal in the small intestine," says Dr. Speckhart. As you eliminate the energy dysfunction, then normal energy flows and immune components, such as the interferons and interleukins, which are held in abeyance by that energy dysfunction, resume their normal operation. Further, we have found that cancer patients are twice as likely to have dental amalgam signals than patients in a control group." This indicates a presumed energy correlation between mercury fillings and cancer.

By combining homeopathic remedies with nutritional strategies and limited use of conventional treatment, Dr. Speckhart has enabled cancer patients, diagnosed at an early stage, to become tumor-detection free, usually within a year. Breast and prostate cancer are reversed more readily with his treatment, possibly due to the lower toxicity of chemotherapy drugs used for these cancers. As with many alternative practitioners, most of Dr. Speckhart's patients have either received or are currently receiving conventional treatments at the time of first consultations with him.

## Homeopathic Remedies Return Therapeutic Energy Signals to the Body

Once the specificities of the energy imbalance are established through EDS investigation and Dr. Speckhart has developed his diagnosis, he uses homeopathic remedies to address the underlying conditions. Some EDS devices are equipped to imprint the desired energy signals corresponding to remedies and nutrients into a carrier medium, such as water; the patient then takes the remedy orally, in small doses of drops, per the physician's prescription. The homeopathic remedies work to restore the EDS readings to close to 50, indicating health and energy balance.

In Dr. Speckhart's experience, it is more effective to prescribe several remedies to be taken concurrently than to prescribe a single remedy. This approach is typical of modern or complex homeopathy. He also finds that high-potency homeopathic remedies tend to be most effective on people with small tumors, i.e., the larger the tumor, the lower the homeopathic potency required. The medicines need to be taken repeatedly until the next visit. Patients with more aggressive forms of cancer visit Dr. Speckhart every 20-30 days, but for milder cancers, a visit once every 2 months is usually sufficient.

Cancer patients who receive conventional treatment tend to recover more slowly under homeopathy, possibly because the strong toxic drug picture of chemotherapy interferes with the more subtle action of the homeopathic remedies, Dr. Speckhart notes. Although chemotherapy agents are toxic and create numerous chemical imbalances, they do not necessarily cancel out the effectiveness of homeopathics. "We can help

QUICK DEFINITION

**Homeopathy** was founded in the early 1800s by German physician Samuel Hahnemann. Today, an estimated 500 million people worldwide receive homeopathic treatment; in Britain, homeopathy enjoys royal patronage. Homeopathy is now practiced according to two differing concepts. In classical homeopathy, only one single-component remedy is prescribed at a time in a potency specifically adjusted to the patient; the physician waits to see the results before prescribing anything further. In complex homeopathy, typified by *Hepar compositum*, a prescription involves multiple substances given at the same time, usually in low potencies .

patients tolerate chemotherapy drugs better by using homeopathic doses of the drugs themselves. This strategy can effectively decrease the biochemical damage caused by chemotherapy if the homeopathic version is given after the chemotherapy effect is complete."

## A Nutritional Program Based on Physiology

Some of Dr. Speckhart's cancer patients benefit from a vegetarian diet, while others seem to do better with a more omnivorous diet, including lean-meat animal products such as fish or poultry, he says. The biochemical individuality and unique physiology of each patient may explain this difference, says Dr. Speckhart. In some cases, patients may need more animal protein, particularly if they have lost a substantial amount of lean body mass.

This is why for Dr. Speckhart dietary prescriptions are less crucial than designating specific measures to enhance organ or digestive-system functioning. "I'm less concerned with the particular foods a person eats than the condition of their liver processing and detoxification capacities, or the status of absorption within the gastrointestinal tract."

Using EDS, Dr. Speckhart can determine which foods are tolerated or utilized by an individual, and which foods act as allergens. Wheat, for example, may cause problems in certain individuals. A disturbance in the energy pattern of the intestine suggests that the body is not responding well to the wheat; however, certain *strains* of wheat may be more easily tolerated than others, and EDS can reveal even this level of specificity.

To suppress the production of free-radicals, known to be a cancer-causing factor, Dr. Speckhart ensures that his patients receive adequate amounts of antioxidant supplements and that they avoid free radical-producing foods.

## The Supportive Role of Chelation in Cancer Therapy

Chelation therapy is used to rid the body of toxic metals such as lead, cadmium, iron, and copper. It is employed by a growing number of U.S. physicians to increase blood flow, thereby helping to relieve or resolve cardiovascular problems. Heavy metal toxicity is implicated strongly as a contributing cause of cancer. "Heavy metals feed free-radical reactions and may also suppress the immune system, making your body less capable of repelling cancer," says Dr. Speckhart. "Since chelation removes metals that can accelerate free radical reactions, it seems likely that chelation treatments can help lower one's susceptibility to cancer."

For more information on **heavy metal toxicity** (pp. 594-600) and **free radicals** (pp. 630-631), see Chapter 25: What Causes Cancer?; for more on **homeopathy**, see Chapter 6: W. John Diamond, M.D.; for more on **chelation**, see Chapter 33: Physical Support Therapies, p. 973.

A **free radical** is an unstable molecule with an unpaired electron that steals an electron from another molecule and produces harmful effects. Free radicals are formed when molecules within cells react with oxygen (oxidize) as part of normal metabolic processes. Free radicals then begin to break down cells, especially if there are not enough free-radical quenching nutrients, such as vitamins C and E, in the cell. While free radicals are normal products of metabolism, uncontrolled free-radical production plays a major role in the development of degenerative disease, including cancer, heart disease, and aging. Free radicals harmfully alter important molecules, such as proteins, enzymes, fats, even DNA. Other sources of free radicals include pesticides, industrial pollutants, smoking, alcohol, viruses, most infections, allergies, stress, even certain foods and excessive exercise.

Chelation refers to a method of binding up ("chelating") and draining toxins and metabolic wastes from the body while at the same time increasing blood flow and removing arterial plaque. In chelation, a nontoxic substance, often EDTA, is intravenously infused over a 1½-3 hour period; usually 20-30 treatments are recommended at the rate of 1-3 sessions per week. Oral chelation is an equally viable approach, although results may take longer to appear.

In 1958, a Swiss study involving 231 adults living near a well-traveled highway showed a higher rate of cancer mortality than other people of the same city who lived in traffic-free areas. The 231 adults also suffered from a higher incidence of nervous disorders, headaches, fatigue, gastrointestinal disorders, depression, and substance abuse.[1] The Swiss researchers suggested that this population's symptoms might be due to a higher level of exposure to lead from automobile exhaust. In 1961, 59 patients from this group received 10 or more EDTA chelation treatments plus vitamins C and B1, while the remaining 172 members of the group were untreated and served as control subjects.

An 18-year follow-up study of the group, conducted by Walter Blumer, M.D., of Nestal, Switzerland, revealed that only 1 of the 59 treated patients died of cancer as compared to 30 deaths (17.6%) among those not treated. Dr. Blumer concluded that EDTA chelation therapy was the only significant difference between the control group and the treated patients.[2] In other words, chelation appeared to produce a 90% reduction in cancer mortality.

The implications of Blumer's research are substantial, according to Dr. Speckhart. "By removing heavy metals through chelation, there is a possibility that you can prevent a cancer recurrence, though this has not yet been demonstrated." He notes that the nutritional supplements typically used as part of chelation therapy may afford an immune-enhancing benefit as well. A wide variety of clinical improvements have been observed among patients treated with EDTA chelation (approximately 26 infusions, extending over about 60 days of therapy) plus multivitamins and trace element supplements.[3] According to Dr. Speckhart, "At the present time, chelation should be viewed as a possible method of cancer prevention where selected metals may be involved in the creation of cancer."

***"By removing heavy metals through chelation, there is a possibility that you can prevent a cancer recurrence, though this has not yet been demonstrated," says Dr. Speckhart.***

## Electrodermal Screening Can Deepen Knowledge about Cancer

Dr. Speckhart proposes that cancer doctors attempt to blend their rational and intuitive faculties, as he has done in his investigations of energy medicine. "If an approach like EDS works, it should be used. Explanations may be formulated later to give us a functional perspective and to find ways to improve the approach."

As already indicated, a major advantage to EDS is that it can help the physician precisely identify which herb or nutrient will be therapeutically useful to an individual cancer patient. For example, EDS may reveal that shark cartilage will be helpful for one cancer patient but not another even when both have the same type of cancer. Studies of Essiac have shown that each of its main components (burdock, Indian rhubarb, and sorrel) has anticancer activity;[4] by testing each component with EDS, Dr. Speckhart can better determine how to combine the ingredients for the individual cancer patient.

As part of his continuing research, Dr. Speckhart uses EDS to gather and analyze data that correlates control measurement points (CMPs, described above) and remedies that might work best for various cancers. Overall the goal is to use EDS to select with more consistency and higher specificity the correct remedies for reversing cancer.

Cancer patients have a higher probability of having signals for the miasmatic conditions called *Syphilinum, Tuberculinum, Psorinum, Scirrhinum, Carcinosinum*, and *Silicea* than people without cancer, Dr. Speckhart says. "We're trying to define the energy characteristics of cancer patients and to identify the most commonly involved points and meridians and which remedies will more often provide balance or show effectiveness on those points. The database we're developing is a statistically valid window on a virtually unexplored dimension of medicine."

EDS gives the attentive physician valuable insights into the nature and origin of cancer, says Dr. Speckhart. "We're finding that energy dysfunction *always* precedes the physical changes. By enabling doctors to identify the dysfunction *before* cancer develops, EDS helps doctors prescribe effective, individualized, preventive measures." This strategy also could be particularly valuable in preventing a recurrence of cancer once an individual has been successfully treated.

The ideal way to treat any disease, says Dr. Speckhart, is to define the energy parameters of the disease before determining a particular treatment. In conventional oncology, CT (computed tomography) scans and MRIs suggest the size, shape, and position of a particular tumor; however, these high-tech approaches are sometimes inadequate, and in any case, they cannot reveal anything about the energy character of the cancer. "EDS will someday be a valuable adjunct for pre-planning surgery and other orthodox strategies."

Dr. Speckhart is also optimistic that EDS and homeopathy will become an integral part of mainstream cancer treatment in the coming decades. The evidence tends to support his optimism. European research confirms the protective effect produced by potentized homeopathic doses of actual carcinogens;[5] homeopathic doses of standard immunotherapy drugs, such as tumor necrosis factor, have been shown to reduce some of the side effects of the drug's crude doses,[6] and homeopathic remedies may also prove beneficial in protecting cancer patients against the adverse effects of radiation treatments.[7]

EDS may one day help explain why the same chemotherapy regimen that causes one individual to become sicker and to deteriorate faster may enable another to get rid of the cancer with little or no side effects. Perhaps, in the latter case, the body's "energy character" is somehow more receptive or "in harmony" with the chemotherapy, speculates Dr. Speckhart. "Using EDS, one could probably develop a dynamic chemotherapy combination for that individual. One would know rapidly and decisively whether there is no longer harmony in the body for a particular drug. The key is to use EDS to identify the correct dose and its frequency by which this imbalance may be eliminated and harmony restored to the patient's meridian system."

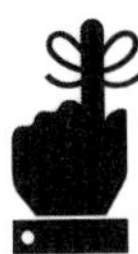

*Cancer survival statistics, flawed and misleading as they are already, do not factor in the far longer survival times commonly produced by physicians using alternative modalities of cancer care. Nor do they account in any way for the radical degree to which alternative medicine applied to cancer care could profoundly shift the outcomes from dismal to successful.*

## CURRICULUM VITAE

# Jesse Stoff, M.D.

Solstice Clinical Associates,
Southwest Professional Plaza,
2122 North Craycroft Road, #112,
Tucson, AZ 85712;
tel: 520-290-4516; fax: 520-290-6403.

Dr. Stoff received his M.D. from New York Medical College in Valhalla, New York. He completed a Fellowship in Clinical Medicine at the Bloomsbury Medical Authority in London, England, and he studied homeopathy at the Royal London Homeopathic Hospital in London, England, from 1982 to 1983. From 1985 to 1991, Dr. Stoff was editor of the *Journal of Anthroposophic Medicine* and from 1986 to1991, he was vice president of the Physicians' Association for Anthroposophic Medicine. Dr. Stoff is a member of 8 professional medical societies and coauthor of the best-selling *Chronic Fatigue Syndrome: The Hidden Epidemic* (HarperCollins, 2nd Edition, 1992).

***"The tumor is not a part of the human organism, but represents a rebellion of the cells against the human organism," Dr. Stoff explains. "Consequently, cancer should be considered a disease of the whole organism, not a disease of cells."***

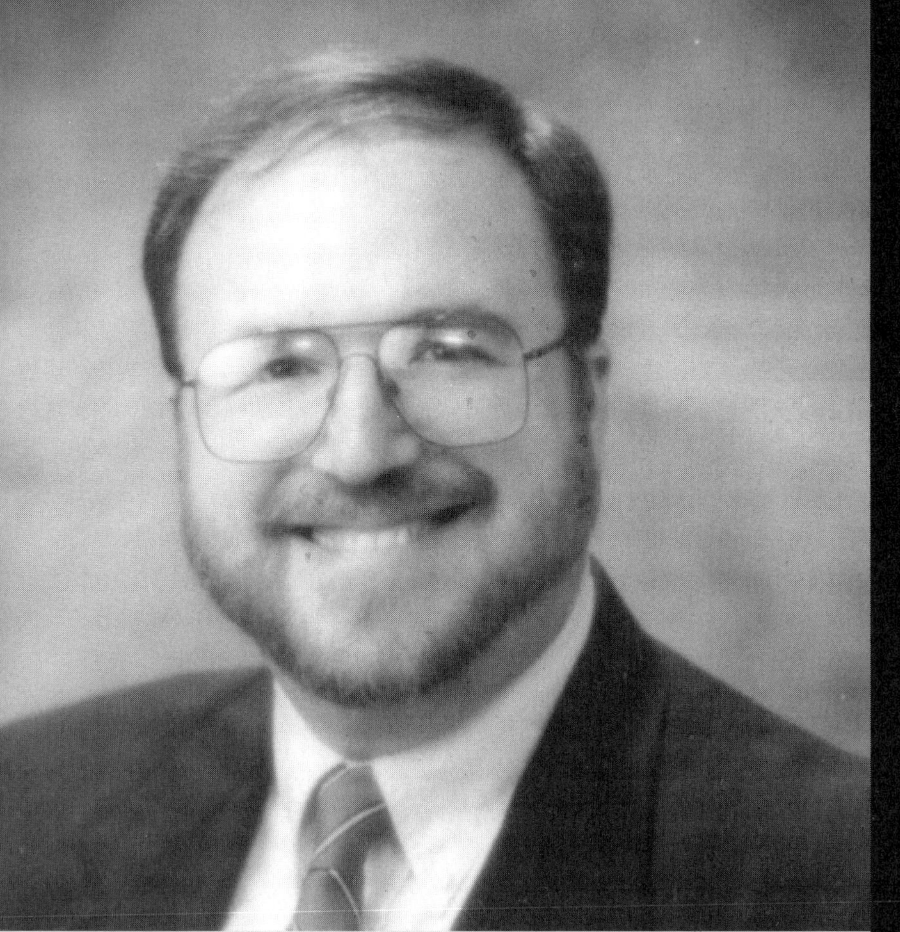

# Chapter 21

# *Jesse Stoff, M.D.*

**ALL ASPECTS OF THE PATIENT'S LIFE,** including body, mind, and emotions must receive therapeutic attention, advocates Dr. Stoff, who prescribes a rich and individualized blend of herbs, nutritional supplements, special homeopathic remedies, dietary changes, detoxification techniques—even music and art therapy—to help patients reverse their cancer.

Early on in his career, Dr. Stoff realized that the mechanistic explanation of human functioning could not adequately explain the dynamic nature of life and health. After completing his conventional medical studies, Dr. Stoff found part of the broader explanation he was seeking in homeopathy, which recognizes the dynamic, if not subtle, side of symptoms and remedies.

**Anthroposophic medicine** is an extension of conventional Western medicine developed by Austrian scientist Rudolf Steiner in the 1920s in conjunction with European physicians. It is based on a spiritual model of the human being and its medicines are extensions of homeopathic remedies. In the U.S., there are about 60 practitioners, all M.D.s, plus many hundreds of nurses and adjunctive therapists, but in German-speaking countries, there are thousands plus several major hospitals in Germany and Switzerland devoted exclusively to this medical approach. **Anthroposophic medicines** are available to physicians (some may be had without a prescription) from Weleda, Inc., 175 N. Rte. 9W, P.O. Box 249, Congers, NY 10920; tel: 914-268-8572; fax: 914-268-8574; or Raphael Pharmacy, 7957 California Ave, Fair Oaks, CA 95628; tel: 916-962-1099.

When he encountered a unique medical system called Anthroposophic medicine, founded by the Austrian scientist Rudolf Steiner (1861-1925), Dr. Stoff knew he had found a way to extend Western medicine into a spiritual perception of the individual. Steiner based his medical views on a larger philosophical system he called Anthroposophy (pronounced ann-throw-POSS-oh-fee) and worked with European physicians in the 1920s to develop its scientific and medical protocols, including the now well-known Iscador, the successful cancer remedy derived from mistletoe.

Between 1986 and 1991, Dr. Stoff served as vice president of the Physicians' Association for Anthroposophic Medicine, and as editor of their *Journal of Anthroposophic Medicine*, he arrived at an appreciation of the deeper psychological, emotional, and spiritual, aspects of disease, including the influence of subtle energies operating within and around the human body, not unlike what is known to practitioners of Chinese medicine and acupuncture. These insights helped Dr. Stoff to discern new possibilities for healing cancer and other serious degenerative diseases and

# Dr. Stoff's Generalized Model for Cancer Treatment

| STRATEGY | DOSAGE/ KEY COMPONENTS | FOR MORE INFORMATION see page # |
|---|---|---|
| **Dietary Plan** | | |
| Primarily vegetarian | cooked grains, beans, and vegetables. If weakened digestive system, avoid raw vegetables and vegetable juices; if low blood cholesterol, 1 egg a day and clarified butter (ghee); if compromised liver function, avoid simple sugars and emphasize high-fiber foods | 749 |
| **Alternative Cancer Therapies** | | |
| Iscador | depending on individual | 830-831 |
| Larix (Ara-6, from the Western larch tree) | 1 tsp. in water or vegetable juice 3X/day; supplement with vitamin C for best results | 831 |
| Ukrain | 5-20 mg every other day; may be used in combination with Taxol | 873 |
| **Botanicals** | | |
| *Gingko biloba* | cleanses blood and enhances circulation 40 mg, 3X/day | 820 |
| Panax ginseng | antioxidant, immune stimulator, 250-1000 mg, 3X/day | 821 |
| Astragalus combinations (GAC, with ginseng, and ligustrum) | immune stimulator 250-1000 mg, 3X/day | 813 |
| Green tea extract | slows down cancer cells Camsin, 2 tablets, 3X/day | 823 |
| *Echinacea* and pau d'arco | protection against infection, 250-1000 mg, 3X/day | 815, 834 |
| Essiac | cleanses blood, especially after chemotherapy or radiation, 1 cup of tea, 3X daily | 815 |
| Aloe vera concentrate | laxative, immuno-modulator; 1-2 ounces in juice or water, 3X/day (at least 1000 mg of the active mucopolysaccharides) | 812 |
| Maitake D-fraction | for weight loss; stabilizes immune system; 10 drops in water or with Ara-6 and glutamine, 3X/day | 833 |

*Continued*

# Dr. Stoff's Generalized Model for Cancer Treatment (cont.)

| STRATEGY | DOSAGE/ KEY COMPONENTS | FOR MORE INFORMATION see page # |
|---|---|---|
| Turmeric | antioxidant, anti-inflammatory inhibits cancer; 100-500 mg, 3X/day | 836 |

## Hormones

| STRATEGY | DOSAGE/ KEY COMPONENTS | FOR MORE INFORMATION see page # |
|---|---|---|
| Melatonin | antioxidant, stimulates immune system, helps reset sleep cycle; 1-10 mg in a long-acting base at bedtime | 941 |
| DHEA | stimulates immune system; 25-100 mg in a long-acting base daily | 939 |
| Thyroid | Armour brand, 1/4 to 3 grains/day | 944 |
| Glandulars (Pituitrophin) | 1-2 tablets, 1-3 times/day | 935 |

## Essential Fatty Acids

| STRATEGY | DOSAGE/ KEY COMPONENTS | FOR MORE INFORMATION see page # |
|---|---|---|
| Flaxseed oil | 2 tbsp/day | 768 |
| Borage oil (GLA 250) | 2 capsules, 3X/day | 770 |
| Fish oils (Super EPA) | 2 capsules, 3X/day (avoid for 3 days before and after surgery) | 768 |

## Supplements

| STRATEGY | DOSAGE/ KEY COMPONENTS | FOR MORE INFORMATION see page # |
|---|---|---|
| Vitamin A | 10,000-100,000 IU/day | 784 |
| Vitamin B-complex | depending on individual | 784 |
| Vitamin B6 (pyridoxine) | 25-300 mg/day (never exceeding 500 mg/day) | 786 |
| Vitamin C | 15-50 g/day | 786 |
| Vitamin E | 400 units 2X/day | 790 |
| Vitamin D | 1000-5000 IU/day | 789 |
| Calcium and magnesium | 800-1000 mg/day of calcium<br>400-800 mg/day of magnesium | 765 |
| Germanium | with vitamin C and Ukrain, 5 ml/day | 771 |
| Selenium | 200-300 mcg/day | 783 |
| Zinc | 30-60 mg/day(only if zinc deficiency) | 793 |
| Coenzyme Q10 | 250-300 mg/day | 766 |
| Amino acids | L-arginine, 5-8 g/day<br>L-methionine, 500 mg, 2-3X/day<br>L-cysteine, 500 mg, 2-3X/day<br>1000-5000 IU/day | 762 |

| STRATEGY | DOSAGE/ KEY COMPONENTS | FOR MORE INFORMATION see page # |
|---|---|---|
| METBAL® | Based on individual needs | 455 |
| **Other Therapies** | | |
| Detoxification | Diet, herbs, Epsom salts, coffee enemas, heat therapy, quercetin (1000-1500 mg, 3X daily) | 949 |
| Exercise | for detoxification, immune stimulation, anticancer effects | 1003 |
| Stress reduction and emotional support | immune-strengthening psychotherapy, support groups, guided imagery, visualization | 459 |
| Music therapy | overall healing | 461 |

to regard illness as an opportunity to take a step on the path toward greater personal growth and awareness.

CAUTION

This chapter includes information regarding actual treatments used by Dr. Stoff only after his careful diagnosis of each patient. All cancer patients are unique. **Do not administer these treatments to yourself or others.** Discuss these treatments with your physician or other qualified health-care professional. Readers should not interpret this material as therapeutic advice, but should see a physician in all cases.

## SUCCESS STORY
### Reversing Prostate Cancer

When Allan, aged 64, was diagnosed with metastatic prostate cancer it had already spread to the lymph nodes surrounding the prostate gland and to the bones. His PSA (prostate specific antigen) reading was over 600, indicating an advanced cancer. Soon after, Allan had surgery and local radiation, including radioactive implants (called brachytherapy). His oncologist had recommended orchidectomy (chemical or physical removal of the testes) and chemotherapy, neither of which Allan wanted to do.

A few months after starting a macrobiotic diet, known to have anticancer effects, Allan consulted Dr. Stoff. Using a unique diagnostic test called the blood crystallization test developed by Anthroposophic scientists, Dr. Stoff gathered substantial information about the functioning of every organ and system in Allan's body. "This test helped me determine what kinds of therapies would be of benefit," Dr. Stoff says. "Based in part

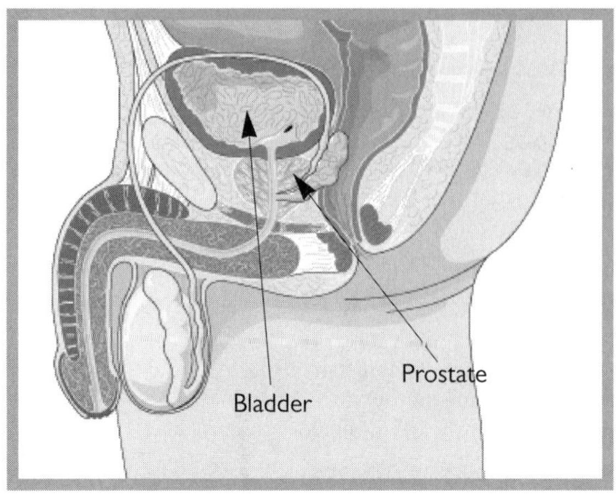

**Figure 21.1—The prostate gland**

on this test, I was able to identify a number of homeopathic medications that might help stimulate Allan's natural healing abilities."

Dr. Stoff administered various homeopathic and Anthroposophic remedies (such as Iscador, *Prostate/Berberis comp*, and *Sabal/Solidago comp*) to Allan and carefully monitored his immune system function, which had been weak. Since the macrobiotic diet had not brought much improvement in Allan's condition, Dr. Stoff prescribed extra nutritional support in the form of high-dose intravenous vitamin C and a balanced array of trace elements. He also gave Allan high doses of minerals, both orally and intravenously, to help make his system less acidic and more alkaline. In addition, a staff psychologist taught Allan various stress reduction techniques.

Allan went into a state of remission within 3 months of his first visit with Dr. Stoff, and 10 years later remains symptom free. His current therapy includes nutritional aides such as arginine, glutamine, vitamin C, *Acidophilus*, antioxidants, maitake, Super-Antioxidant Formula (developed by Dr. Stoff), and thyroid extract. "He's in very good health and we will continue to watch his progress and monitor his immune system," notes Dr. Stoff. "His immune system is evidently strong enough to help keep him in remission. As long as he continues to stay with the recommended program, we expect Allan to remain in remission for the foreseeable future."

## SUCCESS STORY
### Reversing Lymphoma

Peter, aged 45, first consulted Dr. Stoff after receiving a diagnosis of lymphoma. He had been advised to have chemotherapy and radiation, both of which he declined. The lymphoma had spread to his bone marrow, liver, and spleen, and his white blood cell count (a reliable indicator of infection or disease) was 18,000, which is twice the normal level.

Dr. Stoff administered a series of Anthroposophic medicines by injection (Iscador, *Colchicum comp*, and *Chrysosplenium comp*) and gave Peter various nutritional supplements including vitamins C, K complex (a magnesium-potassium solution), Super-Charged Antioxidant, a multivitamin, and flaxseed oil. Within 2 months of starting this program, Peter showed marked progress.

"The medications were effective in lowering his white cell count, bringing it into the normal ranges and allowing his body to push the lymphoma into a full state of remission," Dr. Stoff says. The remission was proven by repeated CT scans. "Peter is definitely in good health and his cancer has been in remission for over 5 years now. We will continue to monitor his progress but we feel confident that he will only continue to get stronger and healthier."

## SUCCESS STORY

### Reversing Leukemia

Theodore, aged 50, came to Solstice Clinical Associates with a diagnosis of chronic lymphocytic leukemia. His conventional doctors were urging a bone marrow transplant and high-dose chemotherapy but Theodore wanted none of that. Dr. Stoff's blood test showed that Theodore's bone marrow was being attacked by cytomegalovirus, a herpes virus which is often active in people with a compromised immune system. This virus was triggering malignant changes in Theodore's bone marrow, thereby producing the leukemia, Dr. Stoff explains. But rather than treating the cancer (leukemia), Dr. Stoff focused his treatment on the virus.

To start off, Dr. Stoff gave Theodore a series of injectable remedies, most notably a preparation used in Anthroposophic medicine called Iscucin (made from *Viscum album*, or mistletoe) to stimulate the natural killer cells of his immune system. Next, he gave Theodore once-daily intravenous infusions of nutrients including vitamin C (50 g), calcium chloride (5 g), vitamin B12 (1000 mcg), vitamin B6 (300 mg), magnesium (2 g), vitamin B complex, adrenal cortex extract, and licorice extract.

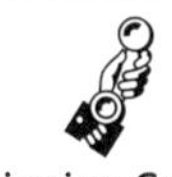

**Aminovirox, Camsin (green tea extract), Aminoplex, and Sof Gel EFA** are available from Tyson and Associates, 12832 South Chadron Avenue, Hawthorne, CA 90250; tel: 800-318-9766; fax: 310-675-4187. **Immune Boosters: Breakfast, Lunch, Dinner** (with different formulations of vitamins, minerals, and botanicals): are available without prescription from Solstice Vitamin Company, 982 Stuyvesant Avenue, Union, NJ 07083; tel: 800-765-7842. **Super-Charged Antioxidant, Super Colloidal Silver, GLA 260** (borage oil), and **Super EPA Fish Oil** are also available from Solstice Vitamin Company.

**Aminovirox™** contains 18 amino acids (excluding arginine, but emphasizing lysine) formulated for rapid absorption primarily for individuals with herpes viral infections, including Epstein-Barr virus. Lysine is believed to be effective in inhibiting the growth of herpes virus. **Aminoplex®** contains a balanced formula of 18 amino acids to help restore nitrogen balance, detoxify heavy metals, reduce the effects of stress, and address amino acid deficiencies. **Green Tea Extract,** made from unfermented tea, contains 4 catechins, crystalline compounds that have been shown in animal studies to be effective against cancer and stroke and to reduce blood composition factors associated with heart disease.

In addition, Dr. Stoff prescribed a series of oral supplements including Aminovirox™ (2 capsules, 3 times daily), Immune Boosters (3 daily, one after each meal), Super Colloidal Silver (one teaspoon, twice daily), folic acid (400 mcg daily), and acidophilus (3 daily doses). Dr. Stoff rotated Theodore through *Acidophilus* in powder, liquid, and capsule form to give him the broadest spectrum of "friendly" bacteria, or beneficial intestinal microorganisms.

Next it was necessary to give Theodore's system high nitrogen amino acids, such as arginine (500 mg, taken 3 times daily), to "feed" the natural killer cells so they could neutralize the cancer. Camsin, green tea extract (2 capsules, taken 3 times daily) also helped here. Further supplements included Super Antioxidant Formula (2 tablets, 3 times daily), borage oil (as gamma linolenic acid, or GLA 240, 2 capsules, twice daily), Super EPA Fish Oil to replenish Theodore's essential fatty acid reserves (2 capsules, twice daily), and a balanced multivitamin.

The synergistic formula paid off. Theodore's lymphocyte count (a measure of his white blood cells) dropped from an extreme high of 60,000 to a more manageable 11,000, but it took the first year to get his white blood cell count down to 20,000. At this point, Dr. Stoff stopped Aminovirox™ and substituted Aminoplex®, a different amino acid formula.

After 6 months on this program, "the virus was gone and Theodore was in remission," says Dr. Stoff. Theodore remains on the supplements and continues to receive the Iscucin injections for 6 weeks twice a year. "He still has leukemia, but it's no longer active and shows no signs of threatening to come out again."

## Cancer Is a Disease of the Whole Organism

According to the anthroposophic medical model, the human being actually comprises 4 "members" or dimensions of energy influence that interact and govern all the organism's life processes. The most condensed level of energy is the physical body, Dr. Stoff explains. The physical body is the presence of the mineral kingdom in the human organism. The physical body comes "alive" or becomes animated by the second member, the field of life energy surrounding it; this "member" reflects the presence of the plant kingdom.

Third, there is the realm of feelings and emotions, which is the presence of the kingdom of animals. The fourth member, unique to humans, is the "Ego," the seat of identity, self-awareness, and consciousness.

"The healthy organism is the result of the cooperation between these 4 aspects of human life," Dr. Stoff says. "The body and all its physical manifestations, including tumors, are manifestations of this complex interaction, which can be influenced through lifestyle, medicines, the mind, or spirit." Consequently, cancer should be considered a disease of the whole organism, not a disease of cells.[1]

Anthroposophic doctors postulate that the form, structure, and growth process of living cells are related to these 4 members of the human organism. The emotional forces oppose and help control the life-energy forces, thereby helping the organism maintain consistency of structure and organization. "The dynamic balance between the forces of growth [life energy] and the forces of breakdown [emotional energy] gives us health in terms of growth, repair and regeneration." When there is a poor integration between these forces, the normal processes of growth and cell metabolism are disrupted and degenerative diseases may develop.

Although it may sound philosophical, the theory Dr. Stoff and his colleagues propose for cancer is rigorously medical in its insight. In cancer, the body's cells and subcellular substances lose their ability to regenerate after decades of having life energy forces acting upon them without restraint. Whereas normally, there is a healthy tension between the life energy forces and the emotional forces, in disease this tension begins to weaken and a new equilibrium with less tension develops. The cells then liberate themselves, evading the body's impulses to shape and form them. Unchecked, they eventually form a tumor.

The tumor is *not* a part of the human organism, but represents a rebellion of the cells against the human organism,[2] Dr. Stoff explains. "Cancer can occur only if the growth process of cells proceeds unchecked. From our perspective, cancer is an expression of a disruption of the patient's growth forces, as well as a failure of the integration of the forces of their Ego, or spiritual identity."

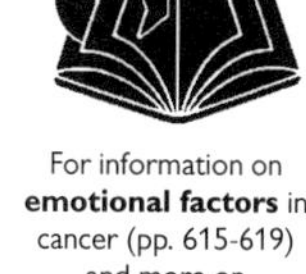

For information on **emotional factors** in cancer (pp. 615-619) and more on **pesticides** and cancer (pp. 568-574), see Chapter 25: What Causes Cancer?

The disruption of the emotional field of the person with cancer is typically the result of a cumulative exposure to toxins, such as free radicals, heavy metals, viruses, and ionizing radiation. Such substances do not support the organism's life force and they lead to a poor integration between it and the emotional field, Dr. Stoff observes. In fact, these factors so weaken the body's life force over time that ultimately they cause the life energy body to begin falling apart. Further, one's self-identity ("Ego forces") can become dissociated through unresolved difficulties and chronic emotional stress, says Dr. Stoff.

Dr. Stoff notes that environmental influences ultimately help cause most cancers through repeated "insults" to the organism. To explain this principle, Dr. Stoff points to Long Island, New York, one of the country's breast cancer "hot spots." The place was once a potato-growing area, but with the advent of modern agriculture, fat-soluble pesticides leached into the groundwater on a regular basis. "Since such a high percentage of a woman's mammary tissue is fat, the breasts tend to accumulate these toxic chemicals more than other body tissues," Dr. Stoff says. "Eventually it becomes a triggering agent for cancer as well as a stimulus for the ongoing promotion and progression of cancer."

***"Since such a high percentage of a woman's mammary tissue is fat, the breasts tend to accumulate toxic chemicals more than other body tissues," Dr. Stoff says.***

In light of these observations, Dr. Stoff believes that cancer therapy needs to correct the regulation of the body's growth forces by assuring an adequate supply of nutrients and other biological response modifiers. "The organism must obtain adequate and appropriate amounts of these nutrients from the plant realm, as this is where the primary elements of health and vitality originate."

At the same time, the powerful emotional forces must be addressed to help control the cells' tendency to proliferate endlessly. It's also important to note that when patients, as individuals, takes steps to find meaning, purpose, and fulfillment in daily life experiences—including the trials and heartbreaks of illness—then they can begin to make an active contribution to the healing process.[3]

"Most people with cancer come to me when everything else has failed and they are so toxic that many of their systems are already extremely weakened," explains Dr. Stoff. "What I try to do is strengthen them in specific areas so that when I detoxify them, they do not become further weakened by the sudden release of yet more toxins into their system."

In approaching the person diagnosed with cancer, Dr. Stoff helps them understand the nature of their illness and feel encouraged to fight it.

"I do not force anything on my patients. I try to develop a caring relationship in which they are aware of my role as a strong ally and as a source of therapeutic support on multiple levels."

The destruction of a tumor is only one of Dr. Stoff's goals. "A more advanced form of therapy aims at balancing the weaknesses and disorders that enable the tumor to thrive within the organism in the first place. This means supporting the life forces in each organ and organ system to the maximum extent possible, recognizing that ultimately the patient's body, not the physician, effects the healing process."

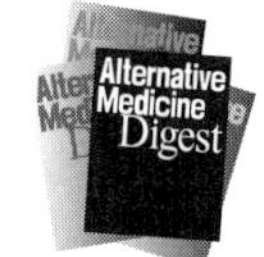


For more on Dr. Stoff's medical protocols, see "Chronic Fatigue and Leukemia," #12, pp. 24-32.

For more information on the **Forcyte System** for breast cancer testing, see Chapter 27: Early Detection and Prevention of Cancer, p. 742.

## Information Is Critical for Successful Therapy

When Dr. Stoff meets with a cancer patient for the first time, he focuses on obtaining information in 3 areas. First, he acquires all the objective disease-related information about the cancer by using cancer markers found in the blood and a test called the Forcyte System, which provides a subcellular portrait of the patient's tumor and its DNA composition. The test enables him to make a quantitative determination of a cancer patient's prognosis. "This information is extremely useful in order to know how aggressive we need to be in attempting to treat this cancer," says Dr. Stoff.

Second, Dr. Stoff gathers extensive blood-related information to assess the person's biochemical balance and immune system functioning. This set of tests includes amino acid levels, cancer markers, lipid peroxide levels, NK cell activation, and other aspects of the body's anticancer defenses. "Measurements of nitric oxide levels and lipid peroxides help us assess ongoing cellular damage as well as the body's ability to deal with such damage," Stoff says. "This information enables us to see exactly where we are and where we need to be. Then the patient and I can sit down and chart a therapeutic course accordingly."

Dr. Stoff uses the lipid peroxide level (the amount of oxidized blood fats, or fats damaged by free radicals) to see whether he needs to increase the individual's antioxidant intake. "There are numerous variables that can affect the lipid peroxide levels. It could be pollution related, fat related, or due to toxins released from the liver that have been stored over the years." In most cases, by reducing the person's exposures to free radicals and increasing dietary antioxidant intake, the lipid peroxide level begins to drop substantially.

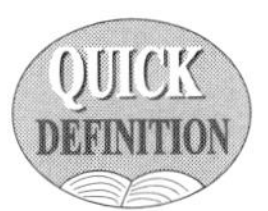

A **free radical** is an unstable molecule with an unpaired electron that steals an electron from another molecule and produces harmful effects. Free radicals are formed when molecules within cells react with oxygen (oxidize) as part of normal metabolic processes. Free radicals then begin to break down cells, especially if there are not enough free-radical quenching nutrients, such as vitamins C and E, in the cell. While free radicals are normal products of metabolism, uncontrolled free-radical production plays a major role in the development of degenerative disease, including cancer, heart disease, and aging. Free radicals harmfully alter important molecules, such as proteins, enzymes, fats, even DNA. Other sources of free radicals include pesticides, industrial pollutants, smoking, alcohol, viruses, most infections, allergies, stress, even certain foods and excessive exercise.

A **cancer marker** refers to any of a variety of blood tests which measure the level of a protein material or other chemical produced by cancer cells. These numbers become elevated in the presence of a cancer or tumor. There are different cancer markers for different kinds of cancer; CEA (carcino-embryonic antigen) test for colon cancer, AFP (alpha fetoprotein) test for liver cancer (primary hepato-cellular carcinoma), PSA (prostate specific antigen) for prostate cancer, CA (carcinoma) 15-3 or 27.29 for breast cancer, and CA 125 for ovarian cancer, to name a few.

Dr. Stoff has observed that cancer markers do not always provide the best indication of the specific character or relative aggressiveness of a cancer. With breast cancer, for example, there are 4 different cancer markers, but it is rare to find a breast cancer that produces more than 2 or 3 of them. "You can have a huge tumor sitting there and any one of these markers can be well within normal range," Dr. Stoff says. There is also a less than adequate correlation between cancer markers and the tumor mass. "You can have people with advanced metastatic disease and only moderately elevated levels of cancer markers, and vice versa," Dr. Stoff says. However, consistent correlations between tumor mass and cancer markers can serve as a rough approximation of how well the battle is going for any one individual, he adds.

When the treatment activates the immune system to respond to the tumor cells, the cancer markers will typically start showing a sudden rise or spike. This is because large amounts of proteins (tumor antigens, or cancer markers) are released as the cancer cells begin to die. "The cancer markers will go through the ceiling at this point," Dr. Stoff says. "One needs to be prepared for this from a psychological point of view." If blood tests are done, cancer patients should realize that the rise will be transient and that it will drop precipitously, usually within 1 to 6 weeks.

During this period, the immune system's scavenging cells, the macrophages, will sweep up the cancer cells' debris. "The take-home lesson is that if you look at cancer markers only, you may get an inaccurate picture of how the cancer is behaving at that time," says Dr. Stoff. "The test should be repeated later on to ensure that the original reading is truly a spike, not an absolute, prolonged rise in the cancer markers."

Third, Dr. Stoff creates a list of all treatment options that may apply or "make biological sense" for this particular cancer. For Dr. Stoff, this may include alternative and conventional treatments as well as combinations of both that might maximize the clinical outcome while minimizing toxic side effects. As it turns out, the majority of his patients have already received extensive conventional treatment and are typically in need of intensive detoxification and immune-enhancing measures. "This individualized approach is why I think I have good results," says Dr. Stoff. "The blood test should reflect changes in the individual's health. If it doesn't, then I know I have to change my strategy."

For more information on the different **immune system cells**, see Chapter 25: What Causes Cancer?, pp. 548-551.

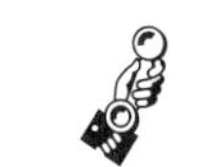

For more information about **Absorbaid**, contact: Solstice Vitamin Co., 982 Stuyvesant Avenue, Union, NJ 07083; tel: 800-765-7842 or 908-810-0909; fax: 908-810-9207.

## A Program of Dietary Support for Cancer Patients

A primarily vegetarian diet is the optimal nutritional strategy for supporting recovery from cancer, Dr. Stoff says. His dietary approach is designed to meet individual needs, determined by objective laboratory tests (blood tests for nutrients, enzymes, hormones, and immune parameters) and subjective measures, such as a person's food tastes and willingness to try a new diet.

The digestive capacities of the individual also must be considered, for they play a fundamental role in determining the body's usage of nutrients. Many of Dr. Stoff's patients come to him with a weakened digestive system, due to the cancer itself or, more often, the toxic effects of previous treatment by radiation or chemotherapy. Cooking foods helps because heating the food breaks down the cellulose, making nutrients more available for digestion.

"We usually begin with foods that are basically predigested, such as cooked grains and cooked vegetables, since the cancer patient's enzyme production in the small intestine is typically poor," Dr. Stoff says. "To consume raw vegetables or vegetable juices will cause additional stress because the patient won't digest it or absorb it. To support the digestive system I often recommend an enzyme formula called Absorbaid."

**Protein—**Although animal products provide accessible protein, as a rule Dr. Stoff encourages his patients to use vegetarian protein sources. The amount of protein they should consume depends, in part, on what the person's kidneys can handle; this is determined by their urinary creatinine and blood urea nitrogen measurements. Creatinine is converted from creatine, an amino acid found in muscle.

Cooking meat, which contains the muscle of animals, results in the conversion of creatine to creatinine; once this is digested, it is rapidly excreted in the urine. Creatinine measurements are a standard medical tool for determining the existence of kidney problems. Nitrogen is the basic element contained in all protein, and the levels of urinary nitrogen reflect how much stress the kidneys are under. Typically, cancer patients should be on a low-protein diet because the breakdown products of animal proteins can be toxic, and this will raise the creatinine levels."

Many people with advanced cancer tend to lose lean-body tissue or muscle mass, a phenomenon referred to as cancer cachexia. "Most people with late-stage cancer are protein malnourished and many show signs of muscular wasting," Dr. Stoff says. "They need plenty of protein in their diet, all in a form and at a pace they can handle without burdening their system. Cooked beans are an excellent way to help meet this need. We may supplement this with amino acids, but the metabolites of vegetable protein tend to be nontoxic."

***"Typically, cancer patients should be on a low-protein diet because the breakdown products of animal proteins can be toxic, and this will raise the creatinine levels," says Dr. Stoff.***

**Fat**—One of the shortcomings of many dietary approaches to cancer, in Stoff's view, is a lack of attention to the blood cholesterol issue. Patients who have received conventional cancer treatment almost always have low blood cholesterol when they first consult Dr. Stoff. This can be detrimental since cholesterol is a critical structural component of cell membranes and is therefore critical to the smooth functioning of all living cells.

"For people with low blood cholesterol, I recommend eating clarified butter also known as ghee, because it is easily absorbed," Dr. Stoff says. Often patients prepare ghee themselves at home. "If they do not have breast or ovarian cancer, I will recommend that they eat one egg a day. On occasion, a cancer patient whose cholesterol is barely over 100 mg/dl may be advised to eat chemical-free steak." To put this in perspective, a healthy cholesterol level is 140-180 mg/dl. The essential point is that a low blood cholesterol level reduces the body's ability to adequately repair and regenerate itself.

Cholesterol also indirectly confers a powerful antioxidant effect, but only at adequate blood levels. If a low-cholesterol bloodstream is awash with free radicals, even large amounts of vitamins C and E and beta carotene may be ineffective. In addition, if the liver is severely toxic, the body's ability to produce cholesterol becomes compromised and blood cholesterol levels decline. "Low cholesterol is often an indication of severe liver dysfunction," Dr. Stoff says. "When someone's liver becomes severely compromised and their cholesterol starts to drop, it must be supplemented immediately [with eggs or other animal products] or their condition will worsen rapidly."

"The cancer patient desperately needs concentrated sources of energy and in substantial amounts, which is partly why fats are an important consideration," Dr. Stoff says. The appropriate use of fats depends on 2 factors: the individual's cholesterol level and the type and quality of fat. For example, the fat in ghee or eggs is better than that in steak.

Dr. Stoff next considers the need for essential fatty acids (EFAs) as indicated by the blood test. Every individual diagnosed with a severe or chronic disease has some form of EFA deficiency. "I have never seen anyone with cancer, lupus, heart disease, AIDS, and many other severe diseases whose EFA panel was not imbalanced in some way," says Dr. Stoff. His typical recommendations for EFAs are flaxseed oil (2 tablespoons per day), borage oil (as GLA 260, 2 capsules, 3 times per day), and fish oils (Super EPA, 2 capsules, 3 times per day).

Depending on the particular type or stage of cancer, a person may need to take larger amounts of EFAs. "A person with prostate cancer may take 8-10 tablespoons of flaxseed oil per day. Someone with breast cancer, depending on their blood EFA panel, may also take 8-10 tablespoons of flaxseed oil or safflower oil."

QUICK DEFINITION

**Lipid** is a biochemist's term for a fat or oil, which is one of the 6 basic food groups. Fats and oils are made of building blocks called fatty acids. Of these long-chain molecules (comprising atoms of carbon, hydrogen, and oxygen) the "fatty" end does not dissolve in water, while the "acid" end does. Fats are also called triglycerides as they consist of 3 (tri) fatty acid molecules joined to one molecule of glycerol, a kind of sugar. Unsaturated fats required in the diet are called **essential fatty acids,** and include linoleic acid (an omega-6 oil), found in corn, beans, and some nuts and seeds, and alpha linolenic acid (an omega-3 oil), found in fish, flaxseed, and walnuts.

CAUTION

The only drawback to taking large amounts of EFAs is that most people will occasionally experience gas, bloating, indigestion, or diarrhea, Dr. Stoff notes. If, at the time of surgery, one takes large amounts of fish oil, the blood may clot more slowly and serious complications may result. For this reason, it is advisable to avoid taking fish oil within 3 days of surgery, both before and after.

**Carbohydrates**—Blood sugar regulation can have a profound bearing on how the body responds to a tumor. When we eat carbohydrate-rich foods, they release sugar which enters the bloodstream as glucose or energy. The pancreas then secretes the hormone insulin, which helps move glucose into the cells. As blood sugar levels drop, the liver responds by releasing its stored glucose (glycogen) into the bloodstream.

This process is important to know because people who have compromised liver function will not be able to carry out this last step efficiently and will tend to develop low blood sugar. "When the blood sugar crashes in this way, the person feels fatigued and depressed; the patient also has anxiety, sweating, and feels dizzy and lightheaded," says Dr. Stoff. "A person in this condition needs to avoid simple sugars and emphasize only the high-fiber foods for a while, until their livers have recuperated. The issue of blood sugar levels is critical because cancer cells thrive on sugar."

There are, however, "backup" systems that can compensate for a weak liver—glycogenic amino acids, for example, amino acids that can be converted into glucose when the body needs it. The most important of these amino acids are serine, glycine, and alanine. According to Dr. Stoff, supplementation with these amino acids helps prevent the blood-sugar rebound effect that would otherwise stress the liver and produce hypoglycemia in the person with cancer. Dr. Stoff often recommends a product called Vital Force (containing amino acids and amino chelated minerals), 4 capsules, 3 times a day between meals.

## The Botanical Route to Immune System Fortification

While Dr. Stoff uses a wide range of botanicals, the 2 he has found indispensable to effective cancer treatment are Iscador (known as European mistletoe or *Viscum album* ) and Larix (or Arabinogalactan). These botanicals work in a complementary fashion to support the body's anticancer defenses, he says.

**Iscador—**From the anthroposophic point of view, Iscador's unique therapeutic value, its specific effect on tumors, lies in its ability to counteract the disorderly proliferation of the carcinoma by strengthening the blueprint of the Ego organization. According to Hans-Richard Heiligtag, M.D., this action results from mistletoe's "strict formative force which expresses itself in its regular rhythmical growth, and on the other hand in its special relation to light and warmth, which enables it to blossom in wintertime. These three factors enable mistletoe to be a cancer remedy."[4]

**Vital Force,** containing 24 amino acids sufficient to meet the body's daily amino acid needs, is part of a 15-item line of nutrient supplements called Doctor's Brand, available from Livingston Health Foods, Inc., 1324 South Sherman Street, Longmont, CO 80501; tel: 800-765-7842.

In other words, the formative force counteracts the revolt of the physical forces which characterizes the malignant cell. At the same time, the ability to counteract the cold of wintertime carries over into mistletoe's ability to counteract the "coldness" that characterizes the cancer-ridden body—cancer patients often complain of feeling cold, but their bodies become warmer after treatment with mistletoe.

Typically, European doctors using Iscador administer the first series of injections to observe any undesirable reactions. The medicine is injected (subcutaneously, as a serum) in the morning, several times per week. Alternatively, Iscador can be taken orally, either as a tincture or in homeopathic form, but only "if the immune system is already somewhat responsive," says Dr. Stoff. If the immune system is weak or severely compromised, he recommends the injection. "The strength that we use for injecting Iscador depends on the energy reserves of the patient and how much immune reserve they have left," says Stoff. "However, all the injections are low potency."

**Larix**—Larch arabinogalactan powder, or Ara-6, is a sweet-tasting medicinal powder highly concentrated in complex carbohydrates or polysaccharides (long-chain sugars) derived from the Western Larch tree (Larix occidentalis). Its special properties include its capacity for stimulating the activity of various types of immune cells. Ara-6 also readily dissolves in water and maintains its chemical stability over a wide range of concentrations, pH, and temperature changes.

Dr. Stoff has seen definitive results with Larix in terms of increasing natural killer (NK) cell activity. "We know that NK activity can help a person with cancer, particularly when trying to prevent new tumors or micrometastases. "Larix seems to stimulate NK activity quite well while also helping to raise the individual's energy level." Ara-6's ability to stimulate the activity of macrophages, another major part of the body's anticancer defenses, may be just as significant as its positive effect on NK activity.

Biochemists have determined that a sugar component of Larix may stimulate NK activity in a manner similar to the sugar component of Viscum album (mistletoe).[5] The combination of these substances could therefore have an additive effect in terms of activating anticancer defenses. Dr. Stoff recommends taking a teaspoon in a glass of vegetable juice or water 3 times a day. Typically people who take Ara-6 are advised to take supplemental vitamin C at the same time because it can enhance the effectiveness of Ara-6.

Depending on the individual treated, Dr. Stoff will invariably use the "normal" dose of an herb along with homeopathic doses (microdilutions) of other herbs. By working in this way, he can optimize the effectiveness of the botanical agent, particularly when a patient does not have the digestive strength to utilize the herbal medicine. The other botanicals most often recommended by Dr. Stoff for helping cancer patients recover from their illness are as follows.

**Ukrain**—Dr. Stoff frequently recommends the use of Ukrain, a derivative of celandine, for the treatment of cancer patients. "I use Ukrain for solid tumors such as breast, lung, and colon, as opposed to leukemia and myeloma," he says. "I have found that it can be beneficial even when used in combination with Taxol. Ukrain also supports liver function in important ways."

***Gingko Biloba***—A member of an ancient family of trees (Gingkoales) no longer found in the wild, for thousands of years, *Gingko* has been a staple of Chinese herbal medicine, recommended for coughs, asthma, and acute allergic inflammations. Recent Western research indicates this herb has useful anticancer properties, including antioxidant activity. Dr. Stoff uses *Gingko* as a blood cleanser and to enhance circulation; his typical dose is 40 mg 3 times daily.

**Panax Ginseng**—For over 2000 years, Chinese doctors have prescribed ginseng, either in the form of powder or extracts, as a general tonic to promote strength, vitality, appetite, emotional stability, and "wisdom."[6] Certain components of ginseng appear to have a distinct immune-stimulating and antioxidant effect. "Ginseng is a potent adaptogenic herb which helps to support the life force," says Dr. Stoff. "On the biochemical level, ginseng exerts a broad-based therapeutic influence, which probably accounts for its consistently supportive role in cancer therapy." He adds that ginseng should never be taken in large doses as it may inhibit immunity.

***Echinacea* and Pau D'Arco**—These 2 herbs have well-known immune-enhancing abilities. According to Dr. Stoff, the primary reason for combining *Echinacea* and pau d'arco is to provide protection against infection. "These herbs should not be considered a primary treatment for cancer," Dr. Stoff says, "but can help immensely in the treatment of associated microbial infections, which are a common problem with advanced cancer."

**Aloe Vera**—"I use quite a lot of aloe vera when someone has trouble with constipation or, specifically, for a failure in the production of secretory IgA (an immunoglobulin, part of the immune system response)," says Dr. Stoff. "This is not common with cancer, but very common with AIDS or chronic fatigue syndrome." Dr. Stoff typically recommends 1 ounce of aloe concentrate in juice or water 3 times a day.

**Maitake Mushroom**—Dr. Stoff prefers to use the maitake D-fraction at 10 drops 3 times a day, mixed in water or with Ara-6 and the amino acid glutamine. "I'm finding that advanced cancer patients who show signs of wasting (serious weight loss) will greatly benefit from this combination. All 3 should be used concurrently to help the individual regain weight and to stabilize the immune system, which can become extremely compromised in the advanced cancer patient."

**Essiac**—"This is an excellent blood cleanser and can help tremendously if someone is toxic from either chemotherapy or radiation," says Dr. Stoff. "Patients seem to feel better taking Essiac; at some level it appears to enhance mood."

***"Essiac is an excellent blood cleanser and can help tremendously if someone is toxic from either chemotherapy or radiation," says Dr. Stoff. "Patients seem to feel better taking Essiac; at some level it appears to enhance mood."***

## A Comprehensive Supplementation Program

**Melatonin**—"The brain hormone melatonin plays a major role in my practice, since it has a definite antioxidant activity, helps reset circadian cycles, and stimulates natural killer cells," says Dr. Stoff. "Melatonin is a potent addition to treatment for a variety of cancers. I have not seen any adverse effect from using this supplement."

Dr. Stoff's endorsement is predicated on the melatonin being the time-release type which is available on prescription. This long-acting melatonin works better than the short-acting form available in health food stores. Dr. Stoff favors melatonin in a microcellulose base without any magnesium and vitamin B6. The optimal melatonin range Dr. Stoff recommends working with is between 1 and 10 mg.

When it comes to cancer treatment, says Dr. Stoff, patients need not take melatonin only at night. "A fairly large number of my patients have irregular daily biological rhythms, (circadian cycles). If you give them melatonin at bedtime, it actually has the opposite effect and makes them wired. They also have unusual secretion patterns for the stress hormone cortisol." Increased stress leads to increased cortisol which then suppresses the immune system. After a few weeks of taking melatonin in the morning, they begin to notice that every time they take it, they feel sleepy. At this point, Dr. Stoff recommends they take it at bedtime, since their circadian cycles have finally shifted to a healthier pattern.

Dr. Stoff coaches his patients in the art of "circadian cycle hygiene," in other words, paying attention to dietary patterns and sleep cycles. People with cancer should go to sleep between 9 and 10 P.M. at the latest and try to rise with the Sun, or at least at the same time each morning. Eating at the same time every day also helps to regulate the body's daily cycles as well.

It's helpful to sleep in total darkness because it maximizes melatonin production, helps regulate the circadian cycles, and has an antioxidant effect, he says. "However, for women, by using a night light at the right time (days 5-28) during the menstrual cycle, you can actually stimulate the production of progesterone and lower the output of estrogen. This, in turn, can greatly reinforce the effect of therapies used for estrogen-sensitive cancers such as breast and ovarian cancers." Certain skin cancers may also benefit by having some night light, he adds.

**DHEA—**This naturally occurring adrenal hormone is a precursor in the synthesis of both testosterone and estrogen. "Unless someone has prostate or testicular cancer, DHEA is the first supplement I hand them," says Dr. Stoff, adding it works "extremely well" in the treatment of breast cancer. "It stimulates immune function and pushes down the levels of cortisol. If someone is under great stress—emotional, toxic, or disease-related—their cortisol level goes up and tends to suppress immune function." Dr. Stoff's typical recommended dosage for DHEA is 25-100 mg in a long-acting base daily.

**Thyroid—**Dr. Stoff monitors thyroid gland function and, when necessary, prescribes thyroid hormone for many of his cancer patients. "I prefer to measure their T3 and T4 levels because the basal body temperature is not a reliable measure in some instances," says Dr. Stoff explains. T3 is the active thyroid hormone. "A low thyroid hormone level can actually result from suppressed pituitary function and not the thyroid. In this case, the goal of therapy should be promoting pituitary function." Dr. Stoff generally prescribes Armour thyroid at a dosage of 1/4 to 3 grains per day, depending on the patient's blood test.

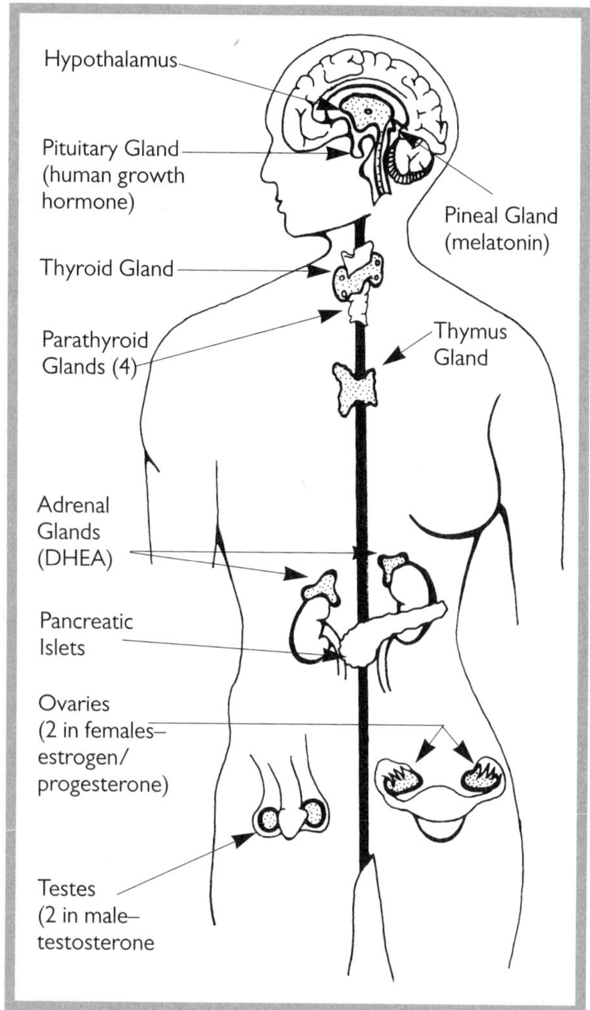


**Figure 21.2—The glandular system**

**Glandulars—**Dr. Stoff uses adrenal cortex, thyroid, and pituitary extracts in addition to homeopathically prepared applications of these glandulars. The pituitary influences many other body systems since it serves as the master gland of the body. "The pituitary is tied into the body's circadian rhythms in intimate ways by virtue of its link to the pineal gland in the brain," says Dr. Stoff. "ACTH and other pituitary hormones can help improve the body's ability to handle all kinds of stress." Dr. Stoff typically uses Pituitrophin, 1-2 tablets taken 1-3 times a day (made by Standard Process and available through Solstice Vitamin Company—see Telephone Icon on page 439).

**Vitamin C—**For cancer patients, Dr. Stoff prefers to administer vitamin C intravenously and will vary the dosage depending on how ill the person is. The range he uses is between 15 and 50 g. He considers it advisable to use Ukrain and other factors in combination with the vitamin C.

**Vitamin A**—Dr. Stoff has found that relatively high doses of vitamin A (10,000-500,000 IU per day) may be effective against cancer, as long as the patient's condition is carefully monitored—a must to avoid toxicity.

**B Complex**—Dr. Stoff uses B complex to maintain optimal functioning of the immune and nervous systems and to reinforce the effects of individual B vitamins, such as vitamins B3, B6, and B12, which he may recommend on an individual basis. Generally, the dose of folic acid should be kept below 400 mcg per day.

**Vitamin B6 (Pyridoxine)**—Dr. Stoff's recommended dosage range for B6 is 25-300 mg per day, depending on individual factors. The dosages should not exceed 500 mg per day. For those who tend to experience severe insomnia at higher doses of vitamin B6, the vitamin can be taken earlier in the day or in smaller doses later in the day, Dr. Stoff advises.

**Zinc**—Dr. Stoff will occasionally recommend zinc as a temporary supplement (30 to 60 mg per day), but only if the person shows definite signs of a zinc deficiency.

**Germanium**—Dr. Stoff often favors the use of germanium to enhance the availability of oxygen to both healthy and cancerous cells. Cancer cells cannot thrive under oxygen-rich conditions. "Giving germanium is part of the Ukrain protocol, along with vitamin C," says Dr. Stoff. "Germanium is one of those compounds that probably used to be more prevalent in our food supply but has been lost because of modern agriculture."

**Calcium**—Dr. Stoff frequently advises his cancer patients to take a calcium supplement, particularly if they are suffering from a cancer that has infiltrated the bones. Dr. Stoff often recommends working within a range of 800 to 1000 mg of calcium daily, and 400 to 800 mg of magnesium. The proper amounts of these nutrients will vary depending on the individual's age, sex, blood chemistry, and other factors.

**METBAL®**—Also known as Cellbal, this natural product is described as a cellular metabolic enhancer or "super vitamin." Made from 4 natural agents (including brown sugar [150 mg], vitamins B3 [20 mg] and C [75 mg], and the amino acid alanine [15 mg]), METBAL was originally developed in Greece in the 1970s by Hariton Alivazatos, a microbiologist and biochemist, to increase the ability of cells to absorb critically needed nutrients. The product is administered intravenously over 5-10 minutes; cancer patients typically receive infusions daily for 28 days; it can also be taken orally as a supplement at the rate of 1 teaspoon 3 times daily. While METBAL does not work specifically against cancer, it appears to increase the cells' ability to assimilate nutrients, trigger the immune system to act against cancer cells, and correct DNA damage by supplying nutrients essential for rebuilding.

***"Counseling helps newly diagnosed cancer patients get over their sense of hopelessness and helplessness; perhaps it even helps them embrace a more assertive, hopeful, fighting attitude," says Dr. Stoff.***

METBAL is not recommended for use during a course of chemotherapy or radiation and at least 4-6 weeks must elapse after these conventional treatments are given before starting it; otherwise, its beneficial effects are neutralized. In addition, patients are to avoid taking birth control pills, hormone replacement therapies, sleeping pills, narcotics, alcohol, and coffee during METBAL treatment, and to follow a prescribed diet. The goal is to make the blood more alkaline, Dr. Stoff explains. METBAL contains a high proportion of niacinamide (vitamin B3), and, as a result, patients often experience a transient flushing or reddening of the skin together with a sense of heightened body warmth. These effects usually last no longer than 3-4 hours and, with each subsequent injection, the reaction times becomes shorter.

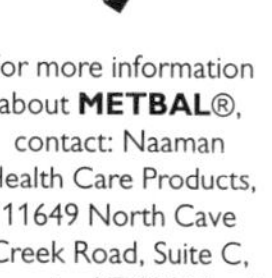

For more information about **METBAL®**, contact: Naaman Health Care Products, 11649 North Cave Creek Road, Suite C, Phoenix, AZ 85020; tel: 602-331-8062; fax: 602-861-1553.

## The Importance of Detoxification in a Cancer Reversal Program

Most of the cancer patients who see Dr. Stoff have already had conventional treatment and are already nutritionally depleted and overloaded with toxins. In this condition, it would be highly dangerous to attempt a strong detoxification program. "To try to detoxify them immediately could literally kill them," Dr. Stoff says. Instead, he stimulates liver function in a gentle and gradual way while supporting the immune system.

Dr. Stoff prescribes foods and herbs to reduce stress on a toxic organ or body region. In the case of an overburdened liver, Dr. Stoff will use botanical medicines such as Essiac, which has "an affinity for the liver and doesn't stress the kidneys." He also frequently recommends silymarin (milk thistle). "This herb is valuable in helping cancer patients recover from the toxic effects of chemotherapy or heavy drug use in general. No other single herb seems to have as much detoxifying, liver-regenerating power."

Dr. Stoff will also recommend various measures to increase the capacity of other organs, namely the kidneys, colon, and skin, to detoxify; this in turn reduces the burden on the liver, which is then freed up for healing.

***An overly toxic liver can be relieved through simple dietary changes such as avoiding oils and high-fat foods and emphasizing raw leafy greens and brightly colored vegetables, says Dr. Stoff.***

Dr. Stoff does not recommend drinking large amounts of carrot juice at first, as is sometimes recommended for cancer patients, because the liver generally cannot fully convert the beta carotene in carrots to vitamin A. The effort alone puts an additional stress on the body. For such individuals, he recommends water-soluble vitamins and minerals so that the liver will not have to work hard. An overly toxic liver can be relieved through simple dietary changes such as avoiding oils and high-fat foods and emphasizing raw leafy greens and brightly colored vegetables.

The toxic kidney is another condition Dr. Stoff commonly sees among his cancer patients, particularly in those who have received extensive conventional treatments. His use of supplements takes into account the organ's specific condition. "If a person has an overstressed kidney, I don't want to provide them right away with amino acids, minerals, and high-dose vitamin C. The reason for this is that these nutrients are all water-soluble and would be eliminated through urination."

If a person has a toxic colon, Dr. Stoff first seeks to determine the reason for the toxicity. A toxic colon or kidney means there is elevated creatinine, constipation, gas, bloating, cramps, and often a skin rash. A heavy meat-eating diet is the number one cause particularly when coupled with a sedentary lifestyle. Starting a regular exercise program and abstaining from eating meat can make an immediate difference.

"When a person comes to me with a toxic colon, we either deal with it from above or below," he says. "Working from above, we would use fiber, Epsom salts, and Chinese herbs (such as San She Dan), all individually determined, to stimulate the colon and help it work better. Working from below, we would use a coffee enema." This is the only detoxifying technique Dr. Stoff uses on a routine basis with his cancer patients. He uses it primarily to stimulate liver detoxification.

**Heat Therapy**—Raising the body temperature, a clinical process called hyperthermia, is another detoxification technique used with some success as part of an alternative cancer treatment program. For example, heat can be localized with the help of medical devices that direct microwaves to the tumor, raising the temperature of the tumor itself to 42° C or 43° C (107.6° F to 109.4° F); this procedure is particularly effective in controlling superficial tumors located on or near the skin. Conventional doctors have used this approach, known by them as diathermy, to lower the effective dosage range of radiation treatment.

***"Heating the body to 40° C (104° F), in combination with taking ginseng or other substances that increase the effect of heat, may be of some value in cancer treatment," Dr. Stoff says.***

As Dr. Stoff explains, cancer cells are more heat sensitive than normal tissues and are more easily killed by heating. Localizing the heat is important, since one cannot raise the whole-body temperature to 42° C or 43° C without lethal consequences.

Another strategy is to raise the whole-body temperature in a more moderate way, from 37° C to 40° C (98.6° F to 104° F). This may be performed by using whole-body wet wraps, saunas, and hot baths. "Heating the body to 40° C (104° F), in combination with taking ginseng or other substances that increase the effect of heat, may be of some value in cancer treatment," Dr. Stoff says. "Taking a hot bath with a cup of Epsom salts and a cup of baking soda mixed into the bath water can heat the body to a moderate degree and provide a gentle detoxifying effect."

One substance that may be combined with hyperthermia to enhance its effectiveness is the bioflavonoid quercetin.[7] This bioflavonoid helps stop

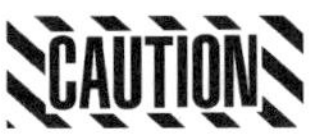


Do not undertake any of these heat therapy strategies alone, but only under professional medical guidance.

A **bioflavonoid** is a pigment within plants and fruits that acts as an antioxidant to protect against damage from free radicals and excess oxygen. In the body, bioflavonoids enhance the beneficial activities of vitamin C, and are often formulated with this vitamin in supplement form. Originally called vitamin P up until 1950, these vitamin C "helper" substances include citrin, hesperidin, rutin, quercitin, epicatechin, flavones, and flavonols. When given with vitamin C, bioflavonoids increase the absorption of vitamin C into the liver, kidneys, and adrenal glands. Acting as antioxidants, they also protect vitamin C from destruction by free radicals.

For more information on **heat therapy,** (pp. 996-1000) **exercise,** (pp. 1003-1005), and **detoxification** (pp. 949-950), see Chapter 33: Physical Support Therapies.

histamine release. Quercetin can inhibit the synthesis of proteins (heat shock proteins) that help tumors resist heat stress;[8] at the same time, quercetin inhibits the transport of lactic acid out of cancer cells.[9] By doing this, it lowers the pH inside the cancer cell and reduces the likelihood that tumor cells will proliferate or metastasize.[10]

Thus, the anticancer effect of quercetin in the context of hyperthermia is twofold: it makes the inside of cancer cells more acidic (lowers the intracellular pH, which helps kill the cell) and makes the cancer cells more vulnerable to the effects of heat. Dr. Stoff's typical dosage is 1000-1500 mg taken 3 times daily.

**Exercise—**To give the body's detoxification systems an added boost, Dr. Stoff will frequently advise his patients to engage in regular stress-free physical activities such as walking, jogging, cycling, or swimming. Gentle games with constant movement such as volleyball and basketball can help stimulate the lymphatic system and overall metabolism, thereby aiding detoxification, Dr. Stoff notes.

Exercise speeds up the neutralization and removal of poisons from the body's cells and tissues through sweating and increased urination and stimulates the activity of natural killer cells and other components of the body's anticancer defenses.[11] A rise in body temperature during exercise tends to increase the production of pyrogen, a substance that enhances the function of white blood cells and thus immune function.[12]

However, as other physicians have noted elsewhere in this book, excessive exercise can be detrimental. Dr. Stoff cautions that it can produce an excess of free radicals and lactic acid, both of which tend to promote cancer. Patients should become involved in an exercise program in a gradual and sensitive manner, respecting their abilities and attitudes. "A fundamentalist Christian will often walk out of your office if you suggest they practice yoga," Dr. Stoff says. "It's important to understand where a person is coming from in their beliefs and to support them; otherwise your recommendations will likely fall on deaf ears."

## Stress Reduction and Emotional Support Must Be Addressed

That there is a definite relationship between emotional stress and weakened immune system activity is indicated by the fact that in the majority of studies reporting significant improvement in the survival of cancer patients, patients were involved in psychotherapy and support groups. As Dr. Stoff sees it, it would almost constitute malpractice for physicians not to emphasize some level of psychological and social support for cancer patients under their care.

All of this explains why Dr. Stoff has a psychologist on his staff to work with patients, helping them deal effectively with the stress and anxiety of cancer. "Most people react to the initial cancer diagnosis with feelings of intense anxiety and fear, as if the disease means sure death. Counseling helps newly diagnosed cancer patients get over their sense of hopelessness and helplessness; perhaps it even helps them embrace a more assertive, hopeful, fighting attitude."

Studies support this conclusion. Longer survival among breast cancer patients (mostly Stage I, some Stage II) has been recorded for those who evince such a fighting spirit, and shorter survival for those with either a helpless-hopeless attitude or stoic acceptance.[16] Cancer patients who were able to express joy or happiness despite their cancer had fewer metastatic sites and tended to live longer than patients who expressed less positive emotions.[17]

It is this attitude of a fighting spirit and joyful, positive frame of mind that Dr. Stoff's

## Emotional Expression and Survival

Stanford psychiatrist David Spiegel, M.D., did a 10-year study of breast cancer patients who had engaged in regular support group meetings. The support group participants shared their fears and concerns in a non-threatening, nurturing setting, and communicated with each other frequently outside the group. They dealt with difficult family issues, concerns about their medical care, and emotional stress regarding their condition and the death of group members. The study showed that breast cancer patients who underwent support group therapy lived nearly twice as long as women with breast cancer who did not.[13]

In another study, patients with lymphoma or leukemia were offered a combination of counseling and home visiting time, in which they could ask questions of the counselor about their condition and treatment options. These patients lived significantly longer than the control group, even when variations in how well they adhered to their medical treatment plan were taken fully into account.[14] Elsewhere, malignant melanoma patients were assigned to 6 weeks of support groups and educational sessions (once a week for 90 minutes) and, compared to patients who didn't participate, they were less anxious and depressed and had significantly lower rates of recurrence and higher rates of survival 6 years later.[15]

psychologist seeks to instill in their cancer patients. Even so, the psychological transformation implicit in the cancer experience cannot be forced and each person must go at her own speed. The goal is to fully support the individual's personal process and world view. "It's their life, their body, their healing," says Dr. Stoff. "You can't impose your beliefs and desires on another person in terms of what they need to do therapeutically. When they choose for themselves, hopefully they choose something they truly believe in. After all, belief, or the placebo effect, carries a lot of therapeutic power."

Patients at Solstice Clinical Associates receive instruction in the use of guided imagery, creative visualization, and meditation. These tools help them cope with stress and get in touch with their inner world. "To identify the right practices for each person requires obtaining a lot of specific information about the person and the disease process." Regarding visualization exercises, one patient may conceive of cancer cells as large and sinister. In this case, the psychologist might suggest visualizing natural killer cells and macrophages to be even larger and powerful enough to engulf the cancer cells. Or one might visualize white blood cells seeking out and attacking cancer cells, seeing these flushed out of the body. The imagery session may end with the patient viewing himself as healthy, full of life, and free of cancer.

> ***It is important to try to work with the imagery the cancer patient—not the doctor—believes to be the best representation of events at the cellular level.***

Alternatively, one might visualize the cancer cells as small, weak, and confused at the outset, easily crushed and disintegrated by the body's anticancer defenses. It is important to try to work with the imagery the cancer patient—not the doctor—believes to be the best representation of events at the cellular level.

According to a study involving 300 cancer patients using imagery, the interpretative evaluation of their images, from a clinical database of thousands of drawings, predicted outcomes with shocking consistency. For example, if the cancer cells' activities were consistently strong, and the immune cells remained weak, then the imagery predicted a poor outcome for the patient. In cases where the patient's cancer went into remission, the evaluation of their images predicted the course of disease with 93% accuracy. For those who died or deteriorated, the test scores predicted that with 100% accuracy.[18]

These dramatic findings suggest that the mind's eye can either improve or worsen the prognosis. In some cases, says Dr. Stoff, it may be helpful to provide more intensive forms of psychotherapeutic support and guidance for patients who continually generate negative imagery of the type described above; suggestions regarding a reorientation of their visualization practice may also be warranted. "We help people learn to deal with such intense and potentially destructive emotions as anger or hostility. In many cases, people with cancer have no idea that they're carrying around a great deal of anger. If they don't vent this anger appropriately, the repressed feelings can undermine their health."

**All therapeutic music needs to be "live" and not from recordings; the belief is that the living sound of the instrument played by a living person imparts the healing benefits.**

## Music Therapy and Curative Art Forms Help Cancer Patients

Expressing one's emotions need not happen by verbal means only, but can occur through movement and artistic exercises, says Dr. Stoff. Artistic therapies form an integral part of the Anthroposophical approach to health and cancer reversal, and this is especially so in the numerous clinics and hospitals in the German-speaking countries of Europe where Anthroposophic medicine flourishes. Indeed, physicians versed in this medical approach will often work with art and dance therapists, knowing that the creative process can serve as a profound healing force in people's lives enabling them to uncover hidden levels of meaning and insight through various forms of expression.

Music, whether self-created or listened to with full attention, can help evoke states of relaxation and pleasure. Sad, mournful music can help stimulate an emotional release, while fiery, lively music can incite an optimistic frame of mind. The music therapist seeks to evoke in the patient a new harmony of body, mind, and emotions through careful selection of fundamental musical elements as is present in various published forms of music. The music therapist also understands that every illness involves disharmony in a certain area of the body, calling for the appropriate instrument to help restore harmony to that area.

The music therapist regards each human being in relationship to the musical instruments—the head corresponds to wind instruments, the chest to string instruments, and the limbs to percussion. Since breast cancer oc-

## How Music Therapy Can Heal

Here is an example of how Anthroposophic music therapy can have a therapeutic role in reversing illness, in this case, asthma. Paul, aged 33, had been suffering from bronchial asthma for seven years. He had frequent asthmatic attacks, especially when he was exposed to cold weather, and it would take him months to recover. Paul had tried all sorts of therapies, including antibiotics, massage, diet, aromatherapy baths, but nothing helped him. Finally he turned to music therapy.

For 30 minutes once a week, Paul worked with a music therapist, alternating between listening to music and playing it. His therapist played live music for him, using wind or string instruments and percussion—but she played it to his back while he listened attentively. The idea is that the live flow of pure musical sounds works therapeutically on his chest and back and thus on his breathing. Paul also learned to play a copper flute which demanded a special breathing technique. Both approaches improved his breathing and reduced stress.

After only a few sessions, he felt more relaxed, his breathing had eased, and his sense of well-being increased. After 6 months Paul told his therapist that music therapy was the only approach that had given him good results. During the 18 months of music therapy, he didn't have a single asthma attack, nor did he have any in the years following.[20]

curs in the chest area, for example, the playing of string instruments is recommended; an ancient Celtic string instrument known as the "crowd" offers particular therapeutic benefit for cancer patients.[19]

All therapeutic music needs to be "live" and not from recordings; the belief is that the living sound of the instrument played by a living person imparts the healing benefits. If the patient plays the instrument, the advice is to play it with attention to breathing rhythms and emphasis on the "warmth" of the notes, tones, and chords. Music therapy can also be done in groups as patients sing, play, or listen together.

Anthroposophic physicians frequently recommend a unique form of art-dance movement called eurythmy (pronounced *your*-RITH-*me*). Eurythmy, which means, literally, "beautiful movements," involves graceful, flowing movements of the hands, arms, and upper torso. European physicians regularly use eurythmy as an adjunct in cancer treatment, contending that it helps generate additional life energy and inner motivation. "These movements engage the entire human; they are done mindfully, requiring one's full presence," Dr. Stoff says. "I believe this is the main reason they carry such healing power."

To locate an **Anthroposophic physician,** contact: Physicians' Association for Anthroposophical Medicine, 7953 California Avenue, Fair Oaks, CA 95628; tel: 916-967-8250; fax: 916-966-5314.

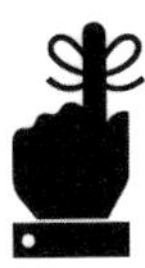

*Depending on a person's biochemical and psychological makeup, certain stressors will play a more primary role in the development of cancer. The key concept is that the cumulative effect of many carcinogens and immune-suppressing agents all acting together is a weakening of the immune system, thereby allowing cancer cells to proliferate.*

## CURRICULUM VITAE

# Jack O. Taylor, M.S., D.C.

Dr. Taylor's Wellness Center, Inc.
3601 Algonquin Road, Suite 801
Rolling Meadows, IL 60008;
tel: 847-222-1192; fax: 847-222-1195.

Dr. Taylor received his chiropractic degree (D.C.) from Logan College in St. Louis, Missouri; he is currently licensed as a nutrition counselor by the State of Illinois, as a certified dietitian by the State of New York, and as a certified clinical nutritionist by the International and American Associations of Clinical Nutritionists. With more than 20 years of experience using nutritional therapies, Dr. Taylor is the author of *Metabolic Assessment from Standard Medical Tests* and *Nutritional Supplements: Use, Formulation, and Production.* Between 1992 and 1993, he served on the advisory board of the Committee on Diet and Nutrition of the National Institute of Health's Office of Alternative Medicine.

***"My goal is not specifically to eradicate disease but to help my patients develop optimal functioning of all body systems and to maintain this optimal health for the rest of their lives," Dr. Taylor says. "If all the body's parts do their jobs, cancer or any degenerative condition will not develop."***

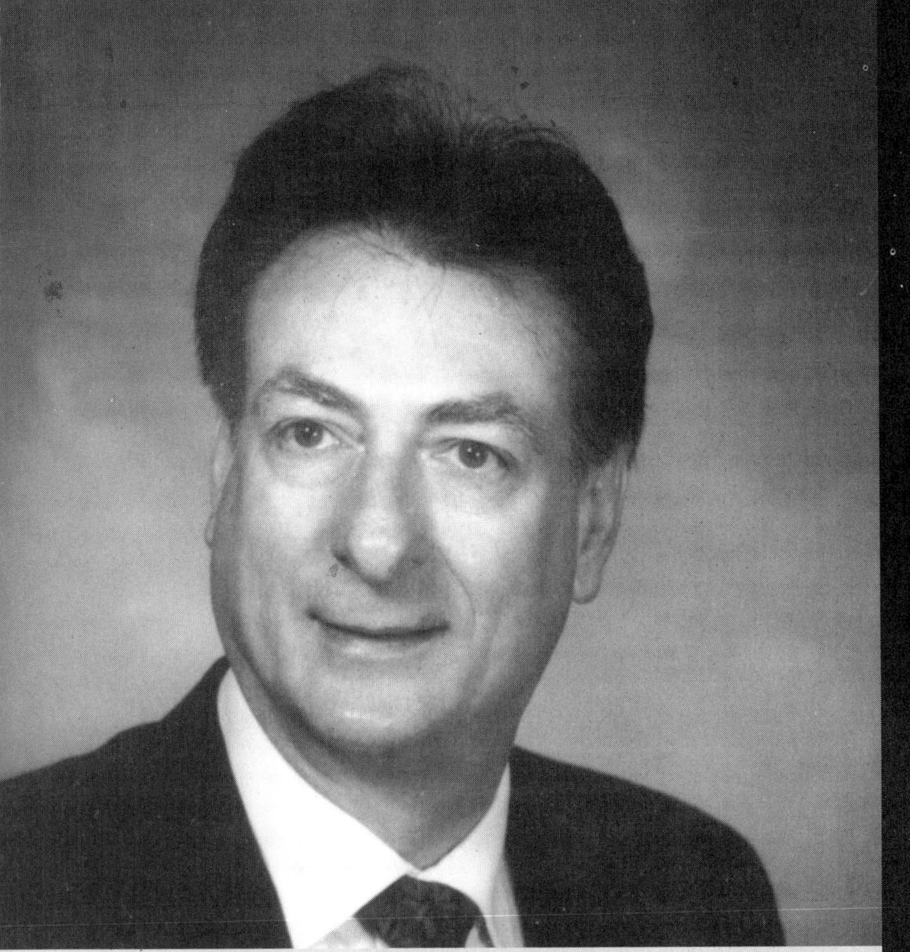

Chapter 22

# *Jack O. Taylor, M.S., D.C.*

**SUCCESSFUL CANCER REVERSAL** depends on working with the "metabolic individuality" of patients, addressing their unique needs as they vary according to genetics, dietary patterns, activity levels, emotional and behavioral patterns, and stress-coping styles, says Dr. Taylor.

For Dr. Taylor, restoring a patient's metabolic balance is a primary therapeutic goal. Dr. Taylor suggests that an individual is healthy only when every part of the body—every organ, gland, muscle, tissue, nerve—is doing the job it should be doing with the least amount of strain or stress to the system. Chiropractic adjustments provide the specific kinds of nerve stimulation that can help guide this process while nutritional and botanical supplements provide additional support.

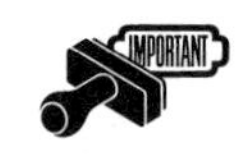


**Jack O. Taylor, M.S., D.C.**, is a chiropractic physician with a master of science in biology and human nutrition and is a licensed nutrition counselor. He was examined by the International and American Associations of Clinical Nutritionists and granted the coveted award of certified clinical nutritionist. In accordance with the laws of the states where he holds licenses, Dr. Taylor does not, and will not, diagnose or treat cancer. As a nutritional counselor, he will accept clients, not patients, for a nutritional assessment, provided their medical condition is supervised and remains the responsibility of a licensed primary care physician. His program supports the overall health of his clients by working toward maximum nutritional efficiency with optimal metabolic balance to enhance the self-healing power of the body.

"Further, as alternative therapies meet with more success in treating crisis situations, particularly cancer and cardiovascular diseases, we see an increasing need for individual follow-up care," says Dr. Taylor. "My goal is not specifically to eradicate disease but to help my patients develop optimal functioning of all body systems and to maintain this optimal health for the rest of their lives."

Although Dr. Taylor's chiropractic training gave him a strong grounding in nutritional principles, early on in his practice he had intuitively felt that something was missing. After several years of dealing with sick people, some of whom he knew were on balanced diets, he began to realize that people were becoming healthy not solely as a result of nutritional *intake*, but also as a result of how the body *processed*

# Dr. Jack Taylor's Support Program for Cancer Patients

| STRATEGY | DOSAGE/ KEY COMPONENTS | FOR MORE INFORMATION see page # |
|---|---|---|
| Vitamin C-mineral complex | 1-20 g/day, depending on individual (DOI) | 786 |
| Vitamin B6 | 25-300 mg/day, DOI | 786 |
| Vitamin B3 | 50 mg, 4-8X/day, DOI | 785 |
| Vitamin B Complex | DOI | 784 |
| Vitamin E | 400 IU, 2X/day | 790 |
| Vitamin A | DOI | 784 |
| Amino acids | DOI | 762 |
| Zinc | 30-60 mg zinc/day, DOI | 793 |
| Selenium | 200-300 mcg/day, DOI | 783 |
| Cesium | DOI | — |
| Coenzyme Q10 | 300-900 mg/day, DOI | 766 |
| Creatine | DOI | — |
| VitaCart | 9 g bovine cartilage/day,DOI | 861 |
| Deodorized shark cartilage | DOI | 863 |
| Essiac tea | DOI | 815 |
| *Acidophilus* | DOI | 762 |
| Marine lipids (fish oil) | 2-4 g of EPA/day, DOI | 768 |
| Flaxseed oil | DOI | 768 |
| Garlic | DOI | 818 |
| Grape seed extract | 200-300 mg/day for 5-10 days, then 60-150 mg/day | 822 |
| Maitake mushroom | DOI | 833 |
| Melatonin | DOI | 941 |
| Pau d'arco tea | DOI | 834 |
| Urea | 5 g, 4X/day, DOI | 874 |
| Haelan 851 | DOI | 824 |
| Hydrazine sulfate | DOI | 868 |
| Support formulas | all DOI: Systems Balance Support Formula 2, Cellular Function Support Formula 1, Immune System Support Formula 14, Digestive System Support Formula 6, Pancreatic System Support Formula 20, | 480 |

*Continued*

## Dr. Jack Taylor's Support Program for Cancer Patients (cont.)

| STRATEGY | DOSAGE/ KEY COMPONENTS | FOR MORE INFORMATION see page # |
|---|---|---|
| | Male Support Formula 12, Female Support Formula 11, Chlorophyll Complex Formula 120 | |
| Glandulars (from New Zealand lamb) | all DOI: spleen, brain, liver, heart, kidney, adrenal, lung, lymph, pancreas, duodenum, thymus, bone marrow, ovary, and prostate | 935 |
| Detoxification, Clearing, and Biogenic formulas | all DOI: Detoxosode O/S, Detoxosode Chemicals, Detoxosode Metals, Detoxosode Virus, Biosode | 472 |

**CAUTION**

This chapter includes information regarding actual treatments used by Dr. Taylor only after his careful diagnosis of each patient. All cancer patients are unique. **Do not administer these treatments to yourself or others.** Discuss these treatments with your physician or other qualified health-care professional. Readers should not interpret this material as therapeutic advice, but should see a physician in all cases.

For more information about **Dr. Kelley's Metabolic Therapy** program, see Chapter 28: Nutrition as Cancer Medicine, pp. 777-779.

these nutrients. It was discouraging and frustrating to prescribe a balanced diet and see dramatic positive responses in some of his patients but no change in others, he says. When he came across the metabolic nutritional theories of William Donald Kelley, D.D.S., everything became clear.

Dr. Kelley was a dentist who, back in 1964, healed himself of pancreatic cancer using his own alternative therapy. Dr. Taylor met Dr. Kelley and observed his systematic investigation of a patient's body chemistry. Dr. Kelley answered all of his questions in great detail and with lucidity. "He reopened doors in my mind that had long been shut," recalls Dr. Taylor. "It was a major turning point in my professional life." Dr. Taylor realized that any help the program provided for people who were diagnosed with cancer was secondary to the balancing of each individual's body chemistry.

Dr. Taylor now regularly applies these principles of "metabolic ecology" to assist people with cancer and other chronic degenerative diseases. His program incorporates all the elements of Dr. Kelley's program but has been brought up to date with new findings and new products, many of which have shown improved clinical efficacy.

He counsels his patients in this way: "You can turn the immune system on with various therapies, but if you don't get out of harm's way —

keep filling it with fat or depleting it with imbalanced nutrition, "street" drugs, air pollution, food additives, hormones, pesticides, and insecticides—you will just further exhaust it. If all the body's parts do their jobs, cancer or any degenerative condition will not develop. We are healthy when every part of our body is functioning optimally, which is the ultimate goal of metabolic therapy."

## SUCCESS STORY

### Reversing Leukemia

When she was 43, Evelyn developed fatigue and depression which gradually worsened over several months. She also lost weight and suffered episodes of severe pain in her right thumb and middle finger. Evelyn consulted her local physician who discovered she had an elevated white blood cell (WBC) count; follow-up bone marrow studies revealed chronic granulocytic leukemia.

> ***"We are healthy when every part of our body is functioning optimally, which is the ultimate goal of metabolic therapy," says Dr. Taylor.***

More laboratory tests showed that Evelyn's WBC count was significantly elevated, at 89,000 compared to the normal range of 4,200-10,000; her platelet count was also high, at 686,000 compared to a normal of 150,000-450,000. Both findings were consistent with the WBC typically seen with leukemia, says Dr. Taylor. Soon after, a bone marrow biopsy and evaluation of the "Philadelphia chromosome," a marker associated with this particular cancer, confirmed that Evelyn had leukemia.

Doctors at the Mayo Clinic in Minnesota recommended the course of chemotherapy standard for chronic granulocytic leukemia, but warned that her prognosis was poor. They also told Evelyn that while they had seen satisfactory control of this disease using this approach, usually they did not manage to reverse it. Evelyn began chemotherapy and within several months, as predicted, the leukemia went into remission; however, since her disease was classified incurable by conventional doctors, she began exploring other options.

When, after completing 10 months of her drug protocol, Evelyn learned of the nutritional-metabolic dietary therapy developed by William Donald Kelley, D.D.S., she began the program under the guidance of Dr. Taylor and discontinued all chemotherapy. She followed the Kelley dietary regimen in full for 7 years. During this time, Evelyn enjoyed excellent health and appeared to be free of cancer. At that point, she began to follow a minimal version of the program because she felt confident her disease was cured.

In the course of a routine checkup Evelyn's hematologist noted an elevated WBC count in the range of 20,000. Six months after she discontinued the Kelley program, a bone marrow biopsy confirmed that she was experiencing a "mild" recurrence of leukemia. When her conventional physicians suggested low-dose chemotherapy, Evelyn agreed while also resuming the Kelley program under Dr. Taylor. "While continuing on our comprehensive nutritional regimen, she again appeared to go into remission, her WBC counts falling in the normal range," Dr. Taylor states. Evelyn eventually died, 12 years after beginning the program with Dr. Taylor, which she followed to varying degrees of intensity that entire time.

Even with aggressive chemotherapy, people diagnosed with chronic granulocytic leukemia rarely survive ten years, notes Dr. Taylor. The invariably fatal prognosis is well-described in the *Merck Manual:* "Average survival time is three to four years from clinical onset; about 20% of patients survive longer than five years, 2% longer than ten years." Clearly, Evelyn surpassed the odds by a great deal and her case offers hope that an integrated nutritional program can help leukemia patients live much longer than "predicted."

## SUCCESS STORY

### Reversing Lymphoma

Roy, aged 64, developed chronic fatigue, experienced mild weight loss, and soon after, suffered a case of pneumonia. Although he quickly recovered, several weeks later lymph nodes in his neck became enlarged. When the swelling did not diminish, Roy was admitted to St. Luke's Hospital in Fargo, North Dakota.

The physician's physical examination of him revealed that Roy had multiple swollen lymph nodes in neck and groin and that his spleen and liver were distended. Biopsy studies of lymph nodes in his neck confirmed that he had "diffuse, poorly differentiated lymphocytic lymphoma." A bone marrow biopsy further proved the presence of the invasive tumor and a lymphangiogram (an analysis of his lymph glands) revealed suspicious nodes along the large arteries of the pelvis. Based on these findings, Roy's doctors concluded that his cancer was "widely metastatic, Stage IVb."

While hospitalized, Roy agreed to participate in an experimental chemotherapy program, but he became extremely ill after this treatment and improved only slowly over several weeks. When after the second round of drugs Roy became weak and bedridden, he decided to halt the chemotherapy even though he was not yet in remission.

While reading about nutritional approaches to cancer, Roy came across the Kelley program, and took it up under the guidance of Dr. Taylor.

Within a few months on the program, many of Roy's swollen lymph nodes completely regressed; Roy continued with the full program for 5 years, before tapering down to a maintenance regimen. Now, more than a decade after his original grim diagnosis, Roy is in good health, with no sign of cancer by all standard medical tests, says Dr. Taylor.

Roy's remarkable outcome is impressive for several reasons, notes Dr. Taylor. Generally, only about one-third of patients with this condition survive 5 years, and prolonged survival is thought to require intensive treatment with multiple chemotherapy agents combined with radiation. But Roy's brief trial with this supposedly standard approach caused him considerable discomfort and did not result in remission.

"This condition is known to be clinically aggressive," says Dr. Taylor.

## Dr. Taylor's Guide to Choosing an Effective Supplement

First, is it a tablet or a capsule? As indicated previously, capsules are preferable to tablets as they offer greater "bioavailability" and thereby enable better utilization by the body, says Dr. Taylor. "Many companies go to great lengths to get good raw materials and assure the proper content only to process a tablet that does not allow for utilization," he says. This does not mean, however, that all tablets are worthless. Dr. Taylor urges people to consider the following issues when selecting their supplements.

- Ask your supplier to furnish you with a certified report of quality control covering dissolution, disintegration, utilization, and content.
- Is the supplement a chemically synthesized compound, or is it derived from food? Though chemists will invariably say otherwise, those supplements that are chemically synthesized are less likely to be utilized in the way nature intended.
- Is the formulation a natural one? Or does it have a brightly colored, dyed sugar coating?
- Is it a sustained-release vitamin? "Remember," Dr. Taylor says, "there are no sustained-release foods, so such vitamins may not necessarily be preferable to those that are immediately available for absorption."
- If the supplement is a glandular, what does it smell like? Is it a fresh, distinctive smell, or does it smell of decomposition? Obviously, in the latter case, the supplement should be considered of questionable quality.

**_Toxins can weaken all vital organs, keeping them from maintaining physical and mental health; toxins in the brain can make one feel depressed, moody, and anxious, thereby interfering with mind/body healing._**

"If you scan the medical literature, the data indicates that long-range survival is possible *only* after the use of aggressive combination chemotherapy, and even then, survival beyond 2 years has been consistently noted only in the minority of patients whose tumors completely disappear." Clearly, Roy's successful outcome with alternative medicine proves the "rules" wrong.

## The Therapeutic Power of Metabolic Ecology

Metabolism is defined as the sum total of physical and chemical processes by which a living organism thrives and maintains itself. Metabolic Ecology therapy guides the organism towards a dynamic, harmonious balance which represents an optimal state of health at the biochemical and physiological levels, explains Dr. Taylor. Metabolic therapy has 4 basic processes:

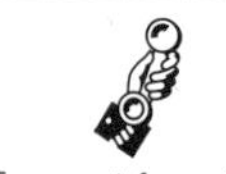

For more information about **Detoxosode** and **Biosode**, contact: HVS Laboratories, P.O. Box 8243, Naples, FL 33941; tel: 800-521-7722 or 941-643-4636; fax: 941-643-7370.

For more information about **detoxification**, see Chapter 33: Physical Support Therapies, pp. 949-980.

### 1. Detoxification of Body Tissues

Removal of toxins from the body can free up the immune system and normalize the functioning of other systems for reversing cancer or from keeping any further development of cancer from taking place, says Dr. Taylor. Toxins can weaken all vital organs, keeping them from maintaining physical and mental health; toxins in the brain can make one feel depressed, moody, and anxious, thereby interfering with mind/body healing.

Dr. Taylor helps his cancer patients detoxify using vitamins, minerals, food supplements, and pancreatic enzymes. Certain micronutrients, including vitamin C, vitamin E, zinc, selenium, and manganese, can bolster the body's antioxidant defenses, while others stimulate the liver's detoxification processes. Dr. Taylor also uses homeopathy for clearing and detoxification and recommends coffee enemas to purge the colon and liver of accumulated toxins, dead cells, or waste products.

Dr. Taylor calls the initial stage of a nutritional program Clearing and Detoxification, noting that "improved health starts with a clean (clear) foundation." Dr. Taylor explains that "residual toxins are a predisposing factor (if not the primary cause) of all physical 'diseases' or metabolic imbalances. To initiate healing, activation or clearing of all vital pathways is essential." All organs involved in elimination—liver, kidneys, intestines, and the blood, immune and lymphatic systems—need to be cleansed and cleared "as a prerequisite for improved metabolism and nutrient assimilation." This is because nutrient assimiliation is essential for nutrient utilization and this, in turn, is required for cellular repair and regeneration. "Healthy cells create a good foundation."

To accomplish clearing, Dr. Taylor has his clients go through a 48-day program, during which they take a series of homeopathic remedies designed for detoxification. Specifically, during the first 12 days, a client typically takes Detoxosode O/S (1 teaspoon, 2X daily, in the morning and evening); during the next 12 days, Detoxosode Chemicals (1 teaspoon, 2X daily, in the morning and evening); for the third set of 12 days, Detoxosode Metals (same dosage); then for the final 12 days, Detoxosode Virus (same dosage).

***"Enzymes help eliminate toxins from the cancer patient's body and assist them in recovering their health; they can also reinforce the benefits of immune-enhancing therapies," says Dr. Taylor.***

Biogenic support is a complementary adjunct to clearing and nutritional supplementation. Biogenic factors for cellular regeneration are the basis of this support, promoting tissue (cell) repair and improving the effectiveness of nutrients. The biogenic support in the form of Biosode should be taken through the above 48-day program and should be continued during nutritional supplementation. The daily dosage is 1 teaspoon (capful) at bedtime.

### 2. Stimulation of Organs and Glands

By giving organs and glands a nutritional or energy boost, they can carry out their specific functions more efficiently. "The boost to organ function can be therapeutic, but should not be considered a lifelong strategy. If wrongly applied, nutritional supplements can actually deplete the body and will build up an energy debt that must be repaid, perhaps in the form of serious disease."

### 3. Substitution for Inadequately Functioning Processes

If the body is not producing a particular chemical in the amount or strength that it should, taking a supplement can help. For example, if the stomach is not producing enough hydrochloric acid, then it can be given as a time-release capsule. Among processes that may be compromised or imbalanced due to inadequate nutrition in the course of cancer are the metabolism of enzymes, eicosanoids (fat components), hormones, and immune components. All these processes can be adjusted by specific nutritional interventions.

### 4. Supplying Nutrients to Rebuild Tissues

Cancer and conventional cancer treatments deplete the body's nutrient reserves and weaken the integrity of cells and tissues. "Supplements can be used as 'concentrated foods' to provide the increased nutritional demand created by the disease or illness," Dr. Taylor says. "They can also help meet the increased nutrient needs for rebuilding a damaged organ or for supporting a particular organ under stress."

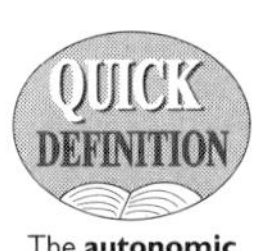


The **autonomic nervous system** has 2 divisions: the sympathetic, or *adrenergic*, nervous system and the parasympathetic, or *cholinergic* nervous system. These two divisions comprise the nerve networks that regulate the actions absolutely essential to life. The autonomic nervous functions must be carried on continuously without interruption, independent of the will. The sympathetic/adrenergic system is closely related to the hormone adrenaline and is primarily a stimulator, or accelerator, of metabolic activities. The parasympathetic/cholinergic system is closely related to the vitamin-like substance choline, and operates mainly as an inhibitor of or brake on metabolic activity. Branches of both sympathetic and parasympathetic nerves send electric impulses to all of our glands and organs. The sympathetic system's basic message is "speed up"; the parasympathetic system's is "slow down."

These 4 aspects of metabolic therapy are incorporated into Dr. Taylor's program of dietary changes, nutritional supplementation, regular exercise, structural and soft-tissue manipulation through chiropractic, and other supportive therapies. While every treatment is tailored to the individual, not the disease, the use of enzymes tends to be consistently applied. "Against a multiplication of abnormal cells, pancreatic enzymes can serve as a powerful countermeasure," says Dr. Taylor. "Enzymes help eliminate toxins from the cancer patient's body and assist them in recovering their health; they can also reinforce the benefits of immune-enhancing therapies." Proteolytic enzymes help identify abnormal protein and act as scavengers to destroy abnormal (degenerative disease) cells.

The metabolic needs of the organism vary greatly from one individual to the next, depending on genetics, dietary patterns, activity levels, and emotional and behavioral patterns, including stress-coping styles, explains Dr. Taylor. This "metabolic individuality" is reflected clearly in the fact that every human body responds differently to foods and environmental cues. "Some people become exhausted quickly while others enjoy a demanding, hectic schedule. Some do better with certain food supplements or types of climatic conditions; some thrive in high-pressure situations, while others do better in more peaceful, low-key situations."

The autonomic nervous system exerts the primary control over metabolism. In most people, based on their genetic makeup, structural, and nutritional factors, either the sympathetic or the parasympathetic system dominates. People with a sympathetic-dominant system tend to have a slow rate of food metabolism and need fast-burning foods such as are found in a primarily vegetarian diet. In contrast, parasympathetic-dominant people tend to have a relatively fast rate of fuel utilization and need food that burns slowly, such as animal products. Some people have a balanced metabolism and need both sympathetic and parasympathetic support.

Given these facts, the systems of some people tend to favor a vegetarian diet while others fare better on animal proteins. According to Dr. Taylor, feeding everyone the same diet would be like dressing everyone in "one-size-fits-all" clothing and could "greatly stifle the development of individual potential," he says.

It is necessary then to determine these biochemical differences to establish each individual's metabolic needs. "Just as petroleum fuels come as regular or high test, leaded or unleaded, each human body needs a different mixture of food fuel." This means that unless your body receives its own properly balanced nutritional supply, optimal health is difficult to establish and maintain.

***"Overall, the appropriate course of treatment addresses* all *problems indicated in the diagnosis as pieces of the 'cancer puzzle'," says Dr. Taylor.***

## Accurate "Metabolic Typing" Is Essential for a Successful Outcome

Individual metabolic requirements should be established before considering cancer therapy of any kind, says Dr. Taylor. "A person with good metabolic levels will respond better to all types of intervention, whether dental, chiropractic, surgical, or medical. Most practitioners realize that the same modality will usually yield different responses or results in different people. The reason for this is that the therapy is applied to different nervous systems and different body chemistries."

## Blood Test Indicators of Metabolic Type

| Blood Component | Metabolic Type If High | Metabolic Type If Low |
|---|---|---|
| Glucose (Blood Sugar) | S/A | P/C |
| Lactate Dehydrogenase | S/A | P/C |
| Thyroxine (T4) | S/A | P/C |
| Carbon Dioxide | P/C | S/A |

These are the key blood readings for metabolic typing. "S/A" signifies a predominance of sympathetic/adrenergic activity; "P/C" signifies a predominance of parasympathetic/cholinergic activity.

The process of "metabolic typing" enables the physician to establish the optimal dietary pattern for a particular individual. Dr. Taylor is able to determine which aspect of the autonomic system is dominant in clients through the metabolic assessment he administers, based on blood chemistry, questionnaire findings, and physical examination. Next is to evaluate the individual's medical history and then determine the status of physiological functions by studying the results of the blood test and the data from urine, electrocardiographic, and fitness testing.

In addition, findings based on kinesiology, reflexology, and iridology (examination of the iris of the eye) can provide a window into the nature of one's disease and indicate the location of specific areas of weakness, says Dr. Taylor. These areas are reflections of the disease process, but Dr. Taylor cautions that "treatment should be applied to the *source* of illness." Physicians can use metabolic therapy without any overt evidence of disease because biochemical imbalances invariably precede overt symptoms. "The best medicine is always preventive."

Overall, the appropriate course of treatment addresses *all* problems indicated in the diagnosis as pieces of the "cancer puzzle," says Dr. Taylor.

### USING THE BLOOD TEST TO ASSESS METABOLIC BALANCE

The "Chem Screen" and "Complete Blood Count" (CBC) tests provide Dr. Taylor with much of the information he needs for determining a course of metabolic therapy. While such tests are standard practice in clinics and hospitals around the country, what is unique about Dr. Taylor's approach is his interpretation of the test results and his translation of these findings into clinical recommendations.

The blood test tells him how much of certain enzymes are present, such as alkaline phosphatase, gamma glutamyl transpeptidase, lactate dehydrogenase, and 2 transaminases. "These enzymes tend to decrease with less than efficient organ function but will actually elevate if organ destruction is occurring," Dr. Taylor says. The blood test also guides Dr. Taylor in assessing different aspects of an individual's metabolic patterning. "Those organs indicating sluggishness or reduced function would suggest a parasympathetic dominance, but those with too much activity would suggest a sympathetic dominance."

The blood study indicates sympathetic and parasympathetic tendencies for the pancreas, kidney, liver, and thyroid. For example, thyroid function is indicated by the relative levels of the hormones thyroxine T4, T3, T7, and TSH (thyroid-stimulating hormone, from the pituitary); of these, the T4 level is the most reliable. Low thyroid activity is an indicator of parasympathetic dominance, while hyperthyroid function indicates sympathetic dominance.

Note that a normal thyroid reading would not necessarily indicate a balance between parasympathetic and sympathetic; other measurements need to be taken into consideration before drawing any conclusions about metabolic type, explains Dr. Taylor. An inefficient fat metabolism is indicated by imbalanced levels of cholesterol, HDL, LDL, and the enzyme SGOT (serum glutamic oxaloacetic transaminase). Either the liver or pancreas could be involved in disordered fat metabolism.

The reference, or "normal" range, is based on healthy volunteers, although normal is not necessarily the *optimal* level. While "healthy" usually means that the volunteer is free of symptoms of illness, the results may be skewed towards a model based on unhealthy people, says Dr. Taylor. Back in 1970, the U.S. Surgeon General stated that "70% of the American population suffers from some degenerative disease" and that "this predicament could be traced directly to poor nutrition." This means if we accept that 70% of our population suffers from some degenerative condition, we are accepting degenerative disease as normal.

Though Dr. Taylor relies heavily on blood analyses to guide his therapeutic protocols, he readily acknowledges the limitations of this perspective. "We need to look at other aspects of bodily function—that is, beyond the blood analysis and metabolic typing, as these provide only a general therapeutic framework."

## A Dietary Program for Different Metabolic Types

Dr. Taylor's basic dietary plan calls for restricting animal protein intake and emphasizing whole grains, fruits, and vegetables, supplemented with proteolytic enzymes and raw juices. As suggested, however, each person has unique capacities for the absorption of food and therefore needs to be dealt with on an individual basis. Dr. Kelley's theory of the various metabolic types ranges from slow-oxidizing vegetarians at one end to fast-oxidizing carnivores at the other. Specific foods are recommended that contain the raw materials needed to improve the blood levels often identified in the testing, and the overall dietary pattern is designed to match the metabolic type of the patient.

Depending on the individual, the proportions of foods can vary widely within this dietary strategy, Dr. Taylor emphasizes. Fruit and vegetable intake can range from 40-85% of daily food consumption; grains, 5-20%; animal flesh, 0-20%; and dairy products, 0-15% (yogurt, cottage cheese, and white, uncolored cheeses, but no processed cheeses or "cheese foods"). As a general guideline, Dr. Taylor advises his patients to derive approximately 60% of their total intake from vegetables and fruits.

"Eat as many of these as possible in raw form or else lightly steamed," says Dr. Taylor. "Green vegetables such as leafy lettuce, green beans, broccoli, spinach, asparagus, mustard greens, or beet leaves are of particular importance, but there are no vegetables that should be restricted from your diet. Pineapples, grapes, apples, and papaya are especially good for you and should be eaten frequently. Citrus fruit intake should be limited to 3 servings per week."

Dr. Taylor usually suggests that any animal product (meat, fish, chicken, lamb, pork) be eaten for breakfast or lunch, so that one does not go to bed with a digestive system laden with animal flesh. "If one eats early in the day, the digestive tract should be clear by the time they go to bed. In this way, the proteolytic enzymes that are produced by the pancreas or taken in capsules can be free to do their scavenger work during the repair, rebuilding, and regeneration time which a restful sleep offers."

Whole grains should make up approximately 10% of total food intake. "Remember to include other grains besides wheat," Dr. Taylor notes. "Rice, oats, barley, millet, rye, and corn should be used in the form of breads, cereals, and pastas. Grains can either be eaten in cooked or sprouted form."

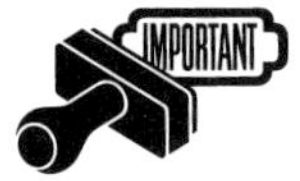


High-protein foods should generally comprise no more than 10% of the diet's total caloric value. "Have a variety of seafood, poultry, and red meats, although red meats such as beef, pork, or lamb should be eaten only about 2 or 3 times per week."

To ensure proper digestion, the protein-rich fare should not be consumed after 1:00 P.M. "As a general rule, one should drink a minimum of 8 glasses of pure water per day," Dr. Taylor says. "Water processed through a reverse osmosis unit is best; spring, mineral, distilled, or other bottled waters are always preferable to tap water."

As for specific foods, Dr. Taylor recommends that patients with "liver overload" (excessive detoxification demands on the liver) eat extra amounts of the bright red and orange vegetables and juices. These foods include beets, carrots, pumpkins, sweet potatoes, yams, and bright squashes. For addressing cases involving "pancreas overload," bright green foods such as sprouts, green onions, broccoli, asparagus, and green beans and leafy greens such as spinach, kale, and Swiss chard are helpful; if anemia is present, the need for green foods and juices is even greater. "Chlorophyll is the 'blood' of a plant and is the best blood builder we can recommend. It is often not advisable to give iron as an isolated supplement, but there appears to be no problem with assimilation of iron found naturally in green foods."

Dr. Taylor advises his patients to uphold the highest standards of purity and quality when making food choices, choosing foods made with whole, natural ingredients whenever possible. When a sweetener is needed, he suggests using honey, molasses, or pure maple syrup; whenever possible, avoid white sugar, white flour, heavily processed, or deep-fried foods, artificial flavorings, colorings, and sweeteners, salted prepared foods, tobacco, nonprescription or street drugs, and soft drinks, while keeping the use of alcohol, coffee, and black tea to a minimum.

## MATCHING THE DIETARY APPROACH TO THE PATIENT'S METABOLIC TYPE

Dr. Taylor's dietary program indicates 3 general patterns based on the style of nervous system involvement. These are, as we explained above, sympa-

## A Primer on Dr. Taylor's Nutritional Formulas

Here is a quick review of the ingredients of some of Dr. Taylor's nutritional formulas.

- Digestive System Support Formula 6: Lipase, protease, and amylase enzymes; magnesium oxide, calcium gluconate, elemental magnesium, zinc citrate, copper, chromium ascorbate; dandelion root, chamomile.
- Pancreatic System Support Formula 20: Pancreas and liver glandular concentrates; lipase, protease, and amylase enzymes; calcium gluconate; orthophosphoric acid.
- Vitamin C Complex Formula 101: Ascorbic acid, mineral ascorbates, bioflavonoids, rose hips.
- Detoxification System Support Formula 17: Vitamin C, sodium and potassium alginates, selenium, apple pectin, garlic, bentonite, aloe vera, L-methionine, chlorophyll, *Cascara sagrada bark,* psyllium seed husks.

thetic, parasympathetic, and balanced. Each of these corresponds to a dietary recommendation.

The first dietary plan is the one many people would expect to apply to all cancer patients, namely, a predominantly vegetarian diet in which 80% of calories derive from raw plant products. According to Dr. Kelly's original theory, however, the basic diet applies only to sympathetic-dominant people; such people are advised to avoid vegetables with a high fat content, such as avocados or deep-fried vegetables. The remainder of the diet consists of cooked cereal grains, lightly cooked vegetables, and occasional small portions of animal products.

In contrast, Dr. Taylor advises parasympathetic-dominant people to get about 20% of their total calories from fatty meats, including large servings of beef, lamb, or pork at least once a day. These high-protein foods should be consumed only in the early part of the day to ensure that they are thoroughly metabolized. Meats (and dairy products) should derive from animals that were fed organically-grown grains and vegetables and not given antibiotics or growth hormones.

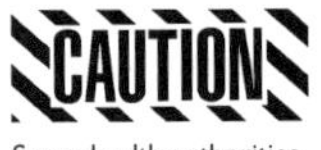


Some health authorities, including nutritionists, might consider some of these recommendations groundless or possibly dangerous given that metabolic types are largely unknown to medical or nutritional science. Dr. Taylor has observed a large number of cancer cases, however, in which adherence to these guidelines, when combined with his specific detoxification and supplementation measures, resulted in definite clinical improvement.

When Dr. Taylor suggests a high intake of animal proteins, he prescribes supplemental digestive enzymes to maximize the absorption of these foods, ample consumption of pure spring or distilled water to flush away toxins produced by animal products and, for similar reasons, moderate exercise.

The third dietary plan is the balanced pattern. Individuals show neither parasympathetic nor sympathetic dominance but a balance of both tendencies. Dr. Taylor advises such individuals to consume a wide variety of plant and animal foods; ideally, all vegetables should be fresh and unprocessed, and meat meals should be alternated with vegetarian meals. Again, the high-protein meal (meat- or legume-based) should be eaten earlier in the day, to enable adequate digestion and detoxification, Dr. Taylor emphasizes.

## Dr. Taylor's Basic Nutritional Support Program

In many instances, changing one's eating habits is not enough to meet the increased nutritional demands posed by cancer or its conventional toxic treatments. That's why Dr. Taylor often recommends the use of antioxidants to help fight "free-radical pathology" and "ensure that there is a proper oxygen-carbon dioxide exchange on a cellular level."

The emotional stress posed by the cancer experience may raise one's nutritional requirements. For this reason, nutritional supplements—he prefers to see them as concentrated foods rather than drugs or medicine—are an integral part of Dr. Taylor's healing program. "These supplements alone cannot cure anything and they can create problems if used haphazardly, but they can be part of a comprehensive therapeutic program."

> ***Since all recommendations are "body-chemistry directed" and not disease-directed, Dr. Taylor says it is impossible to list supplements that apply to every situation.***

The supplement programs Dr. Taylor designs vary widely from one patient to the next. "A person who is in relatively good health may take as little as 6-8 capsules daily, but in contrast, someone diagnosed with cancer or some other degenerative disease may need up to 60-80 concentrated food capsules per day." All supplements are recommended on the basis of blood tests combined with the physician's knowledge of the patient's metabolic type, says Dr. Taylor.

In general, Dr. Taylor finds that supplements in capsule form are preferable to tablets, since the latter tend to contain many inactive ingredients such as binders, fillers, preservatives, and coloring agents. "This nonnutritive material must be detoxified by the liver and other organs and adds more stress to organs already overloaded by disease and inefficiencies," Dr. Taylor says. In contrast, capsules often come with a protein shell with nutritive value and most capsules disintegrate in the stomach in 6 minutes or less.

To make the application of nutritional support most effective, Dr. Taylor developed 4 dozen formulas. Dr. Taylor's basic support program, to be used when there is a diagnosed degenerative disease, including cancer, is taken 4-5 times daily between meals on an empty stomach, such as, for example, at 10 A.M., 2 P.M., 4 P.M., and bedtime. Each round of supplements includes the following: 6 Pancreas Support Formula 20; 2 Digestive Support Formula 6; 1 thymus 213; 1 glandular of the system in question; and 1 Vitamin C 101. Dr. Taylor recommends taking 9 of the Digestive Support Formula 6 at 3 A.M.

Along with these formulas, the following supplements play a pivotal role in Dr. Taylor's approach to helping cancer patients regain optimal physical functioning. He emphasizes that he does not prescribe supplements for disease, but rather for promoting metabolic balance that helps the body resist or reverse disease. "These supplements will push, shove, force, support and strengthen the parts of the body involved in fighting degenerative disease," says Dr. Taylor. "They are not intended as a plan to treat or cure cancer, but as part of a comprehensive *supportive* program."

Since all recommendations are "body-chemistry directed" and not disease-directed, Dr. Taylor says it is impossible to list supplements that apply to every situation. Dosages vary greatly according to age, size, sex, and individual diagnoses of the patient. Here are his comments on selected substances used in his program.

**Vitamin C**—Dr. Taylor prefers to use C complex, which is a mixture of several vitamin C mineral ascorbates (a source of vitamin C superior to ascorbic acid). "The mineral ascorbates have been highly useful in helping cancer patients," says Dr. Taylor. "It appears that the vitamin C is absorbed into cells along with the minerals." He usually recommends vitamin C at the rate of 3-4 g per day, given in 300-400 mg amounts spread throughout the day.

**Vitamin E**—Dr. Taylor recommends the succinate form of vitamin E, 400 units twice a day. This fat-soluble vitamin, one of the body's primary agents for protecting cell membranes, is also among the major nutrients required for a strong immune response.[1]

**B Complex**—Dr. Taylor uses vitamin B complex for maintaining optimal functioning of the immune and nervous systems and to reinforce the effects of vitamin B3.

**Vitamin B6 (Pyridoxine)**—Dr. Taylor insists that any B vitamins be given in a formula containing a base of a whole food source or vitamin B such as concentrated rice powder. Dr. Taylor's recommended dosage for B6 is 25-300 mg per day, depending on individual factors. The dosages should never exceed 500 mg per day. As some people experience severe insomnia at higher doses of vitamin B6, Dr. Taylor advises patients to schedule their supplementation of this vitamin early in the day or to take smaller doses later in the day.

**Selenium**—Dr. Taylor's preferred range is 200-300 mcg per day.

**Zinc**—Dr. Taylor will occasionally recommend zinc as a temporary supplement (30 to 60 mg per day), but only if the person shows definite signs of a zinc deficiency. Zinc supports many aspects of the immune system and its deficiency can potentially make one more vulnerable to certain cancers.[2] Zinc has a close relationship with copper, which is essential to proper functioning of a wide range of immune cell types, including antibody-forming cells, T helper cells, and macrophages, all of which may help the body defend against cancer.[3]

**Maitake Mushroom**—"This is among the more promising therapeutic agents for cancer patients, particularly when taken in addition to a comprehensive nutrition program," says Dr. Taylor. Once again, the intake amount varies according to the metabolic type and condition of the patient.

For **Flax Oil Combination** (the flaxseed/coenzyme Q10 product; from organically raised flax) and other supplements referred to by Dr. Taylor, contact Innovative Therapeutics, 2020 Franklin Street, Carlyle, IL 62231-0512; tel: 888-688-9922 or 618-594-7711; fax: 618-594-7712.

**Marine Lipids (Fish Oils)**—Dr. Taylor recommends supplementation in the range of 2-4 g (2000-4000 mg) of EPA (eicosapentaenoic acid) daily, as indicated.

**Amino Acids**—If the blood levels of albumin, globulin, total protein, or uric acid are outside the optimum ranges or if there is an obvious pancreatic inefficiency present, Dr. Taylor recommends the full complement of free-form amino acids. His recommended dosages for these amino acids are: L-arginine, 5-8 g per day; L-methionine, 500 mg, 2-3 times per day; and L-cysteine, 500 mg, 2-3 times per day.

**Urea**—If tests indicate liver involvement, Dr. Taylor sometimes recommends using about 20 g of urea in powder form, dissolved in 1 quart of water or juice, and consumed over the course of the day, in at least 4 divided doses. He further recommends taking creatine at the same time.

**Flaxseed Oil and Coenzyme Q10**—Cold pressed, unrefined flaxseed oil should not be heated up under any circumstances as this can generate free radicals, says Dr. Taylor. Alpha-linolenic acid (about 60% of the composition of flaxseed oil) works best when mixed directly with sulphur-rich protein food. His recommended amount of pure virgin, cold-pressed, unprocessed flaxseed oil per day is 2-3 tablespoons, depending on the individual's condition; it should be accompanied by a corresponding amount of low-fat or nonfat cottage cheese.

As an alternate, Dr. Taylor suggests taking a flax oil combination product, each tablespoon of which contains coenzyme Q10 (300 mg), vitamin E (300 IU), and L-cysteine (300 mg). The usual daily dosage is 1 tablespoon per 50 pounds of body weight.

**Haelan 851**—While Dr. Taylor's usual recommendations do not include Haelan 851, many patients decide on their own to add this to their program. It is not counter to any of Dr. Taylor's guidelines.

**Melatonin**—Dr. Taylor prescribes the use of melatonin to regulate the body's circadian rhythms. "When our physiological cycles get out of kilter, melatonin can help reset the internal clock." The exact dosage depends on the patient's cancer, overall condition, and any abnormal "body clock" disturbances. Melatonin should always be taken at night, preferably at the same time each night to establish regular physiological timing, says Dr. Taylor.

**Grape Seed Extract**—This extract is high in various phytochemicals (chemicals made by plants), including a variety of bioflavonoids such as the proanthocyanins and anthocyanins. Anthocyanins and other flavonoids extracted from grape seeds are highly effective "scavengers" of harmful free radicals.[4] Though dosages will vary, Dr. Taylor suggests a range of 200-300 mg a day for 5-10 days to saturate the body tissues, followed by a daily maintenance dose of 60-150 mg.

**Garlic—**Dr. Taylor recommends that garlic be included in the diet, either as part of the dietary intake or in supplement form. The amount taken is not as important as the fact that some is consumed daily.

**Essiac—**While Dr. Taylor's usual recommendations do not include Essiac, many patients decide on their own to add this to their program. Again, it is not counter to any of Dr. Taylor's programs.

## CURRICULUM VITAE

# Lawrence H. Taylor, M.D.

Advanced Medicine and Research Center, 1000 Cordova Court, Chula Vista, CA 91910; tel: 888-422-7434; fax: 619-656-1916. (Patients are treated at Allen W. Lloyd Building, Second Floor, Paseo. Tijuana, #406-201, Tijuana, B.C., Mexico.)

Dr. Taylor received a D.O. degree in 1954 from College of Osteopathic Physicians & Surgeons in Los Angeles, and his M.D. in 1964 from California College of Medicine. He has served on the staff of various hospitals and teaching institutions including the University of Vienna Medical School (Austria), University of Amsterdam (Netherlands), Lark Ellen Hospital in West Covina, California, and others, as well as belonging to 8 professional medical societies. Since 1982, Dr. Taylor has actively researched nutrition in cancer therapy, diets and carbohydrate restriction in fungal diseases such as *Candida*, optimum diets for chelating patients, and the relationship between nutrition deficiency and immune dysfunction, among other topics.

***"I am devoting my professional life to improving attitudes and treatment methods in medicine's greatest failure—cancer. Instead of reliance on drugs which usually mask symptoms, since 1982, I have changed the emphasis and direction of treatment," Dr. Taylor says. "I have had success in therapy with allergies, cardiovascular diseases, and cancer by detecting cause-and-effect relationships associated with lifestyles, nutrition, and response behaviors."***

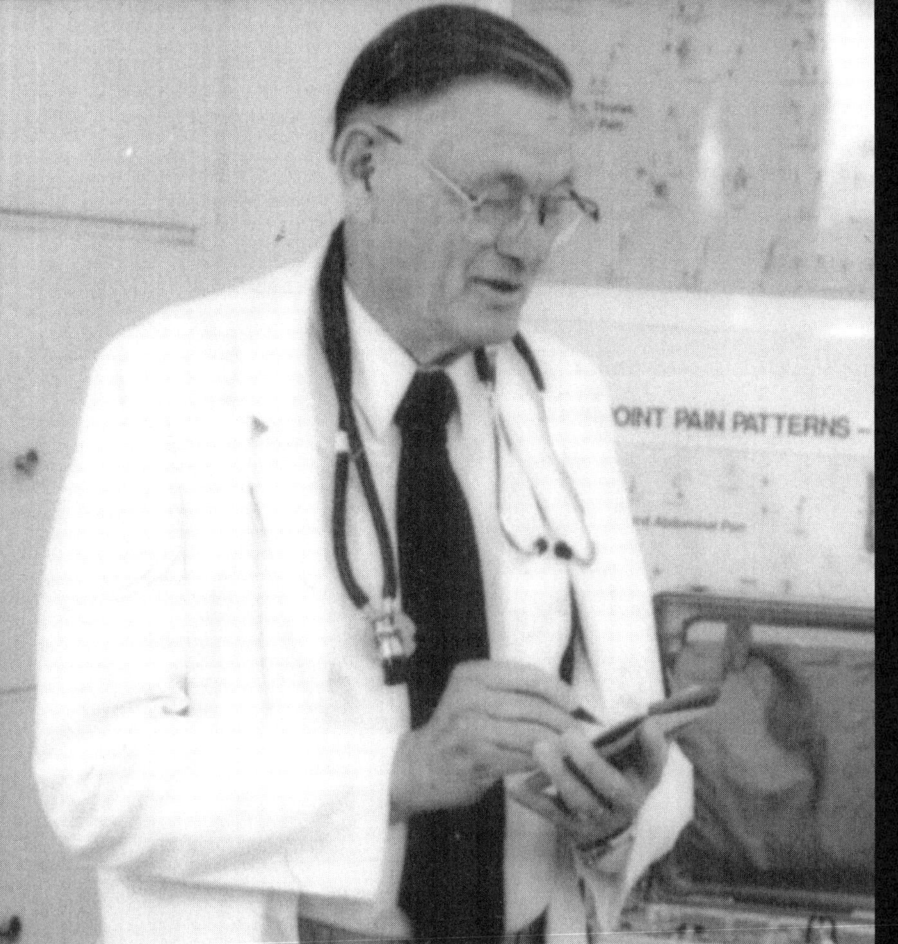


# Chapter 23

# *Lawrence H. Taylor, M.D.*

**SUCCESSFUL OUTCOMES IN CANCER** treatment require a thorough reordering of a patient's body and mind, from immune system support and detoxification to emotional counseling and complete nutritional fortification, even down to the level of DNA, where the cancer mechanism is believed to originate, says Dr. Taylor.

After 4 decades of studying the problem of cancer, Lawrence H. Taylor, M.D., concludes that malignancies are a multifactorial disease. They have multiple causes *and* involve multiple body systems. Malignancies can be reversed, he says, but in most cases a nonlocalized, systemic or whole-body treatment is required. Local treatments can be effective only if the factors known to cause cancer are removed and if all the body systems are working at optimum levels.

For example, cancer of the breast is not limited to the breast. Even before it spreads, other organs and body systems, such as estrogens, progesterone, adrenal secretions, brain hormones, the circulatory and immune systems, are involved in its creation. Malignant and especially pre-malignant changes that have to do with one's genetic constitution, are modifiable with appropriate therapy, says Dr. Taylor. In Dr. Taylor's estimation, 60-80% of cancers are preventable. The war against cancer can be won by prevention alone, he contends, although early detection methods do not constitute true prevention and prevention strategies alone are insufficient as treatments. Nevertheless, long-term remissions cannot be obtained without them.

## The Urgent Need for a New Cancer Paradigm

A new paradigm in cancer treatment is urgently needed, says Dr. Taylor because, as *Scientific American* reported in its September 1996 full issue treatment of cancer, "Twenty-five years of concentrated work have not yet cured the disease that strikes 1 out of every 3 Americans."

# Dr. Lawrence Taylor's Generalized Model for Cancer Treatment

| STRATEGY | DOSAGE/ KEY COMPONENTS | FOR MORE INFORMATION see page # |
|---|---|---|
| **Detoxification** | | |
| Low-fat, high-fiber diet | whole grains, green, leafy vegetables, root vegetables, legumes, and fruits; avoid milk and dairy products; freshly squeezed carrot and other vegetable juices | 749 |
| Sauna or steam bath | gradually building tolerance | 993 |
| Regular exercise | walking or gardening | 1003 |
| Silymarin (milk thistle) | 70-210 mg pills, 2-3 daily | 835 |
| Fluids and electrolytes | drink 5-10 glasses of pure water daily | 791 |
| EDTA chelation | intravenous infusions | 973 |
| Biological dentistry | removal and replacement of mercury amalgam fillings by trained biological dentist | 980 |
| Mental detoxification | positive attitude and asserting one's needs | – |
| **Alternative Cancer Therapies** | | |
| 714X | dosage depending on individual; do not take vitamins E or B12 while undergoing 714X treatment | 871 |
| Amygdalin | dosage depending on individual; intravenously with vitamin C | 812 |
| PolyMVA (DNA nutrient or "metalovitamin," known in U.S. as Polydox) | repairs abnormally altered gene that sets cancer in motion; available only in Mexico. For ill person: 2 tsp in water or juice, 4 times daily for 5 days, then 1 tsp, 4 times daily for 5 days, then 1 tsp daily thereafter. For healthy person: 1 tsp daily for 3 days, then 3-5 drops daily | 506 |
| Shark cartilage | Dosage depending on individual | 863 |
| Thymosin (thymus extract) | 11 mg of peptides from thymus equivalent to 200 mg of dried glandular thymus | 944 |

*Continued*

# Dr. Lawrence Taylor's Generalized Model for Cancer Treatment (cont.)

| STRATEGY | DOSAGE/ KEY COMPONENTS | FOR MORE INFORMATION see page # |
|---|---|---|
| **Supplements** | | |
| General multivitamin | dosage depending on product, but generally for cancer patient, 4-6 tablets daily | — |
| Beta carotene | 25,000 units daily | 764 |
| Vitamin C | 30-60 g intravenously | 786 |
| Vitamin E | 800-1000 units daily | 790 |
| Calcium and magnesium | 800-1200 mg daily of calcium<br>400-1000 mg daily of magnesium<br>If heart or joint problem, ratio of magnesium to calcium should be 1 to 1; otherwise, ratio is 1 to 2 (e.g., 400 mg magnesium to 800 mg calcium) | 765 |
| Selenium | 100 mcg daily | 783 |
| Zinc | 20-50 mg daily | 793 |
| Bioflavonoids | combination of grape seed extract and pine bark (pycnogenol); dosage varies depending on product and individual | 817 |
| Coenzyme Q10 | 250-300 mg daily | 766 |
| Flaxseed oil | 1 tsp daily | 768 |

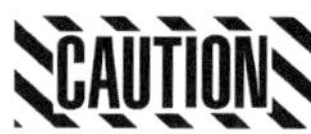


This chapter includes information regarding actual treatments used by Dr. Taylor only after his careful diagnosis of each patient. All cancer patients are unique. **Do not administer these treatments to yourself or others.** Discuss these treatments with your physician or other qualified health-care professional. Readers should not interpret this material as therapeutic advice, but should see a physician in all cases.

These facts come as no surprise to those who seek alternatives in the treatment of cancer and other life-threatening diseases, states Dr. Taylor, who has spent the past 30-plus years pursuing the virtues of nontoxic nutrition-based therapies. "But for scientists and physicians who have chosen to get off the well-worn path of surgery, chemotherapy, and radiation, there are many reasons to be encouraged."

Ironically, one of the biggest rewards of the billions of dollars spent on cancer research in the past 25 years is the growing evidence that cancer can be genetically controlled. There is considerable evidence, Dr. Taylor explains, that genes can be damaged by a variety of factors that range from cellular malnutrition to X-ray exposure, hormonal irregularities, and personality types and emotions. It is on these facts that Dr. Taylor bases his treatment protocols using antioxidants and the newly discovered "polynucleotide reductase" called PolyMVA, discussed below.

Nutrition is still undervalued as a therapy in medicine, says Dr. Taylor. "I am devoting my professional life to improving attitudes and treatment methods in medicine's greatest failure—cancer. Instead of reliance on drugs which usually mask symptoms, since 1982, I have changed the emphasis and direction of treatment. I have had success in therapy with allergies, cardiovascular diseases, and cancer by detecting cause-and-effect relationships associated with lifestyles, nutrition, and response behaviors."

***"How can we cure cancer when the doctor, the community, and the patient all believe that a cancer diagnosis is a death sentence? Fear itself produces hormones that tend to spread the malignant cells," says Dr. Taylor.***

The procedures discussed in this chapter generally fit into 2 classes. First, they correct or modify factors that cause genetic damage. Second, they aim to produce good health. "Successful treatment is hampered by the long history of failure of current methods and by the fear that is generated by these failures," says Dr. Taylor. "Attitudes are restricting advances and progress in cancer therapy. How can we cure cancer when the doctor, the community, and the patient all believe that a cancer diagnosis is a death sentence? Fear itself produces hormones that tend to spread the malignant cells."

Dr. Taylor's approach recognizes this fact and works to reverse cancer through a fourfold strategy: 1) identify and correct gene damage influences; 2) provide treatments that support good health and long life, not only on the cellular and tissue level, but on the organ and systemic or whole-body level; 3) control the tumor burden; 4) develop the patient's sense of personal control and decision-making skills. This fourth category is as important as the other three, Dr. Taylor emphasizes. Extensive European studies indicate that personality is 6 times more important in determining risk to cancer than all the other known risk factors combined.

***"Hope based on facts produces changes in behavior and treatment, thus increasing successful outcomes," Dr. Taylor comments.***

"The development of cancer can be considered, on a psychological basis, as losing control of one's life," says Dr. Taylor. "Couple this problem with the fear factor and there is a poor response to any therapy." Dr. Taylor has found that instilling confidence and decision-making capability in patients will revive their sense of personal control over their life. "The cancer patient who becomes dependent on his physician is never completely cured. Hope based on facts produces changes in behavior and treatment, thus increasing successful outcomes."

> ***"My colleagues and I are opposed to double-blind, placebo-controlled studies in which all patients are given identical treatment," says Dr. Taylor. "The double-blind approach utterly ignores the fact of individual differences and how multiple treatments work together physiologically." Since the characteristics and requirements of the individual are paramount, most double-blind studies are inappropriate under the alternative medicine model.***

## Nutrition, Detoxification, and Immune Support Are Critical

Almost all alternative cancer treatments are based upon nutrition, detoxification, and immune system support. In Dr. Taylor's opinion, successful treatments always begin by carefully considering the individual's biological needs. "Two people with the same type and stage of cancer may require entirely different treatments, and vice versa," he says. "If you don't focus on their unique needs, and think only in abstract terms about the type of cancer they have, your treatment is bound to fail." The medicine of the future, he predicts, will be primarily concerned with an individual's response to treatment, not with what *should* occur based on statistical formulas.

Dr. Taylor offers the following situation as an example of this new thinking. Consider that 3 out of 10 people with an advanced form of cancer respond well to a particular botanical medicine. The fact that only 3 out of 10 responded does not necessarily mean the herbal treatment is a failure. Those 3 who *did* respond in this instance may have had certain key nutritional reserves or strong detoxification abilities. Such factors may need to be present to enable the botanical medicine to work properly.

"My colleagues and I are opposed to double-blind, placebo-controlled studies in which all patients are given identical treatment," says Dr. Taylor.

"The double-blind approach utterly ignores the fact of individual differences and how multiple treatments work together physiologically." Since the characteristics and requirements of the individual are paramount, most double-blind studies are inappropriate under the alternative medicine model.

Dr. Taylor strives to identify the disease-promoting (pathogenic) conditions within each individual, since these conditions must be eliminated to ensure the long-range success of any cancer treatment. If this step is omitted, the factors that encouraged malignant change in the first place may continue to cause its recurrence. Nutrition and toxins are among the most essential yet also the most often overlooked factors in this regard.

In terms of nutrition, Dr. Taylor recommends that his cancer patients consume adequate but not excessive amounts of carbohydrates, fats, and proteins. Unlike micronutrients (vitamins and minerals), these so-called macronutrients usually exist in excessive amounts in the standard American diet. "Too much fat or protein can readily promote cancer," Dr. Taylor says. "Even too much carbohydrate, particularly in the refined or simple forms such as sugar or fruit juice, will also encourage malignancies to expand and spread. The key is balance." In general, he recommends that people follow a strict vegetarian diet, avoiding all animal products, including most dairy products.

***Dr. Taylor strives to identify the disease-promoting (pathogenic) conditions within each individual, since these conditions must be eliminated to ensure the long-range success of any cancer treatment.***

Dr. Taylor observes that conventional treatments are typically used in an abusive fashion by mainstream doctors. For example, chemotherapy destroys the ability of the intestines to absorb and assimilate nutrients, and also tends to destroy enzyme-producing cilia of the small intestine. Therefore, Dr. Taylor assesses the bowel function of all his patients. Conventional doctors tend to overlook the intestinal damage, he says, and they make no effort to supply the nutrients that would either afford added protection against chemotherapy itself or compensate for the nutrient losses caused by chemotherapy.

Another reason conventional treatments fail to reverse most forms of advanced cancer is that they tend to ravage the immune system. Some forms of immune-related imbalance may exist as a consequence of dietary imbalances, or as a result of the cancer itself. Whatever the cause, careful attention must be given to redressing the imbalance. "Our research shows that nearly all types of cancer patients have abnormalities in several immune cells, specifically the T4 and T8, as well as the cytokine called IL-2," says Dr. Taylor. "The use of drugs such as interferon to stimulate these components of the system have generally been unsuccessful, basically because the drugs have been toxic."

In Dr. Taylor's view, oncologists would benefit by using nutritional and hormonal manipulations instead of drugs to support principles of good health. "We need to be extremely gentle and supportive to the body when it becomes sick with an illness as devastating as cancer," says Dr. Taylor. "If we treat it in a crude fashion, loading it up with yet more poisons, we're literally going to be digging our own grave." For the past few decades, he has struggled to help cancer patients recuperate from the dreadful toxic effects of conventional therapies, and to see through the "poison-and-burn" mentality so pervasive among today's orthodox oncologists.

## A 5-Pronged Detoxification Strategy

Detoxification is a priority, Dr. Taylor says, since many cancer patients come to him after having received highly toxic conventional therapies. In addition, many patients have been exposed to a variety of pollutants through their diet and lifestyle. "People on a typical American diet are loaded with toxins," says Dr. Taylor. "Those same toxins, as well as nutrient deficiencies or imbalances in the diet, probably contributed in a direct way to the initiation, promotion, and progression of the cancer. These factors also contribute indirectly by weakening the immune system."

Given that exposure to toxic substances is a key factor in the development of malignancy, identifying and eliminating toxins is a standard procedure in Dr. Taylor's treatment. Free radicals are not often listed as toxins, but their presence in the body encourages cell damage and gene mutation. Treatment for these conditions includes antioxidants, high doses of ascorbic acid, and often EDTA chelation.

Treatment to correct the exposure to the many carcinogens in our environment today cannot begin unless the carcinogen has been identified and recurrent exposure is prevented. Heavy metal toxicity may be a factor indicating the development of cancerous growths, and their presence in the body may prevent or delay healing. Testing hair, urine, blood and teeth provides clues to identifying such problems. Chronic infections, especially those of the gums and teeth, also interfere with healing. Successful treatment produces the death of cancer cells which presumably release harmful toxins, and thus detoxification should focus on eliminating them from the body. Another proven source of internal toxins is the overgrowth of *Candida*, a common bowel fungus. Bowel and systemic candidiasis are common after the excessive use of antibiotics, corticosteroids, and chemotherapy. Bowel and stool testing are necessary in all cases of cancer to determine if *Candida* is a factor.

The main organs of detoxification are the skin, the lungs, the liver, the kidneys, and the bowels. Dr. Taylor's treatment program monitors and improves the function of these waste management systems.

All of Dr. Taylor's cancer patients undergo a 5-7 day program that focuses primarily on bowel and liver detoxification using fiber, enemas, and herbals. The basic components of this program are as follows:

**Low-Fat, High-Fiber Diet—**Whole grains, green, leafy vegetables, root vegetables, legumes, and fruits are balanced nutritionally and also low in fat. Fat tends to suppress the immune system and concentrates fat-soluble toxins. "A low-fat diet therefore supports the immune system's normal functioning and eases the body's toxic burden tremendously," says Dr. Taylor. "It's the kind of diet that gives the liver a chance to function more effectively in detoxification and energy production."

These fiber-rich foods can greatly speed up the detoxification of the colon. Since fiber tends to "sweep out" or bind toxins in the intestines, it can bolster the body's anticancer defenses. Grains, legumes, and some of the more fibrous vegetables are high in cellulose and other fibers that bind bile acids and help keep the bowel clean. Associated with the cellulose are substances called lignans, which show strong anticancer activity, mainly by competing with estrogen for estrogen binding sites.[1] This fact may explain why high levels of urinary lignans (indicating high levels in the blood) are associated with low rates of 2 hormone-sensitive cancers, breast and prostate cancers.

Dr. Taylor notes that obesity and constipation are among the known risk factors for breast cancer, and fiber greatly reduces the risk of developing either of these conditions. "When estrogen is broken down in the liver and expelled into the bile, it will not be adequately excreted if a person has constipation," he states. "Some of those breakdown products are carcinogenic and will be reabsorbed along with the fat molecules."

Modified citrus pectin (derived from citrus fruit) has been shown to inhibit metastasis, or the spreading of cancer cells. One study found that this pectin inhibited the spread of human cancer cells from the prostate to the lungs; specifically, the pectin-treated group had 9 times fewer lung metastases compared to the untreated group.[2] Other research suggests that pectin may be more effective than other fibers in protecting against colon cancer.[3] In some cases of colon cancer, Dr. Taylor may also recommend a modified citrus pectin supplement, 15 g per day.

***"Such toxins as organophosphates and insecticides are most effectively removed by sweating via external heat," says Dr. Taylor. "This is essential yet often overlooked in alternative cancer treatment programs today."***

**Sauna or Steambath—**In order to detoxify the carcinogen-laden fat that gets absorbed by the intestine, Dr. Taylor says that people with cancer need to sweat. Either a sauna, steam bath, or very hot tub bath will work, as long the person sweats. "Such toxins as organophosphates and insecticides are most effectively removed by sweating via external heat," says Dr. Taylor. "This is essential yet often overlooked in alternative cancer treatment programs today." Note that a sauna does not accomplish the same cancer-reversing effects as hyperthermia. This is because in a sauna the body makes adjustments to maintain a steady internal temperature, whereas in hyperthermia, the body "overrides" this restriction.

For people with cancer, the only major precaution regarding the use of saunas or similar heat therapies is to be sure you have a strong heart or adequate cardiovascular fitness. Dr. Taylor suggests starting with a comfortable degree of sauna exposure, and gradually increasing the amount of sauna time as one's heat tolerance increases. Never undertake an extended sauna alone—bring a companion along who can help you exit the sauna should you feel faint or dizzy. For people with high blood pressure, a consultation with a physician is essential for beginning this therapy.

**Regular Exercise—**A second method of removing fat-soluble toxins is through exercise. Vigorous aerobic exercise will induce sweating, thus reinforcing the effects of the sauna; however, in cancer patients, strenuous physical activity may deplete the body's energy and promote lean-tissue wasting (cachexia). Therefore, more moderate forms of exercise are important for both detoxification and general immune enhancement. Dr. Taylor says gentle, practical physical activities—namely walking and gardening—are the ones cancer patients are most likely to adhere to and benefit from.

Hard work outside in the garden is the best exercise for both physical and psychological purposes. "When you're gardening regularly, you get sunshine and fresh air, and many different muscles are used," Dr. Taylor states. "You also have something to show for your endeavors. If you don't have a garden, find someone who has one or perhaps seek out a community garden." These gentle exercises also promote the functioning of the lymphatic system.

Research supports this recommendation. Men who engaged in as little as 1 hour of brisk walking per week (using about 500 calories ) had death rates 15 to 20% lower than men who were almost completely sedentary.[4] Men who walked about 4 hours per week (burning an average of 2000 calories) had death rates that were 35% lower than their inactive counterparts.

**Silymarin—**Also known as milk thistle (*Silybum marianum*), this herb is a potent liver protector and detoxifying agent. "Silymarin is more widely embraced by alternative doctors as a liver cleanser than any other botanical agent," says Dr. Taylor. "The reason for this is that it works very well. The end result is that it enhances liver function, thereby freeing up this organ to more effectively carry out its key healing functions." The usual dosage is 2 to 3 pills daily, in 70- to 210-mg concentrates of silymarin.

**Fluids and Electrolytes—**Drinking plenty of water that is free of chlorine, fluorine, and other toxins, between 5 and 10 glasses daily depending on your thirst and activity level, is important. Spring water is acceptable, since most spring water contains ample amounts of minerals, which need to be replenished after exercising or taking a sauna. Chelated mineral supplements are often beneficial. Sea vegetables and algae supplements, such as kelp powder, cracked chlorella, spirulina, or blue-green algae, can supply other minerals and trace elements in an easily absorbed form.

Overdosing with kelp or algae is not a concern, since in general they provide only trace amounts of organic micronutrients and will not overload the body with minerals and trace elements. In fact, these supplements tend to be far safer than multimineral tablets or other mineral supplements.

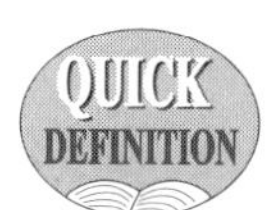


**Chelation therapy** refers to a method of binding ("chelating") an organic substance known as a chelating agent to a metallic ion with a positive electric charge (e.g., a heavy metal) and removing it from the body. One type of chelation therapy involves the chelating agent disodium EDTA given as an intravenous infusion over a 3 1/2-hour period. Usually 20 to 30 treatments are administered at the rate of 1 to 3 sessions per week. Chelation therapy is especially beneficial for all forms of atherosclerotic cardiovascular disease including angina pectoris and coronary artery disease.

**Chelation Therapy—**Heavy metal toxicity may be a factor contributing to the development of cancer. Testing hair, urine, blood, and teeth can help identify the presence of heavy metal toxicity. Chelation with EDTA, DMPS, DMSA, or D-penicillamine can then be used to remove the toxic metals. These chelation agents effectively bind heavy metals and remove them from the body, primarily through the kidneys.

The term heavy metals refers to certain elements such as lead, mercury, arsenic, cadmium, aluminum, and nickel. These substances are toxic to the body at any level and cause dysfunction of various enzyme systems and other cellular functions in the body by competitively binding to enzymes and other proteins in the body at the same sites as magnesium, calcium, or other therapeutic minerals are supposed to bind. However, copper, zinc, manganese, selenium, and certain other minerals required for health can become toxic like other heavy metals when present in amounts that are too high.

For more information on **detoxification** (pp. 949-980), and **biological dentistry** (pp. 980-989), see Chapter 33: Physical Support Therapies.

Chelation has proven particularly effective in removing high levels of the following heavy metals: cadmium, copper, lead, and mercury.[5] DMPS, for example, is often given over a 20-minute period every 3 weeks for 4-12 doses to remove mercury (derived mostly from dental amalgams) from the body.

One chelation expert, John Parks Trowbridge, M.D., of Kingwood, Texas, says EDTA helps to detoxify the body of such poisons as heavy metals, sulfites, growth hormones, antibiotics, and nitrites "by molecular action" and increases the amount of oxygen used by body tissues.[6] By reducing the body's free-radical burden (which would promote tumor growth), chelation probably enhances your ability to fight cancer.[7]

**Biological Dentistry—**Dental amalgams, or "tooth fillings," are about 50% mercury, and this toxic metal has a tendency to gradually leach out of the amalgam and damage our genetic material, paving the way for cancer and immune system suppression. A large body of research demonstrates that mercury from silver amalgams promotes free-radical damage[8] as well as immune-system suppression.[9] Dr. Taylor refers many of his patients to biological dentists who are trained in the careful removal and replacement of silver amalgams with plastic, ceramic, or gold fillings.

## Multiple Antioxidants to Strengthen the System

There are about 50 essential nutrients that must be provided in optimum doses and in forms easily absorbed by the body, says Dr. Taylor. These are the vitamins, minerals, fatty acids, amino acids, and fibers. Chemotherapy destroys the ability of the intestines to absorb and assimilate these nutrients. "Therefore all our patients undergo careful bowel function assessment. As chemotherapy often destroys enzyme-producing cilia of the small intestine, taking enzymes is usually beneficial."

***Chemotherapy destroys the ability of the intestines to absorb and assimilate essential nutrients and often destroys enzyme-producing cilia of the small intestine, so taking enzymes is usually beneficial.***

Dr. Taylor finds that micronutrient testing before and after dietary adjustments is cost effective. These tests demonstrate proper or improper bowel function and the ability to absorb; micronutrient testing can also aid in detecting malabsorption problems caused by a food allergy or sensitivity.

Macronutrients are critical to health and include carbohydrates, fats, proteins, and fibers. The most important medical fact concerning macronutrients is that by controlling the *ratio* of these foods in the diet the physician can control the most important hormone system in the body, prostaglandins, which control inflammatory responses and pain. "The accumulating research shows that nutrition should be the basis for maintaining good health and for the successful treatment of the sick," says Dr. Taylor.

Nutrition can shore up a dysfunctional immune system. The use of the drugs interferon and interleukins by oncologists is based upon the theory that strengthening the immune system will help the body fight the cancer. "Our research shows that nearly all types of cancer patients have abnormalities in several immune cells (specifically, T4, T8, IL2 leukocytes). The clinical reports concerning interferon and interleukins have, in general, been disappointing, so we have adopted more natural methods to support the immune system," says Dr. Taylor.

Beneficial immune system changes can also occur based on shifts in perception and emotions and as a result of nutritional and hormonal manipulations. The use of a darkfield microscope to study live blood cells from the cancer patient can accurately measure responses to treatments.

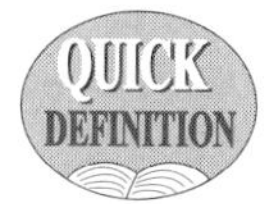

**Darkfield microscopy** is a way of studying living whole blood cells under a specially adapted microscope that projects the dynamic image, magnified 1500 times, onto a video screen. With a darkfield light condenser, images of high contrast are projected, so that the object appears bright against a dark background. The skilled physician can detect early signs of illness in the form of microorganisms in the blood known to produce disease. Blood cells live for about 20 minutes, so the amount of time the blood cell stays viable and alive indicates the overall health of the individual. Specifically, darkfield microscopy reveals distortions of red blood cells (which in turn indicate nutritional status), possible undesirable bacterial or fungal life forms, and blood ecology patterns indicative of health or illness.

An **antioxidant** (meaning "against oxidation") is a natural biochemical substance that protects living cells against damage from harmful free radicals. Antioxidants work against the process of oxidation—the robbing of electrons from substances. If unblocked or left uncontrolled, oxidation can lead to cellular aging, degeneration, arthritis, heart disease, cancer, and other illnesses. Antioxidants in the body react readily with oxygen breakdown products and free radicals, and neutralize them before they can damage the body. Antioxidant nutrients include vitamins A, C, and E, beta carotene, selenium, coenzyme Q10, pycnogenol (grape seed extract), L-glutathione, superoxide dismutase, and bioflavonoids. Plant antioxidants include *Gingko biloba* and garlic. When antioxidants are taken in combination, the effect is stronger than when they are used individually.

Free radicals are not often listed as toxins, but they are among the main by-products of the body's metabolic activities, and their presence in the body encourages cell damage and gene mutation. Antioxidants help neutralize these harmful substances, and in most cases they accomplish this feat in tandem, through various chemical interactions or "synergisms." A synergy occurs when 2 substances combine and produce an effect that is greater than what would be expected if either substance had been analyzed in isolation. In other words, combining the substances multiplies their effectiveness. A classic example of this is vitamin E and selenium.

Dr. Taylor's general recommendations for antioxidants are as follows:

**Beta Carotene—**25,000 units on a daily basis. Beta carotene, a plant pigment found naturally in many fruits and vegetables, is a key antioxidant and precursor to vitamin A. It has repeatedly been shown to enhance the activity of natural killer (NK) cells and other immune cells against tumors.[10,11,12] However, beta carotene may not be advisable for people who have smoked for many years, unless their serum beta carotene levels are already high. "People with low serum levels of beta carotene may be *more* susceptible to lung cancer when they take beta carotene supplements," says Dr. Taylor. "These studies, however, ignore many of the synergisms that exist between beta carotene and other nutrients—you have to have them all to see the anticancer effect."

**Vitamin E—**Between 800 and 1000 units daily. Vitamin E is one of the body's key micronutrients for protecting cell membranes and supporting the immune system's ability to respond to cancer and infection.[13] Vitamin E also increases the effectiveness and specific toxicity of chemotherapy agents on tumors[14] and helps protect against the toxic effects of radiation treatments.[15]

A **free radical** is an unstable molecule with an unpaired electron that steals an electron from another molecule and produces harmful effects. Free radicals are formed when molecules within cells react with oxygen (oxidize) as part of normal metabolic processes. Free radicals then begin to break down cells, especially if there are not enough free-radical quenching nutrients, such as vitamins C and E, in the cell. While free radicals are normal products of metabolism, uncontrolled free-radical production plays a major role in the development of degenerative disease, including cancer, heart disease, and aging. Free radicals harmfully alter important molecules, such as proteins, enzymes, fats, even DNA. Other sources of free radicals include pesticides, industrial pollutants, smoking, alcohol, viruses, most infections, allergies, stress, even certain foods and excessive exercise.

**Selenium**—100 micrograms per day. Selenium has potent synergistic effects with vitamin E, meaning that the ability of these 2 nutrients to enhance the immune system and fight cancer is greater when both are present in adequate amounts.[16] Certain chemotherapeutic drugs as well as heavy metals (cadmium, lead, and mercury) tend to inactivate selenium, rendering it unavailable to the body.[17]

**Bioflavonoids**—The recommended amounts of bioflavonoids will vary depending on the supplement and individual patient factors. Dr. Taylor recommends using a combination of grape seed extract and pine bark (pycnogenol). These substances comprise a group of brightly colored compounds commonly found alongside vitamin C; they aid mainly in blood vessel repair and help prevent bruising. Among the better known bioflavonoids are citrin, hesperidin, rutin, quercetin, and pycnogenol. Many bioflavonoids promote or reinforce the cancer-fighting activities of vitamin C. Some research indicates that quercetin dramatically inhibits the growth of human stomach cancer cells.[18]

**Coenzyme Q10**—250 to 300 mg a day of coQ10 (also known as ubiquinone) is "more of a general antioxidant which supports the function of all the others," says Dr. Taylor. "Its ability to protect the heart and enhance the immune system make it an extremely valuable part of alternative cancer treatment, particularly if the patient is receiving or has received chemotherapy."

## Essential Nutrients That Support the Cancer Reversal Process

All the supplements listed in the previous section serve primarily to bolster and reinforce the body's ability to counteract the effects of free radicals, substances that promote tumor growth and immune system breakdown. Besides free radicals, however, there are numerous other agents and mechanisms that pave the way for the onset and spread of cancer. The following are important in reversing cancer.

**Essential Fatty Acids (EFAs)**—These are nutrients that cannot be manufactured by the body but must be consumed in the food. All EFAs are polyunsaturated fatty acids (PUFAs), but not all PUFAs are EFAs. In fact, *most* PUFAs are *not* essential or required in the diet. There are 2 kinds of EFAs, as determined by certain basic differences in the chemical structure of their molecules: the omega-6 series and the omega-3 series. Most of the omega-6 fatty acids, notably arachidonic acid (animal products except for fish and mother's milk) and linoleic acid (corn oil, safflower oil, and many other vegetable oils) are undesirable because they promote tissue injury, says Dr. Taylor.

***Dr. Taylor advises people to avoid milk and dairy products because they contain omega-6 fatty acids as well as growth hormone residues which further promote the growth of cancer cells.***

The omega-3 fatty acids are the good EFAs. A large body of research shows that the omega-3s help maintain our hormonal balance and cardiovascular health, and support the development of the brain (mother's milk being an excellent source in this regard). What few people realize, however, is that omega-3 fatty acids also play a profound role in the body's anticancer defenses.

For optimal EFA and hormonal balance, Dr. Taylor recommends following the basic proportions of macronutrients outlined in the Sears diet.[19] This diet is composed of 40% complex carbohydrates, 30% fat, and 30% protein, primarily vegetable quality with some lean meats. This fat composition may seem high to many doctors, but Dr. Taylor states that at least half of it must come from omega-3 sources, in order to improve our internal balance of key hormone-like substances called eicosanoids.

Dr. Taylor says the most important omega-3 EFA for fighting cancer is alpha-linolenic acid, which can be obtained from flaxseed oil, one teaspoon per day. "The essential fatty acids are a missing link in most approaches to cancer and inflammatory disorders," he states. "Yet they may be among the most important links because of their effects on eicosanoids. If you don't dramatically curtail your omega-6 intake from red meats, dairy products, and most vegetable oils, your body's synthesis of bad eicosanoids will proceed in such a way as to promote cancer."

At the same time, Dr. Taylor advises people to avoid milk and dairy products because they contain omega-6 fatty acids as well as growth hormone residues which further promote the growth of cancer cells. Sprouts less than 4 days old are also recommended, since these lack the giberellins (naturally present growth hormones) and are high in abscissic acid (cell growth inhibitors).

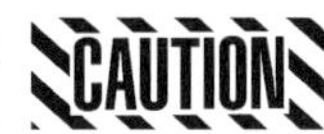

Since copper and zinc are chemically antagonistic, Dr. Taylor advises that their intake be carefully controlled under medical supervision. Ingesting too much copper can readily reduce the body's zinc supply, and vice versa.

**Lipid** is a biochemist's term for a fat or oil, which is one of the 6 basic food groups. Fats and oils are made of building blocks called fatty acids. Of these long-chain molecules (comprising atoms of carbon, hydrogen, and oxygen) the "fatty" end does not dissolve in water, while the "acid" end does. Fats are also called triglycerides as they consist of 3 (tri) fatty acid molecules joined to one molecule of glycerol, a kind of sugar. Unsaturated fats required in the diet are called **essential fatty acids,** and include linoleic acid (an omega-6 oil), found in corn, beans, and some nuts and seeds, and alpha linolenic acid (an omega-3 oil), found in fish, flaxseed, and walnuts.

**Zinc—**Dr. Taylor recommends supplementing with zinc in the range of 20 to 50 mg daily, depending on individual needs as determined by serum zinc levels and T-cell function. Zinc supports many aspects of the immune system, and its deficiency appears to make us more vulnerable to cancer.[20] Zinc has a close relationship with copper, which is essential to the proper functioning of a wide range of immune cell types, including antibody-forming cells, T helper cells, and macrophages, all of which may aid the body in defending against cancer.[21] "Zinc supplementation may be particularly helpful in dealing with prostate problems," says Dr. Taylor.

**Calcium—**The recommended amounts of both calcium and magnesium vary depending on the individual's age, sex, blood chemistry, and other factors. A 19-year prospective study found that calcium deficiency was associated with a higher risk of colorectal cancer.[22] Supplementation should be based on two factors: (1) serum calcium-to-phosphorus ratio (ideally 4 to 1); and (2) the relative amounts of magnesium in the daily diet (ideally 2-to-1 ratio of calcium to magnesium). "Women need more calcium in general to help prevent osteoporosis," says Dr. Taylor. "Though the connection with colon cancer is not definitive, calcium is also needed for numerous other aspects of human health, including heart, muscle, and nerve function." Dr. Taylor's recommended range for supplementation is 800 to 1200 mg per day.

**Magnesium—**The recommended range is 400 to 1000 mg day. If there's a heart or joint problem, magnesium would be taken in a 1-to-1 ratio with calcium (e.g., 800 mg magnesium to 800 mg calcium). Otherwise, it would

## The Benefits of Fresh Vegetable Juice

Vegetable juices of various kinds may be prepared for immediate consumption by a Champion juicer or some form of squeezer-processor. Dr. Taylor recommends starting with carrot juice and drinking it as fresh as possible. "Vegetable juices will oxidize very quickly if you don't drink them right away, such as within 10 to 15 minutes" says Dr. Taylor. "That means that they lose some of their nutritional value unless you drink them fresh." If a surplus of juice is produced, vitamin C crystals (based on the bowel tolerance principle) should be added to prevent oxidation. Dr. Taylor says that these juices should then be placed in the refrigerator for storage. These vegetable drinks typically contain a wide variety of vitamins and minerals, as well as substances that aid in digestion, detoxification, and other key functions.

be one-to-two ratio (e.g., 400 mg magnesium to 800 mg calcium). "It is likely that magnesium reinforces calcium's role in fighting cancer," says Dr. Taylor. "The majority of Americans are magnesium deficient, and that fact has had a profound impact on our nation's overall health." Magnesium assists in the body's uptake of both calcium and potassium, and a magnesium deficiency will promote deficiencies in calcium and potassium.

**Multivitamin**—As an all-purpose supplement, multivitamin pills are used to prevent or rectify nutritional deficiencies during cancer treatment and the recovery process. "Pay attention to the issue of timing whenever you take a multivitamin or other supplements," Dr. Taylor says. "Dr. Emmanuel Revici's concept of anabolic and catabolic nutrients is extremely important in this regard." The cancer patient is typically advised to take 4 to 6 tablets per day, depending on the brand and manufacturer.

**714X**—This substance, developed by Canadian biologist Gaston Naessens, is composed of nitrogen-rich camphor and organic salts. Patients undergoing 714X treatment should not take vitamin E or vitamin B12 at the same time, cautions Dr. Taylor.

For more information about **Emanuel Revici, M.D.,** and his theory of cancer treatment, see Chapter 15; for more information on the **bowel tolerance principle** and vitamin C ingestion, see Chapter 28: Nutrition as Cancer Medicine, p. 788.

**Thymosin**—Dr. Taylor has reported considerable success with this active glandular extract from the thymus gland. The recommended dosage is 11 mg of peptides from thymus, equivalent to 200 mg of dried glandular thymus.

**Cartilage**—Dr. Taylor observes that many cases of advanced cancer have improved when either shark or bovine cartilage was included in the program. Cartilage contains factors that help block the formation of new blood vessels, thereby starving tumors so that they cannot continue to grow. A recent evaluation of 100 case histories suggests that bovine cartilage enhances immune function and the body's ability to resist and reverse cancer.[23]

**Amygdalin—**Dr. Taylor has limited experience with amygdalin, but has seen successful outcomes from Mexican clinics where amygdalin is one of the mainstays of treatment. They report that many patients benefit when amygdalin is administered intravenously, together with vitamin C and other therapeutic substances.[24] He has treated patients who have reported benefits from using this compound.

## Molecular Biology: The Importance of Cellular Nutrition

The next advance in nutrition will be on a cellular and subcellular level. This field, previously known as cellular nutrition, is now called molecular biology.[25] One of its pioneers is Merrill Garnett, D.D.S. Dr. Garnett, a dentist, became an insightful cancer chemistry researcher, combining 2 principles of medicine into the development of unusual compounds that are proving effective against cells whose internal machinery is defective. These defects prevent the cell's normal function, much as cancer cells do.

The first principle of medicine is "do no harm." Dr. Linus Pauling forwarded this principle when he labeled the use of certain essential nutrients as "orthomolecular." His reasoning was that by using compounds needed by the body, such as vitamin C, in varying doses, the cell chemistry could be influenced without injury to the person. After all, the body already knows how to use vitamins, minerals, and amino acids via "established chemical pathways of utilization." A common chemotherapy drug, 5-fluorouracil, has no such pathway and therefore causes damage beyond the destruction of malignant cells. Vitamin C, even in huge doses, rarely causes problems.

The second principle used by Dr. Garnett has nearly been forgotten by physicians who rely upon synthetic drugs for disease control. Yet this principle is used in nearly every biochemical reaction in the body. It is the principle of synergy—multiple substances working together and enhancing one another's effects. Catalysts and enzymes speed up reaction time and can be considered synergists. There is a synergy among vitamins C, A, and E, which work much better together than alone. Vitamin C acts as a transporter of vitamin A to the cell; vitamin A improves the function of vitamin E when inside the cell. By combining certain vitamins and minerals in one molecule, Dr. Garnett put into practice the laws of molecular synergy, and by limiting the combination to orthomolecular (essential) substances, he followed the principle of "do no harm."

**PolyMVA—**This substance represents a new concept in nutritional supplements. Dr. Garnett's patented medicine—it received its patent in October 1995—is a called a "metalo-vitamin." It has effects on the nucleic acid of the gene, helping the gene correct errors in its DNA. Therefore it is also classified as a polynucleotide reductase.[26] A nucleotide is a single unit of DNA, one step in the DNA "spiral staircase;" nucleotides are the basic molecular structure that controls cell division and replication. A reductase is an enzyme that catalyzes a reduction by which a substance gains one or more electrons; enzymes are known to affect DNA repair. Thus a polynucleotide reductase is an enzyme that biochemically affects multiple units of DNA.

***The essence of PolyMVA's action is simple: it repairs the abnormally altered gene that is believed to set the cancer mechanism in motion.***

The thinking behind PolyMVA is gene repair. Molecular biologists point to altered DNA (under the negative influence of a carcinogen or contributing cause) as a factor in the development of tumors. Altered genes in turn produce protein substances that are abnormal. "A major factor in the success of PolyMVA has been to provide an electron energy transfer mechanism from normal metabolic hydrogen carriers to nucleic acids," Dr. Taylor explains. "Nucleic acids are the main constituents of DNA. PolyMVA induces energy-dependent changes in the shape of DNA or RNA as a result of the new reduced state it induces in the nucleotides." Simply put, PolyMVA is a DNA nutrient.

Although the concepts underlying PolyMVA are couched in complex chemical and genetic terms, the essence of its action is simple: it repairs the abnormally altered gene that is believed to set the cancer mechanism in motion.

As a vitamin complex, PolyMVA improves the synergy of other essential nutrients while its metal components activate vitamin B12. The substance also aids in energy transfer inside cells, probably due to its lipoic acid component, which is highly specific for transferring electron energy from a normal metabolic hydrogen carrier to nucleic acids. The synthetic product also contains palladium (an essential trace metal), thiamine, and cyanocobalamin.

As Dr. Taylor explains, free radical damage releases a destructive energy within the cells and this cellular injury contributes to many diseases. "PolyMVA converts this destructive energy into usable cellular energy and DNA is thereby protected. In effect, it converts free radicals to energy. This ability to transfer energy inside the cell provides important functions which stabilize the cell, improve its ability to work, and protect DNA."

The nucleic acids are the backbone of DNA, which contains the estimated 100,000 essential genes of the human body. Carcinogens that alter the chemistry of the gene are major causes of cancer. Detoxification and DNA repair mechanisms, which have been the focus of alternative practices for years, are now the keystone of orthodox cancer research.[27] A new class of enzymes that affect DNA are now being tested in Mexico and Canada. "The development by Dr. Garnett of the first nucleotide reductase can be viewed as the next advance in nutrition on a cellular level," says Dr. Taylor.

***"The development by Dr. Garnett of the first nucleotide reductase can be viewed as the next advance in nutrition on a cellular level," says Dr. Taylor.***

Research on PolyMVA is ongoing in the United States and Mexico, but it is not licensed for use in the United States. The Mexican and Canadian experience with this medicine indicates success in the treatment of certain brain tumors and ovarian and prostate cancers; it has been found to potentiate free-radical scavengers and slow down the aging process. PolyMVA is available only in Mexico where it has received government approval; in the U.S., it is known as Polydox. It is being tested there in 2 groups of patients, says Dr. Taylor. "Some use the PolyMVA as an adjuvant along with standard chemotherapy or radiation. Another group of patients is receiving strictly alternative care, with no chemotherapy or radiation."

Preliminary indications are that PolyMVA is effective against brain tumors, glioblastomas, and lung, ovarian, and breast cancers. In addition,

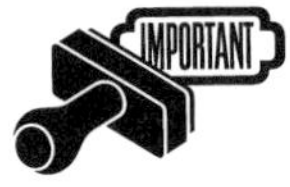


the substance appears to reduce pain, improve appetite, and facilitate weight gain among cancer patients suffering from pain, anorexia, or weight loss from "wasting" (cachexia). Regarding brain tumors, according to Dr. Taylor, "Even in the late stages with extensive symptoms of partial paralysis, memory changes, and ambulatory abnormalities, there was a quick and prolonged return to normal function." As for breast cancers, Dr. Taylor states that "late stages with extensive bone metastasis have reported resolution of the bone loss and reduction of pain."

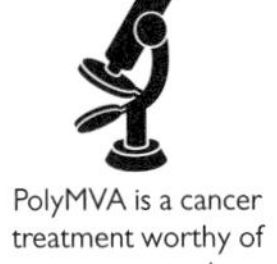

PolyMVA is a cancer treatment worthy of more research.

A recommended dosage for PolyMVA for a person with pain or chronic illness is to start with 2 teaspoons, 4 times daily for 5 days. Follow this with 1 teaspoon, 4 times daily for 5 days, then 1 teaspoon daily thereafter. As a nutritional support and energy source to prevent problems in healthy persons, a recommended dosage is as follows, according to Dr. Taylor: Start with 1 teaspoon daily for 3 days; then go to 3-5 drops daily, mixed with water or juice. The substance is a reddish-brown liquid that does not require refrigeration; no side effects or associated toxicity have been reported over a 2-year period of use.

## Restoring the Art of Medicine to Treating Cancer

In the past, Dr. Taylor has explored a number of "experimental treatments" that he considered worthy of further investigation, including chelation therapy. Because of systematic harassment by the California medical authorities in recent years, however, Dr. Taylor stopped prescribing these substances in the United States.[28] He now sends his patients across the Mexican border to Tijuana, where they can purchase nontoxic medicines and be treated with the best of alternative cancer therapies.

Dr. Taylor, like other alternative medicine physicians, has been systematically harassed, defamed, and subjected to severe financial loss by medical authorities, all without substantial basis. In 1993, Dr. Taylor was arrested and held at $1 million bail; his offices and home were raided by the police, and his medical records and equipment were confiscated. But in August 1995, all 130 charges against Dr. Taylor were thrown out of court as being without legal merit and his medical practice was restored. Even so, California medical authorities continued to seek grounds to revoke Dr. Taylor's M.D. license. They finally succeeded in doing so in 1996.

Despite his years of harassment and oppression by medical authorities, Dr. Taylor remains true to his vision of treating cancer. For him, restoring the art of medicine to the treatment of cancer means restoring faith and compassion, the ultimate powers of healing. These powers may not be measurable by scientific methods, but they are real—and physicians can encourage the cultivation of such powers. The effort must begin from the time of diagnosis, an experience that can be so traumatic as to break the person's spirit. A tremendous amount of courage on the part of the patient is needed to face this diagnosis, says Dr. Taylor. The physician who evinces compassion and an optimistic outlook will help the patient far more than the physician who offers only a grim prognosis.

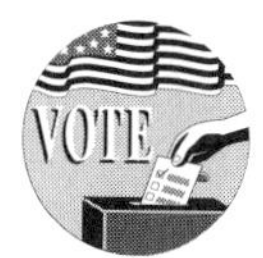


Stop the medical "authorities" from harassing legitimately credentialed M.D.s who are successfully treating cancer. Express your dissatisfaction by contacting your state and federal elected officials.

For more information about the **systematic harassment** of Dr. Taylor, see Chapter 26: How Cancer Politics Have Kept You in the Dark, pp. 694-695.

Dr. Taylor is concerned that many physicians, alternative as well as conventional, become overly fixated on the various tools of cancer treatment, and overlook the profound therapeutic role played by psychospiritual support. "If you don't provide the patient with hope, chances are they will lose touch with their deeper desire to heal in the first place," says Dr. Taylor. "The real art of medicine lies in guiding the person's spirit toward a greater sense of personal meaning and wholeness, a sense that their life is worth living and worth fighting for."

***The physician who evinces compassion and an optimistic outlook will help the patient far more than the physician who offers only a grim prognosis, says Dr. Taylor.***

Fear and depression are generally the result of the standard diagnosis of cancer, Dr. Taylor says. Their continued presence in the emotions of the patient stimulates the production of destructive hormones such as cortisone which in turn *cause* the cancer to spread. "Unless the hope of healing is present, a downward destructive cycle is likely to take place in the patient. False hope is the result of misinforming the patient. It occurs most frequently in the use of radiation and chemotherapy. This is false hope *tripled.*" First, the treatment does no good; second, it causes unnecessary side effects; and third, it is an unnecessary expense. False hope can be avoided by giving the patient and family comprehensive information concerning treatment options, and statistics re-

***"If you don't provide the patient with hope, chances are they will lose touch with their deeper desire to heal in the first place," says Dr. Taylor.***

garding benefits and their possible complications. Incidentally, recommending hospice care before attempting the many benefits of alternative care robs many patients of their final and last hope. Many patients consigned to the hopelessness of hospice care could be successfully treated—as many as 18% according to one famous cancer doctor in Germany.

As the scientific method gained control of medicine, the *art* of practice receded, explains Dr. Taylor. "I contend that a resurgence of the art of medicine will increase the cure rate for cancer. Practitioners of the art will place more emphasis on compassion and understanding and the effects of these emotions on the disease process." They will engender more confidence and hope because many studies indicate that a treatment works better when the patient *believes* in it.

As for the future of alternative cancer therapies, Dr. Taylor points out that a radical transformation in our way of thinking about scientific proof will be needed. Alternative medicine doctors use nontoxic treatments that cannot be "proven" successful under the current scientific model (double-blind, placebo-controlled studies). Dr. Taylor's decades of clinical observation, however, have led him to conclude that these therapies improve the quality of life and, in many cases, extend life as well. "The treatment program I've outlined here is one that supports good health. It may not be a 'miracle' cure, but it is surely good medicine."

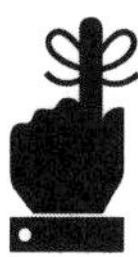

*The concept of a single magic bullet is a conceptual, physiological, and medical mistake. A far more useful clinical model is that presented by alternative medicine: multiple interacting and interdependent factors contribute to the emergence of cancer and multiple modalities, substances, and practitioners contribute to its reversal.*

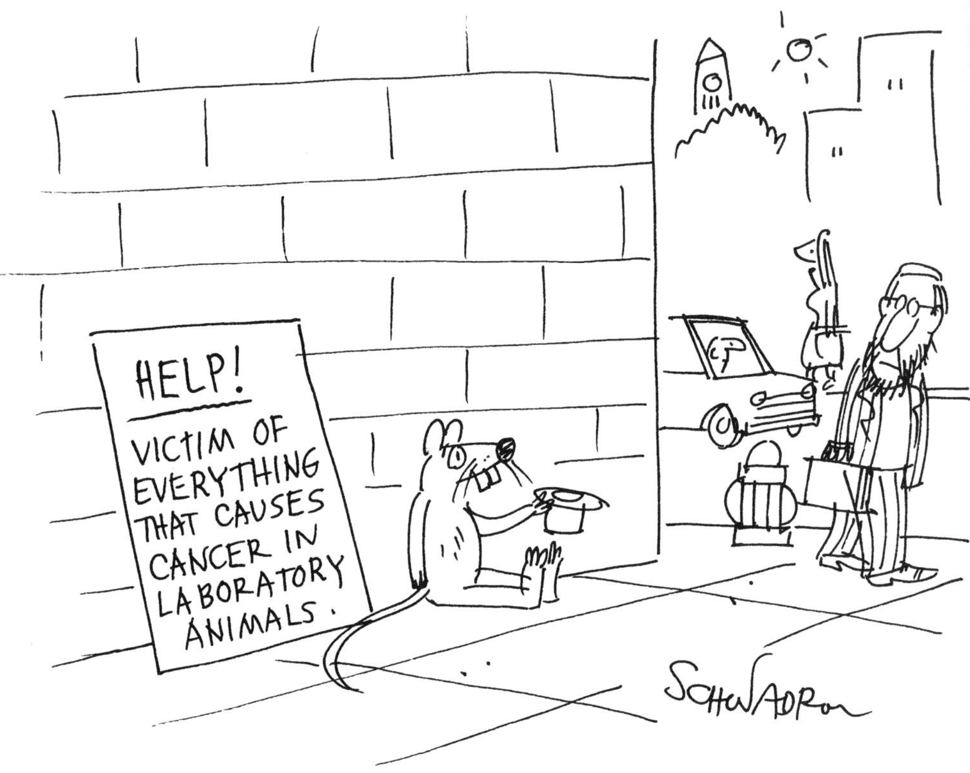
HELP!
VICTIM OF EVERYTHING THAT CAUSES CANCER IN LABORATORY ANIMALS.
SCHWADRON

# *Part Two*

# Criteria for Successful Cancer Treatment

## *Cancer—Its Nature, Causes, Politics, Detection, and Prevention*

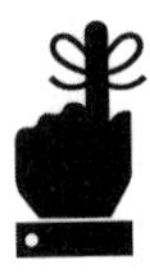

*Curing typically refers*

*to a medical treatment that*

*relieves the patient of the disease.*

*Healing, by contrast,*

*refers to an internal process of*

*"becoming whole," a feeling of*

*harmonious relationship*

*with one's social and familial*

*sphere—indeed, with one's*

*entire environment.*

Chapter 24

# What Is Cancer?

**Despite its seeming chaos, cancer is inherently a rational process that can be defined and explained according to physiological and biochemical principles. Once you understand how the cancer process works, effective therapies can be marshaled to stop it, making life after cancer a medical reality.**

From a biological viewpoint, cancer is fundamentally a rational process. Once its physiological and biochemical mechanisms are understood, however, therapeutic approaches can be successfully deployed against it, in many instances producing stabilizations, remissions, and, practically speaking, life after cancer. Without this understanding, however, appropriate treatments are unlikely, as is the case when rational treatment is approached solely by conventional medical thinking and practices.

## A Chaotic Process within the Rational Order of Biology

Cancer is a disease process in which healthy cells stop functioning and maturing properly. A mishap occurs inside these cells. Perhaps it begins with a change (mutation) in the genetic blueprint, its DNA. The altered DNA makes copies of itself and passes its information and gene sequencing on to other cells, which then become cancer prone. As the normal cycle of cell creation and death is interrupted, the newly mutated cancer cells begin multiplying uncontrollably, no longer operating as an integrated and harmonious part of the body.

In its simplest terms, cancer represents an accelerating process of inappropriate, uncontrolled cell growth—a chaotic process within the order of biology. Cancer cells, when examined under a microscope, are abnormally shaped, inconsistently formed, and disorganized and contain misshapen internal structures—the essence of biological disorder. Cancer, despite its horror for the individual, is a natural phenomenon: it represents the body's response to a continuous attack on its balancing and regulatory mechanisms by numerous factors—33 known contributing causes are discussed in Chapter 25 (What Causes Cancer?).

Cancer may seem to us a modern epidemic, but traces of cancer have been detected in the bones and skulls of mummies from Egypt and Peru embalmed 5000 years ago. Hippocrates (circa 400 B.C.), the renowned Greek physician, first coined the term "carcinoma" to indicate skin cancer; to him, this Greek word (karkinoma, which means "crab") is like a crab because of the way a spreading cancer extends claw-like extensions across the cell, tissue, or skin. What is different today is the incidence of cancer: it is steadily affecting more people each year, specifically 1 out of every 3. It is no longer one serious disease among many, but the disease of our time.

***In its simplest terms, cancer represents an accelerating process of inappropriate, uncontrolled cell growth—a chaotic process within the order of biology.***

The development and growth of a cancer is called carcinogenesis. Physicians now understand that it involves many steps, beginning with specific, undesirable changes in the nucleus of the cell, specifically in its genetic components, the DNA. What distinguishes a cancer process from life-as-usual in the cell is that normally—in a state of health—DNA mutations are repaired or rendered harmless by the immune system, an intricate, multifaceted biochemical defense system. When undesirable genetic alterations remain uncorrected, then a cancer process can potentially escalate to its next stage of uncontrolled rapid growth.

It does this by making copies of itself. This replication, again, is a normal function of DNA, but the trouble here is that it is altered, mutated, and undesirable DNA that is copying itself. As more cancer cells are generated, the process continues to expand and form a tumor. The normal mechanisms of cell growth, replication, differentiation, and maturation then become unregulated, leading to chaos in the body.

Modern oncology (the study of tumors) needs to radically rethink its cancer model, which is based on the Halstead theory of cancer (developed by W. S. Halstead, 1852-1922). G. Zajicek, M.D., of the H. H. Humphrey Center for Experimental Medicine and Cancer Research at Hebrew

University-Hadassah Medical School in Jerusalem, Israel, argues that the Halstead theory, whose central premise is that the primary fact about cancer is the tumor, not the patient as a living organism, must be dropped in favor of a more systemic model.[1]

The fact that the age-adjusted mortality rate for breast cancer has remained virtually unchanged for 60 years (from 1930-1990) means that the standard treatments devised to kill tumors have failed because they are "based on false premises," says Dr. Zajicek. "This hypothesis implies that tumor removal should cure the patient, yet 60 years of intensive effort to remove the tumor did not change the biological outcome of the disease. Obviously, the hypothesis is wrong and should be modified." Focusing medical efforts at removing the tumor is fundamentally a mistake, argues Dr. Zajicek, and will not cure cancer because cancer is "a metabolically systemic deficiency" and "a chronic system disease."[2] Halstead's cancer theory is flawed, says Dr. Zajicek, because it emphasizes the tumor and ignores the patient.

## Cancer Classifications, Types, and Stages

Among the 150 different types of cancer, 5 major groups are conventionally recognized. Carcinomas form in the epithelial cells that cover the surface of the skin, mouth, nose, throat, lung airways, and genitourinary and gastrointestinal tract, or that line glands such as the breast or thyroid. Lung, breast, prostate, skin, stomach, and colon cancers are called carcinomas and are solid tumors.

Sarcomas are those that form in the bones and soft connective and supportive tissues surrounding organs and tissues, such as cartilage, muscles, tendons, fat, and the outer linings of the lungs, abdomen, heart, central nervous system, and blood vessels. Sarcomas are also solid tumors, but sarcomas are both the most rare of malignant tumors and the most deadly.

Leukemias form in the blood and bone marrow and the abnormal white blood cells produced there travel through the bloodstream creating problems in the spleen and other tissues. Leukemias are not solid tumors; they are characterized by an overproduction of abnormal white blood cells.

Lymphomas are cancers of the lymph glands. Lymph glands act as a filter for the body's impurities and are concentrated mostly in the neck, groin, armpits, spleen, the center of the chest, and around the intestines. Lymphomas are usually made up of abnormal lymphocytes (white blood cells) that congregate in lymph glands to produce solid masses. Hodgkin's disease and non-Hodgkin's lymphomas are the 2 most prevalent types of lymphoma in the United States, while Burkitt's lymphoma, rare in the U.S., is common in Central Africa.

Myelomas are rare tumors that arise in the antibody-producing plasma cells or hemopoietic (blood cell-producing) cells in various tissues in the bone marrow.

A key characteristic of cancer cells is their greatly prolonged life spans compared to that of normal cells. It's ironic, given that cancer can potentially prove fatal to its host and thus to itself as an unwelcome "parasite," that cancer cells are essentially immortal. Not only do cancer cells not die when they are supposed to, they also fail to develop the specialized functions of their normal counterparts. Masses of cancer cells may become like parasites, developing their own network of blood vessels to siphon nourishment away from the body's main blood supply. It is this process, that, unchecked, will eventually lead to the formation of a tumor—a swelling caused by the abnormal growth of cells. If the tumor invades adjacent normal tissue or spreads through lymph vessels or the blood vessels to other normal tissues, this tumor is considered malignant.

***It's ironic, given that cancer can potentially prove fatal to its host and thus to itself as an unwelcome "parasite," that cancer cells are essentially immortal.***

Technically, many people carry harmless tumors within their bodies, even until their death from other causes. Such benign tumors are encapsulated by fiber, functionally insulating the body from their otherwise toxic effects. At a certain point, these tumors simply stop enlarging; since they do not "seed" other tumors, they are considered benign. A malignant tumor, which is not encapsulated by fiber, is capable of invading nearby cells and spreading to distant sites within the body. If the cancer cells do not spread beyond the tissue or organ where they originated, the cancer is considered to be localized; if the cancer spreads to other parts of the body, it is then said to have metastasized.

The pathological character of such tumors stems from their cells' ability to invade other tissues and travel through the blood and lymphatic vessels to other areas of the body. Most cancer victims die not from the initial multiplication of these abnormal cells, but as a result of this secondary

## Differentiation in Cancer

Differentiation is a process by which unspecialized cells mature and become specialized to carry out specific tasks. At birth, a human infant has an estimated 5 trillion cells differentiated into about 100 different cell types. Differentiated cells—red blood cells, for example—have a preset life expectancy and are programmed to live, die, and be replaced on a precise schedule. In cancer, there is an abnormal control over the way in which a cell becomes specialized. Generally, a poorly differentiated cancer, in which the tumor cells bear almost no resemblance to normal cells of that particular tissue, is the most virulent and dangerous. Tumors that are moderately differentiated generally pose a more favorable outcome, with survival likelihood, even under conventional medicine, extending into years or decades. A well-differentiated cancer, though less common than a moderately differentiated one, can be indolent and sometimes nonmalignant.

process, metastasis—the spread of cancer to other organs and tissues of the body. This process represents the cancer cells' tendency to break off from the original tumor, float in the bloodstream, and colonize other tissues.

Cancers that metastasize quickly—that is, even when the total number of cancer cells is still small—are generally considered aggressive, which means, more malignant. Aggressive tumors contain cells that are generally less "mature" from a cellular point of view; that is, they are less physically defined and lack some of a cell's standard constituents. It is often said of these cells that they are less well-developed or well-differentiated.

Looking more specifically at the subject of aggressiveness in cancers, oncologists usually allocate the following categories: an aggressive cancer has a doubling time of 60 days or less (meaning how long it takes for the cancer mass to double its size); a moderate cancer doubles in 61-150 days; an indolent cancer doubles in 151-300 days; and a very indolent cancer takes up to 300 days. For a sense of perspective, the average size of a breast cancer when first detected by mammography is about 600 million cells, or about 1/4 inch across; the average size detectable by manual palpation has about 45 billion cells and may be 1 1/4 inches in diameter.

Another characteristic of cells that metastasize is that they exhibit little or no "cell-to-cell adhesion." Most normal cells, by contrast, tend to adhere to one another to form well-defined tissues. The notable exceptions to this are circulating blood cells, which move freely about the body. To a lesser extent, the degree of malignancy depends on the rate at which the cells reproduce and cause tumors to expand. Tumors can either be slow-growing or fast-growing; either way, the tendency is fairly fixed.

In other words, those that grow rapidly and are likely to metastasize will tend to remain aggressive, while those that are less aggressive do not commonly change their behavior; they usually remain slow-growing.[3] Larger tumors—those weighing a few pounds—usually require years to develop, since the body imposes various restraints on cell reproduction. However, prostate cancer is usually slow, but often after treatment, especially conventional treatment, it can become very aggressive.

Once metastasis has occurred, cancer is more likely to be fatal, unless checked or reversed by successful multimodal alternative therapies. Metastasis can lead to the formation of more tumors, which further sap the body's energy supply, weakening (and eventually poisoning) the patient with toxins that make one feel fatigued, achey, depressed, and apathetic. Eventually, the unchecked growth overwhelms other body functions. Whatever the immediate cause, the cancer-related death is usually preceded by metastasis and by the establishment of "secondary cancers" that grow as a result of metastasis from the primary tumor site.

## Staging in Cancer

In terms of tumor size and severity, oncologists (physicians who specifically treat cancer) distinguish 4 different phases, which they call stages. "Staging" refers to an index used by cancer specialists to determine how much cancer exists in the body, its size, location, and containment or metastasis. *Stage I*, the earliest, most curable stage, shows only local tumor involvement. *Stage II* has some spreading of cancer to the surrounding tissues and perhaps to nearby lymph nodes; *Stage III* involves metastasis to distant lymph nodes; *Stage IV*, the most advanced and least easily cured, refers to cancer that has spread to distant organs.

## How the Cancer Process Can Become Life-Threatening

Many, if not most, cancer deaths come as a result of infection by bacteria, viruses, and fungi—microbes that normally would be destroyed by the immune system. In the case of cancer, the immune system becomes severely suppressed, partly because of the systemic weakening brought on by the cancer process and partly because of the negative, toxic effects of conventional cancer treatment—essentially, chemotherapy, surgery, and radiation.

A tumor can directly interfere with the functioning of a vital organ, such as the lungs, liver, pancreas, brain, or kidneys, in effect, strangulating it. When a cancerous mass becomes too large, it steals nourishment from the organ, secreting toxins into it, or causing some form of physical obstruction that effectively shuts the organ down.

## Understanding Clinical Terms: What Is a Cancer "Marker"?

A cancer or tumor marker generally refers to any of a variety of standard laboratory blood tests used to measure the level of a protein material or other chemical produced by cancer cells. These numbers become elevated in the presence of a cancer or tumor. Technically, X rays and scans (such as CT, or computerized tomography) are cancer markers because they can determine with specificity the presence and location of cancer in the body, but the term cancer "marker" usually indicates a blood test.

**Here are a few of the different cancer markers for different kinds of cancer:**

- CEA (carcinoembryonic antigen) test for colon cancer
- AFP (alpha-fetoprotein) test for liver cancer (primary hepatocellular carcinoma)
- PSA (prostate specific antigen) for prostate cancer
- CA (carcinoma) 27.29 for breast cancer
- CA 125 for ovarian cancer

Ideally, after treatment, the numbers go down, indicating that the cancer has been eliminated. If the person is retested some time later and the numbers are again elevated, the indication is that the cancer has either recurred in that area, spread to lymph glands nearby, or metastasized to another organ.

For example, a man's PSA for prostate cancer might test above 4.5 units, which is at the upper end of the acceptable range. After being treated with alternative or conventional methods, his PSA might drop to 0.4 (0 is the bottom of the scale). If, some months later, his PSA jumps to 40, the cancer may have metastasized to the lymph nodes or bone, which are the most common areas of metastasis in prostate cancer. He could then be tested with a nuclear bone scan and/or an alkaline phosphate blood test to determine if the tumor has spread to the bone.

A less specific cancer marker is the AMAS (anti-malignin antibody screen) which detects cancer in the body in general. It has the advantage of being able to detect cancer in its early stages and also screens for all types of cancer (with the exception of leukemia).

For more information about **laboratory tests** to detect the earliest signs of cancer, see Chapter 27: Early Detection and Prevention of Cancer.

Severe malnutrition or emaciation, which is a condition of cellular starvation called cachexia (pronounced cah-CHECK-see-yah) may affect up to 90% of all advanced cancer patients and account for 50% of all cancer deaths.[4] The cancer process effectively starves cancer patients, using up their energy reserves. These effects primarily result from the body's shifting to an inefficient use of fuel sources, as well as the person's loss of appetite.

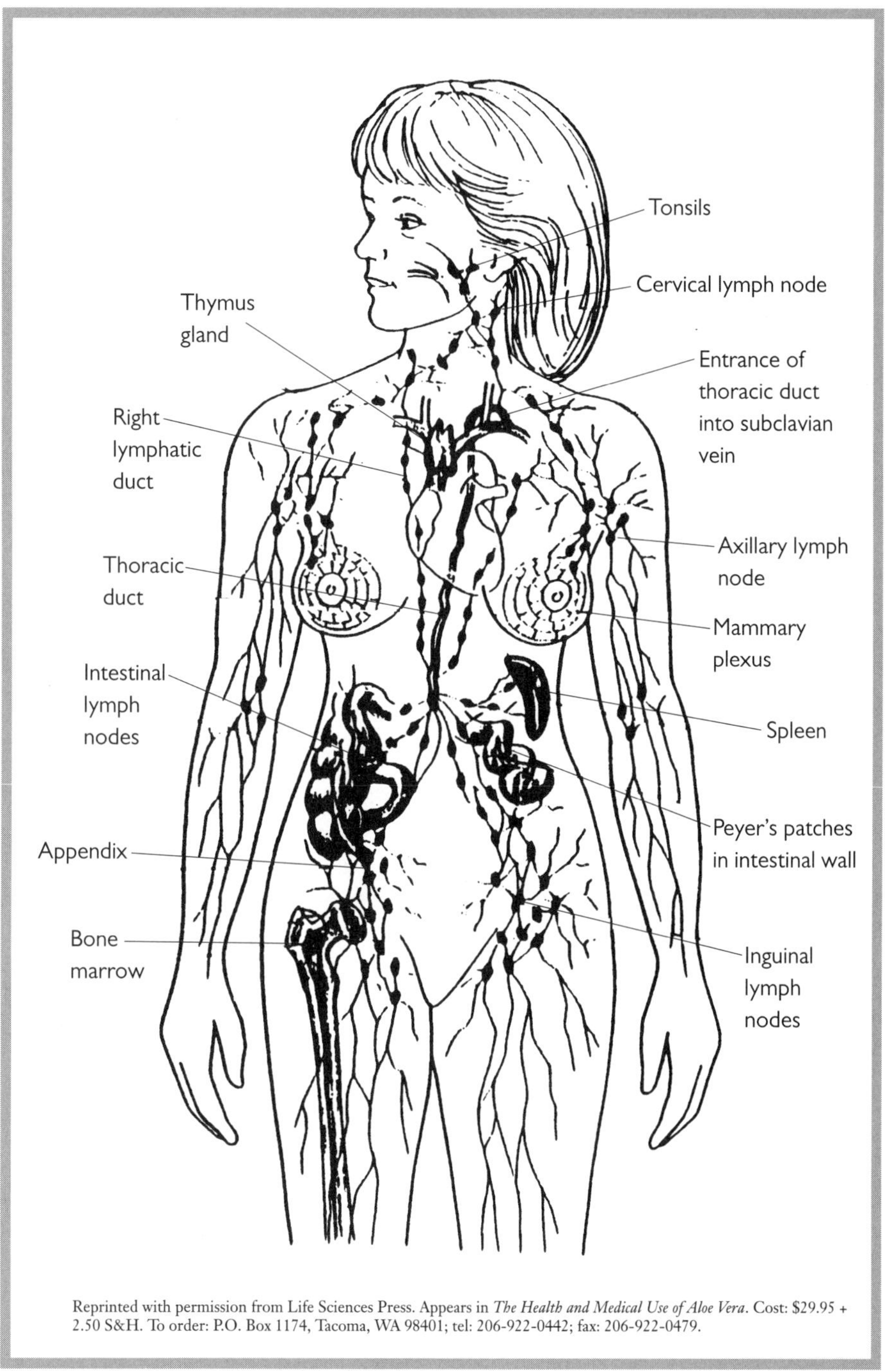


Reprinted with permission from Life Sciences Press. Appears in *The Health and Medical Use of Aloe Vera*. Cost: $29.95 + 2.50 S&H. To order: P.O. Box 1174, Tacoma, WA 98401; tel: 206-922-0442; fax: 206-922-0479.

**Figure 24.1—The lymphatic system, showing the major lymphatic organs and vessels**

# The Major Players in Your Immune System

**Immune System:** The immune system guards the body against foreign, disease-producing substances. Its "workers" are various white blood cells including 1 trillion lymphocytes and 100 million trillion antibodies produced and secreted by the lymphocytes. Lymphocytes are found in high numbers in the lymph nodes, bone marrow, spleen, and thymus gland.

**Antibodies:** An antibody is a protein molecule containing about 20,000 atoms, made from amino acids by B lymphocyte cells in the lymph tissue and set in motion by the immune system against a specific antigen (foreign and potentially dangerous protein). An antibody is also referred to as an immunoglobulin and may be found in the blood, lymph, colostrum, saliva, and the gastrointestinal and urinary tracts, usually within 3 days after the first encounter with an antigen. The antibody binds tightly with the antigen as a preliminary for removing it from the system or destroying it.

**Lymph Nodes:** Lymph nodes are clusters of immune tissue that work as filters or "inspection stations" for detecting foreign and potentially harmful substances in the lymph fluid. Acting like spongy filter bags, lymph nodes are part of the lymphatic system, which is the body's master drain. Cells inside the nodes examine the lymph fluid, as collected from body tissues, for foreign matter. While the body has many dozens of lymph nodes, they are, as noted previously, mostly clustered in the neck, armpits, chest, groin, and abdomen.

Lymph fluid flows in the lymphatic vessels throughout the body, helping to maintain the fluid level of cells and carrying various substances from the tissues to the blood. The human body has 1-2 quarts of lymph fluid, accounting for 1.5%-3% of body weight.

**Thymus and Spleen:** The thymus, located behind the breastbone, secretes thymosin, a hormone that strengthens immune response. It also instructs certain lymphocytes to specialize their function. The spleen is like a large lymph node except that it filters blood rather than lymph fluid.

**Lymphocyte:** A lymphocyte is a form of white blood cell, representing 25-33% of the total count, whose numbers increase during infection. Lymphocytes, produced in the bone marrow and found in lymph nodes, come in 2 forms: T cells, which are matured in the thymus gland and have many functions in the body's immune response; and B cells, which produce antibodies to neutralize an antigen.

**Immunoglobulin:** Each lymphocyte produces a specific antibody or immunoglobulin. There are 5 main types of immunoglobulins, grouped according to their concentration in the blood: IgG, IgA, IgM, IgD, IgE.

**T Cells:** T cells specialize their immune function to become helper (CD4), suppressor (CD8), or natural killer (CD56) cells. Helper cells facilitate the production of antibodies by the B cells. Suppressor cells suppress B-cell activity.

**Natural Killer Cells:** Natural killer (NK) cells are a type of nonspecific, free-ranging immune cell produced in the bone marrow and matured in the thymus gland. NK cells can recognize and quickly destroy virus and cancer cells on first contact. "Armed" with an estimated 100 different biochemical poisons for killing foreign proteins, they can kill target cells without having encountered them previously. As with antibodies, their role is surveillance, to rid the body of aberrant or foreign cells before they can grow and produce cancer. Decreased numbers of NK cells have been linked to the development and progression of cancer, as well as chronic and acute viral infections and other deficiencies of the immune system.

**Macrophages:** Macrophages are a form of white blood cell (originally produced in the bone marrow and called monocytes) that can "swallow" germs and foreign proteins, then release an enzyme that chemically damages, kills, or neutralizes whatever is ingested. The name means "big" (macro) "swallower" or "eater" (phage). Macrophages are the vacuum cleaners and filter feeders of the immune system, ingesting everything that is not normal, healthy tissue, even old body cells or cancer cells.

**Neutrophil:** A neutrophil is a mature white blood cell formed in the bone marrow and released into the blood where it represents 54-65% of the total number of leuokocytes. Leukocytes are white blood cells divided into 6 types (neutrophils, basophils, eosinophils, monocytes, B-lymphocytes, T-lymphocytes) and 2 groups, according to the shape of the nucleus and the presence or absence of granules within the cells; one group includes primarily neutrophils, the other includes lymphocytes. The principal activity of the neutrophil is to ingest foreign particles, especially virulent bacteria and fungi.

**Interferon:** Interferon, familiar to many as a cancer treatment, is a natural protein produced by cells in response to a virus or other foreign substance. Vitamin C and certain herbs can also stimulate its production.

**Interleukin:** Interleukin is a class of proteins with various immune functions including T-cell activation.

Protein-calorie malnutrition is not uncommon among hospitalized patients in general, and can lead to overall weakness, apathy, increases in mortality and surgical failure, a reduction in immunity, and poor responsiveness to treatment. Some cancer patients die from hemorrhage (uncontrolled blood loss from a failure of the blood to clot), which is a frequent cause of death in leukemia, but can also occur when a tumor grows into a large blood vessel. Cancer can impair the blood's ability to form clots and internal bleeding can occur readily and persistently. Cancer can also cause excessive clotting and the formation of thrombi (plural of thrombus, which is a blood clot attached to the interior wall of a vein or artery), cutting off the blood supply to a vital organ.

For information on the **immune system**, see Chapter 25: What Causes Cancer?, pp. 544-551.

## Conventional Medicine Is Losing the War on Cancer

The number of new cancers reported annually has increased steadily since the 1960s, as have cancer-related mortality rates for a variety of cancers.

In 1900, a mere 3% of deaths were attributed to cancer, yet today, that number has jumped by 8 times—to 24%. To put this in perspective, this is an 800% increase in less than a century.

The National Cancer Institute reports a 28% rise in the incidence of childhood cancers from 1950 to 1988. Against some of the more common cancers in the United States—lung, liver pancreas, brain, and bone, as well as advanced cancers of the colon, breast, and prostate—little or no progress has been made in conventional medicine's super-expensive "War on Cancer," since it was declared in 1971 by then-president Richard Nixon.

For information on the **politics of cancer**, see Chapter 26: How Cancer Politics Have Kept You in the Dark.

Cancer is the number one health concern of every American, and for good reason. In 1996, about 1.3 million people in the U.S. will be diagnosed with cancer and more than half this number will probably die from the disease or its treatment. That's about one American life lost to cancer every 45 seconds. "Despite some gains, cancer death rates remain unacceptably high, and the disease will kill 554,740 people in the U.S. this year," wrote J. Madeleine Nash in a special edition of *Time* magazine that summarized conventional cancer treatments.[5]

Cancer now kills more children between the ages of 3 and 14 than any other illness.[6] Of greater concern is the fact that the numbers of both new cancer cases and deaths continue to rise. From 1950 to 1980, there was an 8% increase in cancer deaths,[7] but from 1975 to 1989, the number of new cancer cases reported each year increased 13% and the mortality rate rose 7%.[8] Although mortality rates for a few less common cancers declined, overall rates have continued to rise.[9]

A look at individual cancers paints a more ominous picture. From 1973 to 1987, melanoma (a form of skin cancer) increased by 83%, non-Hodgkin's lymphoma by 51%, and lung cancer by 32%.[10] Of these, lung cancer has become the leading cancer killer among men and women alike, surpassing breast cancer, which was the leading cause of death among women until 1986. In addition, rates of brain, kidney, breast, and prostate cancers have also risen. Specifically, for the incidence of lung cancer in women, between 1973-1990, there was a 100% increase.

Regarding prostate cancer, one estimate cites a 600% increase since 1985 in new cases—"the fastest rise in cancer detection ever recorded." One out of every 5 males born in the 1990s are likely to develop prostate cancer, compared to only one out of 10 females who will probably develop breast cancer.[11] The 30-year trend (1960-62 to 1990-92) for deaths from lung cancer is up 85% for men and up 438% for women; up 29% for prostate; up 4% for breast cancer; up 12% for female pancreatic cancer. The rate of death from some cancers has dropped over this same period: colon and rectum, -9%; male pancreas -5%; male leukemia, -9%; female colon and rectum, -31%; and ovary, -8%.[12]

Breast cancer is perhaps the best example of the changing global picture of cancer. For many years, the incidence and mortality rates for breast cancer have been highest in the U.S. and Northern Europe and lowest in Asia and Africa. In recent years, steep increases have been reported in Asian and Central European populations; thus the size of the differences in rates between such countries as Japan and the U.S. is much less than previously. The annual incidence of breast cancer worldwide is predicted to be more than one million cases by the year 2000.

By the year 2000, scientists expect to see a further increase in cancer mortality rates. They also predict by the year 2000 an estimated 10 million cancer patients and survivors alive in the U.S.[13] The hardest hit will be the elderly, who in the coming decades are expected to experience increases in incidence rates for all cancers, but particularly for those of the colon, rectum, pancreas, stomach, lung, bladder, and prostate; half of these people will probably die within 5 years. Although these are dismal forecasts, they should not be taken as guaranteed outcomes, given that they do not include successful alternative medicine therapies as part of the equation. They do indicate, however, that conventional medicine has failed to stem the tide of this disease.

***Although these are dismal forecasts, they should not be taken as guaranteed outcomes, given that they do not include successful alternative medicine therapies as part of the equation. They do indicate, however, that conventional medicine has failed to stem the tide of this disease.***

According to John C. Bailar III, Ph.D., professor of epidemiology and biostatistics at McGill University in Toronto, Canada, conventional medicine is decidedly losing the war on cancer. In 1993 he declared: "In the end, any claim of major success against cancer must be reconciled with this figure," referring to the steady increase in cancer deaths between 1950 and 1990. "I do not think such reconciliation is possible and again conclude [as he had

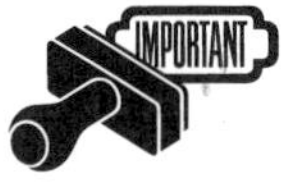

in 1986 when making a similar retrospective review of data] that our decades of war against cancer have been a qualified failure. Whatever we have been doing, it has not dealt with the broadly rising trend in mortality."[14]

Dr. Bailar's data, confirmed by the National Cancer Institute, holds that overall U.S. cancer death rates (adjusted for changes in the size and composition of the population with respect to age) went up by 7% between 1975 and 1990. From 1950 to 1990, the increase was from about 158 deaths per 100,000 people to about 172 deaths. In a review article discussing trends in cancer epidemiology, even as stalwart a defender of the medical status quo as *Scientific American* admitted of cancer that it is "a war not won." The casualty report "from the war on cancer shows that the effort has not slowed deaths from the disease in the U.S."

***The cost to patients and taxpayers for 20+ years of waging "war" against cancer has been 1 trillion dollars as Americans made an estimated 50 million cancer-related visits to doctors.***

Cancer is crippling America's health-care system. Despite spending over $35 billion on cancer research between 1975 and 1995, conventional medicine has made little progress in understanding the underlying causes for the rapid rise of cancer rates or in finding safe and effective treatments. The cost to patients and taxpayers for 20+ years of waging "war" against cancer has been 1 trillion dollars.[15] In pursuit of the elusive goal of a cancer cure, Americans made an estimated 50 million cancer-related visits to doctors and were exposed to countless diagnostic procedures to find out whether they had the disease.

In recent years, about 10% of annual health-care expenditures in the U.S.—an unbelievable sum of $96 billion annually—has been spent on cancer treatment alone.[16] In appreciating these numbers, one must also factor in that the direct cost of hospital care for cancer is considerably higher than the cost of hospital care for other diseases. Most (83%) of the direct expenditures for cancer care are attributable to breast, colorectal, lung, and prostate cancer, in that order.

How does this translate for the person in need of cancer care? The average conventional treatment charge to Medicare (for all types) is $14,205 for the initial 3 months; after this, the cost is just over $800 monthly. For the final 6 months of "terminal treatment" (for cancer patients who don't survive), the average Medicare charge is approximately $23,000.[17] These staggering costs have little to show for them in terms of having successfully stemmed the tide of human death and suffering from cancer.

Spokespersons for conventional cancer care frequently tout 5-year survival rates as indicative of progress and money wisely spent. However, a critical analysis of these numbers reveals such claims to be illusory. The public relations experts of the American Cancer Society claim that more cancer patients are living at least 5 years after their diagnosis than ever before. The facts are that between 1974 and 1976 and 1981 and 1987, the 5-year-survival rates rose only 2%, from 49% to 51%, and for cancers of the liver, lung, pancreas, bone, and breast, 5-year survival rates are about the same as they were in 1965.[18]

***Spokespersons for conventional cancer care frequently tout 5-year survival rates as indicative of progress and money wisely spent. However, a critical analysis of these numbers reveals such claims to be illusory.***

The 5-year mark is used as a yardstick for "cure" by conventional oncologists. It doesn't matter if you die of cancer one day after the 5-year mark, you are still counted among the cases cured. Since many people die not long after 5 years, this can be a highly misleading statistic. For example, the 5-year survival rate for breast cancer is about 75%, but the extended survival rate (beyond 5 years) is less than 50%. Similarly, while the 5-year survival for prostate cancer is about 70%, the 10-year survival rate is only about 35%.[19]

Even the small overall increase in 5-year survival for all cancers may be an exaggeration, since many diagnostic tests in use today enable earlier diagnosis, which makes the survival time only appear longer than in the past. For instance, consider the woman whose breast cancer is diagnosed an average of 3 years earlier because of mammography; today she might live for 7 years. In 1985, using the older diagnostic and treatment tools, this same woman would have appeared to live only 4 years. Nothing has changed in terms of the effectiveness of conventional therapy, and yet the breast cancer patient appears to live longer, owing to the improved screening measures. The "success" exists only on paper.

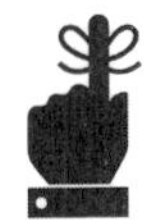

These statistics, flawed and misleading, as they are already, do not factor in the far longer survival times commonly produced by physicians using alternative modalities of cancer care.

These statistics, flawed and misleading as they are already, do not factor in the far longer survival times commonly produced by physicians us-

A PREVENTION PRIMER

## Eight Telltale Signs of Cancer

The message of prevention is that you can beat cancer before it becomes advanced. The key is to detect the presence of cancer early enough so you can treat it with the immune-enhancing, nontoxic treatments of alternative medicine. These methods work best when the body's tumor burden is relatively small—in the earliest phases of the cancer's development.

Here are signs that may indicate the presence of cancer.

1. **A Lump or Thickening in the Breast or Testicles.** Self-examination of the breast and testicles offers women and men the best protection against breast and testicular cancer. A lump or thickening in the breast, or any noticeable change in the testicles, are early warning signs. Such signs are immediate grounds for a medical examination.
2. **A Change in a Wart or Mole.** Changes in warts or moles may be indicative of melanoma or squamous carcinoma. Skin cancers may appear as dry, scaly patches, as pimples that never go away, or as inflamed or ulcerated areas. Warts or moles that grow or bleed should be checked, as should sores in the mouth that persist.
3. **A Skin Sore or a Persistent Sore Throat That Does Not Heal.** Sores that do not heal may also be indicative of melanoma. A persistent sore throat, hoarseness, a persistent lump in the throat, or difficulty swallowing, may indicate cancer of the pharynx, larynx, or esophagus. These cancers are readily treated when caught early.
4. **A Change in Bowel or Bladder Habits.** Continuing urinary difficulties, constipation, chronic diarrhea, abdominal pains, rectal or urinary bleeding, or dark tar-like stools should not be ignored; they should be regarded as signals to seek professional help.
5. **A Persistent Cough or Coughing Blood.** Coughs that become chronic, especially in smokers, should be checked. If there is a cancer in the air passages into the lungs, they may be partially obstructed or irritated or even bleed. Coughing may be a sign of this obstruction or irritation.
6. **Constant Indigestion or Trouble Swallowing.** Difficulties in swallowing, continued indigestion, nausea, heartburn, bloating, loss of appetite, and bowel changes all may be symptoms of colon cancer or cancer of the stomach or esophagus. Unexplained weight loss is also an indicator.
7. **Unusual Bleeding or Vaginal Discharge.** The early stages of uterine endometrial cancer and later stages of cervical vaginal cancer exhibit signs of unusual bleeding or vaginal discharge. Prompt attention to these symptoms means a better chance of catching cancer at its most treatable stage. In the case of cervical cancer, Pap tests can detect problems before the later stages cause bleeding.
8. **Chronic Fatigue.** General feelings of chronic fatigue will often accompany any type of cancer that is rapidly progressing.

If you are experiencing any of these signs and symptoms, contact your physician immediately.

ing alternative modalities of cancer care. Nor do they account in any way for the radical degree to which alternative medicine applied to cancer care could profoundly shift the outcomes from dismal to successful. A rational person will ask why this isn't already so. Powerful economic and political forces are arrayed against alternative medicine—generally and for cancer, specifically—precisely because of its promise of remarkable success at less cost. These forces are delineated in Chapter 26: How Cancer Politics Have Kept You in the Dark Regarding Successful Alternative Treatments.

## You Don't Have to Settle for Conventional "Strategies of Containment"

About the best that spokespersons for the conventional cancer establishment can say in summarizing more than 25 years of cancer research is: "we're making headway." As *Scientific American* editors John Rennie and Ricki Rusting state in their September 1996 issue, entirely devoted to cancer: "There is no way to skirt the fact that the combined death rate for all cancers has yet to come down." Short of finding a "single cure" that would "kill the tumor"—which, *Scientific American* admits, seems unlikely—the article concludes that the current option is to settle for "strategies of containment."[20]

***Powerful economic and political forces are arrayed against alternative medicine—generally and for cancer, specifically—precisely because of its promise of remarkable success at less cost.***

The message of this book is altogether different: You don't have to settle for strategies of containment while you wait for scientists to discover that single magical cure for cancer. The physicians presented in this book offer clinical proof—drawn from their copious patient case records—of successful multimodal alternative approaches to cancer. None of these physicians will ever speak in terms of a "single cure" for cancer. Medically, this is a sophomoric notion, not founded in physiological realities.

These physicians speak about multiple treatments and substances working together—synergistically—to effect major changes in the cancer process, from containment to remission to a life that is cancer free. "Synergy" in alternative medicine treatments means many substances work cooperatively in such a way as to enhance the overall effect, making it stronger than single substances could ever produce alone. More important, even though there are dismaying cancer statistics—see the table on pages 534-537—our doctors insist that you do not have to become a statistic.

Cancer reversal is quite possible, but it requires some effort, commitment, and trust on the part of the person involved, and a comprehensive knowledge by the physician of the modalities available and their effectiveness as proven in clinical practice.

Mortality from certain cancers may seem statistically likely, but that is an illusion compounded by fear and ignorance. It's not only patients who fear cancer outcomes; probably most oncologists are equally in fear of this disease and shield themselves against the disturbing scenarios, statistics, and probabilities they know too well. The physicians represented in this book offer patients the statistics of optimism. Men and women can and do survive cancer, and go on to live long, productive, healthy lives—cancer free.

***The physicians represented in this book offer patients the statistics of optimism. Men and women can and do survive cancer, and go on to live long, productive, healthy lives—cancer free.***

Most of the patient stories in this book present the cancer treatment from the physician's viewpoint. Here is an insightful narrative of the cancer process and its reversal by the person most affected—a woman with cancer.

## Daring to Heal My Cancer with Nutrition—Cheryl Wilkens' Story[21]

Cancer survivor Cheryl Wilkins writes: What prompts a person with cancer to say no to chemotherapy and radiation? As suspicions build today that scientists are misfiring in their battle with cancer, more people like myself are investigating other ways of treatment. One third of Americans are now choosing alternative care, and not just those needing cancer treatment. But if you want to know about cancer, I have a firsthand understanding on why this is so.

My own medical experiences opened my mind to alternative medicine. It all began in July 1991 when a tumor on my knee and 3 moles on my back were surgically removed. The surgeon told me the tumor was merely fatty and the moles were benign. The following month the lump returned to the same place on my knee, but all he said was "it's scar tissue, don't worry about it."

In December, I was back in his office again because the lump had grown dramatically and it felt hot. No longer thinking it was scar tissue, he operated at once. He told me it was a high-grade malignancy, a kind of cancer called histiocytoma. He said he was sure he got it all with his scalpel.

But the next day the lab said he had to cut out an even bigger chunk of my knee, which he did, leaving me with a 15-inch scar, somewhat disabled, and in constant discomfort.

Two weeks later I sat in the oncologist's office. He glanced through my medical file then recommended the maximum treatment of chemotherapy and radiation over the next 6 months to kill any remaining cancer cells. He said he wanted to check with other institutions over the weekend for a second opinion. But when I saw him again the next week and asked him what he had learned, he said he had gone skiing instead. When I told him I'd be seeking a second opinion at the Mayo Clinic in Rochester, Minnesota, and with New York City physician Dr. Nicholas Gonzalez, he abruptly stood up and walked out.

***"When you are diagnosed with cancer, you are introduced to yourself. You find out what you are made of," says cancer survivor Cheryl Wilkens.***

One of the first shocks I got at the Mayo Clinic was that while my surgeon had said there was no evidence of a malignant melanoma, when the Mayo Clinic doctors examined the pathology slides for my moles they called it "a superficial spreading level 3 melanoma." They also told me, for the first time, what the likely side effects of chemotherapy for the histiocytoma might be, such as damage to my kidneys, heart, and gallbladder.

Back home again, my surgeon asked me to visit his office. He "warned" me that I had been the topic of conversation for 15 top cancer specialists and that none of them had heard of Dr. Gonzalez' metabolic-nutritional therapy. They all said I shouldn't waste my time on a New York City "quack." The way the surgeon looked at me would have crushed the hopes of many patients, I'm sure, but when he saw I wasn't convinced, he looked uncomfortable, dropped his surly posture, and changed the subject.

He pulled out a report from the National Cancer Institute that said there basically weren't grounds for believing chemotherapy would be effective for my histiocytoma. Yet here he was telling me I should go through with it because alternative treatments were useless. Meanwhile, my knee wasn't working right because the surgeon had removed my patella tendon. Of course nobody told me about this until much later, when I discovered it by reading through my records. Now my knee wasn't strong enough for me to even walk upstairs.

# Cancer Symptoms and Statistics

| TYPE OF CANCER | POSSIBLE SYMPTOMS (If these occur, see your physician for a physical exam and/or lab tests.) |
|---|---|
| Bladder cancer | Blood in urine, making it look bright red or rust-colored; pain or burning upon urination; frequent urination; feeling the need to urinate but nothing comes out; urine may appear cloudy because it contains pus |
| Breast cancer | A lump or thickening of breast; discharge from the nipple; retraction of the nipple; change in skin of breast, such as dimpling or puckering; redness, swelling, feeling of heat; enlarged lymph nodes under arm |
| Colorectal cancer | Rectal bleeding (red blood in stools or black stools); abdominal cramps; constipation alternating with diarrhea; weight loss; loss of appetite; weakness; pallid complexion |
| Kidney cancer | Blood in urine; dull ache or pain in back or side; lump in kidney area; sometimes accompanied by high blood pressure or abnormality in red blood cell count |
| Leukemia | Weakness, paleness; fever and flu-like symptoms; bruising and prolonged bleeding; enlarged lymph nodes, spleen, liver; pain in bones and joints; frequent infections; weight loss; night sweats |
| Lung cancer | Wheezing "smoker's cough," persisting for months or years; increased, sometimes blood-streaked, sputum; persistent ache in chest; congestion in lungs; enlarged lymph nodes in the neck |
| Melanoma | Change in a mole or other bump on the skin including bleeding, or change in size, shape, color, or texture |
| Non-Hodgkin's lymphoma | Painless swelling in the lymph nodes of the neck, underarm, or groin; persistent fever; feeling of fatigue; unexplained weight loss of more than 10% in a 6-month period; itchy skin and rashes; small lumps in skin; bone pain; swelling in some part of abdomen; liver and spleen enlargement |
| Oral cancer (oral cavity, lip, pharynx) | May often feel a lump in the mouth with the tongue; sometimes a sore spot can be felt while eating or drinking; ulceration of the lips, tongue or other area inside the mouth that does not heal within 2 weeks; dentures may no longer fit well; or in advanced cases, oral pain, bleeding, foul breath, loose teeth, and changes in speech |
| Ovarian cancer | Frequently, few symptoms; abdominal swelling; in rare cases, abnormal vaginal bleeding; women over 40 may experience generalized digestive discomfort |

| POSSIBLE RISKS | 5-YEAR SURVIVAL RATES (all stages) PER CONVENTIONAL TREATMENT | ESTIMATED # OF NEW U.S. CASES FOR 1996 |
|---|---|---|
| Twice as high in whites as in blacks; 2-3 times higher in men as in women; 2-3 times higher in cigarette smokers as in nonsmokers; machinists, truck drivers, and workers exposed to chemicals | 80.7% | 52,900 |
| Increasing age; early menstruation; late menopause; not having a child or having first child after 30; family or personal history; inherited breast cancer gene | 83.2% | 185,700 |
| Polyps, ulcerative colitis, or Crohn's disease; family history; residence in urban or industrial area; specific genetic mutations | 61% | 133,500 |
| Being overweight; twice as high in men as in women; twice as high in cigarette smokers as in nonsmokers; coke-oven and asbestos workers | 57.9% | 30,600 |
| Specific genetic abnormalities (e.g., Down and Bloom syndromes); excessive exposure to ionizing radiation and chemicals such as benzene; HTLV-1 virus exposure | 68.6% | 27,600 |
| Cigarette smoking; secondary smoke; asbestos, radiation, radon, or other toxic exposure | 13.4% | 177,000 |
| Sun exposure, particularly during childhood; sunburning or freckling easily; 40 times higher in whites as in blacks | 86.6% | 38,300 |
| Lowered immune system function as with HIV and HTLV-1 viruses; recipients of organ transplants; possibly exposure to herbicides | 51% | 52,700 |
| More prominent in males, with predisposing factors including tobacco and pipe smoking and chewing tobacco; radiation and other toxic exposures | not available | 28,150 |
| Increasing age; never pregnant; residence in industrial country (Japan excluded); family history of breast or ovarian cancer; inherited breast cancer gene | 44.1% | 26,700 |

## Cancer Symptoms and Statistics (cont.)

| TYPE OF CANCER | POSSIBLE SYMPTOMS (If these occur, see your physician for a physical exam and/or lab tests.) |
|---|---|
| Pancreatic cancer | Upper abdominal pain and unexplained weight loss; pain near the center of the back; loss of appetite; intolerance of fatty foods; yellowing of the skin (jaundice); abdominal masses; enlargement of liver and spleen |
| Prostate cancer | Urination difficulties due to blockage of the urethra; bladder retains urine, creating frequent feelings of urgency to urinate, especially at night; may have difficulty stopping urination; urine stream may be narrow; bladder doesn't empty completely; burning, painful urination; sometimes bloody urine; tenderness over the bladder and dull ache in the pelvis and back |
| Uterine cancer | Abnormal vaginal bleeding of fresh blood, or a watery bloody discharge in a postmenopausal woman (70-75% of all cases are postmenopausal); a collection of fluid may also occur in the uterus; painful urination; pain during intercourse; pain in pelvic area |

*Cancer statistics obtained from *CA—A Cancer Journal for Clinicians* 45:1 (1995), 8-28: Report by the Surveillance Branch of the Department of Epidemiology and Surveillance, American Cancer Society, Atlanta, GA; and "Twelve Major Cancers," *Scientific American* (September 1996), 126-132.

I thought about things. I'm 43. There is cancer in my family. My father, grandfather, and great grandfather all died of cancer. With that kind of history, I thought: maybe it's time to take a different approach to treatment. When you are diagnosed with cancer, you are introduced to yourself. You find out what you are made of. And when you choose an alternative therapy, you find yourself living in a glass house. People watch what you do—they watch everything—and often with a skeptical eye.

In February the next year, or 7 months after my first office visit for my knee problem, I walked into the Park Avenue offices of Nicholas J. Gonzalez, M.D., in New York City for my first 2-hour appointment. I was reassured to learn that he tapes his office visits for future reference. I suppose I wasn't quite as desperate as many of his patients who come to him bearing prognoses of 2-3 months more to live, after having survived un-

| POSSIBLE RISKS | 5-YEAR SURVIVAL RATES (all stages) PER CONVENTIONAL TREATMENT | ESTIMATED # OF NEW U.S. CASES FOR 1996 |
|---|---|---|
| Increasing age; cigarette smoking; higher in countries with high-fat diets; higher in blacks than whites | 3.6% | 26,300 |
| Increasing age; 37% higher in blacks as in whites, with twice the mortality rate | 85.8% | 317,100 |
| **Cervical:** cigarette smoking; sex before 18; many sexual partners; low socioeconomic status; mortality rate twice as high for blacks as whites<br><br>**Endometrial:** Early menstruation; late menopause; never pregnant; estrogen exposure, estrogen replacement therapy without progestin; tamoxifen; diabetes, gallbladder disease, hypertension, and obesity | 68.3% | 49,700 |

successful courses of surgery, radiation, and chemotherapy. Still, the results from his analysis of my blood and hair weren't good news. I had a great deal of cancer in my body, most of it in my lymphatic system.

I saw Dr. Gonzalez again the next day for 2 hours when he laid out the details of his comprehensive program of metabolic therapy. This is based on the 25 years of research by a dentist named Dr. William Donald Kelley who developed a program featuring nutrition, detoxification, and supplements as a way of treating many degenerative diseases, including cancer. Dr. Kelley described 10 categories of metabolic types. As he saw it, there are 10 different body styles of needing and assimilating foods. Nutritional therapy should be based on this, he said. Dr. Gonzalez spent 5 years studying cancer patients in Dr. Kelley's program to be sure it worked.

As I drove back home, I thought that maybe more doctors should ask

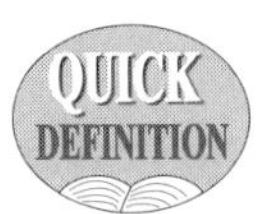


**Kelley's Metabolic Therapy** is a cancer treatment that consists of individualized nutrition, detoxification, and supplementation with pancreatic enzymes. Dr. Kelley, originally a dentist who made his discoveries in the late 1960s while seeking a cure for his own pancreatic cancer, recognized that individuals have different food requirements and ways of digesting and assimilating nutrients. On this basis, he classified 10 different metabolic types for which dietary and nutritional programs must be specifically adjusted. Examples include slow-oxidizing vegetarians and fast-oxidizing carnivores. Specific foods that contain the raw materials needed to improve the blood levels identified in the testing are recommended, and the overall dietary pattern is designed to match the metabolic type.

patients about their bowel movements. All my life I have been constipated. If I went once a week, I considered that normal. Now I see how abnormal and toxic that was, how it contributed to my illness. And I thought: if a body is smart enough to create a disease, then it makes sense that it must be smart enough to cure it, too.

I began to figure out how best I could make Dr. Gonzalez' program work for me. It called for a daily regimen of, literally, 150 vitamins, minerals, and enzymes, starting at 3:30 A.M. I had to do 4 coffee enemas a day, starting at 2 A.M., to help rid my system of the toxins being released as the tumor dissolved. This would especially help my liver and gallbladder, which would respond quickly to the caffeine and contract vigorously, releasing stored wastes.

About once a month I did a special bowel clean-out (Dr. Gonzalez calls it the "clean sweep") using psyllium seed husks and a bentonite liquid. This really scrubbed out my colon. Along with this I did a liver flush (using olive oil, apple juice, ortho-phosphoric acid, and other ingredients) to help purify my liver. Both of these procedures took about a week.

There were other practices I didn't have to do but that Dr. Gonzalez often prescribes to cancer patients. There is a detoxification program Dr. Gonzalez calls the "purge." You drink a mixture of citrus fruit juices and Epsom salts. This is to aid in the rapid removal of metabolic wastes from the body. Dr. Gonzalez also has patients do skin rubs, salt and soda baths, mustard foot soaks, and castor oil compresses—and again, all of this is to draw the toxins out of the body.

I had to start eating organically grown foods and whole grains, only meats produced without hormones or antibiotics, raw vegetables and fresh fruits, fresh juices, especially 8 ounces of carrot juice every day, and no canned, processed, or deep-fried foods.

I figure that by the end of my first year on the Gonzalez program I drank the juice from over 2000 pounds of carrots and an untold amount of apples. I avoided refined sugar out of consideration for my pancreas; I avoided aluminum cooking utensils, as well as aluminum-containing deodorants and lotions. White flour, soybean products, and peanuts also had no place in my diet as part of this program.

# Cancer Information Resources on the Internet

**http://www.casidi.com**
CASIDI (Cancer and Serious Illness Defense Interface) is based upon the most successful principle of medicine: prevention. The site is designed to allow users to assess their cancer risk. This site was developed and maintained by Lawrence W. Taylor, M.D., a physician profiled in Chapter 23 in this book.

**http://cancerguide.org**
Developed by kidney cancer survivor Steve Dunn, this site reviews the clinical merits and research regarding numerous alternative cancer therapies and substances, such as bovine cartilage, Essiac, and antineoplastons.

**http://www.graylab.ac.uk/cancerweb**
This is an England-based multimedia information resource for oncology, providing data on conventional approaches mostly with links to other sites and bibliographic resources.

**http://telescan.nki.nl**
This site is based in the Netherlands and provides information to cancer health professionals, researchers, and patients; it includes ongoing discussions.

**http://cancer.med.upenn.edu** Also known as OncoLink, this site provides information on types of cancer, treatment options, clinical trials, and online patient support services; it offers extensive information-searching tools.

**http://biomed.nus.sg:/Cancer/ biomed.nus.sg/cancer**
Known as CancerNet, this site offers completely conventional medical information about cancer provided by the National Cancer Institute.

**http://nysernet.org/bcic/**
An information clearinghouse on breast cancer with links to numerous conventional medicine organizations (e.g., American Cancer Society, New York State Department of Health), as well as hospitals, libraries, hospices, support groups, and nonprofit agencies.

**http://www.alternativemedicine.com**
This site, maintained by Future Medicine Publishing (the publisher of this book), offers access to all issues and contents of *Alternative Medicine Digest*, an Interactive Index enabling users to research health conditions, and other practical features central to alternative medicine.

**http://www.healthy.net**
Sponsored by HealthWorld Online, this site provides information on both conventional and natural health (alternative medicine) through 11 information centers (e.g., health clinics, books, professional association network, library of health and medicine) and 15,000 electronic pages of health data.

**http://www.allabouthealth.com**
This site embodies a new general health magazine in electronic format by Toronto publisher Terry Borsook. It features the latest research findings, events, trends, books, software, products, articles, commentaries, and numerous links to other relevant web sites.

**http://www.healthoasis.com**
This site bills itself as "the first private health club in cyberspace," comprising a membership that wants to lose weight, improve their health, enhance their spiritual outlook on life, eat better, or develop an exercise program. The site also offers access to 3000 products (nutritional and herbal supplements, books, tapes), as well as news and the latest health information.

Sometimes I had doubts about it all. I would say to myself: "Who do you think you are that you can drink some carrot juice, pop vitamins, do coffee enemas, and get well when there are sophisticated technologies for cancer?" Except they aren't winning the cancer war with these supposed marvels.

My doubts usually came when I wasn't feeling well or was overtired. My husband was a strong support. "It's a done deal," he'd say whenever he saw me in these funks. He meant that, as far as he was concerned, this was the best and only way to whip cancer. That made me able to trudge on. How do you eat an elephant? One bite at a time. The same applies to completing a comprehensive regimen like this one. Just hit away at it one day at a time until it becomes second-nature to you—which took me about 3 years, by the way. Anyway, the alternative to the alternative—conventional medicine—doesn't really work.

***"Looking back at the last 40 years of cancer research, it seems like digging in your pocket for a coin that's not there. The alternative to the alternative—conventional medicine—doesn't really work," Cheryl Wilkens says.***

Looking back at the last 40 years of cancer research, it seems like digging in your pocket for a coin that's not there. Somewhere in my healing journey I took on the attitude of this Chinese proverb: "Man who says it will not work shouldn't disturb man who's making it work." And I thought: Until God opens another door, this alternative treatment is the best for me.

Perhaps my greatest discouragement comes from the fact that a program like this, that works, is not covered by insurance even though it costs less than chemotherapy. I paid for this all out of my own pocket. The supplements ran me about $400 a month and my 2 sessions with Dr. Gonzalez cost $1,800. It was a huge financial burden, yet it was a price I was willing to pay to get well. Of course it meant I had to keep my full-time job as church secretary during this period even though Dr. Gonzalez generally recommends you concentrate your time on healing.

Today, after 3 years on Dr. Gonzalez' program, I am nearly cancer free. According to a standardized blood test used by conventional cancer doctors, I do not have any cancer. But according to the more refined test that Dr. Gonzalez uses, I still have some cancer activity. So I will always have to keep up a nutritional maintenance program.

Am I lucky? Yes, I am lucky—lucky to have taken control of my own health care. Lucky to have been introduced to this form of treatment. Lucky not to have burned up my body with chemotherapy and radiation. Let me tell you something a little grim. In the 3 years I've been on this program, I have known many people with cancer who chose chemotherapy and radiation. They are now either dead or on yet another chemotherapy series for a relapse. Yes, I am lucky!

## Basic Tenets of Alternative Medicine

Although alternative medicine includes a wide range of treatment options of varying approaches, all the therapies are based on a common philosophy that includes the following elements:

- focuses on empowering you to accept responsibility for at least part of the task of recovery and health maintenance in the future
- emphasizes the importance of nutrition as an essential requirement for good health
- considers a balanced lifestyle (proper exercise, sleep, relaxation, and emotional tranquility) a prerequisite for optimum health
- attempts to ensure the efficiency of your body's organs and organ systems (through detoxification, nutritional supplements, and related whole-body approaches)
- recognizes that your musculoskeletal system provides a vital link between nerve transmission and energy pathways and is in direct relationship with internal and emotional states
- treats *you* rather than your symptoms

## What Alternative Medicine Offers Cancer Care

With cancer claiming so many lives each year and bringing sickness and disability to so many more, the search for a cure has become a global industry. Yet, as enticing as the idea of a "magic bullet" for cancer may seem, because of the multiple factors related to the disease, conventional medicine may never find it. As this book explains, the concept of a single magic bullet is a conceptual, physiological, and medical mistake.

A far more useful clinical model is that presented by alternative medicine: multiple interacting and interdependent factors contribute to the emergence of cancer and multiple modalities, substances, and practitioners contribute to its reversal.

For more information on **Kelley's Metabolic Therapy**, see Chapter 28: Nutrition as Cancer Medicine, pp. 777-779.

Alternative therapies offer the advantage of bolstering the patient's own self-healing capacities while avoiding the toxic side effects that accompany conventional medical treatment for cancer. For most alternative medical doctors, the practical starting point is a change in a patient's diet, exercise, and attitudes. By helping to rejuvenate the whole person, these strategies also offer an improved quality of life and a sense of control in the healing process.

***One study found that 88% percent of the spontaneous remission cancer cases involved a significant dietary change, mainly toward vegetarianism.***

Unlike conventional therapies, which actually weaken the body over time, alternative therapies work to support the body's anticancer defenses and detoxification capacities as much as possible. This may explain why the phenomenon of "spontaneous remission—the sudden, unexplained recovery from cancer, without any recognized (i.e., conventional) treatment—is so rare in the typical hospital setting. One study found that 88% percent of the spontaneous remission cancer cases involved a significant dietary change, mainly toward vegetarianism.[22] Many cases also entailed some form of alternative therapy, such as nutritional supplementation and botanical medicine.

A paradoxical situation exists in the language used to describe cancer outcomes. Conventional medicine speaks freely of "cures" when they discuss the fabled magic bullet, but they prohibit (and often punish) alternative practitioners from using the word; yet conventional oncology rarely cures cancer. There is a crucial distinction here, one that has special relevance to the problem of cancer.

***Multiple interacting and interdependent factors contribute to the emergence of cancer and multiple modalities, substances, and practitioners contribute to its reversal.***

Curing typically refers to a medical treatment that relieves the patient of the disease. Healing, by contrast, refers to an internal process of "becoming whole," a feeling of harmonious relationship with one's social and familial sphere—indeed, with one's entire environment. Thus healing pertains to all levels of a person's being, and the most powerful alternative cancer therapies are those aimed at strengthening all these levels at the same time—at reducing the body's toxic burden while also enhancing its multifaceted self-healing capacities and bringing the true character of the individual into focus and healthy expression.

Chapter 25

# What Causes Cancer? Its Origin Is Multifactorial

**If there is a single truth about cancer that is beyond argument, according to the clinical results and testimonies of the many physicians consulted for this book, it is that cancer has multiple, interacting causes. Many interdependent factors—at least 33—in various combinations can contribute to the development of cancer in a given individual.**

If there is a single truth about cancer that is beyond argument, according to the clinical results and testimonies of the many physicians consulted for this book, it is that cancer has multiple, interacting causes. As much as science strives to identify *single* precipitating factors—such as genes or infectious organisms—practitioners of alternative medicine know there is no single cause for cancer, just as there is no single magic bullet therapy or substance to end it. Many *interdependent* factors contribute to the development of cancer. In fact, this chapter will present detailed information on 33 distinct contributing factors that, in various combinations, can begin a cancer process in a given individual.

## A Gradual Systemic Poisoning Then Weakening of the Body

The concept that cancer is the result of multiple factors impinging on an individual's mind, body, and organic systems is actually not a new one, but it is one that has been consistently ignored by conventional cancer doctors. For example, in 1958, Max Gerson, M.D., an alternative cancer treatment pioneer (profiled in this book under Gerson Diet Therapy in Chapter 28: Nutrition as Cancer Medicine) explained in general terms how cancer results.

First, there is a slow buildup of toxicity throughout the body, especially the liver which is responsible for most of the body's detoxification, leading to a functional alteration of most systems including the chemical balance between sodium and potassium in the cells. Next comes a lowering of electrical potentials in the vital organs, a further accumulation of poisons, a reduction in the activity and supplies of oxygen, and the preliminary mutation of some normal cells into cancer cells, said Dr. Gerson. With this, cancer starts, "general poisoning increases, vital functions and energies decrease, and cancer increases," said Dr. Gerson. There next comes a further destruction of the metabolism (energy extraction from food) and liver functioning as the "cancer rules" and spreads.[1]

Today, we talk more in terms of immune system dysfunction and perhaps less in terms of sodium and potassium balances, but Dr. Gerson's basic insight of a progressive, systemic poisoning and weakening is still valid. In fact, it is even more valid today than in the 1950s as we are routinely subjected to far more toxins in our environment today and have become increasingly aware of their harmful effects, particularly with respect to the cancer process.

As Robert O. Becker, M.D., noted authority on the health perils and medical promise of electromagnetic energy, explains, everyone is

## 33 Factors That Contribute to Cancer

- Sunlight
- Chronic Electromagnetic Field Exposure
- Geopathic Stress
- Sick Building Syndrome
- Ionizing Radiation
- Nuclear Radiation
- Pesticide/Herbicide Residues
- Industrial Toxins
- Polluted Water
- Chlorinated Water
- Fluoridated Water
- Tobacco and Smoking
- Hormone Therapies
- Immune-Suppressive Drugs
- Irradiated Foods
- Food Additives
- Mercury Toxicity
- Dental Factors
- Nerve Interference Fields
- Diet and Nutritional Deficiencies
- Chronic Stress
- Toxic Emotions
- Depressed Thyroid Action
- Intestinal Toxicity and Digestive Impairment
- Parasites
- Viruses
- Blocked Detoxification Pathways
- Free Radicals
- Cellular Oxygen Deficiency
- Cellular Terrain
- Oncogenes
- Genetic Predisposition
- Miasm

constantly exposed to substances and energies, from chemicals to X rays, that can potentially start a cancer process. "As a result, we are always developing small cancers that are recognized by our immune system and destroyed." The healthy body can normally handle individual carcinogenic influences, but when they become multiple and cumulative, the body begins to weaken, and this is the point at which harmful influences may gain the upper hand. "Any factor that increases the growth rate of these small cancers gives them an advantage over the immune system," says Dr. Becker, and cancer emerges.[2]

Dr. Becker's observation underscores a key concept involving cancer: cancer cells—an estimated 300, but more if the body has been exposed to carcinogens—are created every day in healthy human beings. What's a mere 300 out of an estimated 30 trillion cells that comprise the human body? Cancer cells, in moderation, are a legitimate part of nature. The difference between a person with cancer and a person with fleeting cancer cells is that in the latter the immune system is able to eliminate the aberrant cells from the system before they are able to do any damage to the body or start an illegitimate growth process culminating in a tumor. As naturopathic physician and educator Joseph Pizzorno, N.D., explains, "When the immune system is not working well, the result is frequent or chronic infections, chronic fatigue, and, eventually, cancer."[3]

On a microscopic level, cancer is Nature's way of removing defective genetic material, says Victor Marcial-Vega, M.D., a cancer doctor profiled in Chapter 13. Cancer reflects a change or mutation in the DNA, a cell's genetic makeup, but this process is defensive and occurs all the time. "The body is creating throughout life and every once in a while something goes amiss. At this point, the body says, 'Oh, this didn't come out that well, let's get rid of it.' The purpose of a cancer cell is to signal the body to get rid of matter in the body that did not replicate normally." The immune response is the body's way of cleaning up defective DNA.

Out of billions of DNA replications occurring in the body each day, several will become abnormal and may lead to cancer. In fact, in an average lifetime, the human body goes through an estimated $10^{16}$ (ten thousand trillion) cell divisions. Those who practice good diet, exercise, and other preventive lifestyle measures may reduce their cancer risk as low as 10%. Despite the astronomic number of cell divisions, the body's cellular defense system is able to hold cancer incidence down to 1 case in every $10^{17}$

cell divisions.[4] "This is the way Nature intended it. When cancer cells occur—and everyone has abnormal cells arising in their bodies throughout the day—they are readily detected and removed by a *healthy* immune system." The immune system helps maintain and revitalize the body by eliminating cancer or otherwise abnormal cells. Only when the immune system weakens can the cancer cells multiply and spread through the body, says Dr. Marcial-Vega.

What makes the immune system weaken is a multiplicity of stress factors, collectively known as carcinogens. Technically, carcinogens refer to chemicals or radiation with cancer-causing potential, but for the purposes of general understanding, we use the term carcinogen more broadly here. Carcinogens as we define them include chemicals, electromagnetic energy, faulty diet, free radicals, genetic predisposition, toxicity, radiation, parasites, strong emotions, and viruses—among others. There are dozens of potential influences, which we will review in this chapter. These are not so much "causes" of cancer, as facilitators: they edge the body into a condition of weakness, vulnerability, and immune dysfunction. In this condition, the ordinary production of a few cancer cells can gain the upper hand in the molecular life of the individual, and a cancer process is initiated.

***"When cancer cells occur—and everyone has abnormal cells arising in their bodies throughout the day—they are readily detected and removed by a* healthy *immune system," says Dr. Victor Marcial-Vega.***

Depending on a person's biochemical and psychological makeup, certain stressors will play a more primary role. The key concept is that the cumulative effect of many carcinogens and immune-suppressing agents all acting together is a weakening of the immune system, thereby allowing cancer cells to proliferate. In this chapter, we'll chart the activity of carcinogens, from ones seemingly removed from the human being (sunlight and electromagnetic energy) to influences closer to the body (pesticides and polluted water), to those that change the nature of the body (food), to ones that work inside the body (free radicals), to ones that may have preceded one's birth (genetic influences).

## Defining a Carcinogen—Initiators and Promoters

The term "carcinogen" is an umbrella term to denote a substance or energy that begins or promotes the cancer process. Literally, the term means to "start" (*genesis*) "cancer" (*carcino*, from the Greek *karkinos* for the crab or cancer). These can be put into 2 categories.

First, there are substances called initiators or triggers that damage genes that normally control the proliferation of cells. When a single cell accumulates various changes or genetic mutations, over a period of months or years, it will eventually escape from the ordinary restraints on cell growth. Defects (changes or mutations) in the DNA become embedded in the genetic materials passed from one cell generation to the next, making it a permanent mutation. The cell grows and produces "offspring" or descendants that are increasingly free of the normal growth constraints. The result is a tumor.

Second, there are cancer promoters. These substances do not damage genes but support the growth of tumor cells or their precursors. After the initiation of the cancer process, the disease will often lie undetected for many years; during this phase, cancer promoters can selectively enhance the growth of tumor cells at the expense of healthy cells. In this way, they further the cellular damage, allowing cancer cells to continue spreading abnormally. Promoters can also hamper the removal of initiated cells by the immune system, make certain tissues a more favorable growth habitat for the tumor, and start the migration of cancer cells to other sites in the body, planting the cancer process like seeds. This later process is called metastasis.

The probability is that if a person gets enough exposure to carcinogens, cancer tumors can and will develop even if the immune system is fairly healthy. This is due to the concept of the total body tumor burden—that is, the sum of all factors suppressing the immune system including the cancer cells themselves. A cancer tumor or leukemia develops when there is either an increased production of cancer cells because of excess facilitators (causes) or a decreased removal of cancer cells from the body because of clogged lymphatic drainage or weakened immunity.

## The Immune System—the First Line of Anticancer Defense

Most tumors never make it beyond the microscopic stage; they disappear before we have a chance to know they exist. In the language of orthodox oncology, these tumors "spontaneously regress." The obvious implication is that certain immune system components stop cancer in its tracks. Could it be that these immune factors largely determine the cancer patient's survival and help explain the anecdotal reports of "spontaneous remission?"

Given that each of us is constantly exposed to carcinogens in our food, air, and water, resulting in the production of cancer cells within the body, and that, normally, the immune system recognizes and destroys these cells before they have a chance to multiply, we can say this means that having abnormal cells develop is probably *not* the critical factor in determining the course of cancer. The primary threat of cancer may result instead from the body's inability to *eliminate* the abnormal cells even when they are few in number.

Many oncologists and medical immunologists now believe that cancer emerges as a result of a functional breakdown or imbalance in the immune system—indeed, as "a prime example of failure of the immune system."[5] The immune system may produce too much of a particular substance and not enough of another, resulting in a diminished ability to resist cancer and other immune-related illnesses.

The immune system has a way to assess whether normal cells have been transformed into cancer cells. This is the job of the specialized white

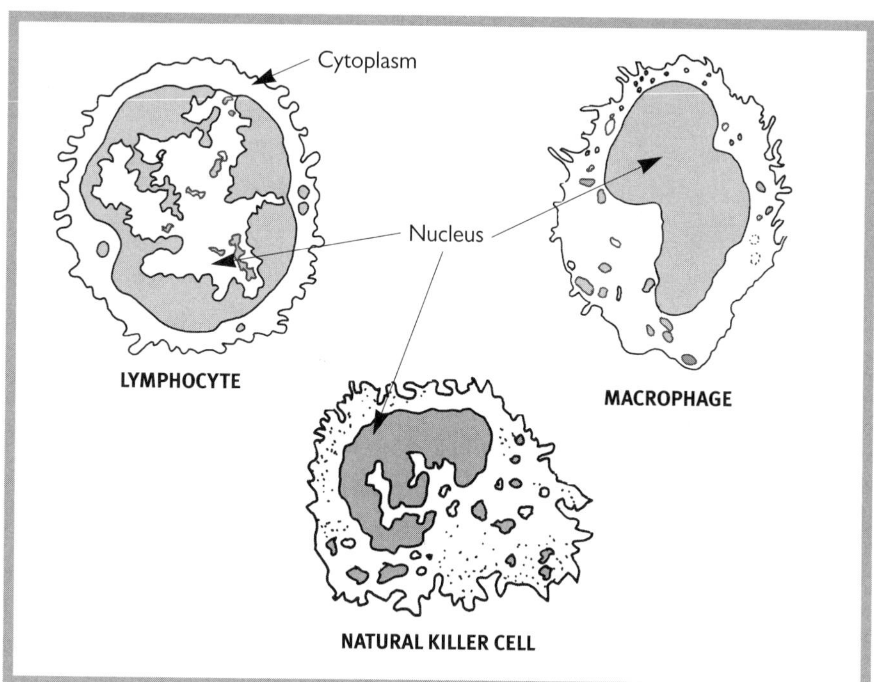


**Figure 25.1— Immune system cells**

**Natural Killer** cells are a type of nonspecific, free-ranging immune cell produced in the bone marrow and matured in the thymus gland. NK cells can recognize and quickly destroy virus and cancer cells on first contact. "Armed" with an estimated 100 different biochemical poisons for killing foreign proteins, they can kill target cells without having encountered them previously. As with antibodies, their role is surveillance, to rid the body of aberrant or foreign cells before they can grow and produce cancer or infection.

**Macrophages** are a form of white blood cell (originally produced in the bone marrow and called monocytes) that can "swallow" germs and foreign proteins, then release an enzyme that chemically either damages or kills the substance. The name means "big" (macro) "swallower" or "eater" (phage). Macrophages are the vacuum cleaners and filter feeders of the immune system, ingesting everything that is not normal, healthy tissue, even old body cells.

blood cells known as T lymphocytes, or T cells. Derived from the thymus gland, these cells travel throughout the body to detect unusual cells and tumor-associated antigens—foreign proteins released by tumor cells. Lymphocytes represent 25 to 33% of the total white blood cell count, which increases during certain infections. Lymphocyte counts may stay the same or decrease slightly in the presence of bacterial infections.

Lymphocytes, produced in the bone marrow, actually come in two forms: the T cells that mature in the thymus gland (behind the breastbone) and have many functions in the body's immune response; and B cells that produce antibodies to neutralize foreign matter in the blood and tissues and are matured by passing through the bursal equivalent in the Peyer's patches surrounding the intestines. Each B lymphocyte produces a single and specific type of antibody. Certain types of T cells signal other white blood cells that cancer cells are present. Some lymphocytes can produce various anticancer chemicals, known to oncologists as cytokines which include tumor necrosis factor, interleukin, and interferon. These are the body's own "chemotherapy," except they don't harm healthy cells as administered chemotherapy does.

Melanoma, a potentially deadly form of cancer, is one of the human tumors most extensively studied for its immunologic characteristics. Evidence for the immune system's involvement in melanoma includes the presence of specific T-cell and antibody responses upon exposure to melanoma cells; also, the more of these T cells present, the longer the melanoma patient's survival.[6] Again, the many anecdotal reports of "spontaneous remission" of cancer among "terminal" melanoma patients suggest that the body naturally has the means to rid itself of this cancer.[7]

One of the body's most immediate and powerful means of protection against cancer results from the action of natural killer (NK) cells. They are a specialized form of lymphocyte capable of migrating to the site of cancer and destroying the malignant cells before they can divide.[8] NK cells afford constant surveillance against cancer. Their "killer" reputation—it comes from the "attack" mentality of conventional medicine—is based on the fact that, without any prior exposure to the abnormal cells, they can cause cells to split or break apart.[9]

In the normal immune system, NK cells will descend directly on a minuscule tumor and begin devouring and disintegrating it. As a consequence, many tumors never make it beyond this asymptomatic stage; however, NK cells have little effect against large tumors. Their main value is in protecting against the spread of micrometastases, those tiny, blood- and lymph-borne accumulations of cancer cells that would otherwise seed new tumor growth.

Macrophages support the body's detoxification channels by scavenging debris and storing wastes. These cells, a major part of the body's first line of defense, destroy cancer cells by splitting them apart and ingesting them; they also regulate cell reproduction as well as the activities of other immune cells. Macrophage function alone can ultimately determine whether tumor cells thrive or die.[10] The increased activity of macrophages has been associated with decreased tumor growth and decreased tumor incidence in animals.[11]

## 33 Factors That Contribute to Cancer

### SUNLIGHT

Solar radiation, or sunlight, particularly ultraviolet-B and ultraviolet-C radiation, is a common carcinogen, accounting for over 400,000 skin cancers of the overall estimated 1 million new cases of skin cancer ocurring annually in the United States. Today even more ultraviolet radiation is present in sunlight because the ozone hole in the Earth's upper atmosphere has expanded, weakening the Earth's natural shield against it.

Skin cancer may take one of 3 forms depending on the type of skin cells involved: melanoma, squamous, and basal. Melanoma (melanocytes are the skin cells here) is generally the most lethal type of skin cancer although it accounts for about 38,000 new cases annually and 7000 deaths in contrast to the other 2 types of skin cancer (squamous and basal) which account for the remaining 962,000 cases and are generally much less deadly because, unlike melanoma, they do not spread to distant body sites.

Scientists believe that the ultraviolet component of sunlight can induce a permanent mutation at a specific point in the DNA (affecting a single gene called the p53 tumor suppressor gene)[12] of skin cells, especially in the skin of people with very fair (whitish) skin, such as the Caucasians of Australia who, constantly exposed to intense sunlight, have the highest rate of all types of skin cancer in the world. Generally, the damaging effects of too much sunlight on fair skin, which produces a temporary but intense immunosuppression, can occur years before an actual tumor appears, often in middle age.

## CHRONIC ELECTROMAGNETIC FIELD EXPOSURE

According to an Environmental Protection Agency study, there is growing evidence of a link between exposure to electromagnetic fields (EMFs)—which are generated by electrical currents—and cancer.[13] An electromagnetic field can be likened to an invisible energy web (shaped somewhat like the contour lines on a topographical map) that is produced by electricity which in turn creates a magnetic field. While EMFs are part of Nature and in fact are radiated by the human body and its individual organs, the quality and intensity (called, respectively, frequency and gauss field strength) of the energy informing this contoured web can either support or destroy health. As a general rule, EMFs generated by human-made technological devices or installations tend to be much more harmful than naturally occurring EMFs.

> ***Electromagnetic changes in the environment can adversely affect the energy balance of the human organism and contribute to disease. As a general rule, EMFs generated by human-made technological devices or installations tend to be more harmful than naturally occurring EMFs.***

Electromagnetic changes in the environment can adversely affect the energy balance of the human organism and contribute to disease. We are surrounded by stress-producing, electromagnetic fields (EMFs) generated by the electrical wiring in homes and offices, televisions, computers and video terminals, microwave ovens, overhead lights, electrical poles, and the hundreds of motors that can generate higher than naturally occurring gauss strengths (magnetic energy measuring unit). EMFs interact with living systems, affecting enzymes related to growth regulation, gene expression, pineal gland metabolism (regulation of the anticancer hormone, melatonin), and cell division and multiplication—all of which can exert a major influence on tumor growth.[14]

The frequency at which an EMF is pulsed determines whether or not it is harmful. For example, the voltage of the electric current used in homes in the United States is 60 Hz (hertz cycles per second). In contrast, the ideal frequencies of the human brain during waking hours range from 8 to 20 Hz, while in sleep the frequencies may drop to as low as 2 cycles Hz. The higher frequencies of EMFs generated by artificial electrical currents may disturb the brain's natural resonant frequencies and, in time, lead to cellular fatigue, according to John Zimmerman, Ph.D., president of the Bio-Electro Magnetics Institute in Utah.

In 1979, Nancy Wertheimer, Ph.D., an epidemiologist at the University of Colorado, found that there was a statistically significant increase in childhood cancers among those who were exposed to the AC (alternating current) EMFs that emanate from the electric power lines that run along many of the nation's city streets.[15] Then in 1987, a large-scale study conducted by the New York State Department of Health confirmed Dr. Wertheimer's findings and added that it causes a reduction in the brain's production of melatonin.[16] This so-called "neurohormone" is an antioxidant and immune-system stimulator that also appears to have many anticancer functions.[17]

## The Leukemia and Brain Tumor Link

Studies have suggested a higher incidence of leukemia and brain tumors among people exposed to electrical fields on the job.[19] Children living near electric power lines may be facing 5 times the risk of all forms of cancer compared to children who do not.[20] Exposure of children to 60-Hz magnetic fields with a strength of only 3 milligauss is correlated with increased cancer incidence, according to epidemiological research at the University of Colorado.

Marjorie Speers, Ph.D., at the University of Texas Medical Branch in Galveston, found that workers exposed to electromagnetic fields showed a 13-fold increase in brain tumors compared to the unexposed group.[21] According to numerous studies examined by Dr. Becker, the scientific evidence is "absolutely conclusive" that 60-Hz magnetic fields cause cancer cells in humans to permanently increase their growth rate by 1600% and to exhibit more malignant features.[22]

According to Dr. Becker, the reason that exposure to electromagnetic fields may be injurious to humans is that they provoke genetic abnormalities when cells divide, thereby activating oncogenes (genes believed to initiate cancer). According to research conducted at the Veteran's Administration Medical Center in Loma Linda, California, and the University of California at Riverside, exposure to EMFs appears to stimulate activity of an enzyme called ornithine decarboxylase, which, in turn, activates another biochemical which is known to accelerate the proliferation of both normal and cancerous cells.[18] "Only a few farsighted individuals, such as Dr. Robert O. Becker, have given much thought to the fact that the new electromagnetic environment created by 20th-century technology may be exerting subtle, yet very important effects upon biology," states Dr. Zimmerman. "This may include alterations in gene expression, immune function, viral pathogenesis, and future genetic tendencies."

David A. Savitz, Ph.D., of the University of North Carolina School of Public Health, looked at cancer risks among children living in proximity to large power lines. His study unveiled the following findings: (1) about twice the risk for all cancers, (2) 2½ times the risk for brain cancer; and (3) 3 times the risk for leukemias.[23] The greater the amount of time spent in EMF-exposing jobs such as that of an electrician, the greater the risk of dying from brain cancer. A 1995 review of the scientific literature confirmed Dr. Savitz's findings with regard to leukemia and other cancers.[24] A 2-year analysis by the EPA concluded that the 8 strongest population studies to date, all involving children, "consistently found modestly elevated risks (some statistically significant) of leukemia, cancer of the nervous system, and, to a lesser extent, lymphomas."[25]

Previously, the same UNC research team had shown that female electrical workers were about 40% more likely to die from breast cancer than women in other occupations.[26] The EMF-breast cancer link is further supported by research showing that lower melatonin levels leave laboratory animals more vulnerable to mammary tumors (the animal equivalent of breast cancer). Rats whose pineal glands (source of melatonin) have been surgically removed are more likely to develop a mammary tumor—and more tumors per rat—than rats with intact pineal glands.

In contrast, rats whose pineal glands have been removed but that are given melatonin injections are no more prone to mammary tumors than other rats.[27] Richard Stevens, Ph.D., at Battelle Pacific Northwest Laboratory, suggests that since melatonin suppresses sex hormones, a low melatonin level would trigger high levels of estrogen and prolactin, thus elevating the risk of breast cancer.[28]

Other studies have linked excessive EMF exposure with increases in suicides,[29] depression,[30] chromosomal abnormalities,[31] and learning difficulties.[32] Dr. Wertheimer has also found that users of electric blankets had a higher incidence of miscarriages.[33]

The EMF exposure from hair dryers, heaters, electric shavers, and other appliances can be injurious to health over time. Food mixers, hair dryers, and vacuum cleaners emit EMFs that are 30 to 100 times greater than the suggested safe limit.[34] Ordinary household appliances tend to generate larger cumulative EMF exposures than power lines. The reason is proximity: most people do not live close enough to power lines to be greatly affected by their EMFs, but the situation is different with kitchen appliances, computers, cellular phones, televisions, even electrical outlets if they're located behind the head of a bed. Although the EMFs from appliances drop off at a distance of about 16 feet, people often stand or sit closer than this to the source of EMFs—typically 18 inches from computers, a few feet from televisions, and almost no distance from cellular phones.[35]

***At the same time, not being exposed to naturally occurring EMFs can have a negative impact on health, for they function as a kind of energy nutrient. Dr. Nakagawa calls this condition "magnetic field deficiency syndrome," noting it can cause headaches, dizziness, muscle stiffness, chest pain, insomnia, constipation, and general fatigue.***

EMFs from these sources are so small that the electrical currents they induce in the human body is actually weaker than those induced by electrical activity in nerve and muscle cells. Yet even these low-frequency EMFs can alter gene expression, the activity of enzymes involved in growth regulation, calcium balance in the cell, and the brain's metabolism of the hormone melatonin.[36] It is also possible that EMFs disrupt hormonal processes and tumor-fighting mechanisms.[37] Any single or combined effect can encourage the multiplication of cancer cells and promote tumor growth.[38]

Studies of human populations have consistently found associations between residential EMF exposure and cancer, particularly in the case of childhood leukemia.[39] Among adults, there is a stronger association between EMF exposure and brain cancer[40] and, to a lesser extent, breast cancer.[41] The National Council on Radiation Protection warned that excessive exposure to EMFs may lead to cancer and that exposure to weak EMFs can disturb the brain's production of melatonin, which may lead to breast cancer.[42] The Council recommended that a maximum exposure limit of 0.2 microteslas (2 milligauss) be set for homes and offices. This level is substantially lower than the field strength of power lines and many common household appliances.

At the same time, *not* being exposed to naturally occurring EMFs can have a negative impact on health, for they function as a kind of energy nutrient. Kyoichi Nakagawa, M.D., Director of the Isuzu Hospital in Tokyo, Japan, observes that the amount of time people now spend in buildings and cars (tightly enclosed spaces) reduces their exposure to the geomagnetic field of the earth and may interfere with their health. Dr. Nakagawa calls this condition "magnetic field deficiency syndrome," noting it can cause headaches, dizziness, muscle stiffness, chest pain, insomnia, constipation, and general fatigue.[43] Another way of explaining this is to say that the beneficial Schumann waves from the Earth itself get deflected by certain human-made devices and overpowered by human-made electromagnetic fields.

***Electromagnetic radiations presumably connected with geological fractures and subterranean water veins, can, when situated underneath homes, have remarkably deleterious effects on the occupants.***

## GEOPATHIC STRESS

Energies from the earth itself can have a carcinogenic effect on humans. Magnetic radiations from the Earth, presumably connected with geological fractures and subterranean water veins, can, when situated underneath homes, have remarkably deleterious effects on the occupants.

The concept of geopathic, or pathogenic, influences from the earth, took root in Germany in 1929 when Baron Gustav Freiherr von Pohl made a systematic tour of the community of Vilsbiburg. It had 565 houses, 3,300 residents, and an unusually high rate of cancer. Von Pohl was acting on a hunch inspired from a survey of Stuttgart in the 1920s that showed a clear correlation between major geological faults in the city and those districts that had the highest cancer mortality rates. His tentative conclusion was that an unknown but noxious radiation emanating from the Earth faults might be an important and overlooked contributory cause of the cancers.

Baron von Pohl located all the major subterranean water veins (lying at a depth of 44-50 meters with a width of 3-4 meters) under Vilsbiburg, then mapped their courses onto the city street plan. Next he cross-checked this with the residences of the 54 recent cancer fatalities and arrived at a startling conclusion: "The completed check of my map confirmed all the beds of the 54 cancer deaths were where I had drawn the radiation currents," von Pohl wrote in 1932 in his now classic *Earth Currents: Causative Factor of Cancer and Other Diseases* .

Eighteen months later, von Pohl returned to Vilsbiburg and found that the beds of another 10 cancer mortalities were situated directly over crossing underground streams. The beds in these "cancer houses" were situated over what von Pohl characterized as geopathic zones marked by "dangerous radiation lines." Geopathology is still essentially unknown in America but since von Pohl's day it is been the subject of considerable research, empirical investigation, and even medical recognition in his native Germany.

***"If one makes sure one's bed does not stand above a strong underground current and one tries not to work above these underground currents, one should not get cancer."—Baron von Pohl, geopathics researcher.***

Von Pohl himself presented dozens of cases in which rapid, perhaps miraculous, cures of numerous complaints, from insomnia to heart spasm, were achieved simply by moving the sleeper's bed out of the geopathic zone situated underneath the house. In the town of Stettin, von Pohl's colleague, Dr. Hager, collated the details of 5348 cancer deaths over a 21-year span and found in each case that a subterranean water vein ran under the cancer patient's house. "Medical science has now a preventative measure which did not exist previously," noted von Pohl. "If one makes sure one's bed does not stand above a strong underground current and one tries not to work above these underground currents, one should not get cancer."[44]

Geopathic stress is almost entirely unacknowledged in the U.S. as a contributing carcinogenic influence. However, European physicians, such as Hans A. Nieper, M.D., medical director of the Paracelsus Silbersee Hospital in Hannover, Germany, are far more aware of this factor as a contributing cause for cancer. According to Dr. Nieper, 93% of all patients with a malignancy have been exposed to geopathogenic influences. As a standard aspect of cancer treatment, he advises "removal of the patient from sites of geopathogenic exposure," noting that such sites may be identified by way of dowsing or a magnetometer (capable of registering abnormal magnetic fields).[45]

There are at least 2 theories attempting to explain the origin of geopathic stress. One theory says it comes from underground; another says from above, through cosmic rays. According to Ludger Mersmann, M.D., a biophysics researcher and inventor, based in Belmont, Massachusetts, the cause of geopathic stress is localized magnetic anomalies—unusual, sudden, local changes and quirks that can upset delicate human physiological balance and create problems.

To prove his hypothesis, Dr. Mersmann invented a device called a geo-magnetometer, which takes precise, local, magnetic field readings in a suspected geopathic zone such as a bedroom. The device then prints a 3-dimensional picture of the disturbed magnetic field. "Geopathic stress consists of several factors, maybe as many as 25, but the main factor is a disturbed magnetic field," says Dr. Mersmann. Here the natural homogeneous magnetic field meets with or turns into a nonhomogeneous field, resulting in a disturbed zone. These geomagnetic anomalies act upon the human organism as stimuli of a localized and chronic nature and, depending on the intensity and length of exposure, lead to impairment of health."

The starting point in Dr. Mersmann's model is a geological factor. It might be a fissure, or fault; the possibly noxious activity of water veins is a secondary factor. The geological factor produces a disturbance in the local magnetic field, which registers as a sharp, sudden, vertical fluctuation in an otherwise smooth, steady field. Dr. Mersmann emphasizes that it is the degree of change in the magnetic field, and the part of the human body (lying in bed) affected by this change, that is of paramount importance. "Different parts of the same body have different intensity lines and this disturbed zone, where the highest gradient is shown, is often the site of the cancer or illness, says Dr. Mersmann.

A second theory explaining the possible origin of geopathic stress points to the sky, specifically, to "a vertical field going from the ground up to the sky," suggests Anthony Scott-Morley, H.M.D., Ph.D., of the Institute of Bioenergetic Medicine in Dorset, England. The vertical field might comprise rays from deep space. "It has been assumed that the vertical field holds the same intensity throughout fairly large areas, but actual readings with the magnetometer indicate wide variability in field strength within short distances." This variability is the origin of geopathic stress. The body is unable to adapt to large changes in field strength within short distances (as few as 6 inches), so its balance, or homeostasis, is upset, immune function can be depressed, and chronic illness can result.

In 1971, the theory of geopathic stress was supported by research showing that water flowing underground, especially subterranean streams that cross, produces measurable increases in magnetic anomalies; these conditions also increase electrical conductivity in the air and soil, and other physical changes. While the changes may be small, though measurable (in the vicinity of 10 inches square), they are still capable of contributing to the development of serious illness, including cancer. One large-scale study by the U.S. government reported that geopathic stress may be a factor in between 40 and 50% of all human cancers and account for between 60 and 90% of all cancers attributed to environmental radiation.[46]

## Geopathic Stress and Feng Shui

Geopathic stress in home and work environments is a key factor in the onset of disease, as well as in the failure of some patients to respond to treatment, even alternative medicine, states Dr. Scott-Morley. Geopathic stress zones may be tiny, but shifting a bed a few feet in a geopathically troubled bedroom, can make, says Dr. Scott-Morley, the difference between cancer and no cancer for the susceptible individual. The growing popularity of feng shui (pronounced FUNG-shway), the Chinese science of landscape interpretation and household exterior and interior design, is bringing the concepts of geopathic stress to a larger audience in the West.

## SICK BUILDING SYNDROME

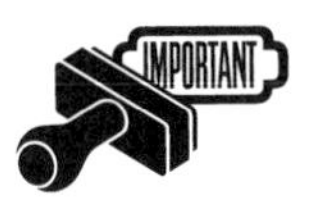


Not only where the house is situated but what is in it and how tightly it is sealed are implicated in cancer risks. In the early eighties, physicians began using the term "sick building syndrome" (SBS) to refer to a host of symptoms produced by low-grade toxic environmental conditions found in living, work, or office spaces. SBS symptoms are numerous: mucous membrane irritation of the eyes, nose, and throat, chest tightness, skin complaints (dryness, itching, abnormal redness), headaches, fatigue, lethargy, coughing, asthma, wheezing, chronic nasal stuffiness, temporary weight loss, infections, and emotional irritability. All of these depress the immune system, rendering the individual susceptible to long-term chronic illness and potentially to a cancer process.

"Indoor air pollution in residences, offices, schools, and other buildings is widely recognized as a serious environmental risk to human health," explains Michael Hodgson, M.D., M.P.H., of the School of Medicine, University of Connecticut Health Center in Farmington. Dr. Hodgson notes that most people in industrialized nations spend more than 90% of their time indoors, that indoor concentrations of pollutants (including toxic chemicals) are often "substantially" higher than found outdoors, and that small children, the elderly, and the infirm are likely to spend all their time indoors, leading to a permanent chronic exposure to low-grade toxic factors.

In most cases, problems with a building's engineering, construction, and ventilation system are the causes. Studies suggest that symptoms occur 50% more frequently in buildings with mechanical ventilation systems. Among 2,000 office workers in Germany with work-related symptoms, there was a 50% higher than average rate of upper respiratory tract infections that were directly traceable to problems with mechanically ventilated buildings, reports Dr. Hodgson. A U.S. study found that 20% of office workers had job-related SBS symptoms, including a subjective sense of being less productive in their work.

***The EPA estimates that indoor radon pollution may cause as many as 10,000 cancers a year in the United States.***

Besides ventilation problems, other sources of indoor toxic pollution include volatile organic compounds released from particleboard desks, furniture, carpets, glues, paints, office machine toners, and perfumes. All contribute to "a complex mixture of very low levels of individual pollutants," states Dr. Hodgson. Bioaerosols are also indoor contaminants and originate as biological agents from mold spores, allergy-producing microbes, mites, or animal danders; then they are distributed through an indoor space by ventilation, heating, or air conditioning systems.

Of buildings classified as sources of SBS, one study showed that 70% have inadequate flow of fresh outside air. It also found that 50 to 70% of such buildings have poor distribution of air within the occupied space; 60% have poor filtration of outdoor pollutants; 60% have standing water that fosters biological growths; and 20% have malfunctioning humidifiers.[47]

According to Dr. Hodgson, the carcinogenic effects of certain indoor air pollutants, such as asbestos, environmental tobacco smoke, radon, and formaldehyde, are well described in the clinical literature and are now considered cancer risk factors. Indoor air pollution, found in offices and homes, often comprises contaminants which lead to cancer. Some examples include formaldehyde fumes from pressed wood furniture; fumes and vapors produced by carpets, cleaning products, air fresheners, paints, office machine toners, hobby supplies (glues, varnishes, etc.), and improperly vented gas stoves and dryers; lead and other chemicals found in drinking and bathing water; office or home air systems that fill the air with bacteria, mildew, and viruses; and radon gas infiltration from the soil.

The EPA estimates that indoor radon pollution may cause as many as 10,000 cancers a year in the United States.[48] Other data suggest that exposure to the radioactive decay products of radon in homes contributes to about 10% of annual lung cancers in the U.S. and that the average lifetime risk of lung cancer from environmental radon is 1 in 1000.

## IONIZING RADIATION

Ionizing radiation consists of high-energy rays that are capable of ripping the electrons from matter, causing genetic mutations that can lead to cancer. This is the type of radiation used in X-ray technology, which may explain why radiologists (people who take many X rays each day) have historically had higher incidences of cancer, as have other workers exposed to low-dose radiation.[49]

> ***"The combined evidence now makes it fully reasonable, scientifically, to infer that* all *kinds of cancer can be induced by radiation," states Dr. Gofman.***

The National Research Council's report, Biological Effects of Ionizing Radiation (BEIR, 1990), concluded that the risk of tumors and leukemias resulting from X rays is 3-4 times higher than was estimated in the 1980 BEIR report. This means that if 1 million people doubled their annual radiation exposure, which would happen with only 5 yearly chest X rays, 5,200 of them would get cancer—4 times more than the 1980 estimate.[50] But this estimate may be too conservative. X rays (or gamma rays) also emanate from fluorescent lights, computer monitors, and television screens, which add additional exposures in the lives of most people.

Medical X rays may cause about 75% of breast cancer, according to estimates made by John W. Gofman, M.D., Ph.D., the director of the Committee for Nuclear Responsibility, Inc., professor emeritus in the Department of Molecular and Cell Biology at the University of California at Berkeley, and the author of 100 scientific papers and several notable books on radiation and health. After investigating the effects of low-level ionizing radiation for 30 years, Gofman concludes that the longer the radiation exposure, the smaller the dose needed to do damage. "The combined evidence now makes it fully reasonable, scientifically, to infer that *all* kinds of cancer can be induced by radiation," states Dr. Gofman.[51]

Dr. Gofman was once Associate Director of the Lawrence Livermore Radiation Laboratory in California, where he conducted research on cancer and chromosomes from 1965 to 1972, until the Atomic Energy Commission stopped supporting his work. Dr. Gofman announced that the official estimates on the cancer risks of radiation exposure had been underestimated by 10 times. These estimates threatened the nuclear power industry and his dismissal soon followed.

In 1995, Dr. Gofman stated: "Our estimate is that about three-quarters of the current annual incidence of breast cancer in the U.S. is being caused by earlier ionizing radiation, primarily from medical sources." The onset of cancer is often a delayed effect, says Dr. Gofman; individuals may live for 10 years following irradiation before a cancer develops. Then new radiation exposures act as a "multiplier" upon the rate at which spontaneous cancers ordinarily occur which, in turn increases with age, Dr. Gofman warns.

This shocker may be good news in disguise because it means potentially 75% of breast cancer could be prevented by avoiding or minimizing exposure to the ionizing radiation from mammography, X rays, and other non-nuclear medical sources such as radiation therapy. Given that 182,000 new cases of female breast cancer occurred in 1995, this means that approximately 136,500 breast cancers might have been linked with diagnostic and therapeutic radiation sources. Even assuming Dr. Gofman's risk estimate is overstated, reducing it by two-thirds still leaves over 45,000 new breast cancer cases that would result annually from unnecessary exposure to medical sources of radiation.

The key to preventing cancer, says Dr. Gofman, is to eliminate this cause, namely, high doses of breast irradiation. Each reduction in breast irradiation today can prevent a possible future breast cancer from developing 10 to 50 years later. If Dr. Gofman's warnings are heeded, the turnaround in mammogram screening policy would have ample precedent. Irradiation of an enlarged thymus gland was practiced routinely between 1911 and 1960, despite dubious results. Dr. Gofman documents the assurances given by doctors to patients regarding the safety and efficacy of relatively high doses of radiation in medicine, now proven to be erroneous. A new series of safety "assurances" are currently in circulation for low doses of radiation, but these are little better than wishful thinking, according to Dr. Gofman, who asserts that "all doses matter."

## NUCLEAR RADIATION

The independent research of the Committee for Nuclear Responsibility has brought attention to the cancer risks associated with living near nuclear power plants. Among the hazards are the small amounts of radioactive gases released daily from nuclear reactors at levels deemed "permissible" by the U.S. Department of Energy. This low-level radioactive pollution returns to us in rainfall which then accumulates in the soils to contaminate the food chain. People who eat dairy products and other foods tainted by these radioactive releases may be unwittingly exposing themselves to dangerous carcinogens. Since dairy products tend to concentrate the radioactive fission products, avoiding such foods may lower your cancer risk.

The global scope of this problem is reflected in studies of the impact of the Chernobyl fallout on the U.S. population. A 1995 study found high concentrations of iodine-131 in the milk produced in Connecticut in the weeks after the Chernobyl accident. The rate of thyroid cancer among children in Connecticut rose sharply after 1989, when cancer increases among children in the area around Chernobyl also began. The age-adjusted rate in Connecticut between 1985 and 1989 and 1990 and 1992 rose from 35 to 43 per million, after 10 previous years of no change. This increase was similar to that seen among children exposed to radioactive milk in the Ukraine.[52]

***In the United Kingdom, a higher rate of leukemia has been reported in children living near nuclear facilities. The incidence of childhood thyroid cancer has increased 100 times in those areas of Ukraine, Belarus, and Russia most acutely exposed to the Chernobyl nuclear accident in April 1986.***

Working or living in the proximity of nuclear power plants presents its special risks as well. In 1991, Steve Wing, Ph.D., an epidemiologist at the University of North Carolina, reported on a study of over 8,000 men working at the Oak Ridge (Tennessee) National Laboratory. Workers who were exposed daily to low-level ionizing radiation had a much higher risk of cancer, particularly leukemia.[53] In the United Kingdom, a higher rate of leukemia has been reported in children living near nuclear facilities. The incidence of childhood thyroid cancer has increased 100 times in those areas of Ukraine, Belarus, and Russia most acutely exposed to the Chernobyl nuclear accident in April 1986, stated experts from the United Nations in

November 1995. Childhood thyroid cancer is the fastest way in which the impact of radiation exposure shows up in the body.

Among the 4,014 white male workers employed between 1951 and 1981 at the Oak Ridge Institute for Science and Education, where uranium is processed, the death rate from lung cancer was 26% higher than in the general U.S. population, and the death rate from stomach cancer was 161% greater. In all, the death rate from all cancers was 21% higher among workers routinely exposed to radiation, reported *The Environmental Times* in July 1996.

Ernest Sternglass, Ph.D., a professor of radiation physics at the University of Pittsburgh, found rising breast cancer rates among women in 268 counties located within 50 miles of nuclear plants. Age-adjusted cancer mortality rates for women living in these areas rose 10% from 1950 to 1989, compared with a 4% increase for the nation as a whole. For the five military plants, the average rate of increase was 41%. The researchers propose that the cancer rates are linked to radioactive iodine and strontium, by-products of nuclear fission which tend to become concentrated in dairy products.[54]

"It takes incredibly tiny amounts of free radicals to kill cells; a single molecule of a free radical can puncture an entire giant cell," explains Dr. Sternglass. "It is as if you threw a dart at a balloon. Free radical oxygen can unzip a lipid cell membrane in a matter of minutes or hours. A 1972 study showed that when cell membranes, taken from lipids in the brain of an ox, were irradiated in water, they burst when given an X ray of a few thousand millirads; but when they were given the same dose over a period of days or weeks or hours, it took only a few millirads to break the membrane."

According to Dr. Sternglass, a prime source of free radicals is low-level radiation, from X rays, background radioactivity, and nuclear reactor fallout. He notes that the Japanese breast cancer rate rose 40% after the atomic bomb was dropped in 1945. "There was no change in pancreatic cancer between 1935 and 1945, then there was a 1200% rise. Did their diet change overnight? Yes, it did. Fallout was added to it. That's strontium-90, strontium-89, cobalt, radioactive iron, iodine-131, radioactive cesium, and 200 other chemicals we are adding deliberately to the environment in order to generate electricity."[55]

The Oak Ridge nuclear power plant in Tennessee provides a vivid example of the harmful effect of nuclear radiation on a local community. For the 7 counties within 40 miles of Oak Ridge, breast cancer rates increased by 39% for women living in 3 downwind areas, in contrast to a 4% decrease among women living in 4 upwind counties.

According to his data, based on studying fission product releases from 90 nuclear plants over 20 years, Dr. Sternglass argues that nuclear radiation plays a major role in the recent rises in breast and other cancers not related to smoking, especially among older persons, and strongly supports the need to replace nuclear reactors with more benign ways to generate electricity.[56] He further states that the conventional risk estimates for "acceptable" chronic, low-dose exposures may be underestimated by 100 to 1,000 times.

Dr. Sternglass' data proves that there is a direct, measurable, and *causal* dose/response relationship between extremely small doses and detectable health impacts; the prime carriers for fission products were municipal water and air, and to a lesser extent, fresh milk and dairy products. In fact, the radiation released by fission products appears to work synergistically (enhancing the negative effects of all factors) with other environmental carcinogens such as air pollutants, diesel fumes, dust, asbestos, cigarette smoke, pesticides, herbicides, and environmental-synthetic estrogens.

Dr. Sternglass also presents further evidence proving the connection between nuclear reactor releases and the rise in breast cancer by the fact that only 4 of 16 industrial countries—New Zealand, Australia, Hong Kong, and Israel—registered declines in breast cancer mortality between 1971 and 1986, while the rates in the other 12 nations rose. The reason for this difference is that these 4 countries did not have large commercial nuclear reactors in operation in or near their borders during this time period, while the other 12 countries did. Chronic exposure to nuclear fission products through the diet and drinking water "may be the single largest factor in the increased incidence of most forms of malignancies" since 1945, says Dr. Sternglass. "In effect, the results presented here represent the outcome of an enormous, unplanned, double-blind epidemiological study in the United States involving some 200 million human beings exposed to fission products for nearly a whole generation," says Dr. Sternglass.

**The Enemy Within**—Since the first atomic bomb explosion in New Mexico in 1945 and the advent of nuclear "power," nearly all of the continental United States has been irradiated by nuclear fallout. Today, 1,321 of the total 3,053 counties in the U.S. are nuclear counties, meaning the residents live within 100 miles of a reactor. In other words, more than 33% of those living in the continental U.S. are regularly exposed to nuclear radiation. These residents suffer higher than average rates of breast cancer, AIDS, and other immune deficiencies, and, among infants, premature births, low birth weights, reduced intelligence, and depressed thyroids.

A former employee of the Environmental Protection Agency, Jay M. Gould bases his conclusions on meticulous research he compiled from data from the National Cancer Institute, state health departments, and the Centers for Disease Control. This data reveals that more than 1.5 million American women have died of breast cancer since the start of the "nuclear age" whereas prior to 1945, the rate of breast cancer incidence was actually declining.

***"There is growing evidence that the nation's present breast cancer epidemic is related to exposure to a wide range of environmental contaminants, including DDT, and other carcinogenic pesticide and estrogenic stimulants," says Dr. Epstein.***

The exposure of an entire generation—Baby Boomers born between 1945 and 1965, the height of nuclear testing—to man-made fission products has led to an unprecedented increase in illness, says Gould. The toxic situation is even worse in heavy rainfall areas—East Coast, Great Lakes, the Northwest—where nuclear radiation combines with chemical pesticides, industrial pollutants, and other environmental toxins in rain. This deadly amalgam enters surface water reservoirs, public drinking water, and thus the human body, faster.

That the New York metropolitan area (including Long Island and southern Connecticut) has the country's greatest concentration of breast cancer mortality is directly attributable to its proximity to 4 nuclear facilities (including Brookhaven National Laboratory) and the deadly confluence of environmental factors cited above, says Gould. Here the breast cancer death rates are as high as 32 per 100,000 compared to 28 in the irradiated Northeast, an average 25.8 for nuclear counties, and 22 in nonnuclear counties. "This means that in the 'nuclear' counties for every 100,000 women, there are nearly 4 more deaths today than in nonnuclear counties—an extraordinarily significant difference," Gould says.

Gould marshals a huge body of health statistics to prove conclusively that those who live in proximity to active nuclear power stations or research facilities (which release radioactive gases, toxic liquid, and solid wastes) have far higher rates of disease than those who do not. The 1,321 nuclear counties account for more than 50% of all breast cancer deaths, says Gould. He also notes that the 14 counties that house the 7 oldest nuclear reactors (maintained by the Department of Energy) had a 37% increase in breast cancer deaths between 1950 and 1989, compared to only 1% for all of the U.S.

Gould's research demonstrates convincingly that negative health effects such as breast cancer mortality are directly related to residential proximity to nuclear radiation. There has been an "overall decline in the health of all age-groups," says Gould, and this cannot be explained without "taking into consideration the great environmental changes" produced by the use of nuclear power. The true cost of winning World War II with nuclear power, says Gould, has been "an uncontrollable epidemic rise in radiation-induced illnesses and in the costs of medical care."

For example, not many people know that in 1945, the Hanford nu-

## Breast Cancer Incidence and Industrial Toxins

As breast cancer incidence rises at a rate of 1.3% annually in the U.S. and Canada, researchers have found that women with the highest levels of the industrial toxins DDE and PCBs in their fat, tissues, and blood were 2-3 times more likely to develop cancer, according to the *Canadian Medical Association Journal* (April 1996).

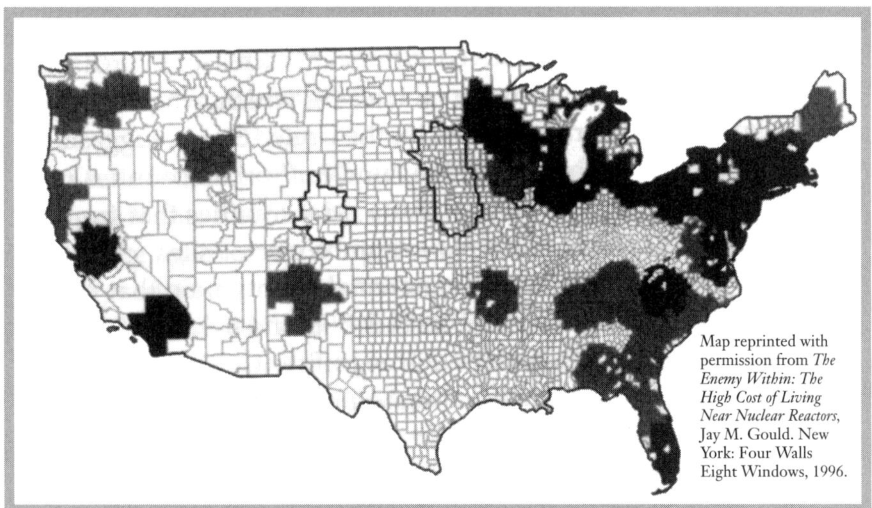
Map reprinted with permission from *The Enemy Within: The High Cost of Living Near Nuclear Reactors*, Jay M. Gould. New York: Four Walls Eight Windows, 1996.

**Figure 25.2—Of the country's 3,053 counties, nearly half, or 1,321, are situated within 100 miles of nuclear reactor sites. The darker areas on the map indicate "nuclear counties" and represent the highest risk areas.**

clear weapons facility in Washington state accidentally released an amount of radioactive iodine into the U.S. atmosphere equivalent to the 1986 Chernobyl nuclear disaster. As a result, 150 million Americans were exposed to the fallout of the nuclear cloud as it drifted across the country.

Since 1945, 184 atmospheric nuclear bombs have been detonated over Nevada, a fire power equal to 15,000 Hiroshima bombs; clouds containing nuclear fallout from these explosions have drifted over nearly all of the continental U.S. Combined fallout from all above-ground nuclear testing by the U.S. and the former U.S.S.R. is estimated to be equivalent to 10,000 Hiroshima bombs.

"The true health effects of ingesting man-made fission products have been withheld from the public for nearly half a century," says Gould. He criticizes mainstream media for ignoring the current large number of class action suits by victims of radiation releases against nuclear facilities. Gould also lambasts the National Cancer Institute's myopic (or willful) distortion of the data in their 1990 report that failed to find any convincing links between radiation exposure and cancer.

"We must press for an end to the production of nuclear weapons and operation of nuclear reactors which destroy the health and economic future of our nation," urges Gould.

## PESTICIDE/HERBICIDE RESIDUES

The scale of the pesticide residue problem is staggering. Since 1945, pesticide use has increased tenfold and, at the same time, crop loss from insects has increased twofold, from about 7 to 13%.[57] After 5 decades of lacing our food supply with these unsafe chemicals, we are using 10 times as much pesticide and losing twice as much to insect pests, according to David Pimentel, Ph.D., professor of insect ecology and agricultural sciences at Cornell University.

Over 400 pesticides are currently licensed for use on America's foods, and in 1995, 1.2 billion pounds were dumped on crop lands, forests, lawns, and fields. This was 100 million more pounds than in 1993. Worldwide, in the past 50 years, some 15,000 chemical compounds and more than 35,000 different formulations have come into use as pesticides.[58] Many of those that are banned in the United States (including DDT) are sold to Third World countries, where they enter food products that are then imported into the U.S., such as coffee, fruits, and vegetables.

"Although these chemicals for the most part have been banned or strictly regulated, they are durable and remain in the environment for a long time," says Samuel Epstein, M.D., Professor of Occupational and Environmental Medicine at the University of Illinois School of Public Health. "Crops grown in soil contaminated with these chemicals will pass on their residue to the animals that are fed them, where they will accumulate in the fatty tissue."

The misuse of pesticides and toxic chemicals in Thailand, for one, has reached a highly dangerous state; 3,672 different pesticides were registered for use in 1994, the highest in all of Southeast Asia, and many farmers pay little attention to the instructions on the pesticide containers. Although Southeast Asia represents only 1.4% of the world's available land for agriculture, it accounts for 3.6% of all pesticide imports. While Thai farmers are dangerously casual in their pesticide use (some foods, such as water chestnuts, are doused with pesticides after harvest), they seem to understand that the result is toxic produce; one poll of 201 farmers showed that 30% of the farmers admitted they didn't eat their own pesticide-laced vegetables. As Thailand exported $8.8 billion worth of agricultural products in 1995, a high degree of pesticide-contaminated fruits and vegetables thereby entered the world market, poised to contaminate eaters.[59]

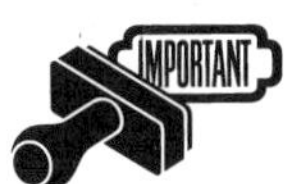


About 50% of pesticide use is nonagricultural, used in building materials (wood preservatives), food containers, golf courses, parks, roadsides, utility rights-of-way, railroad track beds, school grounds and school buildings (as fumigants), restaurants, department stores, office buildings, airplanes, hospitals, mass transit areas, swimming pools, hot tubs, paper mills, and hotels. An estimated 60 million U.S. acres are subjected to herbicidal treatment to curtail vegetation. Home and garden pesticides are another widespread source of contamination; research indicates that fumes from externally applied home and garden pesticides can seep into the home, contaminating residents.

The Environmental Protection Agency (EPA) does not require toxicity testing for many of the chemicals used for these purposes. Of 50 nonagricultural pesticides, EPA had preliminary toxicity data on only 18, and, of these, 17 lacked adequate toxicity information. Of 600 active ingredients in these pesticides, EPA, in 1990, had preliminary assessments on only 194. According to a Government Accounting Office report on this problem, as

## Israel Proves the Pesticide-Cancer Link

In 1978, following public outcry and threatened legal action, Israel banned many toxic chemicals such as DDT and PCBs which had been directly linked in a 1976 study with breast cancer. The study, conducted by the Department of Occupational Health at Hebrew University-Hadassah Medical School in Jerusalem found that when they compared cancerous breast tissue with noncancerous tissue from elsewhere in the same woman's body, the concentration of toxic chemicals, such as DDT and PCBs, was "much increased in the malignant tissue when compared to the normal breast and adjacent adipose tissue."[62]

Once Israel banned these chemicals, they began noting a significant decrease in the level of toxic chemicals found in human breast milk. Over the next 10 years, the rate of breast cancer deaths declined sharply, with a 30% drop in mortality for women under 44 years old, and an 8% overall decline. Interestingly, at the same time, all other known cancer risks—alcohol consumption, fat intake, lack of fruits and vegetables in the diet—increased significantly. Furthermore, worldwide death rates from breast cancer rose by 4%.[63] The only answer scientists could find to explain this anomaly was the greatly reduced level of environmental toxics.

summarized by health researcher John Cary Stewart, EPA "does not have the exposure information it needs to accurately and reliably assess risks for nonagricultural use pesticides."[60]

The crucial point here is quite simple: pesticides leech into public water supplies. Farming areas of the Midwest tend to have the highest concentrations of pesticide residues in their water. In Minnesota, 40% of wells tested had traces of at least one pesticide; in Iowa, 28 out of 70 public drinking wells had one or more pesticides; 70 to 80% of wells and springs tested in northeast Iowa were pesticide-contaminated. Up to 74 different pesticides, derived from agriculture, were measured in various groundwater wells in 38 states. In California alone, 50 different pesticides were detected in groundwater, traceable to direct land application, accidental spills, or leaks. "Groundwater contamination by pesticides and nitrates may be a concern to 53.8 million people."[61]

The Environmental Protection Agency has identified at least 55 pesticides that could leave carcinogenic residues in foods. In a single meal, a person can conceivably consume residues of a dozen different neurotoxic or carcinogenic chemicals, from salad to wine, main dish to dessert. "Many cancer-causing pesticides and industrial chemicals found in the environment and in our foods tend to accumulate in fatty tissues, whether in fish, cattle, fowl, or people," states Dr. Epstein. If people inadvertently choose foods with the highest concentrations of these chemicals, they will build up ever higher concentrations of these same chemicals in their bodies' fatty tissue. This process is called bioaccumulation. According to Dr. Epstein, these fat-soluble carcinogens are found in highest concentrations in the fattiest tissues, such as the brain, sexual organs, and breasts.

Only a fool believes that the EPA's Office of Pesticide Programs is truly protecting the public against pesticide hazards in foods. EPA, when calculating permitted residue levels of a given compound on a single crop, does not take into account individuals' repeated exposure to the same pesticide. The agency sets these levels with "blinders" to the fact that people eat more than one product that has residues of the same compound. EPA scientists have found that, at times, these residues, totaled, can exceed 500% of the allowed daily intake.[67]

Many chemicals in food have not been adequately tested for human safety; even fewer have been tested with the idea of "chemical cocktail syndrome" or multiple chemical exposure in mind. The EPA does not have a scientifically acceptable method for determining the risk for multiple chemical exposure; yet studies of multiple chemical exposure have shown that chemicals act synergistically, that is, enhancing one another's effects. In a classic study, a scientific team tested 3 chemicals on a group of rats, applying one at a time; no ill effects were observed. When they combined and administered 2 at a time, a decline in health was noted and when 3 chemicals were given at once, the rats

## DDT Residues and Cancer

DDT is a prime example of a pesticide residue finding its way through foods into human fatty tissues. Women with the highest blood levels of DDT had 4 times the breast cancer risk of women with the least exposure, according to one study.[64] "This is just one of many studies since the 1970s to associate DDT and other related pesticides and industrial chemicals with breast cancer risk," commented Dr. Epstein. "In fact, there is growing evidence that the nation's present breast cancer epidemic is related to exposure to a wide range of environmental contaminants, including DDT, and other carcinogenic pesticide and estrogenic stimulants."

Anecdotal reports suggest that many conventionally grown coffees carry high DDT residues and enter the human body through regular coffee consumption. Once inside the body, pesticides are strong immune system suppressors. According to environmental medicine expert William Rae, M.D., 81% of 107 cancer patients with measurable exposure to pesticides had much lower than average levels of T and B lymphocytes (white blood cells).[65] DDT is still turning up in strange places in the American environment, such as the San Francisco Bay in California. In 1996, workers dredged 80,000 tons of dirt containing DDT (at 30 parts per million) from Richmond Harbor in San Francisco Bay. This was the former site of a pesticide packaging plant that conveniently (for them) dumped DDT and pesticide residues into the bay. The U.S. government's answer was to move them elsewhere: its Superfund allocated $10 million to enable California to bury the DDT-laced dirt in an Arizona landfill where no doubt it will one day leach into Arizona groundwater.[66]

died within 2 weeks.[68]

The potential of pesticides, alone and in combination, to cause and promote cancer should be of grave concern to all physicians and public health officials. In 1989, the Natural Resources Defense Council (NRDC) announced that the residues of agricultural chemicals on fruits and vegetables eaten during a typical American childhood could be initiating between 5,500 and 6,200 cancers every year. In its study, "Intolerable Risk: Pesticides in Our Children's Food," the NRDC presented a formula for assessing the risk of cancer that took into account the many years that usually elapse between cancer initiation and actual diagnosis. Using this formula, they reported that the exposure to dietary carcinogens before the age of 6 accounts for more than half the lifetime risk of diet-caused cancers.[69]

***In the 10 years after Israel banned many toxic chemicals, such as DDT and PCBs, the rate of breast cancer deaths declined sharply, with a 30% drop in mortality for women under 44 years old.***

The NRDC report estimated that the cancer risk could be as much as 6 times greater for children aged 1-5 than for adults.[70] The greater the length of exposure time, the greater the cancer risk. Cells undergoing rapid growth may be more vulnerable to carcinogenesis than cells that are more static or undergoing slower growth. In light of these facts, a consortium of 75 EPA experts ranked pesticide residues among the top 3 environmentally derived cancer risks.

Of particular concern is the fact that most of these chemicals are fat-seeking (lipophilic), which means they tend to accumulate in fat (adipose tissue) and are seldom discharged by the body, except in the breast milk of nursing mothers.[71] A study comparing levels of chemical residues in breast tissue from women with breast cancer or benign breast conditions found that high levels of PBBs (polybrominated biphenyls) and certain pesticides were found in the fatty tissue samples from those with cancer compared to those with benign breast disease.[72] Research reported in 1991 indicated that men with prostate cancer have a several times higher level of pesticides in their prostate tissue than men with benign prostatic hypertrophy but no cancer.

Another study found a 4 times higher relative risk of breast cancer for women who showed high blood (serum) levels of DDE, a major metabolite of DDT.[73] These preliminary results suggest a role for organochlorine pesticides in the development of breast cancer. More recent research has shown that DDE levels tend to be higher among black women with breast cancer compared to black women without cancer.[74]

The National Academy of Sciences (NAS) estimates that the risk from a lifetime exposure to 28 pesticides in commonly eaten foods could amount to approximately 6 cancers per 1,000 people. Thus, a few of the pesticides currently in use could eventually cause 1.46 million cases of cancer over the average lifetime. The General Accounting Office found the FDA is testing less than 1% of all foods for pesticide residues. According to a 1984 NAS study, 64% of the ingredients in marketed pesticides had not been properly tested for toxicity, although the pesticide industry is legally required to do such tests.[75]

***The National Academy of Sciences estimates that the risk from a lifetime exposure to 28 pesticides in commonly eaten foods could amount to approximately 6 cancers per 1,000 people. Thus, a few of the pesticides currently in use could eventually cause 1.46 million cases of cancer over the average lifetime.***

There is clear evidence that pesticides cause cancers among farmers or agricultural workers, at least if exposure is high enough.[76] Pesticide exposure may result in an increased risk of non-Hodgkin's lymphoma and possibly other cancers. Men in Iowa and Minnesota who handled several pesticide groups or individual insecticides (carbaryl, chlordane, diazinon, dichlorvos, dichloro-diphenyl-trichloroethane, lindane, malathion, and toxaphene) were at least 50% more likely to contract non-Hodgkin's lymphoma compared to nonfarmers.[77]

Men exposed to herbicides more than 20 days per year were 6 times more likely to develop non-Hodgkin's lymphoma relative to nonfarmers. Frequent herbicide users who mixed or applied the herbicides themselves were 8 times more likely to develop this form of cancer.[78] A Swedish study of pesticide applicators found higher risks for testicular cancer, tumors of the nervous system and endocrine glands, and Hodgkin's disease.[79]

Home and garden pesticides—Americans spend an estimated $900 million a year on these products—represent another major source of toxicity. They have been linked to a variety of cancers, including childhood leukemia and brain cancer. Indoor pesticide use was found to result in a risk factor 4 times higher than normal for childhood leukemia; this risk became 7 times higher for the children of parents who used garden pesticides, and continued to climb in both cases as the frequency of pesticide use went up.[80] Childhood brain cancer has been directly associated with adult use of chemical pesticides, such as diazinon and carbaryl, in the garden or orchard, as well as with various herbicides used to control weeds. Pesticides used to control pests in the home have also been implicated in this disease, including those found in no-pest strips, termite pesticides, home pesticide bombs, and flea collars for pets.[81]

No-pest strips may seem innocuous, but they emit continuous vapors of DDVP (the active ingredient used in most strips), a highly carcinogenic chemical associated with an increased risk for all types of cancer in children and adults alike, according to the EPA. People who use these strips as directed and are exposed to them over a lifetime have a greatly increased chance of getting cancer—as high as 1 in 100, which is 10,000 times the risk that the EPA considers to be of significant concern. The EPA also estimates that members of a household using the pest strips face a cancer risk 10 times greater than even pest control workers who apply DDVP thousands of times a year without wearing protective clothing.[82] The cancer danger of garden pesticides extends to pets who come into close contact with contaminated soils, lawns, and plants. Flea collars with DDVP also put pets at an increased cancer risk.[83]

***There are 800 human-made radionuclides (radioactive substances) from the nuclear power industry, of which 200 are believed to be potential drinking water contaminants.***

In recognition of the health hazards of commercial and home use of pesticides, at least 12 states, including Florida, Colorado, California, Pennsylvania, Michigan, Maryland, and West Virginia, now have laws in place requiring commercial users of pesticides (such as organophosphates) to register their uses and spraying schedules in a publicly-accessible database. Individuals sensitive to organophosphates commonly used in lawn and rose sprays are now, in some communities, notified by mail in advance of spraying; in other cases, they may check a database or registry to find out spraying schedules.[84]

## INDUSTRIAL TOXINS

A great number of highly toxic chemicals, materials, and heavy metals are released by industrial processes and find their way into human tissue. Heavy metals, such as lead, arsenic, mercury, aluminum, nickel, cadmium, and many others that have no safe level in the human system may accumulate within the fat cells, central nervous system, bones, brain, glands, or hair, and may have negative health effects.

For example, lead contamination comes from cigarette smoke exposure, ceramic glazes on cooking utensils, canned foods, or lead solder on waterpipes; cadmium can come from cigarettes, instant coffee and teas, nickel-cadmium batteries, some soft drinks, fungicides, and certain plastics; mercury (discussed below) can leak from dental fillings, newer paints, and some fish; and aluminum is in antacids, over-the-counter drugs and douches, aluminum cookware and foil, certain underarm deodorants, and most city water.

The claim that environmental chemicals can cause or promote cancer is supported by the fact that the distribution of toxic-waste dump sites closely correlates with the sites where the highest rates of breast cancer mortality have been registered, according to *Scientific American*, October 1995. Of the 50 highest population centers, Nassau County, near New York City, has the greatest rate, with 70 cases of breast cancer deaths per 100,000 women reported between 1979 and 1992.

A variety of chemicals found in the environment can mimic the activity of estrogen once inside the human body; they are now believed to contribute to many cases of breast cancer. Further, while certain environmental chemicals are known to be estrogenic, generally when found alone they are in such low potencies as to have little measurable effect on biological systems. But when several such estrogenic chemicals are combined, their effect is synergistically enhanced. For example, combining only 2 normally weak environmental estrogens, such as dieldrin, endosulfan, or toxaphene, can produce a result that is 1,000 times more potent.[85]

By 1980, the Environmental Protection Agency had detected over 400 toxic chemicals in human tissue—48 in fat tissue, 40 in breast milk, 73 in the liver, and 250 in the blood. Now, the National Academy of Sciences states that the average American ingests 40 mg of pesticides from food sources alone and carries about one-tenth of a gram permanently stored in body fat. "Virtually anyone willing to put up the $2,000 for the tests will find at least 250 chemical contaminants in his or her body fat, regardless of whether he or she lives in Gary, Indiana, or on a remote island in the South Pacific," state Theo Colborn, Dianne Dumanoski, and John Peterson Wyers. "There is no safe, uncontaminated place."[86]

Dr. Hildegarde L.A. Staninger, Ph.D., medical director of Sunstate Preventive Medicine Institute in Winter Park, Florida, is one of the country's experts in industrial toxicology, which uses a laboratory-based approach that enables physicians to *quantify* the level of dangerous toxic chemicals absorbed into a patient's bloodstream or tissues through external exposure.

For example, Joe, aged 75, was diagnosed with prostate cancer. Dr. Staninger analyzed specimens of this man's cancerous tissue and found abnormally high levels of many carcinogens such as arsenic, chlordane, and DDT. These substances produced a toxic overload on his immune system which led to liver dysfunction and, from there, presumably to the prostate cancer. The prostate is regarded, like female breast tissue, as a kind of reservoir (or dump site) for toxic chemicals in the body. What Dr. Staninger demonstrated by this particular case is the need to perform a split biopsy. Joe's tissue culture was examined both for signs of cancer and carcinogenic toxicity; a biopsy alone without a toxicological analysis would have presented a clinically incomplete picture of his condition.

Industrial workers are routinely exposed to potentially toxic chemicals and substances while on the job. Tanners, oil refinery workers, and insecticide/herbicide sprayers are exposed to arsenic and risk lung and skin cancer. Shipyard workers, demolition experts, and brake-lining mechanics are exposed to asbestos, which places them at risk for lung cancer. Hospital and laboratory staff, as well as those involved in the manufacture of wood products, are routinely exposed to

## What's Causing All the Cancer in Marin County?

The fact that Marin County in Northern California (in the San Francisco Bay Area) has an incidence of breast cancer about 11% higher than the national average has led many physicians in that area to speculate as to what factors may be producing such an abnormally high rate. Marin County is known for its high income and education levels and as having a large proportion of women who have had few or no children, or who have had them late in life. Many women in that area who have practiced a vegetarian diet,exercised regularly and consumed low-fat diets are developing breast cancer; of these women, only about 30% have the known risk factors, including a family history of breast cancer. Representatives from the Marin Cancer Watch and Breast Cancer Task Force in Marin are "convinced something in Marin's environment is contributing to the high incidence." Among the environmental factors suspected by these groups are a glut of electrical devices, overuse of mammograms, and "an epidemic of toxic materials we put into the environment."[87]

formaldehyde. Other carcinogens in the workplace, such as benzene, diesel exhaust, human-made fibers, hair dyes, mineral oils, painting materials, polychlorinated biphenyls, and soot, are linked with specific occupations, routine exposures, and various cancers.[88] It is estimated that 10% of all cancers are attributable to job-related exposure to carcinogens.[89]

## POLLUTED WATER

Tap water from municipal sources is increasingly becoming a health hazard in the U.S. It is not only pesticides and agricultural runoffs that contaminate public drinking water: according to the EPA, the tap water of 30 million Americans contains potentially hazardous levels of lead.[90] In addition, 1 out of every 4 public water systems has violated federal standards for tap water.[91] Municipal water can contain many different contaminants, including disease-causing bacteria, radioactive particles, heavy metals, gasoline solvents, industrial wastes, chemical residues, and synthetic organic chemicals (such as benzene, trichloroethylene, and many more), along with disinfectant by-products.

***What Dr. Staninger demonstrated by this particular case is the need to perform a split biopsy. Joe's tissue culture was examined both for signs of cancer and carcinogenic toxicity; a biopsy alone without a toxicological analysis would have presented a clinically incomplete picture of his condition.***

Groundwater may also contain toxic amounts of radionuclides, naturally occurring radioactive substances such as uranium, radium, and radon that leech into water supplies. A radionuclide is a decay product, called an isotope, from underground rock beds or geological formations; these decay products release alpha particles, which can enter groundwater. In addition, there are 800 human-made radionuclides from the nuclear power industry, of which 200 are believed to be potential drinking water contaminants.[92] According to William L. Lappenbusch, Ph.D., a water toxicologist: "Radionuclides in drinking water cause more cancer than any other stressor in that medium, challenged only by pesticides."[93]

A survey of 100 municipal water systems and suppliers found significant levels of cancer-causing arsenic, radon, and chlorine by-products, reported the Natural Resources Defense Council in October 1995. An estimated 19 million Americans drink water with radon levels higher than federal safety standards, and two-thirds of the 300 major water suppliers and agencies fail to give consumers information on their tap water.

Unexpected pollutants can occasionally find their way into public water supplies, too. Up to 42 homes in San Quentin Village in California found their water supply contaminated with napthalene, a chemical found in mothballs and used in petroleum-based products such as gasoline and paint thinner.[94] A study of 9,500 public drinking-water wells in California revealed that 10% were contaminated with a toxic solvent (perchloroethylene, or PCE) commonly used by the state's 4,000 dry cleaners. This means that about 7.6 million Californians in 37 counties drink water polluted with low levels of a toxic industrial chemical; in 260 of the wells tested, the level of PCE exceeded the state's maximum allowable safety level. The report concluded that PCE is "the most ubiquitous industrial chemical" in California, "tainting more wells than 7 other chemical pollutants combined."[95]

Polluted drinking water can further raise the risk of developing cancer. Water can be polluted by harmful organic and inorganic chemicals, chlorination products, fluoride, radioactive materials, living organisms, and solid particulates, like asbestos. The U.S. Geological Survey examined water samples from 3,351 wells in farming areas and found that 9% exceeded the safety standard for nitrates. Nitrates from decades of heavy fertilizer use seep into the groundwater and can cause fatal oxygen deprivation in infants. The greatest nitrate concentrations in well water were found in the Northeast, Midwest, and West Coast.

Drinking water containing lead can create health problems for both children and adults, including birth defects and learning deficiencies, hypertension, mental deterioration, and impotency. Unless a house has newer copper water lines, lead can leach out of the older water pipes and plumbing into the water. Lead, copper, and other heavy metals found in public water accumulate in body tissues, eventually producing a condition of chronic heavy metal toxicity. It is important to realize that approximately 70% of the toxins from water that enter the body do so through the skin during baths and showers.

## CHLORINATED WATER

While adding chlorine-type compounds to drinking water protects the public from several kinds of harmful bacteria such as *Shigella*, *Salmonella*, and *Vibrio cholera,* chlorine can form cancer-causing compounds in drinking water.

The most taken-for-granted chemical in our water supply is chlorine, which has been used for nearly one hundred years to "purify" drinking water. The disinfection of drinking water with chlorine is standard practice throughout the United States. The amount of chlorine used is particularly high during the summer; since warm conditions favor bacterial overgrowth, chlorination is heaviest in southern parts of the country.

While there is little doubt that chlorine played a key role in eradicating water-borne infectious diseases such as typhoid and cholera, new evidence indicates that drinking chlorinated water increases the risk of cancer for the roughly 200 million Americans who drink it. Consuming chlorinated drinking water is associated with a 20 to 40% increase in the incidence of colon and rectal cancer, according to the results of a Norwegian study published in the *International Journal of Epidemiology* in 1992.

***Consuming chlorinated drinking water is associated with a 20 to 40% increase in the incidence of colon and rectal cancer, according to the results of a Norwegian study in 1992.***

The EPA tries to downplay the cancer risk from chlorinated drinking water by asserting that the known risk of water-borne disease in humans, if water is not disinfected, is much greater than the theoretical risk of developing cancer. However, according to studies conducted jointly at Harvard University and the Medical College of Wisconsin, the consumption of chlorinated drinking water accounts for 15% of all rectal cancers and 9% of all bladder cancers in the United States. That's an additional 6,500 cases of rectal cancer and 4,200 cases of bladder cancer each year. Further, people drinking chlorinated water over long periods of time have a 38% increase in their chances of contracting rectal cancer and a 21% increase in the risk of contracting bladder cancer.[96]

Toxic and carcinogenic chemical compounds called trihalomethanes are formed when chlorine reacts with organic matter in water. Two examples of these compounds are chloroform and trichloroethylene, and both are a grave cause for concern with regard to promoting cancer. Chloroform, once used as an anesthetic, was banned by the FDA in 1976 because of its cancer-causing properties; trichloroethylene is a toxic by-product of many drug manufacturing processes.

Scientists at EPA's Health Effects Research Laboratory have identified 2 other cancer-causing agents that form in drinking water when chlorine interacts with humus, the organic material formed from the decay of plants. One of these, known as MX, has shown up in every chlorinated water source ever tested for it. The EPA lab reports that MX may be the single largest contributor in municipal water supplies of *mutagenicity* (the ability to induce genetic mutations, a rough measure of cancer-causing potential). Another mutagen, called DCA, is known to alter cholesterol metabolism and cause liver cancers in laboratory animals. Many scientists believe these 2 chlorinated acids are among the more dangerous chemicals found in the U.S. water supply.

The dangers from inhaling chlorine can exceed those derived from drinking chlorinated water. The amount of chloroform (the most common trihalomethane in chlorinated water) inhaled or absorbed through the skin during a typical shower may be 6 times higher than that absorbed from chlorinated drinking water, states *International Health News.* This exposure can be cut by 30% or more by using a bathroom fan, keeping the window open while showering, or running the water through an activated carbon filter.

## FLUORIDATED WATER

Fluoride, a poison second in toxicity only to arsenic, has routinely been added to public drinking water and toothpaste since the 1950s, despite mounting evidence of its multiple health hazards. The practice of water fluoridation was first introduced by an aluminum industry lawyer who had become head of the U.S. Public Health Service. Touted as a way to improve the public's dental health, fluoride was also a lucrative way for the aluminum industry to get rid of sodium fluoride, its main toxic waste product. The fluoride compounds most commonly added to water are actually unrefined toxic waste products of phosphate fertilizer production. As early as 1953, scientists proved that fluoridated water did not reduce cavities in children, which had been the rationale for adding it to water and consumable products.

According to the scientific research, fluoride consumption creates multiple hazards with respect to cancer. Fluoride can *produce* cancer, transforming normal human cells into cancerous ones, even at concentrations of only 1 ppm (parts per million). Furthermore, fluoridated water has produced 6 times more bone cancer in males under age 20. Fluoride can increase the cancer-producing potential of other cancer-causing chemicals. Low levels of fluoride can increase the incidence of skin cancers from 12 to 100%, sometimes in only days. As little as 1 ppm of fluoride in water was found to increase the tumor growth rate in mice by 25%. A National Cancer Institute study compiling 14 years of data showed that the incidence of oral and pharyngeal cancer rises with increased exposure to fluoride by as much as 50%, accounting for 8000 new cases per year.

In a now classic study, John Yiamouyiannis, Ph.D., compared the cancer death rates over 30 years in 10 cities with fluoridated water against 10 whose water was not fluoridated. After 17 years of fluoridation, the cancer rate in those cities had climbed by 10%, primarily in people older than 45. While fluoridated water has been outlawed in 14 European countries as well as in Egypt and India as being too toxic for public health, the U.S. still regards up to 4 ppm as a "safe" level. Despite the weight of scientific evidence, the American Dental Association will not endorse any dental product unless it contains fluoride.[97]

Dean Burk, Ph.D., Chief Chemist Emeritus of the National Cancer Institute, estimates that fluoride causes more cancer than any other chemical. Dr. Burk compared the cancer death rates of the largest fluoridated and nonfluoridated cities. These death rates were similar prior to 1953 when the use of fluoride was introduced, then increased markedly among fluoridated cities. According to Burk's estimates, fluoride caused about 61,000 cases of cancer in 1995 and is likely to cause 90,000 cancer cases by 2015.[98]

Note that the fluoride from drinking water adds to other sources of fluoride such as toothpastes, beverages, gels, tablets, and mouth "swish" products. Fluoride becomes *more* concentrated in boiled water but can be removed with reverse osmosis water filters. The metal refining industry releases vast amounts of fluoride compounds into the atmosphere which then rain down on croplands and enter the food chain. Each year, about 143,000 tons of fluoride are pumped into the nation's reservoirs, most of it as recycled industrial waste.

The National Academy of Sciences has found that fluorine (a component of fluoride) slows down vitally important DNA repair activity as mediated by enzymes that normally correct for possible flaws or mutations in the genetic material. These biological effects can be induced by fluoride present even in concentrations as low as 1 ppm, the official "safe" dosage set by the U.S. Public Health Service for drinking water. Even with this "low" standard, the risk of serious chromosomal damage is enhanced; in cell studies, for example, this dosage level has been sufficient to transform normal cells into cancer cells.[99]

## TOBACCO AND SMOKING

Tobacco smoke is *the* top carcinogen, according to Dimitrios Trichopoulos, M.D. and cowriters, as unequivocally stated in *Scientific American.* Dr. Trichopoulos, director of the Harvard Center for Cancer Prevention at the School of Public Health, at Harvard University in Cambridge, Massachusetts, estimates that about 30% of cancer deaths in the U.S. can be attributed to tobacco smoke, making tobacco smoke "the single most lethal carcinogen in the U.S." Passive smoking, or inhaling ambient tobacco smoke, also produces several thousand lung cancer deaths every year, says Dr. Trichopoulos. "Thus, passive smoking is as much a killer as general outdoor air pollution or household exposure to the radioactive gas radon."[100]

***About 30% of cancer deaths in the U.S. can be attributed to tobacco smoke, making tobacco smoke "the single most lethal carcinogen in the U.S."***

It is estimated that 350,000-400,000 deaths occur each year in the U.S. as a result of tobacco use, and about 33% of these deaths occur from smoking-related lung cancer alone. This makes smoking the single major cause of cancer death. Although dietary factors account for a higher percentage of cancer deaths, they do not represent a *single* cause. Smoking has been linked to cancers of the head and neck, mouth, throat, vocal cords, bladder, kidney, stomach, cervix, and pancreas, as well as to leukemia; smokeless tobacco has been linked to cancers of the lip and tongue.[101]

Secondary smoke, or passively inhaled smoke, contains dangerous carcinogens as well, according to the Environmental Protection Agency which listed it in the same category as the known carcinogens, benzene, radon, and asbestos. Indirect, passive exposure causes an estimated 20% of all lung cancers in the United States not attributed *directly* to smoking; that is, it accounts for about 3,000 lung cancer deaths each year among nonsmokers. The risk doubles for nonsmoking spouses living with smokers.[102] Further, long-term exposure to urban air pollution (containing diesel exhaust) increases the risk of lung cancer by about 50%, especially among smokers; cigarette smoking alone increases the risk by 2000%.[103]

Scientists from the Imperial Cancer Research Fund in London, England, found that among women smokers with cervical dysplasia, the number of precancerous lesions was reduced by at least 20% in the women who either quit smoking or cut back by 75% over a 6-month period, as reported in *The Lancet* in 1996. In 4 women, the lesions disappeared entirely, and for 10 women, the lesions were 50% reduced in size. The degree to which women cut back on smoking was directly associated with how much the precancerous lesions shrank. Reading this backwards, you can see how cigarette smoking is directly linked to cancer.

Over 2,000 chemical compounds are generated by tobacco smoke, and many of them are poisons.[104] Carbon monoxide is released during smoking, reducing the amount of oxygen to organs like the brain, lungs, and heart. Nicotine is not only addictive, but also acts as a cancer promoter, making it easier for cancer cells of all types to spread throughout the body.[105]

This fact makes it easy to understand how smoking leads to 2 fundamental health-related problems: (1) production of harmful free radicals and (2) adverse effects on the human immune system. "People who smoke tend to have an extraordinary amount of free-radical activity in their bodies, which can damage their DNA and set the stage for cancer," says Charles Simone, M.D., director of the Simone Cancer Prevention Center in Princeton, New Jersey, and a cancer doctor profiled in Chapter 19 of this book.

"At the same time, the smoke alters the balance of key immune cells and suppresses the natural killer (NK) cells and IgA antibodies, which are a first line of defense against viruses and bacteria," says Dr. Simone. Since NK cells ordinarily would destroy cancer cells in the bloodstream, the suppressive effect on this cell population could explain why smokers are more vulnerable not only to lung cancer, but to other cancers as well.[106]

Tar, which is formed when organic compounds are burned, is the leading cancer-causing chemical found in tobacco smoke. This substance contains extremely carcinogenic hydrocarbons, including nitrosamines, benzopyrenes, benzenes, insecticides, and other toxic compounds, as well as some radioactive compounds like potassium-40 and radium-226.[107] Carbon monoxide is released during smoking, reducing the amount of oxygen to all organs, especially the brain, lungs, and heart. Nicotine, an alkaloid found in tobacco, is not only addictive, but also acts as a cancer promoter, making it easier for cancer cells of all types to spread throughout the body.[108]

Researchers have now not only proven that cigarette smoking is linked to lung cancer, but have demonstrated precisely how, on a molecular level, this happens. Scientists at the University of Texas M.D. Anderson Cancer Center in Houston and the Beckman Research Institute of the City of Hope in Duarte, California, have identified the exact cigarette tar and human gene involved. A tar chemical called benzo(a)pyrene directly damages a tumor suppressor gene called p53 in lung cells; when undamaged, p53 is believed to stop tumor processes from getting under way (see later in this chapter, under "Oncogenes").

***Researchers have now not only proven that cigarette smoking is linked to lung cancer, but have demonstrated precisely how, on a molecular level, this happens. "The damage caused by the carcinogen matches up exactly with the mutations seen in the cancer tissue," stated Gerd Pfeifer, Ph.D.***

As early as 1964, the U.S. Surgeon General declared that benzo(a)pyrene is "one of the two most potent of the seven carcinogens detected in tobacco smoke, and it is present in much larger quantity than any other carcinogen." Scientists also knew that the p53 gene was damaged (mutated) in 3 particular spots in 60-70% of human lung cancers. The missing link is now established: molecules from the breakdown products of benzo(a)pyrene chemically bind to 3 specific locations on the p53 gene (the ones subsequently damaged and found in lung cancer cells), and facilitate the transformation of normal cells into malignant ones. "The damage caused by the carcinogen matches up exactly with the mutations seen in the cancer tissue," stated project director Gerd Pfeifer, Ph.D., at M.D. Anderson Cancer Center.[109]

To make matters worse, smokers tend to have lower blood levels of vitamin C and several other antioxidants that would otherwise scavenge or neutralize the free radicals. As a result, tobacco smoke offers the perfect formula for initiating and promoting cancer: carcinogens, toxins, free radicals, antioxidant deficiencies, and immune suppression.

In addition, a direct link has been found between lung cancer and flue-dried tobacco, especially that to which sugar has been added, whereas no significant correlation between traditional sugar-free, air-dried tobacco and cancer has been established. Studies show that England and Wales, which have the highest male lung cancer rate in the world, also have the highest sugar content in cigarettes, about 17%. France, where tobacco is air-dried and contains only 2% sugar, has one-third less lung cancer; the U.S., where sugar in tobacco averages 10%, has about half the male lung cancer death rate as in great Britain.[110]

Lung cancer escalated from a rare disorder around 1920 (5 cases per 100,000) to a virtual epidemic 50 years later (75 cases per 100,000) and from a handful of deaths in 1920 to 18,000 a year by 1950. In studies of 40,000 male patients, lung cancer was 10 to 30 times more prevalent among those who were smokers; researchers also discovered that the numbers of cancers among smokers went up directly in proportion to how many cigarettes they smoked. Not only was the lung tissue of long-term smokers blackened, but researchers found that the lungs of 93% of smokers exhibited precancerous abnormal cells, compared to only 1% of nonsmokers.

The reason it has taken almost 45 more years for the FDA to get cracking on cigarettes as a true health hazard can be credited to the successful outcome of a meeting of top tobacco industry executives on December 15, 1953, in New York City. There they organized a massive "no harm from cigarettes" public relations campaign to deliver direct attacks on those who were saying that cigarettes cause cancer. "Thus began the conspiracy," explains Philip J. Hilts of Harvard University's School of Public

## The Tobacco-Cancer Cover-up

Tobacco's carcinogenicity was known to tobacco industry officials as early as 1952. In fact, the connection between cigarettes and lung cancer, surprisingly, was also relayed to the public that year in a *Reader's Digest* article called "Cancer by the Carton." Even more convincing was a scientific study published in *Cancer Research* (December 1953). Researchers at the Sloan Kettering Institute in New York City (now called Memorial Sloan Kettering Cancer Institute) painted cigarette smoke condensate onto the skin of mice and found it produced cancers in 44% of the animals.

In fact, the role of inhalants as a carcinogen was demonstrated in 1915 by Katsusaburo Yamagiwa when, presenting his findings before the Tokyo Medical Society, he announced he could produce cancer at will. Yamagiwa painted extracts of coal tar (found in condensed cigarette smoke) on the skin of 137 rabbits every 2-3 days for 3 months. After 12 months, he noted 7 invasive cancers at the sites of application. In 1953, Ernest Wynder, working at the Sloan Kettering Institute, replicated Yamagiwa's work by again producing skin cancer in mice after painting them with, first, condensed coal tar, then tobacco-smoke condensate. In 1949, he had already demonstrated that the risk of lung cancer rose directly in proportion to the number of cigarettes smoked and that smokers had a cancer risk 40 times higher than nonsmokers.

## Hormones Are Linked to Nerve Cell Cancer

A study of 555 mothers revealed that those who took sex hormones for infertility during the time in which they were unknowingly pregnant were 10 times more likely to bear children who developed neuroblastoma within the first 2 years after birth, according to researchers at the Roswell Park Cancer Institute in New York reporting in the *American Journal of Epidemiology* (143: 1996). Neuroblastoma is a malignant tumor of embryonic nerve cells. Those women who took vitamins while on the sex hormones were 72% less likely to have newborns develop neuroblastoma.

Health in Cambridge, Massachusetts.

Money was at the core of the tobacco industry conspiracy, Hilts says, and the strategic use of public relations blocked any serious look at the issue at the time. "The plan was to spend large amounts of money every year indefinitely into the future to prevent, not sworn adversaries, but *scientists and public health officers*, from warning people of a potential hazard in the normal manner."[111] How many thousands of deaths from lung cancer might be laid at the feet of these executives? The bill may finally be coming due to the tobacco industry for the untold deaths resulting from their refusal to be honest with the public regarding the hazards of tobacco smoke. At least 17 states and 12 local governments, including New York City, have filed lawsuits against tobacco companies. New York City, for instance, claims that the health-care costs from smoking amount to $300 million per year for that city; their lawsuit seeks damages for these extreme expenses.[112]

## HORMONE THERAPIES

Drugs given to alter the natural hormonal cycle of women have been selectively implicated as capable of producing cancer. Regarding oral contraceptives, a study showed that women who took birth control pills for more than 4 years were twice as likely as nonusers to develop breast cancer at age 50.[113] For women who start taking birth control pills before age 18 and continue for at least 10 years, the risk of their developing breast cancer before age 35 is 3 times higher, based on a study of 4,212 women, reports *Science News* (June 1995). Women under 35 years of age who had used oral contraceptives for only 6 months still had almost twice the risk of nonusers.

Research reported as early as the late 1960s pointed to serious cancer risks associated with oral contraceptives. As high as 84% of 103 women taking the pill had cervical lesions that were blistered, swollen, engorged with blood vessels, or eroded; such lesions develop in as short a time as one month after taking the pill. More significantly, in 1968, Tilde S. Kline, M.D., of Peter Brent Brigham Hospital in Boston, Massachusetts, reported the results of comparing Pap smears from 1,221 pill users with 16,225 nonusers. Those women on the pill had a 300% higher incidence of cervical dysplasia, usually benign changes in the shape of the cervix that, nonetheless, can be early indicators of possible later cancer.

In the 1960s, Roy Hertz, M.D., then with the National Institutes of Health, made a grim prediction. (Birth control pills had been widely used for about a decade by then.) The year 1971 might be the year in which cancer would begin increasing among women—because of the pill. The full effect of the use of a carcinogen usually takes 10 years to show up, Dr. Hertz advised, then another decade before the cancer is significant enough to produce noticeable symptoms. "Cancer of the breast or of the cervix or of the womb will require from its initiation in the preclinical phase a period of approximately a decade before the clinical manifestation of the tumor," said Dr. Hertz.

His colleague, Georges Mathe, M.D., then director of the French Institute of Cancerology and Immunogenetics, made a more conservative estimate. For Dr. Mathe, the long-term risk of cancer traceable to contraceptives "cannot be dismissed." In 1967, he said, "the incubation time might be 25 years"—which puts the full-fledged cancer epidemic right in our midst in the 1990s.[114] As of 1996, the link between birth control pills and breast cancer remained controversial. Some studies have shown elevated breast cancer rates for women in their 30s and 40s using oral contraception, and a National Cancer Institute study indicated that there was a slightly higher rate in women under 45.

A 1996 study in the journal *Contraception* reported on the results of researchers from 25 countries; they examined 54 epidemiological studies

## Antidepressants Are Linked to Cancer

A recent study involving 7 tricyclic antidepressants and 3 benzodiazepine tranquilizers, including Valium, showed that these drugs could produce higher risks and rates of ovarian cancer. Women of any age who use these drugs regularly have twice the risk of developing ovarian cancer compared to healthy women of the same age who do not use them.

Women who started taking these medications before the age of 50 have the highest risk, which is placed at 2.7 to 3.5 times higher than the average risk. The tricyclic antidepressant desipramine (brand name Norpramin), with 4.6 million annual prescriptions for children with hyperactivity and depression, has been linked to at least 7 cases of sudden death in children using it.[115]

involving 53,297 women with breast cancer and 100,239 healthy women. However, their study also noted that there is a slightly higher incidence of breast cancer in women taking oral contraceptives and for 10 years after they stop taking them; specifically, that increase is 17.5 cases per 10,000 women on the pill (with initial use beginning at age 20-24) compared to 16 per 10,000 women not using oral contraceptives.[116]

The use of hormone replacement therapy and supplemental estrogens for menopausal women has been linked to endometrial and breast cancer. The link was first firmly established in 1989 when Swedish researchers reported the results of a study involving 23,244 women. Those women who had been on estrogen replacement therapy (ERT) for longer than 9 years had a slightly increased risk of breast cancer, they reported, and those who took combined estrogen and progesterone replacement therapy had a higher risk than those women taking either alone. In 1995, Harvard University researchers published the now famous Nurses' Health Study based on data from 1976 to 1992. Their report concluded that women aged 55-59 who took ERT for 5 years or more had a 40% higher risk of developing breast cancer; among women aged 60-64, the risk was 70% higher.[117]

## Blood Pressure Drug May Cause Cancer

According to a study involving 5,000 patients aged 71 and older, conducted by scientists at the University of Tennessee in Memphis, the regular use of calcium channel blockers, the most widely prescribed group of high blood pressure drugs, is associated with a 72% higher rate of cancer. In research published in *The Lancet* (August 1996), this percentage increase is equal to 8 new cancers per 100 people using the drugs for 5 years.

Regarding the risk of endometrial cancer from estrogen replacement therapy, John R. Lee, M.D., women's health expert, educator, and author, based in Sebastopol, California, concludes: "The evidence is overwhelming that natural progesterone [the alternative to ERT] is safe, and only estradiol, estrone, and the various synthetic estrogens and progestins are to be avoided to reduce one's risk of endometrial cancer."[118]

Dairy milk may be another carrier of cancer-producing factors. Ever since recombinant Bovine Growth Hormone (rBGH) was approved by the FDA in 1993 for injecting dairy cows to increase milk yield, consumers have been alarmed about its possible negative health effects and the lack of solid scientific support for its safety. Many have also been outraged by the FDA's failure to require dairies to label milk and milk products as being derived from rBHG-treated cows.

Interest among dairy farmers in using rBGH is dropping off; 87% of those not yet using the hormone do not plan to ever use it and only about 12% of America dairy farms are currently employing it. Meanwhile, the 14-nation European Union has banned its use and Canada has called for a 2-year moratorium on its further use in that country.

So the news that "converging lines of evidence" now incriminate rBGH "as a potential risk for both breast and gastrointestinal cancers" should be the catalyst that gets the FDA to ban the substance from American milk—that is, if they can free themselves from suspected insider connections with Monsanto and several other chemical companies that make rBGH.

In a new study published in the *International Journal of Health Services*, Samuel S. Epstein, M.D., chairman of the Cancer Prevention Coalition and professor at the University of Illinois Medical Center, both in Chicago, Illinois, states that "with the active complicity of the FDA, the entire nation is currently being subjected to ... large-scale adulteration of an age-old dietary staple by a poorly characterized and unlabeled biotechnology product." The result may be major potential public health risks for the entire country, Dr. Epstein suggests.

The problem with rBGH is that it contains a hormone common to cows and humans called IGF-1 (insulin-like growth factor), says Dr. Epstein. IGF-1 causes cells to divide and grow, but when extra amounts enter the human body in the presence of milk protein, the body is unable to destroy it, and it is absorbed by the colon, which is known to have cell receptor sites for IGF-1. The hormone is also known to promote the growth of breast cancer cells. At least 17 scientific studies published since 1991 argue that rBGH milk may have cancer-producing effects.

## Cholesterol Drugs May Cause Cancer

Widely used cholesterol-lowering drugs such as lovastatin (Mevacor) and gemfibrozil (Lopid) can cause cancer in mice and rats and possibly humans, claim researchers at the University of California at San Francisco. Drug exposure that was carcinogenic in rodents was at the same order of magnitude as the maximum dose typically given to humans, reported *Science News* (March 2, 1996). The researchers noted major discrepancies in carcinogenicity in the listings for these drugs in the 1994 versus 1992 editions of the *Physicians' Desk Reference*, supposedly the standard for accurate drug information.

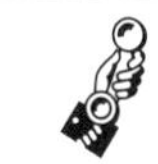

For more information about Dr. Epstein's **rBGH** research, contact: Cancer Prevention Coalition, 520 N. Michigan Avenue, Suite 410, Chicago, IL 60611; tel: 312-467-0600; fax: 312-467-0599.

## Aspirin Is Not Effective against Cancer

Based on an analysis of 2,414 breast cancer cases among 89,528 women participating in a 12-year study, researchers now contend that the regular use of aspirin does not reduce the risk of breast cancer, according to the *Journal of the National Cancer Institute* (July 1996). Rates of new cases were about the same for those taking aspirin as for those who did not.

Monsanto studies prepared for the FDA indicate that the IGF-1 levels in cows injected with rBGH can rise by a range of 25 to 70%. But independent European studies say that rBGH milk may contain a tenfold increase in IGF-1. High IGF-1 levels are particularly dangerous for infants and young children, states Dr. Epstein. "The FDA has dismissed these concerns without investigation and on the basis of unpublished 'confidential' short-term toxicity data, primarily from an industry consulting firm with a tainted track record," Dr. Epstein says.[119]

### IMMUNE-SUPPRESSIVE DRUGS

The widespread, habitual, and chronic use of a great number of conventional drugs, antibiotics, and even vaccinations can have a seriously suppressive effect on the immune system, acting in concert with all the other factors at play to prepare the system for a cancer process. Drugs such as aspirin, acetaminophen, and ibuprofen taken for aches and colds, and glucocorticosteroids (such as cortisone) decrease antibody production and suppress immune vitality.

Vaccinations can suppress the immune system for 1 to 2 weeks. A study of T lymphocyte cells in blood samples from persons before and after typhus vaccinations showed a 50% decrease in the ratio of helper cells to suppressor cells in the immune system; the decrease was most severe between 3 and 14 days after vaccination. A similar drop in T helper cells has been noted in young children following receipt of multiple vaccines, the so-called vaccine cocktails. This might be setting the stage for future immune system depression and the onset of chronic disease, states naturopathic physician Joseph Pizzorno, N.D. "Any suppression of the T helper lymphocytes during this time, even of a transient nature, is undesirable because it may impair proper maturation of their immune systems."[120]

Antibiotics can directly hinder immune activity and increase the intestinal overgrowth of the yeast *Candida albicans*, which then can suppress the immune system. Antibiotics can also upset the balance of microflora in the intestines, leading to a condition called dysbiosis in which "unfriendly," potentially pathogenic, bacteria predominate over the more "friendly," probiotic microflora. According to Carol Jessop, M.D., Clinical Professor at the University of California at San Francisco, 80% of her patients with chronic fatigue syndrome had a history of recurrent antibiotic treatment as a child, adolescent, or adult.

Antibiotics can also lead to food intolerances and allergies, which in turn clog the immune system by creating circulating immune complexes and lowering total lymphocyte counts by as much as 50%. Dr. Jessop also found that a 1-year treatment of her patients with chronic fatigue immune deficiency syndrome with an antifungal drug significantly reduced their fatigue and other symptoms.

Not to be overlooked are cytotoxic agents or chemotherapy drugs used to stop cancerous growth. Given their mission, it is not surprising that they have powerful immune-suppressive effects. They decrease the numbers of neutrophils, and, in effect, render the individual even more susceptible to new, secondary cancers.

### Food Additives to Avoid

**Aspartame:** chemical sweetener used in NutraSweet® and Equal®

**Bromated Vegetable Oil:** emulsifier in foods and clouding agent in soft drinks

**Butylated Hydroxyanisole (BHA) and Butylated Hydroxytoluene (BHT):** prevents fats, oils, and fat-containing foods from going rancid

**Citrus Red Dye No. 2:** Used to color orange skins

**Monosodium Glutamate (MSG):** flavor enhancer used in fast, processed, or packaged foods

**Nitrites:** used as preservatives in cured meats to prevent spoilage

**Saccharin:** artificial sweetener, used in Sweet 'n Low®

**Sulfur Dioxide, Sodium Bisulfite, Sulfites:** preserves dried fruits, shrimp, frozen potatoes

**Tertiary Butylhydroquinone:** used to spray the inside of cereal and cheese packages

**Yellow Dye No. 6:** used in candy and carbonated beverages as a coloring

## IRRADIATED FOODS

Irradiation of food exposes food to the radioactive materials cesium-137 and cobalt-60. Cesium-137 is a by-product of the plutonium-uranium extraction process used in making nuclear weaponry. The intent of food irradiation is to kill insects, bacteria, molds, and fungi, to prevent sprouting, and to thereby extend shelf life, but the results might be injurious to consumers as well. The process of irradiation leads to the formation of toxic substances, such as benzene and formaldehyde, and other toxic chemical by-products that have been scientifically proven to cause diseases that are slow to develop.

*The widespread use of aspartame in soda beverages is hard to believe, given that scientists have evidence suggesting that the artificial sweetener may cause brain tumors.*

A study conducted by Ralston Scientific Services for the U.S. Army and the United States Department of Agriculture found that mice fed a diet rich in irradiated chicken died earlier and had a higher incidence of tumors.[121] The largest animal study done to date resulted in excessively high incidences of both sick and dead animals. In addition, when the herbicides, insecticides, pesticides, fungicides, colorants, antibiotics, steroids, preservatives, and stabilizers in food are irradiated, they transform into what scientists call "Unique Radiolytic Products" (URPs) of unknown toxicity. The FDA estimates that 10% of the chemicals in irradiated food are URPs—that is, not found in normal (nonirradiated) foods and often unknown to science.[122]

Food irradiation may increase the levels of aflatoxin, a deadly carcinogen;[123] it may allow the botulinum toxin (which causes botulism food poisoning) to remain undetected in irradiated foods;[124] over time it may induce some microorganisms to mutate, giving rise to new, dangerous species. Foods that have been irradiated lose much of their nutritional value; the vitamin C content of irradiated potatoes, for example, can be reduced by as much as 50%;[125] in cooked pork, a dose of irradiation equal to one-third the level permitted by the FDA reduced thiamin levels by 17%.[126]

*The process of irradiation leads to the formation of toxic substances, such as benzene and formaldehyde, and other toxic chemical byproducts that have been scientifically proven to cause diseases that are slow to develop.*

As might be expected, the FDA, instead of acting to protect public health, acted to protect the food industry. Even though consumers have a right to know that food has been irradiated, the FDA permits foods exposed to gamma or ionizing radiation to be sold to retail consumers *without* any informational labels. While whole irradiated foods must be labeled with the flowerlike "radura" symbol, irradiated ingredients *within* foods are not regulated. For example, commercially prepared spaghetti sauces may contain irradiated ingredients but not carry any warning.

## FOOD ADDITIVES

Over 3,000 chemical additives are added to the American food supply every year. The vast majority of them have been tested only on animals, not humans. Among the most common are saccharin and cyclamates, both used as artificial sweeteners and linked to greater incidences of bladder cancer; butylated hydroxytoluene, used as a preservative and linked to liver cancer; and tannic acid, found in wines and fruits and linked to liver cancer. Aflatoxins, which are found in milk, cereals, peanuts, and corn, have also been linked to liver, stomach, and kidney cancer.[127]

For more information about **detoxifying** the body of the effects of pollutants, see Chapter 33: Physical Support Therapies, pp. 949-980.

**Aflatoxins** are a group of 16 naturally occurring toxic by-products produced by the fungus *Aspergillus flavus*, often found on peanuts, rice, grain, corn, beans, and sweet potatoes. Aflatoxin B1 (AFB1) shows the highest degree of biological activity and has been linked to higher levels of liver cancer in African and Asian populations where these foods are widely consumed. AFB1 is considered a carcinogen precursor and requires activation before it can produce cellular mutations leading to cancer.

Among the many chemical additives found in supermarket foods that may be linked to an increased risk of cancer are gentian violet, nitrofurans, aldicarb, and aspartame.[128] Gentian violet is a carcinogen used to treat chickens and turkeys for diseases caused by fungus; it is added to poultry feed to inhibit mold. Nitrofurans (nitrofurazone and furazolidone) are added to livestock feed to increase the growth rates, particularly of pigs and poultry. Aldicarb has been associated with altered immune function in women who consume food or groundwater contaminated with small amounts of this additive.

Aspartame is an artificial sweetener made from 2 amino acids, aspartic acid and phenylalanine. It was discovered in 1965 and approved by the FDA in 1981. Today it is found in over 5,000 food products and generates annual sales of $1 billion. Aspartame is 200 times sweeter than cane sugar. The phenylalanine content is a health hazard to those suffering from phenylketonuria (1 out of 15,000 people), an inability to metabolize phenylalanine. Critics claim that the substance can elevate blood pressure, produce insomnia, render one more sensitive to pain, increase the desire for food, contribute to eye degeneration and possibly seizures and mental illness, and perhaps worsen Parkinson's. The widespread use of aspartame in soda beverages is hard to believe, given that scientists have evidence suggesting that the artificial sweetener may cause brain tumors.[129]

Other food additives that may increase the risk of certain kinds of cancer include Blue Dye No. 2, Propyl gallate, and Red Dye No. 3. According to Michael F. Jacobson, Ph.D., of the Center for Science in the Public Interest, which has served as one of the primary watchdog groups for the food industry's use of unsafe additives, there is strong evidence that all these

## Mother's Mercury Passes to the Fetus

German researchers found that pregnant women's mercury amalgams are directly associated with high levels of mercury in their fetuses. The more mercury-based fillings, the higher the levels in the livers of the unborn. The women in the study did not have a history of high mercury exposure from their jobs or from eating fish. German doctors urged reconsideration of the use of mercury amalgams for women during their childbearing years.

additives are linked with cancers.[130] Sadly, the FDA continues to allow the industry to freely add these dangerous substances to our food supply, once again neglecting its charter purpose of protecting the public against dangerous foods and drugs. Consumption of dairy products and meats contaminated with steroids and antibiotics also increases the cancer risk.

### MERCURY TOXICITY

The energy blockages produced by dental problems can also be caused by the "battery" effect of mercury amalgam material most people have as fillings in their teeth. "These so-called silver fillings actually contain 50% mercury and only 25% silver," says Joyal Taylor, D.D.S., of Rancho Santa Fe, California, president of the Environmental Dental Association. These constituents make such fillings especially harmful. Mercury is a noted carcinogen, and has the ability to impair immune function and create blockages in the autonomic nervous system and other tissues.

***As confirmed by a report from the International Academy of Oral Medicine and Toxicology (IAOMT), silver amalgams used in dentistry are 50% mercury and contribute to immune dysfunction and free-radical pathologies, including cancer.***

While all metals used for dental restoration can be toxic, mercury amalgam used for fillings is the most harmful. It is estimated that more than 100 million mercury fillings are placed in the mouths of patients each year in the U.S. One reason for the popularity of amalgam fillings is the relative lack of skill required for its usage. Amalgam is a soft composite comprising an alloy of 2 or more metals—mercury (50%), silver (35%), tin (9%), copper (6%), and a trace of zinc.

"The release of mercury from these amalgams represents the primary source of mercury exposure in people with amalgam fillings," says Stephen Edelson, M.D., medical director of the Environmental and Preventive Health Center of Atlanta, Georgia, and a cancer physician profiled in Chapter 8 in this book. Mercury vapor is readily absorbed into the blood because of its solubility in blood lipids (fatty molecules), Dr. Edelson explains. This process contributes to between 80 and 100% absorption through the lung from which the mercury is then carried to virtually every cell in the body, including the brain.[131]

Evidence now shows that mercury amalgams are the *major* source of mercury exposure for the general public, at rates 6 times higher than that found in fish and seafood. Since mercury vapors are continuously released from amalgam fillings, as long as you have mercury dental fillings, you inhale mercury vapor 24 hours a day, 365 days a year.

After elemental mercury from amalgam fillings is inhaled or ingested, it is converted by the action of bacteria in the body to methylmercury, the organic form of mercury. Methylmercury, because it easily crosses the blood-brain barrier, has been associated with neurodegenerative diseases such as Alzheimer's, multiple sclerosis, and amyotrophic lateral sclerosis. It is important to mention that, as toxic as elemental mercury is, methylmercury is 100 times more toxic.

Mercury is a heavy metal. Heavy metals act as free radicals—highly reactive, charged particles that can cause damage to body tissues if inhaled or absorbed. When present in excess, heavy metals can block the enzymes necessary for the body's detoxification processes, says Daniel F. Royal, D.O., medical director of the Nevada Clinic and the Royal Center of Advanced Medicine, both in Las Vegas, Nevada.[133] Like other heavy metals, mercury has been shown to cause damage to the lining of arteries and nerve bundles (ganglia), particularly those near the prostate, thereby contributing to cancer.

"This means that if amalgam fillings are present, your circulatory sys-

## Mercury Amalgams and Mercury Blood Levels

According to *Occupation and Environment* (1995), people with mercury-based dental amalgams have higher mercury levels in the blood and urine than those without such fillings, and for those not otherwise exposed to mercury through fish products and foods, the levels of mercury in the blood and urine are directly related to the number of their mercury fillings.

***"There have been no studies [in the United States] on the safety of mercury in dental work, but when it leaks from the teeth it can cause both physical and mental problems," states Dr. Joyal Taylor, D.D.S.***

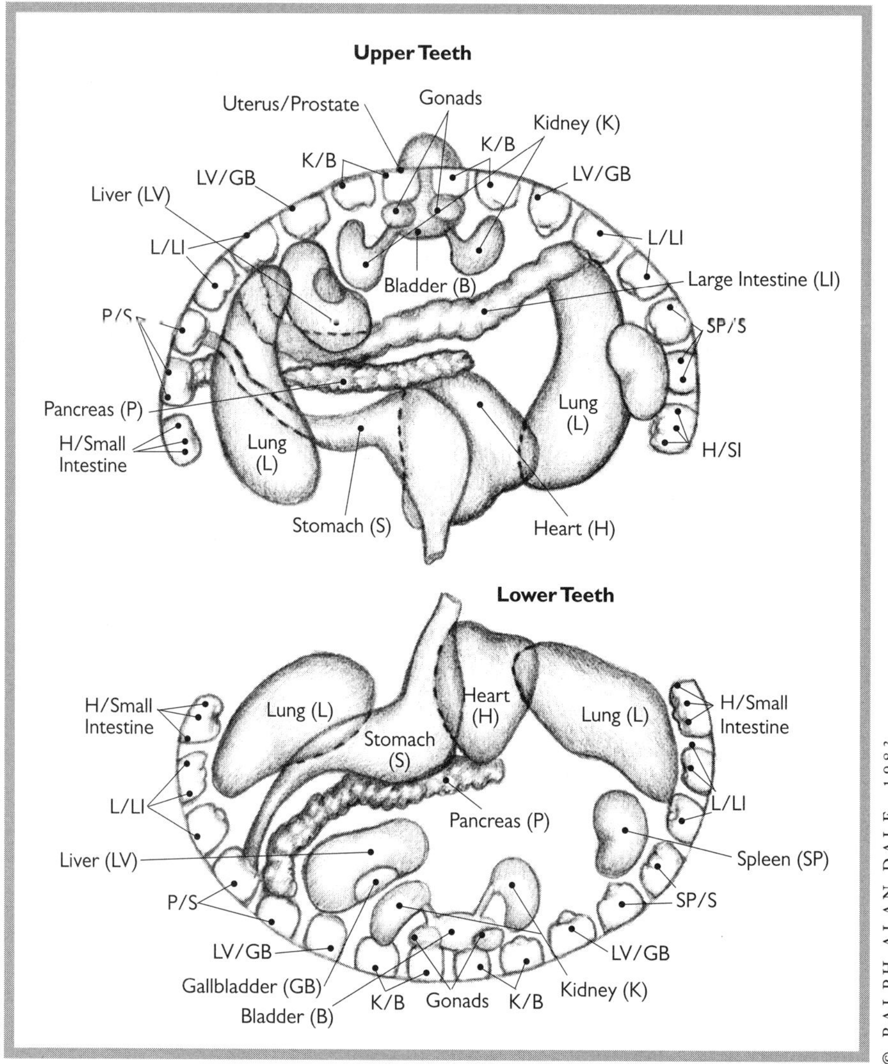



**Figure 25.3—Organ and teeth correspondences on acupuncture meridians in the mouth**

tem is *constantly* being exposed to the damaging effects of this heavy metal and free radical," Dr. Royal explains. "It is interesting to note that cardiovascular disease has become widespread only since the 1920s, about the time of increased use of heavy metals in dental therapy but long after humans began consuming eggs, meat, milk, butter, and cheese, commonly thought to contribute to heart disease."

In his medical practice, based on urine samples taken during a 24-hour period, Dr. Royal has documented many cases of mercury poison-

## The Trouble with Root Canals: Infections under the Teeth

Pockets of infection can exist under the teeth and be undetectable on X rays. This is particularly true for teeth that have had root canals as it is very difficult to eliminate all the bacteria and toxins from the roots during this procedure. These infections may persist for years without the patient's knowledge. When infections are present, toxins can leak out and depress the function of the immune system, leading to chronic degenerative diseases throughout the body. Once the infection is cleared up, many of the symptoms of disease will disappear.

Given the estimated 3 miles of microcanals within a single root canaled tooth, there can be considerable bacterial trouble, according to George E. Meinig, D.D.S., author of *Root Canal Cover-Up.* [132] The bacterial toxins get into the bloodstream near the tip of the tooth root, then circulate throughout the body, wreaking biological havoc, including crippling degenerative diseases. Antibiotics can't kill the bacteria once they're trapped inside the devitalized tooth, so the only way out for the bacteria is down—into the body. "One third of all disease in this country can be either directly or indirectly traced to dental infections," Dr. Meinig asserts.

Dr. Meinig bases his upsetting pronouncements on the 25 years of research by Dr. Weston Price, first published (and ignored) in 1923, whom Dr. Meinig regards as "the world's greatest dentist." Dr. Price's research showed that 25% of patients whose family histories were free of degenerative diseases and who had top-notch immune systems "could expect to have and retain root canal fillings and live without complications arising therefrom through old age," writes Dr. Meinig. But as for the other 75% of patients, root canals could be a significant source of ill health. Dr. Price demonstrated that dead teeth and root canals could make people sick, producing rheumatoid arthritis, heart and kidney disease, and other chronic problems.

In many cases, extraction of the root canaled tooth and a thorough cleaning out of the infected jaw could reverse these conditions in a dramatically short time, usually in a few days. To prove how toxic the removed dental material was, Dr. Price sewed the root canaled tooth under the skin of a laboratory rabbit, and within 3 days the rabbit was dead from the same condition that had made the person ill. In fact, this material was so toxic that Dr. Price could produce the same results in 27 successive generations of rabbits, using the same tooth, even after autoclaving it at high temperatures for 24 hours.

When a tooth with a root canal is removed, the periodontal ligament that attaches the tooth to the underlying bone should also be removed, advises Dr. Huggins, otherwise a pocket of infection can remain. Full removal of the tooth, the ligament, and the surrounding areas of dead jawbone stimulates the old bone to produce new bone for healing. According to Michael Ziff, D.D.S., of Orlando, Florida, there are cases where root canaled teeth should not be pulled. It can be difficult to chew without certain teeth intact and problems can arise if the teeth surrounding the extracted one become misaligned. "The best approach is a conservative one," says Dr. Ziff. "Try other measures first and only remove the tooth as a last resort."

***Evidence now shows that mercury amalgams are the major source of mercury exposure for the general public, at rates 6 times higher than that found in fish and seafood. Since mercury vapors are continuously released from amalgam fillings, as long as you have mercury dental fillings, you inhale mercury vapor 24 hours a day, 365 days a year.***

ing. "Even if amalgam fillings are no longer present in a patient's mouth, mercury levels can often still be detected. It is not unusual to see patients who have had their amalgam fillings removed and replaced as long ago as 10-15 years prior to testing to still have elevated levels of mercury in the body."

Mercury toxicity has been shown to have destructive contributory effects on kidney function, in cardiovascular disease, neuropsychological dysfunction, reproductive disorders, and birth defects, to name a few. Symptoms of mercury toxicity make a very long list: anorexia, depression, fatigue, insomnia, arthritis, multiple sclerosis, moodiness, irritability, memory loss, nausea, diarrhea, gum disease, swollen glands, headaches, and many more. "The preponderance of evidence and medical literature now leaves no doubt that mercury has systemic negative health effects," says Dr. Royal.[134]

The problem of amalgam toxicity is so serious that a growing number of doctors routinely advise their cancer patients to have their mercury amalgams replaced. Mercury amalgams create a constant source of heavy metal toxicity, thus weakening the immune system, and because individual teeth (with their toxic fillings) sit on different acupuncture meridians, it can become imperative for this cancer-contributing cause to be eliminated from a patient's body.

***A Danish study of a random sample of 100 men and 100 women showed that increased blood mercury levels were related to the presence of more than 4 amalgam fillings in the teeth.***

Chronic exposure to mercury may disable the glutathione enzyme system, which plays an essential role in fighting free radicals and preventing injury to DNA and cell membranes;[135] all glutathione system enzymes have shown reduced activity following mercury exposure.[136] Mercury directly inhibits other enzymes, such as catalase and superoxide dismutase, and greatly diminishes the liver's detoxifying capacities.[137] One of the most important contributions of mercury to cancer is through its poisoning of the autonomic nervous system ganglia which then results in arterial spasm and the restricted flow of oxygenated blood to the organs; it also leads to reduced lymphatic drainage from these same organs.

The International Academy of Oral Medicine and Toxicology (IAOMT) cites evidence indicating that dental mercury amalgams are a major contributor to immune dysfunction and free-radical pathologies, including cancer. Among the other potential outcomes of amalgam-related pathology are birth defects, antibiotic resistance, cardiovascular disease, Alzheimer's disease, kidney dysfunction, reproductive disorders and various other health problems.[138] The cumulative weakening effect these toxic "insults" can have on a body makes it more vulnerable to cancer initiation.

Mercury amalgams have been used in dentistry since the 1820s, but not until 1988 did it raise serious enough questions for the Environmental Protection Agency (EPA) to declare scrap dental amalgam a hazardous waste. The American Dental Association, which so far has refused to ban its use, now instructs dentists to "know the potential hazards and symptoms of mercury exposure such as the development of sensitivity and neuropathy," to use a no-touch technique for handling the amalgam, and to store it under liquid, preferably glycerin or radiographic fixer, solution, in unbreakable, tightly sealed containers.[139] All of these cautions are largely for the dentist's safety; as to the dental patient receiving a permanent mercury implant, the ADA has no official comment.

According to the German Ministry of Health, "Amalgam is considered a health risk from a medical viewpoint due to the release of mercury vapor,"[140] which can occur from everyday activities such as chewing and brushing the teeth.[141] Amalgams can also erode and corrode with time. Ideally, they should be replaced after 7-10 years.

***According to the German Ministry of Health, "Amalgam is considered a health risk from a medical viewpoint due to the release of mercury vapor," which can occur from everyday activities such as chewing and brushing the teeth. Amalgams can also erode and corrode with time. Ideally, they should be replaced after 7-10 years.***

Studies by the World Health Organization show that a single amalgam can release 3-17 mcg of mercury per day[142], making dental amalgam a major source of mercury exposure.[143] A Danish study of a random sample of 100 men and 100 women showed that increased blood mercury levels were related to the presence of more than 4 amalgam fillings in the teeth.[144] American, Swedish, and German scientists examining cadavers have also found a clear relationship between the number of fillings and the mercury count in the brain and kidneys.[145]

"There have been no studies [in the United States] on the safety of mercury in dental work, but when it leaks from the teeth it can cause both physical and mental problems," states Dr. Joyal Taylor, D.D.S.[146] In a study of 32 saliva samples taken from individuals with mercury amalgams, Cornelius K. Blesius, M.D., of the Southwest Diagnostic Institute in El Paso, Texas, found that "once a total of 4 amalgam restorations is exceeded, potentially toxic levels of mercury can be expected to be present in human sailva."[147]

***According to Thomas Rau, M.D., medical director of the Paracelsus Clinic in Lustmühle, Switzerland, in about 90% of breast cancer patients he has treated there is a dental factor. This means a problem in a tooth can focus its energy imbalance elsewhere in the body, in this case, the breast.***

## DENTAL FACTORS

The well-documented dangers associated with the use of mercury fillings (amalgams) are only one aspect of the negative health impact that dentistry can have. Practitioners of biological dentistry treat the teeth, jaw, and related structures with specific regard to how treatment will affect the entire body. According to Colorado biological dentist Hal Huggins, D.D.S., "Dental problems such as cavities, infections, toxic or allergy-producing filling materials, root canal, and misalignment of the teeth or jaw can have far-reaching effects throughout the body."

Alternative health practitioners familiar with the principles of biological dentistry have long noted a link between dental problems and degenerative illness. When a tooth is inflamed or infected or otherwise compromised, it can block the energy flow along one or more of the body's acupuncture meridians, causing the deterioration of a corresponding organ or tissue and, in time, leading to cancer. According to Thomas Rau,

M.D., medical director of the Paracelsus Clinic in Lustmühle, Switzerland, in about 90% of breast cancer patients he has treated there is a dental factor. This means a problem in a tooth can focus its energy imbalance elsewhere in the body, in this case, the breast; hence the term "dental focus."

"Each tooth relates to an acupuncture meridian," Dr. Rau states, noting that over the years, he has compiled a dental chart mapping the precise relationship among teeth, meridians, and illnesses. The breast, for example, lies on the Stomach meridian. Accordingly, if you have a problematic tooth (such as a root canal or an infected jaw) situated on this meridian, which passes through the jaw, it blocks the flow of energy and can cause degeneration and eventually cancer. To a lesser extent, a dental focus is also involved in the development of prostate and other cancers.

In a German study, when the teeth of 60 patients (who were not responding well to appropriately indicated therapy) were examined for energetic disturbances using electrodermal screening, it was found that 42 had evidence of both aerobic and anaerobic bacteria of 14 different types including *Aerobacter aerogenes*, *Enterococci*, *Streptococcus viridians*, and *Lactobacilli*; 2 had mostly anaerobic cultures, 5 had exclusively anaerobic, and 6 exclusively aerobic. Of the 60 teeth, only 5 were sterile. In other words, each patient had at least one tooth that was so infected with bacteria that it was sending toxicity signals to other parts of the body as part of a dental focus. "The energetic disturbances noted at these teeth appeared so unfavorable in relation to the illness of the patient and his energetic overall situation that an extraction was performed," commented Joachim Thomsen, D.D.S., a dentist practicing acupuncture in Hamburg, Germany.[148]

## Abortion May Increase Breast Cancer Risk

Researchers analyzing the data from 23 previously reported studies involving 60,000 women claim that there is a slight increase in the risk of breast cancer in women having abortions, according to the *British Journal of Epidemiology and Community Health* (October 1996). An estimated 1.6 million abortions are performed annually in the U.S. While the risk increase is still less a factor than the doubled lifetime risk for women with a strong family history of cancer, in women who are childless and those who had their first child after age 30, the researchers warned that today's rate of abortion could by the year 2040 add 24,500 new cases of breast cancer to the 184,300 now diagnosed each year.

## Prostate Surgery—Leads to High Retreatment Rates

According to a new study issued by Grace L. Lu-Yao, Ph.D., of the U.S. Health Care Financing Administration, surgical removal of the prostate (called prostatectomy) is often not the end stage in treating prostate cancer. In 34.9% of cases (based on a patient study involving 3,494 men treated by prostatectomy), men required further conventional treatment within 5 years, usually radiation, removal of the testes, or hormone supplementation.

According to Dr. Lu-Yao, medical information about low retreatment rates led many men to *believe* that prostate surgery alone would be sufficient for ending the problem. Study contributor Gerald W. Chodak, M.D., of Weiss Memorial Hospital in Chicago, said the likelihood that additional therapy will be required in the future is "an additional piece of information that is not generally provided to patients" at the time a prostatectomy is recommended.

Critics of the study contend that the 34.9% figure is too high and that patients diagnosed since 1996 and the advent of tests for prostate-specific antigen (a prostate cancer marker) will show a lower retreatment rate, possibly in the order of 10%.

SOURCE—L.A. McKeown, "High Retreatment Rates Shown After Prostate Removal," *Medical Tribune* (March 21, 1996), 13.

## NERVE INTERFERENCE FIELDS

Dysfunctions and imbalances in the autonomic nervous system (ANS) can contribute to a cancer process. Imbalances can be caused by skin scars from old accidents or surgeries; poisoned nerve bundles (called ganglia) in the nervous system made toxic from an accumulation of mercury, parasite toxins, solvents, and many other substances; restriction in blood flow (ischemia) to the ANS from strokes or carbon monoxide poisoning; and general trauma to the ANS from events such as gunshot wounds, surgical injury, or skull fracture. Dysfunction in the autonomic nervous system often causes arterial spasm in the part of the body supplied by that ANS ganglia or nerve branch; this in turn starves the tissues of oxygen, and leads to organ or tissue damage and poor flow of lymphatic fluid.

According to Dietrich Klinghardt, M.D., Ph.D., most cases of chronic illness involve changes in the ANS, especially in the electrical activity of the nerve bundles (ganglia) and fibers. A nerve ganglion (meaning "knot") is a group of nerve cell bodies located outside the central nervous system, except for those in the brain, Dr. Klinghardt explains. The majority of the body's ganglia are associated with the ANS. Each ganglion is composed of a mass of neurons and nerve cell bodies enabling it to act as a "little brain" within the body. "Just like thermostats, they can increase or decrease autonomic 'outflow' to the organs they innervate, depending on the needs of the organism."

## Mad Cow and Other Prion Diseases: Another Cancer Link?

Prion diseases (or spongiform encephalopathies), the most commonly known of which are Creutzfeldt-Jakob disease (CJD) in humans and mad cow disease, are fatal neurodegenerative diseases caused by the accumulation in the body of abnormal prion proteins. Prion precursor proteins are normally present in nerve cell membranes. A prion infection produces an abnormal transformation of these precursors. These abnormal prions then destroy neurons, progressively leaving the nervous system full of holes, like a sponge, and death eventually results.

Prion infection may be inherited or transmitted. Mad cow disease (bovine spongiform encephalopathy) has raised the alarming spectre of cross-species transmission. Before mad cow disease was identified in the United Kingdom and steps taken to halt the consumption of diseased cows, house cats and zoo animals who ate food containing bovine by-products contracted the disease. The implications of this for human meat-eating are as yet unknown. However, the U.K. Minister of Health announced in 1996 that 10 new cases of CJD may be related to the victims' being exposed to mad cow disease.

Another prion disease, kuru, appeared in New Guinea among tribes who practiced ritualistic cannibalism. It should be noted that the source of prion infection in the case of mad cow disease was ground-up parts of slaughtered cows added to cow feed. This practice is not limited to the U.K., but is also found in the United States as British cattle have been purchased for breeding in the U.S. in recent years. The risks and the extent of the practice in other meat industries such as poultry, pork, and sheep have yet to be investigated but are likely since poultry and other feeds are protein enhanced with cattle slaughterhouse remains. Meat eaters would be wise to observe caution.[149]

Ganglia are adaptable, Dr. Klinghardt says, which means if an organ or tissue is inflamed, the toxins may be transported to the nearest nerve ganglia, which can then store them, transport them elsewhere, alter them, or create antitoxins to neutralize them. "Although this creates a toxic ganglion which is operating chronically at a higher and more dysfunctional neurological threshold, it saves the organ, and therefore the organism from potential morbidity or mortality." As stated above, illness or a chronic condition can upset the electrical activity of ganglia. "The mass effect is a state of electrical chaos at the spinal cord level with failing control and selection mechanisms. Abnormal neuronal signals are now flooding the brain, leading to disturbances in the central nervous system, autonomic nervous system, and hormonal system."

The source of the abnormal signal and thus all this electrical confusion is a primary lesion called an "interference field" or focus, says Dr.

Klinghardt. In many cases, the focus is the site of an injury ("primary lesion"), such as a scar, or a subclinical illness such as an undetected dental infection; the intestines is a commonly overlooked site for interference fields, but "any part of the body that has been traumatized or ill" can act as one. For example, an acute infection of the upper respiratory tract can leave the sinuses acting as a permanent focus or interference field contributing to chronic illness in an individual.

The **autonomic nervous system** (ANS) can be likened to your body's automatic pilot; it keeps you alive through breathing, heart rate, and digestion, without your being aware of it or participating in its activities. The ANS has 2 divisions: the sympathetic, which expends body energy; and the parasympathetic, which conserves body energy. The sympathetic nervous system is associated with arousal and stress; it prepares us physically when we perceive a threat or challenge by increasing our heart rate, blood pressure, and muscle tension. The parasympathetic nervous system slows heart rate and increases intestinal and most gland activity.

**Neural therapy** uses localized injections of anesthetics, such as lidocaine or procaine, to remove interferences in the body's electrical network and thus relieve chronic pain, reverse injury, and clear energy blockages. The anesthetics are injected into nerve bundles in the autonomic nervous system, acupuncture points, scars, glands, and other tissues. By clearing the local site of interference, neural therapy helps to regulate energy throughout the body.

In fact, 30 to 45% of all illness or pain is caused by an interference field, states Dr. Klinghardt, and "every being is a potential carrier of one or several interference fields."[150] Dr. Klinghardt also estimates that dental factors (such as root canaled teeth, devitalized teeth [from amalgam metal corrosion], impacted teeth, extraction sites) can represent between 50 and 80% of focal areas. Among other bodily sites, these are common focal sites in order of most common to least common: tonsils, sinuses, appendix, scars, reproductive organs, lungs, kidneys, liver, gallbladder, hernia surgery, brain, and bladder.

The approach taken to remove the interference field is called neural therapy and involves the injection of local anesthetics into the site in question. This author (W. Lee Cowden, M.D.) finds that neural therapy, when applied at the right moment in cancer therapy, often causes rapid, dramatic reversal of the cancer. However, neural therapy applied too early can cause cancer to spread.

## DIET AND NUTRITIONAL DEFICIENCES

Rivaling only the role of tobacco and smoking in their ability to trigger and promote, or, when used correctly, reverse cancer, are diet and nutrition. In general, animal proteins and saturated fats are among the prime problems; they are linked strongly to colon, rectal, and prostate cancers. Not only is what we eat potentially a health hazard by introducing carcinogens via various foods into the body, but what we do *not* eat can contribute equally to the initiation of cancer by creating a nutritionally weakened, if not starved, system.

Food can make or break our health and, increasingly, factors related to food—its quality, its nutritional constituents, even how it is grown and processed—are considered a primary agent for contributing to the initiation and promotion of cancer. According to the National Academy of Sciences, 60% of all cancers in women and 40% of all cancers in men may be due to dietary and nutritional factors.[151]

One of the major factors accounting for the steady rise in cancer incidence and mortality rates is nutritional imbalances. The rise of degenerative disease has paralleled the adoption of an overly refined and adulterated, high-protein, high-fat diet over the past 100 years. After World War II, the U.S. population shifted away from regular consumption of whole grains and fresh vegetables, and instead increased its consumption of less wholesome, overly refined foods.

This so-called affluent diet is high in fat, which can more readily concentrate such chemicals as pesticides, preservatives, and industrial pollutants. The National Research Council's extensive 1982 report, titled *Diet, Nutrition, and Cancer*, provided strong evidence that much of the rise in cancer incidence may be related to typical U.S. dietary practices, among other factors.

## Meat Consumption and Lymph Cancer

Researchers at the University of Iowa College of Medicine who studied the eating habits of 35,156 women aged 55-69 over a 7-year period found that those who ate more than 36 servings (4-6 ounces/serving) of red meat per month had a 50% higher risk of developing non-Hodgkin's lymphoma than those women who ate less than 22 servings in a month, according to *The Journal of the American Medical Association*, May 1996.

***One of the major factors accounting for the steady rise in cancer incidence and mortality rates is nutritional imbalances.***

**Excessive intake of animal protein—**The high intake of animal protein is associated with an increased risk of breast, colon, pancreatic, kidney, prostate, and endometrial cancer. Excessive protein may produce large amounts of nitrogenous waste in the intestine, some of which can be converted to the highly carcinogenic compounds, nitrosamines and ammonium salts. Heavy-protein diets may also cause the buildup of metabolic acids in the body and cause large amounts of calcium to leach from the bones, an obvious detriment to women hoping to prevent osteoporosis in later life, but also a serious detriment in the case of bone cancer, when bone-calcium reserves tend to be mobilized and depleted.

A causal relationship between red meat consumption and cancer is supported by several large studies conducted in the U.S. Specifically, women with the highest level of meat consumption had double the rate of breast cancer compared to those who consumed small amounts of meat.[152] Men who ate red meat over a 5-year period were nearly 3 times more likely to contract advanced prostate cancer than men consuming mainly vegetarian fare.[153] High rates of colon cancer have recently been linked to regular intakes of beef, pork, or lamb.[154] In each of these studies, the meat-eating risks are associated with fat intake as well, since American meats are typically high in fat.

The combination of a high-fat diet and preexisting toxic overload (from other multiple sources of toxins, described below) may have a negative effect on health. Fatty foods, particularly red meat, can increase the toxicity of the chemicals that are lodged in them. In several animal studies, chemical carcinogens were more likely to produce tumors in the group that was fed fatty food than in the group fed low-fat foods.[155] Thus, a high-fat diet of animal foods can be especially troublesome because the most potent pesticides are concentrated in fat and the chemical properties of fat itself may actually increase their carcinogenicity. According to William Rea, M.D., director of the Environmental Health Center in Dallas, Texas, non-organic meats have 14 times and non-organic dairy products have 5½ times as many pesticides as non-organic plant-derived foods.

Worldwide, a clear association consistently appears between the highest rates of breast, colon, and prostate cancers and nations that have the fattiest diets.[156] But the link between cancer and meat eaters' exposure to toxic chemicals goes even deeper. All fried and broiled foods contain mutagens, chemicals that can damage cellular reproductive material, but fried and broiled meats have far more mutagens than similarly prepared plant foods. One study indicates that 20% of American meat eaters may have toxic mutagens in their digestive tracts that can be absorbed into the bloodstream where they can attack cells, in contrast to vegetarians who are unlikely to have any mutagens in their digestive tracts.[157]

Smoked, pickled, and salt-cured foods, especially meats, are also implicated in cancer. In parts of China where consumption of smoked and pickled foods are high, cancers of the stomach and esophagus are correspondingly high.[158] These processed foods contain several known carcinogenic substances, including nitrosamines and polycyclic aromatic hydrocarbons, which have been linked in animal experiments to these same cancers of the digestive tract. Additionally, potentially cancer-causing substances are also produced when meat, poultry, or fish are fried, broiled, grilled, or barbecued for a long time at high temperatures.[159]

**Be wary of contaminated fish—**Industrial and agricultural pollution has resulted in chemicals such as mercury, nickel, oil, hydrocyanic acid, and lactronitrile getting absorbed by ocean-borne plankton. From there, the toxins travel up the food chain, becoming concentrated in the tissues of large, fatty predatory fish, like tuna and swordfish. Industrial chemicals such as PCBs (polychlorinated biphenyls) and methylmercury tend to accumulate in significant amounts in some fish and most shellfish. According to toxicologists, it takes only 1/10 of a teaspoon of PCBs to make a person severely ill or possibly cause cancer.

PCB exposure during pregnancy causes delayed brain development in the infant, resulting in slower neuromuscular development and decreased head circumference, birth weight, and gestational period.[161] Such severe adverse birth defects were seen among infants whose mothers ate only 2-3 Great Lakes fish a month over several years. Methylmercury can cause birth defects and may add to a condition of weakened immunity, predisposing some people to cancer.

## California Breast Cancer Rates and Toxicity

White women in the San Francisco Bay Area have the world's highest rate of breast cancer—104 cases per 100,000 women. This statistic is double that of Europe, and 5 times higher than that of Japan, reports the International Agency for Research on Cancer. Fifteen years ago, the Bay Area also led the world in estrogen prescriptions for women. Yet, as two-thirds of the women who get breast cancer have no known risk factors, experts are querying whether exposure to radiation, pesticides, and chlorine-based chemicals may be contributing factors.

Granted, the state has the largest general population in the U.S., but California also leads the U.S. with 17,800 new breast cancer cases and 4,400 mortalities every year, and it also tops the list of America's toxic-waste sites, with 258, nearly 100 more than second-place Alaska and almost 200 more than third-place Maryland.[160]

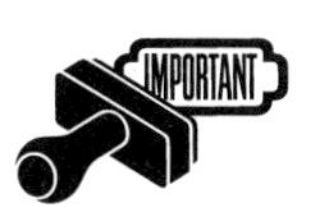


According to a *Consumer Reports* study of fish in the marketplace: (1) 43% of the samples of salmon contained PCBs, a potential carcinogen and reproductive hazard; (2) 99% of swordfish contained mercury, a threat to both the nervous and immune systems; (3) occasional samples of catfish contained DDT, DDE, and DDD, all potentially hazardous; and (4) half of the lakes' whitefish tested contained

PCB residues as well as various pesticides. Most samples of flounder and sole were found to be free of pollutants.[162]

As a rule, it is probably safest to avoid all freshwater fish, including farm-raised catfish, as well as swordfish and shark. Deep-water fish, such as red snapper, halibut, and flounder, are generally safe. Trout and salmon raised in spring-fed water and if not fed animal-derived protein feed, may also be safe and contain sufficient amounts of beneficial fatty acids, the omega-3s that are thought to help stave off cancer.

**Excessive fat intake**—Fat intake, especially animal fat, is one of the key factors consistently implicated in higher cancer rates.[163] The cancers most closely associated with high fat intake include breast, colon, rectum, uterus, prostate, and kidney.[164] Partially hydrogenated vegetable oils, commonly found in processed foods, are considered a major contributor to the carcinogenic effect of fats.[165] A 6-year review of 429 lung cancer cases showed that the dietary intake of saturated fat was the leading cause of lung cancer for people who were lifetime nonsmokers and former smokers. The study was prompted by the fact that in 1992, there were 13,000 cases of lung cancer occurring in U.S. women who were not smokers, therefore another factor must be involved besides tobacco.[166] Some evidence suggests that saturated fat consumption may be a factor.

Saturated fats are comprised of chains of fatty acids (containing carbon, hydrogen, and oxygen atoms) that carry as many hydrogen atoms as possible which results in them remaining solid at room temperature. All animal fats and 2 vegetable oils (coconut and palm) are saturated and, because of their structure (they are sticky) they can contribute to the clogging of blood vessels. Further, as their molecular structure is highly rigid, these fats can seriously alter the normal functioning of cell membranes, including those of immune cells. However, there are no studies that prove that organic coconut or palm oil or organic animal fats create disease if taken with enough polyunsaturated essential fatty acids (EFAs), especially the omega-3s, and antioxidants as well.

With the exception of fish, most of the fats we consume, including all domesticated sources of animal products, are from the omega-6 class. These fats are also found in most plant oils, including corn, safflower, and sunflower. The omega-6 oils, from both plants and animals, appear to be cancer promoters, whereas another class of fats, called omega-3s, found in fish, flaxseed,

## The Toxic Kitchen Cabinet

Many common household items, including cookware, plastics, and cleansers, may be sources of carcinogens and are best avoided.

**Aluminum Cookware:** It is advisable to stay away from aluminum cookware which can release traces of aluminum into the food. These traces can make their way into the bone matrix and create changes in mental functioning.[167] Food cooked in aluminum pans can pick up the element, but as to how much, the research jury is still out,[168] especially with respect to anodized aluminum. "Anodized" cookware is constructed of aluminum that has been placed in an electrolytic solution and subjected to an electric current to seal the pores of the aluminum, a process which lessens—some say eliminates—the aluminum interaction with food. However, the safest cookware is probably glass.

**Plastics:** The safety of plastics used in storing and cooking various foods, particularly when cooking by microwave, is controversial, but it is known that many of the resins used in plastics are cancer-causing substances. Molecules from polyvinyl chloride (PVC), polyethylene (PE), polyvinylidene chloride (PVDC), and plasticizers in plastic wraps can, at the high temperatures achieved in microwave ovens, migrate into foods. Polyethylene terephthalate (PET) trimmer, the thin, mirrorlike, grey stripping in microwave ovens, is the worst offender; it is often used to make microwave pizza crusts brown and microwave popcorn crunchy.

**Kitchen Cleanser:** Many dishwashing liquids, bleaches, chlorinated scouring powders, all-purpose cleaners, and drain cleaners contain petrochemicals. Nontoxic, environmentally-safe alternatives are available in every category of cleanser and detergent. In general, look for products that are water-based, free of phosphates, biodegradable, and free of propellants. Baking soda makes an excellent scouring powder and vinegar added to water can be used for cleaning windows. All detergents are unsafe in that they are absorbed through the skin, then incorporated into the cell membrane bilayer which thereby makes all cells diseased.

pumpkin seed, and walnuts, are beneficial to human health. They appear to be protective against both cancer and heart disease. But even omega-3s must be consumed in moderation with adequate amounts of antioxidant nutrients, as an excess of any type of fat can increase cancer risk.

In breast cancer studies conducted on laboratory mice, tumor growth was enhanced by a high-fat diet only *after* a chemical carcinogen had been introduced.[169] This suggests that fat is probably not an initiator but a promoter of cancer. Studies of fat's suppressive effects on the immune system, as well as fat's ability to generate free radicals (lipid peroxidation), support this interpretation.

**Eicosanoids—**Eicosanoids are hormone-like substances produced from the metabolism of arachidonic acid and other fatty acids. Produced by nearly every cell in the body, eicosanoids are highly potent substances: as little as one *billionth* of a gram can have measurable biological effects.[170] The human body produces a variety of eicosanoids which, in turn, direct a diverse range of functions, including immune-cell activity, platelet aggregation, inflammation, steroid hormone production, gastrointestinal secretions, blood pressure, pain sensation, and the induction of labor.

***Partially hydrogenated vegetable oils, commonly found in processed foods, are considered a major contributor to the carcinogenic effect of fats. A 6-year review of 429 lung cancer cases showed that the dietary intake of saturated fat was the leading cause of lung cancer for people who were lifetime nonsmokers and former smokers.***

Much evidence suggests that one of the eicosanoids, PGE2, promotes the development of various cancers by paralyzing certain key parts of the immune system (specifically the natural killer cells), stimulating inflammatory processes, and promoting the proliferation of tumor cells. Therefore, any agent that inhibits PGE2 synthesis could lower the risk of developing cancer and perhaps even curb the spread of cancer.

Omega-3 fatty acids appear to reduce PGE2-induced inflammation, inhibit tumor cell proliferation, and enhance immune system function, as demonstrated in a study in which omega-3 fatty acids slowed or delayed the development of metastases in breast cancer patients. Specifically, women who had high fatty tissue content of alpha-linolenic acid (the main omega-3 EFA) were 5 times less likely to develop metastases than women with a low content.[171]

One reason doctors may not always observe a beneficial effect of omega-3s on cancer resistance (via eicosanoid production) is that various nutrient cofactors may be missing. Some vitamins and minerals actually encourage the production of the "good eicosanoids" from polyunsaturated fatty acids (PUFAs). These good eicosanoids, which include prostaglandins from the PGE1 series, promote sound immunity and overall well-being. The synthesis of the PGE1 series requires not only the "good" fatty acids (omega-3s), but the presence of zinc, niacin, pyridoxine, and ascorbic acid as cofactors.[172]

Aspirin has also been used to inhibit PGE2 synthesis, and many studies have indicated that aspirin can slow or even block the growth of colorectal cancer.[173,174] Given a choice between aspirin and omega-3 sources (fish oils and flaxseed oil) though, some doctors strongly prefer the latter. For one thing, aspirin use has been associated with reduced kidney function (in geriatric patients), asthmatic tendencies (bronchospasm), fetal resorption (meaning the fetus absorbs some of the aspirin), and other adverse effects.[175]

Most of the doctors featured in this book recommend large reductions in the consumption of dietary fats—with the exception of the omega-3s—to a maximum of no more than 25% of one's total daily caloric intake. The best way to achieve this goal is to avoid all domestic meats, dairy products, eggs, and vegetable oils (with the exception of olive, pumpkin seed, walnut, flaxseed, and sesame oil, the last 4 of which are converted to omega-3). One should cut out margarine, fried foods, oily dressings, and creamy sauces; to be prudent, one's main sources of fat should be fish, nuts, and seeds, and even these should be eaten in moderation.

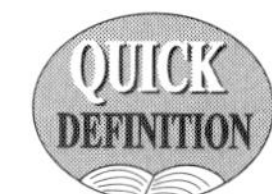


**Lipid** is a biochemist's term for a fat or oil, which is one of the 6 basic food groups. Fats and oils are made of building blocks called fatty acids. Of these long-chain molecules (comprising atoms of carbon, hydrogen, and oxygen) the "fatty" end does not dissolve in water, while the "acid" end does. Fats are also called triglycerides as they consist of 3 (tri) fatty acid molecules joined to one molecule of glycerol, a kind of sugar. Unsaturated fats required in the diet are called essential fatty acids, and include linoleic acid (an omega-6 oil), found in corn, beans, and some nuts and seeds, and alpha linolenic acid (an omega-3 oil), found in fish, flaxseed, and walnuts.

**Excessive intake of refined carbohydrates/sugar—**Sugar and white-flour products are believed to have a direct effect on cancer growth, as well as acting to nullify the positive effects of protective foods such as fiber.[176] In addition, they can significantly add to the risk of breast cancer, says veteran cancer researcher, Wayne Martin, of Fairhope, Alabama. "When someone eats sugar, the body produces insulin, and insulin can promote breast cancer just as estrogen does," he explains.

Sugar is remarkably effective at lowering the immune system's ability to work properly. Eating only 3 ounces (100 g) at one sitting can stunningly reduce the ability of the immune system's white blood cells (specifically, neutrophils) to engulf and destroy bacteria, lowering it from a value of 16 to 10. The immune-suppressive effect starts within 30 minutes after sugar ingestion and can last for up to 5 hours. Neutrophil activity may be reduced by 40% for 2 hours after eating sugar and because neutrophils are responsible for 60 to 70% of the total white blood cells in circulation, this drop means the immune system is working at only half of its intended capacity. Obviously, this situation renders the body vulnerable to infection. As the average American consumes about 5 ounces (150 g) of sucrose (or granular sugar found in various processed foods) daily, it would seem the immune system of many people is chronically suppressed from dietary factors alone.[177]

Tumors are known to exhibit abnormal metabolism that thrives under low-oxygen, high-glucose (blood sugar) conditions—just like a yeast organism in fermenting sugar.[178] Accordingly, if you are sedentary, breathe in a shallow way, and consume a lot of sugar, pastries, and other refined carbohydrate foods, your system may tend to favor the growth of tumors. Keith Block, M.D., profiled in Chapter 2 in this book, notes that sugars also reinforce the "bad fat track" (stimulating prostaglandin E2 production) that promotes inflammation and tumor growth.

**Excessive intake of iron—**Iron overload refers to an excess of body iron. A Danish study found that iron overload significantly raises the risk of developing cancer.[179] Two other recent reports suggest that even moderately elevated iron accumulations in the body may increase cancer risks.[180] Much of the cancer in the U.S. population today may be related to overconsumption of red meat, a rich source of iron.

***"Although it is unclear whether the iron in the meat promotes tumor growth any more than the fat does, iron definitely contributes to free radical production, which only increases one's risk of getting cancer."***

Citing another recent study showing a relationship between high red meat intake and colon cancer,[181] Neal Barnard, M.D., of the Physicians Committee for Responsible Medicine, states: "Although it is unclear whether the iron in the meat promotes tumor growth any more than the fat does, iron definitely contributes to free radical production, which only increases one's risk of getting cancer." Cooking in iron pots or skillets, fortified bread, rice, and pasta products, and multivitamins with iron are further sources of exposure. Iron fortification is largely unnecessary as iron deficiency is uncommon in the U.S., except occasionally in menstruating women.

**Excessive intake of alcohol—**Regular, heavy consumption of alcohol, including beer, is associated with an elevated cancer risk.[182] According to Charles B. Simone, M.D., of Princeton, New Jersey, a cancer doctor profiled in Chapter 19 of this book, an alcohol habit can greatly increase the risk for cancers of the breast, mouth, throat (pharynx, larynx and esophagus), pancreas, liver, and head and neck. Alcohol can accelerate the growth of an existing cancer by suppressing NK cells, those immune cells that would otherwise help repel the cancer.[183]

**Excessive intake of caffeine**—Found in coffee, tea, colas, and chocolate, caffeine is thought to be a factor in the development of cancer of the lower urinary tract, including the bladder. Studies have found the rates for these cancers to be significantly higher in people who drink more than 3 cups of coffee a day.[184] Caffeine can cause damage to genetic material, and impair the normal DNA repair mechanisms, thereby adding to the potential risk for cancer.[185]

For more information on the relationship between **cancer and alcohol consumption**, see Chapter 19: Charles Simone, M.D., pp. 404-405.

***Christiane Northrup, M.D., coined the term "toxic emotions" to indicate the powerful, strongly held, and often unconsciously active beliefs and emotions that help generate symptoms that keep illnesses in place.***

## CHRONIC STRESS

Almost 2,000 years ago, the Greek physician Galen noted that melancholic women were more likely to develop cancer. Today, the mind's mediating role in health and illness is considered powerful, and the effect of emotional stress is increasingly being examined for its links to cancer. Although the concept of stress—being "stressed out" or "under constant stress"—may be commonly discussed today, its role as a contributing factor in many diseases, including cancer, is underappreciated. Estimates suggest that as many as 70 to 80% of all visits to physicians' offices are for stress-related problems. Chronic stress directly affects the immune system and, if not effectively dealt with, can seriously compromise health.

Stress is a pervasive problem among Americans, according to a 1996 poll of corporate executives. For example, 44% of employees polled said their work load is excessive compared to 37% in 1988; 43% are bothered by excessive job pressure; 55% worry considerably about their company's future; 25% of both men and women feel stressed out at work every day, another 12% feel it almost every day, and another 38% feel it once to several days a week.[186]

Research in psychoneuroimmunology, or PNI, has shown that the immune and nervous systems are linked by extensive networks of nerve endings in the spleen, bone marrow, lymph nodes, and thymus gland (a primary source of T cells). At the same time, receptors for a variety of chemical messengers—catecholamines, prostaglandins, thyroid hormone, growth hormone, sex hormones, serotonin, and endorphins—have been found on the surfaces of white blood cells. Such connections serve to integrate the activities of the immune, hormonal, and nervous systems, enabling the mind and emotional states to influence the body's resistance to cancer.[187]

Under emotional distress, the brain may signal the adrenal glands to produce chemicals called corticosteroids, hormones which weaken the immune response. Cancer-related (neoplastic) processes are accelerated in the presence of these chemicals[188] as well as other stress hormones like prolactin.[189] Certain cancers have also been associated with distressing life events. In one study, the risk of developing breast cancer was 5 times higher if the woman had experienced an important emotional loss in the 6 years prior to the discovery of the tumor.[190] Other researchers have reported depressed T-cell activity in spouses whose wives had died of breast cancer[191] and in women who had lost their jobs.[192]

Stress can be defined as a reaction (to any stimulus or interference) that upsets normal functioning and disturbs mental or physical health. It can be brought on by internal conditions such as illness, pain, emotional conflict, or psychological problems, or by external circumstances, such as bereavement, financial problems, loss of job or spouse, relocation, or many of the cancer-contributing factors described in this chapter such as ionizing radiation, geopathic stress, food allergies, electromagnetic fields. Stress, when it becomes chronic, is often unrecognized by the person whose body is experiencing it; one begins to accept it as a fact of life, without being aware of how it is actually compromising all bodily functions and preparing the foundation for illness.

More specifically, research confirms that high levels of emotional stress increase one's susceptibility to illness. Unrelieved, chronic stress begins taxing and eventually weakening, even suppressing, the immune system. Stress can also lead to hormonal imbalances which, in turn, interfere with immune function. Of all the body's systems, stress damages immune function the most. It does so by overly activating the sympathetic part of the autonomic nervous system, the part that controls the "fight-or-flight" response and initiates adrenalin and cortisol release.

According to Leon Chaitow, N.D., D.O., of London, England, psychological and emotional changes in one's life often produce stress. This is manifested in increased adrenalin levels, hormonal changes, and decreased immune function. "Usually, the body can adapt itself, continuing to function during this temporary condition before returning to normal," Dr. Chaitow says. "But when the stress is too severe, or if it becomes chronic, chemical changes begin to occur in the body, creating an environment which may increase the risk of serious disease, including cancer."

Numerous studies have linked stress and its related psychological components to susceptibility to cancer.[193] Several recent studies have even linked stressful changes in a child's life, including personal injury or the loss of health of another family member, with the onset of cancer.[194] Adults who have recently lost a loved one, or been widowed, divorced, or separated, tend to have the highest cancer rates.[195] In addition, a basic inability to cope with stress has been regarded as key to a significant rise in breast cancer incidence.[196] How people deal with illness, especially cancer, also has a dramatic impact on their recovery process.[197]

When hormones (including cortisol and adrenalin) are released by the adrenal glands, they begin to inhibit the activities of white blood cells, decrease the amount of lymphocytes produced, and cause the thymus gland (located behind the sternum in the chest) to shrink. Scientists now know that the T and B cells contain receptors on their cell membranes that recognize and respond to the adrenal hormones released in response to stress.

***More specifically, research confirms that high levels of emotional stress increase one's susceptibility to illness. Unrelieved, chronic stress begins taxing and eventually weakening, even suppressing, the immune system.***

## TOXIC EMOTIONS

Since the late 1960s, Western psychotherapists working with people suffering with serious, even life-threatening illnesses, have acknowledged the power of emotions to contribute to the disease process. Since the 1970s, research in the field of psychoneuroimmunology has documented direct links between emotions and biochemical events in the body, thereby establishing on a scientific basis what folk healers have always known: emotions can manifest themselves as physical symptoms.

Noted women's health expert, Christiane Northrup, M.D., of Yarmouth, Maine, coined the term "toxic emotions" to indicate the powerful, strongly held, and often unconsciously active beliefs and emotions that help generate symptoms that keep illnesses in place. "A thought held long enough and repeated enough becomes a belief," says Dr. Northrup. "The belief then becomes biology."

Dr. Northrup explains that if we fail to work through our emotional distress (which includes damaging beliefs and strong, unexpressed emotions), we set the body for physical distress. Unfortunately, as indicated, many of the foundational beliefs a person holds and many basic emotional traumas are subconscious, active in the brain but beyond our normal awareness. For example, a person may hold the belief that he will never be loved as well as his older brother, or that he is unworthy of being loved; or, a person may have experienced incest, rape, abuse, or other violence as a child and suppressed this knowledge and its attendant pain.

These beliefs and emotions remain active, shaping our biology even if we are oblivious of them. "I know from my practice—and from my life—that most of us aren't aware of our own destructive beliefs that undermine our health," says Dr. Northrup. They become "lodged and buried in the cell tissue." Our personal histories are "stored" throughout the body, in the muscles, organs, and tissues.

That is why, in the view of Dr. Northrup as well as other alternative practitioners working with cancer patients, beliefs and emotions can be legitimate toxins, contributing to an overall weakening of the immune system.[198] This author (W. Lee Cowden) has found the subconscious lack of self-worth or self-esteem to be the most dangerous of all toxic emotions. It can prevent any and all therapy from being effective. Some of the worst emotional stresses contributing to cancer involve events (such as incest or childhood sexual abuse) that the cancer patient experienced as a child and that are "remembered" only at the subconscious level, not in conscious awareness. Many cancer patients cannot recover from their cancer until these memories are discovered and treated. Electrodermal screening can help to indicate and identify hidden emotional traumas of this type.

Although scientists have long debated the role of repressed emotions in cancer, at least 3 studies offer compelling evidence validating that role. In each of these studies, people were followed over time to determine their rates of disease in relation to various behaviors or exposures. Taken together, the results indicate a link between cancer resistance and emotional expression or its suppression.

Emotional repression may also influence one's survival from cancer—that is, how well a cancer patient fares after being diagnosed. In 8 separate studies of patients with various cancers, each reported a significant association between hopelessness or passive coping responses—not taking an assertive position toward one's illness and recovery process—and poor cancer survival rates.[199]

The connection between emotional stress and cancer survival can be explained by recent findings in psychoneuroimmunology (PNI).[200] PNI documents the multiple interactions between the mind (psycho), nervous system (neuro), and cellular dimension (immunology) as it makes or breaks health. Its research suggests that the persistence of cancer cells depends in part on internal body controls that retrain or stimulate tissue growth; psychological factors appear to regulate these controls through neurological, hormonal, and immunologic pathways.[201,202] These and other mind/body links could play a major role in determining a person's ability to survive cancer.

Up to 40% of cancer patients experience clinically significant anxiety and depression; 9 out of 10 of these patients say their distress is linked mainly with the diagnosis and treatment.[203] Married cancer patients live longer than unmarried cancer patients, all other factors being equal (that is, matching subjects for age, sex, education, socioeconomic status, and employment status).[207]

In a controlled study of women with breast lumps, women who had more difficulty expressing anger were more likely to have malignancies at breast biopsy.

## The Role of Emotions in Cancer

In the 1960s, psychotherapist Ronald Grossarth-Maticek administered questionnaires to 1,353 inhabitants of Crvenka, Yugoslavia. After following the subjects for a decade, Grossarth-Maticek concluded that 9 out of every 10 cases of cancer could be predicted on the basis of "an overly rational, anti-emotional attitude" and a tendency to ignore signs of poor health. People with low anti-emotional scores were 29 times less likely to develop cancer than those with high anti-emotional scores.[204]

Patrick Dattore and colleagues followed 200 disease-free individuals for 10 years and compared the psychological tests of 75 veterans who eventually got cancer with the 125 who remained cancer free. Contrary to expectations, those who developed cancer appeared less depressed than the others; however, these same individuals were also more likely to suppress their more intense or upsetting feelings. Again, those who openly expressed their feelings were less likely to develop cancer.[205]

The longest study to date, initiated in 1946, focused on students from the John Hopkins School of Medicine. Pirkko Graves and her colleagues divided 972 of the students into 5 groups based on various psychological measures. Over the course of 3 decades, students characterized as "loners" who suppressed their emotions beneath a bland exterior were 16 times more likely to develop cancer than those who gave vent to their feelings. In an earlier report, based on 1,337 students, cancer death rates correlated significantly with a lack of closeness with parents.[206]

In contrast, women who vented their anger more readily were more likely to have benign lesions.[208]

A strong sense of hopelessness is now ranked as a serious contributing factor in both the emergence of new cases of cancer and heart disease and for death from these diseases. A study of 2,428 Finnish men, aged 42-60 revealed that those with moderate to high hopelessness (based on answers to a questionnaire) died at a rate 2-3 times higher than those who did not feel hopeless; and for those with a "high" degree of hopelessness, the death rate from cancer, heart disease, violence, or injury was 5 times higher, regardless of the presence of other major risk factors.[209]

A 1992 report in *Radiology* from scientists at Boston's Dana-Farber Cancer Institute states, "Optimal care of patients with cancer ... goes beyond technical to emotional and spiritual support."[210] Many physicians now believe that treating an individual's mental and emotional states is as important as treating any cancerous tumors that may be a result of such conditions. The idea that the mind can influence the onset and outcome of many diseases, cancer included, is now increasingly accepted by doctors and patients. With the right attitude and outlook, one can quickly learn to stimulate the immune system and bolster resistance to disease. Deepak Chopra, M.D., an endocrinologist, former chief of staff of New England Memorial Hospital in Stoneham, Massachusetts, and now medical director of the Sharp Clinic in San Diego, California, says the mind is the key to both prevention and treatment of cancer.

According to Steven Locke, M.D., instructor in psychiatry and director of the psychoimmunology research project at Harvard Medical School, science has only skimmed the surface of potential information relating emotions and behavior to immunity in humans. Dr. Locke describes 203 studies covering the period from 1948 to 1985 that treat cancer by "mind/body" methods. Among the methods most often used by cancer patients to reduce anxiety are meditation, prayer, and visualization techniques.

Preliminary studies of biofeedback, meditation, yoga, guided imagery, and other relaxation techniques suggest the mind can enhance immunity against cancer. Deep breathing is a common aspect of relaxation training and probably promotes immune function. By decreasing the intensity of nerve firing and raising the brain's oxygen uptake, deep, regular breathing can help people release worry, anger, and resentment.[211]

## DEPRESSED THYROID ACTION

An underactive or dysfunctional thyroid gland (a key endocrine gland located in the neck) may contribute to a cancer process. Broda O. Barnes, M.D. (coauthor of *Hypothyroidism, the Unsuspected Illness,* in 1976), observed in his clinical practice a myriad of patients with typical hypothyroid (underactive thyroid) symptoms, but whose blood values for thyroid deficiency tested normal. However, he found that if these patients had a low resting temperature in the morning before getting out of bed, they had a high likelihood of responding positively to glandular thyroid replacement therapy, indicating a depressed thyroid condition.

Dr. Barnes presented evidence that suggests a relationship between low thyroid activity and cancer. Research in 1954 by Dr. J.G.C. Spencer from Bristol, England, showed that there was a consistently higher incidence of cancer in areas of 15 countries and 4 continents where goiter (enlargement of the thyroid gland) was more or particularly prevalent among the population than in the non-goiter areas of the same localities. Dr. Barnes noted that Austria, a country with a high incidence of goiter, also had the highest incidence of cancer of any country reporting malignancies at that time, further supporting the proposed link.

Dr. Barnes further noted that if one tried to transplant a cancer from one laboratory rat into another, the grafted malignancy would seldom "take" unless the thyroid gland was first removed from the recipient rat. Patients who had low thyroid function were also susceptible to tuberculosis and viral diseases, Dr. Barnes observed, adding that there was a strong correlation between tuberculosis and lung cancer. Dr. Barnes placed several thousands of his

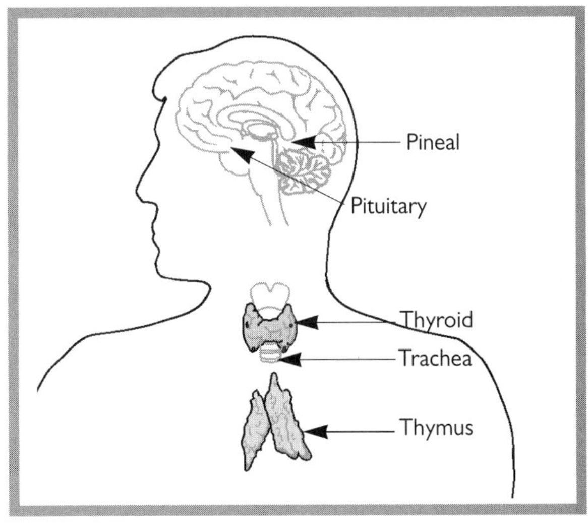


**Figure 25.4—The thyroid gland is the body's metabolic thermostat, controlling body temperature, energy use, and, for children, the body's growth rate.**

# A Primer on the Intestines

**Small intestine**—At about 21 feet long and 1 inch wide, it absorbs about 95% of the fats and 90% of the amino acids we consume as foods. It has 3 parts: the duodenum, which connects directly to the stomach and where most digestion occurs; and the jejunum and ileum, where most of the absorption of nutrients occurs.

The inner surface of the small intestine is expanded by some 600 times through a process of folding into millions of finger-shaped projections and creases called villi, and in-tuckings between the villi, called crypts. The purpose is to increase the area available for nutrient absorption. Each villus is covered by special cells for absorption and contains a tiny lymph vessel called a lacteal. Each villus comprises thousands of microvilli which form a brushlike border; here nutrient absorption occurs at the molecular level.

Average transit time through the small intestine is 2 hours, although 1-6 hours is the range.

**Large intestine**—Digested food passes through the ileocecal valve from the small intestine into the large intestine or colon, which is 5 feet long and 2-1/2 inches wide. Here water is reabsorbed from the digested food, and the remaining contents form the feces; these consist of undigestible cellulose fibers and "friendly" bacteria common to the intestine and representing about 30% of fecal weight. Average transit time through a healthy colon is 12 hours.

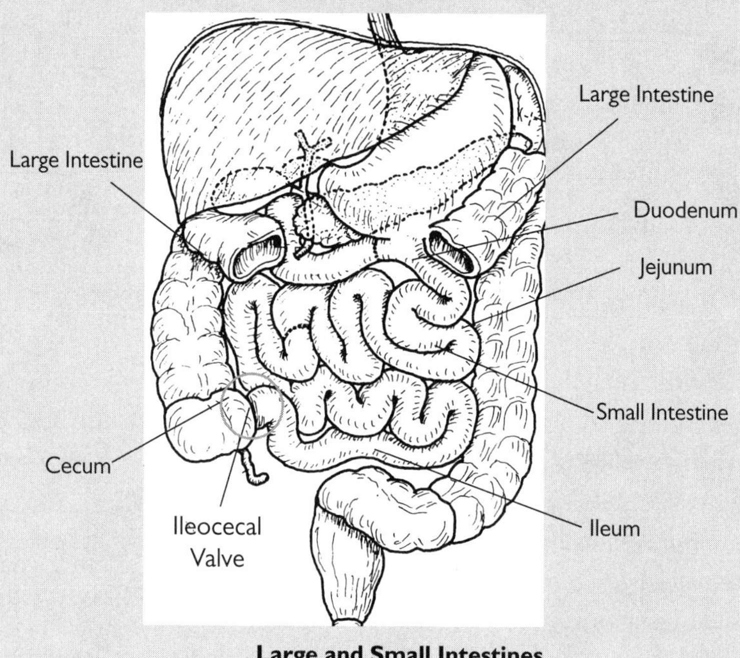


**Large and Small Intestines**

patients on thyroid therapy and not one of them ever developed lung cancer; further, there were only 6 deaths related to malignancies of any type in his practice while, for the same number of people in the general population, at least 20 cancer deaths would have been expected. Subsequent biochemical research has tended to support Dr. Barnes' clinical observations.[212]

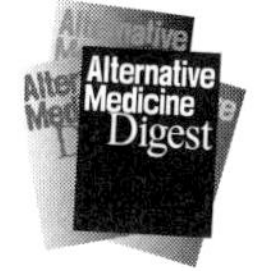


For more about the **thyroid**, see "The Reason Behind," #16, pp. 52-56.

## INTESTINAL TOXICITY AND DIGESTIVE IMPAIRMENT

The intestines, when stretched out, are over 25 feet long. In fact, if the inner surface of the small intestines were smooth and flat rather than convoluted, they would stretch for 2¼ miles or completely cover an area the size of a tennis court. The intestines may harbor the seeds of disease in the form of a false lining that blocks nutrient absorption and creates toxicity. For centuries, physicians across many disciplines have said that health begins and ends in the intestines. Many illnesses, such as a number of cancers, most allergies, infections, liver diseases, acne, psoriasis, and asthma, start in the intestines. The intestines become clogged, toxic, and diseased by what and how we eat and by how poorly we eliminate waste material. Once the bowel is toxic, it creates toxicity for the entire body and an inability to absorb the nutrients necessary for health and healing.

Around 1900, most people in the U.S. had a brief intestinal transit time. That means it took only about 15-20 hours from the time food entered the mouth until it was excreted as feces. Today, many have a seriously delayed transit time of 50-70 hours.

This means there is more time for the stool to putrefy, for harmful microorganisms to flourish, for probiotics to die off, and for toxins to develop and poison the tissues. When you eat mucus-producing foods, this further slows down the transit time. It should now be easier to understand how a toxic bowel can lead to cancer, allergies, and infections. It should also be clear how important it is to prevent and reverse bowel toxicity.

Most people remember, as children, making papier-mâché from refined white flour, water, and paper. Perhaps you pasted the mixture onto a balloon, let it dry, then popped the balloon for a perfect papier-mâché cast of the balloon. A material similar to papier-mâché can develop in the lining of the small and large intestines as a result of eating white flour prod-

Intestinal **dysbiosis** refers to an imbalance between intestinal flora. Specifically, these flora are friendly, beneficial bacteria, called probiotics, such as *Lactobacillus acidophilus* and *Bifidobacterium bifidum*, and unfriendly bacteria in the intestines such as *Escherichia coli* and *Clostridium perfringens*. In dysbiosis, the unfriendly bacteria predominate; they begin fermentation producing toxic by-products such as ammonia, amines, nitrosamines, phenols, cresols, indole, and skatole, which interfere with the normal elimination cycle. Dysbiosis is considered a primary cause or major cofactor in the development of many health problems, such as acne, yeast overgrowth, chronic fatigue, depression, digestive disorders, bloating, food allergies, PMS, rheumatoid arthritis, and cancer.

ucts combined with fluid and cellulose, which is found in vegetables. When you eat other foods that produce mucus, such as dairy products, this causes a rubbery-like material to combine with the papier-mâché lining, and it builds up even faster.

Mucus-producing foods are nearly all foods aside from most vegetables and fruits; however, the most mucus-producing foods are milk products. Other foods include meats, fish, fowl, eggs, soybeans, oily seeds and nuts, and cooked beans and grains (but not beans and grains that have sprouted and grown for 6 days). Fruits and vegetables tend to cause the mucous material in the intestines to break down somewhat and be eliminated.

As this sticky mucoid false lining builds up in the small intestine, it blocks absorption of essential nutrients into the bloodstream and it produces a hiding place in both intestines for bacteria, fungi, yeast, and parasites that are harmful to human health. When these abnormal life forms start growing too freely in the intestines, they kill off *Lactobacillus acidophilus* and other "friendly" bacteria. They also create a situation called dysbiosis (or an imbalance among intestinal microflora) in which the contents of the intestines putrefy and harmful chemicals are generated.

The result is a toxic bowel and a body-wide condition of toxicity as toxins leech out of the intestines into other tissues. The toxins pass through the intestinal wall and accumulate in the lymph vessels. If there are too many toxins, the lymphatic system becomes blocked and overloaded and can no longer drain and filter poisons efficiently. As toxins build up in all the tissues, the result can be swelling of the torso and legs and damage to the immune system, liver, and eventually, the other organs. The inevitable result is illness. As Bernard Jensen, N.D., D.C., documents in *Tissue Cleansing through Bowel Management*, the toxic mucoid false lining of the small and large intestines can and should be flushed out of the body of everyone with chronic degenerative diseases, including cancer patients.

An additional cause of intestinal toxicity results from the decreased production of hydrochloric acid and pepsin in the stomach as people age.[213] This results in the inability to break down protein in the diet. Also with lack of hydrochloric acid in the stomach there is inadequate acid stimulation of the first part of the small intestine (the duodenum) during meals.

The release of the hormone secretin (and possibly cholecystokinin as well) requires acid stimulation in the duodenum.[214] Since secretin and cholecystokinin are responsible for pancreatic secretions, inadequate acid stimulation results in reduced production and release of pancreatic enzymes and bile secretions to aid in the digestive process.

Undigested proteins that pass into the small and large intestines without being broken down into their constituent amino acids produce toxicity. This is because bacteria convert these proteins into nitrosamines and other cancer-causing agents, or because the undigested food proteins are absorbed intact through the intestinal wall into the bloodstream, creating "circulating immune complexes." These complexes put an unnecessary strain on the immune system so that it becomes less capable of identifying and attacking cancer cells. This makes it easier, and more likely, for a cancer process to gain a footing in the organism.

> ***Undigested proteins that pass into the small and large intestines without being broken down into their constituent amino acids produce toxicity and "circulating immune complexes." These complexes put an unnecessary strain on the immune system so that it becomes less capable of identifying and attacking cancer cells. This makes it easier, and more likely, for a cancer process to gain a footing in the organism.***

Certain cells of the stomach (parietal cells) can be damaged by a variety of factors. These include severe emotional or physical stress (especially on a chronic basis), use of tobacco products (either cigarettes, cigars, pipe or chewing tobacco), consumption of alcoholic beverages, consumption of caffeinated beverages including coffee, tea, and sodas, and consuming recognized, or unrecognized, food allergens. Once these cells are damaged, there is a progressive decrease in hydrochloric acid production by the stomach.[215]

The progressive decrease in hydrochloric acid, pepsin, and pancreatic enzymes as people age also results in inadequate amounts of amino acids being broken down from dietary protein. The result is insufficient amounts of amino acids to produce peptide neurotransmitters, peptide hormones, antibodies, structural proteins, metabolic enzymes, digestive enzymes, cell membrane receptors, and a myriad of other protein substances required for health.

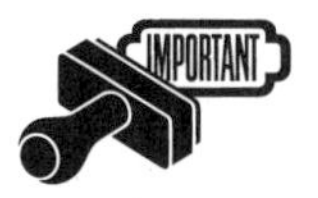

It is important to remember that approximately 50% of the daily utilization of dietary protein goes for the production of enzymes in that individual, a major share of which is for production of digestive enzymes. If there are insufficient amounts of digestive enzymes available to digest food, then extra digestive enzymes from the pancreas will be needed to break down circulating immune complexes or to digest the fibrin coating on cancer cells in the body. This fibrin coating protects the cancer cells from recognition by the immune system.

***"High levels of exposure to carcinogens coupled with sluggish detoxification enzymes significantly increases our susceptibility to cancer," states Joseph Pizzorno, N.D.***

A progressive loss of digestive enzymes and hydrochloric acid also prevents minerals and vitamins from being released from complexes in food. Since these micronutrients are necessary for different enzyme actions inside the body, then ineffective digestion results in dysfunction of a variety of internal bodily functions. These might include food digestion, metabolism, and immune system action. Most minerals require hydrochloric acid in the stomach to convert the mineral into a form which is more easily absorbed; therefore, people who have hydrochloric deficiency do not absorb minerals well. The mineral deficiency that progressively develops results in tissue acidity, because among other things, minerals function in the tissues as binders of metabolic organic acids. Once bound, the mineral salt of the organic acid can be carried out through the kidneys for elimination from the body.

For information on intestinal **detoxification**, see Chapter 33: Physical Support Therapies, pp. 949-980.

## PARASITES

Another factor may be weakening our immune system from the inside and, like toxic emotions, be unknown to us: parasites. The human body may have unwelcome residents that are harmful to health, literally eating us from the inside, using our nutrients and often plugging up our lymphatic vessels. The possible presence of parasites in the body, mostly in the intestines, is a little appreciated but major health problem, according to nutrition educator Ann Louise Gittleman. People assume they are vulnerable to parasites only if they travel in tropical areas, but this is a dangerous misconception, says Gittleman. Anyone can get them (and many probably already have) from merely staying at home.

For more information on **parasite elimination**, see Chapter 33: Physical Support Therapies, pp. 972-977.

Undiagnosed parasitic infections (from microscopic protozoa to various species of worms) may account for a great deal of the otherwise unexplained diseases currently besetting America. One estimate contends that 25% of New York City residents have a parasitic infection and that, by the year 2025, 50% of the projected 8.3 billion world population will have them. Parasites tend to reside in the intestines, but they can also migrate to the blood, lymph, heart, liver, gallbladder, pancreas, spleen, eyes, and brain. While in place, they can produce numerous symptoms: constipation, diarrhea, gas, bloating, irritable bowel syndrome, joint and muscle aches, allergies, anemia, skin problems, sleep disturbances, chronic fatigue, and gradual immune dysfunction.

According to Gittleman's research, parasite damage can be extensive. They can destroy cells faster than they can be regenerated; they can release toxins that damage tissues, resulting in pain and inflammation; and, over time, they can depress, even exhaust, the immune system. Of the dozens of specific parasites of concern to human health, the major groupings include microscopic Protozoa, roundworms, pinworms, and hookworms (Nematoda), tapeworms (Cestoda), and flukes (Trematoda).[216]

According to naturopathic physician Hulda Regehr Clark, Ph.D., N.D., who practices in Tijuana, Mexico, a single parasite—the fluke, a flatworm called *Fasciolopsis buskii*—may be responsible for cancer. Under completely healthy conditions, the body, thanks to the liver, is able to trap and destroy flukes before they have grown large or completed their growth cycle. However, the presence of the solvent propyl alcohol in the body (especially in the liver) makes the immune system unable to destroy the flukes, says Dr. Clark.

Propyl alcohol enters the body through multiple sources: cosmetics, commercial breakfast cereals, shampoo, hair sprays, some bottled waters and fruit juices, rubbing alcohol, mouthwash, shaving supplies, carbonated beverages, decaffeinated coffee, and white sugar. The flukes lay many eggs; once hatched and grown to maturity, the pressure of the fluke population causes the release of a special cell growth factor called ortho-phosphotyrosine, which marks the beginning of the cancer process, Dr. Clark states.

"I see solvent pollution and mycotoxin pollution [such as aflatoxin molds] as the top threats to our health at this time," she explains. Mold

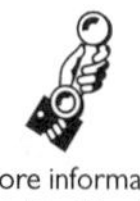

For more information about **Dr. Clark's protocols,** products, and devices for removing parasites, contact: Self-Health Resource Center, 757 Emory Street, No. 508, Imperial Beach, CA 91932; tel: 619-429-4408; fax: 619-429-8042.

toxins prevent the detoxification of solvents, and solvents induce parasites (at least 120 varieties or stages, according to her tests) "to invade animals and tissues that they have never gotten a foothold in before, causing cancer, HIV/AIDS, and a number of other modern diseases."

In her best-selling *The Cure for All Cancers*, Dr. Clark presents 100 case histories illustrating the role of parasites and propyl alcohol in cancer and how an herbal formula (based on black walnut, wormwood, and cloves) helps to eliminate them. Dr. Clark takes the elimination of traces of ortho-phosphotyrosine as an indication of success and cancer reversal. Two studies in the *Annual Review of Biochemistry* (1985, 1988) confirmed that this chemical is a reliable cancer marker for different kinds of malignancies.[217] Ortho-phosphotyrosine is a metabolic by-product of some parasites and a growth factor stimulator for parasites and cancer cells; as such, it can act as a stimulator for the precursors of cancer known as oncogenes (described below).

## VIRUSES

According to some researchers, up to 15% of the world's cancer deaths are attributable to the activities of viruses, bacteria, or parasites. Among the cancer-producing viruses that work through a host's DNA-synthesizing and protein-building mechanisms are human papilloma viruses type 16 and 18 (which are sexually transmitted) associated with cervical cancer, among others, and the hepatitis B virus, associated with liver cancers. Worldwide, viral infections, especially hepatitis, may cause up to 80% of liver cancers. The papilloma viruses 16 and 18 are believed responsible for between 70 and 80% of genital and anal cancers, although up to 30 additional papilloma viruses also may be involved. Epstein-Barr virus, which produces mononucleosis, is also carcinogenic, linked to about 50% of cancers of the upper pharynx, 30% of Hodgkin's, and 10% of non-Hodgkin's and certain gastric cancers.[218]

Researchers at Johns Hopkins University School of Medicine found that when men have sex with up to 21 other partners the risk of their wives' developing cervical cancer increases by 11 times. The risk for wives of men who frequent prostitutes is 8 times higher than average, according to a study of 183 women with cervical cancer and their husbands. Researchers believe this type of cancer is directly linked to human papilloma virus (of which there are 75 strains) spread during sexual intercourse somewhat like venereal disease, reported the *New York Times* (August 7, 1996).

***The single, ultimate root cause of cancer and the source of all its aberrations, Dr. Otto Warburg declared, is life without oxygen, or anaerobiosis. "All normal cells have an absolute requirement for oxygen, but cancer cells can live without oxygen."***

## BLOCKED DETOXIFICATION PATHWAYS

In a healthy individual, the body's normal detoxification systems, especially the liver, are generally able to eliminate toxins and thereby prevent illness. But these systems, including the immune defense, can be overwhelmed by a multiplicity of toxins—any combination of the factors described in this chapter—and become functionally incompetent to complete the vitally necessary detoxification. A blocked detoxification system might involve a clogged lymphatic drainage system in which thickened lymph accumulates dangerously in the lymph nodes without being emptied into the blood circulation for removal from the body. It may also involve chronic intestinal constipation and liver enzyme dysfunction.

For more information about **detoxification**, see Chapter 33: Physical Support Therapies, pp. 949-980.

As Joseph Pizzorno, N.D., explains, to prevent cancer, the liver's detoxification system must be working optimally. When it is not functioning well, it is unable to process and eliminate the multiplicity of carcinogens entering the body, and we become more susceptible to cancer. "High levels of exposure to carcinogens coupled with sluggish detoxification enzymes significantly increase our susceptibility to cancer."

Dr. Pizzorno cites an Italian study of chemical plant workers with an unusually high number of bladder cancer cases. Although all workers in this study had been exposed to equal amounts of toxins, the ones with underfunctioning liver enzyme detoxification systems were the ones to develop bladder cancer.[219]

See also "Intestinal Toxicity and Digestive Impairment" in this chapter, pp. 621-624.

The major players of the immune system—macrophages, natural killer cells and other key components—do not have an unlimited ability to cope with the toxins, carcinogens, and other biological insults imposed by the environment. Four types of system overload may overwhelm the body's anticancer defenses and account for increased susceptibility to cancer:

**1) Metabolic Overload:** Toxins and carcinogens can encourage the cancer process through a mechanism called metabolic overload and secondary carcinogenesis.[220] When we are exposed to high, persistent doses of toxins from various sources—drugs, smoke, alcohol, chemical additives, heavy metals, and many others—a state of metabolic overload can result. The body's natural detoxification mechanisms no longer function optimally. The heavy load of toxins overwhelms enzyme systems that would ordinarily deactivate the toxic form of a substance, turning it into an innocuous form. Since the chemicals are no longer handled normally once the metabolic threshold is reached, the resulting aberrations in metabolic pathways predispose the individual to tumor development.[221]

**2) Endocrine Overload:** Hormones can stimulate abnormal cell growth and proliferation. These substances include growth hormones (found in many animal products), and sex hormones, especially estrogens, testosterone, and estrogen-like substances that mimic the effects of estrogen. Endocrine overload probably occurs as a result of estrogen-like compounds that get into the body and act on susceptible cells, such as the breast cells, thereby causing cancer. Some of these xenoestrogens (foreign estrogens) namely DDT, DDE (a metabolic by-product of DDT), and certain PCBs, have been implicated as a cause of breast cancer.

**3) Free-Radical Overload:** Toxic pollution, tobacco smoke, nuclear and ultraviolet radiation, excessive exercise, and many other seemingly disparate substances and activities can all generate damaging oxygen-free radicals, unstable molecules that circulate within the body. Free radicals (discussed in detail on pages 630-631) are dangerous because they have a tendency to attack and destroy the fragile membranes surrounding cells, thus making the body more vulnerable to various cancer initiators and promoters. In addition, the free radicals themselves may interact with cellular DNA, causing mutations that can lead to cancer formation.[222]

**4) Immune Overload:** The immune system's job is to recognize what is foreign (non-self) and thus potentially dangerous to the body. If the substance encountered by the body is foreign (an antigen), the immune system attacks it and tries to neutralize or destroy it. At the same time, it recognizes and tolerates what is native to the body. This system has the capacity to identify some tumor antigens (foreign proteins on the surface of the tumor) and mount an effective attack that results in tumor rejection.

Unfortunately, sometimes cancer cells retain an identity similar to normal cells and are (mistakenly) immunologically tolerated. At other times, the immune system is overloaded with food allergies and other antigens that form complexes with antibodies; these "immune complexes" inhibit the macrophages' ability to devour and destroy and, as a result, cancer cells can freely multiply.

The tonsils are an integral part of the body's immune and lymph system and need to be functioning in top condition to help the body detoxify itself of the impurities and toxins it encounters every day. Many people unknowingly suffer from chronic tonsillitis (inflammation of the tonsils), a condition largely promoted by the steady stream of toxins produced by infected teeth or by chronically infected paranasal sinuses. These toxins tend to flow through the tonsils via the lymphatic system. At first, the tonsils simply regenerate their tissues after exposure to toxins; increasingly, however, the destroyed tonsil tissue is replaced by inactive scar tissue. The person no longer feels any pain or sensation in the tonsils, which often appear superficially healthy.

German physician and researcher Joseph Issels, M.D., found upon removing degenerated tonsils, that they were surrounded by a thick, callous capsule which required a sharp instrument to pierce. Upon excising the capsule, Dr. Issels and his colleagues typically found "multiple small abscesses as well as up to cherry-sized cysts filled with fluid or thickened pus. The tonsillar tissue was spongy, mushy and had a carcass-like smell."[223] What is important here is that about two-thirds of Dr. Issels' cancer patients had degenerative atrophic tonsils, a fact which highlights yet another source of toxicity which when combined with other factors could lead to cancer growth. A corollary German study revealed that 85% of patients examined had infected tonsils and that the resulting abscesses had drained into the bloodstream, further toxifying the blood.

## FREE RADICALS

A free radical is an unstable molecule with an unpaired electron that steals an electron from another molecule and produces harmful effects. Free radicals are formed when molecules within cells react with oxygen (oxidize), as part of normal metabolic processes. If not controlled by antioxidants, free radicals can then break down cells and damage enzymes, cell membranes, serum lipoproteins, unsaturated fatty acids in cell membranes, and DNA or chromosomes.

Free radicals are produced both by external harmful influences, such as radiation and environmental pollution, and by internal processes, such as metabolism and immune defense. Free radicals are generated by energy production and fat metabolism, from the immune response by white blood cells, and by the liver's own detoxification procedures. However, uncontrolled free-radical production plays a major role in the development of at least 100 degenerative conditions, including cancer, heart disease, and aging. Sources of free radicals include carcinogens, pollution, smoking, alcohol, viruses, radiation, most infections, allergies, stress, low blood supply (ischemia), burns, cold, certain foods, excessive exercise, and inflammation.

In sicknesses marked by an inflammation, even more toxic free radicals are produced by phagocytes activated to scavenge and remove them, because, in doing their job, they set in motion a biochemical cascade that ends up generating more free radicals. The resulting condition is known as oxidative stress or oxidative overload, and describes the ratio between pro-oxidants and antioxidants. (It is a little confusing, but antioxidants are the "good guys" in this ratio and the pro-oxidant free radicals are the "bad guys.")

An antioxidant (meaning "against oxidation") is a natural biochemical substance that protects living cells against damage from harmful free radicals. Antioxidants work against the process of oxidation—the robbing of electrons from substances. If unblocked or left uncontrolled, oxidation can lead to cellular aging, degeneration, allergies, arthritis, heart disease, cancer, and other illnesses. Antioxidants in the body react readily with oxygen breakdown products and free radicals, and neutralize them before they can damage the body. Antioxidant nutrients include vitamins A, C, and E, beta carotene, selenium, coenzyme Q10, pycnogenol (grape seed extract), L-glutathione, superoxide dismutase, and bioflavonoids. Plant antioxidants include *Gingko biloba* and garlic. When antioxidants are taken in combination, the effect is stronger than when they are used individually.

What makes the difference between normal functioning of the immune system, which includes the deactivation of free radicals, and the initiation of a potential cancer process is the amount of antioxidants available in the system. "When free-radical production exceeds the ability of the neutralizing systems, progressive cellular damage occurs," states Dr. Pizzorno.

When this damage becomes chronic, the next step is chronic or serious degenerative disease, including cancer. Although antioxidants are available naturally in foods, to offset intense free radical activity, one often needs to enhance the process with nutritional supplements, especially if one's diet was nutritionally inadequate in the first place. The details on this supplementation with antioxidants comprise significant portions of the treatment protocols offered by many of the cancer doctors appearing in this book.

## CELLULAR OXYGEN DEFICIENCY

One of the most provocative theories of cancer causation was originally put forth by two-time Nobel laureate, Dr. Otto Warburg. He was a German biochemist who won his first Nobel Prize in 1931 for the discovery that oxygen deficiency and cell fermentation are part of the cancer process. "From the standpoint of the physics and chemistry of life, the difference between normal and cancer cells is so great that one can scarcely picture a greater difference," Dr. Warburg wrote.

***Cancer will develop only if the DNA mutates and then goes unrepaired, and this repair mechanism may be impeded by toxic metals such as lead, mercury, and cadmium.***

The single, ultimate root cause of cancer and the source of all its aberrations, Dr. Warburg declared, is life without oxygen, or anaerobiosis. "All normal cells have an absolute requirement for oxygen, but cancer cells can live without oxygen—a rule *without any exceptions.*" Dr. Warburg showed that when you take normal cells from an embryo and force them to grow without oxygen in a Petri dish, they assume the characteristics of cancer cells; they are, in effect, transformed from normal to cancerous by the elimination of their prime nutrient, oxygen. This meant normal cells could be converted to cancerous cells by changing only one variable, said Dr. Warburg.[224]

According to Dr. Warburg's theory, when cells are deprived of oxygen, they can revert to their "primitive" state and enter into glucose reactions, deriving energy not from oxygen, as normal plant and animal cells do, but, rather, from the fermentation of sugar. Oxygen gas, the donor of energy in plants and animals, is dethroned in the cancer cells and replaced by an energy yielding reaction of the lowest living forms, namely, a fermentation of glucose."[225] This primitive survival mode is thought to be the way that organ-

## p53 and the Silence of the Genes

The gene known as p53 is often referred to as the "guardian of the genome," that is, the full complement of human genes arrayed across 26 chromosomes. Under normal conditions, p53 directs cancer cells to stop dividing or to commit cellular suicide, which is why it is described as a tumor suppressor gene. However, a new cancer can actually silence p53 by deleting or mutating the 2 copies of it maintained in most cells. Scientists have found that about 50% of all tumors possess cancer cells devoid of any p53.

What if p53 were deliberately reintroduced into localized tumor masses? Would the tumor begin to regress under the corrective influence of more p53? To test this idea, researchers at the University of Texas M.D. Anderson Cancer Center in Houston packaged p53 into a harmless virus and injected it into lung tumors of 7 cancer patients whose condition had responded to conventional treatment. The virus would insert the p53 genes directly into the tumor.

The gene therapy strategy produced temporary remissions in 3 of the 7 patients and it stopped tumor growth in the other 4; however, all 7 patients eventually died of the cancer.[226]

isms existed first on earth, before they began using oxygen. It is a highly inefficient method, as the rapid reproduction of the cancer cells uses up large amounts of glucose, breaking it down into lactic acid. Lactic acid is a waste product that puts a strain on the body and causes an imbalance in the acid/base ratio, or pH level. As the acidity of the body rises, it becomes even more difficult for the cells to use oxygen normally. Cancerous tumors may contain as much as 10 times more lactic acid than healthy human tissues.[227]

For information on **oxygen** and cancer, see Chapter 32: Enhancing Whole-Body Metabolism, pp. 915-927.

One possible reason for the dramatic increase in cancer rates over the past century, according to Dr. Warburg's theory, may be the decreasing levels of oxygen and the increasing levels of carbon monoxide in urban air. Carbon monoxide (CO) has a higher affinity for hemoglobin (which transports oxygen to the cells) than does oxygen; for this reason, when we breathe in CO, our hemoglobin binds more CO and less oxygen. By contrast, according to this same oxygen deficiency theory, cancer cells cannot exist in an oxygen-rich environment. Therefore, if sufficient oxygen is provided, the frenzied glucose fermentation stops and normal aerobic, or oxygen-requiring, respiration returns.

Humans can become oxygen deficient through several routes, including long-term exposure to air pollution (tobacco smoke, auto exhaust, factory emissions), devitalized foods (overcooked, processed, preserved, all of which deplete oxygen), shallow breathing, and inadequate exercise.

## Oncogenes, Tumor Suppressor Genes, and Their Presumed Cancers

| ONCOGENES | |
|---|---|
| PDGF | glioma brain cancer |
| erb-B | glioblastoma (brain cancer) and breast cancer |
| erb-B2 | breast, salivary gland, ovarian cancers |
| RET | thyroid cancer |
| Ki-ras | lung, ovarian, colon, pancreatic cancers |
| N-ras | leukemia |
| c-myc | leukemia, breast, stomach, lung cancers |
| N-myc | neuroblastoma (nerve cell) and glioblastoma cancers |
| Bcl-2 | cell lymphoma |
| Bcl-1 | breast, head, neck cancers |
| MDM2 | sarcomas |

| TUMOR SUPPRESSOR GENES | |
|---|---|
| APC | colon, stomach cancers |
| DPC4 | pancreatic cancer |
| NF-1 | neuorfibroma, myeloid leukemia |
| NF-2 | meningioma, ependymoma (brain cancer) |
| MTS1 | wide range of cancers |
| RB | bone, eye, bladder, small cell lung, breast cancers |
| p53 | wide range of cancers |
| BRCA1 | breast, ovarian cancers |
| BRCA2 | breast cancer |

Source: Adapted from Robert A. Weinberg, "How Cancer Arises," *Scientific American*, (September 1996), p. 65.

## CELLULAR TERRAIN

The consequences of the multiple factors described above are registered at the cellular level according to factors such as pH (acid/base balance) and oxidation-reduction potential. European practitioners of what is called biological medicine refer to this as the cellular terrain or internal milieu. These terms refer to the general vitality, activity, and biochemical condition of the cells in the body, as measured by certain criteria.

As early as 1952, in his *Hypothesis of Pathogenesis of Cancer*, German cancer researcher Joseph Issels, referred to earlier, outlined the complex series of biochemical changes that result in a "tumor milieu." Dr. Issels defined this as the "primary, humoral precancerous state," that is the biochemical foundations or seed state on which a cancer process could develop. Removing the tumor by surgery or chemotherapy does not affect or eliminate this primary precondition, said Dr. Issels.

Among the original causal factors in cancer, there are prenatal (genetic and constitutional) and postnatal (faulty diet, teeth, tonsils, abnormal intestinal bacteria, and neural disturbances). Any of these factors can create secondary damage at the level of the cell, nervous and hormonal systems, liver, bone marrow, and lymph, and lower immune resistance to create a precancerous tumor milieu. At this stage, there is what Dr. Issels calls "incapacitation of natural resistance" and "complex metabolic disturbance." Psychological or physical triggers can act potently in this milieu. The next step is the emergence of an actual tumor, followed by the manifestation of numerous symptoms.[228]

***Just as Dr. Issels' "tumor milieu" underlies or precedes the appearance of actual cancer tumors, so do Hahnemann's miasms precede activities of the oncogenes.***

At the core of biological thinking is the concept of the body's internal environment, the condition of the cells, known as the terrain, explains Thomas Rau, M.D., medical director of Parcelsus Clinic in Lüstmuhle, Switzerland. When the cell becomes imbalanced, conditions are set for infection, illness, chronic disease, or cancer to begin; when they are rebalanced, conditions are set for healing and a return to health. "As we see it," says Dr. Rau, "sickness is not caused by bacteria, but the bacteria comes *with* the sickness. Bacteria, viruses, or fungi can only develop if they have the suitable cellular conditions. They develop from *within* the organism; they do not invade it from without." Of course, infections may enter the body from outside but if the body is healthy and its cellular terrain balanced, they will not thrive, or even survive.

This idea is known as pleomorphism and, not surprisingly, has been considered heretical ever since French physician and pharmacist Antoine Béchamp (1816-1908), intellectual rival to Louis Pasteur and his germ theory, first proposed it in the 1870s. Béchamp said that microbes—a bacterium, fungus, virus, whatever—can change shape ("morph") and, in fact, take on many ("pleo") sequential shapes that are increasingly pathogenic. It can thereby produce illness from *within* the body.

In contrast, Pasteur's monomorphism holds that bacteria maintain one shape and invade the body from outside, producing infection and illness. Biochemical changes, such as alterations in pH and oxidation-reduction occurring within the cells and blood, initiate this microbiological shape-shifting. Outside influences, such as faulty diet, inadequate nutrition, exposure to carcinogens, chronic organ toxicity, stress, or trauma provide the impetus to throw the cells out of balance, says Dr. Rau. Once imbalanced, disease processes can take root, potentially leading to cancer.

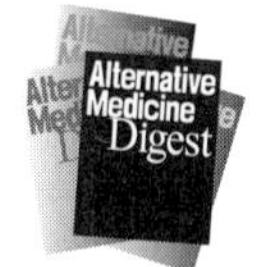


For more about **Dr. Rau's medical approach**, see "Arthritis, Parkinson's, and Fibromyalgia," #13, pp. 24-31.

One of the major breakthroughs in cellular terrain theory came with the development by French biologist Gaston Naessens of an optic microscope called the Somatoscope. The Somatoscope allowed scientists to view *living* organisms at high magnifications. Naessens used this tool to reveal tiny particles in the blood never before seen. He named them somatids, meaning tiny bodies—"the smallest unit of life, the precursor to DNA, capable of transforming energy into matter."

Naessens' research revealed that somatids normally go through a 3-stage microcycle: somatic, spore, double spore. These are nonpathogenic or harmless. But when the immune system becomes stressed or damaged

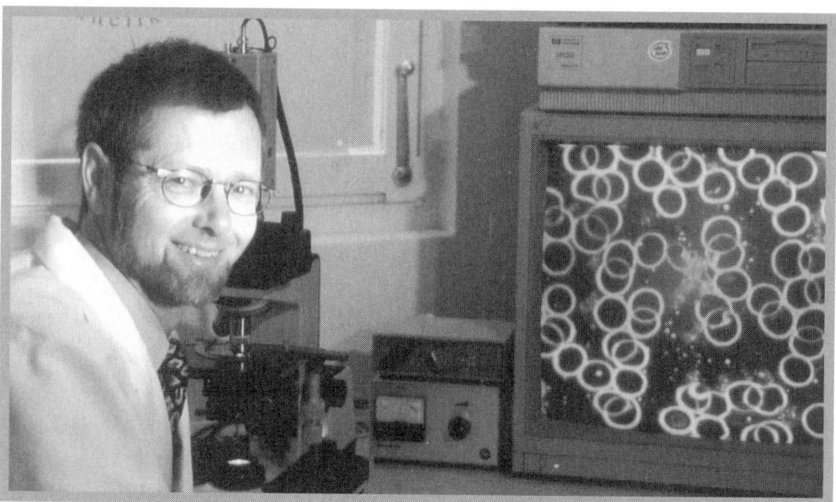

**Dr. Rau examines a live sample of a patient's blood using darkfield microscopy.**

by pollution, sickness, emotional distress, or other causes, the somatids evolve through a macrocycle of 13 additional forms, becoming pathogenic. These various forms have been associated with diseases like cancer, multiple sclerosis, lupus, AIDS, and other disorders. German zoologist and bacteriologist, Guenther Enderlein, M.D., discovered similar microorganisms to Naessens' somatids. He named them *protits*, and found that these tiny, protein-based microorganisms (also known today as L-forms or cell-wall deficient organisms) flourished in the blood cells, plasma body fluids, and tissues, living in the body in a symbiotic or mutually beneficial relationship. Any severe change or deterioration in the body's internal environment, however, caused the protits, like Naessen's somatids, to advance from harmless agents to disease-producing bacteria or fungi.[229]

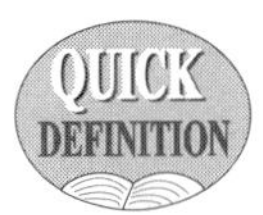

The term **pH**, which means "potential hydrogen," represents a scale for the relative acidity or alkalinity of a solution. Acidity is measured as a pH of 0.1 to 6.9, alkalinity is 7.1 to 14, and neutral pH is 7.0. The numbers refer to how many hydrogen atoms are present compared to an ideal or standard solution. Normally, blood is slightly alkaline, at 7.35 to 7.45; urine pH can range from 4.8 to 7.5, although normal is closer to 7.0. **Acid-base metabolism** refers to the metabolic processes that maintain the balance of acids and bases (alkalines) in body fluids. Acids release hydrogen ions, while bases accept them. The total number of these hydrogen ions present determines the pH of a fluid. Too many hydrogen ions (a pH below 7) produce an acidic state called acidosis, while too few hydrogen ions (a pH above 7) cause an alkaline excess called alkalosis; both can lead to illness. **Oxidation-reduction** refers to a basic chemical mechanism in the cell by which energy is produced from foods. Electrons (negatively charged particles in an atom) are removed from one atom, resulting in "oxidation" of this first atom, and then are added or transferred to another atom, resulting in "reduction" of this second atom. This continual process of energy metabolism is actually a flow of electrons, or a minute electrical current within the cell.

Dr. Enderlein believed that a diet rich in animal fats and proteins could trigger these normally harmless microbes to change into their higher, toxic forms that cause diseases ranging from cancer and leukemia to AIDS. According to his research, radiation and other carcinogenic influences can also initiate this change.[230]

According to Naessens, pleomorphic microorganisms do not directly cause cancer. "They are simply witnesses to a weakening of the natural defenses of the body and signposts that can be used for early diagnosis of disease." Raymond Keith Brown, M.D., a physician and former fellow at the Sloan-Kettering Institute for Cancer Research in New York City, explains: "Pleomorphic organisms are demonstrable as the silent stage of a gamut of infections, and they've been found in not only cancer patients, but those individuals afflicted with arthritis, multiple sclerosis, and other diseases."[231]

## ONCOGENES

The predominant emphasis in conventional cancer research today is to find individual genes capable of causing, initiating, or triggering tumor growth. First identified in the 1970s, these causal genes are referred to as *oncogenes* (meaning the gene that starts the *onkos*, or tumor mass). About 50 different ones have been described to date.

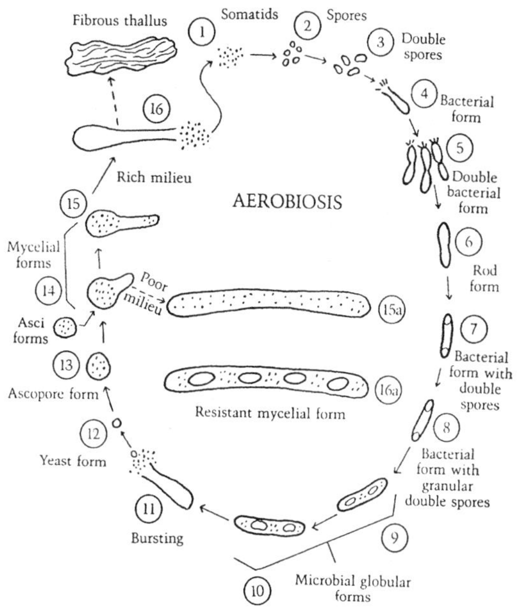

Fibrous thallus
(1) Somatids
(2) Spores
(3) Double spores
(4) Bacterial form
(5) Double bacterial form
(6) Rod form
(7) Bacterial form with double spores
(8) Bacterial form with granular double spores
(9)
(10) Microbial globular forms
(11) Bursting
(12) Yeast form
(13) Ascopore form
Asci forms
(14) Mycelial forms
(15) Rich milieu
(16)
Poor milieu
(15a)
(16a) Resistant mycelial form
AEROBIOSIS

From the book *The Persecution and Trial of Gaston Naessens* ©1991 by Christopher Bird. Reprinted by permission of HJ Kramer, P.O. Box 1082, Tiburon, CA 94920. All rights reserved.

**Figure 25.5—The somatid cycle, according to Gaston Naessens**

For more information on the **pleomorphic theories** of Dr. Enderlein and others, see Chapter 31: New Approaches to Immune Stimulation for Reversing Cancer, pp. 905-909.

An oncogene is a gene believed to transform normal cells into cancer cells, thus initiating the development of cancer. Some of these genes have reportedly been identified in cancer-causing viruses. Proto-oncogenes are genes in a neutral, inactive stage that code for proteins that activate cell division; under certain conditions, they mutate and become oncogenes, which then activate cell proliferation that soon becomes uncontrolled.

Proto-oncogenes are normally active during the development of the embryo and during early childhood when rapid growth is needed; later, they are inactivated by tumor suppressor genes. Numerous external factors can reactivate proto-oncogenes, including mutagens, chemical carcinogens, electromagnetic energy (X rays, sunlight), aflatoxins (mold spores found on peanuts and some other foods), nuclear radiation, viruses, or hormones.

Conventional cancer researchers now consider the oncogene, as a cell that has escaped the normal growth-control mechanisms of the organism, to be the primary causal unit in cancer. Over a long period (often many years), it supposedly evolves through a "sequential accumulation of alterations in the genetic material" into a cancer.[232] Oncogenes are necessary for human survival by stimulating the production of tissue growth factors in the developing human embryo, but when they mutate, they can become cancer-producing agents.[233]

Researchers now believe that about 20% of all human cancers, including cancers of the lung, colon, and pancreas, are partly brought about by mutations in the *Ki-ras* oncogene; members of the *myc* oncogene "family" are also frequently found in cancers, including Burkitt's lymphoma. In about 50% of cancers of the colon and rectum, the ras oncogene has been activated while evidence suggests that the tumor suppressor genes p53 and DCC have been inactivated in 70% of the cases.[234]

***A miasm represents an* energy residue *of an illness from a previous generation, while an oncogene (or inherited genetic mutation) represents a* molecular residue *of an illness from a previous generation.***

The latter belong to another class of genes called tumor suppressor genes or antioncogenes. Under normal conditions, they act to prevent uncontrolled cell growth that could lead to tumors. However, oncogene mutations (technically, when a proto-oncogene becomes a carcinogenic oncogene) inactivate the tumor suppressor genes so that, paradoxically, they actually contribute to tumor growth. Other factors that can inactivate tumor suppressor genes include other DNA changes, chemical carcinogens, and electromagnetic energy. According to cancer researcher Robert A. Weinberg, Ph.D., biology professor at M.I.T. in Cambridge, Massachusetts, a multistep process leads to cancer.

Describing this process in the emergence of colon carcinoma, Dr. Weinberg uses an automotive analogy to make his point: "They [those with colon cancer] carried a stuck accelerator—the growth-promoting *ras* oncogene—and a whole series of defective brakes—inactive versions of the APC, DCC, and p53 genes." In other words, it is not a matter of a single defect capable on its own of precipitating uncontrolled growth. But once multiple control systems were knocked out, the cell had no way of slowing down its growth and returning to normal speed. What follows are repeated cycles of mutations followed by spurts of rapid cell growth, and the appearance of a cell with mutant genes allowing for uncontrolled tumor growth, says Dr. Weinberg.

Cancer will develop only if the DNA mutates and then goes unrepaired. In many cases, the cell manages to repair damage to its own DNA, with the help of DNA-repair enzymes, but this repair mechanism may be impeded by toxic metals such as lead, mercury, and cadmium.[235] Emotional stress has also been shown to adversely affect DNA repair in humans.[236] Unrepaired mutated DNA then raises the cancer risk. Certain substances, such as folacin, zinc, and ginseng, can stimulate the DNA-repair mechanism, thus helping to prevent cancer.[237]

***Dr. Guenther Enderlein believed that a diet rich in animal fats and proteins could trigger normally harmless microbes to change into their higher, toxic forms that cause diseases ranging from cancer and leukemia to AIDS.***

## GENETIC PREDISPOSITION

The theory of gene causation for cancer inevitably leads researchers into speculations about inherited cancers—gene configurations or mutations that might predict if not guarantee that a given individual will develop a particular form of cancer. Here the "cause" of cancer is displaced to a previous generation when, presumably, a genetic mutation occurred that was able to survive the generational leap.

The term "family cancer syndrome" is now used to describe the tendency of particular cancers (such as breast, colon, or ovarian) to show up in succeeding generations of the same family. For example, many scientists now believe that the following inherited cancers may be linked to mutations in certain related tumor suppressor genes: melanoma and pancreatic cancer (MTS1, p16); breast and ovarian cancer (BRCA1); breast cancer (BRCA2); colon and uterine cancer (MSH2, MLH1, PMS1, PMS2); and brain sarcomas (p53). Inheritance of "flawed" genes probably accounts for about 5% of all cancers in the U.S.[238]

Regarding the BRCA1 tumor suppressor gene, women found to have a defect in this gene (through DNA testing) are significantly more *likely* to develop breast cancer. The presence of this gene is not so much a guarantee as an indication of susceptibility. The defective BRCA1 seems to be at fault in the majority of so-called sporadic breast cancers, the nonfamilial tumors that account for 9 out of every 10 breast cancers, or 90% of all breast cancer cases.[239] In 1996, researchers announced in *Nature Genetics* that after studying blood samples from 3,000 Jews of Ashkenazic origin (Eastern and Central Europe), another gene, the BRCA2 mutation, occurs in about 1.5% of the Jewish population but not at all in the non-Jewish population. According to their data, it is estimated that women with the BRCA2 gene have a 30-40% risk of developing breast cancer, and they are at increased risk for ovarian cancer. Like BRCA1, BRCA2 is a normal gene that can initiate cancer when it is mutated.[240]

## MIASM

Predisposition to cancer, and to most major illnesses, involves more than genetic inheritance alone. As the preceding discussion of oncogenes makes clear, genetic changes during one's lifetime and those one might inherit are significant factors in the emergence of cancer. "It is known that the genetic makeup, the DNA, of an individual plays a role in shaping the hereditary predisposition to disease, but this is not the whole story," explains world-renowned homeopath George Vithoulkas.[241]

More than 200 years ago, German physician Samuel Hahnemann, the founder of homeopathy, used the term "miasm" to indicate this deeper predisposition to chronic disease. Just as Dr. Issels' "tumor milieu" underlies or precedes the appearance of actual cancer tumors, so do Hahnemann's miasms precede activities of the oncogenes. Showing remarkable foresight, Hahnemann's concept of miasm accurately prefigures today's description of oncogenes.

According to Hahnemann, 3 miasms underlie all chronic illness, and these parallel broad stages in the history of the human experience with primary disease states. The *Psoric* miasm (from *psora,* meaning "itch") is the earliest and thus the most fundamental predisposing layer. In fact, according to this theory, the *Psoric* miasm is the foundation of sickness underlying all the diseases experienced by humans—cancer, diabetes, and arthritis as well as serious mental disorders such as epilepsy, schizophrenia, and imbecility. The *Syphilitic* miasm came next in the history of human diseases and derives from syphilis. The *Sycotic* miasm, the third layer, arose as a residue of gonorrhea.

Miasms can be thought of as taints or energy residues of previous illnesses. Knowledge of DNA and genes per se was unknown in Hahnemann's time but, even today, most homeopaths understand miasms to be influences that are more subtle and have more of an energy nature than the triggering molecules described by genetics. Homeopaths explain that the miasm can become engrafted onto the fetus as a kind of energy signature or predisposition from a previous generation of that family. As such, it indicates a tendency or susceptibility—but by no means a predictable guarantee—of a person to develop specific types of illnesses.

The miasm is a "maintaining cause," or inherited chronic disease predisposition, while the disease and its symptom picture is the result of the "exciting cause," a stimulus (stress, carcinogens, emotions, thoughts) that provokes or activates the miasm. "It is possible for a parent to acquire an ailment during his life whose influence can be transmitted to the children, even though no known change has occurred in the genetic structure of the parent," Vithoulkas explains. In other words, a miasm represents an *energy residue* of an illness from a previous generation, while an oncogene (inherited genetic mutation) represents a *molecular residue* of an illness from a previous generation. Miasms are broad-focused, predisposing individuals to certain families of illness, whereas oncogenes are coded specifically not only for a single type of illness (cancer) but actual varieties of that illness (breast, ovarian, lung, pancreatic cancers).

As Vithoulkas explains it, "A miasm is a predisposition toward chronic disease underlying the actual manifestations of illness which 1) is transmissible from generation to generation, and 2) may respond beneficially to the corresponding nosode prepared from either pathological tissue or from the appropriate drug or vaccine." Physicians treating cancer with homeopathy often employ *Carcinosin*, a homeopathically potentized remedy known as a nosode made from cancerous tissue.

In a given individual, in most cases there are layers of predisposition, combinations of all 3 miasms, each contributing to the overall symptom picture. According to Vithoulkas, the *Tuberculosis* miasm is actually a combination of the *Psoric* and *Syphilitic* miasms. In recent years, homeopaths have added a *Cancer* miasm to Hahnemann's original 3; the *Cancer* miasm is a combination of the effects (or taints) of the *Psoric*, *Sycotic*, and *Syphilitic* miasms. There is also preliminary discussion about there being a 5th miasm, tentatively called the *Petroleum* miasm, representing, in effect, the inherited energy taints of a century of using petroleum products including gasoline and oil.

For information on **homeopathy** and cancer, see Chapter 6: W. John Diamond, M.D., Chapter 9: James Forsythe, M.D., and Chapter 20: Vincent Speckhart, M.D.

The trouble with miasms, and one that makes them potentially a contributing factor in the onset of cancer, is that they tend to interfere with the action of homeopathic remedies prescribed to reverse illness. As Hahnemann explained, "the vital force is powerless to prevent their [chronic diseases] growth or its own gradual deterioration, resulting in the final destruction of the organism." Vital force in homeopathy is similar to *Qi* in Chinese medicine: it refers to the basic life force or vital energy that directs all the activities of the physical organism.

An untreated miasm can block the action of correctly prescribed homeopathic remedies (and many other treatments as well), thereby preventing "any true and lasting recovery in these chronic maladies," Hahnemann said. It also acts as a layer of interference and illness predisposition. Each of the miasms has a specific, broadly focused homeopathic remedy (nosode) to remove their influence from an individual: *Psorinum* for Psoric; *Medorrhinum* for Sycotic; *Sylphilinum* for Syphilitic.

Chapter 26

# How Cancer Politics Have Kept You in the Dark Regarding Successful Alternatives

**A powerful conglomerate of government agencies, international drug companies, and major cancer treatment hospitals puts profits first. They do not want the public to learn about and pursue effective alternatives. The result is that chemotherapy, radiation, and surgery are the law of the land as cancer treatments—for political, not therapeutic, reasons.**

An important goal of this book is to illuminate the dark fact that most of what you have heard over your lifetime about cancer treatments is not the truth. At the very least, you have received an incomplete picture. If you believe the propaganda you have been fed and you develop cancer, it can cost you your life.

In the United States, economic interests masquerade as therapeutic regimens and scientific concern. Their goal is to own and completely control a disease—cancer—as if it were a commodity, and to quash competition (meaning alternative approaches), so as to maintain a marketplace monopoly.

Money leads politics by the nose. The *financial* interests of drug companies, conventional cancer doctors, hospitals, HMOs, and others in what is known as the Cancer Establishment, have eclipsed the integrity of the Hippocratic Oath; money and politics have proclaimed conventional approaches as scientifically validated and therefore mandated by law. The terrible flaw in this convenient financial setup is that the profits that flow to the cancer establishment are derived from human lives lost to cancer because successful alternative approaches are outlawed or unreported.

To the cancer establishment, a cancer patient is a profit center. The actual clinical and scientific evidence does not support the claims of the cancer industry. Conventional cancer treatments are in place as the law of the land because they *pay,* not heal, the best. Decades of the politics-of-cancer-as-usual have kept you from knowing this, and will continue to do so unless you wake up to their reality.

## The Awesome Financial Success of Cancer, Inc.

Cancer is modern medicine's biggest business. In recent years, the financial burden of cancer has become staggering. In this country alone, over $1 trillion has been spent on treatment, research, and indirect costs since President Nixon's declaration of a "War on Cancer" in 1971. Cancer accounts for at least 10% of the total cost of treating all health problems in the United States, and its share of the total cost of premature death from all causes is about 18%.[1]

The costs continue to rise. A study by the National Center for Health Statistics estimated the overall medical costs for cancer at $71.5 billion for 1985. Of this total, $21.8 billion went to direct treatment costs, $8.6 billion to the cost of lost productivity due to illness (morbidity costs), and $41.2 billion to mortality costs (value of the economic output that is lost from premature death of workers due to disease).[2] But by 1995, the total cost of cancer was $96.1 billion.[3] This is probably a conservative estimate because, in 1990, the National Cancer Institute put the overall costs for cancer at $104 billion.[4]

## Cancer's Annual Treatment Cost (U.S.)

| | |
|---|---|
| Breast | $6.6 billion |
| Colorectal | $6.5 billion |
| Lung | $5 billion |
| Prostate | $4.7 billion |
| Bladder | $2.2 billion |
| Uterine | $1.6 billion |
| Melanoma | $1.1 billion |
| Leukemia | $1.1 billion |
| Kidney | $1 billion |
| Ovarian, Stomach, Pancreas, Cervical | $610 million to $1 billion each[8] |

Consider the cost of non-small-cell lung cancer, which kills more people than any other cancer. Patients—more often, their insurance companies—pay almost $175,000 for one year of treatment for this cancer; over half of this payment goes directly to the cost of chemotherapy drugs.[5] Drug treatments for breast cancer (second biggest killer among women) typically range between $5,000 and $25,000.[6] For "terminal" cases of breast cancer, Medicare payments average between $50,000 and $62,000 per case.[7] Were it not for this immensely lucrative "malignancy market," the medical profession would have abolished slash-burn-and-poison (surgery, radiation, and chemotherapy) treatment long ago because the records of success simply aren't there. But the profits are, and these are too alluring for those in the cancer industry to turn down.

These vast sums of money have not bought much relief for cancer victims. According to Dr. Debra Davis, the Assistant Secretary for the Department of Health and Human Services, "in all age groups cancer incidence is increasing ... and few new effective treatments have been devised for the most common cancers." Mortality rates for the most prevalent cancers continue to rise, and 5-year survival rates have not changed significantly in 25 years. No reasonable person can call this progress, particularly in light of the frequently debilitating effects of chemotherapy and radiation, yet this is the status quo that the cancer industry enforces as scientifically valid and "proven."

Although rising cancer rates are bad news for patients, they are great news for the cancer treatment industry—Cancer, Inc., as some critics have labeled it. In this environment, words that sound scientific and doctorly often mask a different agenda. The phrase "treatment success" can mean profitable, while "dangerous" or "questionable" treatment can refer to therapies that threaten the profits of the cancer industry. When you begin to ferret out the *economic* context and motivations of cancer treatment, it helps you understand why alternative cancer therapies are suppressed or barred from the public's awareness. It helps you see why treatments as dangerous and consistently unsuccessful as radiation and chemotherapy continue to dominate the field of oncology.

***The doctors who perform cancer treatments and the scientists who conduct research are not the ones in control of the cancer field. It is the larger power structure of the cancer establishment that effectively controls the shape and direction of cancer prevention, diagnosis, and treatment.***

The reason alternative cancer treatments are not mainstream has little to do with alleged therapeutic ineffectiveness and far more to do with political control over the therapy marketplace. The politics of cancer have an overriding influence on the science of cancer and, ultimately, on what the public thinks and believes about cancer and what it is able to expect as treatment options. The doctors who perform cancer treatments and the scientists who conduct research are not the ones in control of the cancer field. It is the larger power structure of the cancer establishment that effectively controls the shape and direction of cancer prevention, diagnosis, and treatment.[9]

The field of U.S. cancer care is organized around a medical monopoly that ensures a continuous flow of money to the pharmaceutical companies, medical technology firms, research institutes, and government agencies such as the Food and Drug Administration (FDA) and the National Cancer Institute (NCI), and quasi-public organizations such as the American Cancer Society (ACS). This is "the cancer industry," says Ralph Moss, Ph.D., extensions of which include the corporate media, public relations experts, petrochemical and nuclear industries, corporate scientists, and doctors who specialize in "killing" cancer.[10]

Cancer research has been set up almost entirely in favor of conventional approaches ever since the war on cancer, formalized in 1971 as the National Cancer Act, was first scripted in the 1960s. At that time, Senator Ralph Yarborough (D-Texas) organized the National Panel of Consultants on the Conquest of Cancer. Of its 26 members, 10 came from the American Cancer Society and 4 were affiliated with Memorial Sloan-Kettering Hospital; Benno Schmidt, M.D., the director of Memorial Sloan-Kettering's Cancer Center was the panel's chairman, and Sidney Farber, M.D., former president of ACS, was its vice chairman.

## ROCKEFELLER, I.G. FARBEN, AND THE GLOBAL CARTEL TO ENFORCE DRUG-BASED MEDICINE

In a strange way, the fact that chemotherapy is at the top of the list of accepted— *enforced*—treatments for cancer in the U.S. can be traced to the business interests and manipulations of a giant Germany-based multinational corporation called I. G. Farben and its affiliations with the Rockefeller oil interests, based in New York City but worldwide in its reach. The I.G. Farben conglomerate, first formally organized in 1926 with headquarters in Frankfurt, Germany, controlled nearly the entire German drug and chemical industries during the 1930s. They gained ownership of the technology for producing synthetic fuels from coal, a process called hydrogenation, first achieved by a German chemist in 1913.

I.G. Farben was not so much a discrete, single company as an interlocking web of dozens of companies around the world; in fact, by 1940, not only did I.G. Farben's operations straddle 93 countries, but it was Europe's largest industrial corporation and the world's largest chemical manufacturer. In Germany alone, I.G. Farben controlled 380 companies. In the U.S., I.G. Farben had commercial interests or outright ownership in dozens of major companies, many of them in pharmaceuticals, such as Bayer, Proctor and Gamble, Monsanto Chemical, Dow Chemical, Lederle Laboratories, Hoffman-LaRoche Laboratories, and Squibb and Sons Pharmaceuticals.

The name itself—I.G.—indicates the "cartel" nature of its business operations: *Interessen Gemeinschaft*, means "community of interests." Putting this in perspective, in the oil industry today, OPEC (Organization of Petroleum Exporting Countries) is a cartel whose interests focus around maximizing profits from crude oil. A cartel is a voluntary, often international, combination of independent, private businesses that have similar products or affiliated services for the purposes of limiting their competition, which they do by price-fixing, allocating customers and markets, and exchanging technology. The goal is simple and purely capitalistic: severely curtail the competition to drive up the prices and control the market.

***It was strategically desirable for Rockefeller's oil interests to become linked with I.G. Farben's chemical industry. They understood why and how a global cartel could work to discourage—quash—all small-scale enterprising non-drug-oriented (non-petrochemical-based) approaches to medicine. They would not be able to control the money flow otherwise, and success in an alternative medicinal product—laetrile, Hoxsey herbs, antineoplastons, among many—could eventually undercut their monopoly.***

Long before OPEC, there was I.G. Farben. In the late 1920s, it stood poised to control the entire European petroleum market by offering a less expensive synthetic substitute. This plan might have been desirable to Germany, preparing for war, and for Europe in general, but it was a threat to the hegemony of the multinational oil interests of the Rockefellers, known then as Standard Oil of New Jersey. John D. Rockefeller, Sr. (1839-1937), was the quintessential 19th-century capitalist "robber baron," building up immense wealth by controlling an entire industry—oil. By the 1860s, he already owned the world's largest refinery; in 1870, he founded Standard Oil Company with the intention of "consolidating nearly all oil refining into one giant corporation," explains historian Daniel Yergin in *The Prize*.[11] Already by 1879, Rockefeller's reach was prodigious: he owned 90% of America's oil refining capacity and, in 1899, his new company, Standard Oil of New Jersey, held stock in 41 other corporations.

In 1929, Rockefeller and I. G. Farben cut a deal. Rockefeller would sell oil but not drugs and have the hydrogenation patent for use outside of Germany; I.G. Farben would stay out of oil outside of Germany, and sell only chemicals. I.G. Farben also received 2% of Standard's stock, worth

$35 million. In 1930, the 2 giants established a joint company to develop the oil-chemical field. Over the decades, the Rockefeller/I.G. Farben cartel would reap massive profits from both areas. What better arrangement than to control both drugs and oil? Nearly all manufactured chemicals, including drugs, require coal tar or crude oil as a component (often in the form of petroleum jelly).

It was strategically desirable for Rockefeller's oil interests to become linked with I.G. Farben's chemical industry. They understood why and how a global cartel could work to discourage—*quash*—all small-scale enterprising non-drug-oriented (non-petrochemical-based) approaches to medicine. They wouldn't be able to control the money flow otherwise, and success in an alternative medicinal product—laetrile, Hoxsey herbs, antineoplastons, among many—could eventually undercut their monopoly.

Medical historian and researcher G. Edward Griffin concludes, after poring through reports of U.S. government hearings conducted between 1928 and 1946 to investigate these topics: "The reality, therefore, is that government becomes the tool of the very forces that, supposedly, it is regulating."[12] For "government," substitute NCI, FDA, and the National Institutes of Health (NIH), and you can see why it is axiomatic for these organizations supposedly working *for* the American public to take all possible steps to suppress any innovations that might threaten the global drug (and oil) edifice they represent.

It is also highly revealing to note that, according to Griffin's research, during the 1930s when Nazi Germany was preparing for war, I.G. Farben used its cartel interests in the U.S. to suppress or censure (through canceling advertisements) the publication of any information critical of or unfavorable to Nazi Germany. There is no reason to suppose that such media manipulation stopped with the end of that war. The fact that most mainstream American media consistently and routinely deride, make fun of, or seriously criticize alternative medicine, despite the reality of its successes and clinical efficacy, could be interpreted as meaning that the next generation of I.G. Farben interests may be pulling the strings in editorial offices across the country. The use of alternative medicine runs against the financial interests of the cartel.

There is still another factor that illustrates how a global cartel can strangle alternative medicine. According to Griffin's research, as of 1974,

## Profits for America's Drug Lords Up 23%

**Your Sickness Keeps the Drug Cartel Rich**

While it seems that ever more Americans are becoming ill and finding the cost of insurance, treatment, and medication so increasingly expensive as to bring them close to bankruptcy, America's multibillion dollar drug cartel is reaping enormous profits. Thanks to widespread government support of conventional medicine and FDA's continuing strong-armed interference with free and open marketplace competition among all medical specialties, net profit for Pfizer, for example, for early 1996 jumped 23% while for Johnson & Johnson, it rose by 20.8%.

Among Pfizer's leading profit-making drugs is Norvasc (for angina and high blood pressure), whose sales climbed by 46%, and Zoloft (an antidepressant), whose sales grew by 34%. Sales of Prozac, the popular antidepressant made by Eli Lilly, rose 27%. Overall, Johnson & Johnson's prescription drug sales soared 30.5% higher in this period while their over-the-counter drug sales climbed by 13.2%. Industry analysts estimated that for the entire drug cartel, average profit would grow by 11-13% for the first 3 months of 1996. The next time you reach for a conventional drug, at least you'll have some idea of who's getting rich at your expense. It is not just the Colombians who are making a killing on their drugs.

—SOURCE: Milt Freudenheim, "Drug Makers Raise Profits 20% or More," *The New York Times*, April 17, 1996.

the Rockefeller interests included "vast" stock holdings in the first and third largest insurance companies in the U.S., namely, Metropolitan and Equitable; they also maintained a strong presence (through board of directors' membership) in Traveler's and several other insurers. Rockefeller/I.G. Farben's control in the insurance sector, if it still exists, either actually or camouflaged, could enable the cartel to complete the squeeze on alternative medicine by preventing its practices from being reimbursed by insurance policies across the country.

Open competition among different brands of vitamins, for example, was to be discouraged, as was over-the-counter sale of medicines. Making drugs available only by doctor's prescriptions, Griffin explains, suited the cartel as a long-range strategy because, by this setup, they could continually raise the prices and tightly control the market. Griffin states: "In the specialized field of drugs and pharmaceuticals, the Rockefeller influence is substantial, if not dominant."

The FDA push in the 1990s to reclassify all nutritional and herbal supplements as prescriptive drugs would require massively expensive clinical research, and is a perfect example of a regulatory change that would materially benefit the cancer cartel and help put alternative medicine out of business. Cartels do exist today, as they did during the time of Nazi Germany, Griffin states; the names and ownership lists may have changed, but the interests remain the same. "The pharmaceutical industry, far from being exempt from this influence, has been at the center of it from the very beginning."

These facts practically guaranteed that the American approach to cancer treatment would be dominated, even dictated, by what the Germans were doing prior to and during World War II. I.G. Farben, for example, built the world's largest poison gas industry. Farben was the prime manufacturer of the poison mustard gas used to kill soldiers, and of Zyklon B, the nerve poison used to kill 6 million Jews in the concentration camps of German-occupied Europe. Griffin presents evidence suggesting that I. G. Farben actually controlled the Nazi state and operated many of the concentration camps, including Monowitz, which they built themselves (near Auschwitz, in Poland). At Monowitz, I.G. Farben used both "free" and slave labor, drawing on an estimated 300,000 inmates from the concentration camps as unreimbursed laborers.

***The FDA push in the 1990s to reclassify all nutritional and herbal supplements as prescriptive drugs would require massively expensive clinical research, and is a perfect example of a regulatory change that would materially benefit the cancer cartel and help put alternative medicine out of business.***

"By the time the Nazis began to tool up for war in Europe," Griffin explains, "Farben had gained control over a major portion of America's pharmaceutical industry." Decades earlier, John D. Rockefeller, Sr., had learned from his I.G. Farben colleagues that pharmaceutical drugs could become a source of fantastic profits especially if the competition factor was eliminated from the picture.

The Germans appeared to be pursuing research in 2 related fields: cancer treatment and more effective ways to kill people with chemicals. In a bizarre development, poison mustard gas was simultaneously researched for its ability to kill cancer tumors and soldiers. Some of this research took place at Memorial Hospital (the predecessor to Memorial Sloan-Kettering) and Yale University, mostly under the veil of wartime secrecy.

In 1942, secret research offices in the U.S., Britain, and Nazi Germany were simultaneously studying poison mustard gas as a chemical warfare agent and possible anticancer therapy. Based on the clinical success of treating a single laboratory mouse (which had lymphoma) with a modified mustard gas, human trials began that year. The first human subject died; although his tumor initially regressed, his white blood cell count plummeted from 5,000 to 200 per cubic millimeter of blood. By 1946, at least 160 American patients had been secretly subjected to poison gas treatment for cancer, according to Griffin.

## Memorial Sloan-Kettering Hospital: Treatment Derived from Poison Gas Supports Petrochemical Interests

The history of Memorial Sloan-Kettering Hospital (MSKH) in New York City graphically illustrates how the cancer industry got established and what holds it together. It begins with the Astors, one of New York's superwealthy families in the late 19th century; their money was based on real estate investments made as early as 1809 by family patriarch John Jacob Astor.

In the 1880s, the Astors provided money to found the New York Cancer Hospital. Their lawyer became the hospital's first chairman. Other major contributors also influenced hospital policy. The Douglas family, who made their money in the copper industry, appointed their family physician as medical director and changed the name to Memorial Hospital. James Douglas, of the mining family, was involved in radium extraction from ore mined in Colorado. Radium, of course, is used in radiation therapy. In 1927, Rockefeller invested several million dollars in Memorial Hospital and in the 1930s, gave it a city block for rebuilding the hospital. This act of largesse would also prove to be an imprimatur for Memorial to develop and support chemicalized medicine.

Preliminary successes with chemicalized medicine, as the early mustard gas experiments revealed, foretold vast future profits—especially with government backing. In the 1950s, Memorial Hospital acquired 2 new major investors, both from General Motors: Alfred P. Sloan and Charles F. Kettering, after whom the center was duly renamed. One of the most outspoken proponents of chemotherapy for cancer was Cornelius Rhoads, who had been the leader of the U.S. Army Chemical Warfare Service and a Fellow of the Rockefeller Foundation. In the mid-1940s, Rhoads became head of Memorial Sloan-Kettering's cancer research institute where he became "an evangelist of chemotherapy," according to medical historian James T. Patterson in *The Dread Disease.* Through the case of Rhoads, one can clearly see the revolving-door or interlocking interests of the cancer industry in its formative years.

The salient point here is simple but shocking: the mainstream use of chemotherapy for cancer came directly out of Nazi war science and poison gas weapons research in the interests of further enriching German and American businessmen. The rest followed the predictable venalities of purely profit-centered business development.

In 1987, for example, Memorial Sloan-Kettering owned almost 70,000 shares in 7 major pharmaceutical companies. One of the few cancer writers to document this shady history of the cancer establishment is Ralph Moss, Ph.D., who knows it from the inside. He worked for Memorial Sloan-Kettering in the 1970s in the public affairs department; in 1977, Dr. Moss was fired, he says, for refusing to cover up favorable research data on laetrile.

The opposition of the cancer industry to laetrile, derived from apricot pits and other natural substances, is only one example in a long, depressing saga of big business colluding with the government to suppress therapeutic and commercial alternatives. (You'll learn more about the laetrile controversy in this book, along with stories of similar effective alternatives that were successfully quashed, such as Coley's toxins, hydrazine sulfate, high-dose vitamin C, immunotherapy, Livingston microbial therapy, and antineoplastons, among others.)

***The salient point here is simple but shocking: the mainstream use of chemotherapy for cancer came directly out of Nazi war science and poison gas weapon research in the interests of further enriching German and American businessmen.***

## Restructuring American Medical Education in Favor of Drugs

Rockefeller money was instrumental in eliminating homeopathy and naturopathy and their medical institutions from America for many decades through the infamous Flexner Report published in 1910. Abraham Flexner, a layman, prepared this report, highly damaging to all forms of alternative medicine, while employed by Andrew Carnegie and John D. Rockefeller., Sr. Simon Flexner, Abraham's brother, was president of the Rockefeller Institute for Medical Research.

In 1904, the American Medical Association (AMA) had established a Council on Medical Education whose top priority would be the reform of

U.S. medical schools. It would then work through the state medical licensing boards, controlled by its physician members, to effect changes in its favor at the state level. In 1906, AMA members inspected 160 schools and approved only 82. For political reasons, AMA declined to publicize its findings, so it engaged the Carnegie Foundation for the Advancement of Teaching to replicate the results; the foundation, in turn, hired Simon Flexner's brother, Abraham.

The Flexner report unfairly criticized homeopathic and naturopathic medical colleges for not meeting criteria specific to conventional medical training, and thereby enabled new licensing and accreditation laws to squeeze hundreds of alternative medical colleges out of business, including America's 14 homeopathic schools. "Though a layman, [Flexner] was much more severe in his judgment of particular institutions than the AMA had been in any of its annual guides to American medical schools," comments historian Paul Starr.[13] Thus a nonphysician was able to restructure the U.S. medical training system in favor of drug-oriented conventional medicine, whose harmful effects would last an entire century. The end result of the Flexner study was that U.S. medical schools became intensively drug oriented and all research became focused on developing new drugs. In fact, in the early 1900s, according to Starr's research, the medical research budget of the Rockefeller Institute was "many times larger" than that of the U.S. government's medical research budget.

***Thus a nonphysician was able to restructure the U.S. medical training system in favor of drug-oriented conventional medicine, whose harmful effects would last an entire century. The end result of the Flexner study was that U.S. medical schools became intensively drug oriented and all research became focused on developing new drugs.***

The Institute had been founded in 1902 with a $65 million endowment from John D. Rockefeller, Sr. By 1950, the various Rockefeller foundations had made grants of $821 million for medicine, science, and education. In this way, major investors such as Rockefeller would start seeing a return on their investments in chemicalized medicine and would be assured of at least a 50- to 75-year handicap against the now delegitimated practitioners of what had suddenly become "alternative" medicine.

Beginning in the first decade of the 20th century, conventional medicine guaranteed its domination of the direction of medical research by establishing a number of governmental and private institutes that funded only drug-oriented research, ignoring alternative medicine entirely. The year 1901 saw the founding of the Rockefeller Institute in New York, the Carnegie Institute in Washington, D.C., and the Phipps Institute in Philadelphia. The Food and Drug Administration (FDA) began in 1906, then was greatly expanded in 1938; the U.S. Public Health Service was established in 1912; the National Institutes of Health (NIH) came in 1930 followed by the National Cancer Institute in 1937 and the Communicable Disease Center in 1946 (renamed the Centers for Disease Control, or CDC, in 1970).

After World War II, the NIH would be the conduit for substantial investment of government money in biomedical research focused on drugs and disease entities. All of these developments further entrenched the political dominance of conventional chemicalized medicine in the U.S. In the 1920s and 1930s, yet another measure served to cement conventional medicine in place as *the* medicine of the land. These were the "Medical Practice Acts" enacted state to state "which limited the legal practice of medicine to licensed graduates of the allopathic [conventional medicine] institutions protected from competition by the Flexner Report," states medical historian Harris L. Coulter.

These acts were used, in particular, to prosecute chiropractors, naturopaths, and other drugless practitioners of alternative medicine, says Coulter. The acts still remain in place today in more than 40 states, effectively prohibiting the practice of many forms of alternative medicine.[14]

## The American Cancer Society: A "Temporary" Organization or the Beneficiary of the Cancer Epidemic?

The American Cancer Society, from the beginning, was funded and virtually directed by leaders of the petrochemical industry. The ACS was founded in 1913 at the New York Harvard Club as the American Society for the Control of Cancer. Funds were provided by John D. Rockefeller, Jr. For some years, ACS remained an elite vehicle for charitable contributions of New York's wealthiest individuals and families, such as banking magnate, J. P. Morgan, who contributed $50,000 in the late 1920s.

For decades, ACS used fear of contracting and dying from cancer—"mass cancerphobia," its critics called it—as a prime technique in their advertising and promotions. "The main goal was to urge the general public to consult their physician at the first suspicion of cancer," observes cancer industry critic Ralph Moss. During the 1940s, the society renamed itself the American Cancer Society and radically restructured the organization. The success of the grassroots Women's Field Army in the 1930s as an auxiliary group of the society, had led to a membership exceeding 1 million, compared to ACS' membership of only 986 members. The Field Army's zeal to raise popular awareness of cancer risks and early treatment had encouraged the emergence of alternative treatments and practitioners such as herbalist Harry Hoxsey, who attracted thousands of followers.

This public trend toward alternative treatments for cancer dismayed most of the wealthy patrons of ACS, wedded as they were to petrochemical and pharmaceutical interests. In fact, an ACS representative from Esso (already a giant oil company in the 1940s), allegedly remarked that cancer research was in danger of being "abandoned to quacks and to pseudo-scientific frauds." What he may have meant was that the "quacks"—the alternative practitioners—were achieving enough success and publicity to jeopardize the honeypot of conventional chemical-based cancer treatment. The new organization would put an end to that. Nonmedical representatives from leading pharmaceutical firms such as Hoffman-LaRoche and other businesses were installed as ACS directors, and Madison Avenue-style marketing techniques put ACS' fundraising efforts into high gear.

ACS described itself as a "temporary" organization that would cease to exist once cancer had been eradicated. Now, nearly a century later, the society is the richest private medical-oriented charity in the world, with no sign of going out of business. For fiscal year 1991, the ACS held fund balances of $491.7 million, enough to cover operating costs for approximately 1 year. In addition, ACS holds tens of millions of dollars in stocks, bonds, commercial paper, and U.S. government bonds.

ACS headquarters is housed in a lavish office building in Atlanta, Georgia, almost directly across the street from the U.S. Centers for Disease Control. The organization consists of a national society with 57 chartered divisions (members of divisional boards of directors, both medical and lay, in all states plus 5 metropolitan areas) and over 3,500 community-based units. These are volunteer groups that direct the society's programs in counties throughout the United States.[15] Curiously, although *nationally* ACS bills itself as primarily volunteer based, the single most important spending category at the *state* level is for staff salaries, ranging from 45% to 60% of the total budget.

According to ACS brochures, the charity's programs are devoted to research, detection and treatment, prevention, and communications with the public. Fundraising and management of the national ACS (salaries and overhead costs) comprise nearly one-quarter of the society's total annual budget—quite a sum of money for a "volunteer organization." Research comprises another quarter, while prevention comprises only about one-fifth of the budget. Other costs go to patient services (about 14%), detection and treatment (about 10%), and community services (about 7%).[16]

In the 1970s, the ACS was accused by the independent research group National Information Bureau of hoarding millions of dollars' worth of publicly contributed funds, well beyond the society's operating expenses, in interest-generating bank accounts.[17]

***We believe the American Cancer Society in effect is an unofficial and primary public relations arm for the mainstream cancer industry. Since ACS is privately funded, a great deal of effort is devoted to producing—one is tempted to say "tailoring"—messages about cancer, stirring up fears about cancer, and getting people to donate money in response to this fear.***

Even though ACS claimed that it reached an estimated 71 million Americans in 1991 with its public education programs (a 12.6% increase over the previous year and 21 million more people than in 1988), the death rate from cancer during that same period did not decline but rose by 5.3%, from 497,500 deaths in 1988 to 524,100 in 1992. "Surely an *effective* education campaign reaching tens of millions of people year after year would produce more promising results," comment James T. Bennett, professor of economics at George Mason University, and Thomas J. DiLorenzo, professor of economics at Loyola College, "yet cancer remains a killer on the rampage."

Supporting public education is a cornerstone of ACS' fundraising appeal, yet the advice of the self-styled "nation's health nanny," the authors add, is "nothing more than common sense, which is defined as normal native intelligence independent of specialized knowledge or training. Should tens of millions of dollars be spent each year to teach the public common sense?"[18]

We believe the American Cancer Society in effect is an unofficial and primary public relations arm for the mainstream cancer industry. Since ACS is privately funded, a great deal of effort is devoted to producing—

one is tempted to say "tailoring"—messages about cancer, stirring up fears about cancer, and getting people to donate money in response to this fear. Much of this work is done by influencing writers and editors to present information according to the ACS party line. Efforts to solicit support are stepped up around the cancer deaths of major public figures, such as Mickey Mantle and Gilda Radner. Nor does ACS hesitate to sell its name as a product endorsement. In 1996, needing cash to boost its "cancer-fighting programs" at a time when membership donations were stagnating, ACS accepted $4 million to exclusively endorse Florida orange juice and NicoDerm antismoking patches.

ACS propagandists have always understood the value of linking negative emotions (fear of dying from cancer) with appeals for financial support. The ACS's fundraising maneuvers in the 1940s and 1950s focused on the idea that cancer kills. Advertisements featured morbid images such as gravestones and coffins and the terrifying "beware of cancer" message. This was invariably followed by a message of hope—"we can beat cancer, we can cure it in your lifetime—"and this was followed by an appeal for funds.[19] When President Nixon declared war on cancer in 1971, the ACS took up more belligerent language and regularly offered reports signifying "progress" in the official war.

Several years ago, a group of 60 independent scientists and doctors strongly criticized the ACS for a lack of leadership in cancer prevention. They stated that ACS and other parts of the cancer enterprise had "continuously minimized the evidence for increasing cancer rates which it has largely attributed to smoking and dietary fat, while discounting or ignoring the causal role of avoidable exposures to industrial carcinogens in air, food, water and the workplace."[20]

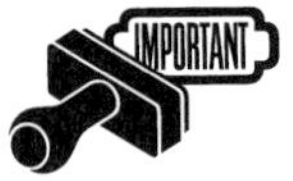


Evidence suggests that ACS is not the public's best health advisor when it comes to issues that might conflict with its clear financial interests. Throughout the 1980s, the ACS kept silent when the Reagan and Bush administrations rolled back regulations on industrial carcinogens, and it failed to warn the public about avoidable exposures to environmental carcinogens. The society also refused to join a coalition including the March of Dimes, American Heart Association, and American Lung Association to support the Clean Air Act. It refused to support the Toxic Substances Control Act and never once entered the fight for clean water legislation. ACS opposed the FDA's ban on saccharin;

1 year earlier, the society had accepted a grant from Coca-Cola (a manufacturer of saccharin-sweetened soda).

Finally, ACS has opposed or failed to support occupational safety standards, efforts to reduce radiation exposure, and other forms of environmentally oriented cancer prevention.[21] Looking at the evidence, we wonder if ACS actually benefits from the *promotion* of cancer.

For decades, ACS has lobbied vigorously to suppress innovative cancer therapies within the medical community. It has consistently blacklisted, even vilified, people who use such therapies, mainly through the publication of its pseudoscientific journal, *CA: Cancer Journal for Clinicians.* Its official blacklist, "Unproven Methods of Cancer Management," was changed during the 1980s to "Questionable Methods of Cancer Management," but this change was mere window dressing. In the early 1990s, the society changed the name again to "Alternative and Complementary Methods of Cancer Management." Evidently, when medical journals began publishing surveys showing that as many as 50-60% of cancer patients used alternative therapies, the ACS decided to get with the program—as minimally as possible, of course.

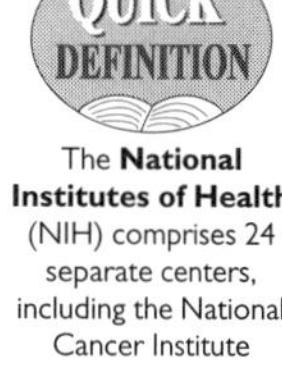


The **National Institutes of Health** (NIH) comprises 24 separate centers, including the National Cancer Institute (founded 1937; $2 billion annual budget). With a total annual budget of $10 billion, the NIH, founded in 1887, is one of 8 health agencies within the Public Health Service, which is a division of the U.S. Department of Health and Human Services. The Office of Alternative Medicine is currently within the NIH.

The ACS is a powerful influence on cancer research, the acceptance of new therapies, and the inner workings of the cancer industry. "The Society now has tens of millions of dollars to distribute to those who favor its hegemony, and many powerful connections to disconcert those who oppose it," says Ralph Moss.[22]

## The National Cancer Institute: A Cure for Cancer Is Not in Its Interests

The National Cancer Institute is part of the National Institutes of Health (within the Department of Health and Human Services) and holds primary responsibility for funding the so-called war on cancer. Although NCI, as a taxpayer-funded organization, supposedly represents the government's position on cancer, its policies are guided largely by 2 smaller, privately-run organizations: the American Cancer Society and Memorial Sloan-Kettering Cancer Institute in New York City.[23] The ACS and NCI work together as partners, with the ACS being more actively involved in "education" (i.e., media manipulation and propaganda) and fundraising efforts.

According to Samuel Epstein, M.D., of the University of Illinois Medical Center, the NCI's objectivity toward cancer-related issues has long been compromised by serious conflicts of interest. "For decades, the war on cancer has been dominated by powerful groups of interlocking professional and financial interests," Dr. Epstein explains, "with the highly profitable drug development system at its hub—and a background that helps explain why 'treatment,' not prevention, has been and still is the overwhelming priority, as indeed it is for most physicians."[24] A revolving door operates between NCI and its friends in the pharmaceutical industry. Dr. Epstein cites numerous examples, among them that of Stephen Carter, head of drug research and development at Bristol-Myers Squibb, a former director of NCI's Division of Cancer Treatment.

In addition, Dr. Epstein notes that "NCI has apparently never initiated any scientific or other intervention in legislative, regulatory or public arenas designed to prevent or reduce avoidable exposures to any carcinogens other than tobacco."[25] A relatively small amount of funding is devoted to research on carcinogens found in food, air, and water. One of its most dubious forms of "prevention" is what NCI refers to as "chemoprevention," which includes the use of highly toxic and carcinogenic agents like tamoxifen for preventing breast cancer. Use of this drug for "prevention" has been shown to increase the risk of uterine and other reproductive cancers.[26]

NCI's *real* politics are clearly revealed in the following example. In February 1996, the World Health Organization formally designated tamoxifen as a carcinogen. Tamoxifen is a synthetic hormone and the most widely prescribed drug given to prevent breast cancer recurrence. Studies show that women taking tamoxifen after surviving breast cancer then have a high propensity to develop endometrial cancer. The National Cancer Institute and Zeneca Pharmaceuticals, which makes the drug, then aggressively lobbied State of California regulators to keep them from adding tamoxifen to their list of carcinogens, according to *Science News*, March 2, 1996.

***Studies show that women taking tamoxifen after surviving breast cancer then have a high propensity to develop endometrial cancer. The National Cancer Institute and Zeneca Pharmaceuticals, which makes the drug, aggressively lobbied State of California regulators to keep them from adding tamoxifen to their list of carcinogens.***

One of NCI's primary functions is to approve grants for research, an area in which NCI shows preferential treatment for conventional approaches. Applicants who propose new chemotherapy protocols are whisked through the grant approval process much faster than applicants who propose unconventional or complementary cancer treatments (e.g., nutrition combined with chemotherapy). Established cancer treatment centers are far less likely to be scrutinized than a new applicant or one suggesting a controversial therapy.

After the experts' visit, one of NCI's committees, the National Cancer Advisory Board (NCAB), assigns the project a priority rating. The final decision is made by NCI's Grant Management Office, which rarely overrules the powerful NCAB. It is almost unheard of that NCI will fund research that could, in any way, threaten the cancer treatment industry's arsenal—chemotherapy, radiation, surgery, and certain orthodox forms of immunotherapy. Doctors with excellent credentials and research staff are regularly turned down if they propose projects that involve a more complementary or integrated way of approaching cancer. This routine practice explains why the majority of studies of herbal medicines used in conjunction with chemotherapy and radiation have come from other countries, notably China.

NCI officials also keep the money flowing the way they want it by staying closely involved in coordinating the research protocols and "managing the data" generated by a research project. A prime showpiece for how NCI handles research of unorthodox cancer treatments is the Burzynski case, explained later in this chapter. As with ACS, you cannot look to NCI for genuine innovations in cancer therapy.

Follow the money trail and you'll see why it is this way. Most cancer research is funded by the pharmaceutical industry, and large clinical trials are both costly and time-consuming; the cost of establishing a new drug can run to $250 million. Even so, for patentable products such as chemotherapy agents, an investment is good business because it is likely to pay off, especially with government-mandated use. By definition, a profit-oriented pharmaceutical company is not going to pursue nonpatentable products such as laetrile, maitake mushroom, and most other alternative medicines, because they cannot be registered as patented drugs and thus controlled in the marketplace. "Pharmaceutical manufacturers are loath to fund research on therapies that aren't patentable," states Adriane Fugh-Berman, M.D., in *Alternative Medicine: What Works*.[27] The drug mentality rules.

The funding problem is a blatant example of how the medical establishment stifles important investigations of alternative medicine. In 1993, the Office of Alternative Medicine was established within the National Institutes of Health and given a mere $2 million research budget, yet that same year the NIH spent $68 million—remember, this is taxpayer money—on a single trial of one drug. In other words, a single chemical drug trial received 34 times more funding than an entire research department.

***By definition, a profit-oriented pharmaceutical company is not going to pursue nonpatentable products such as laetrile, maitake mushroom, and most other alternative medicines, because they cannot be registered as patented drugs and thus controlled in the marketplace.***

## FDA: *The Cancer Industry's Rabid Attack Dog*

The Food and Drug Administration (FDA) was originally mandated to monitor and regulate the presence of harmful substances in foods and drugs. During its early years, from 1906 to 1938, the FDA was "undermined by the combined political influences of the food and drug industry," reports Raymond Keith Brown, M.D. In 1938, Congress re-enlivened the FDA with new legislation in response to 100 deaths from a contaminated antibacterial drug called sulfanilamide. From then on, new drugs would have to pass safety tests established by the government.

Then in 1962, the thalidomide disaster in England and Germany, in which this sedative prescribed for pregnant mothers led to horrible birth defects in their infants, gave the FDA's role enhanced importance. At the time, FDA had not approved thalidomide for use in the U.S., thereby averting a repetition of the European tragedy. In the 1960s, the Kefauver-Harris amendment—the result of "good intentions, politics, and misguided scientism," says Dr. Brown—set FDA on the road of legitimated repression. "This gave autonomous police powers to the FDA to make and enforce decisions on drug safety," comments Dr. Brown. "More crucially, proof of efficacy, in addition to that of safety, became mandatory for the licensing of new drugs."[28]

Although the FDA is supposed to block harmful or useless treatments, devices, and substances from entering the marketplace, it has failed miserably in this function. The FDA routinely allows extremely toxic drugs to enter the medical marketplace. Its record is so poor it is as if the FDA legitimates products only if they later can be (and are) proven toxic. The FDA claims that "the benefits far outweigh the risks" with regard to these products, but such a claim is clearly in question, given the dismal failure of conventional cancer treatment and the stunning escalation of cancer cases.

The FDA's enforcement of potentially hazardous treatment methods has been inexcusably one-sided. "It has come down hard on practitioners of unconventional medicine, often unfairly branding them as quacks," notes Ralph Moss. "At the same time, it has been extraordinarily lax in the treatment of the largest [pharmaceutical] companies. It is hard to escape the impression that this agency, once considered the triumph of progressive consumerism, now exists primarily to serve the interests of the industry majors."[29]

One reason that helps explain the FDA's unwavering allegiance to conventional medicine, despite its demonstrated ineffectuality in treating cancer, is its back-door connection with the drug companies. One study found that almost 50% of high-ranking FDA officials had been employed by major drug companies immediately before joining the FDA. The study further disclosed that half of these officials upon leaving FDA took up executive jobs in pharmaceutical companies.[30]

In fact, as early as 1974, disgruntled FDA scientists testified before Congress that their agency was a pawn of the pharmaceutical industry. Soon after, the FDA spent $200,000 preparing a whitewash of this testimony, conveniently exonerating the agency of these claims. Around the same time, Congress discovered that 150 FDA employees owned stock in 27 of the companies they were supposed to regulate.

Indeed, the FDA has a long record of harassing doctors who use alternative cancer therapies. In the 1950s, they raided the offices of Wilhelm Reich, M.D., and accused the Austrian doctor of harming cancer patients. It was Reich's work with an energy accumulating device, the "orgone accumulator," which brought him into direct conflict with the FDA and led to his eventual imprisonment and the burning of his books. Dr. Reich had concluded that cancer involved a "bio-electric disturbance" within the organism, and he claimed that the orgone accumulator could help resolve this disturbance. He documented numerous cases of significant pain relief and even total remission of advanced cancers using this device.[31]

Ozone is another target in FDA's sights. Ozone therapy, for example, remains in the medical underground—too promising to be ignored and too novel to gain mainstream acceptance. The FDA's claim against ozone therapy is that no scientific evidence exists to back the claims for its efficacy, yet the FDA has 600 research papers from Germany detailing ozone's therapeutic value. In the United States, where the drug industry may lose profits if this nonpatentable, inexpensive approach is followed, the use of oxygen therapies remains severely restricted. FDA testimony before a House Judiciary Subcommittee in 1993 singled out ozone therapy as a "scam" perpetrated by "classic snake-oil salesmen."[32]

***In May 1992, the FDA stormed the offices of Jonathan Wright, M.D., partly in an effort to get him to stop using oxygen therapy. "The FDA won't spend a dime on ozone research, but they have spent over $1 million intimidating, harassing, and persecuting me alone," says Dr. Wright who was eventually vindicated.***

In May 1992, the FDA stormed the offices of Jonathan Wright, M.D., partly in an effort to get him to stop using oxygen therapy. "The FDA won't spend a dime on ozone research, but they have spent over $1 million intimidating, harassing, and persecuting me alone," says Dr. Wright who was eventually vindicated.[33]

Behind the fact that the FDA is highly selective in how it implements policy directives lies a serious discrepancy. For example, a 1992 study published in the *Wall Street Journal* revealed that 60% of drug advertisements in medical journals actually violated FDA guidelines, yet FDA did nothing about these violations.[34] An even deeper explanation for the FDA bias in favor of conventional medicine is found in activities it undertook in 1985. At that time, the FDA teamed up with the Pharmaceutical Advertising Council (a lobbying arm of numerous drug companies) to use drug industry funds to combat "quackery" in medicine—alternative medicine. The FDA and the council jointly issued a statement addressed to the presidents of advertising and public relations firms around the U.S. asking for their cooperation in the crusade against fraud and quackery in medicine. "The FDA is supposed to regulate the pharmaceutical industry, but instead they are teaming up to work on an antifraud campaign against an industry that some could construe to be an economic competitor," explains Mark Blumenthal, executive director of the American Botanical Council in Austin, Texas.

Not all therapies are subjected to such repressive action by the FDA. Shark cartilage has recently come under FDA scrutiny as a potentially useful cancer treatment. In recent years, in fact, the FDA has granted full approval for several clinical trials treating advanced cancers with cartilage. This action would *seem* to indicate a shift in its traditionally repressive attitude toward alternative therapies but, on closer analysis, we see that it is actually a ploy to discredit alternative medicine. Why does the FDA seem willing to research shark cartilage? In many of the studies now under way, shark cartilage is given only to patients for whom conventional treatment has failed. As an example, a study being conducted by researchers at St. Barnabas Hospital in Livingston, New Jersey, focuses on patients with advanced prostate or breast cancer who did not respond to conventional therapies—either radiation or chemotherapy, or a combination of the two.[35]

"This means that many of the patients in the studies have been subjected to extremely toxic treatment beforehand, without the benefit of naturopathic therapies to mitigate the toxic side effects," says Martin Milner, N.D., who has helped coordinate shark cartilage research. "This represents a built-in bias against the scientific assessment of the efficacy of alternative approaches such as shark cartilage. Many of these patients are already beyond the point of recovery once they start cartilage therapy." The FDA knows that when consumers read negative findings regarding shark cartilage, the

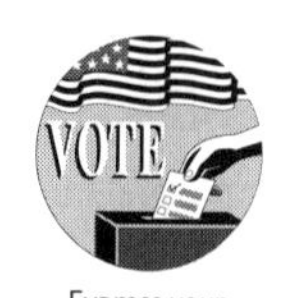


Express your dissatisfaction with FDA police tactics by contacting your Congressional representatives and demanding they reform the FDA.

## The Truth about Quackery

The derisive term "quackery" does not originate in any therapeutic gaffes committed by alternative practitioners but in the field of conventional dentistry. In 1840, U.S. dentists formed the American Society of Dental Surgeons. Members were required to sign "pledges" promising *not to use mercury* in dental fillings. Several members were suspended from the dental society in New York City in 1848 for "malpractice for using silver mercury fillings."

Mercury was called "quicksilver" in this country and "quacksalver" in some European countries. A "quack" is one who pretends to cure disease, and a "salve" is a substance for application to wounds or sores. The derogatory term "quack" was first used in reference to anyone using mercury preparations on the skin to "cure" diseases. Today, ironically, conventional dentists brand as quacks any dentists who report that mercury fillings are harmful and should not be used.

A quack, as defined today, is one who talks pretentiously without having sound knowledge of his subject. A quack makes vain and loud pretensions of medical ability, boasting of unfounded medical expertise. A major intention of this book is to revert this term to its rightful owners: the purveyors of conventional cancer treatments.

therapy will be regarded a failure and disappear from public attention. It is a clever but venal way of appearing to support something while working to repudiate it.

There is another reason the FDA is focusing all current studies of shark cartilage on patients with late-stage cancers. "The FDA is steeped in the thinking that conventional intervention for early-stage cancer is effective," Dr. Milner says. "But clearly they're also afraid of the possibility that alternative therapies could be just as effective, perhaps more so, with early-stage cancers. That's just too much of a threat to the pharmaceutical industry."

## The AMA: *Looking after Conventional Medicine's Special Interests*

Another major player in the politics of keeping American medicine conventional is the largest physicians' trade group and lobbying arm, the American Medical Association, now headquartered in Chicago, Illinois. In large part, the AMA was established in 1847, four years after American homeopaths first organized their association, to counter the marketplace success of homeopathy in America. "The rapid growth of homeopathy during these very years was furthered by the same atmosphere of public hostility to orthodox medicine," comments medical historian Harris Coulter. "Introduced into the United States in 1825, by the 1840s, [homeopathy] was offering severe competition to orthodox medicine."[36]

As early as 1850, AMA was politically maneuvering against alternative medicine; at that time, AMA's Code of Ethics ordered its members to boycott all homeopathic physicians and to avoid all consultations or even social contact with them. This regulation remained in effect until 1900. After the publication of the Flexner Report (mentioned earlier), the question of consulting with homeopaths would be moot, as there would be almost none left in the U.S.

You may not realize it, but the AMA, representing about 41% of American M.D.s, has its hands in many aspects of your everyday life. The AMA now looms as a monolithic communicator of medical information—and biases.

Each week their public relations staff sends out news releases to 4,000 medical journalists, video news releases to 800 TV outlets, and taped medical reports to 5,000 radio stations. There is probably no other organization on earth that distributes more words about conventional medicine to doctors and the public than the AMA. Ever wonder why commercial television and most mainstream magazines are so sarcastic and skeptical about alternative medicine? Just follow the paper trail out of the editor's office back to the AMA.

The AMA also works hard to keep certain other works from reaching the public, such as denying public access to the National Practitioner Data Bank. Run by the U.S. government, it lists all M.D.s who have committed malpractice, crimes, or ethical violations. For you, the citizen, this information is off limits. To the AMA also goes a fair amount of credit for blocking health care reform in 1994.

Fortunately, the American public is waking up to the AMA's monopolistic control over information and medical practice. M.D.s are no longer the "Marcus Welby" heroes they once were. Polls show that the AMA's public approval rating fell from 59% in 1986 to 43% in 1993. The number of Americans who thought the AMA was a reliable source of information on health declined from a low of 31% in 1989 to a trough of only 23% in 1993. Polls from that year also showed that 70% of Americans are beginning to lose their faith in conventional doctors.[37]

***Only 23% of Americans think the AMA is a reliable source of health information and 70% are losing faith in their conventional doctors, says a 1993 poll.***

It is highly unlikely the AMA will do it, given their history, but the polls seem to be saying it is time the AMA started looking after patients' interests for a change.

## Why the "Most Remarkable Anticancer Agent I Have Come across in My 45 Years of Experience in Cancer" Was Suppressed by NCI

This statement was made by Dean Burk, M.D., at the time he was head of cell chemistry research at the National Cancer Institute (NCI) in the 1970s. Some of his colleagues considered Dr. Burk to be "the world's greatest biochemist." The object of Dr. Burk's glowing praise was a substance called hydrazine sulfate, an inexpensive, nontoxic, easily available chemical that promised to reduce cancers faster, more safely, and more dependably than any known chemotherapeutic agent. True to an apparent mission of preventing effective cancer cures from being discovered, NCI worked skillfully to discredit hydrazine sulfate and to keep any knowledge of it from the general public.

Preliminary animal studies supported Dr. Gold's idea and, by the end of 1973, about 1000 people were using hydrazine sulfate. Soon after, the FDA issued a few Investigational New Drug permits to physicians allowing them to legally experiment with or administer the substance to patients. Dr. Gold organized the Syracuse Cancer Research Institute to handle the development of the product and its protocols.

The American Cancer Institute and NCI had no comment about the research, although NCI's Dr. Burk shared his enthusiasm for hydrazine sulfate with colleagues at Memorial Sloan-Kettering Hospital in New York City. In late 1973, the hospital started clinical trials with Dr. Gold's substance, but soon it became clear to him that they were setting things up to scuttle his research and discredit hydrazine sulfate. Dr. Gold specified the appropriate test dosages and the criteria governing dosage increases; MSKH ignored these specifications, however, and administered doses at levels far higher than what Dr. Gold considered safe or advisable. The result was that hydrazine sulfate not only failed to work properly, it produced negative, even dangerous results, such as "serious nervous system toxicities," according to an MSKH scientist.

The drug's contrived "failure" at Memorial Sloan-Kettering conveniently allowed the other gatekeepers of conventional cancer treatment, such as ACS, to put hydrazine sulfate on their list of "unproven" methods—perhaps the decision those concerned wanted in the first place. After all, hydrazine sulfate posed 2 major threats: first, it worked, and second, it hardly cost anything—about $25 to $50 for a year's supply. Could the cancer industry allow a new substance to compete with its comfortable drug monopoly?

In the USSR, however, it was different. Scientists at St. Petersburg's N.N. Petrov Research Institute of Oncology, Ministry of Health, produced research supporting hydrazine sulfate on 6 important counts. Specifically, they found that it could stop the growth of animal cancers, that it was relatively nontoxic, and that it could control cancer growth in human subjects. Even better, hydrazine sulfate produced objective, measurable improvements in about 33% of cancer patients studied and subjective improvements in 58%.

Lydia Danova, M.D., Petrov Institute's clinician most experienced with hydrazine sulfate, unhesitatingly declared her support for the value of this substance to journalist Jeff Kamen when he personally visited their facilities in 1994. "I recommend that American doctors use it to treat lymphoma, especially Hodgkin's, and brain tumors," said Dr. Danova. "Hydrazine sulfate prevents progression of tumors in the brain, prolonging the life of brain cancer patients—and providing the only treatment for inoperable nonmalignant tumors of the brain as well. You can see concrete results." This is why the Pharmacological Committee of the Russian Ministry of Health, equivalent to America's FDA, fully approved hydrazine sulfate for use in adult cancer patients.

However, Petrov Institute was dependent on NCI funding for various projects and, as Kamen observed, its staff appeared to be "intimidated by the mere mention of the NCI from which they still hope to get some badly needed assistance." On Kamen's first day of visiting, Petrov staff members, including Kaydo P. Hanson, M.D., its director, were "amazingly candid" in their discussions of the merits of hydrazine sulfate; but the next morning, they were fearful of NCI reprisals for their forthrightness. "It is important," Dr. Hanson told Kamen, "that you do nothing which suggests that we are criticizing [NCI]. NCI is very important, and we must not offend them." The old KGB couldn't have frightened Hanson any better.[38]

Even though officials in NCI and ACS ignored or disparaged the Russian

## How Hydrazine Sulfate Works

As an independent physician and researcher based in Syracuse, New York, Joseph Gold, M.D., identified hydrazine sulfate as the most likely chemical agent to fulfill his new theory of cancer reversal. More people die from the side effects of the cancer process than from the invasiveness of the tumor itself, Dr. Gold reasoned. Chief among these cancer side effects is cachexia, which means weight loss due to loss of lean tissue and muscle mass. The cachexia or wasting process begins as soon as the first cancer tissue appears in the body, and it speeds up the concentration of toxins in the body and the rate of opportunistic infection.

Cancer cells are somehow able to recycle their waste products, but they do so at the energy expense of their host, the human; the constant energy drain literally uses up the body's muscle and tissue reserves. The cancer uses sugar (glucose) from the body as fuel and releases lactic acid as a waste product, which is released into the blood. Then the body has to detoxify the lactic acid in the kidneys and liver and reconvert it back into glucose. This new glucose is once again taken up by the cancer, and the cycle continues.

With this in mind, Dr. Gold reasoned that there might be a better approach to cancer than chemotherapy, which depends on highly toxic substances to kill cancer cells. What if, he postulated, you try to block the cancer cells from doing damage to the human body through cachexia by supporting the individual's metabolism? Studying the medical literature in the early 1970s, Dr. Gold came upon a reference to hydrazine sulfate, an easily synthesized substance, that supposedly could block a liver enzyme from converting lactic acid into glucose.

research, by 1978, an estimated 5,000 patients were taking hydrazine sulfate under the guidance of their doctors. Subsequent Russian research in 1981 showed that of 225 patients treated with hydrazine sulfate, 65% experienced a positive subjective response. This finding means that, in the opinion of the individual cancer patient, hydrazine sulfate had beneficial effects.

Joanne Daniloff, D.V.M.D., and professor at Louisiana State University in Baton Rouge, explained in a letter to Jeff Kamen in 1994 how hydrazine sulfate had saved her life. At the time, she had survived 7 years after receiving surgery and hydrazine sulfate for her glioblastoma multiforme (grade IV) brain cancer, one of the fastest growing and most untreatable kinds. "You understand, then, that I am appalled by the [NCI's] design of studies that result in claims that hydrazine sulfate has little or no effect on cancer treatment. I find it difficult to understand how any study with such obvious flaws can claim any result or be published in any reputable journal."[39]

## NCI Director Vows to Take Off His Gloves on Hydrazine Sulfate

Rowan Chlebowski, M.D., Ph.D., of Harbor-UCLA Medical Center in Los Angeles heard about the Russian research and organized a research program at the hospital to study hydrazine sulfate. The result was 4, double-blind, placebo-controlled studies—completely by the "scientific" book—demonstrating the efficacy of the substance against lung cancer. In 1981, NCI's director, Vincent DeVita, M.D., appeared on ABC News where he flippantly discounted hydrazine sulfate as being "a very low-priority thing" and "unexciting."

The Russian research did not impress him: "I'm very unexcited—we throw away drugs that are better than hydrazine sulfate." Two years later, Dr. DeVita told Dr. Chlebowski: "I'm going to take off my gloves on hydrazine sulfate," and he branded it an "unproven method" in the next edition (1985) of his influential textbook, *Cancer: Principles and Practice of Oncology*. In June 1989, FDA agents raided the offices of 2 U.S. distributors of the product, seizing supplies and documents.

When Dr. Chlebowski published his results in the *Journal of Clinical Oncology* in 1990 demonstrating how hydrazine sulfate extended the survival rates of lung cancer patients, a guest editorial by Steven Piantodosi, M.D., of Johns Hopkins Oncology Center in Baltimore tore it to shreds, claiming that clinical trials with such a small number of patients—Dr. Chlebowski used 65—was not valid science. The inference of course was that Dr. Chlebowski was a second-rate scientist as well. Apparently Dr. Chlebowski, discouraged by this editorial savaging despite his 10 years of earnest research and his conclusion that hydrazine sulfate might potentially have saved the lives of millions of cancer patients, dropped his research and abandoned the field.

During the 1980s, the American Association for Cancer Research (AACR) prevented the Russian scientists (notably Michael L. Gershanovich, director of medical oncology at the Petrov Research Institute of Oncology in Leningrad) from publishing their results in the leading American cancer journals or from presenting their results at the AACR meeting. AACR's action made it impossible for NCI to sponsor any further drug tests on hydrazine sulfate, given that the Russian research results had not been officially reported to the U.S. scientific community.

It is not surprising: The success of hydrazine sulfate contradicted claims and commitments at ACS, MSKH, and AACR, where chemotherapy was the law of the land.

Notwithstanding continued official cancer industry opposition, information about hydrazine sulfate's anticancer effects managed to appear in *The Lancet*, *Cancer*, and the *Journal of Clinical Oncology*. In 1991, Petrov Institute scientists reported that hydrazine sulfate stopped tumors in nearly 50% of its patients, including tumors of the breast, ovaries, cervix, vulva, and endometrium. A smaller but still significant number of patients had even better results, with their tumors disappearing altogether. NCI did not follow up on the Russian studies, which had involved 740 patients over 15 years, and American cancer officials dismissed it as "poorly done work ... not up to our standards."

During the period 1992-1993, clinical trials were conducted on hydrazine sulfate in the U.S. but without the input of Dr. Gold and in violation of his specific protocol warning that it not be used in conjunction with incompatible substances such as alcohol, sleeping pills, or tranquilizers. Patients were allowed to ingest these substances, in effect scuttling the test results, which were inconclusive. "NCI is up to its usual tricks," Dr. Gold had commented in 1988, as if foreseeing the con-

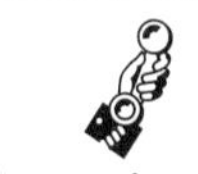

For more information about **hydrazine sulfate,** contact: Joseph Gold, M.D., Syracuse Cancer Research Institute, 600 East Genesee Street, Syracuse, NY 13202; tel: 315-472-6616.

tinuation of its obstructive attitude 5 years later.

There are many reasons why NCI and its cancer industry colleagues did not and still do not want hydrazine sulfate, or any other effective, inexpensive, easily made and administered cancer treatment, to flourish, or even take root, in the U.S. Again, follow the money and you begin to understand why hydrazine sulfate drew "such terrible fire from those now dining at the trough of cancer cash," as journalist Jeff Kamen explained in a major exposé on the subject.[40]

Here is what would likely happen if hydrazine sulfate were thoroughly, fairly, tested, proven to be effective, and allowed to be used:

- NCI's $2 billion annual research budget would be curtailed.
- Prominent cancer treatment centers such as Memorial Sloan-Kettering, M.D. Anderson, and Mayo Clinic would have dramatically fewer patients; the need for ACS and other "charitable" cancer organizations would disappear.
- Pharmaceutical industry income would be reduced, as would the income of hospitals, oncologists, and other health professionals working in the cancer industry. Finding a cure for cancer is absolutely contraindicated by the profits of the cancer industry's chemotherapy, radiation, and surgery cash trough.

***Dr. Chlebowski, discouraged by this editorial savaging despite his 10 years of earnest research and his conclusion that hydrazine sulfate might potentially have saved the lives of millions of cancer patients, dropped his research and abandoned the field.***

Looking back over nearly 3 decades of work and concern about the fate of hydrazine sulfate as an anticancer treatment, Dr. Gold tallies up the numbers of Americans who are virtually assigned to needless suffering because of NCI's tactics. The data from the UCLA-Harbor Hospital trials indicates that of the 1 million new cases of cancer every year, about 50% would be helped and some patients would achieve considerable extensions in their survival rates, lessening of pain, and improvement in the quality of their lives. The Russian data also showed that about 50% of cancer patients would experience significant improvement in symptoms, while 40% would show a stabilization or regression of tumor growth.

NCI's actions with respect to hydrazine sulfate, characterized by intimidation, coercion, steadfast opposition, and possibly clinical trial-rigging, are "truly one of the most shameful, scandalous medical undertakings in this country's history," says Dr. Gold, "depriving vast numbers of people of their health, happiness, and lives."

## The Politics of Laetrile: The Chemotherapy Monopoly Didn't Want Patients to Have It

Perhaps no other supplement stirred up as much controversy in the 1970s as vitamin B17, also known as amygdalin or laetrile. Amygdalin is found widely in nature in all the seeds or kernels of apricots, apples, cherries, plums, and peaches, as well as in buckwheat, millet, and other foods. Even though amygdalin's critics in the cancer establishment believe it has been discredited, among alternative physicians, amygdalin is one of the most widely used supplements, and for good reason.

> ***NCI's actions with respect to hydrazine sulfate, characterized by intimidation, coercion, steadfast opposition, and possibly clinical trial-rigging, are "truly one of the most shameful, scandalous medical undertakings in this country's history," says Dr. Gold, "depriving vast numbers of people of their health, happiness, and lives."***

Evidence of amygdalin's cancer-fighting ability was established by Kanematsu Sugiura, Ph.D., a biochemist (1892-1979) at Memorial Sloan-Kettering Hospital who had studied cancer since 1912 and worked at the hospital since 1917. On the basis of considerable research, Dr. Sugiura was able to contend in 1974 that amygdalin stopped the growth of small tumors and could dramatically reduce the spread of breast cancer in laboratory animals. This pronouncement, however, was for Memorial Sloan-Kettering's ears only; Dr. Sugiura's research was not made public. According to his research, whereas 80% of laboratory animals with mammary cancer developed lung metastases, only 20% of those treated with amydgalin developed lung metastases.[41] He also reported that amygdalin delayed the development of spontaneous mammary cancers for 3-4 months.[42]

During the years 1973 and 1974, other positive reports of amydalin's therapeutic effectiveness against cancer were published, reinforcing Dr. Sugiura's claims. Apparently, this was not the kind of news Memorial Sloan-

Kettering wanted to hear. Perhaps officials there realized that their institution would lose a tremendous amount of money from the chemotherapy industry if the amygdalin findings continued to be publicized. A number of "top experts" were hired; not surprisingly, they discredited Dr. Sugiura's claims. As with hydrazine sulfate, it seems the cancer industry closed ranks.

One study at the Mayo Clinic, sponsored by the National Cancer Institute, allegedly proved amygdalin to be worthless. But according to Michael Schachter, M.D., a complementary physician profiled in Chapter 17 in this book, the Mayo Clinic study had serious flaws.

First, the researchers used isoamygdalin, a relatively inactive form of amygdalin. Second, most of the patients chosen for the trial were considered "terminal" and had already run the medical gauntlet of surgery, chemotherapy, and radiation treatment. Aside from the immune-depressing effects of these therapies, the patients' disease states may have become too severe for *any* therapy to have an effect. Third, the cancers of 70% of the patients were stabilized during the 3 weeks they received amygdalin intravenously. When intravenous treatment was discontinued, however, and only oral amygdalin was used, the patients' health declined.

In other words, the "scientific" clinical trial was set up in such a way as to produce damaging, even negative, results for amygdalin. Certainly, as Dr. Schachter put it, "One must wonder what the results of the Mayo Clinic study would have been if patients with less advanced cancers had been used, if a proper quality of amygdalin had been used, and if the patients had been given a longer trial of intravenous amygdalin."

## Making a Medical Outcast of a Cancer Pioneer: *The Case of Stanislaw Burzynski, M.D., Ph.D.*

The hydrazine sulfate story gets repeated all over again in the concerted effort to suppress another alternative cancer therapy involving the use of antineoplastons. Follow the details of the National Cancer Institute's case against Stanislaw Burzynski, M.D., Ph.D., and you'll see how the politics of cancer can suppress a promising, alternative cancer treatment because its success threatens the cancer establishment.

The original focus of Dr. Burzynski's research was the biochemistry of peptides, which are chains of amino acids, the building blocks of proteins. Noting that people with chronic kidney failure rarely develop cancer, Dr. Burzynski proposed that this finding could relate to a superabundance of peptides within their blood, a fact that distinguishes these patients from cancer patients. Based on this insight, he proceeded to investigate the potential cancer-repelling role of these peptides, which he called antineoplastons, meaning substances that work against (anti) a neoplasm (an abnormal growth of new tissue, such as a tumor).

Beginning in the 1960s, Dr. Burzynski applied the standard medical model to his research and medical practice.[43] He conducted his research according to prevailing scientific standards, publishing his findings in peer-reviewed journals. Dr. Burzynski originally identified and isolated 5 different antineoplastons in the urine of healthy humans. He determined that these molecules have a strong anticancer effect at a genetic level: they appear to stimulate the activity of "tumor suppressor genes," genes that literally turn off the activity of certain oncogenes (genes that promote tumor growth).[44] By this action, antineoplastons can actually stop cells from multiplying out of control and eventually producing a tumor mass, said Dr. Burzynski. One might think cancer results from a *deficiency* of antineoplastons.

***The "scientific" clinical trial was set up in such a way as to produce damaging, even negative, results for amygdalin.***

The scientific rigor of his work was such that, in 1974, Dr. Burzynski secured a research grant from the National Cancer Institute (NCI), an impressive accomplishment. Shortly after, he became director of the Peptide Research Project in the Department of Anesthesiology at Baylor College of Medicine in Houston, Texas. In 1977, Dr. Burzynski was unable to secure the continuation of NCI funding and was told by Baylor officials that he must either discontinue his cancer research or pay his own way.

That same year, Dr. Burzynski published "Antineoplaston A in Cancer Therapy" in *Physiological Chemistry and Physics.* The study focused on 21 cancer and leukemia patients, most of whom had advanced-stage disease and were considered untreatable by conventional means. The patient received antineoplastin therapy. Over the course of 9 months, 4 patients achieved a complete remission while 4 others achieved partial remission (defined as a 50% or greater reduction in tumor size). In 6 cases, the disease was said to have "stabilized" (neither advancing nor regressing), and 2 patients discontinued the treatment after obtaining less than partial remission. Only 5 patients died from complications resulting from their original disease.[45]

At this point, Dr. Burzynski was convinced that antineoplaston therapy could save the lives of cancer patients, and he had the preliminary evidence to prove it. In his mind, he had both a practical and a moral imperative to continue with the research. He decided to launch an independent cancer treatment facility—the Burzynski Research Institute—and began the practice of charging his patients for what he called an "experimental treatment." Without the financial backing of his patients and their insurance companies, Dr. Burzynski would not have been able to carry on his research. Did the National Cancer Institute pick up the tab for completing his research? Did the American Cancer Society help with favorable publicity? Of course not.

***What made Dr. Burzynski a threat to the cancer industry from the beginning was the prospect that antineoplaston therapy represented a successful alternative to toxic and dangerous chemotherapy drugs, upon which most of the cancer industry's profits depend.***

In selling an "experimental treatment," Dr. Burzynski opened himself up to charges of unethical conduct and to the suspicion that he had become a "merchant of false hope."[46] He was, with increasing frequency, barred from publication in conventional medical journals. At the same time, popular magazines began touting Dr. Burzynski's therapeutic results and criticizing the cancer establishment for suppressing the information. The reports questioned why tax dollars and charitable donations were often misused by the NCI, ACS, and FDA, which, they claimed, were too quick to dismiss the efforts of innovators like Dr. Burzynski.[47]

From the late 1970s to the present, every available government, state, and medical agency aligned with the cancer industry has done its best to put Dr. Burzynski out of business. What made Dr. Burzynski a threat to the cancer industry from the beginning was the prospect that antineoplaston therapy represented a successful alternative to toxic and dangerous chemotherapy drugs, upon which most of the cancer industry's profits depend. Since the approach was grounded in scientific research, antineoplaston therapy could not easily be labeled as just another alternative approach predicated on minimal "medical intervention."

Even though he knew that getting an intrinsically biased government agency such as NCI to cooperate fairly in a clinical trial of nontoxic cancer treatment was a dubious long shot, Dr. Burzynski also knew NCI validation was necessary for the future of his antineoplaston therapy. In 1991, the NCI conducted a "best-case series" review to evaluate the clinical outcomes of a group of patients treated at Dr. Burzynski's Houston clinic. There were problems from the beginning and in August 1995, NCI shut down the cancer trials and blamed the failure on Dr. Burzynski. However, a careful study of the correspondence between him and NCI officials reveals how NCI deliberately and craftily scuttled the research trials, then tried to cover its tracks with bureaucratic backfilling and misleading statements. NCI wasn't clever enough because it left a smoking gun.

## HOW NCI MANIPULATED FACTS BY SLEIGHT-OF-HAND

In October 1995, NCI released a statement to the press and public called "Cancer Facts," explaining why the antineoplaston trials, part of its official Cancer Therapy Evaluation Program (CTEP), were closed. NCI's "facts" were more sleight-of-hand and outright misrepresentation than fact.

First, NCI said that out of Dr. Burzynski's "entire clinical experience, he was able to select only 7 brain tumor patients who had benefited from antineoplastons." The inference, of course, is that for the several thousand other patients, the therapy had been ineffective. According to Dr. Burzynski, he prepared "dozens of cases for the NCI reviewers;" they had seen only 7 because they budgeted only one day to visit his office.[48]

Second, NCI claimed Dr. Burzynski had not included all available patient information. The opposite is true, says Dr. Burzynski who notes that an NCI official actually commended him on "how complete and well-organized" his patient studies were.

Third, specific protocols had been established by Dr. Burzynski: at the dosage level to be tested, only patients with a tumor of a specific size would be included in the study. On October, 26, 1993, Dr. Burzynski informed NCI's Michael A. Friedman, M.D., associate director of NCI's Cancer Therapy Evaluation Program (CTEP), that he would ship the antineoplastons needed for the clinical trials once NCI made his requested corrections in the protocols.

According to a letter dated November 2, 1993, from Dr. Friedman, NCI reluctantly agreed to Dr. Burzynski's exclusion requests:

> We have substantial factual disagreements and scientific reservations with

> many of the comments made in your October 26th letter, including your preposterous claim that NCI wasted eight months. Nonetheless, we will accede to all modifications that you have stipulated. We do so because we are committed to beginning the clinical studies as quickly as possible.... The dose and schedule will be modified exactly as you require. We believe this to be the dose and schedule found in your protocol BT6....

Specifically excluded from the trials would be tumors larger than 2 inches (5 cm), patients with multiple tumors, patients with cancer that had spread to the spinal cord, and patients with a Karnofsky performance score (a technical parameter) of less than 70%. A few months later, it all changed. On March 23, 1994, Dr. Burzynski received a letter from Mario Sznol, M.D., head of the Biologics Evaluation Section, Investigational Drug Branch, within CTEP:

> As you know, the NCI-sponsored trials of antineoplastons have been initiated and some patients have been enrolled. However, a great many more have sought access to the trial but have not been allowed to participate because of their inability to meet all the eligibility criteria. Because of this, there is strong interest on our part and that of the investigators to broaden the eligibility criteria. While we recognize the need for and the value of clear eligibility criteria, we believe that the protocol now excludes some patients who would otherwise be good candidates for the trial.

Dr. Sznol informed Dr. Burzynski that he proposed lowering the Karnofsky performance status from 70 to 60, allowing tumors up to 8 cm in size, and allowing multiple tumors or ones that had spread to the spine. Writing on April 19,1994, Dr. Burzynski declined, commenting that "to expand the trials now through admission of such difficult cases is premature" and that "such patients should be involved in a separate trial for large and multifocal tumors and treated and evaluated according to a modified protocol."

Dr. Burzynski rejected this change in his study's research design because it would require a stronger dose, not agreed upon in the original plan for the study. Dr. Burzynski knew that the clinical future of his antineoplastons was at stake, and wanted to give them a test equal to their therapeutic abilities. He was also beginning to doubt that anyone at CTEP or NCI wanted authentic proof to emerge that antineoplastons worked.

By January 31, 1995, however, NCI had evidently ignored Dr. Burzynski's request not to change the protocols. Mark Malkin, M.D., of Memorial Sloan-Kettering Cancer Institute in New York, wrote a letter to John L. Lewis, M.D., chairman of the hospital's Institutional Review Board, saying that the exclusionary protocols had been changed to allow for larger or multiple tumors, those that had spread to the spine, and patients with a Karnofksy score of 60%.

These sweeping changes, wrote Dr. Malkin, "have been made at the request of NCI." They certainly were not made at the request of Dr. Burzynski. "Without informing me, NCI changes the rules to allow patients with *any size* or number of tumors, low performance scores and spinal cord metastases," says Dr. Burzynski in March 1995, when he learned of NCI's actions. "In other words, NCI was accepting patients whose brains and spinal cords were literally consumed by large malignant tumors—patients so advanced as to have no chance whatsoever."[49]

***Did the National Cancer Institute pick up the tab for completing Dr. Burzynski's research? Did the American Cancer Society help with favorable publicity? Of course not. The minute NCI saw evidence of antineoplastons working, they distorted the data by withdrawing the 2 successful patients and thus the evidence.***

When Dr. Burzynski demanded that NCI explain its actions, Dr. Sznol passed the buck back to Memorial Sloan-Kettering. Anyone versed in the history of how NCI discredited hydrazine sulfate by changing the trial design prejudicially against it, would certainly recognize the pattern at this point. According to Dr. Sznol:

> At the investigators' request, the amendments to modify the eligibility restrictions ... have been approved. These amendments were initiated by the investigators when it became apparent that many good candidates for the study were being excluded because of what we perceived to be overly stringent and unnecessary eligibility restrictions... In the meantime, we will allow the amendments to stand, since all evidence you have provided to date indicates that these newly eligible patients may have a chance for benefit without undue risk of harm, and are appropriate candidates for evaluation of the drug.

## Oncologists Critical of FDA

A July 1995 survey of 140 conventional cancer doctors (oncologists) revealed that 76% believe that the FDA should not restrict information about new uses for drugs and devices, 61% favored the FDA allowing physicians to use unapproved drugs and devices, and 21% had a totally unfavorable opinion of the FDA, according to the Competitive Enterprise Institute (1001 Connecticut Ave. NW, Suite 1250, Washington, D.C. 20036).

In July 1995, Dr. Burzynski protested NCI's summary actions. He insisted that "NCI either honor our agreement or change the Informed Consent statement (which patients must read and sign) to reflect the fact that I, the drug's discoverer and developer, felt that the treatment was unlikely to be effective in such advanced patients in the doses being used."

NCI's response was to close all antineoplaston studies under way at Memorial Sloan-Kettering and the Mayo Clinic. A public statement later issued by NCI as part of their CancerNet Fact Sheet declared: "On August 18, 1995, the studies were closed because a consensus could not be reached with Dr. Burzynski on the proposed changes in the protocol to increase accrual, and there was no hope of completing the studies in a timely manner." According to National Institutes of Health (NCI's parent organization) legal advisor, Robert B. Lanman: "Although NCI clearly prefers to conduct or sponsor studies with the ongoing support and cooperation of a drug's inventor, the permission of such an individual is not required." In effect, NCI was saying they can change the research rules anytime they want, and that Dr. Burzynski could do nothing to stop them.

***NCI's conduct toward Dr. Burzynski is a striking example of how an agency presumed to be objective can set up a study that will either prove or disprove anything it wants. In this case, there is clear evidence that NCI wanted to prove antineoplastons didn't work.***

Later, Dr. Burzynski learned that at some point before the termination of the studies, NCI had disqualified 2 patients from continuing in the study. One patient no longer had any detectable cancer cells; the second had skin reactions, not from antineoplastons, but from a different drug. Actually, this skin condition had improved under antineoplastons. In other words, the minute NCI saw evidence of antineoplastons working, they scuttled the data by withdrawing the 2 patients and thus the evidence.

In their final report, the NCI reviewers said there was "presumptive evidence of antitumor activity." The evidence was not presumed; it was visible, tangible, and provable. This gross misstatement is a blatant example of how top NCI officials—not the scientists within the Institute, but the policy purveyors for the cancer industry—routinely turn reality on its head in order to satisfy their own agenda. The report from the NCI scientists who actually reviewed the patient records was diametrically opposite to the above statement. This report, documented in the minutes of the Decision Network Committee meeting, offered the following statement: "The site visit team determined that antitumor activity was documented in this best-case series and the conduct of Phase II trials was indicated to determine the response rate."[50]

By scientific standards, the NCI should have continued with the next phase of studies. Instead, however, NCI dropped the antineoplaston research because "there was no hope of completing the studies in a timely manner." After 30 years of failing to find a cancer cure, the NCI had suddenly decided to impose a time limit on saving human lives. The net result of NCI's shady backroom maneuvers is that the trials were halted and Dr. Burzynski's antineoplastons are no closer to government approval than they were in 1974, when Dr. Burzynski received his first research grant from NCI.

Frank Wiewel, director of People Against Cancer, has strongly criticized the actions of the CTEP. In his opinion, "It had no intention of doing a fair evaluation of Dr. Burzynski. It allowed the protocols to be violated for every single patient of the Burzynski group. That's why Dr. Burzynski decided to stop the trial, and it is what any self-respecting, well-trained scientist would have done."

## A CANCER AGENCY DEDICATED TO SUPPRESSING CURES FOR CANCER

NCI's conduct toward Dr. Burzynski is a striking example of how an agency presumed to be "objective" can set up a study that will either prove or disprove anything it wants, or simply defer the potential validation of a new therapy into the indefinite future. In this case, there is clear evidence that NCI wanted to prove antineoplastons didn't work.

Changing the eligibility criteria for subjects in a study is like fixing a horse race because you have bet heavily on a lame horse (chemotherapy and radiation) that would otherwise not even place. Then, when the strong horse (antineoplastons) did poorly, NCI could claim they had "scientifi-

## Cancer Research Dead End: Cancer Research's False Model of Biology

Imagine if the prevailing theory in astronomy were still the incorrect notion that the sun revolves around the earth, and that we all trusted the findings and techniques that came out of this mistaken view. Yet for the last 40 years, with 500,000 dying from cancer every year, the medical establishment continues to wage its costly and ineffectual "war against cancer" based on just such a distorted model.

That model is based on studying cancer cells in a petri dish, far removed from their context, the living human body. This procedure is called "cell lines" and has been favored by cancer researchers for decades. Cell lines represent a unique new form of life; the trouble is, they have nothing to do with the reality of cancer within the body or with human biology. Cancer cells implanted in a petri dish do things cells never do anywhere else: they don't die. Their behavior is completely different from that of cells in a living body. And some of those used for research purposes are more than 40 years old.

In 1951, cells from the cancerous cervix of Helen Lane were removed from her body after her death at Johns Hopkins Hospital in Baltimore, Maryland. They were placed in a petri dish and allowed to grow. This was the first cell line, now called HeLa, and 44 years later, cancer researchers around the world are still using descendants (cell lines) from her original tumor. In other words, hardly any cancer research is done on freshly obtained malignant cells.

Virtually the entire multibillion dollar cancer research edifice is founded on this erroneous model of biology, reports researcher Gerald B. Dermer, Ph.D., in *The Immortal Cell: Why Cancer Research Fails*.[51] Not only that, many cancer researchers know the cell line model is incorrect but don't wish to lose their funding by admitting it publicly. This explains why the leading cancer "therapies," such as chemotherapy, immunotherapy, and radiation, based on the cell line model, work so poorly. The contradictions between the real world of cancer in living men and women and the artificial, theoretical world of cancer in a glass dish is the core of the scandal and the grand deception in cancer research.

Meanwhile, scientists keep the truth under wraps to keep the research dollars flowing. This is the secret of the astonishing failure of cancer research. As one researcher privately admitted, "The bottom line is dollars."

cally" evaluated them. In fact, however, the antineoplastons would have come up short only on paper. As the documents suggest—this is a convincing and damaging paper trail, a true "smoking gun" revealing NCI tactics at every stage—the outcome was *predetermined* by special interests working through the NCI.

If NCI had been genuinely interested in finding a nontoxic alternative to conventional cancer treatment, it would have worked with Dr.

## The Drug Industry—America's Nonstop Profit Center

In case you're wondering what is driving U.S. annual health-care costs over the unbelievable $1 trillion mark, take a look at recent drug industry statistics to see a major contributing factor.

According to information reported in 1993, drug prices outside the U.S. were 10%-70% lower than those charged for the same drugs in America; prescription drug prices rose about 3 times higher than inflation between 1980 and 1990 as drug makers boasted annual profits 3 times higher than the national average for Fortune 500 companies. Further, drug companies spend about $13,000 per U.S. physician in marketing, about 22% of their total sales (about $75.2 billion worldwide) on promotion, and $231 million to develop and patent a single drug.

It is not as if the exceptionally high drug profits are making life any easier for the sick. Patients pay exorbitantly for these "modern medical miracles." For example: a diabetic woman's monthly drug cost is $150; a heart transplant patient shells out $50 a day for antirejection pills; a Gaucher's disease patient needs $270,000 a year for drugs. Herbs are mostly unpatentable and thus far less profitable, so it is in the interests of drug companies to suppress rather than support them. That is what keeps "The Club," or the organized conventional medicine establishment, highly profitable, says medical researcher and activist Michael L. Culbert, D.Sc.

"While the American expression of the Drug Trust is the focus ... the international nature of the pharmaceutical octopus cannot be overlooked," writes Culbert, "for it has played a role, both openly and behind the scenes, not only in endlessly producing toxic synthetic compounds for human consumption, but in helping bar the development, use and distribution of natural therapies at every turn."[52]

Burzynski, the expert on antineoplastons, to assure that antineoplaston therapy was tested under optimal conditions. This is precisely what it does for the purveyors of chemotherapy drugs: the primary investigators (those who conducted the preliminary research), not NCI, are the ones who set the study's parameters and overall design. But the lucrative chemotherapy market is directly threatened by the advent of antineoplaston therapy and NCI works like a chemotherapy hired gun to ensure that the business remains profitable.

The FDA got into the act with a vengeance as well. On March 24, 1995, Dr. Burzynski was on *CBS This Morning*, presenting 3 of his cancer patients who had recovered using antineoplaston therapy. That same morning, the FDA raided his medical office and seized 15 patient records, claiming that Dr. Burzynski was illegally shipping his medicines interstate. FDA conveniently overlooked the fact that it had already granted Dr. Burzynski,

## The Cancer Industry Suppresses the Rife Frequency Generator

An energy medicine device that arrived in the world with a great deal of therapeutic promise and ingenuity was the Rife Frequency Generator, the creation of Raymond Royal Rife of San Diego, California. During the 1920s, working at his Rife Research Laboratory in Point Loma, California, Rife produced 5 different microscopes (comprising 14 lenses and prisms, a quartz crystal illumination unit—5,682 working parts in all) with magnification capabilities ranging from 5,000 to 60,000 diameters and a resolution of 31,000 diameters.

We must bear in mind that in Rife's time, the best resolution available through any other microscopic system was only 2,000 diameters, so his "Rife Universal Microscope" was an outstanding achievement. Even today's electron microscopes, which have resolutions of about 25,000 diameters and magnifications up to 200,000, cannot work with live specimens. Working with resolutions of 17,000 diameters, Rife was able to study a sub-microscopic layer of biology that had never before been visible, including 20,000 laboratory cultures of living cancer cells obtained from a nearby hospital.

In the 1940s, the possibilities for this instrument sent shock waves through the cancer industry when Milbank Johnson, M.D., conducted the first and only study of the Rife Frequency Generator as a potential cancer treatment. Dr. Johnson coordinated the study in conjunction with the Medical Research Committee of the University of Southern California.

Dr. Milbank's test involved the use of the Rife Frequency Generator for daily treatments of 3 minutes' duration, at 3-day intervals, as it had been shown previously that allowing this time to elapse between treatments produced better results. The group treated with the Rife device were 16 patients with various types of advanced cancers, all of whom had been declared "terminal" or "incurable." After 3 months of the Rife treatment, 14 of these "hopeless" cases were declared clinically cured and in good health by a staff of 5 M.D.s and by Alvin G. Ford, M.D., group pathologist.[53]

Unfortunately, the cancer industry sought to discredit Dr. Rife and all Rife devices were later outlawed by the FDA. No subsequent research was ever conducted. The American Cancer Society never once mentioned this one-and-only study of the Rife Frequency Generator in its critique of electronic devices.[54] This convenient omission is entirely consistent with the ACS's "coverage" of alternative cancer therapies.

as a special clinical investigator, the legal right to ship these medicines interstate. In its zeal to quash all successful alternatives, the FDA does not hesitate to break its own rules. On June 21, 1995, the FDA again raided Dr. Burzynski's clinic and seized 800 X rays and CT scans, leaving Dr. Burzynski unable to treat his patients.

Today, Dr. Burzynski's antineoplastons are often referred to as a form of nontoxic chemotherapy intended to reinforce the body's natural defense system against cancer. He has continued to synthesize the antineoplastons in his

47,000-square-foot government-approved facility in Texas. For Dr. Burzynski's 3,000 patients, antineoplaston treatment is a lifesaver; among prominent alternative physicians, the treatment is gaining respect and credibility. Outspoken alternative medicine advocate Julian Whitaker, M.D., for example, has stated: "This is a treatment I would try if I discovered I had cancer."

## The Medical *Media* Monopoly: Don't Trust Everything You Read in the Mainstream Press

Do you think the newspapers, magazines, and television news reports present medical information fairly and objectively? Think again. Medical propaganda is rampant in the United States. Its goal is to mislead, confuse, and coerce you into supporting conventional medicine and enhancing the cancer industry's spoils of war.

With respect to cancer, this propaganda includes messages such as "You must have a regular mammogram for early detection of breast cancer," even though the evidence does not support this claim. The problem begins with the American Cancer Society and extends to the distributors of cancer-related information—the news market and publishing houses that control the information.

According to Ben Bagdikian, University of California at Berkeley dean emeritus in journalism and author of *The Media Monopoly*, 50 corporations controlled more than half of the media in 1982; by December 1986, this number had shrunk to 29 corporations; 6 months later, it was 26. Today, some 15 corporations control almost all of the country's newspaper circulation and a handful of firms control the television networks. TV coverage is increasingly restricted by a small but powerful elite. A listing of the directors of the 3 major TV networks—NBC, ABC, and CBS—reveals a tight interlocking of banking and industrial connections.

This centralization of our mainstream information delivery system translates into one simple fact: the power to *shape* the nation's news and popular culture is in the hands of a few who are most sensitive to the money flow. "Objective" news is up for sale to the highest bidder. Corporate interests increasingly shape how Americans think and what they believe about health care. If the American Cancer Society (ACS) decides that chemotherapy needs promoting, prevention needs downplaying, or alternative medicine needs bashing, the desired message can be easily broadcast to large segments of the population. Sensational stories—a perfect example is the recent "Beta carotene supplementation leads to higher lung cancer rates" garbage—can receive top billing, while stories touting the cancer-repelling benefits of beta carotene are ignored.

For example, the ACS regularly sponsors a Science Writer's Forum to assist writers in "understanding cancer." The main function of these seminars is to program the media with carefully tailored messages about cancer. It is reported that during these seminars, the Society tends to exaggerate the ability of conventional medicine to treat and cure cancer. Such claims are generally based on an initial reduction in tumor size (tumor response) rather than on prolongation of survival.[55] In addition, the quality of life, often seriously jeopardized by toxic treatments, is rarely discussed.

Media experts within the ACS are in effect the "consensus-making machinery" of the cancer industry. Wielding the power to influence the media and public on a massive scale, the Society issues reports and press releases. Critics call these documents medical propaganda. ACS focuses a "blame the victim" perspective for cancer causation, focusing almost exclusively on lifestyle choices such as smoking, drinking, and high-fat diets, while trivializing or giving scant attention to *avoidable* causes from daily exposure to external carcinogens in air, water, food, and the workplace.

Some of the disturbing messages come from physicians who work visibly in the health market. A prime example is KGO's Dean Edell, M.D., whose "To Your Health" column in the *Edell Health Letter* (published by *Health Magazine*) has frequently maligned proponents of alternative medicine. In a 1992 editorial, "Declare War on Cancer Quackery," Dr. Edell delivered the standard "arguments" against alternative cancer treatments: any benefits people get must be due to the placebo effect; none of the treatments have been carefully tested; and "most of these treatments are pretty useless, which makes them costly."[56] Dr. Edell appears on radio and television in many cities throughout the United States, so his opinions, whether or not based on fact, reach millions of people regularly. At the end of the editorial, he advises listeners with questions or concerns about alternative cancer treatment to dial the free telephone number for the American Cancer Society.

## Medical Propaganda Masquerading as Objective Reporting

In case you thought the prestigious *New York Times* could be counted on to report the news objectively, an analysis of how it recently covered the subject of alternative medicine and cancer treatment—how it buried it in pejoratives, to be more precise—should convince you that even such highly regarded newspapers often serve the propagandistic agenda of conventional medicine.

In articles appearing on the front page on June 17 and 18, 1996, the *Times* seemed to represent both sides of the discussion, presenting the views of alternative medicine experts and their critics. But the way it framed the discussion, the context in which it presented the information, and the words it used clearly reflects its strong bias against alternative medicine.

Alternative medicine and its "untested" therapies are thriving on the "fringes" of health care, said the *Times* in its headline. And note how the following words or phrases used by the *Times* serve to establish doubt and skepticism about alternative medicine:

> alarming, escaping scrutiny, outlawed, once obscure treatments, folk remedies, based on whims or discredited science, dangers, Orwellian newspeak, snake oil, anecdotal evidence, not met scientific standards, ill advised, mavericks, quackery, selling misbeliefs, outside mainstream, drawn guffaws, questionable standards, dubious studies, unproven ideas.

If you don't see through this deceptive linguistic smokescreen, you remain subject to the propaganda trance that keeps unfavorable attitudes about alternative medicine in place.

At the same time, by strongly praising conventional medicine with powerful, almost hypnotic phrases, the *Times* doubles its disparaging slam against alternative medicine. It accomplishes a kind of brainwashing. The uncritical reader ends up assuming that conventional medicine *must* be the voice of authority.

By comparison, note how reassuring, even paternal, the words and phrases used to refer to conventional medicine come across in contrast to the words of warning and derision cited above: "medical experts;" "reached unsurpassed heights of technical sophistication;" "rigorous scientific tests;" "advising the public on risky therapies." Here are phrases used in reference to alternative medicine: "government officials sharply criticize;" "Dr. Caplan is gravely concerned;" "rejecting the rules for clinical trials;" "denounced such therapy."

The clever editor then selects quotes from opponents of alternative medicine—some of them industry-supported "experts" parading as concerned "quackbusters"—and allows them to further disparage alternative therapies without implicating the editor or newspaper in the mud throwing. The effectiveness of the propaganda depends on how well the reader's thoughts can be shaped by the *subtext*—the clever use of words, tones, and nuances designed to frame the material in the desired way. Although the main text of the article seems to examine both sides of the topic, fairly quoting authorities from both positions, the subtext is more subliminally powerful in weighting the conclusion in favor of one side and against the other.

For example, a third article on the antineoplaston cancer treatment of Stanislaw Burzynski, M.D., appeared in the *Times* in late July with the usual slant. Here the boldfaced subheadlines framed the attitude for the reader: "the evidence is lacking;" "the opposition is widespread;" "hope may be all that is offered." The article disparaged Dr. Burzynski's antineoplastons because their efficacy was "unproven" and the treatment was "expensive." The article did not mention, in contrast, the great unproven honeypot of cancer treatment chemotherapy, which is effective in fewer than 10% of cancer cases and is extraordinarily expensive.

With the *New York Times* a widely read and respected national newspaper whose stories are picked up by numerous smaller papers, medical propaganda favoring conventional medicine is being shamelessly distributed throughout the country in the guise of objective news reporting.[57]

Similarly, how "scientific" is *Scientific American* when out of a 184-page special issue devoted to cancer in September 1996, only 2 pages were given to alternative cancer treatments? Evidently it is scientific only when it is not inconvenient for the cancer industry. According to French psychiatrist Jean-Jacques Aulas, who wrote the 2 pages, of alternative medicine's 80 "unconventional medical techniques, ranging from acupressure to macrobiotic Zen," those used for diagnosis have no rational basis. "Many consist of a mixed bag of general laboratory tests and sorcery, and not one has been shown the least official value for detecting any form of cancer. I believe these techniques should be banned or that the 'institutes' that use them should supply prospective patients with objective information about their effectiveness."

Apparently, *Scientific American* is more intent on upholding the party line than doing any diligent research outside its bailiwick, for it commits the usual factual mistakes and research omissions. For example, Aulas states that according to "several independent evaluations of case records," Gerson Therapy has no "discernible effectiveness." Here Aulas ignores the retrospective independent British study of Gerson Therapy demonstrating 5-year survival rates, depending on cancer type, ranging from 39% to 79% compared to 6% to 39% for conventional methods.

Aulas also declares that only "modest improvements" have been documented for hydrazine sulfate; evidence presented in this chapter disproves that and explains how the politics of medicine downgraded "substantial" to "modest." Aulas is similarly misguided regarding orthomolecular therapy and megadose vitamin C therapy. In his estimation, such approaches fared no better than placebos, according to NIH research. He conveniently ignores the results of 12,986 clinical studies on vitamin C (as of 1996), many of which clearly demonstrate highly beneficial results. Citing FDA research, Aulas dismisses 714X (developed by Canadian biologist Gaston Naessens) as nothing more than camphor and water. This is not true. Our research shows that *Scientific American*'s material on alternative medicine is flawed. To us, a disturbing bias is apparent in its coverage.

***How "scientific" is* Scientific American *when out of a 184-page special issue devoted to cancer in September 1996, only 2 pages were given to alternative cancer treatments? Evidently it is scientific only when it is not inconvenient for the cancer industry.***

If conventional treatments have been "exhausted," Aulas states patronizingly, then patients may try unconventional ones to increase their sense of control and well-being "even if they do not lengthen survival." Once again, evidence documented in this book unarguably demonstrates that alternative cancer approaches considerably lengthen survival times far in excess of anything conventional medicine can muster. Aulas also brazenly asserts that "no alternative treatment for cancer has a definite influence on the course of the disease." We suggest he talk to the numerous cancer survivors discussed in this book.

The copious footnotes in this book, citing clinical research mostly drawn from conventional medical journals, should convince the reader that *Scientific American* is wrong. We believe the article in question is irresponsible.[58]

## Doubt Is Their Product: When Science Becomes Public Relations

One of the prime reasons that our protracted war on cancer has turned into an unwinnable "medical Vietnam," says Robert N. Proctor, history of science professor at Pennsylvania State University, is that cancer research and the reporting of its results has become a predominantly *political* issue. And when you link politics with medicine, you suddenly enter a perilously dark territory in which truth recedes and special interests rush to the forefront.

As an estimated 538,000 Americans now die of cancer every year, a "cure" grows ever more remote and even clarity about prevention gets increasingly obscured by the financial interests of the conventional medical establishment. You have "islands of agreement separated by deep seas of controversy," writes Proctor. Cancer research is *big* business and unless you are a discriminating, resourceful reader, most likely you have been subjected to the clever, often deceitful, promotional efforts of corporate trade association "science." In 1986, at least 1,700 associations spent $2 billion on "issues management, advocacy, communication, and image advertising"—on smokescreens, in other words, but not the bare truth.

Trade associations (notably tobacco, petrochemical, and asbestos) adeptly combine research and advocacy—sometimes as "a mixture of scientific fact and fiction," says Proctor—to produce a culture of doubt and uncertainty in which they are carefully insulated from charges of bias or legal liability. In this ambiguous new world of propaganda, manipulation, and public-opinion shaping, "rhetorical strategies of avoidance" reign supreme. In Proctor's view, "all [associations] share a desire to absolve their constituent clients' substances ... of blame for an alleged nuisance"—especially if it is a cancer cause. If suspected cancer causes are in doubt from conflicting studies or inconclusive results, this becomes the perfect excuse, if you're a regulatory body, for doing nothing to change it.[59]

## Scenarios the Cancer Industry Doesn't Want You to Know About

There is a great deal that the worldwide cancer industry and its U.S. representatives do not want you to know about medicine. The following story is typical, only one among many.

In February of 1994, Dustin Kaufmann, aged 2½, was diagnosed with a highly aggressive form of brain tumor known as medulloblastoma. Three-quarters of the tumor was surgically removed, but the remaining portion was inoperable. Dustin's doctors encouraged his parents to enroll Dustin in a study at the University of Minnesota to test various regimens of chemotherapy followed by radiation.[60] This therapy had "a success rate of 20-40%," according to a resident pediatric oncologist, whom we shall call Dr. A. They were also told that the therapy might enable Dustin to live another 5 years, but that he would likely end up in a wheelchair, with stunted growth and learning disabilities.

When the Kaufmanns asked for names of parents whose children had undergone the treatment, no names could be provided. Then they asked to talk with parents of *any* child treated for brain cancer at the University of Minnesota, but no names came back. The 20-40% success rate began to look like a sham. Knowing it was possible that Dustin could die or end up severely debilitated by conventional treatment, the parents began seeking alternatives. They left the university offices without signing the consent form for Dustin's participation in the experimental program.

A few weeks later, returning to pick up Dustin's medical records, they were ushered into a room for an unscheduled conference with Dr. A. and 2 other members of the pediatric oncology department (including its chairman), 2 interns, and a social worker. The doctors told the Kaufmanns that their opinions take precedence over parents' opinions and that the doctors might have to ask the courts to allow them to start treatment on Dustin, regardless of what the parents wanted for him.

As a result of their independent research, the Kaufmanns had heard that many brain cancer patients were having good results with the antineoplaston treatment of Stanislaw Burzynski, M.D., in Houston, Texas. When they mentioned this to Dr. A., she said their chances of success with antineoplastons were zero; at the same time, Dr. A. admitted she had nothing to support her contention.

Undaunted, the Kaufmanns started Dustin on antineoplastons in April 1994. About 6 weeks later, MRI (magnetic resonance imagery) scans revealed that the tumor had undergone a complete remission. Dustin stayed on Dr. Burzynski's treatment for 1 year, and felt healthy and robust during this time. When a subsequent MRI showed that the tumor had returned, Dustin's dose of antineoplastons was increased, leading to a second remission—an outcome unheard of in orthodox medicine.[61] Dustin's most recent

MRI, taken on January 6, 1996, showed only a tiny fragment, probably scar tissue from the vanished tumor.

Sometimes the cancer industry authorities prevent patients from even reaching the office. In 1995, Adrian Chavez, aged 6, of Contra Costa, California, had a recurrence of leukemia. Doctors at Children's Hospital in Oakland resumed his chemotherapy, but when Adrian's white blood cell count continued to increase (an indication that his leukemia was getting worse), the mother took Adrian to an expert herbalist.

***A doctor called Adrian's mother the next week and demanded that she bring him in the next day. When she refused, a sheriff's deputy and a Children's Protective Services worker went to her home and forcibly took Adrian to Children's Hospital and forced him to undergo chemotherapy—against the mother's and the child's wishes.***

A doctor called Adrian's mother the next week and *demanded* that she bring him in the next day. When she refused, a sheriff's deputy and a Children's Protective Services worker went to her home and forcibly took Adrian to Children's Hospital and *forced* him to undergo chemotherapy—against the mother's and the child's wishes. According to an *Associated Press* report, "In general, the agency will take sick children from their homes if doctors warn their lives are in danger." [63] The danger here is the cancer industry's unchallenged status as the treatment of first and *only* resort.

Another example of how local medical authorities can shut down a respected cancer doctor because he has tried something innovative is the case of Sharon Smith, a 40 year-old woman diagnosed with breast cancer that had metastasized to the bone. All conventional cancer treatments had failed, and she had been told nothing more could be done. This dismal prognosis left her little choice but to seek out alternatives to chemotherapy and radiation.

In October of 1993, she went to Lawrence H. Taylor, M.D., an alternative medical practitioner based in San Diego, California (and profiled in Chapter 23 of this book). Dr. Taylor treated her with his multifaceted program and intravenous administration of "Immunostim" (also known as 714X), a nontoxic combination of ammonium compounds, camphor, phosphors and salts of silicate, all of which have been used in medicine for years. None are individually on the FDA's restricted drugs list, although 714X is not FDA approved. Based on his clinical observations, Dr. Taylor estimated that 80% of his patients underwent at least partial remissions (measurable reductions in tumor size) after taking Immunostim.

After showing some signs of relapse in December, Sharon then returned to Dr. Taylor's clinic and received her second series of treatments in January, 1994. Sharon's X rays at this time revealed that her cancer had stopped spreading to the bones. She had gained weight, her appetite was improved, and her pain was gone. "Her oncologist looked at the X rays, saw that the tumors were getting smaller, that her pain was gone and appetite had returned," says Dr. Taylor. "He told her something was definitely going on, though he did not quite understand why she was improving. She told him about the Immunostim and other treatments, but he was incredulous."

In March of 1994, however, the city police of San Diego raided and closed Dr. Taylor's offices. Meanwhile, Sharon's oncologist called the office for more Immunostim, but none was available, since authorities had confiscated his drugs and refused to release any of the medicine she had been using. Despite petitions by Sharon's attorney and oncologist to obtain more Immunostim, all requests were denied. The oncologist then issued a request to study Immunostim at a local university, but the inquiry came too late for Sharon. Within 2 weeks of being denied her nontoxic medicines, Sharon became increasingly fatigued and began to lose her appetite. Six months after the shutting down of Dr. Taylor's practice, Sharon died.

While no one can tell whether Immunostim would have saved Sharon's

## Running Away from Chemotherapy

Here's a scenario with implications the cancer industry prefers not to discuss. In the summer of 1994, Billy Best, aged 16, caught the nation's attention by running away from home to avoid chemotherapy for his Hodgkin's disease. For 1 year, Billy received alternative cancer treatment consisting of a healthy diet, Essiac herbs, and a therapy called 714X, given as injections. At the end of that year, Billy was cancer free.

Dana Farber Cancer Institute in Boston, Massachusetts, a major authority on conventional cancer treatments, was clearly embarrassed by the media attention that followed. They issued a statement trying to downplay the implications of Billy's outcome. Declaring that Billy had no evidence of cancer according to CT scans and other diagnostic tests, they called his recovery a case of spontaneous remission.[62] What was embarrassing was that the Institute and other chemotherapy centers had long cited Hodgkin's disease as a perfect example—the real fact is that Hodgkin's is one of a very few examples—of chemotherapy's success. Billy Best thought differently, and probably owes his life to having rejected conventional medicine.

life, her greatly improved condition under the Immunostim treatment, followed by her deterioration when it was withdrawn, attests to the power of this alternative therapy. "There was definite evidence of remission before her Immunostim was taken away," says Dr. Taylor. "Her dramatic improvement in health, together with the objective reduction in tumor size, suggest that Sharon would have continued to improve under our care."

Sharon's case is a tragic example of how the politics of cancer can threaten patients' lives. Nontoxic medicines, despite their clinical efficacy as attested to in thousands of testimonials, are considered "dangerous" and "unproven" by the medical establishment. Meanwhile, the highly toxic medicines that are killing cancer patients remain the only officially sanctioned treatment and, as such, continue to receive virtually all the research funding. "The main reason we don't see research on nontoxic agents is that they're nonpatentable, so they represent no profit to the pharmaceutical industry," says Dr. Taylor. "Human greed continues to perpetuate a great deal of death and misery. Cancer is the medical profession's most lucrative business, and most oncologists aim to keep it that way." As a result of his use of Immunostim and under FDA pressure, Dr. Taylor's California medical license was revoked in February 1996.

### Cancer Site Diagnoses Unnecessary

Detailed cancer site diagnosis may be a waste of money, according to *Archives of Internal Medicine* (October 1995). In 400 tests conducted to find the primary tumor site in 56 cancer patients—at an average cost of $17,973 per patient—tests correctly identified the sites for only 4 patients. Of these patients, 81% died within a year. With 1.2 million new cancers occurring each year, the cost of tests that are inaccurate, unsuccessful, and do not contribute to patient survival, is $1.5 billion annually.

For information on **Dr. Lawrence Taylor's cancer approach**, see Chapter 23: Lawrence H. Taylor, M.D.

## The System Punishes Good Physicians: *The Case of Glen Warner, M.D.*

Now in his 70s, Glen Warner. M.D., is an oncologist who practices in Seattle, Washington. He has treated approximately 20,000 cancer patients over his lifetime of practice. Dr. Warner combines conventional treatment, such as chemotherapy, with dietary prescriptions, psychological counseling, and the use of other alternative techniques aimed at stimulating the immune system. Increasingly, conventional doctors in Washington state decided Dr. Warner's approaches were too far from the mainstream for their comfort.

*"Human greed continues to perpetuate a great deal of death and misery. Cancer is the medical profession's most lucrative business, and most oncologists aim to keep it that way," says Dr. Taylor.*

In July 1995, the Washington State Medical Quality Assurance Commission (MQAC) stormed his offices and demanded his medical license and all controlled medicines. They ordered him to clear his crowded waiting room of all patients and to assign them to other doctors. All complaints of "medical negligence" against Dr. Warner were filed by other doctors, not patients. They claimed he had deviated too much from accepted cancer practices, despite his 20 years of peer-approved cancer work. Doctors, not patients, had complained to MQAC about 6 patients Dr. Warner had treated in the previous 5-10 years; the complaint was that their cancers had not responded to his treatment.

Even though none of the doctors on the board were cancer specialists or oncologists—meaning they were not professionally qualified for the job—they were assigned to review all records pertaining to charges made against Dr. Warner. More outrageous was the statement by an attorney for the MQAC that cancer patients are "unqualified" to know whether or not they are receiving appropriate care.

*For the cancer industry, the trouble with Dr. Warner is that he places a premium on medical* **science** *instead of medical* **business.** *His brand of oncology does not help fill the coffers of the chemotherapy industry. "[Chemotherapy] is an incredibly lucrative business for doctors, hospitals, and pharmaceutical companies."*

As Patrick McGrady, director of CANHELP and a public ally of Dr. Warner, sees it, "Probably no other doctor in the Seattle community can claim to match Dr. Warner's 1000-plus surviving cancer patients." And these are loyal patients, too, for when Dr. Warner's license was seized, 350 patients wrote letters of protest; in the ensuing months, says McGrady, hundreds more followed suit.[64] "Denying patients freedom of choice, abruptly interrupting doctor-patient relationships, and imposing a rigid standard of care is no way to develop the best medical care," says Dr. Warner. As of August 1996, Dr. Warner's medical license was permanently revoked following an unsuccessful court appeal.

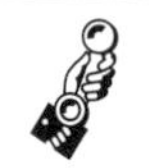

For more information about **CANHELP** and a copy of Patrick McGrady's "Cancer Patient's Bill of Rights," contact: CANHELP, 3111 Paradise Bay Road, Port Ludlow, WA 98365; tel: 206-437-2291.

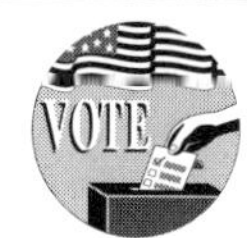


Express your dissatisfaction by writing: NIH, Office of the Director, Harold Varmus, M.D., Room 126, NIH 1, Bethesda, MD 20892; tel: 301-496-1766; or National Cancer Institute, Richard D. Klausner, M.D., Director; Building 31, tel: 301-496-5615; fax: 301-402-0338; e-mail: klausner@helix.nih.gov. Help change the politics of cancer by supporting political action groups, such as: Citizens for Health, P.O. Box 1195, Tacoma, WA 98401; tel: 206-922-2457; fax: 206-922-7583; American Preventive Medical Association, 459 Walker Road, Great Falls, VA 22066; tel: 800-230-2762; fax: 703-759-6711; and National Health Federation (publishers of *Health Freedom News*), 212 W. Foothill Blvd., Monrovia, CA 91016; tel: 818-357-2181; fax: 818-303-0642. Stay informed about FDA activities and tactics with: *FDA Hotline*, P.O. Box 161132, Altamonte Springs, FL 32716; tel: 407-628-1377; fax: 407-628-9935; 12 issues/$187.

Ironically, at the same time as he lost his license, data from 13 western Washington counties compiled by the Fred Hutchinson Cancer Research Center of Seattle showed that "in the most intractable cases, Dr. Warner's cancer patients fared no worse than others in western Washington. At best, Dr. Warner's patients enjoyed up to 9% greater survival rates over 10 years compared to the 13 reported counties." Specifically, of Dr. Warner's patients, 48% enjoyed a 5-year survival rate compared to 46% for the 13 counties; 34% had a 10-year survival compared to 30%, and 25% had a 15-year survival compared to 21% for patients receiving conventional care.[65]

Dr. Warner is another example of a physician who has been punished for deviating from the (ineffective) conventions of mainstream cancer treatment. For 20 years he served on the staff of Seattle's Swedish Hospital Tumor Institute, he ran a private practice in Seattle for 15 years, and he is the only physician who has registered all his cases in the database of the epidemiology section of the Fred Hutchinson Cancer Center (FHCC), regarded as one of the most prestigious cancer research centers in the world.

Concurrently, Dr. Warner and his associates, in collaboration with the University of South Carolina School of Medicine's Immunology Section, spent 15 years investigating appropriate tumor markers for breast cancer. His research team has also been involved with the John Wayne Cancer Center of UCLA in immunotherapy of 6 cancer patients. With credentials and affiliations of this caliber, one wonders how members of the Washington State Medical Disciplinary Board justified their actions.

It is not as if Dr. Warner's patients complained; on the contrary, many of them survived cancer, thanks to Dr. Warner's methods. For example, Patricia Montsini, aged 62, was diagnosed with advanced ovarian cancer and received a "terminal" diagnosis. Her doctors insisted she have chemotherapy, even though they didn't expect it to improve her chances of survival. Patricia consulted Dr. Warner and began his program. After 1 year, she had a complete remission. "I have never had a day since when I did not feel better than the day before," Patricia says of her recovery. "Dr. Warner gives hope." Louise Berry, aged 51, had advanced-stage breast cancer that had spread to her bones. Her condition was considered inoperable, but after undergoing Dr. Warner's treatment, Louise recovered completely and is now cancer free.

"Molecular biology has shown that the most successful approach is to use immune-enhancing substances that our body ordinarily makes to fend off cancer," says Dr. Warner. "Healing comes from the body itself, not from anything the doctor actually uses. We only assist in the process." For the cancer industry, the trouble with Dr. Warner is that he places a premium on medical *science* instead of medical *business.* His brand of oncology does not help fill the coffers of the chemotherapy industry. "[Chemotherapy] is an incredibly lucrative business for doctors, hospitals, and pharmaceutical companies," Dr. Warner says.

There is tremendous institutional resistance to anyone who attempts to practice and scientifically document the effectiveness of complementary approaches in oncology. In Dr. Warner's words, "The medical establishment wants everyone to follow the same exact protocol. They don't want to see the chemotherapy industry go under, and that's the number one obstacle to any progress in oncology."

Dr. Warner's is one among *many* cases that might be presented to make the same point. Our government agencies, chartered supposedly on behalf of the public's health, seem intent on preventing effective alternative treatments from reaching the public. Nothing is likely to change unless every citizen, every *potential* cancer patient, takes political action today and speaks out against the travesty of the cancer industry.

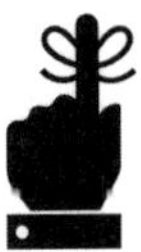

*A strong immune system can stop cancer in its tracks by identifying cancer cells and mounting an effective attack against tumors and small groups of renegade cells that have spread from the original or primary tumor.*

Chapter 27

# Early Detection and Prevention of Cancer

**Detecting signs of cancer at the earliest stages, even before any traces of pathology are apparent, is both desirable and practically possible. It is also the key to cancer prevention. A variety of innovative "early warning" diagnostic tests are now available to make very early detection entirely feasible.**

One of the hallmarks of the alternative medicine approach to treating and reversing cancer is to detect signs of cancer at the earliest possible time and to take all practical steps to prevent its recurrence, or to keep it from developing in the first place.

**Cancer Detection and Prevention Tests Profiled in This Chapter**

- AMAS
- PSA
- Pap Smear
- PAPNET
- Mammography
- Hemoccult Test
- Darkfield Microscopy
- Biological Terrain Assessment
- CBC Blood Test Report
- Maverick Monitoring Test
- ToxMet Screen
- Individualized Optimal Nutrition (ION)
- Oxidative Protection Screen
- Pantox Antioxidant Profile
- FORCYTE Cancer Prognostic System
- T/Tn Antigen Test
- Lymphocyte Size Analysis

Prevention is the most important and reliable cancer-fighting tool that exists today. The fact that cancer can be treated and reversed and that it can be detected early and prevented are *the* most important messages of this book. Foremost among the preventive measures is to maintain a strong and healthy immune system. This can be accomplished in a number of ways, such as maintaining a diet that ensures the optimal intake of immune system-enhancing nutrients and decreasing your intake of immune system-suppressing foods. Living a life free from constant emotional or mental distress is also important, as is avoiding carcinogenic toxins, geopathic zones and harmful electromagnetic fields in your home and work environment.

The following case study perfectly illustrates how early detection and prevention work well together in keeping cancer at bay.

## Cancer Antibodies Act as an Early Warning Signal

Sue, aged 35, felt a stinging sensation on her shoulder blade as she reached to scratch it in the shower. When a spot of blood appeared on her washcloth, she realized she had chafed a mole slightly wider than the diameter of a pencil eraser. Upon closer inspection, she saw that one half of it was shaped differently than the other and had slightly jagged edges.

Several weeks later, when the mole still appeared to be irritated, Sue decided to consult a physician who was a proponent of alternative medicine. The physician examined the mole carefully, then advised Sue to have it removed and sent to the lab for analysis. Noting her pale complexion and low energy levels, he placed Sue on a low-fat, high-fiber diet, and nutrient supplement program.

A few days later, Sue's doctor informed her that she had malignant melanoma, a potentially deadly form of skin cancer. Upon removing the tissue around and under the mole, the surgeon had determined that this cancerous lesion had penetrated several layers of skin and the underlying layer of fat. According to biopsies at the time, the cancer had apparently not spread to the lymph nodes—good news for Sue. Sue underwent a complete series of nutrient and enzyme tests to provide optimal support for her body's anticancer defense systems. However, her physician recommended that she take the AMAS (anti-malignin antibody screen) test, which is designed to pick up cancers well in advance of other signs and symptoms.

The result from the AMAS test, which was repeated twice, revealed that cancer still existed in Sue's body. Furthermore, the nutrient and enzyme tests indicated several deficiencies that could compromise her body's ability to fight the cancer. Since the cancer was still at an early stage, the doctor recommended that she try a vegetarian diet based on the Gerson therapy, which has shown considerable success in the treatment of malignant melanoma. He also expanded her supplement program, which had included vitamins C and E, coenzyme Q10, selenium, and zinc, to now include germanium and various enzymes, glandulars and botanical medicines such as Essiac tea, *Echinacea*, and maitake mushroom.

Ten months later, Sue's AMAS test indicated that she no longer had cancer. All her nutrient and enzyme levels had returned to the optimal range and her doctor declared her to be in excellent health. She continued with the nutrient treatment regimen for several months longer and decided to maintain a primarily vegetarian diet and regular exercise program thereafter. At the same time, she decided to spend less time in the bright sun, exposure to sun being a risk factor in developing melanoma.

Fortunately, Sue caught the cancer early. Malignant melanoma is now the most common cancer among women ages 25-29 and second only to breast cancer in ages 30-34. From 1975 to 1992, the overall number of melanoma cases reported annually in the United States has tripled, increasing more than any other cancer; the disease now claims at least 7,000 American lives each year and accounts for 75% of all skin cancer deaths. Finally, it is more likely than other skin cancers to spread to other parts of the body, making it more difficult to arrest and cure.

In light of these facts, Sue's emphasis on early detection and prevention serve as an excellent example for others to follow. Sue took 2 crucial steps that gave her excellent chances for long-term survival: First, she took action *early*, embarking on a nutritional and botanical program to strengthen her immune system at a point when the melanoma had not yet grown to a dangerous degree.

Second, after the cancer had apparently been eliminated from Sue's body, she adopted an active *preventive* strategy. In other words, she made a conscious decision to reevaluate aspects of her former lifestyle and environment that could have contributed to the weakening of her immune system. She opted to stay with her new diet program, to exercise regularly, to reduce her exposure to sunshine, and to generally monitor her stress level. These important changes enabled Sue to keep the cancer at bay for good.

### AMAS

## Accurate Blood Test for Early Cancer Detection

Until recently, there was no single blood test that could reliably and accurately indicate whether cancer was present, either for an initial diagnosis or for monitoring a recurrence. The tests available were sometimes positive when cancer was not present (a false positive), and sometimes negative when it was known that the person had cancer (a false negative).

Many oncologists and cancer specialists use blood tests called cancer markers, which detect substances present in abnormal amounts in the blood or urine of a person with cancer. But cancer markers can be unreliable for a variety of reasons. Some fail to indicate the presence of the new, previously undetected cancers and show only whether known cancers are shrinking or expanding. Others register levels of substances that could be produced by diseases other than cancer. Still others are not sensitive enough to pick up cancers in a certain percentage of patients.

For many years, researchers have been hoping for a cancer marker that could serve as a reliable indicator for a variety of cancers. Possibly the most accurate cancer marker was unveiled in the 1990s, thanks to the efforts of Harvard-trained biochemist and physician Sam Bogoch, M.D., Ph.D., who labored for 20 years before finally uncovering the secret to detecting *all* forms of cancer in its earliest stages. Known as AMAS (anti-malignin antibody screen), the test analyzes a sample of blood to reveal whether antibodies to cancer are present.

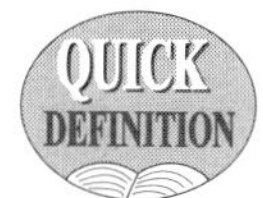


An **antibody** is a protein molecule containing about 20,000 atoms, made from amino acids by B lymphocyte cells in the lymph tissue and set in motion by the immune system against a specific foreign protein, or antigen. An antibody is also referred to as an immunoglobulin and may be found in the blood, lymph, colostrum, saliva, and the gastrointestinal and urinary tracts, usually within 3 days after the first encounter with an antigen. The antibody binds tightly with the antigen as a preliminary for removing it from the system or destroying it.

An **antigen** is any biological substance (a toxin, virus, fungus, bacteria, amoeba, or other protein) that the body comes to regard as foreign and dangerous to itself. As such, an antigen induces a state of cellular sensitivity or immune reaction that seeks to neutralize, remove, or destroy the antigen by dispatching antibodies against it.

Generally speaking, the test is called an immunoassay, which means it measures the amount present of a specific antibody, in this case, anti-malignin, an antibody that acts against the inner protein layer of a cancer cell, called malignin. Dr. Bogoch found that the anti-malignin antibody serves as a reliable marker for cancers of *all* kinds. "If there are any cancers that don't respond to the [AMAS] test, we haven't found them yet," says Dr. Bogoch. "Aside from being an invaluable tool for early detection, if a person goes into remission, this is a useful test for determining that a person is staying in remission."

Although it was approved by the FDA in 1977, it wasn't until late 1994 that the clinical trials with 4,278 patients were completed, validating the test's effectiveness. Now this patented, FDA-approved anti-malignin antibody screen is available to doctors, worldwide, through Dr. Bogoch's Oncolab. According to Dr. Bogoch, AMAS is 95% accurate on the first test, and 99% when repeated; the test can detect cancer up to 19 months before conventional medical tests for cancer can find it.

AMAS can monitor the degree of remission following treatment, so we now have an objective way of measuring the effects of alternative cancer treatments. It also means, obviously, that lives can be saved. Approximately 35% of those who die from cancer could be saved with an earlier diagnosis followed by prompt treatment.

The advantage of the new blood test, states Dr. Bogoch, is that it "gives a much more accurate answer at a fraction of the cost and inconvenience" of standard cancer tests. When the last malignant cancer cells are destroyed in the body, the anti-malignin antibody levels return to normal, and the cancer

***The advantage of AMAS, states Dr. Bogoch, is that it "gives a much more accurate answer at a fraction of the cost and inconvenience" of standard cancer tests. When the last malignant cancer cells are destroyed in the body, the anti-malignin antibody levels return to normal, and the cancer can be considered cured.***

can be considered cured. In fact, a new study by Dr. Bogoch involving 1,175 breast cancer patients proved that clinical remission, whether after 1 or 30 months, is directly correlated with normal AMAS levels.

However, it must be pointed out that end-stage cancer patients (especially those who have undergone extensive immunosuppressive therapies such as high-dose radiation and/or high-dose chemotherapy) cannot produce enough anti-malignin antibody to make the test positive, which means the test results will be meaningless.

The AMAS test is valuable for *early* detection of breast and prostate cancers, which are notoriously hard to catch at this stage. When tiny tumors are found in the milk ducts of breasts, many women panic and opt either for total breast removal (mastectomy) or for the more conservative procedure—removal of a lump of tissue (lumpectomy). The increased use of mammography during the 1980s caused the number of diagnoses of these small tumors to soar. This type of tumor, called ductal carcinoma in situ, is too small to feel but can be picked up by a mammogram. It is impossible, however, to determine from a mammogram which of these small tumors are dangerous and which are not.

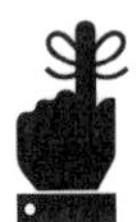

The AMAS test is most suited to detecting cancers in their earliest developmental stage, before gross tumor masses are observable, and for determining whether all signs and activities of cancers have disappeared following treatment. It is *not* suitable for detecting advanced cancers with severe immune suppression.

The AMAS test resolves this dilemma and helps patients avoid unnecessary anxiety and unnecessary medical treatment. A positive AMAS reading indicates that malignant tissue is present and that a lumpectomy or mastectomy may be warranted. "If you have a change in a very small area of a benign breast tumor, this is enough to trigger an antibody response," says Dr. Bogoch. "You could have malignant tissue present in only 1-2 ducts in a large area of an otherwise benign tumor and this would show up in the AMAS test." A tumor the size of only 1-10 mm is picked up readily by one AMAS test whereas most other means used, including mammography, do not pick up cancer at this level.

In the case of prostate cancer, the AMAS has also shown value. The false positive rate for prostate specific antigen (PSA) can be as high as 75%, or 3 out of every 4 PSA tests results—in other words, it can be as low as 25% correct. In contrast, the false positive rate for the AMAS is only 5%, meaning that only 1 in 20 tests tend to give a false reading.

This means that the AMAS test is 95% reliable, except in advanced stages of cancer, in which, as Dr. Bogoch explains, "the antimalignin antibody is wiped out," meaning there is nothing for the test to pick up. The person who is initially diagnosed with advanced-stage cancer typically *appears* ill or will show various outward physical signs of disease.

In these advanced cases, other types of medical testing are recommended—cancer markers (but not the AMAS), biopsies (surgical samples of cancerous tissue to determine the degree of malignancy), and various scans, depending on the type of cancer. With brain cancer, for example, CT (computerized tomography scans) and physical examination are typically used, and an MRI (magnetic resonance imaging) scan can give even more specific information. X rays and bone scans are useful for detecting metastases to the bone; ultrasound and liver scans can be used to detect metastases in the liver.

Ultrasound, in general, is one of the least invasive and most helpful ways to diagnose tumors of the kidney, uterus, ovaries, gallbladder and pancreas; ultrasound is able to detect very small tumors. It is also useful in detecting cancer in younger women, whose breast tissue is dense.[1] Unlike X rays or mammograms, ultrasound delivers no harmful radiation that could either seed cancer or further its course. But all of these tests fall short when it comes to revealing tiny tumors and none surpass the AMAS for picking up cancer in its earliest phases of development.

QUICK DEFINITION

A **cancer marker** refers to any of a variety of blood tests which measure the level of a protein material or other chemical produced by cancer cells. These numbers become elevated in the presence of a cancer or tumor. There are different cancer markers for different kinds of cancer: CEA (carcino-embryonic antigen) test for colon cancer, AFP (Alpha fetoprotein) test for liver cancer (primary hepato-cellular carcinoma), PSA (prostate-specific antigen) for prostate cancer, CA (carcinoma) 15-3 or 27.29 for breast cancer, and CA 125 for ovarian cancer, to name a few.

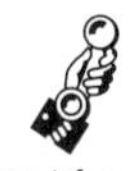

For more information about **AMAS,** contact: Oncolab, 36 The Fenway, Boston, MA 02215; tel: 800-922-8378; fax: 617-536-0657. The test costs $135 (follow-up, $85) and can be ordered by any physician who is licensed to order clinical laboratory tests.

## Orthodox Screening Methods and Their Relevance to Prevention

In most cases, cancer takes years or even decades to develop into a *visible* tumor. But even if a tumor is not yet visible by conventional means, it is still active as cancer and a serious health threat waiting to announce itself. Knowing that early detection of the growing tumor allows for early treatment and better chances of survival, holistic-minded physicians have begun seeking ways, such as the AMAS test, to diagnose *precancerous* conditions—those that precede the actual appearance of the cancer.

Although there are many ways to detect cancer early and keep it from gaining a foothold in the body, not all the tests are useful in detecting cancer in an early, treatable stage. For example, both chest X rays and sputum samples have been used to detect the presence of bronchial carcinoma, a form of lung cancer. By the time the cancer can be detected by these tests, however, it has already advanced to a stage that may be extremely difficult to cure.

In addition, as indicated previously, some screening tests can yield false results—either false negatives or false positives. In the case of false negative results, the person experiences great relief that no cancer appears to be present when, in fact, cancer does exist. A false positive test may make an individual anxious enough to opt for unnecessary treatment when no cancer is present.

Two common statistical measures of the usefulness of a screening test are sensitivity and specificity. Sensitivity refers to the probability that a test will show a positive result when cancer exists; specificity is the probability that a negative test result occurs when cancer is absent. A test that has high sensitivity and high specificity is far more useful than one with low readings for either or both of these measures. For example, PSA (prostate specific antigen, a specific marker for potential prostate cancer) has low sensitivity (68%) and specificity (60%).[2] In contrast, recall that the AMAS has high sensitivity (95%) and specificity (95%).[3]

A fundamental difference between the AMAS test and other diagnostic tests is that the AMAS detects all types of cancer whereas most other tests target only one kind of cancer. For example, PSA detects only prostate cancer and the Pap smear picks up only cervical cancer, albeit at any early stage of the disease. By using a test that picks up all cancers early on, it is more likely to catch cancers that would otherwise be missed by the more specific tests. We'll briefly review the 3 most common screening methods for the early detection of cancer—PSA, Pap smear, and mammography—and show how they can be used, misused, and misinterpreted.

## PSA

### Prostate Specific Antigen: Early Detection and Prevention of Prostate Cancer

Prostate cancer is the second leading cause of cancer-related deaths among American men and the most frequently diagnosed malignancy (other than skin cancer) in this segment of the population. An estimated 244,000 new cases of prostate cancer were diagnosed in 1995,[4] and the incidence of prostate cancer is increasing at an accelerated pace—in 1994, rates were 21% higher than in 1993.[5] The number of new cases almost doubled from 1990 (106,000) to 1994 (200,000).[6] The important point here, however, is that this surge of new cases appears to be related to the increased popularity of prostate cancer screening via the use of a prostate cancer marker, the prostate-specific antigen, or PSA.

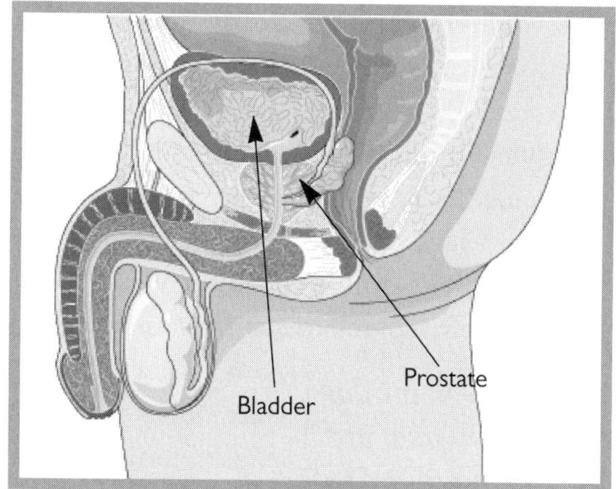

**Figure 27.1—The prostate gland**

In recent years, doctors have looked to the PSA as a way to catch prostate cancer early. The disease can develop and spread with little or no warning signs, and many cases are discovered too late, that is, after they have spread beyond the prostate and are extremely difficult to reverse. In fact, the conventional medical establishment believes that "there is no cure for prostate cancer once it has spread beyond the gland."[7] However, as the numerous alternative physicians in this book explain through their vivid case histories, this belief is incorrect; nearly any kind of cancer can be reversed or at least contained using multimodal alternative approaches.

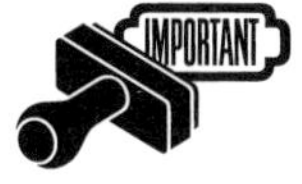


Although the PSA may help detect tumors too small to raise a bump on the prostate, the test is fraught with problems. To begin with, a high PSA reading (a positive or "high" result is greater than 4) is by no means proof that cancer is present, since factors other than cancer—an enlarged prostate (benign prostatic hyperplasia), mechanical pressure on the prostate, or inflammation of the prostate (prostatitis)—can cause the level to rise. Not surprisingly, then, the so-called false positive test results for PSA are extremely common, occurring in approximately 50% of all PSA test results. On the flip side, many men who actually have cancer may show a low or normal PSA reading at the time of testing.[8]

PSA may still have value when used in conjunction with other methods, namely digital rectal examination and ultrasound-guided biopsy of the prostate. When combined with these diagnostic techniques, PSA improves early detection, albeit by only 25%.[9] It is possible that the PSA now may be unnecessary as an initial screening device, thanks to the existence of the AMAS which picks up all early signs of cancers, not just prostate.

Prostate cancer is generally classified as: (1) latent or benign; (2) moderately progressive; and (3) rapidly progressive and extremely malignant. Some experts now believe that the PSA screening is valuable only for the moderately progressive form, stating that "tumors of the first form need never be detected and tumors of the third form progress so rapidly that timely screen-detection is nearly impossible, and, when accomplished, may be valueless."[10]

***Roughly 12 million American men are walking around today with microscopic signs of prostate cancer. For most of these men, the PSA may cause unnecessary worry and premature treatment because it picks up prostate tumors that are likely to remain inactive for life. In other words, men with this form of the disease die with prostate cancer, not from prostate cancer.***

The latent, harmless form of prostate cancer is the most prevalent. Autopsies of thousands of men who died suddenly from automobile accidents, heart attacks, or other non-cancer-related causes have found that approximately 15% of men in their 50s have some cancerous cells in their prostates.[11] The number jumps to 40% for men in their 70s, and to 50% for men 80 and older.[12] If you apply these estimates to the current U.S. population, this means that roughly 12 million American men are walking around today with microscopic signs of prostate cancer.

For most of these men, the PSA may cause unnecessary worry and premature treatment because it picks up prostate tumors that are likely to remain inactive for life.[13] In other words, men with this form of the disease die *with* prostate cancer, not *from* prostate cancer. Thus, by definition, their survival cannot be extended by early detection. Consequently, the only consequence of early detection for this "silent majority" of prostate cancer patients is a great deal of undue anxiety. The cancerous cells in most men's prostates tend to grow so slowly that the majority of prostate tumors never become large enough to be visible or palpable. "Only about 1% of the [cancer] cells ever develop into full-blown prostate cancer, and only about 3 in 1,000 [prostate] tumors have been shown to cause death."[14]

When prostate cancer is detected in its early stages, prevention should be emphasized before treatment. At this juncture, the wise physician will recommend "watchful waiting," which entails careful observation and monitoring to assure that small, slow-growing tumors remain so. Watchful waiting is considered appropriate for men in their upper 60s and older, who have a high PSA reading or positive result on the digital rectal exam, but are likely to die of another cause before their prostate tumor becomes a grave threat. Watchful waiting (compared to treatment) has lowered the death rate from prostate cancer among men with non-metastasized prostate tumors.[15] This fact underscores the point that many U.S. men are being *overtreated* for a prostate condition that may never be life threatening.

***Fewer than 10% of all doctors who recommend surgical removal of the prostate (prostatectomy) even discuss watchful waiting as a viable option with their patients. This profit-driven situation persists despite excellent data supporting the practice of watchful waiting and despite the fact that incontinence, impotence, and other side effects too frequently follow prostate surgery.***

Unfortunately, since treatment in the form of surgery and radiation generates huge amounts of money for conventional physicians and hospitals, watchful waiting is not always encouraged. Fewer than 10% (1 in 10) of all doctors who recommend surgical removal of the prostate (prostatectomy) even discuss watchful waiting as a viable option with their patients.[16] This profit-driven situation persists despite excellent data supporting the practice of watchful waiting and despite the fact that incontinence, impotence, and other side effects too frequently follow prostate surgery.

If you do have an elevated PSA (a reading greater than 4), then a repeat test and a digital rectal exam are needed. Since the digital rectal exam can raise the PSA, have the blood drawn *before* the rectal exam. It may be advisable to also undergo an ultrasound or sonogram of the prostate and a prostatic acid phosphatase blood test which increases the accuracy of the PSA and digital examination in finding prostate cancer. During a prostate sonogram, a blunt probe about the size of a thumb is inserted into the rec-

## Recommendations for Prevention of Prostate Cancer

In taking active steps to prevent prostate cancer from developing, the following represent key findings to keep in mind:

- Vegetables rich in beta carotene—including broccoli and other green vegetables, carrots, and squashes—may lower the risk of prostate cancer.[19]
- Foods containing tomatoes appear to reduce prostate cancer rates by 45% for those who have at least 10 servings a week.[20]
- Fish oil supplementation (containing eicosapentenoic acid, or EPA) may suppress the growth of prostate cancer cells[21] and inhibit the promotion of prostate cancer.[22]
- Selenium inhibits the growth of carcinoma cells in the prostate[23] and also blocks the stimulatory effects of the heavy metal, cadmium, on prostate cancer.[24] Zinc also blocks the effect of cadmium.
- Soy foods, by virtue of their high genistein content, may help keep latent prostate cancer from developing into an invasive form.[25]
- Modified citrus pectin was found to reduce the number of metastases in laboratory animals injected with prostate cancer.[26]
- Physically active men have a much lower risk of prostate cancer than their less active counterparts for the same age group.[27] The deep breathing of oxygen and the 15-fold increase in lymph fluid flow caused by exercising may explain the benefit of exercise on the prostate.
- Being overweight, smoking, and consuming alcohol may increase the risk of prostate cancer.
- A large body of evidence suggests that chemical toxins combined with poor nutrition may overwhelm the detoxifying mechanisms of the liver—in particular, the activity of an enzyme called glutathione S-transferase, or GST—and that GST may play a key role in defending normal prostate cells against carcinogenesis.[28]
- Reducing one's exposure to toxins (mainly by eating a low-fat, vegetarian diet) and attending to other risk factors can improve the chance of surviving prostate cancer when diagnosed early.

tum and sound waves from the probe create "echo" images of the prostate on a TV screen so that tumors may be seen. Prostatic acid phosphatase is an enzyme made from protein in the prostate gland and becomes elevated usually when the prostate develops cancer, infections, inflammation from toxins, or benign prostatic hypertropy.

If these tests also indicate prostate cancer, an ultrasound or guided needle biopsy will usually provide the definitive diagnosis. If the cancer is confirmed at this point, it is also advisable that you immediately adopt a low-fat, high-fiber diet, among other important lifestyle changes.

Many studies have shown that people who eat diets high in fat, especially animal fat, are more likely to develop prostate cancer.[17] U.S. men have prostate cancer rates that are 30-40 times higher than men in China and about 6-10 times higher than men in Japan; Asian males consume less than half the saturated fat eaten by their U.S. counterparts who get their fat mainly from red meats and dairy products.[18] Men consuming meat 5 times a week were 2 to 3 times more likely to develop invasive prostate cancer than those who eat meat once a week.[29] This increased risk of prostate cancer from eating meats and dairy may be at least in part related to the high pesticide content of these foods, as there is a 14 times higher pesticide level in meat and a 5½ times higher pesticide level in dairy products compared to plant-derived foods, according to William Rea, M.D., director of the Environmental Health Center in Dallas, Texas.

The low-fat, mainly vegetarian diet recommended here for prostate cancer patients stands in contrast with the one recommended by the National Cancer Institute. The NCI says that most cancer patients should eat high-calorie diets—that is, high in fat and sugar—to counteract the risk of cancer-related malnutrition; the American Cancer Society (ACS) seconds this view in its free 94-page guide, *Eating Hints for Cancer Patients.*[30] The NCI/ACS position on diet for cancer patients is extremely misguided. A growing number of cancer specialists and researchers say that a calorie-rich diet of this kind probably *promotes* prostate cancer as well as most other cancers.

Many cancer experts contend that the diet that apparently helps prevent cancer—one low in fat and high in fiber and antioxidants—will tend to slow or even block cancer's development. This line of reasoning is summarized by noted cancer epidemiologist Lawrence Kushi, Sc.D., who states: "If we believe that dietary factors act as *promoters* of carcinogenesis, then the influence of diet on tumor growth and spread should not necessarily be much different before or after clinical expression of the tumor." Dr. Kushi continues by noting that, specifically, one can make a strong case that "the time of clinical presentation of cancer is fairly arbitrary. This is particularly so when one considers the evolving technology and acceptance of screening procedures. Of course, there will be cases where caloric support is paramount, but for the otherwise healthy cancer patient ... the same dietary approach for prevention, broadly speaking, could be used for treatment as well."[31]

Regarding conventional treatment of prostate cancer, called androgen ablation, new research suggests that suppressing the male sex hormone may be counterproductive. Since the 1950s, oncologists have believed that prostate cancer cells require testosterone, the primary male sex hormone or androgen, to grow, so that by blocking or removing testosterone, this should cause prostate cancers to shrink. However, physicians note that in about 80% of cases treated with anti-testosterone therapy (androgen ablation: either the testicles are removed surgically or a chemical is administered to block the male hormone action), while the cancers initially disappear, they almost always return in 1-3 years.

**Differentiation** is a process by which unspecialized cells, while maturing, become specialized for designated tasks, thereby expressing only specific bits of genetic information. At birth, a human infant has an estimated 5 trillion cells differentiated into about 100 distinct cell types. Differentiated cells—red blood cells, for example—have a preset life expectancy and are programmed to live, die, and be replaced on a precise schedule. Cancer cells are cells that fail to differentiate or specialize in a normal way, which also means that their life spans are prolonged and they become virtually immortal.

More worrisome has been the discovery that the prostate cancer cells, after this 1-3 year period, can now grow independently of testosterone and no longer respond to ablation therapy. According to Shutsung Liao, Ph.D., a biochemist at the University of Chicago, the use of anti-testosterone drugs may be a dangerous mistake because it "may stimulate cancer growth by preventing testosterone from killing tumor cells that are androgen-independent but sensitive to the hormone's lethal effects in small amounts."

Dr. Liao recommends a repeated cycling of therapies, alternating androgen ablation with testosterone administration when the prostate cancer becomes androgen independent. Nobody expects a cure from this convoluted approach, but rather only "disease control." The example does show the kinds of knots conventional physicians can tie themselves into by forgetting the interdependent wholeness of the body and focusing on its minute particularities.[32]

If the PSA is persistently elevated (a reading of 10 or higher) after 2 months of the "watchful waiting" strategy noted above, a prostate needle biopsy can indicate the status of tumor cells. The cell patterns are graded from 1 to 5, where a score of 1 indicates highly differentiated cells (meaning a relatively benign tumor) and 5 shows very poor differentiation (meaning a highly aggressive tumor). In this case, surgery combined with hormone therapy may be needed, together with the alternative strategies outlined in this book. Conventional strategies such as surgical removal of the prostate and/or radiation therapy in these cases should be considered a "last resort."

**Pap Smear vs. PAPNET**

## Early Detection and Prevention of Cervical Cancer

An estimated 15,700 women will develop cervical cancer in 1996, and nearly 5,000 might die from it.[33] Even so, cervical cancer accounts for only about 3% of all new cancer cases in the U.S. and about 2% of all cancer-related deaths. The early form of the disease, called cervical dysplasia, is almost always reversible; however, once it becomes invasive or malignant, the cure rate drops by 50%.

The precancerous condition called cervical dysplasia is detected in about 2.5 million women in the U.S. each year and, of these cases, the most advanced or severe form translates into the greatest risk of continuing on to cervical cancer. When cells of the cervix undergo changes, initially they are not malignant; over time, however, particularly if toxins and poor nutritional conditions prevail, the altered cells lead to cervical cancer. Fortunately, nutritional, botanical supplements, and certain other alternative medicine techniques can often convert the premalignant cervical cells back to normal cells, thus averting the development of cervical cancer.

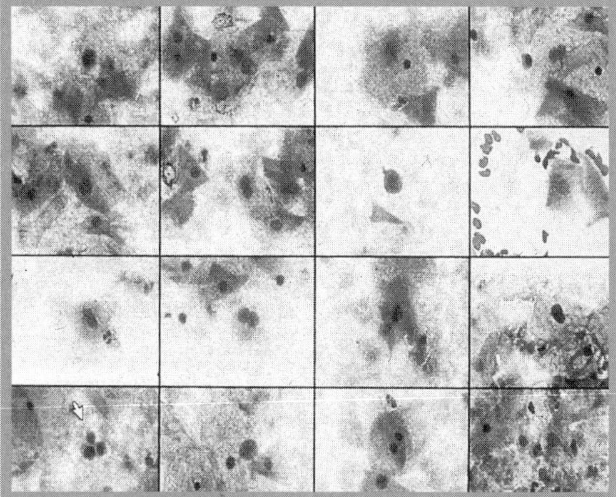

The PAPNET system presents 128 "cell scenes" from the original Pap smear, 16 of which are highlighted (top); also shown are details of a single scene (bottom).

The traditional Pap smear, introduced some 50 years ago (by George N. Papanicolaou, M.D., Ph.D.) for early detection of cervical cancer, generally means about 70% fewer deaths from cervical cancer. The Pap smear examines stained cells from the mucous membrane of the cervix for precancerous changes in cells. It is estimated that one-third of the women who die from cervical cancer do so because it was not accurately detected soon enough for successful treatment.

## Smoking and Cervical Dysplasia

Women smokers with cervical dysplasia should stop smoking immediately. Heavy smokers may be 4 times more likely to develop cervical cancer: light smokers have about twice the risk.[34, 35] A British study drew the following conclusions about the effect of smoking on cervical dysplasia and cervical cancer:

- Precancerous lesions of (cervical dysplasia) CIN shrank by at least 20% in most women smokers (82%) who either quit smoking entirely or greatly reduced the number of cigarettes they smoked.
- The lesions disappeared in 4 out of 28 women who quit smoking or cut back on the habit, and shrank by 50% in 10 of 17 who quit smoking altogether.
- About 1 out of every 3 women who kept on smoking showed a continual increase in the growth of precancerous lesions.
- Lesions did not disappear in any of the women who continued smoking.[36]

Of course, smoking should be avoided for other reasons as well. For instance, the risk of dying from lung cancer is 12 times higher in women who smoke than in those who have never smoked.[37]

Unfortunately, false negatives are common with this test, occurring in about 30% of all cases. According to the medical journal *Acta Cytologica*, the error rate for cervical cancer may be as high as 50%. A woman may have several false negative Pap tests in a row before falling ill and finding out that she has actually developed cervical cancer. The Pap smear registers between 50,000 and 300,000 cells in a single smear but those indicating potential cancer may be limited to a dozen or fewer cells. It is no wonder that identifying these few cells amidst many thousands is a formidable task that can result in false negatives. The situation with false *positive* Pap tests is serious. They have led to unnecessary hysterectomies, costing women their reproductive potential and often causing them profound misery.

A screening procedure developed in the late 1980s, called PAPNET Testing successfully identifies abnormal cells in 97% of cases. Using an automated microscope, a full-color camera, and a high-speed image-processing computer, the PAPNET system meticulously screens slides for evidence of abnormalities. Once abnormal individual cells or cell clusters from a single Pap smear have been pinpointed, their images are stored in the computer. When the entire Pap smear has been rescreened, the 128 "cell scenes" judged as most significant by the PAPNET computer are selected for visual evaluation by trained technicians.

Researchers at the University of California at Los Angeles proved that PAPNET is more accurate at reclassifying potential positive Pap smears than manual, visual evaluation. When lab technicians studied 62 Pap smears by standard manual methods, 31% of negatives needed further review; PAPNET reclassified 83% of them and found about one half to be abnormal. To date, PAPNET has been applied to 400,000 Pap smears in laboratories in 15 countries. In the U.S., at least 100 laboratories use the PAPNET system, charging an average of $40 per rescreening.[38] Dorothy L. Rosenthal, M.D., and colleagues reported in *Acta Cytologica* that in reducing screening errors PAPNET is saving lives.

***Unfortunately, false negatives are common in Pap smears, occurring in about 30% of all cases. According to the medical journal* Acta Cytologica, *the error rate for cervical cancer may be as high as 50%. A woman may have several false negative Pap tests in a row before falling ill and finding out that she has actually developed cervical cancer.***

If you are diagnosed as having evidence of cervical dysplasia—consider yourself fortunate. A balanced nutritional program alone often results in cancerous cervical cells reverting to normal, or "re-differentiating." Again, nutritional changes generally call for a predominantly vegetarian, low-fat, high-fiber diet.

Results from a study of 30 patients with this precancerous condition indicated that supplementing with beta carotene (30 mg orally per day for 6 months) suppressed cervical dysplasia; in addition, local application of a form of vitamin A (B-trans retinoic acid) was found to reverse moderate but not severe cervical dysplasia.[39] Research suggests that regular supplementation with vitamin C, vitamin E, and selenium, helps protect against cervical dysplasia and cervical cancer.[40]

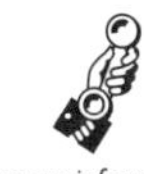

For more information about **PAPNET** and labs that use the system, contact: Neuromedical Systems, Inc., 2 Executive Blvd., Suffern, NY 10901; tel: 914-368-3600 or 800-PAPNET-4; fax: 914-368-3896.

Supplementation with folic acid alone has been shown to reverse cervical carcinoma in situ.[41] Folic acid seems to inhibit the incorporation of human papilloma virus (HPV, a sexually transmitted co-carcinogen that greatly increases a woman's chances of developing cervical cancer) into the DNA. Folic acid may act as a cancer *promoter*, so women should take it only in later stages of the disease under professional guidance and with regular monitoring.

Women are also advised to avoid oral contraceptives and douching with any liquid other than water. Oral contraceptives increase the risk of cervical dysplasia by 50% and of cervical cancer by 20%.[42] Douching with anything but water (or water plus vinegar) may increase the risk of cervical cancer by as much as 4 times.[43] Keep in mind, however, that the poten-

## Basic Guidelines for Breast Self-Examination

Beginning at age 20, women should practice regular breast self-examination, using both visual inspection and palpation of each breast. Look for anything unusual, including swelling, breast enlargement, dimpling, and skin or nipple changes.

Firmly press the breast tissue against the chest wall with the fingers in circular patterns from the outer edges of the breast toward the nipple. Palpate first superficially, then deeper. Be sure to examine the entire breast, covering the area up to the collarbone and over to the shoulder, and around the armpit where numerous lymph nodes lie. Do the examination while standing, and again while lying down, preferably with the arm on the side being examined held above the head in order to flatten the breast tissue against the chest wall.

Premenopausal women are advised to examine their breasts 5-7 days after they begin menstruating or shortly after their period ends. At these times, the breasts are least likely to be tender or swollen. Postmenopausal women should choose a specific date to do the self-examination once each month—perhaps the first day of the month—to ensure consistent checking. Women who have had a mastectomy or lumpectomy should inspect the incision to feel for any nodules or skin changes.

tial impact of all these risk factors can be amplified or mitigated by the type of diet one maintains.

### Mammography

## Early Detection and Prevention of Breast Cancer: The Problems with Mammography

Breast cancer is the second leading cause of cancer-related death among women, and for women diagnosed between the ages of 15 and 54, it is the most common cause of cancer-related death. In 1992, the last year for which accurate statistics are available, 43,068 breast cancer deaths were reported. It is estimated that in 1996, 184,300 new cases of breast cancer will be diagnosed in U.S. women and 44,300 will die from the disease.[44] In fact, in the United States, every 15 minutes, 5 new cases of breast cancer are diagnosed and at least 1 woman dies of the disease.[45]

Remember, though: this is the cancer world according to conventional medicine. Given the right combination of therapy and prevention, far more people can survive cancer and live long, productive lives than conventional cancer experts would ever deem possible. Quite simply, they are wrong, and this book should convince you of that.

The most basic way to detect breast cancer early is through self-examination. Most women do not check their breasts regularly for lumps and many lumps are found by accident.[46] Not surprisingly, women at the highest risk for breast cancer are those least likely to examine their breasts, probably owing to

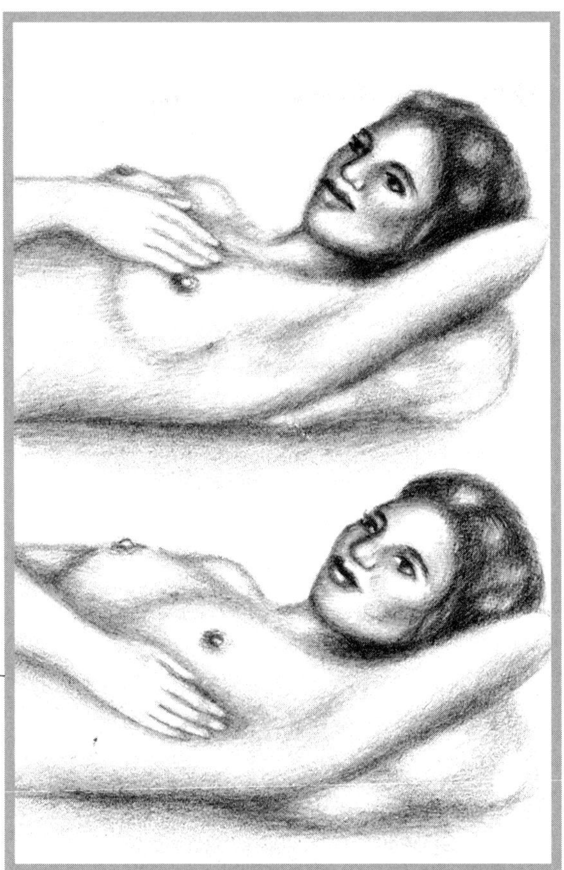

Figure 27.2—Breast self-examination

the anxiety associated with breast cancer.[47] This situation would change if women realized that *the majority of breast lumps are benign.* By regular breast self-examination, women can greatly increase the chances of detecting breast cancer at a stage when it is easiest to reverse. Also, avoiding caffeinated beverages and chocolate reduces the size and number of benign breast lumps thereby making the self-examination for breast cancer more reliable.

Breast self-examination has its limitations. If the tumor is pea-sized and located deep within the breast tissues, it may go undetected no matter how diligent the woman is with her self-examinations. For this reason, conventional doctors in the U.S. encourage women to undergo mammography on a regular basis. Although it is an imperfect technique with serious limitations, mammography can detect most tumors approximately 6 months to 3 years before they are physically palpable. A survey of 281 women by Breast Cancer Action in San Francisco, California, revealed that of the 226 women (of whom 70% were aged 40-59) who had breast cancer, 44% discovered this through breast self-exam, 37% through mammograms, and 8% through a physician's exam.[48]

About 90% of breast cancers can be detected by mammograms; the remaining 10% are obscured by dense surrounding breast tissue. Given the hazards of long-term radiation exposure, the possibility of its stimulating tumor growth in high-risk women (those with a family history of the disease, for example), not to mention the often unnecessary secondary expenses involved, mammography should be used with prudence.

Approximately 25% of breast cancers detected by mammography are in the earliest stage, meaning they have an overall 5-year survival rate of greater than 95%.[49] Simply put, early detection makes early treatment possible. Some research indicates that mammography does extend and save lives in older women.[50] Statistics in this population, according to the cancer establishment, may explain the recent decline in breast cancer mortality. It is also possible, however, that other factors have come into play, such as more attention to nutrition and exercise, which could augment the effects of breast cancer therapy.[51]

As a screening method, mammography has been widely abused. Some women, after receiving notice that they are to return for a repeat mammogram, become so distraught that they cannot continue to function normally at home or in the workplace. The fear is usually unfounded (although its strain on the nervous and immune system is unavoidable) since, as we have said before, 70-80% of all positive mammograms do not, on biopsy, show any presence of cancer.[52] Furthermore, in 90% of these "callbacks," the first readings were simply not clear because of dense, overlying breast tissue that interferes with the results.[53]

If the biopsy does reveal a tumorous growth, a woman may rush to the conclusion that she has cancer, even though the tumor may, in fact, be benign. Overreactions of this kind can lead to unnecessary treatment, typically, surgery followed by radiation and chemotherapy. Summarizing 2 decades of research on mammography and insights gleaned from his own 35 years of clinical practice, David Plotkin, M.D., concludes that "Mammography is only leading physicians to diagnose an ever-larger number of harmless tumors. Patients who otherwise would never have known they have a tumor may needlessly suffer through the unique pain, anxiety, disfigurement, and expense associated with modern medicine and cancer."[54] He further notes that despite all the "hopes" pinned on mammography, "it has had little impact on women's health—indeed, it may have had none." However, let us not be fooled by the term "benign." Fundamentally, all cancer is malignant.

Dr. Plotkin draws our attention to the fact that although the incidence of breast cancer is rising steadily, the rate of actual deaths has not changed since 1935: then it was 26.2 per 100,000 and as of 1992, it was still 26.2 cases per 100,000. What has increased is the *risk* of having breast cancer diagnosed but not the likelihood of dying from it. However, that these figures have remained static for almost 60 years does not mean conventional treatments have been successful, says Dr. Plotkin; if anything, they indicate that chemotherapy, radiation, and surgery have failed to change the mortality outcomes for cancer. "To my way of thinking, the constancy of the death rate in the face of rising incidence and aggressive treatment is a strong hint that we need to approach the disease in another way."

***That these figures have remained static for almost 60 years does not mean conventional treatments have been successful, says Dr. Plotkin; if anything, they indicate that chemotherapy, radiation, and surgery have failed to change the mortality outcomes for cancer.***

What has changed, says Dr. Plotkin, is the type of breast cancer itself. Increasingly, women are developing breast cancers that are slow to grow, that have slow tumor "doubling" rates. For example, based on a study of 448 women with tumors originally detected by mammography, a tumor may double in volume in as little time as 10 days or it may take 7,051 days (almost 20 years), while the average doubling time was 260 days. The incidence of in-situ tumors (less than 1/2 inch across, located within the ducts and lobules of breast tissue) made up 1-2% of all breast cancers in 1976, but in 1996, they comprised 10%, which is a 5- to 10-fold increase. The significance of this increase is that this type of cancer tends to be well-differentiated, slow-growing, and less of a life-threatening tumor.

While a mammogram may accurately indicate a tumor, it cannot in itself tell the physician what the doubling time is; if a cancer will not double for 15-20 years and the woman is already in her 60s—the median age for diagnosis of breast cancer is 64—then the woman may well live into her late 70s or early 80s, in effect, coexisting with her cancer without the need for toxic intervention such as chemotherapy, radiation, or surgery. Dr. Plotkin speculates that perhaps the chief result of the surge in mammography since the 1980s "has been to disguise our inability to cure the old cancer, by burying it in cases of new cancer."

***Based on 40 years of studying the effects of low-dose radiation on humans, John W. Gofman, M.D., Ph.D., a renowned authority on the health effects of ionizing radiation, estimates that 75% of breast cancer could be prevented by avoiding or minimizing exposure to the ionizing radiation from mammography, X rays, and other medical sources. Dr. Gofman believes strongly that there is no "safe threshold" for exposure to low-level ionizing radiation.***

The use of mammography for women under 50 years of age has been a subject of controversy. According to the highly regarded journal *The Lancet*, for women over the age of 40 it does more harm than good. That is because, of the 5% of mammograms that suggest further testing, up to 93% are false-positives—i.e, follow-up biopsies indicate no cancer. Regarding mammograms for women in this age group, the researchers concluded, "The benefit is marginal, the harm caused is substantial, and the costs incurred are enormous, [so] we suggest that public funding for breast cancer screening in any age group is not justifiable."[55] Despite the evidence and expert arguments, the American Cancer Society and many conventional doctors continue to recommend that all women over age 39 be screened by mammography.

*The Lancet* report also noted that, even among women over age 50, the presumed benefits—a 30% reduction in mortality—were based on early trials, with scant attention paid to later trials showing no significant benefit in any age group. In addition, the report presented a compelling case for more restricted use of mammograms, given the following facts: "(a) the great majority of positive screenings are false positives; (b) screening leads to many unnecessary investigations and useless surgery; (c) a 'negative' screening does not mean the absence of breast cancer; (d) in the large majority of women whose breast cancer is diagnosed by screening, the outcome is unchanged."[56]

For more on the health hazards of **low-level ionizing radiation,** see Chapter 26: What Causes Cancer? pp. 561-562.

Regarding this last point, *Lancet* authors stated that, in most cases, breast cancer has been present for many years before it is detected by mammography. Moreover, about 40 replications or doublings of the breast cancer cells create a potentially lethal burden, yet mammography cannot detect a mass until 25-30 such doublings have already occurred.[57] By this time, the cancer is far less treatable than it would have been after 15-20 doublings.

The potential damage incurred by low-level radiation exposure (typically from medical X rays) directly to the breast tissue is another area requiring further scientific scrutiny. For ethical reasons, it is unlikely that a randomized, prospective study will ever be conducted to investigate this issue. Mammograms involve small amounts of ionizing radiation but its proponents like to say that the benefits of mammograms outweigh radiation-related risks.

However, based on 40 years of studying the effects of low-dose radiation on humans, John W. Gofman, M.D., Ph.D., a renowned authority on the health effects of ionizing radiation, estimates that 75% of breast cancer could be prevented by *avoiding* or *minimizing* exposure to the ionizing radiation from mammography, X rays, and other medical sources.[58] Dr. Gofman believes strongly that there is no "safe threshold" for exposure to low-level ionizing radiation.

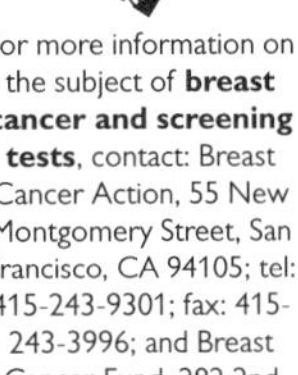

For more information on the subject of **breast cancer and screening tests**, contact: Breast Cancer Action, 55 New Montgomery Street, San Francisco, CA 94105; tel: 415-243-9301; fax: 415-243-3996; and Breast Cancer Fund, 282 2nd Street, 3rd Floor, San Francisco, CA 94105; tel: 415-543-2979; fax: 415-543-2975; tbcfund@aol.com

Another potential concern about the mammogram is that it may, on occasion, help *spread* an existing mass of cancer cells. During the procedure, considerable pressure is placed on the woman's breast, as the breast is firmly squeezed between 2 flat plastic surfaces by the mammography technologist. According to Lorraine Day, M.D., a pathologist and former breast cancer patient, this compression could cause existing cancer cells to move (metastasize) from the breast tissue. "When you have a mammogram, the breasts are squashed down fairly hard. If there are cancer cells, they are more likely to spread to other parts of the body, so that now you have cancer cells circulating in the bloodstream." A woman can and should request reduced compression if it becomes too intense or painful, Dr. Day adds.

This subject was addressed in *The Lancet* in April 1994 where J. P. van Netten of the Royal Jubilee Hospital in London reported that mammography can rupture in-situ cysts in the breast and spread cancer cells into surrounding tissue. They based this conclusion on a study of 110 women, average age of 39, noting that this type of tissue injury could account for the development of "overt invasive cancer" and metastases.[59] Since mammographic screening was introduced in 1983, the incidence of a form of breast cancer called ductal carcinoma in situ (DCIS), which represents 12% of all breast cancer cases, has increased by 328%, and 200% of this increase is due to the use of mammography, reported *The Lancet* in July 1995.

Estrogen therapy, if ongoing at the time of mammogram screening, can confuse the test results. According to a study of 8,800 postmenopausal women aged 50 and older, the use of estrogen replacement therapy (ERT) leads to a 71% increased likelihood of receiving a false-positive result on mammogram screening, according to Mary B. Laya, M.D., M.P.H., study leader at the University of Washington at Seattle, who published the results in the *Journal of the National Cancer Institute* in 1996. Dr. Laya also found that women on ERT were more likely to get false-negative readings. In both cases, faulty mammogram results lead to expensive and unnecessary tests in addition to exacting a heavy emotional toll.

***The annual mammographic screening of 10,000 women aged 50-70 will extend the lives of, at best, 2-6 of them; and annual screening of 10,000 women in their 40s will extend the lives of only 1-2 women per year.***

Mammograms are grossly cost ineffective. As they range in price from $50 to $200, it would be necessary to screen 20,000 women annually at an estimated cost of $1.2 million to benefit a *single* woman in terms of accurate early detection of breast cancer, according to *The Lancet* (July 1995). Similarly, Russell Harris and Linda Leininger of the University of North Carolina at Chapel Hill reported in the *Annals of Internal Medicine* (April 1995) that the annual mammographic screening of 10,000 women aged 50-70 will extend the lives of, at best, 2-6 of them; and annual screening of 10,000 women in their 40s will extend the lives of only 1-2 women per year.

## THE AMAS TEST COMPARED TO MAMMOGRAPHY

Our view is that mammography is, indeed, overused and should not be a routine part of breast cancer screening. Instead, the AMAS test should be a first choice. This test has been extensively evaluated with respect to early detection of breast cancer.[60] As noted earlier in this chapter, unlike mammography, which does not distinguish between benign and malignant breast tumors, the AMAS detects malignant growth *only* and has far greater sensitivity and specificity than mammography. If the AMAS is *positive*, a mammogram or ultrasound may be done to ascertain the location of the tumor for surgical purposes and a needle biopsy (perhaps with ultrasound) may be recommended. If 2 consecutive AMAS test results are *negative*, then a mammogram is unwarranted.

Frankly, we believe mammography is no longer needed as a primary screening tool. Instead, it should be used *only* to confirm suspicions of the breast self-examination and AMAS results. Additional mammograms, performed to clarify the probability of malignancy, become unnecessary with the AMAS. Moreover, the AMAS can be used to follow breast cancer patients who are in remission, since the AMAS returns to normal within 3 months after the breast tumor (and metastases, if present) are removed or eradicated.[61]

In summary, early detection via mammography is meaningful mainly if the cancer is caught very early, prior to any metastasis. Unfortunately, the mammogram cannot be relied upon to do either. Therefore, for women older than age 49, we advocate the use of monthly breast self-examination and an annual AMAS. The AMAS will greatly reduce the need for mammography and spare many women unnecessary grief. After this, treatment options will have to be carefully weighed.

Clearly most women would be better off taking aggressive preventive measures to lower their cancer risk rather than relying on the debatable results of mammograms. There are many ways to reduce one's risk of developing breast cancer. If you have an immediate family relative (such as mother, sister, or daughter) with breast cancer—especially more than one—you should take an active role, now, to modify these risk factors. Your risk is particularly high when breast cancer occurred in your mother, especially if your mother had cancer in both breasts or was premenopausal when the cancer was diagnosed.[62]

## Mammograms—Too Many False Positives

Mammography can also create problems in the form of false positive test results. A Swedish study of 60,000 women, aged 40-64, who were screened for breast cancer revealed that of the 726 actually referred to oncologists for treatment, 70% were found to be cancer free. For women under 50, the number of false positives for breast cancer was 86% of those referred for more testing. In addition to the needless anxiety produced, the clinical follow-up for false positives accounted for almost 33% of the total cost of the entire screening program, according to the *British Medical Journal* (February 1996).

***For women older than age 49, we advocate the use of monthly breast self-examination and an annual AMAS test. The AMAS will greatly reduce the need for mammography and spare many women unnecessary grief.***

Women who wish to keep their risk of breast cancer to a minimum should pay attention to the following established risk factors:

**High-Fat Diet and High-Caloric Intake—**Evidence shows that high-fat diets and high-calorie diets—fat is high in calories, so the 2 factors are typically inseparable—raise the risk of breast cancer.[63] All studies that suggest high-fat diets are not a risk factor for breast cancer have had 1 or more critical flaws in their clinical design, thus invalidating them as evidence.[64] Fat is a source of estrogens, free radicals, and (invariably) pesticides, all of which can promote breast cancer. The *ideal* fat content is 10-20% of the diet's total calories—the balance achieved in a predominantly vegan diet. High-fat diets, because they increase breast density, tend to create difficulties in interpreting mammograms, as we have pointed out before.[65]

**Estrogen Replacement Therapy (ERT)—**This is often recommended for postmenopausal women as a way to reduce the risk of osteoporosis, yet 2 evaluations of multiple studies determined that long-term use of ERT can significantly increase the risk of developing breast cancer.[66] The use of estriol, a relatively harmless form of estrogen, and natural progesterone may help resolve this problem.[67]

**Pesticides and Other Organohalogen Compounds—**Many risk factors exist that are not included in conventional risk-factor studies. Higher breast cancer rates have been found in the offspring of women who took DES (diethylstilbestrol) and among women with high breast-tissue concentrations of PCBs (polychlorinated biphenyls) and DDE (dichloro-diparacholophenylethylene: a metabolite of the infamous DDT pesticide).[68] DDE levels tend to be higher among African-American breast cancer patients than African-American women without cancer.[69] Higher levels of PBBs (polybrominated biphenyls) and certain pesticides have been found in fatty tissue samples from women with breast cancer compared with women who had benign breast disease.[70]

The difficulty in calling these pesticides and other organohalogen compounds "risk factors" is that chronic low-level exposure is prevalent in the general population; about 90% of the organohalogen exposure that has been linked with breast cancer is traced to food, either as deposits on the food or as residues from food chain concentration.[71] Pesticide use

For more information about **pesticides** (pp. 568-574), **high fat diets** (p. 604), and **hormone therapies** (pp. 586-590), see Chapter 25: What Causes Cancer?

represents a "hidden killer" because these chemicals not only directly promote tumor growth, but can suppress the immune system, thereby increasing susceptibility to disease.[72]

**Other Key Risk Factors**—Among the strategies for reducing your risk of developing breast cancer are the following:

- minimize exposure to low-level ionizing radiation
- increase intake of dietary antioxidants (from fruits, vegetables, and vitamin supplements)
- exercise regularly but in moderation
- have a baby (pregnancy reduces a woman's lifetime estrogen exposure)
- breastfeed your baby (lactation helps discharge pesticides and other toxins from the breast)
- avoid magnetic fields from power lines, electrical appliances, computers, geopathic lines, as these electromagnetic fields may alter the brain's healing and repairing, protein synthesis, and melatonin production; melatonin appears to help protect against breast cancer.[73]

### The Hemoccult Test

## Early Prevention and Detection of Colorectal Cancer

Colorectal cancer (cancers of either the colon or rectum) is the second most common cancer in the United States and surely one of the deadliest. In fact, about 1 out of every 5 cancer deaths (20%) in the U.S. is attributed to colorectal cancer and almost half of all colorectal patients will probably die, according to conventional medical statistics. One reason for this heavy death toll may be that the majority of colorectal cancer cases are diagnosed at a late stage of the disease.

Detected early, progression of this disease is entirely preventable. Among the more reliable early signs of colorectal cancer is blood on the surface of or mixed in feces. If not visible to the eye, colorectal blood can be detected by chemical tests. In some cases, pain and tenderness are felt in the lower abdomen but often, however, no symptoms appear until the tumor grows so big that it causes obstruction or rupture of the intestine; at this point, surgery and aggressive forms of treatment become necessary.

For this reason, many doctors now recommend the hemoccult (guaiac) test, in which a sample of feces is applied to a card imprinted with a solution of guaiac, a plant gum. In the laboratory, the presence of hemoglobin, hence the name, *hem*occult (i.e., blood in the feces) is indicated by a color change (usually to blue) on the card; this happens when a liquid hemoccult developer is applied to the feces on the guaiac card. The test will sometimes yield false positive results if the person has recently consumed fresh fruits or vegetables, red meat, iron tablets, aspirin, nonsteroidal inflammatory drugs, or vitamin C supplements, so you will be advised to avoid these for at least 24 hours before taking the test.

A positive finding with the hemoccult test warrants having a sigmoidoscopy, another tool used to detect polyps and tumors. This procedure involves the use of a flexible tube, about the diameter of a pencil, that is inserted to a maximum of 10 inches into the colon. Using this lighted instrument, the physicians explores the lower interior portion of the colon, called the sigmoid. Research indicates that 2 out of every 3 cases of colorectal cancer are accessible to detection by this means.[74]

To lower the risk of colorectal cancer, those over age 50 who have a poor diet and heavy meat-eating background should consider switching, if they haven't already, to a more vegetarian diet. Many oncologists recommend sigmoidoscopy at least every 3 to 5 years once people reach age 50, however, if you are physically active, have a normal 2-3 bowel movements daily, follow a sound low-fat, high-fiber diet, and have no symptoms, this practice should not be considered necessary.

If colorectal cancer is detected early, dietary treatment along with the other alternative therapies described throughout this book may constitute the best line of attack. The number one risk factor for colorectal cancer is the consumption of red meat (but not fish or white meat) and refined sugar-containing foods or white flour products; a diet low in fruits and vegetables also increases the risk.[75] Dietary antioxidants (notably vitamin E), calcium, vitamin D, and the B-vitamin folic acid (folate) may also reduce the risk or even aid in reversing this cancer in its early stages.

Regarding calcium and vitamin D, while the research does not support a link between low intake of dairy products (high in calcium and vitamin D) and the development of colorectal cancer,[76] it is still advisable to remove all dairy from the diet, except for low-fat yogurt on an occasional basis. A diet rich in cereal grains, fresh vegetables and fruits, legumes, and fish will be the healthiest strategy for anyone at risk for colorectal cancer or already diagnosed with the disease. Garlic, onions, chives, and cruciferous vegetables (broccoli, Brussels sprouts, cabbage, bok choy, etc.) are the most protective.[77]

For more information on the health hazards of **chlorinated water**, see Chapter 25: What Causes Cancer? pp. 579-580.

Along with avoiding red meat, dairy, and processed meats, one should abstain from alcohol and smoking, both of which have been shown to significantly amplify the risk of initiating or promoting colorectal cancer, or of causing a recurrence.[78] Several Norwegian studies have found that people who consume chlorinated drinking water have a higher incidence of colorectal cancers; chlorinated water is associated with a 20-40% increase in the incidence of colon and rectal cancers.[79]

### Darkfield Microscopy

## See Disease First in the Living Blood

Until recently, scientists assumed that the only diseases generated by microbes were infectious disorders such as AIDS, influenza, or tuberculosis. It was assumed that blood contained no living organisms that could contribute to cancer since the use of standard microscopes had failed to detect any sign of such microbes. When the powerful electron microscope is used, live organisms are placed in a vacuum and subjected to deadening protoplasmic changes induced by a barrage of electrons—meaning it is virtually impossible to observe *living* organisms under an electron microscope.

Based on the findings from more sophisticated light microscopes, there is now compelling evidence that such microbes do exist and may play a major role in cancer. Even better, this advance now enables forward-thinking physicians to see signs of cancer in living blood, even if it is only energetic traces or indications, *before* it manifests as a palpable tumor. French Canadian biologist Gaston Naessens invented an optic microscope called the Somatoscope, which enabled him to view tiny particles in the blood never before seen. He called these particles somatids, which means tiny bodies.

"I have since become convinced that the somatid is the smallest unit of life, the precursor to DNA, capable of transforming energy into matter," Naessens says. What Naessens called "somatids," the German bacteriologist Gunther Enderlein called "protits" and Virginia Livingston Wheeler, M.D., called *Progenitor cryptocides.* Many researchers believe these are essentially variations of the same microbe. Whatever the name, the research

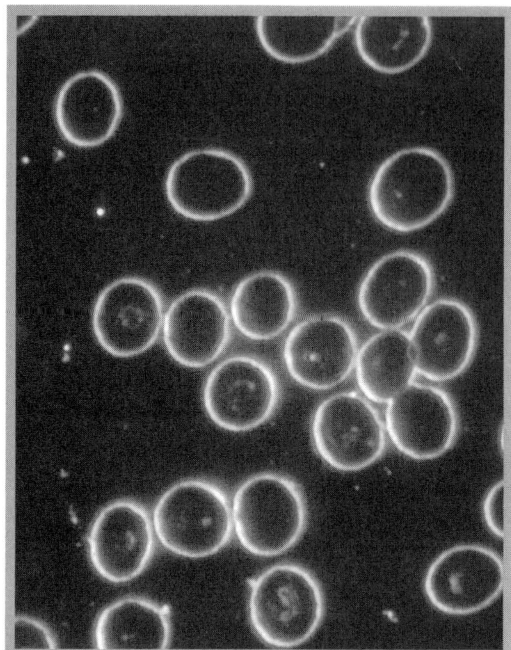

Darkfield view of normal blood

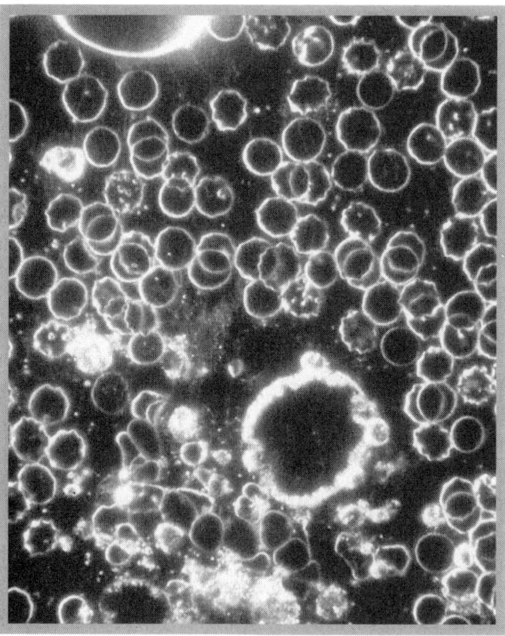

Darkfield view of blood of someone in early stages of cancer

cited here tends to confirm the pleomorphic or form-changing nature of microorganisms believed to underlie the cancer process.

The use of darkfield microscopy was a major change in the diagnostic routine of Maarten Klatte, M.D., a Dutch homeopathic physician and founding director of Vitality Research in The Hague, Netherlands. Like many physicians, he had assumed that all the essential components of blood could be detected by an electron microscope. "Instead of looking at blood, I looked at numbers," Dr. Klatte says. "These days, I look at the form and motion of the blood components, which include living organisms. I now realize that the old blood analyses, based on measurements, told us relatively little about the true condition of the blood." For Dr. Klatte, the difference between standard blood analysis and the darkfield method is "like the difference between night and day."

To illustrate the value of the method, Dr. Klatte cites the example of taking the white count of a cancer patient who has come to see him for the first time. The white count is a measure of the concentration of neutrophils (a type of white blood cell) in the blood. The standard procedure is to obtain a total white count and then compare it to the so-called "normal range;" if the patient's white count falls within the normal range, it is presumed to be normal. Using the darkfield microscope, what is normal quantitatively can be abnormal in a qualitative or "functional" sense, says Dr. Klatte. Even though the white cell count in a particular patient is normal, he maintains, the condition of the white blood cells may be revealed by the darkfield microscopy to be far from healthy.

***"When the pleomorphic cycle appears, we can take action and reverse the cycle with therapy," says Dr. Klatte. "If the cycle does not reverse, we know that the therapy is not working."***

The darkfield microscope enables Dr. Klatte to view neutrophils and describe cells with "ragged" cell walls, cytoplasm leaking out of the cells, and cells that seem immobilized or lifeless. "If most of the cells look paralyzed and broken," says Dr. Klatte, "then the 'normal' cell count means nothing. Motion tells me a lot more about the cells' function. Form tells me whether the cells are damaged by free radicals or whether there are

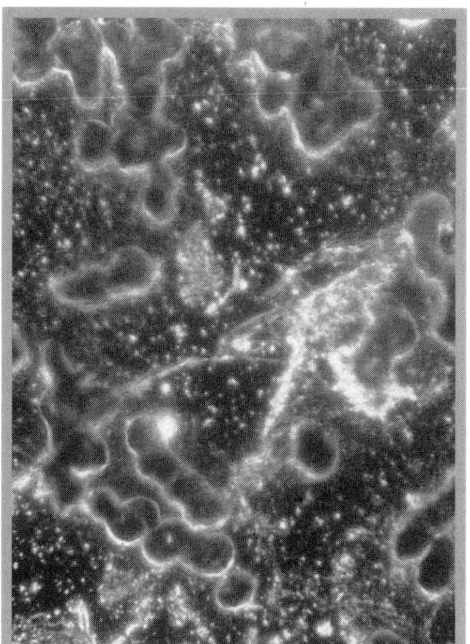

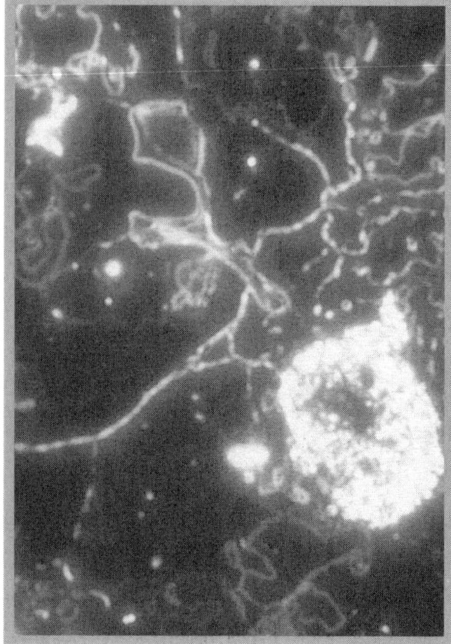

**Darkfield view of blood of a person with advanced cancer (left) and another with very advanced cancer (right)**

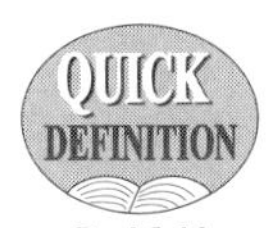


**Darkfield microscopy** is a way of studying living whole blood cells under a specially adapted microscope that projects the dynamic image, magnified 1500 times, onto a video screen. With a darkfield light condenser, images of high contrast are projected, so that the object appears bright against a dark background. The skilled physician can detect early signs of illness in the form of microorganisms in the blood known to produce disease. Blood cells live for about 20 minutes, so the amount of time the blood cell stays viable and alive indicates the overall health of the individual. Specifically, darkfield microscopy reveals distortions of red blood cells (which in turn indicate nutritional status), possible undesirable bacterial or fungal life forms, and blood ecology patterns indicative of health or illness.

For more information on the application of **darkfield microscopy** and **pleomorphic theory** to cancer treatment, see Chapter 31: New Approaches to Immune Stimulation for Reversing Cancer, pp. 905-909.

cell-wall deficiencies that need to be corrected nutritionally." A cell-wall deficiency means that the membrane surrounding the cell is porous or perhaps fragmented, allowing inappropriate or foreign substances to enter and exert harmful effects. Poor cellular function is indicated by a lack of responsiveness to foreign microorganisms.

Dr. Klatte, like many physicians, used to think that in healthy people, the blood and urine are basically sterile. Through the darkfield microscope, he has become aware that the blood is full of living microorganisms. "Thanks to Gaston Naessens, Guenther Enderlein, and others, we now understand much more about the *living* particles in our blood," says Dr. Klatte, who has worked with Naessens and confirmed the form-changing cycle of Naessens' somatids.

In fact, this cycle reveals the physical states of health and disease, according to Dr. Klatte. The somatid cycle indicates early signs of cancer, usually 6-18 months before the onset of clinical symptoms such as a swollen lymph node or lump in the breast. "When the pleomorphic cycle appears, we can take action and reverse the cycle with therapy. If the cycle does not reverse, we know that the therapy is not working." In the physician's hands, the darkfield microscope is an early detection tool and a way to evaluate the effectiveness of a therapy. Dr. Klatte routinely invites his patients to look at their blood before, during, and after treatment. "They now regard their blood as a living part of who they are, rather than as an abstraction, which is the perception they got from viewing numbers [blood measures] instead of seeing blood in its live condition." As the patients watch their blood improve over time, the darkfield images serve as a kind of psychobiological feedback providing positive reinforcement for positive changes.

Douglas Brodie, M.D., a cancer physician profiled in Chapter 3 of this book, makes use of darkfield microscopic principles by way of a simple yet versatile procedure called live blood analysis (LBA). Dr. Brodie uses LBA for obtaining a quick and accurate assessment of his patient's blood composition and viability. With a single sample, taken by a pinprick of the fingertip, LBA is able to provide a composite of numerous factors from living blood.

The darkfield technology allows doctors to observe multiple vitamin and mineral deficiencies, toxicity, and relative degrees of oxygenation as well as tendencies toward liver weakness, excess fat, clotting, and arteriosclerosis. Tendencies toward allergic reactions—including those that may be delayed or hard to determine based on external symptoms—can also be detected using the LBA.

With our increasing awareness of the importance of a strong immune system, the LBA is a valuable tool, providing dynamic assessment of the degrees of cancer resistance a person possesses. LBA permits problems to be detected and treated *before* more serious complications arise. Physicians can use it to determine blood imbalances that do not show up in the conventional procedure, known as the complete blood count (CBC). "In many cases, the live blood analysis provides information that enables us to predict which direction the cancer patient's body is heading," says Dr. Brodie. "We then make specific adjustments in nutrition and other modalities to optimize the healing process."

***Dr. Klatte routinely invites his patients to look at their blood before, during, and after treatment. "They now regard their blood as a living part of who they are." As the patients watch their blood improve over time, the darkfield images serve as a kind of psychobiological feedback providing positive reinforcement for positive changes.***

Furthermore, new technological developments enable patients to see the results of their LBA as they are revealed on screen. "I have my patients view their own drop of blood to keep as a reminder to maintain their prescribed nutritional program," says Dr. Brodie. "This is a powerful way to reinforce their own disciplined adherence to the program." The LBA picture also provides a basis for comparison on the next examination; typically, evaluation of the LBA results takes about 20 minutes. Additional lab tests can then be performed to confirm the results and to provide a more comprehensive clinical picture of the individual's condition.

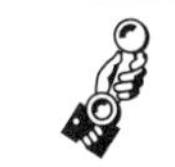

For more information on the **Live Blood Analysis** system used by Dr. Brodie, contact: NutriScreen, Inc., James R. Privitera, M.D., director, 105 North Grandview, Covina, CA 91723; tel: 818-966-1618; FAX: 818-966-7226. Dr. Privitera provides detailed instruction manuals in darkfield microscopic interpretation and nutritional prescribing to licensed health-care professionals.

### Assessment of Biological Terrain

## Biochemical Information Is Paramount

French biologist Louis Claude Vincent, Ph.D., discovered that the key to healing was not the use of powerful drugs, but, rather,

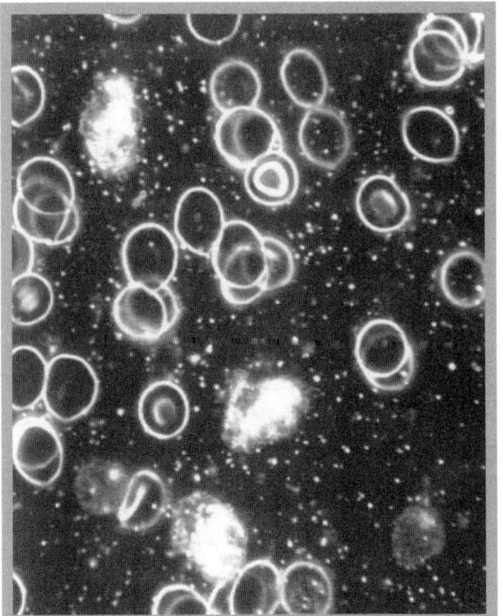

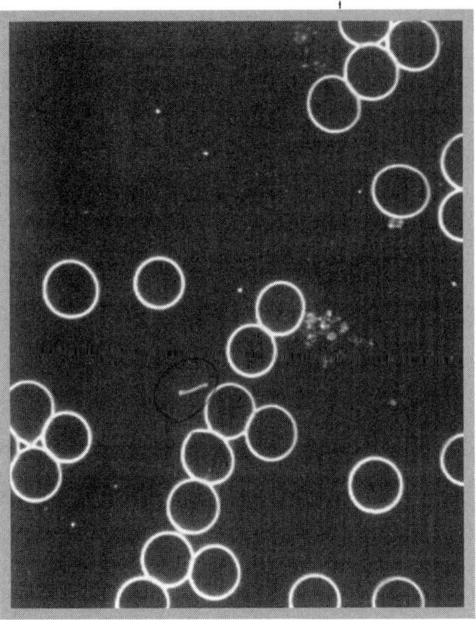

**Darkfield microscopy photographs of 2 patients—a 49-year-old female suffering from osteoblastic metastasis (left) and a 66-year-old female suffering from primary lung carcinoma (right)**

knowing the patient's biochemistry and the optimal conditions or "terrain" for body function. In 1958, Dr. Vincent was hired by the French government to determine why people living in certain regions of France had high cancer rates. This assignment led him to examine the relationship between the external environment—molded by a person's emotional and physical stress exposure, dietary choices and other lifestyle habits—and the internal environment of the body. Dr. Vincent also showed that water quality is an important factor to evaluate in clusters of cancer cases.

"Biological terrain" is a phrase used to describe the conditions, general health, and activity level of cells. This includes the status of microorganisms at the cellular level: some are beneficial to life and health, others are not. Each type of bacteria, fungus or virus thrives in a precise biochemical medium. Viruses require a fairly alkaline environment to function, whereas fungi favor a more acidic environment; bacteria can thrive under various conditions, but their growth is best stimulated in high-sugar conditions. An excess of toxins in one's diet and environment tends to increase the production of acid within cells, forcing the body to compensate by producing a strong alkaline chemical reaction in the blood

For more information on **biological terrain,** see Chapter 25: What Causes Cancer? pp. 633-636.

which, in turn, tends to favor the growth of cancer cells (which generate and tolerate large amounts of acid) and fungi.

Dr. Vincent concluded that the components of the blood, urine, and saliva afford insight into the way the body functions. By monitoring biochemical changes in these fluids and by making appropriate changes in diet, lifestyle, and medical treatment, health can be reestablished and disease processes retarded or possibly reversed.

In the pioneering tradition of Dr. Vincent, Robert Greenberg, D.C., of the Whole Health Centre in Chesterfield, Missouri, developed an approach to assessing health known as biological terrain assessment, or BTA. This test enables him to determine the optimal conditions for a specific patient's internal environment. According to Dr. Greenberg, the healthy body must satisfy 3 criteria to function at the highest level: (1) optimal pH (acid-base balance); (2) optimal oxidation-reduction potential; and (3) resistivity (the opposite of electrical conductivity). Through BTA, these factors are measured in blood, urine, and saliva, to yield a total of 9 measures.

Before we learn how BTA does this, let's review these 3 factors in more detail. "The pH reading tells us whether enzymatic activity in the body is occurring properly and if digestion and absorption of vitamins and other nutrients is adequate," says Dr. Greenberg. "It can also alert us to the potential presence of environmental or industrial contaminants, substances that prove very damaging to the body's delicate chemistry." In general, the urine is a better indicator of pH changes than the blood

## A Primer on Cellular Terrain

The term **pH,** which means "potential hydrogen," represents a scale for the relative acidity or alkalinity of a solution. Acidity is measured as a pH of 0.1 to 6.9, alkalinity is 7.1 to 14, and neutral pH is 7.0. The numbers refer to how many hydrogen atoms are present compared to an ideal or standard solution. Normally, blood is slightly alkaline, at 7.35 to 7.45; urine pH can range from 4.8 to 7.5, although normal is closer to 7.0. **Acid-base metabolism** refers to the metabolic processes that maintain the balance of acids and bases (alkalines) in body fluids. Acids release hydrogen ions, while bases accept them. The total number of these hydrogen ions present determines the pH of a fluid. Too many hydrogen ions (a pH below 7) produce an acidic state called acidosis, while too few hydrogen ions (a pH above 7) cause an alkaline excess called alkalosis; both can lead to illness. **Oxidation-reduction** refers to a basic chemical mechanism in the cell by which energy is produced from foods. Electrons (negatively charged particles in an atom) are removed from one atom, resulting in "oxidation" of this first atom, and then are added or transferred to another atom, resulting in "reduction" of this second atom. This continual process of energy metabolism is actually a flow of electrons, or a minute electrical current within the cell.

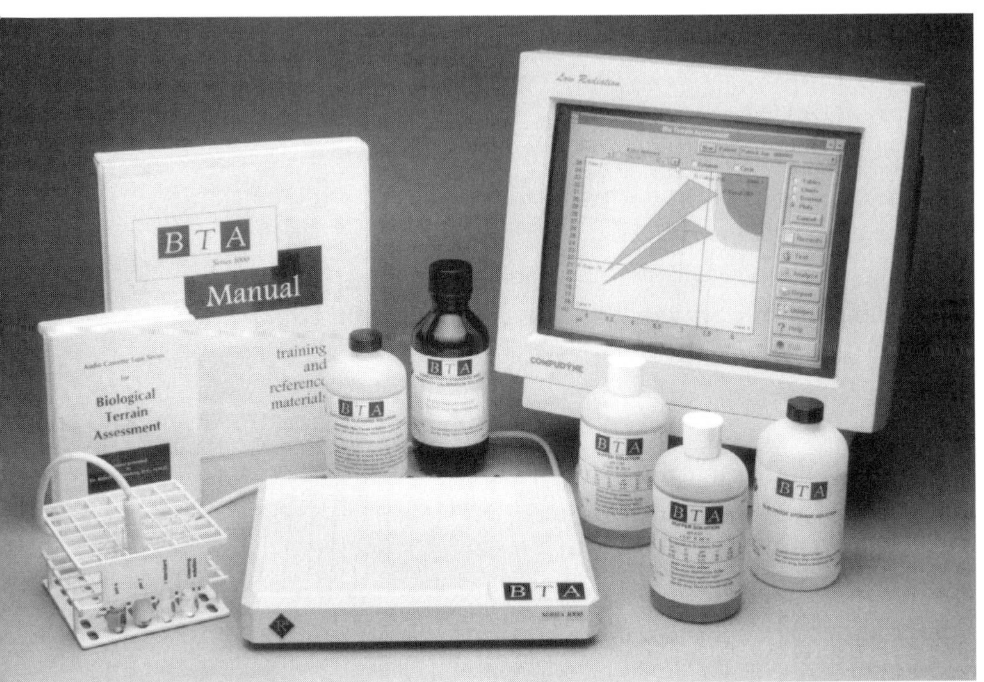


**The Biological Terrain Assessment unit analyzes blood, urine, and saliva samples and displays information about an individual's cellular health on its monitor.**

because the blood's pH level is very tightly controlled; however, both measures together, along with salivary pH, give a more complete picture of the body's chemical balance.

Oxidation-reduction potential (abbreviated as redox) refers to the degree of "oxidative stress" on the body, or how much free-radical burden (oxidation of tissues) the body is exposed to. "Because of the effects of stress, poor air, poor food quality, and lack of aerobic exercise typical of most Americans, these values are generally much lower than they should be to sustain a healthy body," says Dr. Greenberg. "If the values remain low for extended periods of time, the person will be more susceptible to cancer and other illnesses."

The third factor, resistivity, is a measure of a tissue's resistance to the flow of electrical current, as opposed to conductivity which indicates the ability to transmit or conduct electrical current through a cell, nerve, or muscle. With low resistivity (high conductivity), there is typically a congestion or buildup of mineral salts. High resistivity (low conductivity) means a lack of minerals, which indicates the need to further evaluate the individual for specific deficiencies of these vital elements.

The BTA analysis is carried out in only 10 minutes by a computerized device called a BTA S-1000. The device uses a pen-shaped microelectrode to determine pH, resistivity, and redox values in blood, saliva, and urine. A sample of blood (0.5 ml) and saliva (0.5 ml), and first morning urine is obtained following a 12-14 hour fast. If a person eats an acid-producing, alkaline-producing, salty, or antioxidant food just before the BTA, the testing reflects more about the ingested food than the body's baseline condition.

"Urine is a good indicator of the body's secretory ability and toxic load on cells," says Dr. Greenberg. "Blood is a good indicator of toxicity and oxygen balance, while saliva offers insight into a person's digestive capacities." Taken together and analyzed by means of the BTA S-1000, Eames claims that these measures provide a benchmark for determining whether or not someone is getting healthier or sicker.

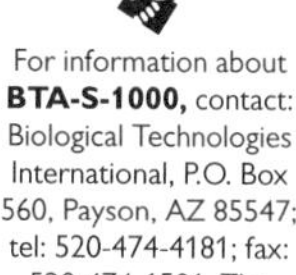

For information about **BTA-S-1000,** contact: Biological Technologies International, P.O. Box 560, Payson, AZ 85547; tel: 520-474-4181; fax: 520-474-1501. The approximate cost of the equipment is $10,550.

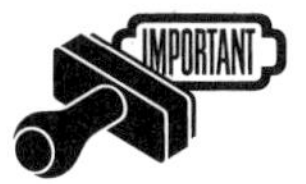


For cancer patients, the test provides insight that can guide the physician in redirecting biochemical parameters in the patient, using nutrition, botanical medicines, exercise, and other approaches. "The goal is to move the body toward the optimal benchmark, which is the same regardless of age, weight, and sex," says Dr. Greenberg. "We find that people who attain these benchmarks seem capable of maintaining sound health indefinitely."

The therapeutic approach indicated by BTA findings will vary greatly from one cancer patient to the next, and even for people with the same type and stage of cancer. "When the patient's body chemistry is balanced and maintained with a healthy diet, proper vitamin and mineral supplementation, adequate amounts of exercise and rest, the body can remain healthy and nourish a vibrant immune system to protect and sustain it. The BTA may uncover inadequate enzymatic secretions in one person and chronic and degenerative stress in another. As a result, they are placed on different nutritional and lifestyle modification programs and require unique nutritional support or therapies."

Many patients who undergo a BTA came into their doctor's offices with reports of "normal" laboratory values, based on the CBC and other standard tests. Yet these same individuals *display* illness both objectively and subjectively, even though their standard blood results do not show it. "Often potent influences exist within the patient's system which can include pollutants, environmental poisons, parasites, viruses, fungi, invasive microbes, lack of adequate vitamins and minerals, lack of oxygen, and excessive carbon dioxide," says Dr. Greenberg. Most standard laboratory tests are incapable of detecting these elements and, as a result, many patients remain sick; meanwhile, their doctors contend that nothing more can be done, and thus advanced cancer patients frequently find themselves written off as terminal.

In our clinical practice, we the authors have found BTA to be a highly useful tool for determining general susceptibility to cancer as well as for helping assess changes that need to be made in the course of the treatment program.

### The CBC Blood Test Report

## Reading Health Status in the Blood

Whether you are a conventional physician, naturopath, or chiropractor—or their patient—knowing as much as possible about the biochemical status of a person is an invaluable guide to developing the most effective, individually tailored supplement program. With this in mind, in 1985, Mark A. Schauss developed a new method for making optimum, practical use of information revealed by the standard blood test.

Now, through his Carbon Based Corporation, the CBC Blood Test Report inexpensively offers both doctors and patients several user-friendly formulations of blood test analysis information, opening "a therapeutic window" to one's unique biochemistry, says Schauss. It also empowers patients to take more control of their health care by being able to make more informed decisions. According to CBC medical director Patricia Kane, Ph.D., the CBC Blood Test Report can "depict a patient's potential disease patterns, i.e., whether abnormalities in their blood indicate a predisposition toward a certain disease. On the lookout for that disease, a physician can further investigate, perhaps stopping the disease before it strikes. By predicting these patterns, the test offers a new outlook toward *preventive* medicine."

For more information about the **CBC Blood Test Report,** contact: Carbon Based Corporation, 153 Country Club Drive, Suite 5, Incline Village, NV 89451; tel: 702-832-8485; fax: 702-832-8488.

The Basic Status Report alphabetically lists the amounts detected of about 44 substances normally found in the blood. But it also ranks these items, such as cholesterol, lymphocytes, sodium, and bilirubin, according to their relative deviation from the mean. Schauss calls this ranking "% Status:" this demonstrates by what percentage the client's readings are higher or lower than a statistical norm.

For example, normal sodium levels range from 135 to 145, so a one-point deviation is substantial as there are only 10 points for normalcy, Schauss explains. On the other hand, normal triglycerides range from 0-250 so a one-point change here is not significant. The idea is to provide a statistical context and normative comparison for the tests results as measured against agreed-upon standards of what's normal, Schauss says. The analysis also offers a Panel Report. This groups the results according to 14 biochemical functions, such as electrolytes, kidney function, acid or alkaline pH, nitrogen and protein. "You can review each of the panels at a glance for an unbalanced pattern in your patient's blood chemistry," says Schauss.

A particularly innovative feature is the Disease Indicators Report, in which the total blood status is compared with the known indicators of any of 140 diseases. Here, known disease patterns, as revealed in a blood analysis, are correlated with the individual's results. For example, the test might indicate a 62.5% match for myasthenia gravis, a 40% match for folic acid deficiency, and a 33.33% match for angina pectoris. This is *preventive* information of high value.

The Drug Interactions Report identifies potentially aggravating effects if the patient were to use any of hundreds of conventional drugs. For example, if one's total bilirubin is out of balance, the use of aspirin, pencillin, niacin, streptomycin, among many others, is contraindicated because these would further the imbalance. Finally, the Biochemical Pharmacology Report suggests which supplements are indicated for the given abnormal blood chemistry; the exact dosages are left to a physician to determine. Carbon Based Corporation delivers the 5-part report to clients within 2-36 hours (although 48-72 hours is standard) at a cost to practitioners of about $100, including blood test fees.

## Tests That Enable You to Know Your Heavy Metals Toxicity Levels

Increasingly, practitioners of alternative medicine find that low-level but chronic exposure to a variety of toxic heavy metals pose serious health dangers if the metals are allowed to stay in the body. These toxins are now commonly found in our food, water, and air, as well as cooking utensils, cosmetics, auto exhaust, tobacco smoke, and many of the building materials and fabrics in our work and living environments, pesticides in our foods, and dental materials in our teeth (mercury fillings).

Typical symptoms of heavy metal toxicity can include nervous system disorders, depression, fatigue, skin rashes, high blood pressure, hyperactivity, nausea, irritability, headaches, and more serious conditions including autism, intelligence deficits, and cancer. But before you can remove heavy metals from a person, you need first to determine which ones are present and in what amounts.

## Maverick Monitoring Test

If you suspect toxicity as a contributing factor in cancer, first you must identify the toxins, explains Hildegarde A. Staninger, Ph.D., medical director of Sunstate Preventive Medicine Institute in Winter Park, Florida. Dr. Staninger is one of the country's experts in industrial toxicology, which uses a laboratory-based approach that enables physicians to quantify the level of dangerous toxic chemicals absorbed into a patient's bloodstream or tissues through external exposure.

To test for the damage level of toxin activity, Dr. Staninger relies on the Maverick Monitoring Test (MMT), an innovative protocol she developed to measure body levels of toxic agents that create harmful free radicals. These measures provide scientifically based indications for treatment.

The Maverick Monitoring Test is actually a nontechnical name for a test to measure malondialdehyde (MDA) levels, the chemical end result of heightened free radical activity and cellular damage, the oxidation of lipids (fats), and an irregular combination of fats and proteins. Maverick determines how much MDA is present in the patient's body by analyzing urine or a blood sample. If necessary, Maverick can screen for up to 22 related chemical compounds.

For information on **Maverick**, contact: Hildegarde L. A. Staninger, Ph.D., Sunstate Preventive Medicine Institute, 2699 Lee Road, Suite 303, Winter Park, FL 32789; tel: 407-628-3399; fax: 407-628-1061. For information on **ToxMet**, contact: MetaMetrix Medical Laboratory, 5000 Peachtree Industrial Blvd., Suite 110, Norcross, GA 30071; tel: 770-446-5483 or 800-221-4640; fax: 770-441-2237.

Maverick specifically looks at the compounds normally inside a cell that, when the cell wall is broken down and the compounds interact with substances outside the cell, will cause free radical pathology. "This is what starts disease," Dr. Staninger explains. "It ends with the death of the cell." The amount of MDA tells the physician how much free-radical damage the body has sustained; it can also indicate how well the patient is responding to a nutritional antioxidant program, based on how much MDA levels decreased.

The screen, which costs $56, can also measure the effects of chemotherapy and radiation and then determine the best dosages of antioxidants to counteract these effects. Even better, "Maverick detects a potential health problem *before* it occurs," says Dr. Staninger. Maverick does not diagnose a specific disease; rather, it highlights the possible *preconditions*, in terms of free-radical activity, that may lead to or already be contributing to an illness.

### ToxMet Screen

The ToxMet screen from MetaMetrix Medical Laboratory provides an inexpensive but detailed analysis of the levels of specific heavy metals in a patient's system, based on a urine sample. The test typically costs about $100 and is ordered by a physician.

ToxMet tests for levels of 4 highly toxic heavy metals, including arsenic, cadmium, lead, and mercury; it also reports on levels for 10 potentially toxic elements, such as aluminum, bismuth, boron, nickel, and strontium. Finally, information is gathered on a patient's status regarding 14 essential metals and minerals, such as copper, calcium, chromium, molybdenum, selenium, and vanadium.When tests results exceed limits believed to be safe, the report indicates a "high" concentration. For example, one patient was high in arsenic (65 units compared to a high limit of 40) and cadmium (3.7 compared to the limit of 2). ToxMet also indicated that this patient had high levels of calcium, magnesium, manganese, and zinc.

On the basis of this information, a physician is able to develop an individualized nutritional prescription and detoxification program to both eliminate the toxic metals from the system and to rebalance the amounts of essential nutrients. A preventive intervention such as this is both wise and practical; when you can see the potential for illness in a metal toxicity or imbalance, you can take immediate steps to prevent this from developing into a serious health problem.

## Laboratory Tests That Measure Antioxidant Protection

### Individualized Optimal Nutrition

The comprehensive information provided by Metametrix's ION (Individualized Optimal Nutrition) Panel can be used preventively to catch imbalances and potential illness in their earliest stages. ION, which measures 150 biochemical components, is also highly useful for physicians who need detailed biochemical assessment, based on a blood and urine sample, of patients who might already have cancer, chronic fatigue, or other immune disorders, heart disease, learning difficulties, obesity, or multiple chemical sensitivities.

Specifically, ION checks for nutritional status in categories including vitamins, minerals, amino acids, fatty and organic acids, lipid peroxides, general blood chemistries (cholesterol, thyroid hormone, glucose), and antioxidants. In each category, a patient's levels are compared with predetermined limits. In one patient, phenylalanine concentration was 47 units compared to the accepted range of 55-140; her tryptophan was also low at 16 compared to the range of 20-60. In the 10 essential amino acid derivatives, this patient tested out of range on taurine, at 48, instead of 50-250.

Based on the individual's test results, ION can provide supplement recommendations. For the antioxidant panel, for example, ION provides the precisely tailored blend of 16 substances from coenzyme Q10 and copper citrate to beta carotene and vitamin C. Finally, ION summarizes the test results into 9 categories according to disease risk, such as cardiovascular, liver function, intestinal balance, energy, digestive disorders, and thyroid status. In each case, an individual's biochemical status is contrasted against a healthy norm. The total ION test of 7 panels typically costs between $600 and $1000, although individual panels may be ordered.

## Oxidative Protection Screen

Introduced in November 1995, the Oxidative Protection Screen from Antibody Assay Laboratories of Santa Ana, California, can provide your physician with an actual biochemical analysis of how well your body is handling free radicals. This information, in turn, is valuable for a physician in assessing a patient's overall health, the degree of antioxidant "protection" one has, and the possible need for further nutrient supplementation. The test cost to patients is about $96.

When lipids (fatty acids, steroids, and other oily organic compounds) are damaged by free radicals, they form lipid peroxides which circulate in the blood. Using a drawn blood sample from a patient, the lab test determines the amount of lipid peroxides in the plasma; these numbers vary with age and gender. For a 20-year-old woman, for example, the normal range is 1.5-1.99 micromole/liter but for a 60-year-old female, it is 2.15-2.82 micromole/l. An elevated amount, beyond this range, indicates a high production of free radicals, while the lower the amount of lipid peroxides, the stronger the antioxidant protection.

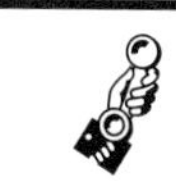

**Oxidative Protection Screen** must be ordered by a licensed health-care practitioner. For information, contact: Antibody Assay Laboratories, 1715 E. Wilshire, #715, Santa Ana, CA 92705; tel: 714-972-9979 or 800-522-2611; fax: 714-543-2034. **The Pantox Antioxidant Profile** also must be ordered by a physician. Contact: Pantox Laboratories, 4622 Santa Fe Street, San Diego, CA 92109; tel: 800-PANTOX 6, 619-272-3885, or 800-726-8696; fax: 619-272-1621. For more information about **ION**, contact: MetaMetrix Medical Laboratory, 5000 Peachtree Industrial Blvd., Suite 110, Norcross, GA 30071; tel: 770-446-5483 or 800-221-4640; fax: 770-441-2237.

The Total Oxidative Protection Index™ will indicate your system's overall ability to withstand the "attack" of free radicals and thus your individual degree of oxidative protection. The normal range here is 45-63%; ranges above 63% indicate a high degree of antioxidant protection and health.

## The Pantox Antioxidant Profile

Based on a blood sample of 5 ml, this diagnostic screen measures the status of 20 factors determining the body's antioxidant cellular defense system, in comparison with a database of 4,000 other normal and healthy profiles. On the basis of this precise biochemical information, both physicians and patients can take nutritional steps to prevent disease from developing. The test cost to patients is $250 prepaid and is reimbursable by almost all insurance companies, Medicare assignments, and managed-care groups.

Specifically, the screen reports on the biochemical presence of lipoproteins (cholesterol, triglycerides), fat-soluble antioxidants (vitamins A and E, carotenoids, coenzyme Q10), water-soluble antioxidants (vitamin C, uric acid, bilirubin), and iron balance. The test helps answer the question: are you getting the *right* antioxidants in the *correct* amounts? The Pantox profile is displayed in bar graphs with accompanying explanatory medical text, telling you if your levels of a specific nutrient are low and pose a health risk.

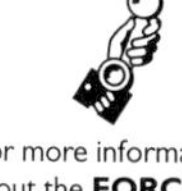

For more information about the **FORCYTE Cancer Prognostic System**, contact: Dianon Systems, 200 Watson Boulevard, Stratford, CT 06497; tel: 800-328-2666 or 203-381-4000; actual lab tests are performed by Cytology Technology, Inc., 8058 El Rio, Houston, TX 77054; tel: 713-748-6800.

It is important to realize that just because you consume a nutrient, does not mean your body has assimiliated it and that it is present and active in your bloodstream. Stress produced by the heightened activity of free radicals can seriously deplete your reserves of antioxidants, despite a healthy diet and imprecise nutritional supplementation, explains Pantox Laboratories Director Charles A. Thomas, Jr., Ph.D. The practical goal, says Dr. Thomas, is for "an individual to take steps to change one's levels so as to join others who are experiencing a *lower* rate of degenerative diseases."

## The FORCYTE Cancer Prognostic System

### Assessing the Details of a Tumor

Starting with a surgical or fine needle biopsy specimen of a tumor, the FORCYTE Cancer Prognostic System provides the oncologist with information useful in making predictions about treatment outcome. The FORCYTE system creates a subcellular portrait of a tumor by way of a 3-dimensional multiparameter histogram. These parameters include information about cell subpopulations, their respective cell cycle phase, and DNA synthesis rate (or cell size).

More specifically, the histogram displays information about G1 diploid cells, G1 tumor cells, S-phase cells, and S-cycling and S-noncycling cells, a cell subpopulation that tends to be highly resistant to conventional therapies. FORCYTE provides objective indicators closely related to actual tumor cell activity with which a physician can decide which kind of treatment will be most effective.

***"What is unique about the T and Tn antibody test is that it enables detection of the majority of cancers before any biopsy can pick up the presence of cancer," says Dr. Springer.***

## Dr. Georg Springer's T/Tn Antigen Test

Georg Springer, M.D., an immunologist who founded the Heather Bligh Cancer Research Laboratories at the Chicago Medical School, uncovered evidence that certain proteins (antigens) on the surface of blood and skin cells can be identified by the immune system (antibodies). Dr. Springer recognized that the T and Tn antigens are specifically associated with cancers of all kinds and that the T and Tn antigens are found in places where cancer has spread but not in benign breast tumors.[80]

Dr. Springer further discovered that the concentration of T and Tn correlates with the aggressiveness of the breast cancer.[81] In other words, the T and Tn antigens serve as specific markers for the presence of cancer; in the case of breast cancer, the more markers, the more advanced or aggressive the cancer. "What is unique about the T and Tn antibody test is that it enables detection of the majority of cancers before any biopsy can pick up the presence of cancer," says Dr. Springer. "We find that people without any previous cancer, who show positive test results, consistently develop cancer later on."

In general, the less aggressive cancers produce a higher proportion of T than Tn antigens, while Tn predominates in more aggressive primary cancers. The relative concentrations of these antigens, however, will vary depending on the cancer type and stage. For example, an association between the T antigen and human colon cancer with metastasis to the liver has been found;[82] this antigen is also an indicator marking the recurrence of bladder cancer.[83] In contrast, uterine cancer with metastasis has shown a closer relationship with the Tn antigen concentration,[84] yet, as Dr. Springer notes, both T and Tn antigens may be elevated in cancers of the lung, ovary, pancreas, and colon.[85]

***It is important to realize that just because you consume a nutrient, does not mean your body has assimilated it and that it is present and active in your bloodstream. Stress produced by the heightened activity of free radicals can seriously deplete your reserves of antioxidants, despite a healthy diet and imprecise nutritional supplementation.***

The identification of these T and Tn antigens enabled Dr. Springer to develop a skin-prick test to predict or indicate the likely future development of breast and other cancers. The test result, which is determined 1-2 days later, is positive when an area of skin greater than 4 mm turns reddish and hardens. Dr. Springer's skin-prick test depends on the body's "delayed hypersensitivity reaction" to the injected antigens, meaning it takes the body some time to "decide" how it will react to these foreign proteins.

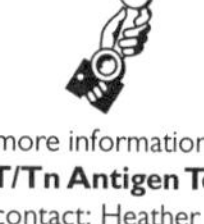

For more information on the **T/Tn Antigen Test**, contact: Heather Margaret Bligh Cancer Research Laboratories, Georg F. Springer, M.D., Director, Finch University of Health Sciences, The Chicago Medical School, 3333 Green Bay Road, North Chicago, IL 60064; tel: 847-578-3435; fax: 847-578-3432.

If a person tests positive, there is delayed immunity which means these antigens are already present in the body, causing the immune reaction to an existing cancer to be present unless the person has had the skin test performed before. In this case, the present positive skin test may be only a memory reaction to the previous skin antigen application.

In a study of T/Tn antigen test, positive test results occurred in the following:

- 94% of lung cancer patients (15 out of 16 people)

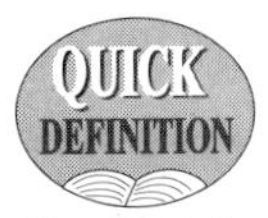


A **lymphocyte** is a form of white blood cell, representing 25-33% of the total count, whose numbers increase during infection. Lymphocytes, produced in the bone marrow, come in two forms: T cells, which are matured in the thymus gland (behind the breastbone) and have many functions in the body's immune response; and B-cells, which produce antibodies to neutralize an antigen (foreign and potentially dangerous matter in the blood). Each B-cell produces a single and specific antibody.

- 80% of breast cancer patients (20 out of 25 people)
- 7% of patients with benign (nonmalignant) tumors (26 out of 349 patients)
- 0% of healthy people (0 out of 148 people) in the control group.[86]

A delayed skin reaction to T and Tn antigen does not occur in healthy people, but is usually found to be highly typical among cancer patients, where it indicates a sluggish or dysfunctional immune system.

Dr. Springer's skin-prick/blood test can predict the onset of cancer, on average, 6 years in advance of other tests, and sometimes as much as 10 years. "We have shown that 78% of patients with preclinical breast lesions [benign tumors] showed positive tests months to years before their biopsy or X ray turned positive [malignant]," says Dr. Springer.[87] Dr. Springer found that 84% of 506 patients with a variety of cancers of all stages reacted positively and that the test could detect preclinical cancers with 90% accuracy.[88] Based on these small numbers of patients assessed thus far, the skin-prick test for cancer is extremely sensitive and specific.

## Lymphocyte Size Analysis

Russian immunologist Valentin Govallo, M.D., recognized that lymphocytes, or white blood cells, could be classified as either normal or enlarged. Lymphocytes tend to swell and increase in size among cancer patients compared to healthy people. Using a microscope, you can measure the diameters of lymphocytes and count the numbers of swollen versus normal cells in a sample of a patient's blood. Dr. Govallo calls this a "lymphocytogram." If the number of swollen lymphocytes is excessive, then cancer will most likely develop. The test's diagnostic accuracy for various types of cancer is 90%.[89] Dr. Govallo states that lymphocyte diameters vary within broad limits among individuals. In healthy, noncancerous individuals, about 25% of the lymphocytes are small (7-7.5 microns in diameter) which means the ratio of large to small lymphoctes is 3:1. According to Dr. Govallo, the ratio quickly shifts to 6:1, 7:1, or greater, among cancer patients—even

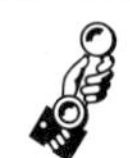

For more about **Dr. Govallo's approach**, contact: People Against Cancer, Box 10, Otho, IA 50569; tel: 515-972-4444. Also contact: Dr. Coulter about licensing VG-1000 for other locales: Harris L. Coulter, Ph.D., Empirical Therapies, Inc., 4221 45th Street, N.W., Washington, D.C. 20016; tel: 202-362-3185 or 202-364-0898; fax: 202-362-3407.

among those who have not yet developed overt signs of cancer, such as palpable tumors.

In cancer patients who have developed visible tumors or who are predisposed to developing a tumor, small lymphocytes practically disappear from the blood whereas the number of enlarged lymphocytes increases dramatically. After observing many cancer patients and measuring their ratios of swollen to normal lymphocytes, Dr. Govallo concludes: "When this ratio is out of balance, the patient *will* develop cancer. It is only a matter of time."

For information about **lymphocyte treatment**, see Chapter 31: New Approaches to Immune Stimulation, pp. 886-888.

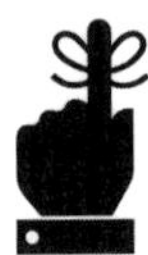

*Given the right*

*combination of therapy*

*and prevention, far*

*more people can survive*

*cancer and live*

*long, productive*

*lives than*

*conventional cancer*

*experts would*

*ever deem possible.*

# *Part Three*

# A Complete Guide to Innovative Approaches to Cancer Treatment

## *Nutrition, Botanicals, New Pharmacologicals, Immune Stimulators, Metabolic Factors, Physical and Energy Support Therapies*

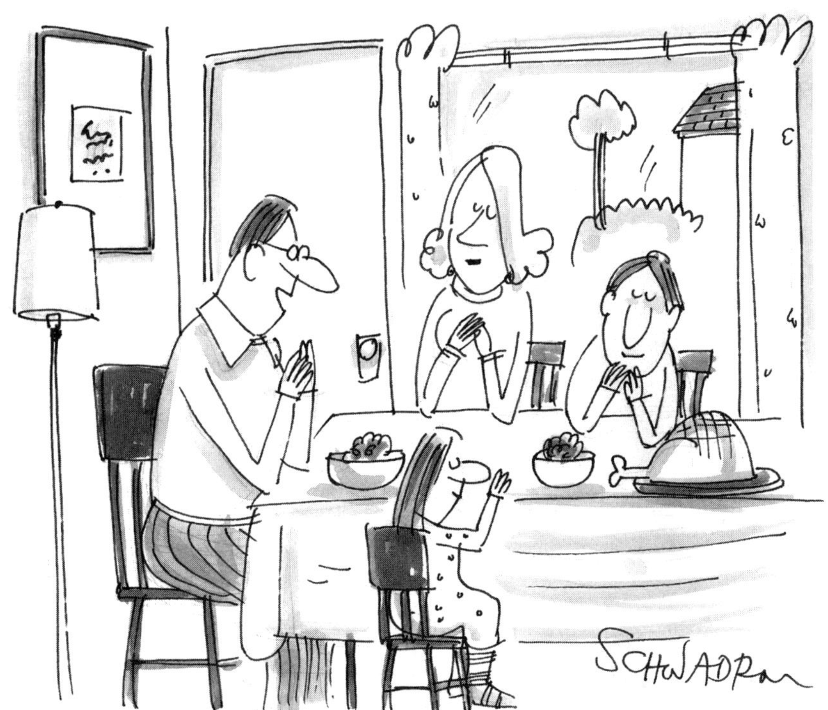


"BLESS THIS FOOD, AND PROTECT US FROM THE PESTICIDES AND ADDITIVES THEREIN."

Chapter 28

# Nutrition As Cancer Medicine

## *A Complete Guide to Dietary Changes and Anticancer Nutritional Supplements*

**Nutrient deficiencies, which are prevalent today, can contribute to an overall weakening of the body and its immune defenses, making a person more vulnerable to cancer onset. This is why nearly all alternative cancer physicians use nutritional supplementation as a frontline approach in treating cancer, most often combining several dozen substances in a complete nutritional package.**

As the numerous physicians in this book have explained, diet and nutrition both are at the core of cancer etiology and its successful treatment. The leading nutritional problem in the United States today is "overconsumptive undernutrition," or the eating of too many empty-calorie foods, says Jeffrey Bland, Ph.D., a biochemist and nutrition expert. Studies have concluded that almost two-thirds of an average American's diet is made up of fats and refined sugars, and thus have low or no micronutrient density.

Consequently, the remaining one-third of the average diet is counted on for 100% of the essential nutrients needed to maintain health. This contributes to nutrient deficiencies that can rob the body of its natural resistance to disease and promote premature aging while weakening its overall physiological performance.

The United States Department of Agriculture found that a significant percentage of the population receives under 70% of the RDA for vitamins A, C, and B-complex, and the essential minerals calcium, magnesium, and iron.[1] A separate study found that most diets contain less than 80% of the RDA for calcium, magnesium, iron, zinc, copper, and manganese, and that the people most at nutritional risk are young children and women from adolescence to old age.

While a cumulative lack of essential nutrients can contribute to illness, including cancer, the correct fortification with these nutrients can start reversing chronic conditions. However, it is important to appreciate that nutrients work together and act according to various biochemical relationships.

Vitamins and minerals help regulate the conversion of food to energy in the body, explains Dr. Bland. As such, they can be separated into 2 general categories: energy nutrients, which are principally involved in the conversion of food to energy; and protector nutrients, which help defend against damaging toxins derived from drugs, alcohol, radiation, environmental pollutants, or the body's own enzyme processes. "The B-complex vitamins and magnesium are examples of energy nutrients because they activate specific metabolic facilitators called enzymes, which control digestion and the absorption and use of proteins, fats, and carbohydrates. These nutrients often work as a *team*, their mutual presence enhancing the other's function."

In the process of converting food to energy, free radicals are produced that can damage the body and set the stage for degenerative diseases, including cancer, arthritis, heart disease, and premature aging. Protector nutrients such as vitamin E, beta carotene (a nutrient from which vitamin A is made), vitamin C, and the minerals zinc, copper, manganese, and selenium, play a critical role in preventing or delaying these degenerative processes.

Vitamins and minerals in effect "drive" the biochemical and electrical circuitry of the body. The body's functioning is therefore profoundly affected by how nutrients either work together or against each other. Nutrients taken simultaneously can inhibit each other. Iron, for example, is best absorbed when taken separately from pancreatic enzymes and should also not be taken with vitamin E.

### Nutritional Substances and Therapies Covered in This Chapter

- *Acidophilus* (the *Lactobacilli* family)
- Amino acids
- Beta carotene
- Calcium
- Chromium
- Coenzyme Q10
- Copper
- Eicosapentenoic acid (EPA fish oils)
- Flaxseed oil
- Gamma linolenic acid (GLA)
- Germanium
- Gerson Diet Therapy
- Inositol
- Iodine
- Kelley's Metabolic Therapy
- Manganese
- Molybdenum
- Orthomolecular Medicine
- Potassium
- Selenium
- Vitamin A
- Vitamin B complex
- Vitamin B3 (niacin)
- Vitamin B6 (pyridoxine)
- Vitamin C (ascorbic acid)
- Vitamin D
- Vitamin E
- Vitamin K
- Water
- Zinc

> **Nutritional Rating of Americans**
>
> A new Healthy Eating Index study of 4,000 Americans, conducted by the U.S. Department of Agriculture, reveals that 88% of the population does not get good grades for proper nutrition. More than 80% eat too much saturated fat and too little fruits, vegetables, and fiber-rich grains. The worst eaters are aged 15-39. Overall, the American diet of the 1990s achieves only 63% of what the USDA considers good nutrition.

There are also nutrients that enhance the effects of other nutrients. For example, vitamin C taken with iron facilitates the maximum absorption of the iron. Similarly, clinical studies have shown a relationship between low intakes of beta carotene (pro-vitamin A), vitamin E, and vitamin C and higher incidences of cancer.[2] Robert Cathcart, M.D., has documented the effective use of vitamin C in treating various infectious diseases, including the common cold, flu, pneumonia, and hepatitis, among other infectious disorders;[3] infection among cancer patients is a common cause of death.

In addition to disease control, specific nutrients can help people cope with specific lifestyle, environmental, and emotional/psychological factors. For example, when recovering from cancer surgery, a person may need higher levels of zinc;[4] individuals who are exposed to smog or other pollutants require higher levels of the protector nutrients such as selenium, vitamin E, and vitamin C;[5] and anyone under heavy emotional or physical stress, typical of the cancer experience, will need higher intakes of all the B vitamins.[6]

## Benefits of a Whole-Foods, Mainly Vegetarian Diet

In light of this knowledge of nutrition and its specificity, there are 2 primary ways to gain the needed nutrients: through a carefully constructed diet or through an equally specific nutrient supplementation program. We'll consider the merits of improving the diet first.

A whole-foods diet promotes health by decreasing fat and sugar intake and by increasing the consumption of fiber and nutrients, particularly the numerous antioxidants and other phytochemicals ("phyto" means plant) that have been identified as beneficial anticancer nutrients. Fiber is found in plant foods, such as brown rice, broccoli, oatmeal, or almonds but not in animal products like meat, cheese, milk, eggs, and butter. Fiber is the transport system of the digestive tract, moving or "sweeping" food wastes out of the body before they have a chance to form potentially cancer-causing and mutagenic chemicals. These toxic chemicals can cause colon cancer or pass through the gastrointestinal membrane into the bloodstream and damage other cells.

A vegetable-based, whole-foods diet is typically much lower in fat. On a percentage-of-calories basis, most vegetables contain less than 10% fat and most grains contain from 16-20% fat; by comparison, whole milk and cheese contain 74% fat; a rib roast is 75% fat; eggs are 64% fat; low-fat milk or a skinned, baked chicken breast still has 38% fat. Not only do animal foods have more fat, but most of these fats are saturated, which research has shown raises blood cholesterol levels. A low-fat, whole-foods diet also means fewer calories, since an ounce of fat contains twice as many calories as an ounce of complex carbohydrates (as found in vegetables). Studies have shown that a diet containing fewer calories is associated with reduced DNA damage, thus lowering cancer risks and increasing longevity.[7]

**Lipid** is a biochemist's term for a fat, which is one of the 6 basic food groups. Fats and oils are made of building blocks called fatty acids. Of these long-chain molecules (comprising atoms of carbon, hydrogen, and oxygen) the "fatty" end does not dissolve in water, while the "acid" end does. Fats are also called triglycerides as they consist of 3 (tri) fatty acid molecules joined to one molecule of glycerol, a kind of sugar. Unsaturated fats required in the diet are called **essential fatty acids**, and include linoleic or gamma-linolenic acid (omega-6 oils), found in corn and beans, and in many seeds, nuts, and grains; and alpha linolenic acid or eicosapentanoic acid (omega-3 oils), found in fish, flaxseeds, and walnuts.

Plant foods are richer sources of micronutrients than their animal counterparts. Compare wheat germ to round steak: ounce for ounce, wheat germ contains twice the vitamin B2, vitamin K, potassium, iron, and copper; 3 times the vitamin B6, molybdenum, and selenium; 15 times as much magnesium; and over 20 times the vitamin B1, folate, and inositol. The steak contains only 3 micronutrients in greater amounts: B12, chromium. and zinc.

These differences have practical ramifications. Eating more nutrient-dense plant foods tends to decrease one's desire to consume processed sugars; lower sugar consumption then decreases overall calorie intake. At the same time, the extra nutrients increase our protection against cancer. A cup of broccoli, for example, provides 70 mg of vitamin C, more than any other vegetable except green peppers; vitamin C blocks the formation of cancer initiators called nitrosamines and may also keep cancer cells from growing into deadly tumors. Broccoli contains more fiber and calcium on a per gram basis than most other vegetables, which may account for its protective effects against colon cancer. It is also a rich source of folate, a B vitamin that seems to protect against cervical cancer, and of beta carotene, the famous plant pigment that probably helps fight lung cancer in the *early* phases of development.

In fact, among individual vegetables, broccoli may offer particularly strong anticancer potential. In a study of the diets of 1,200 people over 66 years old, those people who consumed the most green vegetables had a significantly lower cancer risk than those who ate the least; people who ate broccoli less than once a week had increased their risk of developing cancer by 20%.[8] In a second study, 2 groups of rats were fed organically grown broccoli, which made up either 10% or 25% of their diet; a third group received no broccoli.[9] All 3 groups were then exposed to the carcinogenic chemical, benzopyrene. Upon measuring levels of liver enzymes that stop benzopyrene from causing cancer, the researchers found the broccoli-fed rats had significantly more than the non-broccoli-fed rats.

There are compelling reasons for adopting a more plant-based diet. First, important antioxidant nutrients, including vitamin C, beta carotene, vitamin E, and many cancer-fighting substances known as phytochemicals, are found in fruits, vegetables, and grains. These antioxidant nutrients are considered the best *protection* against cancer and other environmental-related diseases. As mentioned above, the high-fiber content of plant foods helps keep the digestive tract clean by absorbing and eliminating many potentially dangerous toxins.

A primarily vegetarian diet will not only tend to keep the body less burdened by toxins, but it will directly support the body's anticancer defenses. A landmark study of vegetarians was conducted by researchers at the Institute for Experimental Pathology, German Cancer Research Center, in Heidelberg, Germany.[10] The blood from a group of male vegetarians was drawn and compared to the blood from a group of male, age-matched nonvegetarians.

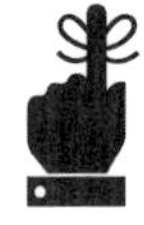

The researchers proposed that "the enhanced natural cytotoxicity may be one of the factors contributing to the lower cancer risk shown by vegetarians."[11]

The vegetarians' blood contained significantly higher levels of carotenes, creatinine and an enzyme called glutamine-transferase. Carotenes are components of vitamin A (as in beta carotene), while creatinine is a substance found in the urine as a result of creatine metabolism, related to muscle activity. At the same time, the vegetarians' natural killer (NK) cell activity was twice as high as the meat eaters' NK cell activity. NK cells are among the immune system's prime cancer-fighting cells.

### A Quick Review of Nutritional Factors in Reversing Cancer

**Beta carotene**—The precursor of vitamin A, beta carotene is found in carrots, sweet potatoes, spinach, and most leafy green vegetables. A diet high in carotenes, especially beta carotene, is protective against all cancers but beta carotene is particularly important for women as a deterrent to cervical cancer.[12] Beta carotene has also been shown to protect the lungs against tobacco smoke and smog, thus inhibiting the development of lung cancer.[13] Ex-smokers who ate green and yellow vegetables high in beta carotene every day decreased their risk of stomach and lung cancer.[14]

## Longevity and a Vegetarian Diet

Vegetarians live longer than meat eaters, concludes the British Medical Association. Vegetarians have a 28% lower risk of dying from heart disease and a 39% reduced chance of dying from cancer, according to a 12-year research program involving 5,000 British meat eaters and 6,100 vegetarians.

**Vitamin B6**—Found in bananas, leafy green vegetables, carrots, apples, organ meats, and sweet potatoes, vitamin B6 is essential for maintaining optimal immune function and also helps maintain the health of the mucous membranes, which line the respiratory tract and provide a natural barrier to pollution and infection. Vitamin B6 also affords valuable protection against cervical cancer.[15]

***A landmark German study found that vegetarians' natural killer (NK) cell activity was twice as high as the meat eaters' NK cell activity. NK cells are among the immune system's prime cancer-fighting cells.***

**Vitamin C**—Found in citrus fruits, cantaloupe, broccoli, green peppers, and many other fruits and vegetables, vitamin C is integrally involved in the maintenance of a healthy immune system, as well as protecting against a variety of cancers.[16]

**Vitamin E**—Found in dark green vegetables, eggs, wheat germ, liver, unrefined vegetable oils, and some herbs, vitamin E is a powerful antioxidant that can directly reduce the damage done by ozone and other substances found in smog. It can also help protect against bowel cancer.[17]

**Selenium**—An essential trace mineral found in fruits and vegetables, selenium helps the body produce glutathione, an enzyme essential for detoxification. Low dietary levels of selenium have been correlated with higher incidence of cancer; accordingly, supplementation of this nutrient acts as a deterrent against cancer in general.[18]

**Folic Acid**—This substance protects against cervical cancer in particular, and is necessary for proper synthesis of RNA and DNA. It is found in beets, cabbage, dark leafy vegetables, eggs, dairy products, citrus fruits, and most fish.[19]

**Calcium**—This mineral protects against colon cancer and is vital for proper bone and tooth formation, blood clotting, and cellular metabolism.[20] It is found in dark green vegetables, most nuts and seeds, milk products, sardines, and salmon.

**Iodine**—Available in seafood and sea vegetables such as kelp, dulse, and iodized salt, iodine protects against breast cancer and is needed for proper energy metabolism as well as the growth and repair of all tissues.[21]

**Magnesium**—Found in most nuts, fish, green vegetables, whole grains, and brown rice, magnesium protects against cancer in general and is necessary to maintain the pH balance of blood and tissue, as well as the synthesis of RNA and DNA.[22]

**Zinc**—This mineral protects against prostate cancer and is necessary for the formation of RNA and DNA, as well as for healthy immune function.[23] It is found in whole grains, most seafoods, sunflower seeds, soybeans, and onions.

**Garlic**—Garlic or its components can help lower the risk of tumors in the stomach, colon, lung, and esophagus.[24] Research from China has reported that those who eat a great quantity of garlic have much lower rates of stomach cancer than the rest of the population.[25]

**Omega-3 Fatty Acids**—These fats, essential for the proper functioning of all tissues and cells in the body, may inhibit cancers, especially breast cancer.[26] They're found in fish such as salmon, mackerel, sardines, haddock, and cod as well as flaxseed oil.

**Fiber**—Whole grains and other fiber-rich foods are essential to any anti-cancer diet, as fiber helps facilitate the prompt removal of toxins from the digestive tract. It is important to include a wide variety of these whole grains in the diet because different whole-grain foods contain different kinds of fiber.[27] Consume at least 25-30 g of fiber a day, equivalent to 6 or more servings of grains and 5 or more servings of vegetables (including legumes) and fruits.[28]

## A Beginner's Guide to Nutritional Supplements

In addition to gaining needed nutrients through a carefully constructed whole-foods diet, the well-considered use of nutritional supplements can reliably fortify your body with the essential nutrients. Today, an estimated 46% of adult Americans take nutritional supplements, many on a daily basis, indicating that more people are taking a proactive approach to their own health care.[29] A 1996 survey showed that annual U.S. expenditures for vitamins was an estimated $1.15 to $1.26 billion.[30]

While it is recommended that a person try to obtain as many nutrients as possible through eating a variety of nutrient-dense foods, this can be impractical sometimes due to several factors. These include a reduced calorie diet; dislike of certain foods; loss of nutrients in cooking; variable quality of food supply; lack of knowledge, motivation, or time to plan and prepare balanced meals; and nutrient depletion caused by stress, lifestyle, and certain medications. This is where nutritional supplements can play an important role in filling nutrient gaps.

Research has demonstrated that diet alone is usually not sufficient to supply the nutrients necessary for overall good health. While most experts agree that nutritional supplements are vital for a variety of illnesses, injuries, and age-related problems, vitamin and mineral supplements can also help to maintain optimal physical and psychological health, promote longevity, and prevent chronic disease.

Nutritionists Jeffrey Bland, Ph.D., and D. Lindsey Berkson, M.A., D.C., offer these recommendations for taking nutritional supplements:

- Take supplements with meals to promote increased absorption. Take fat-soluble vitamins, such as vitamin A, beta carotene, vitamin E, vitamin D, and the essential fatty acids (linoleic, or gamma linolenic, and alpha linolenic acid or eicosapentenoic acid) with the one daily meal that contains the most fat.

- Take amino acid supplements on an empty stomach at least an hour before or after a meal; take with fruit juice to help absorption. Whenever using an increased dosage of an isolated amino acid, be sure to supplement it with an amino acid blend.
- If you become nauseated when you take tablet supplements, consider taking a liquid form, diluted in a beverage.
- If you become nauseated or ill within an hour after taking nutritional supplements, consider a bowel cleanse or rejuvenation program prior to beginning your nutritional supplementation program.
- If you are taking high doses of supplements, do not take them all at one time; divide them into smaller doses and take throughout the day.
- Take digestive enzymes with meals to assist digestion. If you are taking pancreatic or other enzymes for other than digesting food—for eliminating toxins, for example—be sure to take them on an empty stomach between meals.
- Take mineral supplements at a different time than your highest fiber meal of the day, as fiber can decrease mineral absorption. Zinc's absorption is especially impaired by the phytates found in beans, cereals, bread, and pasta.
- Whenever taking an increased dosage of an isolated B vitamin, be sure to supplement with a complete B-complex.
- When taking nutrients, be sure to drink adequate amounts of purified water or fresh vegetable or fruit juice to mix with digestive juices and prevent side effects.

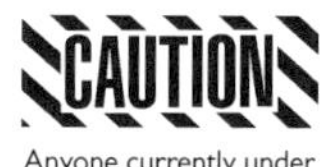


Anyone currently under medical care, taking medications, or having a history of specific problems should always consult with a physician (preferably one knowledgeable about diet and supplemental nutrients) before making any changes in diet or lifestyle, including the use of supplements. To eliminate guesswork and frustration, consult a qualified health professional trained in nutritional biochemistry to help assess individual needs and develop an effective, personalized program.

Nutritional supplements are not a panacea, however, and it is important to be aware of certain potential risks. Prolonged intake of excessive doses of vitamins A, D, niacin and possibly B6 may produce toxic effects. Other vitamins, minerals, and accessory nutrients can sometimes cause side effects when they interact with conventional drugs or interfere with a person's biochemical individuality. Nutritional supplements should also never take the place of proper dietary habits or appropriate medical care when warranted.

## Food Nutrients Can Complement Conventional Cancer Treatments

Research shows that nutrients and other biological response modifiers (BRMs) can directly impede tumor growth and metastases.[31] According to Keith I. Block, M.D., profiled in Chapter 2 of this book, at least 5 lines of BRM research offer solid evidence that alternative therapies need to become integrated into conventional cancer care:

- Natural killer (NK) cells can stop the spread of cancer cells (micrometastases). Research has shown that NK activity is amplified by supplementation with selenium,[32] germanium,[33] and ascorbic acid.[34] As mentioned earlier, vegetarians may have double the NK activity of their meat-eating counterparts.[35]
- Omega-3 fatty acids from fish oils, flaxseed, and certain plants tend to inhibit certain tumor-promoting substances, the "bad" eicosanoids. Women with high concentrations of omega-3 fatty acids in their breast tissues are 5 times less likely to develop deadly metastases than other women.[36] These "good fats" have recently been proposed as a standard addition to the treatment of liver cancer.[37]
- Soybeans and other legumes contain daidzein and genistein, naturally occurring "phytoestrogens" which may block the action of estrogen, thus slowing the growth of hormonally-dependent tumors.[38] Genistein can block the activity of certain oncogenes (cells believed to initiate cancer) and has antioxidant, antiestrogenic, and antitumor activity.[39]
- The essential oils of citrus fruits, spices and herbs contain a substance called limonene, which stimulates the 2 primary phases of liver detoxification. Limonene and its derivative, perillyl alcohol, may block both tumor promotion and progression by inhibiting a specific oncogene.[40]
- The nutrients zinc, selenium, and folate have been shown to stimulate or "upregulate" DNA repair enzymes.[41] A lack of these nutrients could be detrimental, then, since unrepaired mutated DNA in

QUICK DEFINITION

An **oncogene** is a gene believed to transform normal cells into cancer cells, thus initiating the development of cancer. Some of these genes have reportedly been identified in cancer-causing viruses. Proto-oncogenes are genes in a neutral, inactive stage that under certain conditions become oncogenes. Oncogenes are necessary for human fetal development and have been present in life forms for an estimated 500 million years; when they mutate, they become cancer-producing agents. Among the estimated 48 different oncogenes thus far identified, here are their believed correlations with some of the types of cancer they tend to precipitate: erbb2 (breast); fos (lung); jun (lung); hras (pancreatic); kras (colon); nras (lung, others); myc (breast, colon, small-cell lung).

## More Antioxidants Mean Less Cancer

In an Italian study, the dietary habits of 2,569 women, aged 20-74, with breast cancer were compared to 2,588 women in the same age range without cancer. Researchers found that the women with cancer had significantly lower intakes of the antioxidants beta carotene, vitamin E, and calcium than the cancer-free women; to a lesser extent, lower intakes of riboflavin, iron, and potassium were also observed in the women with breast cancer, according to the *International Journal of Cancer* (1996).

cancer-inhibiting (suppressor) genes can raise the cancer risk.

### The Future of Nutritional Medicine in Cancer Care

There is still some prejudice among conventional physicians regarding nutritional therapy for cancer and other diseases. Little research has adequately addressed the use of nutrition as an adjunctive treatment for cancer therapy. Although more than 70 controlled trials have evaluated the use of nutritional support for cancer patients, a 1994 review of these trials indicated many had serious shortcomings in study design which limited the ability to draw solid conclusions.[42]

For this reason, the technical indications for using nutrition therapy adjunctively in cancer care remain controversial. Counterbalancing this situation, however, is the empirical fact that many physicians have used nutritional therapies successfully against cancer and other serious diseases and have the patient outcomes on record to prove their efficacy.

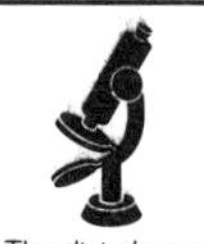

The clinical use of nutritional therapies as part of a cancer treatment program should be further researched to validate and substantiate clinical results.

Increasingly, we are seeing strong consensus regarding the *preventive* role of diet. This emphasis should be applied directly to the prevention of cancer recurrence after the initial tumor-killing therapies have been successfully employed. Many scientists have begun to outline a scientific rationale for dietary guidelines that may reduce the risk of some types of cancers, such as breast, colon, and prostate.[43] Among the more exciting trends in innovative cancer care is the growing interest in the use of nutritional supplements (primarily antioxidants) and in changing the quantity and quality of dietary fat as an adjunct to breast cancer treatment. According to the New England Deaconess Hospital at Harvard Medical School, the use of fish oils or other sources of omega-3 fatty acids may change "tumor protein breakdown rates and inhibit the proliferation potential of tumors."[44]

Further, there is considerable evidence that antioxidants, by protecting against free-radical-related tumor promotion, can help inhibit some forms of cancer from developing, as well as bolster many components of the immune system.[45] One of the key insights is that the immune system itself, in mounting its response against cancer cells, toxins, and microbes, can produce highly potent and potentially harmful substances such as cytokines (an immune cell) and oxidant molecules (e.g., hydrogen peroxide, lipid peroxides, and hypochlorous acid). Antioxidants are required in sufficient supply to protect the body against these "side effects" of the immune response.[46]

What's holding back greater acceptance of nutritional supplementation in cancer treatment? In most medical schools, students receive only a few hours of instruction on nutrition. As a result, most new doctors have little knowledge of the power of nutrition against disease. Without this knowledge, some feel threatened by patients who begin adopting nutritional strategies outside of their prescribed medical treatment. Further, since conventional medicine has a history of rejecting nutritional intervention, most doctors are discouraged from thinking along these lines and, consequently, do not incorporate nutrition in their practices.

***Among the more exciting trends in innovative cancer care is the growing interest in the use of nutritional supplements (primarily antioxidants) and in changing the quantity and quality of dietary fat as an adjunct to breast cancer treatment.***

Abram Hoffer, M.D. (profiled in Chapter 10 of this book), foresees a change. "It takes approximately 40 years for innovative ideas to be incorporated into mainstream thought. I expect and hope that orthomolecular medicine within the next 5-10 years will cease to be a specialty in medicine and that all physicians will be using nutrition as an essential generalist's tool in treating disease."

Richard P. Huemer, M.D., of Vancouver, Washington, a colleague of Dr. Linus Pauling and himself a pioneer in the field of orthomolecular medicine, agrees. "We need a paradigm shift, and I think it's beginning to occur. Nutrition needs to be looked at not as a means of preventing specific deficiency diseases, but as a means of contributing to the overall health of the person and their resistance to chronic diseases. We have to start looking for the optimum levels of nutrients necessary for optimum health instead of the minimum amount needed to prevent diseases."

## A Glossary of Nutritional Supplements for Fighting Cancer

### ACIDOPHILUS

*Acidophilus* is a generic term for the *Lactobacilli*, or "friendly bacteria" (probiotics) that naturally inhabit the healthy intestine. These bacteria consist mainly of the species *L. acidophilus* or *L. bulgaricus* and *L. casei;* they can markedly enhance nutritional status and have specific and important therapeutic roles.[47]

Among their many health-promoting functions, they: (1) exert direct activity against tumors; (2) prevent cancer by detoxifying or preventing the formation of carcinogenic chemicals; (3) reduce the level of cholesterol, which indirectly aids in cancer resistance; (4) help produce important B vitamins which assist in immunocompetence; (5) curb or destroy potentially pathogenic bacteria and hostile yeasts such as *Candida albicans*, thereby freeing up the immune system for surveillance against cancer cells; and (6) through their production of lactic acid, preserve and enhance the digestibility of foods which are fermented with them, such as soy products (miso, tamari), sauerkraut, and pickles.[48]

For more information about **friendly bacteria/probiotics** as part of a detoxification program, see Chapter 33: Physical Support Therapies, pp. 962-964.

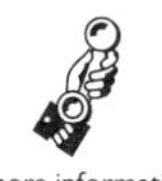

For more information about ***Lactobacillus acidophilus***, contact: The Torrance Company, P.O. Box 242, Portage, MI 49081; tel: 800-327-0722 or 616-327-0722; fax: 616-327-0763.

One of the main anticancer effects of *Lactobacilli* is the conversion of harmful substances called primary bile acids into secondary bile acids. Researchers at Tufts University found that *L. acidophilus* significantly lowers the cancer-triggering activity of certain compounds in the feces of meat-eating animals;[49] these same friendly bacteria reduce the number of colon tumors even after animals receive a potent carcinogen.[50] A study of 138 patients with bladder cancer found that those given 1 g of *Lactobacillus (L. casei)* 3 times a day for 12 months were significantly less likely to develop a recurrence of bladder cancer than those patients receiving the placebo.[51] Other research showed that a cell wall derivative of *L. abulgaricus* improved survival among 100 advanced cancer patients.[52] One of the most effective and powerful Lactobacillus species used to date on humans is probably *L. plantarum*.

### AMINO ACIDS

Amino acids, the building blocks of protein, can have specific applications for cancer therapy. In humans, we find 20 amino acids that make up proteins (long chains of amino acids) and peptides (short chains of amino acids). Of these, 8 are considered to be essential and cannot be made within the body and the rest are considered nonessential, as they can be synthesized within the body from the essential 8 amino acids. Some amino acids, such as glutamine, may be considered to be conditionally essential amino acids. This means that although the body is capable of making glutamine under certain stress situations, it cannot make enough glutamine for the body's needs. Under such a situation, the person can greatly benefit from supplementation with significant amounts of glutamine.

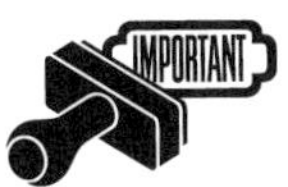


Since amino acids work as a team, as do the other nutrients in the body, it is important not to be deficient in any of them. A test called a fasting plasma sample determines amino acid deficiencies. If any of the essential amino acids is found lacking, steps should be taken to correct the deficiency either with appropriate food or with amino acid supplementation. In addition, there are a few particular amino acids which play a special role in cancer treatment.

The amino acid L-arginine may enhance the anticancer activity of cytotoxic T cells, NK cells, and other key immune components.[53] Animals fed a low-arginine diet showed an inability to increase their NK activity; however, when given arginine supplements, their NK activity increased.[54] Other types of white blood cells involved in the body's anticancer defenses are also stimulated by dietary enrichment with arginine.[55] Methionine, a sulfur-containing amino acid, when combined with choline, significantly increased the survival of mice with aflatoxin-induced liver cancer.[56]

Another sulfur-containing amino acid, cysteine (especially if given as N-acetyl cysteine) assists in various detoxification processes and reduces the toxic side effects of both chemotherapy and radiation treatments.[57] N-acetyl cysteine is a precursor for the production of glutathione, which serves in the key antioxidant system called glutathione peroxidase. Blood levels of glutathione peroxidase tend to decrease after the sixth decade of life and are typically lower in patients with malignant cancers.[58]

Reduced L-glutathione (the active form) is often depleted in persons with mercury toxicity (such as those with amalgam dental fillings) which probably increases cancer risk and cancer progression.[59] Glutathione reduces free-radical damage to DNA and prevents depletion of other antioxidants, helps metabolize various carcinogens, activates certain immune

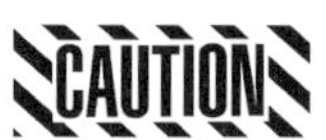

As with all the other supplements, it is essential to consult your doctor regarding supplementation with arginine and methionine. The clinical use of electrodermal screening can provide information as to appropriate supplementation levels.

**Amino acids** are the basic building blocks of the 40,000 different proteins in the body, including enzymes, hormones, and the key brain chemical messenger molecules called neurotransmitters. Eight amino acids cannot be made by the body and must be obtained through the diet; others are produced in the body but not always in sufficient amounts. The body's main "amino acid pool" consists of: alanine, arginine, asparagine, aspartic acid, carnitine, citrulline, cysteine, cystine, GABA, glutamic acid, glutamine, glycine, histidine, isoleucine, leucine, lysine, methionine, ornithine, phenylalanine, proline, serine, taurine, threonine, trytophan, tyrosine, and valine.

cells, helps synthesize and repair DNA, and may inhibit angiogenesis, a blood vessel-forming process required for tumor growth.[60] Like cysteine supplements, glutathione supplements also diminish the toxic side effects of conventional radiation and chemotherapy treatments.[61]

While the research remains preliminary, both methionine and arginine may actually *promote* the development of cancer under some circumstances. Certain types of cancer seem to require methionine for growth, thus restricting one's intake of this amino acid may actually inhibit their growth.[62] In animal studies, arginine stimulated metastasis and tumor growth in both colon and breast cancers.[63] Supplementation with arginine above 5 g per day—the therapeutic range—may activate the growth of some viruses.[64] However, this stimulation of viruses can be prevented often times by taking L-lysine along with the arginine.

## BETA CAROTENE

Beta carotene, classified as a carotenoid, is the pigment that accounts for much of the color in the plant world and is the dominant plant pigment in most fruits and vegetables. It is converted to vitamin A in concert with the body's own needs for the vitamin. As an antioxidant and precursor to vitamin A, beta carotene can enhance the activity of natural killer (NK) cells and other immune cells against tumors.[65,66,67]

A review of the scientific literature on vitamin A and beta carotene shows that beta carotene has antioxidant and immune-enhancing properties that are not found in vitamin A.[68] The immune system changes caused by beta carotene include a significant increase in T- and B-cell numbers, macrophage activity, interleukin production, and NK cell tumor-killing (tumoricidal) abilities.[69]

There are over 500 naturally occurring carotenoids, of which a large number have been found to be pharmacologically active, such as phycopene, lycopene, and others. These carotenoids are thought to work together, so taking high doses of any one of them could offset the activities of the others. For this reason, it may be preferable to supplement with a natural carotenoid complex, such as Betaplex or Carotenoid Complex.

## Unraveling the Beta Carotene Controversy

In 1996, 3 widely publicized studies reported on the results of using beta carotene as a cancer-prevention protocol for high-risk groups. In the first study involving Finnish smokers, researchers reported that beta carotene supplementation led to slightly increased lung cancer mortality. The second study examined the preventive action of beta carotene and retinol (vitamin A) against cancer and heart disease in people who smoked or who had been exposed to asbestos. This study was halted before completion because of an increase in the rate of new cancers and mortality in the group receiving supplementation. In the third study, involving physicians rated as being low risk, beta carotene appeared to have no effect on either morbidity or mortality.

On the basis of these studies, mainstream media published articles denouncing beta carotene supplementation as worthless, along with warnings about its potential health risks. In the ensuing months, experts in the field of nutrition and alternative medicine explained the flaws in all 3 studies. For one, the studies evaluated a synthetic beta carotene, and synthetic vitamins have been demonstrated to work differently (or less effectively) than natural ones. For another, the studies evaluated only a single nutrient acting in isolation, a condition never advised by experienced health-care practitioners.

"The results of these 3 trials point to the important and not unexpected conclusion that the *total* diet and all its constituents may be the most important consideration in determining nutrient factors related to cancer risk incidence," commented Jeffrey Bland, Ph.D., a prominent nutrition researcher and director of HealthComm International in Gig Harbor, Washington. The studies overlook the fact that balancing antioxidant intake (vitamins C and E, selenium, *and* beta carotene) is of paramount importance in cancer prevention diets rich in vegetable products.

Hundreds of other clinical studies have already demonstrated the preventive role of carotenoids from dietary or supplemental sources. It would be "irresponsible," states Dr. Bland, to use these 3 flawed studies as a basis for regulating or restricting the use of beta carotene.[70]

## CALCIUM

Cancer patients may need to take a calcium supplement, particularly if they are suffering from a bone cancer that is causing bone-calcium losses. A 19-year prospective study found that calcium deficiency was associated with a higher risk of colorectal cancer.[71] Numerous animal studies have found that calcium may inhibit colon cancer, and human studies indicate that the mineral may reverse the rapid growth (hyperproliferation) of colon cells.[72] Note that magnesium is involved in the body's uptake of both calcium and potassium, and a magnesium deficiency tends to promote deficiencies in calcium

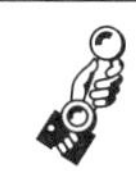

For more information about **Beta-plex**, contact: Scientific Botanicals, P.O. Box 31131, Seattle, WA 98103; tel: 206-527-5521; fax: 206-526-7948. For **Carotenoid Complex** (containing beta carotene, alpha carotene, gamma carotene, lycopene, lutein, capsanthin, and other carotenoids), contact: Solgar Vitamin and Herb Company, 500 Willow Tree Road, Leonia, NJ 07605; tel: 201-944-2311; fax: 201-944-7351.

and potassium. For this reason, when taking calcium supplements (which are best absorbed at bedtime), it is generally a good idea to also supplement with magnesium as well (which is better taken in the morning).

## CHROMIUM

Chromium supplements (either chromium picolinate or chromium polynicotinate) may help people regain normal thyroid function, which can in turn bolster thyroid function. Chromium forms part of the glucose tolerance factor (GTF), a molecule that assists in the control of blood sugar levels. In fact, chromium itself appears to act more like a hormone than an element. Diabetics appear to be unable to effectively produce GTF from chromium, and should take chromium in the form of GTF. Anything that helps better regulate blood sugar levels could substantially improve immune function and cancer resistance since sugar promotes the "bad" eicosanoids which in turn promote cancer growth.

***A 19-year prospective study found that calcium deficiency was associated with a higher risk of colorectal cancer. Numerous animal studies have found that calcium may inhibit colon cancer, and human studies indicate that the mineral may reverse the rapid growth (hyperproliferation) of colon cells.***

The United States appears to be a chromium-deficient nation, probably due to our overindulgence in refined grain products. In one study, Asian peoples averaged 4.5 times as much and other nationalities also had markedly more chromium in the blood compared to Americans.[73] Refined foods such as white sugar and white flour are extremely low in chromium since it is lost through refining processes. In grains, for example, chromium is contained in the outer bran portion, so much is lost in the production of white flour. In this case, there is also an additive effect since our body's chromium needs increase in proportion to blood-sugar levels; thus higher intakes of simple sugars tend to deplete the body of chromium.[74] Finally, excessive iron intakes (either from red meat or iron supplements) can deplete chromium levels by causing excessive chromium losses in the urine.[75]

## COENZYME Q10 (COQ10)

CoQ10, also known as ubiquinone, is one of a family of brightly colored substances, called quinones, which are widely distributed in nature because they are essential for generating energy in living things that use oxygen. The body produces its own coQ10, but usually produces less with aging; therefore dietary sources are important for this coenzyme, especially for older people. It is found in fairly high concentrations in fish (especially sardines), soybean and grapeseed oils, sesame seeds, pistachios, walnuts, and spinach.[76]

There is evidence that endurance athletes may need more dietary coQ10 than others, and that sedentary people do not use coQ10 as efficiently as people who are physically active. CoQ10 plays an important part in the body's antioxidant system. When combined with vitamin E, selenium, and beta carotene, coQ10 can significantly reduce free-radical damage in the liver, kidney and heart tissues.[77] Another beneficial effect in cancer patients is to increase macrophage activity.[78]

In one study, 90 mg of coenzyme Q10 were given daily to 32 breast cancer patients for 2 years. All patients survived and 6 had partial remissions. One of the partial responders then received a high dose of 390 mg of coQ10 daily; within 3 months the tumor had completely regressed. The researchers then gave 300 mg of coQ10 to a second breast cancer patient, who showed no evidence of tumor growth or metastasis after 3 months. One of the authors commented that in treating almost 7,000 cases of breast cancer during a 35-year period, he had "never seen a spontaneous complete regression of a 1.5-2 centimeter breast tumor, and has never seen a comparable regression on any conventional antitumor therapy."[79]

More recent findings substantiate the view that supplementation with coQ10 can cause complete regression of tumors in advanced breast cancer, including one patient with numerous metastases to the liver.[80]

## COPPER

This trace element is essential to proper functioning of a wide range of immune cell types, including antibody-forming cells, T helper cells, and macrophages, all of which may help the body defend against cancer.[81] Copper functions as a cofactor for many important enzymes, called cuproenzymes, which speed up the body's energy-yielding (oxidation) reactions. It is intimately involved in healing processes, excretion of certain toxins (purines), maintaining connective tissues, and formation of red blood cells. A deficiency of this element results in a lowered resistance to infections and to a shortened life span following infection.[82] Copper also affects inflamma-

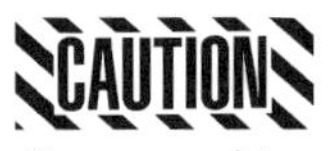


Since copper and zinc are chemically antagonistic, Charles B. Simone, M.D., (profiled in Chapter 19 of this book), advises that their intake be carefully controlled under medical supervision. Ingesting too much copper can readily reduce the body's zinc supply and vice versa.

Since EPA fish oil retards normal blood clotting, high doses (more than 5000 to 6000 mg daily) are contraindicated for people anticipating surgery.[88] In addition, long-term supplementation with EPA may induce a deficiency of vitamin E, unless supplements of vitamin E are added. This situation may occur because EPA is highly unsaturated, thus requiring vitamin E for its preservation. Polyunsaturated fats are more vulnerable to rancidity and free-radical activity, and vitamin E helps prevent these effects. Patrick Donovan, N.D. (profiled in Chapter 7 of this book), suggests including 400 IU of vitamin E for every 2500 mg of EPA. A minimum of 1000 mg of EPA is required to produce anticancer effects. It is also important that EPA be provided in proportion to GLA (gamma linolenic acid) in a ratio of 5 parts EPA to 1 part GLA, to encourage the production of beneficial eicosanoids for immune-system enhancement.[89]

tion—sometimes stimulating, other times inhibiting the process—and bears a close relationship with zinc.

## EICOSAPENTENOIC ACID (EPA FISH OILS)

Essential fatty acids, required for health and proper metabolism, include linoleic acid and alpha linolenic acid (ALA). These essential fats are found in flaxseed oil and the oils of certain other seeds, nuts, and vegetables. They play an important role in reducing heart disease and in preventing and treating various cancers.[83]

Lipids are the biochemist's term for fats. Although most animal fats are harmful to human health, some, such as those found in fish, are actually helpful. Eicosapentaenoic acid, or EPA, is the primary fatty acid found in most fish oils. Classified as an omega-3 fatty acid, EPA helps maintain the proper levels of beneficial eicosanoids, hormone-like substances that mediate the body's response to cancer and other disease processes. There is good evidence that EPA slows tumor growth[84] and reduces the invasiveness of human tumor cells in culture.[85] In addition, EPA improves the response of tumor cells to hyperthermia and chemotherapy agents by altering properties of the tumor cell membrane.[86] Recent research suggests that EPA may have a beneficial role as an adjunctive treatment for breast cancer.[87]

## FLAXSEED OIL

About 58% of flaxseed oil (also known as linseed oil) is alpha-linolenic acid (ALA), one of the omega-3 fatty acids our bodies need for good health. This makes flaxseed the richest source of ALA. This particular omega-3 helps maintain the levels of health-promoting eicosanoids (biological activators that regulate all biological activities and inhibit the production of tumor-promoting eicosanoids). ALA enhances immune function and cellular oxygen use, thereby helping to dissolve tumors.

A study involving 121 women with localized breast cancer found that those who had low levels of ALA were more likely to have their breast cancer spread to lymph nodes around the armpit and to have tumors that exhibited an "invasive" quality. After a period of 31 months, researchers found that the 21 women in this group who developed postsurgical metastases into other body tissues were conspicuously low in ALA. In their estimation, a low level of ALA was the most important contributing factor in the spread of the breast cancer.[90] The results from this study suggest that supplementing the diet with flaxseed oil "may help prevent breast cancer, tumor invasiveness, and metastasis," concludes Michael Murray, N.D.[91]

A $20 million study by the National Cancer Institute (NCI) in 1990 found that flaxseed oil, but not fish oil, reduced the growth of breast cancers and metastases in laboratory animals when compared to cancerous growth in animals receiving corn oil.[92] Although the NCI study was halted before completion, it determined that flaxseed oil exerts a strong anticancer effect provided the particular oil is high in lignans. Flaxseed oil has been found to contain up to 100 times more lignans than many other plant foods. Animal studies showed that test subjects receiving flaxseed oil experienced a significant reduction in tumor size and numbers (greater than 50% reduction) after only 1-2 months.

***A $20 million study by the National Cancer Institute in 1990 found that flaxseed oil, but not fish oil, reduced the growth of breast cancers and metastases in laboratory animals when compared to cancerous growth in animals receiving corn oil.***

Once in the gastrointestinal tract, lignans are converted into enterolactone and enterodiol, which are believed to be the compounds in flaxseed with an anticancer effect. Researchers have found that lignans can bind to estrogen receptors in the body and usefully obstruct the cancer-enhancing effects of estrogen on breast tissue. "Lignans are probably one of the protective factors against breast cancer in vegetarian women," explains Dr. Murray. He also reports that women with high levels of lignans in their urine tend to have much lower rates for breast cancer.[93]

German biophysicist Johanna Budwig noted that high concentrations of both oxygen and essential fatty acids (such as alpha linolenic acid, ALA) exist in rapidly growing tissues. However, in tumors, though a mass of rapidly growing cells, the opposite is true: ALA concentration and oxygen are always depressed. "Dr. Budwig stated that the tumor mass resulted from waste accumulations the body cells could not remove because they lacked the en-

**CAUTION**

Since flaxseed oil is highly unsaturated, it readily oxidizes when exposed to the open air. If the oil becomes highly oxidized and rancid, it can be dangerous for cancer patients. It has a short shelf life and must be purchased as fresh as possible and always kept tightly sealed in the refrigerator. Never heat or cook cold-pressed (unrefined) flaxseed oil under any circumstances. If these guidelines are not followed, the resulting rancidity makes this oil unfit for human consumption. Vitamins A (or beta carotene), C, and E, and the minerals zinc, selenium, and sulfur-containing amino acids (such as cysteine) are among the substances most required to protect the essential fatty acids from destruction by oxygen and free radicals.[96]

ergy necessary to do so," says Dr. Etienne Callebout, M.D. (profiled in Chapter 4 of this book). "This energy is supplied by electrons donated from ALA and oxygen, along with other essential nutrients." ALA enhances immune function and cellular oxygen use, thereby helping to dissolve tumors.[94]

Based on the work done by Dr. Budwig, we now know that ALA works best when mixed directly into sulfur-rich protein foods.[95] A typical recommended amount of pure virgin, cold-pressed flaxseed oil per day is 1-2 tablespoons, depending on the individual's condition.

## GAMMA LINOLENIC ACID (GLA)

The 2 classes of essential fatty acids are omega-3 and omega-6. These names refer to their chemical structure. All fatty acids consist of a chain of carbon atoms. Each carbon is connected to at least one other carbon atom by a single or a double chemical bond. The last carbon of the chain is the omega carbon, reflecting the name of the last letter of the Greek alphabet, which is omega. Omega-3 fatty acids have their first double bond on the third carbon from the omega or last carbon, while the omega-6 fatty acids have their first double bond on the sixth carbon from the omega carbon.

Gamma linolenic acid, a member of the omega-6 family, can stimulate he production of "good" eicosanoids (such as PGE1) which in turn can impede the growth of tumors. GLA can be converted into PGE1 and other "good" eicosanoids or into PGE2 and other "bad" eicosanoids, depending on how much EPA, insulin, and sugar there is in the body at the time of conversion. One study found that GLA supplements provided both subjective and objective improvements in 21 cases of untreatable cancer.[97] When combined with vitamin C, GLA supplementation led to a doubling of the mean survival time for patients with liver cancer (primary hepatic carcinoma).[98] Combinations of GLA and EPA (eicosapentaenoic) seemed to enhance the destruction of cancer cells, possibly by altering the characteristics of the tumor cells themselves.[99]

Under healthy conditions, the human body produces its own GLA through the body's conversion of linoleic acid (LA) to GLA. This essential conversion process is inhibited, however, by the following factors: (1) a diet containing high-cholesterol foods such as eggs, beef, and dairy products; (2) alcohol consumption, (3) zinc deficiency, (4) trans-fatty acids (from margarine, processed oils, and junk foods), (5) viral infections, and (6) the aging process.[100] High-sugar diets may also interfere with the mobilization of GLA from fats stored in our bodies.[101]

By consuming GLA as a supplement, we can bypass the conversion process of LA to GLA, thus ensuring the production of the protective eicosanoids. The richest sources of GLA are borage oil, black currant oil, evening primrose oil, and mother's milk. GLA has often been lumped in the same category with alpha-linolenic acid, which is found in flax, pumpkin seed, soybeans and walnuts, and is a member of the omega-3 family. Although these fatty acids are similar in structure, they have different properties and are *not* interchangeable. The transformation of GLA into the good eicosanoids (e.g., PGE1) is promoted by zinc, vitamin C, and vitamins B3 and B6.

## GERMANIUM

This unusual trace element enhances the availability of oxygen to both healthy cells and cancer cells. The latter cannot thrive under oxygen-rich conditions. One of these compounds, germanium sesquioxide, blocks or slows the growth of tumors and significantly lengthens survival times in laboratory animals.[102] A major study in Japan found that people with inoperable lung cancer who were treated with germanium as well as chemotherapy and/or radiation showed a higher response rate and better survival times, particularly for small-cell lung carcinoma.[103] Not only were metastases reduced, but patients also reported an enhanced quality of life with fewer side effects from drugs or other treatments.

## GERSON DIET THERAPY

Max Gerson, M.D. (1881-1959), emigrated from Germany to the United States in the 1930s. Shortly after graduating from the University of Freiburg in 1909 where he specialized in internal medicine and physiological chemistry, Dr. Gerson began to experience severe migraine headaches. By 1919, with his medical practice well established, Dr. Gerson had also found a cure for his migraines by reworking his diet to eliminate salt. After succeeding in this, he found that he was able to successfully treat arthritis, pulmonary tuberculosis, and lupus patients with diet alone; then, in 1928, he took the next leap—treating cancer with diet.

"The ideal task of cancer therapy is to restore the function of the oxidizing systems in the entire organism," Dr. Gerson explained. To accomplish this, 3 factors had to be addressed: first, detoxify the body; second, fortify the system with minerals from the potassium group; and third, continuously introduce oxidizing enzymes until the body's own ability to produce them is reactivated.

The important concept here is oxygen and oxidation. Dr. Gerson understood that cancer cells grow in conditions of limited or no oxygen and through fermentation. "The malignancies in human beings continuously fall back deeper and deeper into fermentation," he said. Regarding potassium, Dr. Gerson stated that in a sick body, and particularly in one that has cancer, potassium is inactive, and sodium and related minerals exist in an unfavorable chemical state.[104]

***"Cancer is not a single cellular problem; it is an accumulation of numerous damaging factors combined in deteriorating the whole metabolism, after the liver has been progressively impaired in its functions," said Dr. Gerson.***

A key element in the Gerson dietary plan is to reestablish the correct cellular balance between sodium (Na) and potassium (K). "It is my opinion that K and Na also play an important role in the cancer problem." As he explained it, in chronic diseases such as cancer, sodium and calcium invade particular organs and cause their potassium to leech out, disrupting the appropriate balance between the two. "From my own clinical experiments, I have learned that it is not only necessary to change the metabolism in one or another substance [such as potassium and sodium], but it is also necessary to change the intake of proteins, enzymes, vitamins, etc., simultaneously to activate all natural healing forces which we need for our therapy."

Dr. Gerson further noted that cancer is not caused by a single deficiency, such as of hormones, vitamins, or enzymes. "Cancer is not a single cellular problem; it is an accumulation of numerous damaging factors combined in deteriorating the whole metabolism, after the liver has been progressively impaired in its functions." This slow poisoning of the entire organism, a lowering of the electrical activity in vital organs, and the weakening of the liver, the prime organ of detoxification, creates a "cancerous body that is anergic," says Dr. Gerson. This means that "it cannot prevent cancerous growth nor respond and defend itself against it." Treatment must restore these functions so that the body's immune response, including the liver, can function appropriately again, Dr. Gerson said. Fundamental among these functions is the "production, activation and reactivation of oxidizing enzymes" capable of raising the level of oxygen in the cells.[105]

Dr. Gerson believed that cancer would not occur in bodies with a properly balanced and functioning liver, pancreas, thyroid, and immune system. In his approach, thyroid extracts seem to enable the body to fight cancer more effectively by stimulating liver and thyroid function. Coffee enemas are used as needed for pain reduction, appetite stimulation, and liver detoxification; patients take 3-4 coffee enemas a day for detoxification and pain relief. Enemas of chamomile tea or castor oil are also used. "Only a detoxified body has both power of resistance and healing," said Dr. Gerson.

***Of patients with Stage IVa melanoma, 39% of Gerson therapy patients survived for 5 years, compared with 6% of patients treated by conventional medicine.***

There is also supplementation with pepsin (an enzyme), potassium, iodine, niacin, pancreatin (a digestive enzyme culled from bovine pancreas), and vitamin C. The Gerson program also includes salt and sodium restriction and potassium supplementation; high doses of micronutrients, especially through raw fruit and vegetable juices; severe restrictions on fat intake; and a reduction in protein intake by adopting a vegetarian diet. Dr. Gerson also restricted tobacco, sharp spices, tea, coffee, cocoa, chocolate, alcohol, refined sugar and flour, all processed or canned foods, nuts, mushrooms, soybeans, pickles, cucumbers, pineapples, and all berries (except red currants).

Regarding potassium supplementation, Dr. Gerson recommended 4 teaspoons in juice 10 times daily in a specific chemical formulation he developed on the basis of 300 experiments. Dr. Gerson also recommended high doses of Lugol's solution (iodine plus potassium iodide) and thyroid extract, which he believed went directly to the tumor.

With his low-fat, nearly vegan (no animal products, including eggs or dairy) dietary regime, Dr. Gerson found that he could reverse the majority of cancer in patients that came to him. Small amounts of dairy products are permitted on this diet. The caloric limit is 2600-3200 calories per day. Patients on the Gerson program supplement their main diet 10 times a day

***In most medical schools, students receive only a few hours of instruction on nutrition. As a result, most new doctors have little knowledge of the power of nutrition against disease and are discouraged from thinking along these lines and consequently do not incorporate nutrition in their practices.***

with freshly cut fruit (primarily apple) and vegetable juices (primarily carrot), taken at hourly intervals. This inundates the body every day with the living nutrients from nearly 20 pounds of fresh, organic foods. In fact, Dr. Gerson once estimated the average quantity of fresh, raw vegetables, mostly as juice, that a typical patient might consume in a year on his diet: 1800 pounds carrots, 1300 pounds apples, 350-450 pounds calf's liver juice, 145 heads of red cabbage, 400 heads lettuce, and 125 pounds of green peppers. In addition, there would be large amounts of oranges, grapes, grapefruits, and tomatoes.

As mentioned previously, Dr. Gerson discovered that cancer patients had an excess of sodium far outweighing the potassium in their bodies; the 2 normally exist in a specific balance to each other. Sodium acts as a poison in the body because it is an enzyme inhibitor, whereas potassium is an enzyme activator. The fruits and vegetables in the Gerson diet help correct the sodium and potassium imbalance which, in turn, helps revitalize the liver so it can again rid the body of malignant cells. The coffee enemas then aid in the elimination of these dead cancer cells.

**Staging** in cancer terminology is a relative index of how much cancer exists in the body, its size, location, and containment or metastasis. Stage I, the earliest, most curable stage, shows only local tumor involvement. Stage II indicates some spreading of cancer to the surrounding tissues and perhaps to nearby lymph nodes. Stage III involves metastasis to distant lymph nodes. Stage IV, the most advanced and least easily cured, means the cancer has spread to distant organs.

Many of Dr. Gerson's cancer patients, whom he treated in the 1940s and 1950s, are documented to have lived in good health for many decades after their treatment period. For example, a woman in her early forties was diagnosed with advanced melanoma and cervical cancer. Six months after beginning the Gerson therapy, a second biopsy revealed that her cervical cancer had completely disappeared. Similarly, her melanoma vanished. That was over 12 years ago, and she has been free of cancer ever since.

A study of 5-year survival rates highlights the profound therapeutic value of the Gerson program for treating malignant melanoma, one of the most deadly cancers. Today's oncologists agree that melanoma is among the cancers most responsive to measures that enhance immune system function, yet conventional treatment does not do so.

In this study, Gar Hildenbrand of the Gerson Research Organization and Shirley Cavin from the University of California at San Diego's Cancer Prevention and Control Program compared 5-year melanoma survival rates of Gerson therapy patients to rates found in comparable, conventionally treated groups in the medical literature. The study examined 153 white adult cancer patients, 25 to 72 years of age, in various stages of melanoma.[106] Here is a summary of the results of Hildenbrand and Cavin's work:

- Of patients with Stages I and II melanoma (localized), 100% of Gerson therapy patients survived for 5 years, compared with 79% of patients receiving conventional treatment.
- Of patients with Stages IIIa melanoma (regionally metastasized), 82% of Gerson therapy patients were still alive at 5 years, compared with 39% of the conventionally treated patients.
- Of patients with Stages IIIa and IIIb melanoma (regionally metastasized), 70% of Gerson therapy patients were still alive at 5 years, compared with 41% of the conventionally treated patients.
- Of patients with Stage IVa melanoma (a new classification proposed by the authors to cover distant metastases), 39% of Gerson therapy patients survived for 5 years, compared with 6% of patients treated by conventional medicine.[107]

These results are stunning. Even considering possible weaknesses in the study's design, the substantial differences in survival between the Gerson patients and conventional patients is too great to be dismissed. Although Dr. Gerson died in 1959, his work is carried on by his daughter, Charlotte

## American Eating Trends

A U.S. Department of Agriculture survey of what Americans ate in 1994 shows that Americans consumed 33% of their calories from fat, down from 40% in 1977, but that 30% of Americans are overweight (up from 22%), are eating 6% more calories per day, 22 pounds of salty snacks per year compared to 17.5 pounds, and that children aged 5-16 drank 23% more soft drinks than in 1977. Almost 25% of the vegetables eaten by American children ages 2-18 are French fries, 50% eat less than a single serving of fruit and 30% eat less than one serving of vegetables each day, according to a survey of 3,148 children published in *Archives of Pediatrics and Adolescent Medicine,* January 1996.

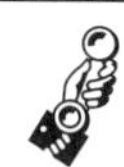

For more information about the **Gerson Therapy** there are 2 organizations you can contact. The Gerson Research Organization, 7807 Artesian Road, San Diego, CA, 92127-2117, tel: 800-759-2966; fax: 619-759-2967. Their clinic is the Max Gerson Memorial Cancer Center of CHIPSA, 670 Nubes, Playas de Tijuana, Mexico. The Gerson Institute, headed by Charlotte Gerson is PO Box 430, Bonita, CA 91908-0430; tel: 619-585-7600; fax: 619-585-7610. Their bimonthly Gerson Healing Newsletter is available for $25. Their clinic is Meridian, Calle de la Lava #2971, Playas de Tijuana, Mexico.

## American Nutrition Shows Improvement Over 3 Decades

Researchers at the University of North Carolina compared the eating habits of 32,406 Americans from 1965 to 1991 and found that still only 25% eat a healthy diet as defined in 1989 by the National Academy of Sciences. The study examined healthy eating practices according to income groups and ethnicity. The strongest gains in healthy eating were among wealthy whites with a 156% increased consumption in soybeans and legumes, 256% increase in low-fat milk, 157% in poultry, 44% in vegetables, and a 99% drop in whole milk, 52% drop in eggs, and 89% drop in red meats. In 1965, only 4.7% of wealthy whites ate a healthy diet compared to 20% in 1991.

In contrast, in 1965, 16.4% of poor blacks ate a healthy diet compared to 1991 when the figure rose to 23.5%. At the same time, the number of low-income whites eating healthy diets grew from 9.3% to 19.9%. It appears that higher-income whites did the most to reduce their consumption of high-fat foods. Although many Americans in all socioeconomic groups made dietary changes to lower fat, we are eating higher amounts of processed fast foods, such as pizza, tacos, and pasta, with high levels of hidden fats, according to a report published in *The New England Journal of Medicine* (September 1996).

Gerson Strauss, and her staff at the Gerson Institute in Tijuana, Mexico.

## INOSITOL

This natural substance, an unofficial member of the B vitamin family, is found in virtually all body cells where it plays important roles in sending signals between cells and their environment. Inositol hexaphosphate is a key phytochemical present in high-fiber foods containing phytic acid and can be isolated from legumes, cereal grains, and citrus fruits. In the body, inositol helps the liver remove excess fat from its tissues; this in turn prevents liver stagnation from fat and bile buildup.

John Potter, Ph.D., a researcher at Fred Hutchinson Cancer Research Center in Seattle, Washington, has identified inositol hexaphosphate as one of 15 different classes of phytochemicals that have shown anticancer activity.[108] In fact, phytic acid may be one of the key reasons for why a high-fiber diet has a protective effect against cancer.[109]

## IODINE

Iodine has anticarcinogenic properties[110] and may help protect against breast cancer.[111] Iodine may also lower one's cancer risk by fortifying the thyroid gland.[112,113] Iodine deficiency is the second most common malnutrition in the world, with about 400 million people suffering from this condition. Iodine is part of the structure of the thyroid hormones, T3 and T4, which in turn regulate our body's energy usage and numerous body functions.

Iodine's effects are far-reaching, since the metabolism of all the body's cells—except for brain cells—is influenced by thyroid hormones. Activated neutrophils (a frontline-of-defense type of white blood cell) may use the conversion of iodide to iodine to produce free radicals, which help kill infectious organisms.[114] This process is particularly important in the case of advanced-cancer patients, many of whom die from infections (e.g., pneumonia) because their immune systems are depressed.

## KELLEY'S METABOLIC THERAPY

Individualized nutrition, detoxification, and the use of pancreatic enzymes make up the therapy advanced by William Donald Kelley, D.D.S. A dentist by training, Dr. Kelley developed his protocol in response to his own pancreatic cancer, which he faced and reversed in the late 1960s. Dr. Kelley called his program "metabolic ecology" to indicate that the patient's entire way of life must be changed. "The person who has the disease should be treated, not the disease that has the person," he explained. "We call our system of cancer therapy Ecological because the total person and his total environment must be considered in order to give proper treatment." Dr. Kelley likened his approach to that of a fine watch: "Each part must be there and be working properly or it does not work at all. Each step of the ecological treatment must be followed exactly or there will not be any relief of the symptoms."[115]

One of the main points of Dr. Kelley's therapy is that cancer is often caused by the body's inability to effectively metabolize protein; this inability can be linked to improper amounts of proteolytic enzymes.

According to Dr. Kelley, these protein-digesting pancreatic enzymes, rather than the immune system, are the body's first defense against tumors. This led him to declare that, fundamentally, cancer is a deficiency of pancreatic enzymes; this deficiency then leads to a disordering of protein metabolism, and from there, to the proliferation of abnormal cells. In addition, an imbalance in mineral metabolism underlies immune dysfunction, which again, is a steppingstone to cancer, says Dr. Kelley. He believed that excessive protein intake is the most significant cause of pancreatic enzyme deficiency.

Dr. Kelley's theory is supported by research which has shown that not only does the pancreas secrete digestive enzymes into the small intestine, it also secretes them into the bloodstream where they can reach all cells in the body, including cancer cells, which they digest and subdue.

## The 10 Metabolic Types

Dr. Kelley classified patients into 10 different metabolic types, with slow-oxidizing vegetarians at one end and fast-oxidizing carnivores at the other, and, more precisely, according to the quality of involvement and efficiency of operation of the sympathetic or parasympathetic nervous system, and with respect to their operating relationship. These classifications may be generalized as follows:

- extreme sympathetic dominant, but efficient
- extreme parasympathetic dominant, but efficient
- balanced but inefficient
- balanced and efficient
- inefficient sympathetic
- inefficient parasympathetic
- requiring cooked foods
- average/healthy, requiring well-balanced meals
- sympathetic dominant (but less strongly so than earlier similar category)
- parasympathetic dominant (again, less strongly so than earlier similar category)

His metabolic detoxification therapy calls for coffee enemas, restricting of protein intake, and emphasizing a diet of whole grains, fruits, and vegetables supplemented with proteolytic enzymes and raw juices. Dr. Kelley advised cancer patients to altogether avoid pasteurized milk, peanuts, white flour and sugar, chlorinated water, and all processed foods. In general terms, he recommended that the diet consist of about 70% raw foods, such as fresh raw salads, to maximize the consumption of living enzymes. Dr. Kelley developed a line of 25 nutritional formulations for hard tumors (solid mass cancers) and 29 for soft tumors (leukemia, lymphoma, melanoma) which the patient takes until they are cancer free for 2 years. However, as each person has a different capacity for absorbing nutrients, the therapy needs to be carefully individualized.

Nicholas Gonzalez, M.D., of New York City, a classically trained immunologist, currently employs a cancer treatment, which to a large extent, is based on Kelley's therapy. Dr. Gonzalez' protocol includes 6 basics first put forward by Dr. Kelley: a diet appropriate for each individual; intensive nutritional support; protomorphogens (raw beef organs and glands); digestive aids such as hydrochloric acid; proteolytic enzyme supplementation; and thorough detoxification.

Dr. Gonzalez did not just blindly adopt Dr. Kelley's work. Rather, his belief that Kelley's protocols are valid comes as a result of his 5-year study of Dr. Kelley's cancer patients. Dr. Gonzalez originally tracked 50 patients, ranging in age from 21 to 71, all of whom were diagnosed as "terminal" or with an extremely poor prognosis. Their cases encompassed 25 different types of cancer. Dr. Gonzalez found that many of the patients in this group survived 10 years or longer.

To further test Dr. Kelley's results, Dr. Gonzalez tracked 22 patients who had been diagnosed with pancreatic cancer, since this form of cancer tends to have a 5-year survival rate with conventional medical therapies of nearly 0%, as well as a life expectancy of only 2-3 months. Ten of the patients who consulted with Dr. Kelley once and then did not follow his treatment program survived only an average of 67 days, or just over 2 months; 7 who followed his program only partially survived an average of 233 days, or nearly 8 months. But the 5 patients who followed his program closely had a median survival rate of 9 years. As of 1987, 4 of the 5 were still alive; the 5th had died of Alzheimer's disease.[116] In his own practice today, Dr. Gonzalez claims that about 80% of his patients do well on his application of Dr. Kelley's therapy.

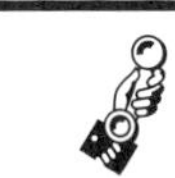

To contact **Dr. Gonzalez, M.D.**, 36A East 36th Street, Suite 204, New York, NY 10016; tel: 212-213-3337; fax: 212-213-3414.

For more about the **Kelley** program in action, see Chapter 22: Jack Taylor, D.C.

***Dr. Kelley advised cancer patients to altogether avoid pasteurized milk, peanuts, white flour and sugar, chlorinated water, and all processed foods. In general terms, he recommended that the diet consist of about 70% raw foods, such as fresh raw salads, to maximize the consumption of living enzymes.***

According to Dr. Gonzalez, the National Cancer Institute is reviewing his patient records. "The ultimate goal for all of us is to try to get trials so we can get our therapies tested. Then if it does work, the world will have the documented facts to confirm it." Dr. Gonzalez says that each of his patients comply close to 100% with their individual program and that most of his patients have already received radiation and chemotherapy and been told by their previous physicians that they have only a few months to live.

For example, a 28-year-old lawyer suffering from leukemia was brought to Dr. Gonzalez. Her leukemia was in its most advanced stage, referred to as "blast crisis," and she had been told by her previous doctors that she had only a few days to live. Dr. Gonzalez not only kept her alive but, after 3 months on his protocol, she became noticeably better. A year later, she was in complete remission and resumed her career.

## MANGANESE

Manganese helps maintain the structural integrity of heart and kidney cell membranes and promotes tissue oxygen uptake, food absorption, neurotransmitter synthesis, fertility, insulin synthesis, fat (lipid) and carbohydrate metabolism, and homeostatic blood-clotting mechanisms.[117] It is part of the main antioxidant enzyme, superoxide dismutase, and there is some evidence that it may help to counteract the immune-suppressive effects of stress hormones called corticosteroids. Manganese may increase the binding ability and other activities of white blood cells.[118] Finally, this element is a cofactor in various enzyme systems.

***Biochemist Roger J. Williams, Ph.D., realized that each individual is nutritionally unique and requires variations in nutrient intake to function optimally. His concept of biochemical individuality sparked the emergence of new preventive diagnostic procedures.***

## MOLYBDENUM

This trace element is required in tiny amounts for human health—the official recommended daily allowance (RDA) is 150-500 mcg daily. Molybdenum is an essential part of at least 3 key enzyme systems and supports the liver's detoxification of sulfites (in many preservatives), alcohol (in beverages and medications), aldehydes (a toxic byproduct of metabolizing various chemicals), and copper-containing compounds.[119] A molybdenum deficiency, which can be detected by a urine or blood test, is associated with cancer of the esophagus.[120]

## ORTHOMOLECULAR MEDICINE

In 1968, Nobel Prize-winner Linus Pauling, Ph.D., coined the term "orthomolecular" to describe an approach to medicine that uses naturally occurring substances normally present in the body. *Ortho* means "correct to normal," and orthomolecular physicians recognize that in many cases of physiological and psychological disorders health can be reestablished by properly correcting, or normalizing, the balance of vitamins, minerals, amino acids, and other such substances within the body.

Most conventional physicians still disregard the relationship of correct nutrition to health. The prevalent notion is that a "balanced" diet will provide all the nutrients one needs, but what is overlooked here is that most of the U.S. food supply is grown in nutritionally depleted soil, then highly processed. Orthomolecular physicians recognize these factors and know that biochemical individuality can play a crucial role in health.

The concept of biochemical individuality is based on the work of Roger J. Williams, Ph.D., a pioneering biochemist who discovered vitamin B5 (pantothenic acid) in the 1930s. In treating his patients, Dr. Williams realized that each individual is nutritionally unique and requires variations in nutrient intake to function optimally. His concept of biochemical individuality sparked the emergence of new preventive diagnostic procedures, such as nutritional assessment and risk-factor analysis. These procedures rely on physiological data, as well as personal and family health history, dietary intake analysis, and scientifically advanced biochemical screenings to help determine a person's unique biochemical and nutritional status.

Although meeting RDAs for nutrients may prevent incidences of severe deficiency that lead to disease, orthomolecular physicians contend that these levels do not provide for optimal health, and people may need many more times the RDAs. For example, studies of guinea pigs show a 20-fold variation in their requirement for vitamin C. Similar human studies showed that the elderly may require more vitamin B12, men may need more zinc, and that children have varying needs for vitamin B6. Richard Kunin, M.D., of San Francisco, California, summarizes the principles of orthomolecular medicine in this way:[121]

- Nutrition comes first in medical diagnosis and treatment, and nutrient-related disorders are usually curable once nutritional balance is achieved.
- Biochemical individuality is the norm in medical practice; therefore universal RDA values are unreliable nutrient guides. Many people, because of their genetic disposition and/or the environment in which they live, require an intake of certain nutrients far beyond the RDA suggested range (often called a megadose).
- Drug treatment is to be used only for specific indications and always mindful of the potential dangers and adverse effects.
- Environmental pollution and food adulteration are inescapable facts of modern life, and avoiding them is a medical priority.
- Blood tests do not necessarily reflect tissue levels of nutrients.
- Hope is the indispensable ally of the physician and the absolute right of the patient.

## American Attitudes about Nutrition

While 80% of Americans recognize the importance of good nutrition, 36% are reluctant to give up their favorite foods to achieve it, says a study of 800 adults by the American Dietetic Association, released in September 1995. The study also found that 71% of consumers pay some attention to nutritional labeling and 50% say new label information is easier to understand than it used to be.

The basis of orthomolecular medicine lies in creating a thoroughly *healthy* diet. Junk foods, refined sugar, and food additives are eliminated; every effort is made to eat nutritious whole foods, high in fiber and low in fat. Depending on the health condition, vitamins, minerals, and other nutrients are taken as supplements; the types and amounts of these nutrients are determined by blood tests, urine analysis, and nutrient-level assays. Frequently, supplementation is based not only on a patient's symptoms, but on results reported in medical journals and, quite commonly, the clinical experience of the doctor.

For more on **orthomolecular medicine**, see Chapter 10: Abram Hoffer, M.D.

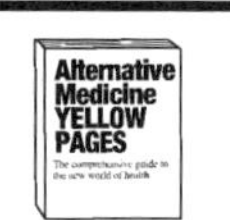


See "Diet," p. 113; "Nutritional Therapy," p. 187; and "Orthomolecular Medicine," p. 196.

Prescribed doses of vitamins are sometimes injected to speed the initial response, and follow-up treatment usually consists of vitamin pills several times a day until adequate dosage is achieved. Mentioned above, this dosage has often been called a "megadose" because the amounts of nutrients taken are often far greater than the levels needed to prevent deficiency. As a result, orthomolecular medicine has also been called "megavitamin therapy."

One argument against megavitamin treatment put forward by conventional doctors is that high doses of certain vitamins are toxic and may cause certain reactions. A major study, however, indicates that the total number of fatalities from overdoses of major pharmaceutical drugs for the 8-year reporting period from 1983 to 1990 equals 2,556 whereas the total number of fatalities resulting from high doses of vitamin supplements during the same period is zero.[122]

Nevertheless, orthomolecular physicians are aware of the problems associated with megavitamin therapy, and if symptoms arise, the dosage of the offending vitamin is reduced. In some cases, these reactions are carefully observed as an indication that the body has been saturated with the vitamin. When this occurs, the dose is lowered until the symptoms disappear and the body is supplied with optimal levels of the nutrient. An example is the method of administering vitamin C to bowel tolerance for the common cold, flu, and other conditions as pioneered by Robert Cathcart III, M.D., of Los Altos, California.[123] The bowel tolerance test is widely used by proponents of vitamin C for cancer treatment. Among the cancer doctors profiled in this book, Abram Hoffer, M.D., is an outstanding practitioner (and educator) in the field of orthomolecular medicine.

## POTASSIUM

As pioneering cancer doctor Max Gerson, M.D., found, raising the body's potassium supply seems to help counteract tumor growth. In addition, research shows that by controlling the types of salt and water content at the cellular level, cellular function, energy production, and overall biological integrity can be improved or restored. Chinese studies indicate that high-potassium, low-sodium environments can partially return damaged cell proteins to their normal undamaged configuration. According to Freeman Cope, M.D., "the damage in other tissues, induced by toxins and breakdown products from the cancer, is probably partly repaired by the Gerson therapy through this mechanism." [124]

## SELENIUM

This trace element has a synergistic, or cooperative, relationship with vitamin E, meaning that the 2 nutrients mutually reinforce the body's anticancer defenses. An integral part of the body's antioxidant enzyme system (glutathione peroxidase), selenium has key effects on DNA metabolism, cell membrane integrity, and optimal functioning of both the liver and pancreas. As such, it can interfere with both the initiation and promotion phases of cancer development. Glutathione peroxidase protects tissues against free radical damage, and its anticancer effects are greatly dependent on the availability of selenium.[125]

According to biochemist Gerhard Schrauzer, Ph.D., selenium is often deficient in cancer patients.[126] This fact is significant, since even small doses of selenium have been found to greatly enhance the cancer-fighting activity of Natural Killer (NK) cells in laboratory animals.[127]

For more on **selenium**, see Chapter 15: Emanuel Revici, M.D., p. 313.

Selenium supplements have been shown to impede the reappearance of tumors in animals whose tumors regressed following ovariectomy.[128] Many chemotherapeutic drugs and various heavy metals (lead, mercury, cadmium) tend to inactivate selenium, making it unavailable to the body.[129]

He analyzed the blood-bank data from 17 countries and reported that areas with low levels of selenium in the diet had higher levels of leukemia and cancers of the colon, rectum, prostate, ovary, breast, and lung.[130] A study in Finland found that subjects with serum selenium levels less than 45 mcg/liter were three times more likely to develop cancer as subjects with serum selenium levels above 45 mcg/liter.[131]

Researchers at the Chinese Academy of Medical Sciences Cancer Institute in Beijing, China, found that when members of a family with high rates of liver cancer took at least 200 mcg of selenium daily for 2 years, it significantly reduced the development of new cases of liver cancer, according to *Biological Trace Element Research* (1991).

## VITAMIN A

This fat-soluble vitamin, which exists primarily in the form of retinol, has repeatedly been shown to enhance the activity of immune cells against tumor cells.[132,133,134] Most of the research seems to indicate that vitamin A's greatest benefit is in preventing cancers or recurrences of cancer. Accutane (13-cis-retinoic acid) is a pharmaceutical derivative of vitamin A, and has proven effective "in preventing second primary tumors in patients who have been treated for squamous-cell carcinoma of the head and neck, although it does not prevent recurrence of the original [type of] tumor."[135]

In one study, 9 men with an untreatable form of lung cancer (metastatic, squamous cell lung carcinoma) were given vitamin A palmitate or 13 cis-retinoic acid (a form of vitamin A) without other medical intervention. Fifteen months later, the men's immune function had improved and significant progress against the tumor had been made.[136] A study by Frank Meyskens, Jr. at the University of Arizona Cancer Center in Tucson, found that vitamin A provided protection against stage I and stage II malignant melanoma when combined with BCG injections (Bacillus Calmette-Guérin is a vaccine commonly used against tuberculosis ).[137]

## VITAMIN B COMPLEX

This group of B vitamins, which includes B1, B2, B3, B6, folic acid, and pantothenic acid, acts as a biochemical team to help speed up chemical reactions as catalysts and support overall energy metabolism. Deficiencies of any one or more of the B vitamins inhibit the immune system's ability to fight cancer.[138,139] Both pantothenic acid and vitamin B6 have been shown to inhibit the growth of tumors.[140] A B6 deficiency depresses numerous aspects of immune function, including T-cell activity, antibody responsiveness, and other factors.[141] Cancer patients are frequently deficient in folic acid, which has been shown to inhibit the growth of chemically induced tumors.[142]

IMPORTANT

A major side effect of niacin supplementation is a tingling or flushing in the skin, beginning in the face or neck. If the sensation becomes intolerable, Abram Hoffer, M.D. (profiled in Chapter 10 of this book), suggests switching to the ester form of the vitamin, inositol hexanicotinate. This form is expensive but provides inositol with only minimal flushing.

Vitamins B1 (thiamin) and B2 (riboflavin) are more indirect immune-system supporters and primarily serve in the maintenance of mucous membranes, formation of red blood cells, and metabolism of carbohydrates, the body's most efficient energy source. The B-complex vitamins are typically used to maintain proper functioning of the immune and nervous systems and to reinforce the effects of B vitamins taken separately.

***Deficiencies of any one or more of the B vitamins inhibit the immune system's ability to fight cancer. Both pantothenic acid and vitamin B6 have been shown to inhibit the growth of tumors.***

## VITAMIN B3 (NIACIN)

There is growing evidence that vitamin B3, also known as niacin or nicotinic acid, may increase the therapeutic efficacy of cancer treatment. This vitamin exists in nature primarily in the form of 1 of 2 coenzymes, NAD and NADP, both of which are required by more than 150 enzymes involved in respiration and the transfer of electrons. Without these enzymatic reactions, our body's energy production would shut down in the blink of an eye.

Max Gerson, M.D., founder of the Gerson Therapy (see Gerson Diet Therapy, p. 771), successfully treated many cancer patients with a dietary regimen that included 50 mg of niacin 8-10 times per day.[143] Good dietary sources of niacin include brewer's yeast, fish, asparagus, and whole grains. Coffee beans contain a biologically inactive derivative of niacin, which is then converted to the active form of niacin by ordinary roasting procedures; thus coffee drinkers tend to receive a substantial amount of niacin.[144] Coffee is not recommended for cancer patients, however.

## VITAMIN B6 (PYRIDOXINE)

The immune and nervous systems are strongly influenced by the systemic supply of this B vitamin, which aids in DNA/RNA synthesis, fat and protein metabolism, hemoglobin function, and tryptophan metabolism (which in turn affects mood and level of alertness).[145] Vitamin B6 has been shown to inhibit the growth of various tumors[146] including liver cancer.[147]

Like vitamin C, vitamin B6 is also essential in the production of prostaglandin E1, which is necessary for normal thymus function and regulation of T cells. When vitamin B6 was given to 33 bladder cancer patients, there was a marked reduction in recurrence rates compared to the control group.[148] There is also considerable evidence that vitamin B6 helps protect against the toxic side effects of radiation treatment for cancer.[149]

***Other research shows that vitamin C enhances the anticancer activity of some chemotherapy drugs, including Adriamycin; the vitamin enhances the effects of radiation treatment and protects healthy tissues (skin and bone marrow) during such treatment.***

## VITAMIN C (ASCORBIC ACID)

Found in citrus fruits, broccoli, green peppers, and many other fruits and vegetables, vitamin C is involved in the maintenance of a healthy immune system as well as protecting against a variety of cancers.[150] There is now solid evidence that this vitamin is essential for optimal functioning of the immune system.[151] Among those immune components most actively involved in fighting cancer are the natural killer (NK) cells, which are only active if they contain relatively large amounts of vitamin C.[152] Vitamin C also boosts the body's production of interferon, which has anticancer activity.[153]

Hugh Riordan, M.D., director of the Center for Human Functioning in Wichita, Kansas, notes that vitamin C increases intracellular peroxidases, enzymes that help protect the cell against harmful free radicals.[154] Dr. Riordan also states that vitamin C is 20 to 30 times more toxic to cancer cells than to normal cells. Cancer patients taking vitamin C report an improved appetite and mental outlook, as well as a decrease in pain and the need for painkilling drugs.[155] Other research shows that vitamin C enhances the anticancer activity of some chemotherapy drugs, including Adriamycin;[156] the vitamin enhances the effects of radiation treatment and protects healthy tissues (skin and bone marrow) during such treatment.[157]

Specifically, Dr. Riordan's research showed that ascorbic acid and its salts are toxic to tumor cells in vitro (in a test tube) and in vivo (in the living body) when given at high enough levels to maintain blood concentrations above the levels known to be toxic to tumor cells. Ascorbic acid has the potential to selectively kill tumor cells in a manner similar to other chemotherapy agents, Dr. Riordan concluded.

According to Stephen Edelson, M.D. (profiled in Chapter 8), who uses megadoses of vitamin C, "Most studies of ascorbic acid in cancer have not utilized high enough doses to maintain a plasma concentration sufficient to kill tumors, yet the evidence suggests it is feasible to use ascorbic acid as a cytotoxic (cell-killing) chemotherapeutic agent and that it can be successful with no side effects. We are using this therapy successfully in our center. However, further clinical research is necessary to determine all the details concerning the long-term effectiveness of ascorbic acid in killing cancer cells."

***A daily dose of 10 g of vitamin C spread throughout the day significantly extended the survival and improved the quality of life in 100 "terminal" cancer patients.***

This water-soluble vitamin has shown an ability to selectively kill tumor cells in a manner similar to other chemotherapy drugs.[159] Vitamin C combined with various B vitamins may significantly limit tumor growth without harming the body's normal tissues.[160] A daily dose of 10 g (10,000 mg, spread throughout the day) of vitamin C significantly extended the survival and improved the quality of life in 100 "terminal" cancer patients in Scotland.[161] A larger dose (at bowel tolerance level) further extended the survival and quality of life in another large group of terminal cancer patients in Canada. Linus Pauling, Ph.D., offered several reasons why subsequent studies have not found such positive results. First, the dosages were too low; second, the supplements were discontinued prematurely; third, patients who had been heavily pretreated with chemo- and radiation therapy were beyond the point of recovery. Biological limits need to be recognized—there's a point where terminal cancer patients can no longer respond to even the best therapies.

The mechanisms of action by which vitamin C aids cancer patients are many, says Michael N. Schachter, M.D. (the subject of Chapter 18). They include bolstering various elements of the immune system and stabilizing

## Vitamin C's Cancer Protection

Current studies lend strong support to the importance of vitamin C in slowing the development of cancer, cataracts, and heart disease. A recent study, conducted by James E. Enstrom, M.D., an epidemiologist at the University of California at Los Angeles, suggests that men who consume vitamin C every day, at levels that are 500-666% of the U.S. RDA, live about 6 years longer than men who do not.[162]

A separate review by Gladys Block, Ph.D., an epidemiologist of the National Cancer Institute's Divison of Cancer Prevention and Control, found a statistically significant benefit in 33 of 46 studies.[163] She concluded that vitamin C affords added protection against cancers of the colon, rectum, pancreas, bladder, lung, larynx, oral cavity, esophagus, stomach, cervix, brain, endometrium, and breast.

and strengthening the connective tissue surrounding solid cancers in order to help prevent the spread of the cancer. These effects may be obtained from the administration of either oral or injectable vitamin C. Another effect of vitamin C, which was demonstrated years ago but generally ignored until the 1990s, is that vitamin C in high concentrations can actually kill cancer cells and leave normal cells alone, Dr. Schachter says. "This cancer cell-killing effect may be obtained *only* with intravenous infusions of vitamin C; one cannot reach these blood levels by oral intake."

Vitamin C is usually started at between 4-6 g a day, in divided doses. This daily dosage is then increased until bowel tolerance is attained. The dosage is then reduced to just below that level and maintained for several months or preferably lifelong.

In addition to suffering temporary diarrhea, a small percentage of people experience gastric distress, such as gas and bloating. According to nutritional biochemist Ross Pelton, this problem can be alleviated by switching to the less acidic calcium ascorbate salt.[164] Author W. Lee Cowden, M.D., prefers equal parts of calcium ascorbate and magnesium ascorbate as long as kidney function is normal. If sodium ascorbate is administered intravenously or orally, transient fluid retention will occasionally result (from the sodium overload); this can be problematic for people with hypertension or heart problems.

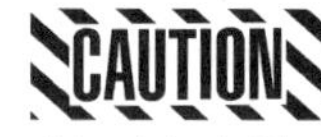


Although vitamin C has extremely low toxicity even at high doses, certain side effects may occur.

For more information on **vitamin C**, see Chapter 10: Abram Hoffer, M.D., pp. 215-217.

On rare occasions, cancer patients with rapidly growing malignant tumors and a heavy tumor load will show a sudden increase in tumor necrosis (the death of cancer cells causing toxic accumulation), a potentially fatal complication calling for careful treatment.[165] One study found that vitamin C enhanced leukemia development in some human leukemia cell lines, though it had the opposite effect in other leukemia cell lines.[166] Until more is known, patients with leukemia should be cautious about taking vitamin C, particularly in large doses. We recommend careful monitoring by a physician.

For many years, the medical community promoted the erroneous belief that vitamin C supplementation eventually causes kidney damage. Studies by Hoffer, Cameron, and others have shown that high doses of vitamin C do *not* cause kidney damage, even when cancer patients use the vitamin in high doses over many years.[167]

After 2 decades of discounting Linus Pauling's work, the medical establishment finally embraced vitamin C as an anticancer agent. In September of 1990, at a symposium sponsored by the National Institutes of Health, scientists reviewed evidence for the vitamin's role in the prevention and treatment of cancer.[168] They concluded that vitamin C demonstrates a consistently protective effect on a variety of human tumors.

## Antioxidants Stop Spread of Cancer

A Scottish study of 50 men, half of them cigarette smokers, demonstrated clearly that nutritional supplementation with antioxidants such as vitamins C, E, and beta carotene for up to 20 weeks had a "highly significant moderating effect" on DNA damage done by free radicals, according to *Cancer Research,* March 15, 1996. In particular, the antioxidants were able to stop the spread of cancer (metastasis) caused by the generation of hydroxyl free radicals. DNA taken from invasive, spreading cancer was shown to have twice as much free radical-caused DNA damage.

## VITAMIN D

This vitamin, also classified as a hormone, appears to have cancer-killing (antitumor) properties.[169] Though research findings are still preliminary, vitamin D and its metabolites may increase the number of vitamin A receptors on cells ("up-regulating"), inhibit the formation of new tumor blood vessels (angiogenesis), induce the conversion of cancer cells back to normal cells (cell differentiation), and induce "cell suicide" (apoptosis) in cancer cells.[170] Researchers in Australia concluded that vitamin D may protect the body against prostate cancer. They based this conclusion on the fact that there are far more cases of prostate cancer in northern areas such as Iceland, Denmark, and Sweden, where there is limited natural sunlight, compared to areas of more intense, sustained sunlight.[171]

**CAUTION**

In general, vitamin D should be reserved for cancer patients with low vitamin D levels; moreover, the patient must be carefully monitored to avoid toxicity.

The vitamin D supplement may be given in the range of 400 to 1000

**_Vitamin E boosts the effectiveness of chemotherapy agents on tumors, but lack of vitamin E increases the toxic effects of Adriamycin (a common chemotherapy agent) on heart tissue. Supplementation with vitamin E helps protect against the toxic effects of radiation treatments._**

IU daily. Note that vitamin D manufactured in the skin by the influence of sunlight will not cause toxicity, no matter how much sun exposure an individual receives. The body automatically shuts down its own vitamin D production once the requirement is reached, typically within 15 minutes of exposure to sunshine.

## VITAMIN E

This fat-soluble vitamin, one of the body's primary agents for protecting cell membranes, is also among the major nutrients required for strong immune responses to cancer and infection.[172] One study found that, for 43 patients with oral leukoplakia (a premalignant condition) who were given 400 IU of vitamin E twice daily for 24 weeks, nearly half (46%) showed significant clinical improvement.[173] In animal studies, the vitamin has reversed the development of chemically induced tumors[174] and has even been shown to *prevent* tumor development, suggesting a role in warding off recurrences of cancer.[175]

Vitamin E boosts the effectiveness of chemotherapy agents on tumors,[176] but lack of vitamin E increases the toxic effects of Adriamycin (a common chemotherapy agent) on heart tissue.[177] In addition, the supplementation with vitamin E helps protect against the toxic effects of radiation treatments.[178] Many physicians have begun to recommend the succinate form of vitamin E, which seems to enter cells more readily.

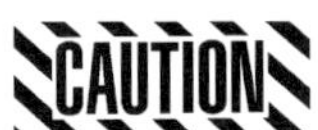


The injectable form of vitamin K that is administered to all babies born in U.S. hospitals contains phenol, a known allergen and carcinogen. Unless you have a hereditary tendency toward blood coagulation problems, we do not recommend using injectable vitamin K, as there is some evidence that this may contribute to an increase in childhood cancers.[180] Japanese doctors use the oral form of vitamin K, and many European physicians are increasingly following suit.

## VITAMIN K

This vitamin's primary function is as a coagulating factor, a nutrient that aids in blood clotting. There is some evidence that vitamin K, probably in the form of vitamin K-3 (menadione), is effective as an anticancer agent. This form of the vitamin can be toxic, in contrast to the preferred nontoxic form, vitamin K-1 (phylloquinone or phytonadione). A growing body of evidence indicates that vitamin K-1 supplements enhance the antimetastatic effects of anticoagulant factors in the body.[179] In addition, severe vitamin K deficiency has been found in cancer patients receiving prescription antimicrobial antibiotics. A 1-mg-per-day oral dosage of vitamin K-1 (phytonadione) should not represent any hazard to patients receiving anticoagulant therapy.

## WATER

While water is not a nutritional supplement, the need for pure water is recognized and advocated by physicians profiled in this book. Pure water is an integral part of anticancer nutrition. Here are practical guidelines:

First, determine the quality of water in your home by asking the water department for standards and analysis. Verify the condition of your home's water lines because lead can leach out of the soldering on older water pipes and plumbing into household tap water. Drinking bottled water is a viable alternative, but be careful about the source—many waters are simply repackaged city supplies. Buying water in glass bottles is best but hard plastic bottles are usually better than soft plastic. Choose only those waters that provide a full analysis of their contents and sources, and look for waters that are Canadian glacial melt or that have been purified through deionization. Such brands are known as "distilled" or "purified by reverse osmosis."

There are 3 basic types of filtration systems:

**1. Solid block carbon filters** appear to be much more effective in removing organic chemicals such as solvents and trihalomethanes than activated granular carbon filters. If you prefer to leave dissolved minerals in your water, carbon block filters are recommended because they do not remove these inorganic compounds.

**2. Reverse osmosis** systems force water under pressure through a membrane. They are most effective against inorganic pollutants like nitrate and against metals like lead; deionization resins are also used to accomplish this purpose.

**3. Distillation** purifies water by boiling and condensing it. Metals and inorganic compounds are effectively removed in this way because they are heavier and have a much higher boiling temperature than the water, but some organic compounds have nearly the same boiling temperature as water and may not be removed.

The best systems combine several methods of filtration for optimal pollutant removal, such as carbon block filtration combined with reverse

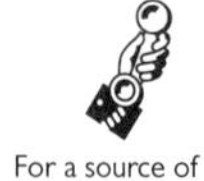

For a source of a **KDF showerhead filter**, contact: Health Restoration Systems, P.O. Box 832267, Richardson, TX 75083: tel: 214-480-8909; fax: 214-480-8807.

osmosis, which is effective against organic and inorganic pollutants, as are carbon block and distillation combinations. These can range in price from $150 for an under-the-sink model combining carbon filtration with reverse osmosis, to $1,500 for a whole-house filter that will purify even the water for your shower. Since it has been estimated that approximately 70% of all pollutants that enter the body from water come in through the skin during bathing or showering, it would be wise to use a good quality showerhead filter (with a combination carbon and KDF ion resin) if a whole house filtering system cannot be employed.

***"I expect and hope that orthomolecular medicine within the next 5-10 years will cease to be a specialty in medicine and that all physicians will be using nutrition as an essential generalist's tool in treating disease," says Abram Hoffer, M.D., Ph.D., a pioneer in orthomolecular medicine.***

**Microwater—**This is a new water filtration system with potential therapeutic benefits, originally developed in Japan. Microwater uses a technology that filters and enhances the quality of water by making the size of water molecules smaller. It is already a $700-million-a-year industry in Japan and is now being introduced in the U.S. The Microwater unit, hooked up to a faucet, uses a carbon-activated filter to remove impurities from the water, then it injects a small electrical charge into the water that separates the water into 2 kinds: Flowing out of one tube is an acidic water (with positive ions) useful for topical, external uses; out of another tube comes alkaline water (with negative ions) for drinking. It makes this separation at the rate of 1 gallon per minute.

The applications of the acidic portion of Microwater are numerous and quite surprising. According to the research, and based on early reports from African and South American users, acidic Microwater acts as a "superoxidant" to disinfect and sterilize surfaces, skin, wounds, even surgical instruments. It can kill bacteria and viruses, it can promote the healing of acne, eczema, wounds, sore throats, and blisters, and it can improve skin quality. When used on foods, it can retard spoilage or act as a bacterial cleanser for meats; it can be used by dentists to sterilize the mouth during dental procedures; and you can use it as a mouthwash when you brush your teeth.

Regarding the alkaline Microwater, here the smaller size of the water molecules shows its advantage. Acording to Hidemistu Hayashi, M.D., one of Japan's foremost Microwater researchers, alkaline Microwater can act as a powerful antioxidant in the body, destroying harmful free radicals, just as do antioxidants such as vitamins A, C, and, E. Although the reports are still, strictly speaking, anecdotal, in those who drank Microwater every day for several months Dr. Hayashi reports that he and his colleagues have seen improvements in diabetes, constipation, ulcers, blood pressure, allergies, circulation, migraines, obesity, osteoporosis, and menstrual irregularities. Not surprisingly, the use of Microwater as a preventive medicine technology is reportedly expanding in Japanese clinics and hospitals.

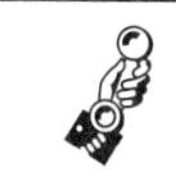

A kitchen-model **Microwater** unit costs around $1,500 and can be easily installed in 10 minutes. For information, contact: Mizutek International, 335 Countyview Drive, Mill Valley, CA 94941; tel: 800-456-4520; fax: 415-383-9078; or Tomoe USA Inc., 379 Oyster Pt. Blvd., Suite 6, South San Francisco, CA 94080; tel: 800-794-7947.

CAUTION

High zinc levels in the blood may be associated with higher mortality rates from cancers of the colon, breast, ovary, lung, bladder, prostate and oral cavity. These findings may be related to heavy meat-eating practices, since red meat typically contains large amounts of zinc. Caution should be exercised whenever using zinc as part of a cancer treatment program. It is well established that zinc is antagonistic to both copper and selenium; supplementation with zinc should therefore be carefully monitored by the appropriate health professionals.

Once Microwater gets absorbed by the body's cells, says Dr. Hayashi, it helps to dissolve acidic wastes that have accumulated there over many years and reduces the chronic dehydration common in many people. In effect, thanks to the smaller molecular size, more water is absorbed by the body and more water actually penetrates all the cells and tissues; when the body has more water to work with (and in this case, a more refined form of it), it is better able to deliver nutrients to all the cells, tissues, and organs.

The water tastes unusually smooth and soft due to its high concentration of negative ions (typical of pure mountain springs), and so it can be quite refreshing. "We are advancing the theory that the most effective and economical source for an antioxidant is ordinary tap water *after* it is filtered and treated with a Microwater unit," says Dr. Hayashi.

## ZINC

This trace element is occasionally recommended as a temporary supplement (30 to 60 mg per day), but it should never be used routinely by itself. Like selenium, zinc supports many aspects of the immune system, and its deficiency can potentially make us more vulnerable to certain cancers.[181] Zinc is necessary for the free-radical quenching activity of superoxide dismutase (SOD), a powerful antioxidant enzyme which breaks down the free-radical superoxide to form hydrogen peroxide. A deficiency of zinc can lead to depressed activity of NK cells and other white blood cells.[182]

As mentioned earlier, Zinc has an antagonistic relationship with copper—an excess of one can cause a deficiency of the other. Both, ironically, are essential to proper functioning of a wide range of immune cell types, including antibody-forming cells, T helper cells, and macrophages, all of which seem to help the body defend against cancer.[183]

Chapter 29

# Botanicals As Cancer Medicines

## *A Complete Guide to Anticancer Herbal Supplements*

**In the physician's effort to bolster the body's natural immune defenses against cancer, employing the nontoxic biochemical components of herbs is a prime approach. Once the basis of ethnic healing traditions, botanicals are now proving their value in cancer treatment to Western science.**

Herbs, or botanicals, contain a large number of naturally occurring chemicals that have biological activity. In the past 150 years, chemists and pharmacists have been isolating and purifying active compounds from plants in an attempt to produce safe and effective pharmaceutical drugs. Examples include digoxin (from foxglove, *Digitalis purpurea*), reserpine (from Indian snakeroot, *Rauwolfia serpentina*), colchicine (from autumn crocus, *Colchicum autumnale*), morphine, (from the opium poppy, *Papaver somniafera*), and many more.

According to Andrew Weil, M.D., herb and plant derivatives reach the bloodstream and target organs by an indirect route, which means that their effects are usually slower in onset and less dramatic than those of purified drugs administered by more direct routes. "Doctors and patients accustomed to the rapid, intense effects of synthetic medicines may become impatient with botanicals for this reason," Dr. Weil states.

But this delayed response is a relatively minor issue compared to what botanical medicine has to offer when used to facilitate healing in chronic health problems. Through skillful selection of an herb (or herbs in combination) targeted to the individual patient, major changes in health can be effected with less danger of the side effects inherent in drug-based medicine. However, the common assumption that herbs act slowly and mildly is not necessarily true; adverse effects can occur if an inadequate dose, a low-quality herb, or the wrong herb is prescribed.

In recent years, a great deal of pharmaceutical research has gone into analyzing the active ingredients of herbs to find out how and why they work—an effect referred to as the herb's action. Herbal actions indicate the ways in which the remedy affects human physiology. In some cases the action is due to a specific chemical present in the herb or it may be due to complex synergistic interactions among various constituents of the plant. In the case of cancer, botanical agents work by:

- stimulating DNA-repair mechanisms (via sulfur-containing compounds)
- producing antioxidant effects (via the quenching of free radicals by carotenoids and the scavenging of oxygen radicals by ascorbic acid and polyphenols)
- promoting induction of protective enzymes, e.g., proteases (via indoles)
- inhibiting cancer-activating enzymes (via some flavonols and tannins)
- inducing oxygenating effects (via flavonols and rare elements such as germanium)

**Botanical Substances Covered in This Chapter**

- Algae (chlorella, sea vegetables, green concentrates)
- Aloe vera
- Amygdalin/laetrile
- Astragalus
- Cat's claw
- *Echinacea*
- Essiac
- Flavonoids
- Garlic
- *Gingko biloba*
- Ginseng
- Grape seed extract/pycnogenols
- Green tea
- Haelan 851
- HANSI
- Hoxsey herbs
- Iscador (mistletoe)
- Larch arabinogalactan
- Maitake mushroom
- Pau d'arco
- Pectin, modified citrus
- Silymarin
- Turmeric

## The Herbal Foundation of Effective Cancer Therapy

Herbal medicine, also known as botanical medicine, phytotherapy, or phytomedicine, is the science of using plants medicinally. An herb can be the whole plant, leaf, flower, stem, seed, root, fruit, bark, or any other part deemed useful for its medicinal, food flavoring, and/or fragrant property. In many traditional medical systems, the different parts of each plant are known to have specific therapeutic properties, which were discovered only after many centuries of trial-and-error observation.

James A. Duke, Ph.D., a former U.S. Drug Administration researcher, notes that more than 25% of prescription drugs and other medications used today are derived from (or at least based on) substances naturally found in plants.[1] Out of an estimated 250,000 to 500,000 plants in existence today, only about 5,000 have been extensively studied for their medicinal applications. "[This] illustrates the need for modern medicine and science to turn its attention to the plant world once again to find new medicine that might cure cancer and many other diseases," says Norman R. Farnsworth, Ph.D., Professor of Pharmacology at the University of Illinois at Chicago. "Considering that 121 prescription drugs come from only 90 species of plants, and that 74% of these were discovered following up native folklore claims," Farnsworth adds, "a logical person would have to say that there may still be more jackpots out there."

***Out of an estimated 250,000 to 500,000 plants in existence today, only about 5,000 have been extensively studied for their medicinal applications. "[This] illustrates the need for modern medicine and science to turn its attention to the plant world once again to find new medicines that might cure cancer and many other diseases," says Norman R. Farnsworth, Ph.D.***

For example, the conventional anticancer drugs vincristine sulfate and vinblastine sulfate are alkaloids derived from the Madagascar periwinkle (*Catharanthus roseus*) traditionally used in whole, dried form by native healers of Madagascar. Though *Catharanthus* is not employed directly as herbal medicine for cancer, some physicians have begun to use it in homeopathic and "microdose" forms.

Another herb that has been incorporated into the chemotherapy arsenal is the dried root of the mayapple (*Podophyllum peltatum*) and Himalayan mayapple (*Podophyllum hexandrum*). A derivative of this plant has been administered intravenously in treating testicular and ovarian cancers, lymphomas, small-cell lung cancers, and certain forms of leukemia.[2] Sales of the drug, called podophyllotoxin, reached $100 million a year in 1990—the same year the plant was listed as an endangered species. Only 2 years later, sales had jumped to $275 million. Now that the Himalayan mayapple is endangered, the drug company that owns the patent on podophyllotoxin may need to seek alternative sources.

Among the more recent entries onto the anticancer herbal stage are the following:

**Betulinic Acid from Birch Trees**—This substance blocked the growth of human melanoma tumors that were transferred to mice, all without harming normal cells (no toxicity).[3] Tests in human cancer cell cultures indicated effectiveness against cancers of the lymph, lung, and liver as well.[4] Betulin, a compound that can be converted to betulinic acid, is a major constituent of white-barked birch trees, which are found in abundance throughout the northern hemisphere.

***Thuja* Tincture from "Tree of Life"**—*Thuja occidentalis* (arbor vitae, or Tree of life) has served as a successful adjunctive herbal therapy for many cancer cases. An 86-year-old woman had been suffering for 14 years from a large orange-sized tumor in her right breast. It had spread to the lymph nodes and doctors labeled it "inoperable, stage 3 breast carcinoma with lymph metastases." The tumor had never been treated. The woman was given tamoxifen, an estrogen blocker, as well as a tincture of *Thuja* herbal extract (20 drops, 3 times daily), *Echinacea* (1 tablet, 3 times daily), and various vitamins and minerals. She also applied *Thuja* cream locally and later took comfrey, passionflower, sweet violet, cleavers (bedstraw), and chickweed. After 1 month on this program, the abnormal lymph nodules had disappeared and the tumor was softening; 6 months later the tumor had shrunk by 25%, and after another 6 months, no sign of cancer remained.[5]

**Bromelain from Pineapple**—Bromelain, a mixture of proteases and other enzymes isolated from pineapple stems and fruits, has been used for centuries to treat inflammatory disease and other health problems. More recently, its anticancer activity has attracted the interest of scientists. Bromelain has been shown to induce differentiation of 3 leukemia cell lines (in culture) as well as to stimulate the anticancer defenses (monocyte and macrophage cell-killing activity) and to inhibit cancer cell growth.[6] The report cites these effects as a possible explanation for the observed tumor-killing potential of bromelain when combined with chemotherapy treatment, and notes that such effects are seen in cancer patients even after oral administration of bromelain (suggesting that the stomach does not break it down). However, rectal administration of bromelain may still be preferable for greatest effect.

**Phenolic Antioxidants from Mint**—Members of the mint family contain special antioxidant compounds that seem to be even more effective than vitamin E (perhaps the premier antioxidant) in helping to prevent recurrences of tumors. An example of these phenolic compounds is rosmarinic acid, which is found in high levels in some mints, including the wild self-heal (*Prunella vulgaris*), long deemed by Native Americans and traditional Chinese doctors to be a major herbal medicine.[7]

**Centella Extract from *Gotu Kola* (*Hydrocotyle centella*)**—This nutrient-rich herb is said to neutralize and remove toxins, improve mental functioning, and help people prevent a nervous breakdown (or cope better following a breakdown).[8] Scientists at the Amala Cancer Research Center in Kerala, India, found that *Gotu kola* (*H. centella*) showed a strong ability to kill cultured cancer cells. They also showed that *centella* extract more than doubled the lifespan of mice with tumors and showed a remarkable lack of toxicity even in doses far in excess of those used for therapeutic benefit.[9]

**Perillyl Alcohol from Lavender Flowers**—The oil of lavender contains a cancer-fighting component called perillyl alcohol. This substance, which also happens to be a metabolic derivative of the citrus oil compound limonene, has been shown in animal studies to inhibit more than 80% of all chemically induced breast cancers (mammary carcinomas). It is thought that the compound probably blocks tumor growth by inhibiting the gene believed to initiate cancer (the p21 ras oncogene).[10]

**Pollen from Honeybees**—Pollen is the male sex cell from a plant; bees pick up this substance when they enter flowers in search of nectar. Research dating back to 1948 and published in the *Journal of the National Cancer Institute* found that animals whose normal diets were supplemented with bee pollen had a significantly lower tumor incidence than animals fed the normal diet alone.[11] A study in *Nature* reported that royal jelly (derived from pollen) protected all mice injected with cancer cells for longer than 12 months, in contrast to those in the control group, injected with the same number of cancer cells, all of which died within 12 days.[12] In studies of women suffering from inoperable uterine cancer, those given bee pollen were found to maintain strong immune systems and to suffer far less from nausea, hair loss, and fatigue compared to the control group receiving a placebo. Similar results have been reported in studies of cancer patients undergoing radiation treatment.[13]

**Other Herbs**—Other herbal medicines have been identified as potentially useful adjuncts to cancer treatment. These include: pearl barley (*Hordeum vulgare*); reishi mushroom (*Ganoderma lucidum*); shiitake mushroom (*Lentinula edodes*); cauliflower (*Brassica oleracea*); wax gourd (*Benincasa hispida*); calendula (*Calendula officinalis*); chaparral (*Larrea divaricata* and *Larrea tridentata*); white mulberry (*Morus alba*); Japanese pepper (*Piper futokadsura*); thyme (*Thymus serpyllum*); Chinese cucumber (*Trichosanthes kirilowii*); and stinging nettle (*Urtica dioica*).[14]

Rather than consider herbal treatments as alternatives for early or follow-up cancer care, cancer researchers are more likely to investigate the use of herbs as an adjunct conventional treatment. Botanicals have been shown to directly counteract the dangerous effects of chemotherapy and radiation that are toxic to the body, suppress the immune system, and can cause serious mutations and/or damage to cells. Certain botanicals enhance immunity whereas others stimulate the body's detoxification and antioxidant systems. Still others may block the activity of tumor-stimulating hormones, such as estrogen and prolactin. The use of botanical agents in tandem with conventional treatment may not necessarily be the optimal strategy in every case. What is very important, however, is that combining these 2 divergent approaches affords a way for conventional medicine to begin making the transition to a more sensible and ultimately more effective way of treating cancer.

## Low Cost of Herbs

A major reason for the current government-level interest in herbs is to lower health care costs, according to the *Medical Tribune* (January 1995). Botanicals can treat migraines at 10¢-25¢ per day compared to $2-$8 for conventional prescriptions. For lowering cholesterol, coated garlic tablets cost 15¢ per day compared to $4 for a prescription drug. Given that no new conventional anticancer therapy has emerged in over 20 years of dedicated research, looking to botanicals may "provide some light in the otherwise dark cancer tunnel."

Some 3,000 or more plant species have been used in alternative and traditional treatments of cancer; the bulk of these remedies come from the rich history and practice of traditional Chinese medicine. Given the gross lack of funding for alternative medical research, however, it may be decades before these herbs are definitively tested as anticancer agents. In the meantime, people with cancer would stand to benefit from the seasoned advice and insights of doctors who are knowledgeable about the medicinal use of botanicals.

## Traditional Chinese Medicine and Herbal Cancer Treatment

Traditional Chinese medicine (TCM) is an ancient system of medicine that

***The* Journal of the American Medical Association *reported that life expectancy doubled for patients with rapidly advancing cancers when* Fu Zhen *was added to their treatment plan: "Patients who received* Fu Zhen *therapy survived longer and tolerated their treatment better than those patients who were treated by Western medicine alone.***

combines the use of herbs with acupuncture, food therapy, massage, and therapeutic exercise. TCM regards energy imbalances as causing the patterns of disharmony in the body that lead to disease. Viewing each patient as unique, the goal of all treatment is to restore balance to the whole person. Dr. Pan Chen-lian of the Zhejiang Research Institute of Traditional Chinese Medicine, states: "The clinical anticancer therapies are based on principles such as clearing away heat and toxic materials, treating toxifying diseases ... activating blood to remove stasis, softening and resolving hard lumps and invigorating *qi* [life energy]."[15]

Research has shown that TCM can effectively complement conventional medicine when the 2 systems are used in concert against cancer and other life-threatening diseases.[16] In China, a combination of TCM and Western medicine has been shown to be more effective for treating liver cancer than conventional Western medicine alone.[17] TCM can also reduce or minimize the toxic side effects of chemotherapy and radiation treatments while reinforcing their cancer-killing effects. Conventional oncologists who use herbs have been surprised to find that their patients not only suffer far less from nausea, hair loss, and depressed immunity, but also that their rate of recovery increases to an unexpected degree.

**Fu Zhen Therapy—**Among the better-studied Chinese anticancer herbal treatments is *Fu Zhen* therapy. A favorite anticancer adjunctive treatment in many Chinese hospitals, *Fu Zhen* features the following herbs: ginseng, ligustrum, astragalus, codonopsis, atracylodes, and ganoderma. *Fu Zhen* helps restore energy levels, enhances digestion, and strengthens the immune system by increasing the activity of the nonspecific immune cells (e.g., macrophages) and cytotoxic T cells, both integral parts of the body's anticancer defenses.[18]

The *Journal of the American Medical Association* reported that life expectancy doubled for patients with rapidly advancing cancers when *Fu Zhen* was added to their treatment plan: "Patients who received *Fu Zhen* therapy survived longer and tolerated their treatment better than those patients who were treated by Western medicine alone." In addition, the 5-year survival rate was twice as high among patients with nasopharyngeal (nasal passage and pharynx) cancer (53% versus 24%).[19]

Conventional Western doctors would do well to explore *Fu Zhen* and incorporate it into their treatment plan.

In a study of Stage II primary liver cancer, 29 of the 46 people receiving *Fu Zhen* therapy along with conventional treatment survived for a year, and 10 survived for 3 years. Meanwhile, in the control group, 6 of the 30 patients who received only radiation or chemotherapy survived 1 year; by the third year, all were dead.[20] In laboratory studies, *Fu Zhen* botanicals have been found to prevent the growth of transplanted tumors.[21] In light of such impressive findings, one might expect *Fu Zhen* to become a standard part of conventional cancer care; sadly, this has not been the case.

***Liu Wei Di Huang* (“Six Flavor Tea”)**—Those diagnosed with small-cell lung cancer may enhance the benefits of conventional treatment by taking a traditional Chinese kidney tonic known as Six Flavor Tea, *Liu wei di huang*, or *Jin Gui Shen Qi* (Gold Book Tea). Researchers at the Beijing Institute for Cancer Research found a significantly higher incidence of both tumor reduction and survival among cancer patients taking the teas.[22] Median survival for the group receiving both treatments was 16 months compared to 10 months for the conventionally treated (control) group.

***Rabdosia rubescens***—A study of 115 patients with inoperable cancer of the esophagus showed that patients taking *Rabdosia rubescens* in combination with conventional chemotherapy treatment showed a 3-fold increase (41.3%) in survival rates compared to patients receiving only conventional treatment (13.6%).[23]

**Other Chinese Anticancer Herbs**—A Chinese herb called *jian-pi yi-qi li-shui* was shown to reverse chemotherapy-caused kidney failure by 93%.[24] A commonly used herb, Chuling (*Polyporus umbellatus*), stimulated immune activity around tumor sites and increased the life span of tumor-bearing test animals by about 72%.[25] The anticancer drug cyclophosphamide resulted in significantly improved antitumor activity and reduced toxicity

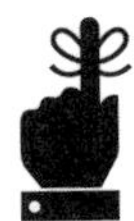

The use of electrodermal screening as a research tool could significantly extend clinical knowledge of the suitability of previously unstudied Chinese herbs for cancer treatment.

when combined with another traditional Chinese herb, *Buzhong Yiai*, or Central Qi Pill.[26] Chinese doctors often recommend using actinidia root in cancer treatment; this root contains a complex sugar (polysaccharide) called ACPS-R, which has both immune-enhancing and antitumor properties.[27]

Recent reports out of China suggest that Chinese herbal knowledge provides an untapped cornucopia of therapeutic possibilities for cancer patients everywhere. In the landmark medical text, *Anticancer Medicinal Herbs*, Dr. Min-yi Chang describes the clinical effectiveness and practical use of 256 anticancer herbs that he has used since 1982 in treating 5,000 cancer patients. Again, the best choices are those that have dual effects: reducing the tumor and strengthening the body's immune capacities. Dr. Chen-lian Pan, his colleague, reports that, using Chinese herbs alone, 300 cases of advanced cancer were shown to have a survival rate of 51%, with the longest survival period being 11 years.[28]

***The herb-treated cancer patients had twice the survival advantage after 1 year, and 4 times better survival after 2 years, compared to the chemotherapy patients. Readers in the West are unlikely ever to see such results published in American medical journals, which are funded primarily by the pharmaceutical industry.***

Researchers at Longhua Hospital of Shanghai Traditional Chinese Medical College selected 60 patients with advanced squamous (oral and lung) cancer and randomly divided them into 2 groups of 30 patients each. One group was treated with traditional medicinal herbs and the other with chemotherapy. The average length of survival for the herbal group was 465 days while that of the chemotherapy group was only 204 days.[29] The survival rates after 12 and 24 months were 67% and 13% for the herbal group, and 33% and 3%, respectively, for the chemotherapy group.

In other words, herb-treated cancer patients had twice the survival advantage after 1 year, and 4 times better survival after 2 years, compared to the chemotherapy patients. These dramatic findings were published in a 1985 issue of the *Chinese Journal of Modern Developments in Traditional Medicine*. Readers in the West are unlikely ever to see such results published in American medical journals, which are funded primarily by the pharmaceutical industry's advertisements.

**Kampo**—No discussion of TCM approaches to cancer therapy would be complete without some mention of kampo, the Japanese version of Chinese herbal medicine. The botanicals used in kampo medicine are typically taken in groups of 10 or more plants. Though there are over 140 different kampo preparations, most of the research has focused on *Shi-un-hou*, *Juzen-taiho-to*, and *Sho-saiko-to*. *Shi-un-hou* has been particularly effective in blocking the formation of skin tumors in animals.[30] *Juzen-taiho-to*, which consists of astragalus, angelica, cinnamon, foxglove, ginseng, licorice, nettle, peony root, and other herbs, may dramatically boost the anticancer activity of natural killer cells for several months after administration.[31] In addition, kampo medicines have proved more effective than conventional Western medicines in treating chronic, intractable prostatitis.[32]

***In a study of Stage II primary liver cancer, 29 of the 46 people receiving Fu Zhen therapy along with conventional treatment survived for a year, and 10 survived for 3 years. Meanwhile, in the control group, 6 of the 30 patients who received only radiation or chemotherapy survived 1 year; by the third year, all were dead. In light of such impressive findings, one might expect Fu Zhen to become a standard part of conventional cancer care; sadly, this has not been the case.***

*Sho-saiko-to* is composed of the following traditional Chinese herbs: *Bupleurum* root, pinellia tuber, scutellaria, jujube fruit, ginseng, licorice, and ginger. This kampo medicine appears to override the inhibition of macrophage immune cells by the "bad" eicosanoid (a component of an essential fatty acid) PGE2, thus enabling the macrophages to more effectively fight cancer.[33] A study of 260 patients with cirrhosis (a risk factor for liver cancer) was conducted to evaluate the preventive effect of this herbal formula. Half the group was randomly assigned to the combined kampo/conventional treatment, while the other half received only conventional treatment. The group using combination therapy had a higher survival rate than the patients using only conventional drugs: after 5 years, 78% of the patients in the combined therapy group were still alive compared to 68% of patients in the group receiving conventional pharmaceuticals alone.[34]

## Herbs Can Complement Low-Dose Chemotherapy

When chemotherapy must be employed, the strategic use of certain herbs known to Chinese medicine can mitigate its effects.

- For stomach cancer patients receiving Chinese herbs, there is improved natural killer cell (anticancer) activity and a significant improvement in the ability to tolerate chemotherapy compared to patients not receiving herbs (95% vs. 79%). The herb-treated patients reported higher energy levels, improved weight gain, and better overall quality of life.[35]
- Survival rates are improved for patients with lung, breast, throat, and nasopharyngeal cancers who used Chinese herbs in combination with chemotherapy or radiation, versus conventional treatment alone.[36]
- Despite several cycles of chemotherapy, there was no significant drop in immune cell counts in a group of breast cancer patients using Chinese herbs.[37]

## Ayurvedic Medicine's Herbs for Cancer Treatment

Practiced in India for the past 5,000 years, Ayurvedic medicine (pronounced *eye-your-vade-ick* and meaning "science of life") is a comprehensive medical system that combines natural therapies with a highly personalized approach to the treatment of disease. Ayurvedic medicine places equal emphasis on body, mind, and spirit and strives to restore the innate harmony of the individual.

Ayurvedic physicians regard cancer as a product of internal disharmony caused by the interaction between a person's constitutional tendencies and various dietary and environmental factors that lead to an accumulation of toxins, or impurities, that eventually weaken the body's ability to defend against cancer. A person's constitution, or how a specific individual's mind/body is composed and designed to function, is the touchstone of Ayurvedic medicine. It refers to the overall health profile of the individual including strengths and susceptibilities. Identifying a person's constitution, therefore, is the first critical step in the Ayurvedic process; once established, it becomes the foundation for all clinical decisions.

To determine an individual's constitution, Ayurvedic doctors first identify the patient's metabolic body type or *dosha*, which may be any 1 of 3 types: *vata*, *pitta*, and *kapha*. The dosha is akin to a blueprint that outlines all of the innate tendencies built into a person's system. Ayurvedic medicine, for example, considers distinctions of physique, such as being thin, muscular, or fat, to have far greater influence on a person's health and well-being than physical attributes alone. Understanding a person's *dosha*, for example, helps clarify why that individual will have no reaction to milk, chili, loud noise, or humidity, whereas another will not be able to tolerate them. Cancer is regarded by Ayurvedic doctors as the end result of specific components of the dosha interacting with accumulated toxins.[38]

By rebuilding and rejuvenating the body and all its systems, each of the Ayurvedic herbs helps bring the *doshas* back into harmony. The Ayurvedic herbs that may offer the most promise for treating cancer are called *rasayana* or rejuvenation herbs. They are used in a program of tonification, which means enhancing the body's inherent ability to function. Ayurvedic physicians say that *rasayana* extends longevity by slowing down the biological clock and retarding the aging process—a process associated with the development of cancers. *Rasayana* is also used to restore vitality to the reproductive system, countering sterility and infertility, improving sexual performance, and assuring healthier newborn babies.

The herbal formulations of choice for cancer therapy include Maharishi-4 (M-4) and Maharishi-5 (M-5). These little-known preparations actually have been studied at numerous institutions, such as Ohio State University, Columbus; Indiana University, Indianapolis; University of Kansas, Kansas City; South Dakota College of Pharmacy, Brookings; and the University of Colorado, Denver. Both M-4 and M-5 were found to reduce the incidence of chemically induced breast cancer (mammary carcinoma) in up to 88% of laboratory animals. In the animals that did not receive the *rasayanas* prior to the chemical induction of breast cancer (the control group), subsequent administration of the herbal medicines M-4 and M-5 caused up to 60% of fully formed tumors to regress.[39]

In another study, M-4 was shown to reduce the formation and proliferation of tumors in laboratory rats exposed to the carcinogen, DMBA. Again, nearly two-thirds of the mice showed marked regression of tumors within 1 month of using M-4.[40] In a third report, M-4 prevented lung cancer metastases in up to 65% of the treated animals.[41] Researchers reported that M-5 also induced conversion of cancerous cells to normal cells (cell differentiation) in 75% of neuroblastoma cells in culture.

Researchers at the Institute of Medical Sciences at Banaras Hindu University in Varanasi, India, reported on over 400 cases of cancer patients undergoing Ayurvedic treatments alone or in combination with conventional treatment. The groups were divided as follows: (1) patients who underwent radiation treatment, supplemented by Ayurvedic medicines fol-

## Use of Herbal Remedies

A survey of 251 persons living in rural Mississippi found that 75% had used plant-derived herbal remedies over the past year, according to researchers at the University of Mississippi in 1995. Use of herbal remedies (including, most frequently, lemon, aloe, castor oil, garlic, poke, and sassafras) was highest among those aged 45-64.

For a list of sources and information about **Ayurvedic herbs,** contact: Maharishi Ayur-Ved Products International, Inc., 1115 Elkton Drive, Suite 401, Colorado Springs, CO 80907; tel: 719-260-5500; fax: 719-260-7400.

lowing surgical removal of their tumor(s); (2) patients who received chemotherapy, supplemented by Ayurvedic medicines; (3) patients maintained solely on Ayurvedic medicines (all previous therapy had failed, or the patient had come to the institute in an advanced stage); (4) patients who received combined therapies—chemotherapy, radiation, and Ayurvedic medicines; and (5) patients who had chemotherapy alone.[42]

The patients who received Ayurvedic medicines alone, such as *Amora rohitica*, *Glycerriza glabra*, and *Semecarpus anacardium*, achieved the most favorable results. These 3 formulas were effective in bringing about remissions, in controlling the growth of malignant cells, and in improving the quality of life.[43] An example cited by the researcher is the case of a young man, aged 30, who had non-Hodgkin's lymphoma that had infiltrated the lymph nodes in his abdomen. After 3 months of herbal treatments, his lymph nodes had returned to normal and there was no sign of cancer. The patient recovered his appetite and now leads an active, healthy life.[44] Those receiving chemotherapy alone had poor survival rates during a 10-year follow-up. When the Ayurvedic formula was combined with chemotherapy, however, the survival span increased significantly—2 to 3 times.

## A Glossary of Botanicals, Biological Response Modifiers (BRMs), and Nontoxic Pharmacological Agents

Numerous botanicals can be used to intervene therapeutically at various stages of the development of cancer. In addition to traditional botanicals, here we examine the biological response modifiers (BRMs) as well as nontoxic pharmacologic anticancer agents currently in use among innovative cancer physicians today. BRMs are substances derived from both plants and animals that have definite biological activity in the human body. Many of these have also been called phytochemicals, which means "chemicals made by plants." Some BRMs stimulate immune function directly, while others modulate the activities of hormones, enzymes, and other biological components which, in turn, can alter the course of cancer.

## ALGAE (CHLORELLA, SEA VEGETABLES, GREEN CONCENTRATES)

Algae are simple microscopic organisms that grow in masses in water and contain an abundance of nutrients.

**Chlorella**—In Japan, *Chlorella pyrenoidosa*, a freshwater single-celled green algae, is more popular as a regular supplement than vitamin C. There, an estimated 5 million people use this medicinal algae every day. Chlorella contains 60% protein, including all the essential amino acids, and high levels of vitamin A and chlorophyll.

It is chlorella's high chlorophyll content (more chlorophyll per gram than any other plant) to which many researchers (and enthusiastic users) attribute its broad-spectrum health benefits (amply researched by Japanese scientists), but new research from Japan suggests that chlorella's secret might lie elsewhere—in its albumin. Continually secreted by the liver, albumin is the most abundant protein found in the blood, where it acts as a major natural antioxidant, contributing an estimated 80% of all neutralizing activity against free radicals that would otherwise damage cells and tissues.

Albumin transports key nutritional substances and detoxifies the fluid surrounding cells in the connective tissue. But most important, at least 38 scientific studies have demonstrated the strong relationship between high blood levels of albumin and a longer cell life span. This research, says Tim Sara, president of Nature's Balance, a major U.S. supplier of chlorella, "has confirmed that serum levels of albumin are extremely accurate indicators of overall health status and that low albumin levels exist at the onset and progression of virtually every nonhereditary, degenerative disease process, including cancers and cardiovascular heart disease."

The chlorella connection is simple, says Sara, who uncovered it in Japanese research data. A series of studies with rats demonstrated that chlorella supplementation increases albumin levels by 16-21%. Another study showed that of 50 people with Alzheimer's, aged 70-90, taking 6 g daily of chlorella for 6 months, 68% experienced at least a 30% improve-

## Chlorella as a Detoxifier

Chlorella is considered a first-string detoxifying agent, capable of removing alcohol from the liver and heavy metals (such as cadmium and possibly mercury) as well as certain pesticides, insecticides, and polychlorbiphenyls (PCBs) from the body's tissues. A Japanese study showed that taking 4-6 grams of chlorella before consuming alcohol can prevent hangovers 96% of the time—even after a night of heavy drinking. Chlorella can also absorb toxins from the intestines, help relieve chronic constipation, favorably alter the bacteria flora content of the bowel, and eliminate intestinal gas. It is also effective in healing skin wounds, both mild and severe.[45]

ment. Both scientific documentation and reliable anecdotal reports indicate that chlorella is effective in helping to reduce the symptoms of numerous types of cancers, diabetes, low blood sugar, arthritis, AIDS, pancreatitis, liver cirrhosis, hepatitis, peptic ulcers, viral and bacterial infections, anemia, and multiple sclerosis. Chlorella isn't a cure-all," says Sara, "but albumin is."

Chlorella contains more than 20 different vitamins and minerals and 19 amino acids, including large concentrations of lysine, which is helpful against viruses associated with cancer (e.g., leukemia and cervical cancer). Chlorella is often used in combination with other "green foods," such as spirulina, barley greens, and wheat grass, which have similar properties. Japanese scientists have conducted extensive research on the antitumor activity of chlorella, which has shown strong promise for the treatment of leukemia and breast cancer.[46] Researchers in India recently fed spirulina, a type of blue-green algae, to 44 people who had precancerous mouth lesions from chewing tobacco; after 1 year, the patches disappeared in 20 of those who ate the algae, and 5 others showed significant improvements.[47]

**Sea Vegetables—**Also known also as marine algae or seaweeds, sea vegetables have strong anticancer activity. Tumor growth in mice with implanted sarcomas was inhibited in the range of 89% to 95% when mice were fed with a seaweed called kombu.[48] Overall, tumors underwent complete regression in more than half of the mice of each treated group.[49] Other animal research found that a diet containing 5% kombu significantly delayed the inducement of breast cancer (mammary carcinoma).[50] It has been suggested that seaweed may be an important influence on the low rates of certain cancers in Japan where sea vegetables constitute about 5% of a woman's total food intake. On average, Japanese women have 3 to 9 times less breast cancer than American women.[51]

Scientists at McGill University in Canada have found that the most common edible seaweeds, such as kelp and kombu, contain a substance called sodium alginate, which can reduce the amount of radioactive strontium absorbed through the intestine by 50-80%.[52] The researchers stated that marine algae may aid "in preventing absorption of radioactive products of atomic fission" and it could possibly be used as a natural decontaminator.[53]

**Green Concentrates**—Also known as "green drinks" or the "super-vitamin," green concentrates typically include combinations of chlorella, wheat and barley grass, spirulina, blue-green algae, and other nutrients. Green grasses such as wheat, barley, alfalfa, and oat provide complete proteins.

One green concentrate product, ProGreens, is a dry green powder containing 33 nutritional substances at a cost of $40. It is taken in water or juice, 1-2 times daily, on an empty stomach. Packaged in a plastic tub representing a 30-day supply, ProGreens is a complete herbal multivitamin. The benefits of the ingredients in ProGreens, according to company president Stephen Levine, Ph.D., include immune system support, antioxidant protection, gastrointestional fortification, energy boosting, and overall nutrient supplementation.

Among the 4 algae in the product, chlorella is known as the "unpoisoner" because it can detoxify the body of heavy metals such as cadmium and lead and of uranium radiation. The "probiotic" or friendly bacterial cultures (about 5 billion organisms from 8 dairy-free sources) regulate and balance the intestines. The product also contains natural fibers (flaxseed meal), bioflavonoid extracts (milk thistle, bilberry), herbs (ginseng, *Echinacea*, licorice root), and other high-nutrient foods (lecithin, bee pollen, beet juice powder).[54]

Another product, Green Magic is a drinkable green superfood containing 16 ingredients. Its benefits include nourishing the body, strengthening the immune system, and detoxifying the blood. In addition to chlorella, spirulina, and wheat, barley, and kamut grasses, the product contains coenzyme Q10 (benefits the cardiovascular system and increases cellular energy), superoxide dismutase (neutralizes toxins), and Jerusalem

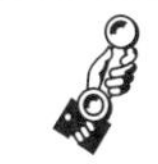

For **ProGreens**, contact: Nutricology, Inc., Allergy Research Group, P.O. Box 489, 400 Preda Street, San Leandro, CA 94577; tel: 510-639-4572 OR 800-545-9960; fax: 510-635-6730. For **Green Magic**, contact: New Spirit Naturals, Inc., P.O. Box 3300, San Dimas, CA 91773; tel: 800-922-2766, 714-592-4445, or 909-592-4445; fax: 909-599-4035. For **chlorella** information and product, contact Nature's Balance, Inc., 10705 North Main Street, Suite 307, Archdale, NC 27263; tel: 910-434-4102; fax: 910-434-3119; orders: 800-858-5198. Also contact: Sun Wellness, Inc., 4025 Spencer Street, Unit 104, Torrance, CA 90503; tel: 800-829-2828 or 310-371-5515; fax: 310-371-0094. For information about **Green Vibrance**, contact: TAAG, Vibrant Health, 432 Lime Rock Road, Lakeville, CT 06039; tel: 800-242-1835 or 860-435-3506; fax: 860-435-3576. For **Pure Synergy**, contact: Synergy Company, P.O. Box 2901, CVSR, Moab, UT 84532; tel: 800-723-0277 or 801-259-5366; fax: 801-259-2328.

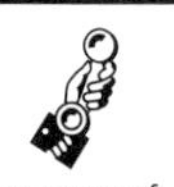

For a source of **medicinal aloe** named Mannapol® (containing aloe leaf gel and dioscorea from Mexican wild yam), contact: Mannatech™ Inc., 2010 North Highway 360, Grand Prairie, TX 75050; tel: 214-641-8829; fax: 214-623-1902. For information on **Caraloe Classic aloe vera juice**, contact: Carrington Laboratories, 2001 Walnut Hill Lane, Irving, TX 75038; tel: 800-444-2563 or 214-518-1300; fax: 800-358-5233 or 214-550-7556.

artichoke flour (stabilizes blood sugar and supports colon health). Green Magic comes in powder form and can be used daily (1-3 tablespoons) as a source of multiple nutrients.[55]

## ALOE VERA

Aloe is a garden succulent that has long been used medicinally for symptom relief and healing of cuts, burns, and various skin problems, as well as for infections and constipation. Certain aloe-containing seeds contain a chemical, called aloe emodin, which shows significant pharmacologic activity against leukemia.[56] Some studies indicate that aloe bolsters the tumor-fighting activity of macrophage immune cells.[57] Recent research by Russian scientists shows that aloe juice reduces new tumor mass and the frequency of metastases at different stages of the cancer's development.[58]

Acemannan, a water-soluble compound found in Aloe vera, is a potent stimulator of immune function. While the therapeutic efficacy of acemannnan for human cancer remains to be proven, the compound has demonstrated some anticancer activity in animals.[59] The antitumor activity of aloe vera gel seems partly due to its ability to inhibit angiogenesis, platelet aggregation (hence, potentially blocking metastasis), production of harmful eicosanoids (e.g., PGE2), and inflammatory reactions.[60]

## AMYGDALIN/LAETRILE (VITAMIN B17)

This substance, highly concentrated in the pits of apricots and other fruits, allegedly was used some 3,500 years ago by Chinese doctors for the treatment of tumors. The noted biochemist Ernest Krebs, Jr., Ph.D., first specifically identified amygdalin as an anticancer agent. His discovery was based on a theory that cancer grows from misplaced trophoblast cells; these are cells found in a pregnant human uterus that multiply rapidly during the first few weeks after conception. Under normal, healthy conditions, trophoblast cells are destroyed by the pancreatic enzyme, chymotrypsin; if they escape destruction, they can lodge in the embryo and remain there, dormant, for decades, waiting to develop into a tumor when the pancreas becomes dysfunctional.

Amygdalin has been found to have strong cancer-fighting potential, particularly with regard to secondary cancers, including a 60% reduction in lung metastases.[61] Epidemiologic studies, animal studies, and clinical studies all show evidence of amygdalin efficacy. Research indicates that it can extend the lives of both breast and bone cancer patients.[62] Ralph Moss, Ph.D., previously cited in Chapter 26, How Cancer Politics Have Kept You in the Dark, was discharged by Memorial Sloan-Kettering Hospital when he revealed an apparent cover-up by authorities there of positive findings about amygdalin. According to Moss, subsequent research findings on amygdalin have been consistently suppressed by the pharmaceutical industry, presumably because the substance is nonpatentable.

Amygdalin is one of many nitrilosides, which are natural cyanide-containing substances found in numerous foods, including all the seeds of the prunasin family (apricots, apples, cherries, plums, and peaches), buckwheat, millet, and cassava melons. Amygdalin consists of 2 sugar molecules, a benzaldehyde and a cyanide radical. In the body, the 2 sugar molecules are split off in the liver by the enzyme beta glucosidase and are replaced by glucuronic acid. This results in a selective toxicity to cancer cells and relative nontoxicity to normal cells because the enzyme glucuronidase, which splits off the glucuronic acid, is high in cancer cells and low in normal cells. Once glucuronic acid is split off, the remaining benzaldehyde spontaneously splits off cyanide, which is toxic to the cancer cell.

For the story of the political suppression of **laetrile** by the cancer industry, see Chapter 26: How Cancer Politics Have Kept You in the Dark, pp. 673-674.

Studies show evidence of benzaldehyde's anticancer activity. Prolonged survival among those with advanced inoperable cancers has been observed following intravenous benzaldehyde treatment,[63] and antitumor responses were seen in patients with various forms of advanced metastatic cancers (lung, liver, stomach, prostate, lung and bone.)[64]

An additional mechanism that protects normal cells from cyanide is that they contain an enzyme known as rhodanase or sulfur transferase, which adds a sulfur atom to any free cyanide to form thiocyanate, a relatively harmless substance. Cancer cells do not have significant amounts of this enzyme. Blood thiocyanate levels may be used to help monitor the proper dose.

Amygdalin may be given orally or intravenously.

## ASTRAGALUS

In recent years, astragalus has captured the interest of many conventional doctors because of its ability to reduce the toxic effects of conventional cancer treatment. For example, astragalus appears to protect the liver against the harmful toxic effects of chemotherapy and may be effective in treating terminally-ill liver cancer patients.[65] In a study conducted at the Peking Cancer Institute, researchers observed a much higher survival rate among advanced liver cancer patients when they were treated with both radiation and astragalus compared to those treated with radiation alone.[66]

Clinical research in Japan indicates that a ginseng-astragalus combination (GAC) may have a "biphasic" or regulatory effect on natural killer (NK) cell function, increasing it if NK activity is low and decreasing it slightly if the activity is excessive.[67] Similarly, GAC has also been shown to decrease levels of the stress hormone cortisol when the hormone was high (in the case of ulcer), and to increase cortisol levels when it was chronically low (in the case of "psychovegetative syndrome").[68] When GAC was used in laboratory animals as an adjunct to chemotherapy before and after treatment, various immune cell counts and the usually observed chemotherapy-induced decreases in key blood measures were significantly prevented and toxic side effects were reduced.[69]

In China, physicians frequently combine astragalus with another Chinese herb called ligustrum. Research at Loma Linda University in California found that astragalus and ligustrum when taken together enhance each other's immune-stimulating properties; ligustrum has been shown to increase the number and activity of various immune cells, whereas astragalus helps increase NK activity and interferon levels.[70] Swainsonine, a derivative form of astragalus, can inhibit the development of distant metastases of malignant melanoma, a deadly form of skin cancer.[71] We now know that the potent antimetastatic activity of this substance not only extends to other tumor types as well but that it is not limited to experimentally induced metastases.[72]

## CAT'S CLAW (*UÑA DE GATO*)

The indigenous peoples of Peru have traditionally used this rain forest vine as a tribal medicine for cancer, arthritis, and other diseases. The name, cat's claw, derives from the fact that the thorns found on this vine resemble the claws of a cat. Recent studies indicate that the plant, *Uncaria tomentosa*, contains substances that have immune- and digestion-enhancing properties.[73] These beneficial constituents of cat's claw include several types of antioxidant compounds (polyphenols, triterpines, and the plant steroids beta-sitosterol, stigmasterol, and campesterol).[74] The presence of these compounds may, in turn, account for the antioxidant and antitumor properties of cat's claw.[75] According to several unpublished studies, cat's claw treatment has been shown to lead to the remission of brain tumors and other tumors.[76]

## *ECHINACEA*

This herb has well-known immune-enhancing abilities. *Echinacea* was found to increase NK cell activity by 221% in patients with inoperable metastatic esophageal or colorectal cancer.[77] Patients with inoperable, far-advanced liver cancer showed a 90% increase in their NK activity when *Echinacea* was combined with a thymus-stimulating agent (thymostimulin).[78] In addition, a natural chemical substance in *Echinacea*, arabinogalactan, stimulates the tumor-killing activity of macrophages.[79] The primary role of *Echinacea* is to provide protection against infection, a common and sometimes deadly complication in advanced-stage cancers.

## ESSIAC

In the 1920s, a Canadian nurse named Rene Caisse introduced a nontoxic herbal tea for treating cancer. The tea was originally named *Lasagen* by the Ojibway, a Native American tribe based in Ontario, Canada. Caisse obtained the formula for this natural herbal combination from a breast cancer patient who had been healed by an Ojibway medicine man; she renamed it Essiac (which is Caisse spelled backwards) and used it to treat thousands of cancer patients until her death in 1978.

Although Essiac has never undergone randomized clinical trials, Caisse and her associates recorded many impressive case histories attesting to its efficacy. Canadian radio producer and broadcaster Elaine Alexander of Vancouver, British Columbia, collected testimonials from cancer patients who had achieved complete remission or remarkable improvement using Essiac. The recoveries encompass cancers of the pancreas, breast, ovaries, esophagus, bladder, bones, and bile ducts, as well as lymphoma and malignant melanoma.

In 1937, Caisse was introduced to Dr. John Wolfer, then director of the cancer clinic at Northwestern University Medical School. Wolfer arranged for Caisse to treat 30 terminal cancer patients with Essiac under the supervision of 5 doctors. After 18 months, the doctors concluded that Essiac had relieved pain, shrunk tumors, and improved the survival odds of these patients.

Also in 1937, Emma Carson, M.D., spent 24 days inspecting the Bracebridge Clinic in Ottawa, Canada, where Caisse had done most of her work. Dr. Carson reviewed over 400 cases of cancer patients who had been treated with Essiac and recorded notes of indisputable improvements. She declared: "I could scarcely believe my brain and eyes were not deceiving me on some of the most seriously afflicted cases ... The vast majority of Miss Caisse's patients are brought to her for treatment after [conventional treatment] has failed to be helpful, and the patients are pronounced incurable. Really the progress obtainable and the actual results from Essiac treatments and the rapidity of repair were absolutely marvelous and must be seen to convincingly confirm belief."[80]

Among the most compelling anecdotal success stories was the case of Charles Brusch, M.D., cofounder of the prestigious Brusch Medical Center and former physician to President John F. Kennedy. After Brusch's recovery from advanced colorectal cancer, he signed a notarized statement testifying that he endorsed Essaic: "For I have in fact cured my own cancer, the original site of which was the lower bowels, through Essiac alone."[81]

When she was 70, Caisse traveled to the Brusch Medical Center in Massachusetts, where she treated terminal cancer patients under the supervision of 18 doctors. After several months, Dr. Brusch and his research director, Dr. Charles McClure, again offered a statement: "Clinically, on patients suffering from pathologically proven cancer, [Essiac] reduces pain and causes a recession in the growth; patients have gained weight and shown an improvement in their general health ... Remarkably beneficial results were obtained even on those cases at the 'end of the road' where it proved to pro-

## Essiac's Anticancer Benefits

According to a report issued in 1993, Essiac tea: (1) strengthens the immune system; (2) reduces the toxic side effects of many drugs; (3) increases energy levels; and (4) diminishes inflammatory processes.[82] Studies of some of Essiac's main components—burdock, Indian rhubarb, sheep sorrel, slippery elm—have each demonstrated a significant amount of anticancer activity.[83] Emodin, one of the main constituents in rhubarb, has been shown to inhibit various cancer cell lines[84] and to reduce tumor cell numbers and increase survival time in leukemic mice.[85] Japanese researchers have identified a potent factor in burdock that can block cell mutation without the need for "metabolic activation."[86]

long life and the quality of that life ... The doctors do not say that Essiac is a cure, but they do say it is of benefit."[87]

In a letter dated August 3, 1991, Dr. Brusch further stated: "I have been taking this [Essiac] myself since 1984, when I had several cancer operations, and I have every faith in it. Of course, each person's case is different as well as each person's own individual health history ... Someone may respond in a week; someone else may take longer, and whether or not someone is cured of cancer, Essiac had been found to at least prolong life by simply strengthening the body."[88]

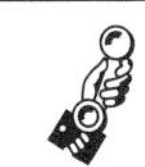

For information about **Essiac**, contact: Essiac USA, Inc., 26 Union Street, Newburyport, MA 01950; tel: 508-462-4976; fax: 508-465-8214. Also: Green Leaf Herbs, 1080 East Sandy Lake Road, No. 85, Coppell, TX 75019; tel: 800-770-1080; fax: 972-437-9954.

Keith I. Block, M.D., director of Cancer Care at the Edgewater Medical Center in Chicago (see Chapter 2), is among those physicians who do not regard Essiac as particularly powerful against cancer. It is possible that Essiac is less effective today than it was decades ago. Certainly our diet and environment have become increasingly polluted since the early 1900s, and that places a growing burden on the body's immune and detoxification systems. These major social changes have made the regression of cancers a more difficult task; the prospect of a magic bullet for cancer—whether herbal or pharmaceutical—seems more remote than ever before. To obtain the best results, we recommend combining Essiac (made from all organically grown ingredients) with other anticancer agents and other cancer-fighting modalities. Many of the physicians interviewed for this book share this view.

A **bioflavonoid** is a water-soluble pigment within plants and fruits that acts as an antioxidant to protect it against damage from free radicals and excess oxygen. In the body, bioflavonoids enhance the beneficial activities of vitamin C, and are often formulated with this vitamin in supplement form. Called vitamin P up until 1950, these vitamin C "helper" substances include citrin, hesperidin, rutin, quercitin, epicatechin, flavones, and flavonols. When taken with vitamin C, bioflavonoids increase the absorption of vitamin C into the liver, kidneys, and adrenal glands. Acting as antioxidants, they also protect vitamin C from destruction by free radicals.

## FLAVONOIDS

This class of phytochemicals is responsible for many of the bright colors in fruits and vegetables, and they are also among the most beneficial substances found in these cancer-fighting foods. Among the better-known flavonoids are such bioflavonoids as citrin, hesperidin, rutin, and quercetin; other flavonoids include the proanthocyanins and anthocyanins. Studies indicate that quercetin dramatically inhibits the growth of cancer cells in the stomach.[89] Anthocyanins and other flavonoids extracted from citrus and grape seeds are highly effective "scavengers" of free radicals—highly reactive and unstable molecules that promote tumor growth.[90]

## GARLIC

Long appreciated as a folk remedy believed to benefit the immune system and to help ward off colds, cumulative scientific research now highlights garlic's proven ability to work as a cancer inhibitor and as a valuable adjunct to alternative cancer therapy. Much of this progressive research began in the 1950s in Japan, a country known for its medicinal use of garlic. In 1954, a German researcher joined forces with Manji Wakunaga, a garlic expert. Together they established a method of growing a high potency garlic organically, free of pesticides, chemical seed treatment, and inorganic fertilizers, in the virgin woodlands of Hokkaido, Japan. Wakunaga then perfected a 20-month cold-aging process by which garlic's offensive odor was naturally removed and its healing properties strengthened.

The result was Kyolic® Aged Garlic Extract™, for which Wakunaga received a special industry award from the Japanese government in 1991. The product is now widely available in liquid, tablet, or capsule form—but why take a garlic pill when you can eat fresh raw whole garlic? Evidence suggests that the cold-aging process may actually enhance garlic's medicinal qualities.

Specifically, the aging process removes garlic's harsh, irritating, and toxic compounds and its strong odor; it also converts certain components (such as alliin and allicin) into valuable, safe, and stable compounds (such as thioallyl). "These compounds represent the activated, predigested, readily bioavailable, and effective forms of garlic's active principles," says Brenda Lynn Petesch, Kyolic's research and development nutritionist. With these facts in hand, Wakunaga appropriately dubbed his product Kyolic (from kyo, Japanese for "powerful" and *garlic*).

Data supporting garlic's medicinal claims come from human, animal, and cell studies, says Petesch. Studies of eating habits in China and Italy where garlic consumption is high established that the risk of stomach cancer declined by about 50% among those people with a high raw garlic intake. Residents of Cangshan County in China regularly ate 20 g of garlic daily and had the lowest death rate due to stomach cancer in China while residents in Qixia County, where garlic consumption was minimal, had a death rate from stomach cancer that was 13 times higher.

Animal studies have shown that aged garlic extract appears to stop the growth of cancers of the breast, bladder, skin, and colon, and the initial development of malignant tumors of the esophagus, stomach, and lungs. One study involving mice who received 20 once-weekly injections of diallyl sulfide, a garlic constituent, reduced the frequency of colon and rectal cancer by 74%.

Research involving human cell cultures indicate that garlic may inhibit the proliferation of breast, skin, and nerve cancer cells. Further, a study at the National Medical Center Hospital in Japan showed that garlic extract (with vitamins B1 and B12 and liver extract) produced a "moderately effective" response in 70% of patients. Garlic helped reduce anorexia and fatigue, side effects of radiation and chemotherapy for patients with head and neck tumors, and the toxic effect on the heart of a cancer drug called Doxorubicin. According to chief researcher Minoru Toriyama, it also enhanced "the patient's will to fight against his disease."

***Research involving human cell cultures indicate that garlic may inhibit the proliferation of breast, skin, and nerve cancer cells. Further, a study at the National Medical Center Hospital in Japan showed that garlic extract (with vitamins B1 and B12 and liver extract) produced a "moderately effective" response in 70% of patients.***

According to Petesch, Kyolic Aged Garlic Extract may produce these anticancer benefits by speeding up the excretion of chemical carcinogens from the cells, protecting DNA from carcinogenic damage, enhancing the activity of enzymes that detoxify poisons, and boosting the vitality of the immune system. Garlic protects DNA by blocking the toxic effects of aflatoxin, a fungus found on peanuts and grains, which would otherwise help precipitate genetic mutations.

**Aflatoxins** are a group of 16 naturally occurring toxic by-products produced by the fungus *Aspergillus flavus*, often found on peanuts, rice, grain, corn, beans, and sweet potatoes. Aflatoxin B1(AFB1) shows the highest degree of biological activity and has been linked to higher levels of liver cancer in African and Asian populations where these foods are widely consumed. AFB1 is considered a carcinogen precursor and requires activation before it can produce cellular mutations leading to cancer.

Research on the clinical use of Kyolic garlic to date has been conducted at 50 universities, hospitals, and institutes worldwide, while the Japan-based Wakunaga Pharmaceutical Co., Ltd., maintains 20 Ph.D.s with a $10 million annual research budget. Other proven health benefits attributable to Kyolic, says Petesch, include an ability to promote energy, protect against free radicals in the blood, detoxify and protect the liver, minimize immune suppression as a result of radiation, curtail the growth of the yeast *Candida albicans*, reduce the secretion of stress hormones, increase levels of beneficial intestinal bacteria, and protect the heart by inhibiting inappropriate blood clotting.

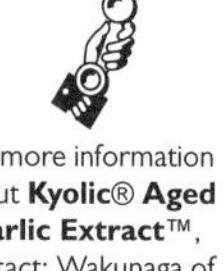

For more information about **Kyolic® Aged Garlic Extract™**, contact: Wakunaga of America Co., Ltd., 23501 Madero, Mission Viejo, CA 92691; tel: 714-855-2776; fax: 714-458-2764.

During the late 1980s, there were so many reports on the anticancer effects of garlic that scientists organized the First World Congress on the Health Significance of Garlic and Garlic Constituents. The Congress concluded that "garlic in various forms, from cooked garlic, garlic oil, raw garlic juice, to products of garlic powder and aged garlic extract, can provide health benefits of reducing cardiovascular and cancer risks."[91]

A recent review indicates that components of garlic inhibit the initiation and promotion phases of oncogenesis; in addition, garlic seems to strengthen various aspects of the immune system's response to tumors.[92] More specifically, garlic extract appears able to enhance natural killer cell activity, improve the therapeutic ratio between helper/suppressor T cells, stimulate macrophages to greater activity, and enable lymphocytes to become even more cytotoxic (cell-killing) against tumors. Garlic may also block the adhesion of cancer cells to the surface of blood vessels, thereby helping to prevent metastases.[93] Therefore, anyone who already has cancer may benefit from garlic. Many of the commercially available garlic supplements, however, are devoid of the volatile oils that contain anticancer factors, so one must select garlic supplements discerningly.

## *GINGKO BILOBA*

*Gingko biloba* is a member of an ancient family of trees (*Gingkoales*) no longer found in the wild. For thousands of years, *Gingko* has been a staple of Chinese herbal medicine, recommended for coughs, asthma, and acute allergic inflammations. Ginkgolide B, one of the active compounds in *Gingko*, apparently works by interfering with a chemical in the body known as PAF (platelet activating factor); PAF may affect the cancer process by acting as a tumor-promoting agent, and may affect tumor growth by stimulating inflammation and inducing angiogenesis.[94] PAF levels tend to be markedly higher in patients with malignant breast tumors compared to those with benign breast tumors (or healthy subjects).[95]

British research has shown that Ginkgolide B is effective in treating kidney disorders and counteracting a number of toxins.[96] A study at Loma Linda University found that *Ginkgo biloba* extract (GBE) is a highly effective antioxidant that may greatly curtail the free-radical damage that naturally accompanies the anticancer activity of macrophages.[97] Other studies have found that GBE halts lipid peroxidation[98] (another major source of free radicals) and can dramatically lessen the damage to normal cells that is typically associated with the chemotherapy drug, Adriamycin.[99]

**CAUTION**

All forms of ginseng should be taken in moderate doses based on the product's ginsenoside content. As a general rule of thumb, a standard dose is 4 to 6 g daily; be careful of doses larger than this as they may inhibit immunity.

## GINSENG (PANAX )

For over 2,000 years, Chinese doctors have prescribed ginseng, either in powder or extract form, as a general tonic to promote strength, vitality, appetite, emotional stability, and "wisdom."[100] Panax ginseng, a small perennial woodlands plant is different but related to Siberian ginseng (*Eleutherococcus senticosus*), a medium-sized shrub that is more widely distributed in terms of where it is found in Nature. Ginseng contains a number of active constituents, including saponins, essential oils, phytosterol, amino acids, peptides, vitamins, and minerals.

Over a dozen saponins have been identified as the most active therapeutic constituents in ginseng.[101] Ginseng saponins have been shown to stimulate macrophage and NK cell activity, as well as to promote antibody production and restore sexual behavior in stressed animals.[102]

A report in *Free Radical Biology and Medicine* states that Panax ginseng has a wide range of beneficial actions, including antiaging, immune enhancement, antistress, and antitumor effects.[103] Most of these effects may be attributed to ginseng's ability to protect against "peroxidized fatty acids" which, in turn, generate free radicals from the unsaturated fatty acids in cell membranes.[104] Peroxidized fatty acids are those in the cell membrane that have been attacked by free radicals, in turn producing peroxides; these cause a chain reaction producing even more free radicals.

In a study of aflatoxin-induced cancers, those animals receiving ginseng had a 75% lower rate of liver cancer and a 29% lower rate of lung cancer compared to animals that did not receive ginseng.[105] Japanese scientists have also observed strong inhibitory effects of ginseng on human ovarian cancer cell growth in test animals.[106] Gastric carcinoma cells treated with ginseng oil in culture also appeared to halt the growth of the cancer cells, thought to be due to an effect on the cells' DNA and carbohydrate (energy) metabolism.[107]

Regular use of Panax ginseng can cut one's cancer risk in half, according to Korean researchers T. K. Yun and S. Y. Choi who conducted a survey of 1,987 pairs of individuals, each pair including a person *with* cancer, age- and sex-matched to a person *without* cancer. People who had used ginseng for 1 year had a 36% lower cancer rate than nonusers; those who used ginseng for 5 years or more had a 69% lower cancer rate.[108] Siberian ginseng stimulates the anticancer activity of NK cells and may also help regenerate NK cells destroyed by toxins or by conventional treatments.[109]

## GRAPE SEED EXTRACT/ PYCNOGENOLS

Grape seed extract is high in various phytochemicals (chemicals made by plants), including a variety of bioflavonoids such as the proanthocyanins and anthocyanins. Anthocyanins and other flavonoids extracted from grape seeds are highly effective "scavengers" of harmful free radicals.[110] The antioxidant components of grape seed extract seem particularly helpful in curbing free-radical damage (from peroxidation) which can alter fats and lipids (low-density lipoproteins) circulating in the bloodstream and embedded in cell membranes.[111]

An **antioxidant** (meaning "against oxidation") is a natural biochemical substance that protects living cells against damage from harmful free radicals. Antioxidants work against the process of oxidation—the robbing of electrons from substances. If unblocked or left uncontrolled, oxidation can lead to cellular aging, degeneration, arthritis, heart disease, cancer, and other illnesses. Antioxidants in the body react readily with oxygen breakdown products and free radicals, and neutralize them before they can damage the body. Antioxidant nutrients include vitamins A, C, and E, beta carotene, selenium, coenzyme Q10, pycnogenol (grape seed extract), L-glutathione, superoxide dismutase, and bioflavonoids. Plant antioxidants include *Gingko biloba* and garlic. When antioxidants are taken in combination, the effect is stronger than when they are used individually.

Pycnogenols have been shown to be up to 50 times more effective than vitamin E and 20 times stronger than vitamin C in free-radical neutralizing power. That is why many researchers contend that pycnogenols might be the most powerful antioxidants yet discovered. European scientists call it the "youth nutrient" because it helps slow cell mutation and keep collagen (the fibrous part of connective tissue) healthy and flexible. A British scientist calls pycnogenols the "arteriosclerosis antidote" because they help maintain the integrity of arteries and enhance circulation. In 1986, Dr. Masquelier found that grape seeds produce an even better pycnogenol antioxidant than pine tree bark. Among the benefits claimed for grape seed extract, is its ability to:

- improve blood and lymph circulation
- reduce thickening of the arteries
- improve eyesight
- improve skin quality
- dramatically improve peripheral circulation
- protect central nervous system tissues

- block the release of enzymes that produce histamines (the culprit in allergy attacks)
- help restore elasticity, flexibility, and strength to the body's connective tissues
- help tone skin and restore flexibility to joints, arteries, capillaries, and other body tissues.

## An Antioxidant Discovered in 1534

One of the most powerful antioxidants, the predecessor of grape seed extract, was discovered in 1534 when Canadian natives showed French explorer Jacques Cartier how to make a nourishing tea from pine tree bark and needles. Even though these substances had little vitamin C, somehow the brew kept Cartier's crew from dying of scurvy. The mysterious lifesaving ingredient in pine tree bark is now known as a bioflavonoid, which enhances the action of small amounts of vitamin C. In the 1940s, Dr. Jacques Masquelier gave this pine tree bark bioflavonoid a special name, pycnogenol (pronounced pick-NAH-jen-all) and began explaining how the extract could scavenge free radicals in the body even better than the "experts," vitamins C and E.

Grape seed extract is now widely prescribed in France and Italy, where grapes are abundant. There doctors suggest grape seed for improving blood flow to the brain and heart, treating varicose veins, certain skin discoloration, tingling in the extremities, bleeding gums, glaucoma, hemorrhoids, excessive menstrual bleeding, and hardening of the arteries. Researchers suggest saturating the body tissues with a dosage in the range of 200-300 mg a day for 5-10 days, followed by a daily maintenance dose of 60-150 mg a daily. The substance is absorbed almost immediately by the body (in about 20 minutes) and produces no side effects.

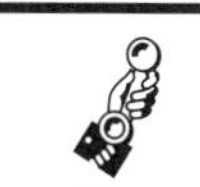

Sources of **grape seed extract** include: Flanagan Microclusters® from Carotec, Inc., P.O. Box 9919, Naples, FL 33941; tel: 800-522-4279 or 941-353-2348; fax: 941-353-2365. As Pronogenol™, from Prolongevity Ltd., P.O. Box 229120, Hollywood, FL 33022; tel: 800-544-4440 or 954-766-8433; fax: 954-761-9199.

## GREEN TEA (CATECHINS)

Green tea (*Camellia sinensis*) is a highly popular beverage among the Chinese and Japanese who consume, on average, 2-10 cups daily. Green tea contains a substance called epigallocatechin gallate, which inhibits the growth of cancers and lowers cholesterol.[112] This is one of a number of chemical compounds known as "polyphenolic catechins," which are many times stronger than vitamin E in defending the body against free radicals.[113] The catechins found in green tea support the immune system's responsiveness and have demonstrated powerful anticarcinogenic effects.[114] Studies have indicated that green tea consumption can reduce the risk of cancers of the liver and throat (esophagus).[115] Green tea flavonols (the active bioflavonoids in the tea) may offer substantial cancer protection if consumed on a regular basis.

## HAELAN 851

This liquid soybean concentrate is rich in zinc, selenium, vitamins A, B1, B2, B12, C, D, E and K, as well a variety of amino acids. The soybeans used to make Haelan 851 are grown in special, mineral-rich soils, and harvested at the peak of ripeness to ensure maximal nutrition. A fermentation process then splits (hydrolyzes) many of the soybean proteins into amino acids and compounds that are rich in nitrogen and by-products (through fermentation) of naturally occurring substances called isoflavones, protease inhibitors, saponins, phytosterols, and other compounds.

***The researchers reported that Haelan greatly improved the patients' physical functioning and quality of life, helped resolve "vital energy deficiencies," strengthened the immune system, improved appetite, and "by means of supporting healthy energy and lowering toxicity," relieved side effects caused by conventional treatments.***

The formulation was developed in China by a microbiologist at Fujien Provincial Agricultural College. Haelan is an Old English spelling for healing, and 851 refers to the year (19*85*) and month (*1*, or January) it was discovered.

Studies of Haelan indicate that when Haelan is combined with chemotherapy in laboratory animals with liver cancer, survival is significantly increased.[116] In addition, Haelan has demonstrated effectiveness against gastric cancer, immune dysfunction, and free-radical damage (lipid peroxidation).[117]

Chinese researchers conducted a clinical study of Haelan in combination with other treatments on 239 people who had been diagnosed with various cancers—of the lung, stomach, esophagus, intestines, and lymphatic system. The researchers reported that Haelan greatly improved the patients' physical functioning and quality of life, helped resolve "vital energy deficiencies," strengthened the immune system, improved appetite, and "by means of supporting healthy energy and lowering toxicity," relieved side effects caused by conventional treatments.[118] Nutritional biochemist Ross Pelton, Ph.D., has recorded many "terminal" cancer cases that were reversed with Haelan treatment.[119]

The apparent efficacy of Haelan 851 underscores the nutritional, even therapeutic, benefits of soybeans and soy products. To illustrate how important this can be, Michael Schachter, M.D. (see Chapter 18) cites recent research on isoflavones, the most studied of which is genistein, found in high concentrations in soy products. As Dr. Schachter explains, these products may help to fight cancer in several ways including the following:

First, they can induce apoptosis, which refers to programmed cell death. If this is done with cancer cells, it speeds up the death of unwanted cancer cells. Second, genistein is a tyrosine kinase inhibitor. Tyrosine kinase is an enzyme which helps platelets to aggregate or cluster together. Platelet aggregation is essential in stopping bleeding. However, excessive platelet aggregation can lead to clot formation which, in turn, can lead to heart attacks and help cancer gain a foothold and spread. Thus, using genistein to inhibit excessive platelet aggregation may help to prevent or treat our 2 greatest killers.

Third, genistein inhibits another enzyme known as DNA topoisomerase II, which in turn slows down the synthesis of DNA and cell division. The result is a slowing down of the growth of cancer, whose cells are dividing and thus multiplying too quickly. Fourth, genistein and other isoflavones inhibit angiogenesis. Angiogenesis means new blood vessel formation. Solid cancers, such as breast, prostate, lung, and colon (as opposed to cancer of the blood—leukemia), require new blood vessel formation in order to grow. Without angiogenesis, a cancer will not grow any larger than the size of a pencil point. This is the same angiogenesis function that is believed to be interfered with by shark cartilage (discussed later in this chapter).

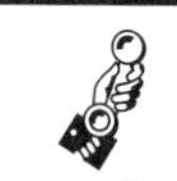

For a source of **Haelan 851**, contact: Haelan Products, Inc., 3220 Severn Avenue, Suite 120, Metairie, LA 70002; tel: 504-885-2776 or 800-542-3526; fax: 800-258-2173. For a source of **Yang's 851**, contact: Beso® Biological Research, Inc., 13139 Ramona Blvd., Suite #G, Irwindale, CA 91706; tel: 800-898-2376. For a source of **Genista**, or **soy protein isolate**, contact: Cartilage, USA, 200 Clearbrook Road, Elmsford, NY 10523; tel: 800-700-REAL or 914-345-6300; fax: 914-592-7166.

For **Ecogen 851 Soy Drink**, contact: ecoNugenics, Inc., 65-J Koch Road, Corte Madera, CA 94925; tel: 800-308-5518; fax: 415-927-1128; http://www.econugenics.com

Fifth, under conditions of excessive sex hormone stimulation, genistein appears to inhibit the availability of the sex hormones, thus helping women with hormone-sensitive breast cancer and men with hormone-sensitive prostate cancer. Sixth, isoflavones appear to induce differentiation of cancer cells, which means they help to move cancer cells back toward normalcy. This helps in the overall goal of alternative cancer therapy to control the cancer. Thus you can see that genistein and the other isoflavones may play an important role in preventing and treating cancer.[120]

## HANSI

The name HANSI refers to a series of homeopathically prepared herbs that have been proven effective in the treatment of cancer and chronic fatigue. The product was developed by Argentinian biologist Juan Jose Hirschmann who named it after his childhood nickname "Hansi," which is German for "little John." But the initials also stand for Homeopathic Activator of the Natural Immune System which concisely describes the product. When Hirschmann first introduced HANSI in Buenos Aires, Argentina, in July 1990, so great was the demand for this alternative cancer formula that even with 40 physicians on staff, his clinic reached operating capacity in its first week, registering, at peak time, 1,200 patients a day.

Since then, an estimated 100,000 cancer patients have used HANSI with good results, indicated most notably in dramatic increases in levels and activity of natural killer cells, central to the immune response to cancer, says David C. Christner, managing director of Hansi International, Ltd., in Sarasota, Florida. "A large amount of evidence is leading to the conclusion that HANSI is a powerful enhancer of the human system," Christner says.

The basic product starts with about 10 components, then is adjusted according to whether it will be delivered orally or by injection and whether it is to address cancer, chronic fatigue, AIDS, asthma, or other conditions, Christner says. For example, the basic HANSI contains low-potency homeopathic dilutions (4X to 11X) of mostly rain-forest and desert plants such as *Cacti grandiflora* (cactus), aloe, arnica, lachesis, licopodium, and others, in a 2-8% alcohol base tincture. HANSI variations include these plus *Colocinthis*, *Pulmonaria reticulosa*, *Berberis vulgaris*, and silica.

Hirschmann and Christner emphasize their company's commitment to performing the "hard science" to provide physicians with "incontrovertible evidence" that HANSI gets results. In a landmark study in 1992 involving 87 patients with advanced pancreatic cancer (which is usually fatal within 3-6 months and presents a cure rate of 1%), 60 of the patients taking HANSI daily remained alive 1 year after the study began. Two years later, more than 50% of the patients were still alive and well, according to study director, Cesar Bertacchini, M.D. of the Instituto de Medicina Integracion in Buenos Aires.

Further, appetite remained stable in 57% of the cases and increased in 7%, 73% had no pain or only mild pain, 56% reported no nausea or vomiting, and 36% experienced a reduction in these symptoms. HANSI was able to stop weight loss (which is typical of advanced cancer) for 34% and 11% gained some weight. Patients receiving HANSI did not have chemotherapy or radiation during this treatment.

IMPORTANT

Several studies have shown conclusively that HANSI has no toxicity or secondary effects for patients, said Dr. Bertacchini. Subsequent studies indicate that HANSI produces a greater tolerance for radiation and chemotherapy, both subjectively and in terms of the return of a patient's blood to "normal" or pretreatment status. Early results from a 1995 study at the Goodwin Institute for Cancer Research in Plantation, Florida, involving breast cancer in mice demonstrated that HANSI treatment produced a 40% decrease in tumor size in 30 days.

Hansi International is presently engaged in several key research projects in conjunction with the University of California at Irvine, College of Medicine, where HANSI's efficacy in treating chronic fatigue syndrome will be evaluated. Chief researcher, Darryl M. See, M.D., comments: "Over the past 2 years I have been involved in screening various herbs and homeopathic preparations for *in vitro* immune-stimulating effects. Among the 200 or so I have tested, HANSI proved to be among the most effective in increasing natural killer cell function." Natural killer cells are key cancer fighters in the immune system.

For more information about **HANSI**, contact: Hansi International, Ltd., 2831 Ringling Blvd., Suite A-102, Sarasota, FL 34237; tel: 941-953-4863; fax: 941-366-2023. The approximate U.S. price for a 30-day supply of oral HANSI J and H together is $100

HANSI for injection or intravenous infusion is available in the U.S. in accordance with the FDA's "Personal Use Exemption" which permits importation by individuals of a 3-month supply. On the other hand, HANSI oral formulas ("Rejuvenator Formula 'J' and 'H'" for chronic fatigue, arthritis, or immune boosting) are, technically, available to anyone as over-the-counter remedies without restrictions, says Christner. However, oral HANSI is absorbed more slowly and dissipates faster than the injected form. At present, HANSI in all applications is fully legal in Mexico, the Bahamas, Argentina, and Hungary.

## HOXSEY HERBS

Harry Hoxsey was an herbal folk healer who eventually attracted a devoted following of cancer survivors after he developed an herbal therapy that

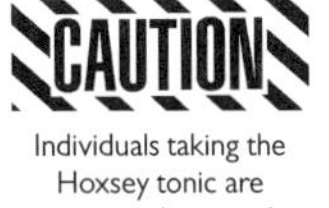


Individuals taking the Hoxsey tonic are cautioned to avoid tomatoes, alcohol, processed flour, and vinegar because they can negate the tonic's effects.

originated with his great-grandfather. The elder Hoxsey bred horses in Illinois in the 1840s. One of his horses had cancer on its leg and was put out to pasture to die. The horse began grazing on certain plants and soon after experienced a spontaneous remission. Hoxsey's great grandfather formulated the plants the horse had grazed on into a salve and used it to treat other horses. Hoxsey's father, who was a veterinarian, also used the salve and passed the formula on to his son, Harry Hoxsey.

The classic Hoxsey formula comes in a potassium iodide solution and contains the following herbs: red clover (*Trifolium pratense*), buckthorn bark (*Rhamnus purshianus*), burdock root (*Arctium lappa*), stillingia root (*Stillingia sylvatica*), barberry bark (*Berberis vulgaris*), chaparral (*Larrea tridentata*), licorice root (*Glycyrrhiza glabra*), Cascara amarga (*Picramnia antidesma*), and prickly ash bark (*Zanthoxylum americanum*).

Today, the Hoxsey therapy consists of a mix of herbal preparations for internal and external use, and an emphasis on diet, vitamin and mineral supplements, and personal counseling. The external formula (but not the internal one) includes *Sanguinaria canadensis*, also known as bloodroot, which has been used by Lake Superior Native Americans to treat cancer.

Wide-ranging laboratory research has found definite biological activity in the various ingredients of the Hoxsey herbal formula. Studies have shown antitumor effects with components of prickly ash and stillingia,[121] burdock,[122] and extracts of barberry.[123] In addition, the genistein found in red clover may be responsible for a wide range of anticancer activities, including antioxidant activity (blocking free radicals, which promote tumor growth), anti-estrogen activity (slowing tumor growth in some cancers), and inhibition of new blood vessel formation (promoting anti-angiogenesis, which blocks tumor growth).[124] Licorice (*Glycyrrhiza uralensis*) has a variety of immune-stimulating properties and direct antitumor effects;[125] it also demonstrates a unique ability to block estrogen's cancer-stimulating effects.[126] Not all studies have been able to demonstrate anticancer effects for these ingredients, however, and different types of cancers react differently to the formula.

Cancers that have responded favorably to the Hoxsey combination include lymphoma, melanoma, and skin cancer. A 5-year preliminary study followed patients with advanced cancer who were treated at 3 alternative cancer treatment clinics. Six of 16 patients treated at the Hoxsey clinic remained alive and were reported to be disease free after 5 years. Two of these patients had cancers that are normally considered incurable or "terminal." In contrast, all patients from the other 2 clinics, where Hoxsey herbs were not used, had died at the end of 5 years.[127]

Hoxsey therapy is practiced at the Bio-Medical Center in Tijuana, Mexico, where, based on patient records, an estimated 80% of patients who use the Hoxsey formula benefit substantially. According to Mildred Nelson, R.N., who has singlehandedly carried on the challenging work of Harry Hoxsey since 1963, many of today's cancers are more difficult to treat with the Hoxsey therapy than they were decades ago. "People's bodies are more toxic today because the environment is more polluted. They also tend to develop multiple types of cancer over time, whereas in the past it seemed that we would only see people with one type of cancer, and that was it. Also, metastases were less common as well."

The Hoxsey approach includes a psychological component, whose objective is to encourage patients to maintain a strong fighting spirit toward their cancer. "After over 4 decades of observing cancer patients, I have consistently seen that mental attitude makes a big difference in who tends to live after a diagnosis of advanced cancer," says Nelson. "The people who make it are typically the ones who decide they're going to fight this cancer, and they're great about taking their medicines, staying on the diet, and doing the things that help them get well and stay well." Generally, patients take the herbal tonic daily and begin to feel more energetic and vital within a few weeks. Typically, they will continue the treatment for several years, at which point they usually feel their health has been restored.

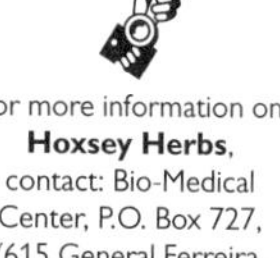

For more information on **Hoxsey Herbs**, contact: Bio-Medical Center, P.O. Box 727, (615 General Ferreira, Colonia Juarez), Tijuana, Tijuana, B.C. Mexico; tel: 52-814-9011 or 52-814-9132.

Examples of long-term survivors from the Bio-Medical Center's patient files include: a 62-year-old man with terminal malignant melanoma, whose disease had continued to spread after surgery; he is now in stable condition and still improving 3 years later; a 75-year-old man diagnosed with metastatic prostate cancer now lives with no sign of cancer; a 56-year old woman sent home to die after her surgeons found a tumor the size of a ping-pong ball in her right ovary. In the last example, exploratory surgery had shattered the tumor into several pieces, causing it to spread to the colon and liver, yet 14 years after receiving a death sentence from her doctor, she remained vigorously healthy.

## ISCADOR (MISTLETOE)

**Anthroposophic medicine** is an extension of conventional Western medicine developed by Austrian scientist Rudolf Steiner in the 1920s, in conjunction with European physicians. It is based on a spiritual model of the human being and its medicines are extensions of homeopathic remedies. In the U.S., there are about 60 practitioners, all M.D.s, plus many hundreds of nurses and adjunctive therapists, but in German-speaking countries, there are thousands plus several major hospitals in Germany and Switzerland devoted exclusively to this medical approach.

For information on **anthroposophic medicine**, see Chapter 21: Jesse Stoff, M.D.

Iscador is the trade name for a mistletoe preparation that has been used by European physicians since 1920. Iscador consists of fermented extracts of European mistletoe (*Viscum album*), some forms of which are combined with small amounts of metals to produce certain desired, anticancer effects.[128] Originally conceived by Rudolf Steiner (1864-1925), Austrian scientist and founder of anthroposophic medicine, the therapeutic success of Iscador has been reported in nearly 5,000 case studies. In animal experiments, Iscador has been found to kill cancer cells, stimulate the immune system, and significantly inhibit tumor formation.[129]

The activity of various immune cells, including NK cells, increases significantly within 24 hours of injecting Iscador.[130] These effects might explain various findings that Iscador selectively inhibits the growth of different types of tumor cells.[131] Two reviews of the clinical research on Iscador have concluded that treatment with Iscador increases both the length and quality of life, stabilizes the cancer, causes tumors to shrink, and improves the overall condition of the patient.[132,133]

As reported in the *Journal of Anthroposophic Medicine* and in *Anthroposophical Medicine and Therapies for Cancer*, Iscador's potential as a cancer therapy is strongly supported by the following findings: (1) significantly more breast cancer patients treated with Iscador were alive after 10 years compared to patients who received no Iscador; (2) people with cervical cancer who had a combination of surgery, Iscador, and radiotherapy showed an 83% survival rate after 5 years compared to a 69% survival rate for those who received radiation alone; (3) normally 50% of bladder papillomas become malignant in 3 years, but with Iscador, only 3 out of 14 did; (4) among bronchial cancer patients, 75% of those given Iscador were still alive after 4 years compared to only 35% of those without Iscador; and (5) the survival rate after 3 years for skin cancer patients on Iscador was 80% compared to 65% for those without it.[134] In addition, Iscador has successfully extended the lives of individuals with cancers of the lung, breast, stomach, colon, ovaries, and cervix.[135]

A recent study of 36 patients with stage III ovarian cancer by Richard Wagner, M.D., of Stuttgart, Germany, proved that the use of Iscador can produce results at least comparable to chemotherapy for this type of cancer. All 36 patients had already received chemotherapy at the time of the trial. Specifically, Dr. Wagner found that 15 patients experienced a halt in tumor growth or a "no change" status for at least 6 months, as verified by sonography and tumor-marker analysis. Also, 8 patients had a partial remission, and 3 patients had full remission for 6 months; 10 patients experienced a tumor progression.

Patients receiving Iscador had an "excellent quality of life" with no side effects other than a coin-sized area of redness at the injection site. "Comparing the side effects," concludes Dr. Wagner, "it is immediately apparent that patients given mistletoe treatment have better survival quality [than those on chemotherapy], with the survival period presumably the same. We would therefore always prefer mistletoe treatment in this particular situation."

Dr. Wagner further noted that patients who received only chemotherapy had a 50% survival rate after 7 months while those who took Iscador after chemotherapy had this rate after 14 months. If chemotherapy were as effective as stated in the literature, Dr. Wagner said, his patients would also have reached 24 months' survival with it, "but at the cost of side effects such as alopecia, neutropenia, pyrexia, edema and allergic reactions."[136]

Despite the wealth of clinical and research data demonstrating the benefits of Iscador, it is not currently licensed by the FDA for sale in the United States.

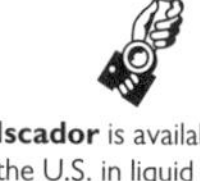

**Iscador** is available in the U.S. in liquid form (*Viscum compositum*) to qualified health-care practitioners. Contact: Biological Homeopathic Industries (BHI), 11600 Cochite SE, P.O. Box 11280, Albuquerque, NM 87123; tel: 505-293-3843; fax: 505-275-1672; BHI has Iscador in 3 potencies called Mite, Medium, Forte, each containing *Viscum album*, CANP (adenosine monophosphate), and homeopathic mercury. Also contact: Weleda, 175 North Route 9W, Congers, NY 10920; tel: 800-241-1030 or 914-268-8572; fax: 914-268-8574; M.D.s and D.O.s may order from Weleda. For Iscador in a form suitable for subcutaneous injection, physicians must order from Europe; Weleda can provide more information. For referrals of physicians practicing anthroposophic medicine, contact: Physicians' Association for Anthroposophical Medicine, 7953 California Avenue, Fair Oaks, CA 95628; tel: 916-967-8250; fax: 916-966-5314.

## LARCH ARABINOGALACTAN (LARIX, ARA-6)

This immune enhancer is a sweet-tasting medicinal powder highly concentrated in complex carbohydrates or polysaccharides (long-chain sugars) derived from the Western Larch tree (*Larix occidentalis*). It was first identified and developed from a paper byproduct by naturopathic physician Peter D'Adamo in 1992. While there were, at the time, 50 patents on larch for somewhat crude formulations, Dr. D'Adamo holds exclusive rights for the use of larch (as pharmaceutical grade Larix) as a "nutraceutical," that

## Green Tea Inhibits Lung Cancer

In a laboratory experiment, scientists induced lung cancer in 104 rats by injecting them with 2 known carcinogens over a 3-month period. Of those rats that received an extract of green tea (*Camellia sinensis*), only 8 cases (16%) of cancer developed compared to 25 cases (46%) among the rats that received none. In addition, the survival time for rats on green tea increased by a highly significant 133 days, according to *Biomedical Environmental Science* (1995).

is, as a plant-derived therapeutic agent.

The large size of the sugars in Larix is thought to account for its special properties, including its ability to stimulate the activity of various types of immune cells. Larix also readily dissolves in water and maintains its chemical stability over a wide range of concentrations, pH, and temperature changes. According to Dr. D'Adamo, Larix enhances the delivery of other medicinal agents, including chemotherapy drugs. It is presumed to make capillaries more permeable for microabsorption and to stimulate the liver to produce antibodies.

The role of Larix as a modulator of immune system activity is not surprising since several major immune-enhancing herbs are known to contain significant amounts of arabinogalactans, such as *Echinacea purpurea*,[137] *Baptisia tinctoria*,[138] *Thuja occidentalis*,[139] *Angelica acutiloa*[140] and *Curcuma longa*.[141] In addition, many edible plants are rich sources of arabinogalactans, including carrots, radishes, tomatoes, wheat, maize, pears, coconuts, and many other foods.[142]

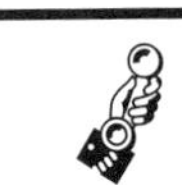

**Larix** is available to qualified physicians only from: North American Pharmacal, 10 Morgan Avenue, Norwalk, CT 06851; tel and fax: 203-866-7664.]

At least 2 animal studies have demonstrated that Larix can inhibit liver metastases and prolong survival times.[143] In a third animal experiment, arabinogalactans blocked highly metastatic lymphoma cells from colonizing the liver.[144] Dr. Peter D'Adamo notes that Larix may be used in conjunction with modified citrus pectin, since both polysaccharides work in the same way—by inhibiting the attachment of metastatic cells to liver tissues (parenchyma).[145]

The immune-related effects that have been seen with Larix include stimulation of the NK cells and macrophages. In one study, the enhanced tumor cell-killing (cytotoxicity) of NK cells was not a direct effect of Larix, but was due to stimulation of other immune cells (monocytes); these cells increased their production of various immune-enhancing chemicals known as cytokines, including gamma-interferon and interleukin-2.[146] This research is still preliminary, however, and wide variations were seen in Larix's ability to stimulate NK activity.[147] Biochemists have determined that it may be a sugar component of Larix that stimulates NK activity in a manner similar to that of the sugar component of Viscum album (mistletoe).[148] Since the 2 sugars appear to occupy the same receptor,[149] they may compete with each other to stimulate NK activity.

Larix appears to be totally safe for regular daily use. Less toxic than methyl cellulose, the component of many fiber supplements, Larix (Ara-6) has been approved as a dietary supplement by the FDA and the Canadian Governor-in-Council. One study fed laboratory animals a diet comprised of 50% Larix for 6 months without finding any ill effects.[150]

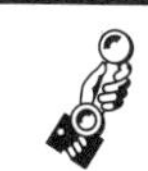

For a source of **maitake** mushroom under the Grifron® brand, contact: Maitake Products, Inc., P.O. Box 1354, Paramus, NJ 07653; tel: 800-747-7418 or 201-229-0101; fax: 201-229-0585.

**CAUTION**

Concern has been raised by Canadian researchers that the commercially available lapachol products do not contain adequate amounts of the active pau d'arco substance.[155] To resolve this problem, it may be helpful to contact the supplier to determine whether the product has been analyzed by an independent laboratory. The clinical use of electrodermal screening can enable a physician to determine if a given product has therapeutic efficacy for a given patient.

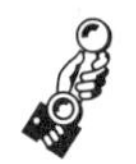

For a source of **pau d'arco** as *Tahebuia* liquid extract, contact: Phyto Med, P.O. Box 279, Sandy, oR 97055; tel: 503-668-4000; fax: 503-668-7800.

## MAITAKE MUSHROOM (*GRIFOLA*)

According to researchers at the National Cancer Center in Japan, complete tumor elimination was experienced in about 80% of cancer-induced animals fed extracts from maitake, shiitake, and reishi mushrooms.[151] Compounds in each of these mushrooms increase the tumor-fighting activity of NK cells and improve antibody responses, but maitake seems to have the strongest and most consistent effect.

Maitake exhibits potent activity against cancer, inhibiting both carcinogenesis and metastasis, according to Hiroaki Nanba, Ph.D., of the Department of Immunology at Kobe Women's College of Pharmacy in Kobe, Japan. Animal research suggests that maitake supplements increase the body's ability to kill tumors.[152] When maitake was compared to a common form of chemotherapy, the maitake "D-fraction" demonstrated superior ability to inhibit the growth of tumors (about 80% versus 45%).[153] Unlike other mushroom extracts, the maitake extract shows strong anticancer activity even when administered orally. Dr. Nanba reports that maitake increases the NK cell's tumor-killing ability and enhances other immune cells' production of interleukin-1, a protein that aids in defense against cancer and viruses.[154]

## PAU D'ARCO

**Modified citrus pectin** is available without a prescription as Pecta-Sol™ in 800-mg capsules from ecoNugenics, Inc., 65-J Koch Road, Corte Madera, CA 94925; tel: 800-308-5518; fax: 415-927-1128; http://www.econugenics.com and from Allergy Research Group, 400 Preda Street, P.O. Box 489, San Leandro, CA 94577; tel: 800-545-9960 or 510-639-4572; fax: 510-635-6730.

This herbal extract from the inner bark of trees of the *Tabebuia* genus, found in South American rain forests, offers another herbal option in treating cancer. The main active ingredient is a substance called lapachol, a substance whose molecular composition makes it uniquely suited to induce strong biological activity against cancer.[156] Nine patients with various cancers (liver, kidney, breast and prostate adenocarcinomas, and squamous cell carcinoma of the palate and uterine cervix) were given pure lapachol in 250-mg capsules with meals.

All 9 patients showed a shrinkage of tumors and reductions in tumor-related pain; 3 patients experienced complete remissions, and there were no adverse side effects.[157] In studies of mice injected with leukemia cells, the life span of animals given lapachol was 80% greater than that of the control group.[158] Other investigators have reported that lapachol is well tolerated and causes no severe side effects. Nausea, vomiting, and slow clotting have occurred only at very high oral doses.[159]

## PECTIN, MODIFIED CITRUS

This substance is a special pH-altered form of citrus pectin, a type of fiber that lowers blood cholesterol levels. The research on modified citrus pectin indicates that its therapeutic potential for helping to prevent cancer metastases is quite strong. Apparently, a compound called rhamnogalacturonan found in modified citrus pectin has a "bridging effect" that enhances the cell-killing (cytotoxic) ability of T cells, which play a critical role in the body's immune response to cancer.[160] Another study indicates that NK cell and macrophage cytotoxic activity are also enhanced by modified citrus pectin.[161]

A specially modified form of citrus pectin has provisionally been shown to be effective in halting the spread of cancer cells in rats with prostate cancer. This study demonstrated that modified citrus pectin, when administered at the rate of up to 1% (weight/volume) in the rodents' drinking water for 3 weeks, significantly reduced the spread of cancer from the prostate to the lungs and lymph nodes.[162] Specifically, while 15 out of 16 control animals developed a secondary lung cancer, 7 of 14 rats did not, presumably because of the action of modified citrus pectin. While 55% of the rats developed secondary lymph node cancer, of those on modified citrus pectin only 13% had lymph node metastasis.

Six other clinical studies suggest that the substance also enhances the anticancer effect of certain immune system cells. Human studies are now under way to see whether modified citrus pectin can similarly act to stop the spread of cancer in the human body. At the same time, a handful of progressive physicians are already incorporating modified citrus pectin in their anticancer supplement program.

## SILYMARIN (MILK THISTLE)

The liver is our primary filter for poisons circulating in the bloodstream, converting potentially toxic substances into innocuous or excretable substances. Highly toxic chemicals can overwhelm the liver, resulting in its dysfunction, which is why, for centuries, European herbalists have used silymarin for restoring liver function. German researchers, for example, have found silymarin highly effective in the treatment of toxic liver damage consequent to deadly amanita mushroom poisoning.[163]

The herb has served as a supportive treatment for cirrhosis (associated with liver cancer) and hepatitis, as well as fatty degeneration of the liver caused by alcohol and other chemicals.[164] A review of double-blind studies concluded that silymarin is a therapeutically useful medicinal plant that accelerates the process of regeneration of damaged liver tissue.[165] Rich in antioxidants and bioflavonoids, silymarin appears to reduce the levels of various liver enzymes found in the blood of patients with chronic liver disease, suggesting a liver protective effect.[166]

***A specially modified form of citrus pectin has provisionally been shown to be effective in halting the spread of cancer cells in rats with prostate cancer. Six other clinical studies suggest that the substance also enhances the anticancer effect of certain immune system cells.***

Some clinicians (including this author, W. Lee Cowden, M.D.) believe that silymarin should always be given in conjunction with sublingual L-glutathione because silymarin can induce a particular enzyme (cytochrome P 450) action in the liver which sometimes produces excessive oxidized free-radical by-products that use up available amounts of L-glutathione.

## TURMERIC

This East Indian herb of the ginger family, a major ingredient of curry powder, appears to exert powerful antioxidant effects, sufficient to reduce carcinogenesis. Research indicates that turmeric can inhibit cancer at various stages of cancer development.[167] After 1 month, smokers who took 2 tablets containing 750 mg of turmeric daily had a significant reduction in the level of urinary mutagens (indicating damage from cigarette smoking) whereas the control group's urinary mutagen level remained unchanged.[168] In another study, turmeric was shown to decrease the formation of abnormal DNA (DNA adducts) after exposure to the well-known carcinogen, benzoapyrene.[169] Turmeric combined with betel leaf was found to be more effective against oral cancer than when either ingredient was used alone.[170]

The main active component of turmeric is a yellow pigment called curcumin, which possesses both anti-inflammatory and antioxidant properties. Recent animal studies indicate that curcumin inhibits skin cancer and the formation of skin tumors.[171] One study of 62 patients focused on those with skin cancer (squamous cell carcinoma) or ulcerating oral cancers that had not responded to conventional therapies. After topical treatment of a vaseline containing 9.5% curcumin, all 62 patients showed significant reductions in the size of their cancerous lesions, as well as decreased itching, pain, odor, and drainage (exudate).[172]

In addition, dietary administration of curcumin suppresses colon tumor size significantly (by more than 57%) and may also inhibit the progression of the cancer.[173] Part of this therapeutic effect may be that curcumin helps reduce the production of PGE2 and other "bad" eicosanoids that promote tumor growth.[174] Curcumin also plays a role in the production of the carcinogen-detoxifying enzyme, glutathione-S-transferase.[175]

Chapter 30

# The New Pharmacology for Treating Cancer

## *A Complete Guide to Innovative Anticancer Substances*

**While chemotherapy, radiation, and surgery have been touted (and enforced) as the modalities for cancer treatment, the research evidence fails to support the oncologists' claims. Rather, it highlights the dangers of generally trusting full-strength chemotherapy as it can destroy the immune system while reversing, at best, 7-15% of a few cancers. Forward-looking cancer physicians now rely on new substances such as 714X, cartilage, Carnivora, Ukrain, and hydrazine sulfate, as well as new approaches, such as very low-dose chemotherapy, producing better results than full dose and with fewer side effects.**

Before introducing innovative anticancer substances used by cancer doctors who are forging a new approach to a nontoxic pharmacology, it is important to explain the manifold limitations and dangers of conventional chemotherapy and radiation. While these methods remain the norm for conventional cancer treatment, there is no conclusive body of evidence or data demonstrating long-term successful outcomes or reasonable rates of remission to support these standard practices.

As some oncologists and alternative practitioners suggest, however, perhaps less is more. Perhaps a highly weakened or diluted dose of chemotherapy might produce cancer-cell-killing effects without creating dangerous toxicity throughout the body. In fact, on the forefront of this new approach, physicians are experimenting with (1) low-dose chemotherapy, (2) chemotherapy combined with protective nutritional and botanical supplements, and even (3) homeopathically prepared chemotherapy.

Chemotherapy may be clinically necessary to control tumor mass (as opposed to being routinely prescribed) in some patients. Low-dose chemotherapy is preferable to what is presently regarded as today's normal dose, and can have a place when used with alternative modalities in the hands of an experienced physician. What needs to be strongly challenged is the prevailing concept that *only* chemotherapy in full strength is a viable way to treat cancer.

There are techniques, such as darkfield microscopy of live blood and electrodermal screening (both discussed throughout this book), that enable the trained physician or oncologist to assess the potential appropriateness or inadvisability of chemotherapy, in whatever dose or combination, based on specific indications from an individual patient. Surely this approach is preferable to the flying-blind, "one-drug-fits-all" approach of high-dose chemotherapy routinely prescribed by oncologists.

The physician and the patient must always remember that the decision to use chemotherapy or to employ the alternatives, or to do both, is patient driven. The best we can do as responsible researchers and physicians is to report the data and help guide the individual patient to an informed choice of treatment.

**Anticancer Substances Covered in This Chapter:**

- Alkylglycerols
- Antineoplastons
- Carnivora®
- Cartilage, bovine
- Cartilage, shark
- Cesium
- DMSO
- Glutathione and N-acetyl cysteine
- Hydrazine sulfate
- Indocin
- Mellitin
- Nucleic acids
- 714X
- Sodium butyrate
- Staphage lysate
- Tagamet®
- Ukrain
- Urea

## A Toxic Treatment Feared Almost as Much as Cancer Itself

Today's conventional cancer treatment will be remembered as a crude and often inhumane technique that causes extensive damage to the body. Surgery excises normal tissue along with malignant tissue and often compromises the lymphatic and other systems vital to the body's resistance to disease. Surgery is generally the lesser of 3 evils, for the damage caused by radiation and chemotherapy may be far more grievous, given that both destroy normal cells as much as cancer cells and actually increase one's risk of eventually dying from cancer. It is well known that all chemotherapeutic agents are cytotoxic, or poisonous to cells,[1] and that their cell-killing ability is not specific.

*What needs to be strongly challenged is the prevailing concept that only chemotherapy in full strength is a viable way to treat cancer.*

When technicians drop the chemotherapy "bomb" inside a living human body, a great deal of "collateral damage" results. The body's rapidly dividing cells found in the bone marrow (the source of all immune cells), the lining of the gastrointestinal tract, and the hair follicles bear the brunt of chemotherapy-induced damage, giving rise to side effects such as diarrhea, nausea, hair loss, anemia, and suppressed immunity.

Other common side effects include mouth sores, infections, nervous system problems, skin rashes, and problems with the lungs, kidneys, and liver—the body's primary detoxification organs. So morbid are people's associations with this sickening form of treatment that the mere thought of having another chemo treatment can trigger the vomit reflex, a phenomenon known as anticipatory vomiting.[2] Victims of the chemical assault feel sick and tired on a regular basis—probably much sicker than they would have felt had they been left untreated.

***The rationale for chemotherapy and radiation is that cancer is an enemy that must be killed or destroyed, even when the treatment causes the person great discomfort, perhaps even death. Chemotherapy drugs originated out of mustard gas, designed as a poison for use in warfare. No wonder chemotherapy is feared almost as much as cancer itself.***

It is this long list of toxic effects, which may in fact become life-threatening, that makes chemotherapy a highly questionable method. According to Howard Greenwald, M.D., "The patient may become exhausted because loss of appetite has led to malnutrition; bone marrow poisoning may undermine resistance to infectious disease; lung damage, kidney dysfunction, and hemorrhage may occur."[3] The rationale for chemotherapy and radiation is that cancer is an enemy that must be killed or destroyed, even when the treatment causes the person great discomfort, perhaps even death. Remember, chemotherapy drugs originated out of mustard gas, designed as a poison for use in warfare. No wonder chemotherapy is feared almost as much as cancer itself.

Virtually all the FDA-approved anticancer drugs are markedly *immunosuppressive*, because they ruin a person's natural resistance to disease, including cancer. Ulrich Abel, Ph.D., of the Heidelberg Tumor Center in Germany, conducted a comprehensive review of the world literature on survival among cancer patients receiving chemotherapy. He found that chemotherapy can help only about 3% of the patients with epithelial cancers (e.g., cancers of the breast, lung, prostate, and colon).[4] These cancers account for about 80% of all cancer deaths. In a study of chemotherapy-treated breast cancer patients, the researchers concluded, "Survival may even have been shortened in some [breast cancer] patients given chemotherapy."[5] In general, chemotherapy's effectiveness is seen only with small, early tumors, not with large tumors.

One of the ironic "side effects" of chemotherapy or radiation is an increased likelihood that cancer will reappear later on as secondary tumors or that it will eventually spread to other parts of the body (metastasis).[6] When chemotherapy and radiation are used at the same time, secondary tumors occur about *25 times more* than the expected rate.[7]

Despite the aggressive, even militaristic "kill-or-cure" zeal of today's oncologists, chemotherapy's success record is dismal. It can achieve remissions in about 7% of all human cancers;[8] for an additional 15% of cases, survival can be "prolonged" beyond the point at which death would be expected without treatment. This kind of survival is not the same as a cure or even restored quality of life. The statistics show us that chemotherapy is useless in treating about 80% of malignant tumors, in particular those that occur most frequently, such as cancers of the lungs, breast, colon, pancreas, and bladder.[9] Chemotherapy has had little or no impact on survival in the vast majority of tumors;[10] in fact, as of 1988, more than 40 years since its introduction, chemotherapy was still considered an "experimental treatment" in a majority of patients with lung cancer.[11]

***One of the ironic "side effects" of chemotherapy or radiation is an increased likelihood that cancer will reappear later on as secondary tumors or that it will eventually spread to other parts of the body (metastasis).***

Chemotherapy's 7% "cure" rate is all the more pathetic when you consider that it typically refers to survival for only 5 years and thus overlooks the risk of "secondary cancers" or recurrences. In *The Facts about Chemotherapy*, Paul Reich, M.D., and Janice Metcalf, M.S., rather breezily discuss the risk of deadly recurrences as one of the known "side effects" of treatment. "Some drugs can cause secondary malignancies, usually years after the patient completes treatment. Secondary malignancies commonly occur as leukemia, lymphoma, or sarcoma. They can be treated with chemotherapy, but their cure rate is low."[12]

For more information about the history and political aspects of **chemotherapy** for cancer and the absence of adequate double-blind, controlled, clinical studies proving or disproving its efficacy, see Chapter 26: How Cancer Politics Have Kept You in the Dark.

The attitude oncologists have toward these second malignancies seems to be that they are of minimal importance. In a tone that seems cynical, Dr. Reich comments: "Almost always, the expected benefit of therapy will outweigh the risk of a second malignancy ... It is important to try to cure the patient, and certainly you cannot worry about a second malignancy if the pa-

# Common Chemotherapy Drugs

| BRAND NAME | GENERIC | COMPANY |
| --- | --- | --- |
| **Antibiotic Derivatives** | | |
| Adriamycin | doxorubicin hydrochloride | Adria Labs |
| Blenoxane | bleomycin sulfate | Bristol Labs |
| Cerubidine | daunorubicin hydrochloride | Chiron Thera |
| Cosmegen | dactinomycin | Merck & Co. |
| **Antiestrogen** | | |
| Nolvadex | tamoxifen | Zeneca Pharmaceuticals |
| **Antimetabolites** | | |
| Efudex | fluorouracil | Roche Labs |
| Folex | methotrexate sodium | Adria Labs |
| FUDR | floxuridine | Roche Labs |
| Intron A | interferon alpha-2b | Schering |
| Leucovorin Calcium | glutamic acid | Lederle Labs |
| Methotrexate | | |
| sodium injections | methotrexate sodium | Chiron Thera |
| tablets/parenteral | methotrexate sodium | Lederle Labs |
| Mexate | methotrexate sodium | Bristol Labs |
| Mithracin | plicamycin | Miles Pharmaceuticals |
| Purinethol | mercaptopurine | Burroughs Wellcome |
| Roferon-A | interferon alpha-2b | Roche Labs |
| Thioguanine | 6-thioguanine | Burroughs Wellcome |
| **Cytotoxic Agents** | | |
| BiCNU | sterile carmustine, BCNU | Bristol-Myers Squibb |
| CeeNU | lomustine, CCNU | Bristol-Myers Squibb |
| Cytosar-U | sterile cytarabine | Upjohn |
| Cytoxan | cyclophosphamide | Bristol-Myers Squibb |
| Emcyt | estramustine phosphate sodium | Adria Labs |
| Hydrea | hydroxyurea | Bristol-Myers Squibb |
| Matulane | procarbazine hydrochloride | Roche Labs |
| Mutamycin | mitomycin | Bristol-Myers Squibb |
| Myleran | busulfan | Burroughs Wellcome |

| BRAND NAME | GENERIC | COMPANY |
| --- | --- | --- |
| Neosar | cyclophosphamide | Adria Labs |
| Platinol | cisplatin | Bristol-Myers Squibb |
| Vincasar | vincristine sulfate | Adria Labs |
| **Hormones** | | |
| Depo-Provera | medroxyprogesterone acetate | Upjohn |
| Emcyt | estramustine phosphate sodium | Adria Labs |
| Estrace | estradiol valerate | Bristol-Myers Squibb |
| Megace | megestrol acetate | Bristol-Myers Squibb |
| Stilphostrol | diethylstilbestrol diphosphate | Miles Pharmaceuticals |
| TACE | chlorotrianisene | Merrell Dow |
| Teslac | testolactone | Bristol-Myers Squibb |
| **Nitrogen Mustard Derivatives** | | |
| Alkeran | melphalan | Burroughs Wellcome |
| Leukeran | chlorambucil | Burroughs Wellcome |
| Mustargen | mechlorethamine (nitrogen mustard) | Merck & Co. |
| **Steroids and Combinations** | | |
| Celestone Soluspan | betamethasone sodium phosphate acetate suspension | Schering |
| **Other** | | |
| DTIC-Dome | dacarbazine | Miles Pharmaceuticals |
| Elspar | asparaginase | Merck & Co. |
| Lysodren | mitotane | Bristol-Myers Squibb |
| Oncovin | vincristine sulfate | Lilly |
| Velban | vinblastine sulfate | Lilly |
| VePesid | etoposide | Bristol-Myers Squibb |

SOURCE: Adapted from *1995 Physicians' Desk Reference* (Montvale, NJ: Medical Economics) and *1996 Physicians' GenRx* (New York: Mosby).

tient does not survive the first."[13] In other words, cancer recurrence is considered an acceptable side effect of chemotherapy treatment for cancer.

One of the often touted examples of the "success" of chemotherapy is Hodgkin's disease (lymphoma), for which chemotherapy claims a "cure rate" of 80%. Once again, long-range effects are ignored. "Cure" means that 80% of patients entering a study are, typically, alive and free of cancer 3 years after their chemotherapy is completed; the reason 3 years is used as a cut-off point is that the majority of Hodgkin's disease patients who have a relapse do so within 2-3 years after the treatment. The statistics conveniently ignore secondary cancers associated with this conventional strategy.

***Despite the aggressive, even militaristic, "kill-or-cure" zeal of today's oncologists, chemotherapy's success record is dismal. It can achieve remissions in about 7% of all human cancers; for an additional 15% of cases, survival can be "prolonged" beyond the point at which death would be expected without treatment. This kind of survival is not the same as a cure or even restored quality of life.***

One sincerely wonders on what intellectual (or humane) grounds these often ineffective, toxic approaches are so casually labeled "therapies."

The failure of conventional oncology is well-documented in the medical literature yet not widely covered by the mainstream press. A striking example of this seemingly deliberate disregard for the (damaging) facts of research is a report in the *British Journal of Cancer*. In a study of 78 patients who had undergone surgery for colorectal cancer, one group was subsequently treated with chemotherapy while another received a placebo (no treatment). For the first 5 years, survival rates were similar in the 2 treatment groups, although the chemotherapy-treated group suffered from such side effects as significant nausea, skin rash, and suppression of the immune system, according to the report.

Beyond the 5-year mark, the chemotherapy-treated group showed a sharp *increase* in deaths while the group receiving no treatment showed no increase. The placebo group's long-range survival (68%) was nearly double the chemotherapy group's survival (38%). For patients who survived 5 years from the time of surgery, the no-treatment group (placebo) had a significantly better chance of survival (100%) compared to the chemotherapy group (57%).[14] This study never received any coverage in the mainstream press; instead, the reports that typically receive the most coverage are those that speak glowingly of chemotherapy's results after 2-3 years of treatment.[15]

On September 15, 1993, the *Journal of the National Cancer Institute* published the results of a major study examining the effectiveness of chemotherapy for all types of cancer. The results were dismal. Chemotherapy provided a "durable response" in only 3% of cases, while another 4% of the patients had "a significantly long survival period." In other words, at best, only 7% of patients benefited from chemotherapy in any way.[16]

Keep in mind that the 5-year mark is still used as the official guideline for "cure" by mainstream oncologists. Statistically, the 5-year cure makes chemotherapy look good for certain kinds of cancer, but when you follow cancer patients beyond 5 years, the reality often shifts in a dramatic way. Ralph Moss, Ph.D., formerly employed at Memorial Sloan-Kettering, the largest cancer treatment center in the U.S., provides the following criteria for measuring the effectiveness of a given cancer treatment. "If it only temporarily shrinks tumors, with a probable loss in well-being, then it is at most entirely experimental and unproven, and should not be represented as anything else. At worse, it could be not just ineffective, but painful, destructive—even fatal."[17]

***In* The Facts about Chemotherapy, *Paul Reich, M.D., and Janice Metcalf, M.S., rather breezily discuss the risk of deadly recurrences as one of the known "side effects" of treatment. The attitude oncologists have toward these second malignancies seems to be that they are of minimal importance. In other words, cancer recurrence is considered an acceptable side effect of chemotherapy treatment for cancer.***

When we ran a Medline computerized search for the clinical trials testing the effectiveness of chemotherapy agents over the past decade, we did not find even one double-blind, placebo-controlled trial. The only such trials were those designed to study which supportive agents could help prevent or minimize chemotherapy-associated nausea and vomiting. Ironically, among the most recent "agents" to have proven efficacy is ginger.[18] How can the cancer establishment get away with claiming that most herbal medicines (as well as other alternative therapies, for that matter) are "unproven" when the effectiveness of their own chemother-

## Radiation Therapy Speeds Up Prostate Cancer Doubling Time—Media Ignores Facts

According to the *Cancer Communication Newsletter*, mainstream television media are dangerously misrepresenting conventional medical procedures for prostate cancer, including radiation, by not disclosing the serious side effects.

Radiation therapy—implanting radiation seeds in the prostate gland—routinely given for early signs of prostate cancer can actually hasten the development of that cancer. Prostate cancer cells can double in as little as 1.2 months after radiation treatment while unradiated prostate cancer cells may take an average of 4 years to double. Similarly, it will take up to 20 years for the average untreated prostate cell to double 5 times but if treated with radiation therapy, it can double 5 times in only 6 months—40 times faster, said *Cancer Communication Newsletter*.

Meanwhile, despite these facts or perhaps unaware of them, urologists send thousands of patients with suspected prostate cancer to radiation therapists every year. According to medical statistics culled from *Urological Nursing*, *Family Urology*, and other sources, and published in the *Cancer Communication Newsletter*, about 30-40% of men in their 50s have signs of prostate cancer, but of these, only about 8% will ever feel the effect of this disease in their lifetime, and less than 3% will die from it.

Yet if a man in his 50s has an elevated prostate specific antigen (PSA, a standard prostate cancer marker) and undergoes prostate surgery, he has a 20% risk of the following scenario happening: The surgery can actually release cancer cells into the blood, and from 6 months to 5 years later, he will again have an elevated PSA, indicating cancer.

Research reported in *Family Urology* indicates that while 50% of male radiation patients may experience a drop in their PSA, it is sustained in only 20%; this means only 10% of the total radiation patients have a sustained decline in PSA. It also means that about 90% are likely to have cancer cells that, owing to radiation, now double 40 times faster than unradiated prostate cells.

The point is brought more keenly home by realizing that for the man who initially had a 92% likelihood of having no ill effects from latent prostate cancer, now, as a result of surgery or radiation treatment, is likely to become incontinent or impotent, and have to deal with a rapidly growing cancer.

In light of this evidence, men should seriously consider all their medical options before undertaking radiation therapy for prostate cancer. Men are further encouraged to demand of their conventional physicians that they investigate these research results and take them into consideration in designing a treatment program.

SOURCE—*Cancer Communication Newsletter* 12:4 (September 1996), 15-16; *Family Urology* (Spring 1996), 11; *Journal of American Medical Association* 275:4 (January 24/31, 1996), 289; *Urological Nursing* (March 1994), 14.

apy drugs are unsubstantiated by the very clinical trials they regard as standards?

## Why Chemotherapy Kills More Patients Than It Cures

Researchers at Stanford University recently gained an insight into why chemotherapy is such a dismal failure.[19] Aside from burdening the body's detoxification system and suppressing the immune system, chemotherapy can cause a mutation in the gene that is supposed to protect the body against cancer. This "tumor suppressor gene" (also known as the p53 gene) normally codes for a protein that stops the growth of potential cancer cells by binding to key sites on the cells' DNA and thereby blocking the process of cell division.

Here is where chemotherapy wreaks even worse damage than is commonly understood. Chemotherapy kills cells by damaging their DNA. All malignant tissues harbor some cells that have a natural resistance to many chemotherapy agents, just as bacteria exposed to antibiotics develop resistance to those drugs. Although the chemotherapy agents initially affect most cancer cells, those that are resistant survive and eventually they develop into an even more dangerous tumor. This process is accelerated by the tendency of cancer cells to mutate with ever greater frequency as the tumor develops.[21]

To make matters worse, some of the cells develop mutations in their p53 genes, and the defective p53 protein can no longer do its job. These mutated cells have an enormous competitive advantage and eventually dominate the tumor. When the p53 gene mutates, the tumor's growth spins out of control. Since their p53 is no longer effective, the mutated cancer cells refuse to die and continue to multiply, while the rest of the body suffers from the poisons of chemotherapy. This biological scenario helps explain why most cancer patients treated with standard chemotherapy are worse off than they would have been without the drugs.

This is why many now claim that the "success" of conventional can-

## Chemotherapy Breeds More Cancer

Patients who take chemotherapy for Hodgkin's disease are 14 times more likely to develop leukemia as a result, according to experts from 14 cancer centers who studied 10,000 cases. Use of chemotherapy also increased the risk of bone, joint, and soft-tissue cancer by 6 times, according to the *Journal of the National Cancer Institute* (May 1995). Radiation therapy increased the risk of developing respiratory cancer by 2.7 times and female genital cancers of the uterus and ovaries by 2.4 times.[20]

***Highly aggressive chemotherapy actually shortens survival times compared with patients in whom chemotherapy was delayed or administered less aggressively, says Ulrich Abel, Ph.D.***

cer treatment is often illusory. German cancer researcher Ulrich Abel, Ph.D., observes that the temporary shrinking of a tumor mass—defined as either a partial or complete remission—is not necessarily a good sign, because the remaining tumor cells often grow much faster and more virulently after the first series of chemotherapy treatments.[22] Highly aggressive chemotherapy actually shortens survival times compared with patients in whom chemotherapy was delayed or administered less aggressively, says Dr. Abel. Paradoxically, patients whose tumors showed no response to chemotherapy actually survived longer than patients who did respond.[23]

***A study of over 10,000 cancer patients shows clearly that chemotherapy's supposedly strong track record with Hodgkin's disease is actually a lie. Patients who underwent chemotherapy were 14 times more likely to develop leukemia and 6 times more likely to develop cancers of the bones, joints, and soft tissue than those patients who did not undergo chemotherapy.***

A related insight is that free-radical damage to DNA increases the risk of cancer cells spreading. It is the metastases that typically kill cancer patients. Human DNA from invasive, spreading cancer (metastases) contains twice as much damage due to free radicals as DNA from noninvasive tumors.[24] This fact explains why patients who manage to survive chemotherapy and radiation tend to develop more deadly cancers later on, because both chemotherapy and radiation generate free radicals in abundance. On the basis of this research, there are strong grounds for advising that, with rare exceptions, chemotherapy should be avoided or its use minimized to keep your DNA intact and your immune system functioning optimally.

According to the recommendations of the physicians in this book, if you have already received conventional chemotherapy and radiation, you can start mitigating the damage by boosting your body's antioxidant supply. Studies have shown that supplementation with antioxidants can bring about a significant increase in survival for breast cancer patients[25] and prevent recurrences of bladder cancer;[26] in addition, decreasing the consumption of dietary fat, another common source of free radicals, increases the survival rates of breast cancer patients.[27]

## Biological Response Modifiers and Low-Dose Chemotherapy

Nutrients and numerous other "biological response modifiers" (BRMs) can directly impede tumor growth and metastases.[28] According to Keith I. Block, M.D., (see Chapter 2), BRM research offers solid evidence that alternative therapies need to become integrated into sensible cancer care:

- A number of herbs have proven to be effective when used in complement with fractionated chemotherapy, a form of low-dose chemotherapy (LDC) that entails very small doses spread out over a longer period of time.
- For stomach cancer patients receiving Chinese herbs, NK cell (anticancer) activity improved and the ability to tolerate chemotherapy improved significantly compared to patients not receiving herbs (95% vs. 79%). The herb-treated patients reported higher energy levels, improved weight gain, and better overall quality of life.[29]
- Survival rates improved in patients with lung, breast, throat, and nasopharyngeal cancers who used Chinese herbs in combination with chemotherapy or radiation, versus those who relied on conventional treatment alone.[30]
- No significant drop in immune cell counts was observed after several cycles of chemotherapy in a group of breast cancer patients using Chinese herbs.[31]

## Breast Cancer Surgery and the Menstrual Cycle—Timing Enhances Survival

If surgery for breast cancer is medically unavoidable, choosing the time within a woman's menstrual cycle for the operation can make a crucial difference in survival. A study of 289 premenopausal women undergoing mastectomy or lumpectomy revealed that those who had the surgery between days 18 and 20 of their cycle fared the best, with a 76% better survival rate (up to 18 years of follow-up) than women having surgery during days 3 to 12 of their cycle.

The difference is progesterone: its levels increase steadily as the menstrual cycle progresses, but especially after ovulation until about day 23. The desirable level of progesterone was placed at 4 nanograms/ml. Matching surgery to menstrual cycles doubles the survival rate for cancers involving the lymph nodes.[32]

Combining the LDC approach with strategic use of Chinese botanicals, nutraceuticals (food-derived BRMs), and phytochemicals (plant-derived BRMs), reduces the toxic potential of chemotherapy to the point where adverse side effects are entirely avoided, says Dr. Block. His patients frequently eat, read, even converse while undergoing the fractionated chemotherapy program. Hair loss and nausea are virtually nonexistent—an outcome unheard of in conventional oncology.

LDC protocols appear to offer the side benefit of stimulating the immune system. As Wolfgang Kostler, M.D., another physician using highly reduced (fractionated) preparations of chemotherapy, states, "Low-dose chemotherapy is very activating to the immune system."[33] Stanislaw Burzynski, M.D., embattled pioneer of antineoplastons, uses low-dose methotrexate and has observed a similar enhancement of immune function. With judicious use of detoxifying and immune-stimulating BRMs as a complement to reduced-dose chemotherapy, these specialists are slowly transforming the field of cancer treatment.

## Making Chemotherapy Use Rational: The Ex Vivo Apoptotic Assay

Conventional cancer treatment routinely administers powerful and toxic chemotherapy drugs to cancer patients based on statistical probabilities that these drugs will have some effect. Yet often patients find out that particular cancer drugs are ineffective for them only after taking them and enduring their toxic side effects. A new lab test takes the guesswork out of conventional and alternative cancer treatments. It is called the "Ex Vivo Apoptotic Assay" and was developed by Robert A. Nagourney, M.D. Dr. Nagourney, a board-certified oncologist, hematologist, and pharmacology professor, is founder and medical director of Rational Therapeutics of Long Beach, California, which provides the test.

Apoptosis (pronounced *ap-op-TOW-sis*) is a clinical term that means "programmed cell death." The concept of apoptosis underscores an important fact about cancer, says Dr. Nagourney. "In terms of what defines cancer, it is not that cancer cells grow too much; it is that they die too little. The entire hypothesis of modern cancer research has been largely focused on cancer as a disease of cell proliferation and cancer treatment as a mechanism for inhibiting this proliferation. In simplistic terms, cancer drugs were designed as birth control pills for cancers. More correctly understood, what you need to do in a patient is not stop the cells from growing as much, as to actually stop the cancer cells from living. Instead, you must arrest their viability, stop them in their tracks, and make them die as they are programmed to do."

Dr. Nagourney's test is a short-term measure of the ability of a substance to produce cancer cell death. "Our role is to inject some logic and sense into a rather hectic and haphazard administration of therapies," says Dr. Nagourney. "We call our approach 'rational therapeutics' because we think it is a very intelligent way to deal with cancer."

Let's say your physician tells you that the use of Adriamycin (a chemotherapy drug) induces remissions in 38% of women with breast cancer. How can you tell *in advance* if you're part of the 38% for whom it works or the 62% for whom it has no effect? "We can now painlessly determine things in a test tube for a patient that they would only be able to find out if they went through the treatments," Dr. Nagourney says. "This is crucial since I've never seen a correctly administered chemotherapy for an 'average' patient."

***"We can now painlessly determine things in a test tube for a patient that they would only be able to find out if they went through the treatments," Dr. Nagourney says. "This is crucial since I've never seen a correctly administered chemotherapy for an 'average' patient."***

Based on their cumulative results, Dr. Nagourney's team has compiled a bell-shaped data curve that shows the range of sensitivity and resistance to different drugs among individuals with the same kinds of cancer. From this he now knows that out of 100 women with breast cancer, perhaps 35 will have cancer cell death taking 0.15 mcg/ml of doxorubicin, while 25 will require only 0.05 mcg/ml, and still others will need 1.0 mcg/ml. His test can determine the likely effect on human cancer tissue from any of about 70 chemotherapy drugs, given singly or in combination. It can also test botanical substances such as betulinic acid (from white birch bark), Alvium (a 12-herb formula), antineoplastons, interferons, or, theoretically, any substance capable of killing cancer cells. All that is required is a living tissue sample of cancer cells obtained from the patient by biopsy, or a blood sample in the case of leukemias.

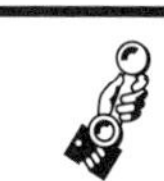

For more information about the **Ex Vivo Apoptotic Assay,** contact: Rational Therapeutics, Cancer Evaluation Center, 3601 Elm Avenue, Long Beach, CA 90807; tel: 310-989-6455; fax: 310-989-6454; Internet web site address: **http://www.Rational-T.com**. The Assay generally costs $2000 for lab studies, and $2500 with a consultation with Dr. Nagourney.

The goal is to see which substances produce cancer cell death during a 72-96 hour process in which the cancer is grown in a test tube. The result *objectively* indicates the likely human response of an *individual* patient to a specific drug, says Dr. Nagourney. On this basis, the physician can then tailor a customized treatment plan with a fair measure of assurance that it will be effective.

On the average, Dr. Nagourney says, a patient that is found "sensitive" (responsive) to an identified drug or substance is 2-3 times more likely to respond favorably when that drug is given clinically. This also means that the test can produce 2-3 times better outcomes in patients than the national averages reported by the National Cancer Institute, Dr. Nagourney notes. Generally, the assay's ability to predict outcomes was scored at 19 out of 21 in a test published in the *Journal of Hematology Blood Transfusion* in 1990, while between 85% to 95% of specimens submitted provide successful studies.

***"Our data shows that people undergoing oncological basic therapy do far better than conventionally treated patients. We see much lower rates of recurrences and metastases with our approach compared to chemotherapy or radiation treatment," says Dr. Kostler.***

For example, a man with colon cancer was tested for sensitivity to 16 chemotherapy drugs. The results indicated his system was "resistant" (unresponsive) to 6 drugs, such as carmustin, nitrogen mustard, and taxol, and that it had an "extreme drug resistance" to doxorubicin "with a near-zero response probability to that agent." The assay also indicated the Ex Vivo Best Regimen, in this case, a combination of 2 drugs whose effects would be strengthened for this individual when applied together.

While Rational Therapeutics does not prescribe medicines for cancer, as a complement to the test results, clinicians will suggest "a carefully developed antioxidant and nutrition program designed to aid in the patient's recovery and minimize the toxic side effects of chemotherapy treatments," says Dr. Nagourney. It is a holistic approach in that "we make a global or 'whole person' assessment of each patient," so that treatment can be objectively individualized. In this way, says Dr. Nagourney, the field of cancer treatment can be "advanced by studying the most rational and reliable indicators of positive cancer response: each patient's own cancer cells."

## Wolfgang Kostler, M.D.—Preventing Breast Cancer Recurrences with Oncological Basic Therapy

A high degree of success in preventing recurrences or metastases of breast cancer is possible, says Dr. Wolfgang Kostler, when you correct the inner environment of the body, strengthen the immune system, detoxify the cells, and neutralize the negative effect of free radicals. If you change the cellular terrain and its biochemical conditions, breast cancer will not recur.

Dr. Wolfgang Kostler bases his perspective on cancer on the premise that it is not the primary tumor that kills the patient, but the recurrences and metastases. "There are body conditions that favor the cancer's ability to thrive. This means we have a cancer-*prone* environment inside the body. If you don't focus on this internal environment, you can't effectively treat cancer because the cancerous internal milieu still elicits the creation of the tumor."

***"The post-surgical period is the time to be most vigilant, since surgery itself can create metastases at the microscopic level, setting the body up for much more dangerous conditions later on," Dr. Kostler says.***

President of the Austrian Society of Oncology, Dr. Kostler studied medicine at the University of Vienna and continued his studies in oncology at Lainz Hospital in Vienna, Austria. In 1977, he opened a private practice in Vienna, where he continues to treat patients and conduct research. In 1986, he cofounded a modern cancer treatment clinic in Vienna called the Sanatorium Dobling, where he is chief of the ambulatory care unit. From 1984-1988, Dr. Kostler lectured at the University of Vienna, in the Institute of Nutritional Sciences, and served as president of the Austrian Hospital, a humanitarian medical association.

Prevention of metastases and cancer recurrences is the area of oncology that affords the greatest opportunity for winning the war against cancer, says Dr. Kostler. He and his colleagues have demonstrated that if strong immune function is maintained and free-radical damage (e.g., lipid peroxidation) is minimized, then the cancer patient will not relapse and new tumors or metastases will not form.

The careful timing of specific kinds of intervention is essential for achieving the best results. If a person receives the appropriate measures at the right time, the chances of recurrences after surgery are greatly minimized. Making dietary and lifestyle changes *before* surgery gives the body a head start and prepares it for the stress unavoidably caused by surgery. "The operation is only the removal of a symptom, which is like a red flashing alarm light," says Dr. Kostler. "It is just the end product of a very toxic situation." In principle, any tumor's growth can be halted and effectively reversed if the right treatment choices are made at the right time, Dr. Kostler contends.

***"Breast cancer can be easily treated if you do the right things at the right time. If you change the internal environment—the cellular terrain and its biochemical conditions—breast cancer will not recur," says Dr. Kostler.***

Dr. Kostler is dismayed that many oncologists adopt a passive, anti-prevention attitude toward the cancer patient's prognosis. "The key is to take an active stance against the possibility of recurrences and metastases, not to succumb to the old wait-and-see policy which allows these processes to take place and push the cancer out of control." Following surgery, Dr. Kostler recommends therapeutic strategies that will likely prevent recurrences and metastases. "The postsurgical period is the time to be most vigilant, since surgery itself can create metastases at the microscopic level, setting the body up for much more dangerous conditions later on."

## WORKING AGAINST ALL KNOWN TUMOR-CAUSING FACTORS

The goal of Dr. Kostler's Oncological Basic Therapy (OBT) is to prevent recurrences and metastases by identifying and compensating for all known tumor-causing factors. This large, multifaceted program includes the following components:

- **Antioxidant Therapy:** Free radicals damage (oxidize) the membranes of the mitochondria inside cells. "The mitochondria are the energy generators or power plants of the cell," says Dr. Kostler. "If the energy of the cell is decreased, then disorganized processes will follow. This means that the suppressor genes will not work and will not block the oncogenes that form cancer." Free radicals are unavoidable, but the body's main radical-scavenging mechanisms are supported by vitamins E and C, beta carotene, copper, zinc, manganese, and selenium.
- **Biological Dentistry:** Biological dentistry calls for the removal of

infected teeth and mercury amalgams to restore healthy functioning of soft tissues.

- **Regulation of Intestinal Balance:** The use of probiotics (e.g., *Lactobacilli*) helps create an optimal balance of intestinal microbes.
- **Detoxification of Heavy Metals:** In addition to dental mercury amalgam removal, selenium supplementation (selenium counteracts mercury overload), chelation, heat therapy, and other techniques can aid in this process.
- **Nutritional Therapy:** Supplementation with minerals, trace elements and vitamins, as well as dietary adjustments, may be needed.
- **Immune Modulation:** Imbalances in various types of immune cells can be rectified through nutritional, botanical, and BRM supplementation.
- **Hormone Therapy:** The use of tamoxifen and other hormone blockers can help curb tumor growth.
- **Antiviral and Antimycotic Therapies:** Viral and fungal infections (mycosis) can be sources of free radicals and contribute to cancer, so they need to be effectively countered.
- **Psychotherapy:** Music, meditation, relaxation, and activities that create pleasure and happiness can help activate the immune system.
- **Physical Therapy:** Massage and other aspects of physical therapy are helpful for patients whose physical condition has deteriorated. Physical training and exercise strengthen the anticancer defenses.

Dr. Kostler's therapies work best when they can be started before surgical removal of the tumor; he recommends surgery in most cases. The initial goals of his therapies are to detoxify the body, stimulate the immune system, and block estrogen activity. The use of tumor-killing therapies such as chemotherapy and radiotherapy are in most cases ineffective in helping the cancer patient because the elimination of the tumor does

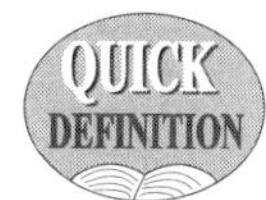


**Biological dentistry** stresses the use of nontoxic restoration materials for dental work and focuses on the unrecognized impact that dental toxins and hidden dental infections can have on overall health. Typically, a biological dentist will emphasize the safe removal of mercury amalgams; in many cases, either the avoidance or removal of root canals; the investigation of possible jawbone infections (cavitations) as a "dental focus" or source of bodywide illness centered in the teeth; and the health-injuring role of misalignment of teeth and jaw structures.

**Friendly bacteria,** or probiotics, refer to beneficial microbes inhabiting the human gastrontestinal tract where they are essential for proper nutrient assimilation. The human body contains an estimated several thousand billion beneficial bacteria comprising over 400 species, all necessary for health. Among the more well known of these are *Lactobacillus acidophilus* and *Bifidobacterium bifidum*. Overly acidic bodily conditions, chronic constipation or diarrhea, dietary imbalances, overly processed foods, and the excessive use of antibiotics and hormonal drugs can interfere with probiotic function and even reduce their numbers, setting up conditions for illness.

For more information about restoring **intestinal balance** and colonic detoxification, see Chapter 33: Physical Support Therapies, pp. 949-980; for more on **biological dentistry**, see Chapter 33: Physical Support Therapies, pp. 980-989; and Chapter 25: What Causes Cancer? pp. 594-602.

***Dr. Kostler's breast cancer patients have shown much better survival rates than patients who have undergone lumpectomy or mastectomy followed by radiation. The median survival is 5-6 years without any recurrences.***

nothing to change the environment that allowed the tumor to grow. If such therapies are employed, it is crucial to have an aggressive oncological basic therapy (OBT) program before, during, and after treatments, Dr. Kostler emphasizes.

Dr. Kostler prefers to work with people who have not undergone conventional measures, including lumpectomy "Breast cancer can be easily treated if you do the right things at the right time. This means that you improve the environment inside the patient—the same environment that once allowed the cancer to grow—before the body is subjected to a surgical procedure of any kind." If you change the internal environment—the cellular terrain, its biochemical conditions—breast cancer will not recur.

## HIGH POSTSURGICAL SURVIVAL RATES FOR BREAST CANCER CASES

To contact **Dr. Kostler**, write: Wolfgang Kostler, M.D., Sofienalpanstrasse 17, A-1140 Wien, Austria.

Few doctors can claim the therapeutic success rate Dr. Kostler has achieved with prevention of breast cancer recurrences and metastases. Based on his experience with 250 women who have received his protocols for breast cancer since the early 1980s, Dr. Kostler is confident in claiming that recurrences can be prevented with his approach.

However, there is no way to guarantee the prevention of recurrence or metastasis if the tumor diameter is greater than 4 mm; that is because angiogenic factors (which promote formation and growth of new blood vessels critical to a tumor's survival) are produced in cancers of this size, and they enable cancer cells to spread through the blood and lymph. In addition, the breast cancer patient must receive OBT *before* the surgery to prevent recurrences or metastases.

If the hormonal factors are blocked and the immune system is stimulated, the body has a much stronger chance of fighting off any further development of cancer. To block hormonal estrogen activity, Dr. Kostler uses tamoxifen and has not observed any adverse effects of this treatment, despite evidence linking tamoxifen use for breast cancer to the later appearance of endometrial cancer. Tamoxifen is typically prescribed after breast cancer surgery to block the regrowth of remaining cancer cells. The drug blocks the activity of estrogen, the hormone that would otherwise stimulate this growth.

"We don't see the kinds of adverse effects with tamoxifen that other doctors have seen in other parts of the world, says Dr. Kostler. "In 6 years of use, not one of our patients has developed uterine cancer or any of the serious side effects that people have associated with tamoxifen. We are very careful in our use of this hormone blocker." Tamoxifen is important because it blocks both estrogen and prolactin; prolactin levels are high in breast cancer patients and this hormone is an even more potent stimulator of tumor growth than estrogen.

Though the use of radiation following lumpectomy has recently been touted as a sure way to treat many kinds of breast cancer and prevent recurrences, Dr. Kostler disagrees with this practice. Radiation is a source of free radicals that can damage DNA and predispose the body to later cancers. "It may eliminate the cancer initially, but not in the long run." This is true even if a person receives a great many antioxidants prior to the radiation. "You can't take enough antioxidants to protect you against radiation. It is like trying to stop the damage caused by the bombing of Hiroshima. There is no way to safeguard against the potential harm to the DNA."

Dr. Kostler has compared his data with published research findings on lumpectomy with radiation, examining incidence for both recurrences and metastases. His breast cancer patients have shown much better survival rates than patients who have undergone lumpectomy or mastectomy followed by radiation.[34]

"Our data shows that people undergoing oncological basic therapy do far better than conventionally treated patients. We see much lower rates of recurrences and metastases with our approach compared to chemotherapy or radiation treatment. It seems clear that we should make every effort to minimize free-radical damage, not increase it with those modalities." Among those breast cancer patients who have attended Dr. Kostler's clinic, those with the longest survival have been free of cancer for 13 years; the median survival is 5-6 years without any recurrences.[35]

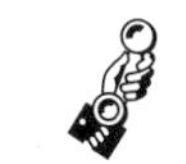

For a source of **shark liver oil**, or alkylglycerol, contact: Scandinavian Natural Health & Beauty Products, Inc., (Alkyrol® brand), 13 North Seventh Street, Perkasie, PA 18944; tel: 215-453-2505; fax: 215-453-2508.

For more information about the political aspects of **antineoplastons** and the cancer industry's organized suppression of **Dr. Burzynski**, see Chapter 26: How Cancer Politics Have Kept You in the Dark, pp. 671-605.

An **oncogene** is a gene believed to transform normal cells into cancer cells, thus initiating the development of cancer. Some of these genes have reportedly been identified in cancer-causing viruses. Proto-oncogenes are genes in a neutral, inactive stage that under certain conditions become oncogenes. Among the oncogenes identified with the type of cancer they tend to precipitate are: erbb2 (breast); fos (lung); jun (lung); hras (pancreatic); kras (colon); nras (lung, others); myc (breast, colon, small-cell lung).

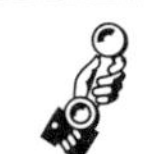

For more information about **antineoplastons** and Dr. Burzynski, contact: Burzynski Research Institute, Inc., Stanislaw Burzynski, M.D., 12000 Richmond Ave., Suite 260, Houston, TX 77082; tel: 713-597-0111; fax: 713-597-1166]

## A Glossary of New Pharmacological Substances for Treating Cancer

### ALKYLGLYCEROLS (SHARK LIVER OIL, MOTHER'S MILK)

A group of compounds called alkylglycerols (pronounced all-kill-gliss-ser-alls) can bolster anticancer defenses and protect the body against the harmful effects of radiation-induced injury.[36] The richest source of these special fats (also called "ether lipids" or "alkyllyso-phospholipids") is shark liver oil,[37] but these fats are found to a lesser extent in mother's milk, which contains 10 times more alkylglycerols than cow's milk.[38]

Animal studies have indicated that alkylglycerols have antitumor activity, probably mediated through certain immune cells (macrophages) in the form of direct and selective destruction to cancer cells.[39] Cell culture studies have shown that alkylglycerols are "selectively toxic against cancer cells" and this "selection" seems to be affected by the cholesterol concentration of the cancer cell; as the cholesterol level drops, the cancer cells die more rapidly.[40]

Extracts of shark liver oil may help people tolerate both chemotherapy and radiation. The administration of alkylglycerols prior to radiation treatment was found to cause advanced tumors to regress toward less advanced stages;[41] alkylglycerols also caused reversal of tumor growth in animal studies.[42] A possible explanation for these findings is that this substance can inhibit a variety of tumor-promoting substances, including the "bad" eicosanoids and platelet-activating factor (PAF).[43] One potential area of concern, however, is contamination of shark liver oil by ocean pollutants. No published research, to our knowledge, has yet addressed this issue nor have the potential toxicities at normal doses been adequately studied.

Scientists at Johns Hopkins University School of Medicine found that a synthetic form of squalamine, originally derived from shark liver, is effective in controlling the growth of brain tumors in rats and in extending their lives. The substance suppresses the formation of new blood vessels in the tumor, thus preventing it from growing, reports the *New York Times* (May 1, 1996).

## ANTINEOPLASTONS

Beginning in the 1960s, Stanislaw Burzynski, M.D., isolated several peptides (chains of amino acids, the building blocks of protein) from human urine and found them to be effective in controlling the growth of certain types of cancer. Dr. Burzynski originally identified and isolated from the urine of healthy humans 5 different antineoplastons (meaning substances that work against [anti] a neoplasm [an abnormal growth of new tissue, such as a tumor]). He determined that these molecules have a strong anticancer effect at a genetic level: specifically, they appear to stimulate the activity of "tumor suppressor genes," genes that literally turn off the activity of certain oncogenes (genes that promote tumor growth).[44] By this action, antineoplastons can actually stop cells from multiplying out of control, eventually producing a tumor mass, said Dr. Burzynski. It is almost as if cancer results from a deficiency of antineoplastons.

Dr. Burzynski has successfully used antineoplastons, which he produces himself in an FDA-approved manufacturing facility in his Houston, Texas, clinic. Currently, he has 65 different treatment protocols using 2 antineoplaston formulas. The protocols differ according to type and size of tumor, although best results appear to come from treating brain tumors, metastatic breast cancer, and non-Hodgkin's lymphoma.

As part of a study, he used antineoplastons to treat 20 patients who had advanced-stage astrocytoma, a particularly fast-growing type of brain tumor that tends to occur in young children. Nearly 80% of them responded favorably, and a number of them were tumor free 4 years later.[45] Animal studies in Japan indicate that low doses of orally administered synthetic antineoplaston A10 help prevent cancers of the breast, lung, and liver.[46]

At the Ninth International Symposium on Future Trends in Chemotherapy in March 1990, Dr. Dvorit Samid stated, "Antineoplaston AS2-1 profoundly inhibits oncogene expression and the proliferation of malignant cells without exhibiting any toxicity toward normal cells."[47] Based on clinical results of 7 studies presented at the conference, Dr. Samid concluded: "Antineoplaston therapy restores to the body those natural com-

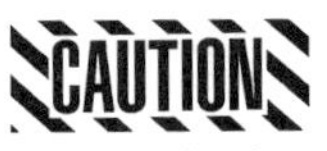


Known side effects from Carnivora® are minimal: taken orally without dilution, it can sometimes produce nausea or vomiting; when injected, it can produce a temporary increase in body temperature. Ninety-day studies with rats in which the rodents received doses 30-60 times higher than the recommended human dose showed no toxic reactions.

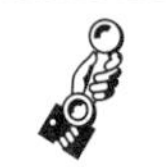

For more information about **Carnivora**®, which is available as drops or injectable ampules, contact: Carnivora-Forschungs-Gmbh, Postfach 6, Lobensteiner Strasse 3, D-96365 Nordhalben, Germany; tel: 09267-166; fax: 09267-1040.

pounds that have anticancer activity. Because they are natural compounds, the body tolerates them well, and therefore we minimize the problem of adverse effects. Antineoplastons could be a very valuable, effective, and safe approach to cancer therapy."[48]

According to scientific reports presented at the 86th Annual Meeting of the American Association for Cancer Research in March of 1995, Dr. Burzynski's antineoplastons increase the activity of tumor suppressor genes.[49] At this time, there is no other treatment available that is directed to this critical mechanism in the development of cancer. Ironically, instead of being acknowledged for this Nobel Prize-worthy discovery, Dr. Burzynski has been repeatedly harassed by the FDA and the Texas medical board.

## CARNIVORA®

This extract of the meat-eating plant Venus' flytrap (*Dinoea muscipula*) was introduced into cancer therapy by German oncologist Helmut Keller, medical director of the Chronic Disease Control and Treatment Center in Bad Steben, Germany. Dr. Keller has conducted extensive studies of the intravenous delivery of Carnivora as used in German cancer clinics. The medicine contains one-third pressed Venus' flytrap juice, one-third alcohol, and one-third purified water. Dr. Keller has treated over 2,000 cancer patients with Carnivora, so named in honor of the plant's well-known insect-eating ability. One of the active ingredients appears to be a chemical called plumbagin which has anticancer properties;[50] when topically applied, it can lead to a total reversal of skin cancer.[51]

Although Dr. Keller's work has not been published in peer-reviewed journals, his laboratory studies indicate that Carnivora directly inhibits the metabolic activity of cancer cells. In a clinical study of 210 cancer patients for whom conventional treatments had failed, each received 50-60 drops of Carnivora orally 5 times a day plus one intravenous infusion daily. The results were excellent: 16% of patients showed tumor remission and 40% had no further tumor progression; in the remaining 44% no improvement was noted, although about one-quarter of these patients experienced a palliative effect. This means they felt a decrease in subjective complaints and pain and an increase in appetite, vitality, and positive attitude, according to Dr. Keller. The study showed that more than half, or 56%, experienced either a tumor remission or their cancer development became stable and did not worsen.

In a second study, again after previous conventional therapies had failed, 57 patients (average age 51, with malignancies or chronic immune disorders) took 2 ml of Carnivora daily for 116 days. At the end of this trial period, reports Dr. Keller, 57% reported an improvement in their condition, 25% showed no change, and 18% worsened. In those with malignancy, 45.5% of patients experienced tumor remission; in 34.5%, the tumors became stationary; in 20%, there was no change.

Carnivora is an immunomodulator, which means it stimulates the activity of T helper cells. This in turn enables the body to wage a more vigorous defense against the illness, explains Dr. Keller. Carnivora appears to target tumor cells and bolster the immune system. After the intravenous program is completed, intramuscular injections may be carried out several times a week until the treatment program is finished. People should not attempt to produce their own Carnivora, however, since it first must be purified of naturally occurring plant toxins that would otherwise cause fevers and other adverse reactions.

***In a clinical study of 210 cancer patients taking Carnivora, more than half, or 56%, experienced either a tumor remission or their cancer development became stable and did not worsen.***

## CARTILAGE, BOVINE

In 1954, John F. Prudden, M.D., discovered that bovine cartilage had a remarkable ability to help wounds heal faster. Today, bovine tracheal cartilage is one of the few substances proven to accelerate wound healing, which is why most surgical textbooks mention it. But Dr. Prudden became deeply intrigued with the wider therapeutic potential of this obscure substance. When he watched it dramatically shrink a breast tumor and reduce the malignant ulceration of the chest wall of a desperate patient, he was hooked for life.

The development of new blood vessels (angiogenesis) is a prerequisite for tumor growth, yet this process can be stopped by cartilage from either cows or sharks. Bovine tracheal cartilage (BTC) causes a general activation of the body's anticancer defenses and has demonstrated effectiveness against cancers of the ovary, pancreas, colon, and testes;[52] a BTC extract inhibited the growth of tumor cell lines from 22 patients with various cancers.[53] Since the 1950s, Dr. Prudden has sponsored more than $7 million worth of clinical studies. Since 1972, Dr. Prudden has used BTC to successfully treat 110 cases of advanced cancer; the partial and complete response rate, taken overall, is approximately 30% within a 7-month treatment period.[54] Not surprisingly, William Lane, Ph.D., the proponent of shark cartilage, acknowledges that Dr. Prudden is "the father of cartilage therapy." A quick look at Dr. Prudden's casebook helps make the point.

In a now classic study released in 1985, Dr. Prudden reported on the results of a trial with 31 cancer patients all of whom had failed to respond to conventional therapies or had a cancer that was not treatable at all. After starting a regimen of cartilage—typically 9 g daily, taken orally in 3-gram installments 3 times daily—90% of the patients had a partial or complete response. Dr. Prudden also reports success in causing a large rectal tumor to disappear, leaving the patient cancer free for 18 years after treatment. Bovine cartilage produced a complete healing of breast cancer after all other therapies had failed; this patient remained free of cancer for 10 years until her death from other causes. A man with prostatic cancer that had spread to the bones had a complete remission. An elderly woman, aged 79, with kidney cancer that had spread to her lungs and liver, survived 4 years with much improved conditions.

As impressive as these early results sound, bovine tracheal cartilage is not a cancer cure but a very successful palliation. It is not, strictly speaking, a cure because patients who respond to it must continue taking it at the rate of 9 g daily for the rest of their lives to avoid a possible remission. It also takes up to 4 months for the initial positive effects to show up in the system, Dr. Prudden advises. In more than 25 years, he has never observed any toxic side effects from using bovine cartilage, even with doses 3 times as high as the therapeutic dose.

Bovine cartilage is similar to fetal mesenchyme, the basic tissue from which all muscle, bone, tendons, ligaments, skin, fat, and bone marrow develop as the fetus grows. Dr. Prudden considers the bone marrow to be the heart of the immune system, the basic prototype for all healthy tissue. Bovine cartilage also contains large sugar molecules called mucopolysaccharides that appear to block cell division in the cancerous cells. If the cells cannot divide, they cannot multiply, which means the cancer doesn't spread. Bovine cartilage also seems to stimulate the activity of macrophages, those immune cells that "eat" all foreign materials in the body, including cancerous cells. In addition to stimulating the immune system, the cartilage works to decrease the size and population of malignant cells, thus normalizing the renegade cancer cells.

Certain other facts about bovine cartilage recommend it as a worthy contender in the cartilage-against-cancer field, according to physicians cited in this book. For example, it takes about 70 g of shark cartilage to get healing results in contrast to 9 grams of bovine cartilage. For the therapeutic dose needed, bovine cartilage is 4 times less expensive than shark cartilage. In addition, shark cartilage is 22% calcium, which puts 14 times the normal RDA for calcium into your system, which might be too much. Bovine cartilage at therapeutic dosage has only 10% of the calcium RDA and it contains a chelating substance that helps remove excess calcium from your system.[55]

***Bovine cartilage also seems to stimulate the activity of macrophages, those immune cells that "eat" all foreign materials in the body, including cancerous cells. In addition to stimulating the immune system, the cartilage works to decrease the size and population of malignant cells, thus normalizing the renegade cancer cells.***

## CARTILAGE, SHARK

The popularity of shark cartilage is largely due to William Lane, Ph.D., an agricultural biochemist who published 2 popular books, *Why Sharks Don't Get Cancer* (1992) and *Why Sharks Still Don't Get Cancer* (1996). Researchers at Massachusetts Institute of Technology put cartilage on the treatment map in the mid-1970s when they demonstrated in rabbits and mice implanted with tumors that an infusion of calf cartilage stopped tumor growth with no sign of toxicity 20 days after the infusion. In fact, the average maximum blood vessel length had been reduced by 75%.

In a Cuban study, 14 out of 29 "terminal" (untreatable) cancer patients survived after receiving shark cartilage; of those who died, 9 actually died of cancer and 6 others died of other causes. The survivors were leading normal lives nearly 3 years later. The results of the Cuban trial have been widely disseminated both in the media, through presentations to the public, and by the conventional and alternative medical communities. The

For more information about **shark cartilage**, see Chapter 14: Martin Milner, N.D., pp. 301-302; Chapter 18: Michael B. Schachter, M.D., pp. 377-378; and Chapter 19: Charles B. Simone, M.D., p. 402.

For information on **bovine tracheal cartilage**, contact: The Foundation for Cartilage and Immunology Research, 104 Post Office Road, Waccabuc, NY 10597; tel: 800-910-4701. For information on **Vita-Cart**®, a commercial preparation using bovine cartilage, contact: Vita-Cart, 1117 East Putnam Avenue, Suite 286, Riverside, CT 06878; tel: 800-947-8482; fax: 203-661-6653. For information on **shark cartilage**, contact Cartilage Technologies (Cartilade® brand), 200 Clearbrook Road, Elmsford, NY 10523; tel: 800-700-7325; fax: 914-592-7166. For information on **Benefin**™ and **Immunofin**™ (organically-processed shark cartilage products), contact: Lane Labs USA, Inc., 172 Broadway, Woodcliff Lake, NJ 07675; tel: 800-526-3005 or 201-391-8600; fax: 201-391-8601.

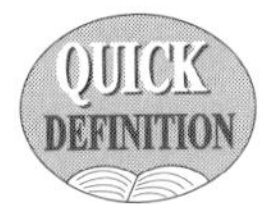


The term **pH**, which means "potential hydrogen," represents a scale for the relative acidity or alkalinity of a solution. Acidity is measured as a pH of 0.1 to 6.9, alkalinity is 7.1 to 14, and neutral pH is 7.0. The numbers refer to how many hydrogen atoms are present compared to an ideal or standard solution. Normally, blood is slightly alkaline, at 7.35 to 7.45; urine pH can range from 4.8 to 7.5, although normal is closer to 7.0.

Cuban study is ongoing. At 23 months, which was 4 times the expected life-span, half (14) of the original group of 29 patients were still alive, doing well, and enjoying completely normal lives. After 33 months of receiving no treatment other than a modest holding dose of shark cartilage daily, no new deaths had been reported.[56]

According to Dr. Lane, ovarian cancer responds the most consistently to shark cartilage, while uterine, cervical, and central nervous system cancers respond positively. According to X rays, "no regrowth of central nervous system tumors that had been surgically removed was found." Further, Dr. Lane reports that shark cartilage is "highly effective" against advanced prostate tumors, achieving tumor reduction rates of 15 to 67%. It is also capable of significantly lowering PSA counts in 12-16 weeks. Generally, shark cartilage works best against solid tumors; pancreatic cancers, provided they are not too advanced, also respond well.[57]

In 1990, T. Oikawa further confirmed the clinical benefit of shark cartilage by finding a "significant inhibition of angiogenesis" with the substance.[58] One substance found in sharks, called squalamine, has recently demonstrated the ability to attack tumors via antiangiogenesis. According to researchers at John Hopkins University, animal studies of squalamine suggest a potential therapeutic benefit for patients with brain cancer.[59]

Shark cartilage's major effect may come from its protein component, which has antiangiogenesis properties as do genistein and other isoflavones, says Michael B. Schachter, M.D. (see Chapter 18). Shark cartilage is a tissue which does not contain blood vessels, he explains. It has proteins which prevent new blood vessel formation. "Thus the administration of relatively large doses of shark cartilage powder either orally or by rectal retention enema appears to be effective for some cancer patients in controlling cancer growth and even causing regression of the cancer."

Although shark cartilage inhibits abnormal angiogenesis (as during cancer progression), it does not appear to interfere with normal angiogenesis necessary for healing. "In fact, it may actually promote new blood vessel formation," says Dr. Schachter. This was seen in the pathology slides of the Cuban shark cartilage study in which the blood supply within the cancerous tissue was cut off, while the connective tissue surrounding the cancer had an increase in blood vessels. "Consequently, it is not necessary to limit the use of shark cartilage following a surgical procedure (when angiogenesis is necessary for healing) or in heart patients who need the development of collateral circulation as part of the healing process."

Several shark cartilage products indicate on the label that the product should not be used postoperatively or in cardiac patients. These labels were written before it was known that shark cartilage does not appear to interfere with healthy blood vessel formation and, in the opinion of Dr. Schachter, may be ignored.

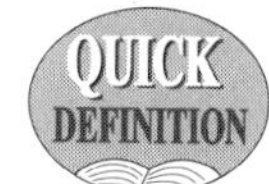


**Chelation therapy** refers to a method of binding ("chelating") an organic substance known as a chelating agent to a metallic ion with a positive electric charge (e.g., a heavy metal) and removing it from the body. One type of chelation therapy involves the chelating agent disodium EDTA given as an intravenous infusion over a 3 1/2-hour period. Usually 20 to 30 treatments are administered at the rate of 1 to 3 sessions per week. Chelation therapy is especially beneficial for all forms of atherosclerotic cardiovascular disease including angina pectoris and coronary artery disease.

## CESIUM

This nonradioactive form of cesium, a rare alkali metal widely distributed in the Earth's crust and listed in the periodic table of elements, has been used with some success as an alternative cancer therapy. Interest in cesium therapy began when scientists observed that areas with low cancer rates had high concentrations of alkali metals in the soils (such as lithium, sodium, or potassium).[60] As early as 1927, Japanese researchers identified cesium as having antitumor activity. It was then suggested that alkalinizing the body fluids could, in turn, push the normally acidic (low) pH of the cancer cell toward a weakly alkaline (high) pH, promoting the cancer's demise.[61] Thus cesium emerged as a high pH-inducing therapy.

***Dr. Lane reports that shark cartilage is "highly effective" against advanced prostate tumors, achieving tumor reduction rates of 15 to 67%. It is also capable of significantly lowering PSA counts in 12-16 weeks.***

A study reported that cesium chloride, when combined with chelation therapy and nutritional supplements, led to significant improvement in about half of all "terminal" cancers of the breast, colon, gallbladder, liver, lung, lymphoma, pancreas, prostate, and pelvis, most of which had not responded to conventional therapy. The cesium treatment consistently resulted in the disappearance of pain within 3 days; autopsies revealed the absence of cancer cells in most cases, which is why the doctors involved in this study called this "a remarkably successful outcome of treatment."[62]

*As reported in the* **American Journal of Surgery,** *researchers found that DMSO combined with lowered doses of anticancer drugs can produce "the same cytotoxic [cell-killing] effect as a full dose of drugs without DMSO, and with less systemic toxicity."*

There appears to be an intracellular relationship or balance between cesium and potassium that promotes the destruction of cancer cells.[63] Cesium is similar to potassium, which may explain why it is taken up so easily by cancer cells;[64] this uptake is enhanced when supported by vitamins C and A, and the minerals zinc and selenium.[65] These supplements, along with a high-potassium diet, may also help eliminate the potential toxicity of cesium.[66] Ironically, cesium has been used in cancer therapy for many years, but in the form of radioactive isotopes or "seeds" implanted in cancer patients as part of radiation therapy.

**CAUTION**

High and potentially toxic concentrations of DMSO may be needed to induce cancer redifferentiation, but this often results in bad breath and a skin odor similar to that from high consumption of garlic. Other potential side effects include occasional nausea, headaches, and dizziness; localized skin rashes may develop when DMSO is applied directly to the skin (especially with concentrations of DMSO greater than 50%). Never mix DMSO with any chemical or drug and apply it to the skin; the proper DMSO dosage for such a combination is unknown. As with other pharmacologic substances, consult your doctor regarding proper usage of DMSO.

## DMSO (DIMETHYLSULFOXIDE)

This substance is present in small quantities in grains, fruits, and vegetables and is naturally present in small quantities in the human body.[67] It is more commonly known as a solvent derived from coal, oil, and lignan, a structural material in plants. Although the primary clinical use of DMSO has been to treat inflammation, it is also known to induce the differentiation of malignant cells—that is, it causes them to become benign.[68]

Some researchers propose that DMSO may be particularly beneficial to cancer patients who require bone marrow transplantation, since it causes differentiation of malignant bone marrow cells.[69] DMSO has demonstrated effectiveness in slowing or halting the progress of cancers of the bladder,[70] colon,[71] ovary,[72] breast,[73] and skin.[74] Malignant leukemia cells have been observed to revert to normal or benign cells following DMSO treatment.[75] One of the most exciting aspects of DMSO is its apparent ability to help deliver anticancer substances to the site of the cancer[76] where it seems to enhance the effects of various cell-killing agents while simultaneously reducing the toxicity of conventional treatments.[77]

DMSO stimulates various parts of the immune system and scavenges hydroxyl radicals, the most potent of free radicals.[78] Since free radicals promote tumor growth, this may be one of the mechanisms by which DMSO interferes with the development of cancer. It may also explain why patients who receive DMSO while undergoing either chemotherapy or radiation—both of which *generate* free radicals in order to kill cancer cells—are far less prone to such side effects as hair loss, nausea, and dry mouth.[79]

When DMSO is present in a water solution, each water molecule will bond preferentially to DMSO rather than to other water molecules. Biochemists at the Institute for Theoretical Biology, in Theresa, New York, have noted that DMSO increases the flow of essential mineral ions (cations) across cell membranes and may decrease the effect of carcinogens by "cleansing" the cell membrane.[80] It is probably owing to this unique chemistry that DMSO is able to help deliver anticancer substances to the site of the cancer.[81] For example, agents effective against lung tumors could be more effectively transported in the presence of DMSO.[82]

The late Eli Jordan Tucker, M.D., of Houston, Texas, found in the late 1960s that by combining DMSO with hematoxylon (a laboratory staining agent) and administering it intravenously and topically to a variety of terminally ill cancer patients that 38% showed marked improvement with DMSO/hematoxylon alone, and 70% showed marked improvement when the combination was used with surgery, radiation, and/or chemotherapy.[83]

These DMSO-related activities may explain why this substance seems to increase the potency of various therapeutic agents against cancer.[84] Since DMSO is a free-radical scavenger and enables smaller doses of drugs to be used, it can greatly reduce the toxicity of conventional treatments. For instance, as reported in the *American Journal of Surgery*, researchers found that DMSO combined with lowered doses of anticancer drugs can produce "the same cytotoxic [cell-killing] effect as a full dose of the drugs without DMSO, and with less systemic toxicity."[85] The same researchers also reported that DMSO may similarly aid in the treatment of ovarian cancer.[86] In studies with rats, DMSO had no effect when used alone against prostate cancer but, again, when combined with other therapeutic agents, the doses could be lowered and the same effects achieved.[87]

## GLUTATHIONE AND N-ACETYL CYSTEINE (NAC)

For complete information about the political aspects of **hydrazine sulfate** and the efforts of the cancer industry to suppress this substance, see Chapter 26: How Cancer Politics Have Kept You in the Dark, pp. 667-674.

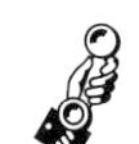

For more clinical information about **hydrazine sulfate**, contact: Syracuse Research Institute, Joseph Gold, M.D., 600 East Genesee Street, Syracuse, NY 13202; tel: 315-472-6616. The general public may obtain hydrazine sulfate from Great Lakes Metabolics, 1724 Hiawatha Court N.E., Rochester, MN 55904; tel: 507-288-2348; fax: 507-285-4475.

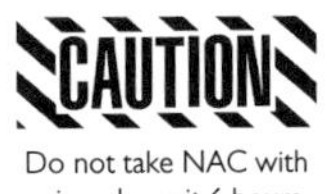


Do not take NAC with minerals; wait 6 hours after taking NAC to take minerals.

Glutathione is a protein that contains the amino acids cysteine, glycine, and glutamic acid; NAC, a derivative of cysteine, is an amino acid precursor for the body's production of glutathione. Cysteine accounts for glutathione's antioxidant activity and its role in the key antioxidant enzyme, glutathione peroxidase. Blood levels of glutathione peroxidase tend to decrease after the sixth decade of life and are typically lower in patients with malignant cancers.[88] Supplementing regularly with a combination of glutathione and NAC may be especially important for older people who have been exposed to numerous toxins in their diet and environment.

Glutathione reduces free-radical damage to DNA and prevents depletion of other antioxidants. It also helps metabolize various carcinogens, activates certain immune cells, helps synthesize and repair DNA, and may inhibit angiogenesis, a blood vessel-forming process required for tumor growth.[89] Glutathione is also a component of glutathione-S-transferase, an enzyme that assists in the liver's metabolism of drugs and toxic chemicals (xenobiotics). That is why this enzyme is important to the liver's phase II detoxification mechanisms, which complete the detoxification of these toxic compounds. Glutathione and NAC supplements have been found to diminish the toxic side effects of chemotherapy and other conventional treatments.[90]

Glutathione is most effective if absorbed under the tongue at a dose of 100-500 mg daily rather than being swallowed; this is because stomach acid and digestive enzymes can degrade it. NAC is best taken as 1200 mg every other day for a 150-pound person, and less for people under that weight.

## HYDRAZINE SULFATE

This experimental synthetic chemical developed by Joseph Gold, M.D., seems to inhibit the loss of protein or body mass caused by cancer, while at the same time exerting indirect antitumor effects. In clinical trials, the compound significantly improved the nutritional status and survival of lung cancer patients.[91]

A study of 740 cancer patients (200 with lung cancer, 138 with stomach cancer, 66 with breast cancer, 63 with Hodgkin's disease, 31 with melanoma, and others) reported tumor stabilization or regression in about 51% of patients, while 46.6% of the patients reported symptomatic improvements, such as fewer respiratory problems and a decrease in fever.[92] Decreased pain was noted even in cases of metastatic bone cancer, and some patients improved so markedly that they were once again able to walk and care for themselves. In one study, the compound significantly improved the nutritional status and survival of lung cancer patients;[93] it may also aid in treating cancers of the breast, lung and larynx, as well as Hodgkin's disease, desmosarcoma, and neuroblastoma."[94,95]

Hydrazine sulfate improves appetite, increases a patient's sense of well-being, results in weight gain in those who have lost weight, and may contribute to a shrinkage of tumors. It seems to work by interfering with the liver's ability to produce glucose from lactic acid, a process known as gluconeogenesis. Cancer cells thrive on glucose: they metabolize glucose to lactic acid, which enters the bloodstream and travels to the liver. The liver then converts this lactic acid to glucose which, in turn, enters the bloodstream and goes back to the cancer cells where it is metabolized. This process allows the cancer to grow quickly while normal cells in the body break down. This destructive cycle may continue, resulting in a wasting away of the lean mass of the patient, until death ensues.

By blocking a particular enzyme in the liver and interfering with gluconeogenesis, hydrazine sulfate inhibits the cancer while allowing normal cells to thrive, thus reversing the vicious cycle. The bulk of the research indicates that hydrazine sulfate leads to significant subjective improvements (notably in pain control) as well as to favorable clinical outcomes for many types of cancer.[96] Although the substance is inexpensive and nonpatentable, the FDA has made it illegal for chemical companies to sell hydrazine sulfate to the public.

## INDOCIN (INDOMETHACIN)

This substance is a member of the family of nonsteroidal medications and has about the same contraindications as aspirin, the worst of which is bleeding or perforated ulcers; either can be a surgical emergency. By inhibiting the production of the "bad" eicosanoid, prostaglandin E2, indocin effectively slows tumor growth, permitting more macrophages to enter the tumor.[97] A growing body of research indicates that indocin may be effective against various cancers.[98]

## MELLITIN

This substance is derived from the "sting" of honeybees. Increasingly used as a "folk remedy" for rheumatoid arthritis and multiple sclerosis, the honeybee's venom has recently shown promise as an anticancer agent as well. Immunologist and pathologist Robert Raison, Ph.D., of the University of Technology in Sydney, Australia, found that bee venom can be combined with certain antibodies to target cancer cells without damaging normal cells. The venom's main poison, mellitin, killed tumor cells by damaging their outer membrane, causing them to break open.[99]

***In animal studies, 714X was effective against bone and breast cancer. In humans, researchers reported a shrinking of the tumors, weight gain or weight stabilization, reduction or elimination of pain, and extended survival.***

## NUCLEIC ACIDS (2LC1 AND 2LCL1)

The use of homeopathically potentized nucleic acids is based on the collaborative work of Maurice Janaer, M.D., president of the Belgian Homeopathic Medicine Federation, and Bernard Marichal, M.D., honorary president of the Italian Medical Association for Immunotherapy and coauthor of *Theoretical and Practical Treatise on Immunotherapy at Infinitesimal Doses*. These physicians discovered novel homeopathic strategies for helping cancer patients.

Dr. Janaer has long asserted that toxicity was the main factor limiting the use of nucleic acids and various biological response modifiers (BRMs) in conventional treatment protocols. To prevent toxic side effects from pharmacologic doses, Dr. Janaer conceived of applying the homeopathic principles of dilution and energization (potency). In so doing, he was able to demonstrate their effectiveness in "re-balancing" the immune systems of large numbers of patients.[100] Drs. Janaer and Marichal diligently investigated the clinical usefulness of homeopathic doses of nucleic acids and BRMs. In terms of cancer therapy, Janaer and Marichal have observed consistently strong clinical benefits with the use of 2 homeopathic blends, called 2LC1 and 2LCL1.

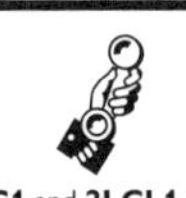

**2LC1** and **2LCL1** can be obtained from: Labo-Life Espana SA, Ctra Palma-Inca, Km 17.8, 07330 Consell (Majorca) Espana; tel: 34-71-14-20-17; fax: 34-71-14-20-69; or from Labo-Life, La Rambourgere Sainte-Marie, 79160 La Chapelle-Thireuil, France; tel: (011) 33 49 0422 12; fax: (011) 33 49 0422 13.

This innovative approach is based on synergistic interactions among 3 fundamental principles: (1) perilingual absorption, which helps bypass the disadvantages posed by the action of digestive juices and slow assimilation via the oral route; (2) infinitesimal dilutions, which bypass the toxic side effects associated with normal, pharmacologic doses; and (3) sequential treatment, which means spreading the administration of active agents over a certain period of time instead of prescribing the same substance or combination of substances each day. Using this approach, Dr. Marc Patte, director of medical communications for LaboLife in Spain, has documented numerous recoveries from a wide variety of advanced cancers, including metastatic liver cancer, breast cancer, leukemias, and others.[101]

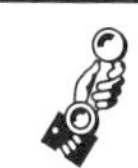

To obtain **714X** within Canada, a physician must request permission from the Emergency Drug Release Program (part of the Health Protection branch of the federal government) in Ottawa for authorization. To contact them: Emergency Drug Release Program, Bureau of Pharmaceutical Assessment, Holland Cross, Tower B, 1600 Scott Street, Ottawa, Ontario, Canada K18 1B8; tel: 613-941-2108; fax: 613-941-3194. To obtain 714X outside of Canada, contact: Cose, Inc., 5240 Mills Street, Rock Forest, Quebec, Canada J1N 3B6; tel: 819-564-7883; fax: 819-564-4668.

## 714X

This unique compound, discovered by French Canadian biologist Gaston Naessens, consists of nitrogen-rich camphor and organic salts. Dr. Naessens discovered that tumor cells produce a substance, cocancerogenic K factor (CKF), which paralyzes the immune system. 714X seems to neutralize CKF, thereby enabling the immune system to more readily identify and destroy cancer cells. In animal studies, 714X was effective against bone cancers (osteosarcomas) and breast cancer (mammary gland malignant tumors). In humans, researchers reported a shrinking of the tumors, weight gain or weight stabilization, reduction or elimination of pain, and extended survival.[102] Dr. Naessens has collected hundreds of human case histories in which 714X was effective against melanomas, carcinomas, lymphomas, osteosarcomas, and other types of cancer.[103]

For more about the clinical uses of **nucleic acids**, see Chapter 4: Etienne Callebout, p. 113.

For more about **Dr. Naessens**, see Chapter 27: Early Detection and Prevention of Cancer, pp. 727-731.

The usual treatment course involves 3 consecutive series of injections of 714X directly into the lymph nodes of the groin. The injections are given once daily for periods of 21 consecutive days, followed by a break of 2 days to allow the patient to rest while the natural defenses of the body are restored. People with advanced cases of cancer can receive more intense and prolonged therapy, since 714X has no harmful side effects, other than burning sensations at or around the site of injection. In general, patients undergoing the 714X treatment should not take vitamin E or vitamin B12 at the same time.

## SODIUM BUTYRATE

Butyrate is another term for butyric acid, an oily substance present in cow's butter; technically, it is a short-chain fatty acid produced by bacteria in the colon. Widely used as an artificial flavoring in liqueurs, syrups, and candies, sodium butyrate has also been investigated as a treatment for various forms of cancer, notably colon cancer.[104] The primary effects seem to include an ability to convert malignant cells to benign cells and to trigger cancer cell death. Since butyric acid degrades quickly, however, some researchers believe its usefulness is limited.[105]

Caution should be exercised since sodium butyrate actually seemed to promote the development of colon cancer in laboratory animals;[106] to counterbalance the effects, potassium, magnesium, or calcium supplements may be needed. The paradox of the use of this substance is that in other contexts, as an artificial flavoring, sodium butyrate is considered a potential carcinogen; yet here, in a different (therapeutically correct) context it demonstrates therapeutic merit.

## STAPHAGE LYSATE

This vaccine consists of remnants of a common bacterium called *Staphylococcus aureus* (as well as viruses which attack the bacterium) and appears to be useful as a general immune booster, a stimulator of macrophage production, and an inducer of interferon.[107] Robert E. Lincoln, M.D., of Medford, Massachusetts, first pioneered the use of staphage lysate in the 1940s and developed a large practice in which this substance had a prominent role, including as a cancer treatment. By 1952, the use of this substance had become so controversial and politicized—not, apparently, from any therapeutic shortcomings—that Dr. Lincoln was expelled from the Massachusetts Medical Society and staphage lysate was listed with the American Cancer Society (ACS) as an "unproven" method. In 1975, staphage lysate was quietly reinstated by ACS.

In 1987, Dr. Cecil E. Pitard of the University of Tennessee School of Medicine proposed making staphage lysate a standard adjunctive treatment for cancer.[108] The basic principle of its operation is that the immune system is "tricked" into producing cells that would target and eliminate not only these foreign substances found in the *Staphylococcus aureus*, but also any cancer cells in the system. Staphage lysate increases delayed cellular immunity and other immune functions that play a role in cancer resistance.[109,110] Staphage lysate is not currently available in the United States owing to FDA obstruction.

## TAGAMET® (CIMETIDINE)

This common prescription drug is best known for its ability to inhibit the formation of stomach acid, thereby aiding in the treatment of duodenal ulcers. Since the side effects are generally mild or quite rare (diarrhea, headaches, and occasional allergic reactions), Tagamet seems worthy of consideration. As early as 1978, scientists noted that tumor cell growth could be inhibited with Tagamet;[111] Tagamet seems to bolster the cancer-fighting activity of natural killer cells,[112] and increase the number of T helper lymphocytes as well as their ability to use zinc and magnesium.[113] At the same time, it helps reduce the activity of suppressor T cells (which suppress other immune functions).[114]

However, since Tagamet reduces gastric acid production, it likely impairs absorption of essential minerals and amino acids and, secondarily, impairs the formation of important hormones, enzymes, neurotransmitters, antibodies, cell membrane receptors, and structural proteins. It may also increase toxic undigested protein in the bowel and blood.

***Ukrain alters the oxygen consumption of cancer cells in an irreversible manner. Since the cancer cells stop "breathing" (called cell respiration) at this point, after 15 minutes of Ukrain treatment, they die.***

## UKRAIN

This substance is derived from a combination of a common plant called celandine (*Chelidonium majus*) and thiophosphoric acid (also called thiotepa, one of the original chemotherapeutic agents). The combination of the 2 appears to neutralize the toxic effect of the alkaloids contained in thiophosphoric acid; by this method, Ukrain has been rendered almost completely nontoxic such that Ukrain does not harm the body's healthy tissues and anticancer defenses but actually fortifies them.[115]

Clinical research has shown that Ukrain improves the overall condition and extends the survival of "terminal" cancer patients by giving their immune systems a boost and by blocking tumor growth.[116] In 2 studies of Ukrain treatment, significant clinical benefits (objective tumor regression) occurred for both lung cancer[117] and cervical cancer patients.[118] Ukrain helps

## Cancer Remissions with Ukrain

Scientists at the Ukrainian Anticancer Institute in Vienna, Austria, have carried out clinical studies of Ukrain over a 10-year period on 206 patients with cancers at various stages of development. Total remissions were achieved even in cases of advanced metastatic cancer; the best success rate with Ukrain (93%) was achieved with cancer patients starting treatment at the earliest stage of tumor development (no metastasis). For those starting therapy in stage II (minimal metastasis), the success rate was 72%, and for those in stage III (advanced, metastatic cancer), the success rate was 30%.[123]

fortify the immune system in people with a variety of cancers;[119] it consistently increases the number of T helper cells, which coordinate key immune-related activities. At the same time, Ukrain alters the oxygen consumption of cancer cells in an irreversible manner by increasing the oxygen (O2) consumption in both normal and malignant cells. In normal cells, the O2 consumption rate then stabilizes within 15 minutes; in cancer cells, however, O2 consumption drops down to zero.[120] Since the cancer cells stop "breathing" (called cell respiration) at this point, after 15 minutes of Ukrain treatment, they die.

Ukrain also inhibits the synthesis of genetic material and protein in cancer cells, but not in normal, healthy cells.[121] This may account for the findings supporting Ukrain's ability to completely inhibit growth in 57 of 60 human cell lines representing cancers of the lung, colon, kidney, ovary, breast, and brain, as well as melanoma and leukemia.[122] (These are the same 60 cancer cell types the NCI uses to screen effective cancer medications and determine research funding eligibility.) Only 2 leukemia cell lines and one brain cancer cell line were not inhibited by Ukrain. At high concentrations (100 mcg per ml), however, Ukrain causes "100% growth inhibition" in all 60 human cancer lines.

Finally, Ukrain possesses a strong attraction (cytotoxic selectivity) for cancer cells, and when exposed to ultraviolet light, it glows. For these reasons, it can be used to determine whether a suspicious growth is malignant.[124]

## UREA

One of the natural by-products of protein digestion (nitrogen) is urea, a natural diuretic (which means it induces urination) compound which also shows strong antioxidant activity. Approximately 1 ounce of urea is excreted daily in human urine. Urine-derived products have been used in cancer treatment since the 1940s, although they remain controversial.

When given orally, urea reaches high enough concentrations in the liver to inhibit cancer growth. Specifically, urea appears to work against solid tumors by destabilizing components called fibrin stroma; it also works against the formation of new blood vessels in tumors.

Observations made over an 11-year period by the physicians Evangelos Danopoulos, professor at the Medical School of Athens University and a member of the governing board of the Hellenic Anticancer Institute, and his daughter Iphigenia Danopoulos, both of Athens, Greece, indicate substantial clinical benefits from using urea to treat liver cancer.[125] Significant healing responses were reported in 15 of 22 patients diagnosed with cancer that had metastasized to the liver.[126] Since the liver is the only organ that shows high concentrations of urea after oral administration—the substance is rapidly excreted via the kidneys—this therapy may not be effective against cancers other than those of the liver.

***Significant healing responses were reported in 15 of 22 patients diagnosed with cancer that had metastasized to the liver. Since the liver is the only organ that shows high concentrations of urea after oral administration—the substance is rapidly excreted via the kidneys—this therapy may not be effective against cancers other than those of the liver.***

More specifically, in 1954, Dr. Danopoulos announced that urine had anticancer properties. He proposed that the active component was urea, a by-product of protein metabolism secreted by the liver and the main substance excreted in the urine. Dr. Danapoulos found that injections of a 50% urea solution directly into a mass of large, fast-growing tumors was effective, and that injections around the tumor site were even more effective.[127] The theory behind urea therapy is that it alters the chemical properties of the cellular surfaces around malignant tumor cells, and thereby disrupts the processes necessary for uncontrolled cellular growth.[128] Dr. Danapoulos also reported that when 46 patients with large cancers around the eye received urea injections and surgical removal of the tumors, this combination therapy was effective for 100% of these patients.[129]

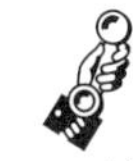

**Urea** is available in powder form (in a formula with creatine monohydrate) from: Innovative Therapeutics, 2020 Franklin Street, Carlyle, IL 62231; tel: 888-688-9922 or 618-594-7712; fax: 618-594-7711.

Dr. Danapoulos then found, in the 1970s, that oral administration of urea was effective against liver cancer. In a study of 18 patients who were given 2 to 2.5 g of urea orally 4-6 times per day, the patients survived an average of 26.5 months—5 times longer than expected. In a separate study, 11 patients with primary liver cancer and 17 with metastatic liver cancer were treated with 10 to 15 g of urea daily. Again, survival among this group was superb, averaging nearly 26 months.[130] Dr. Danopoulos stated that as urea goes directly to the liver when introduced into the human body, if the liver is more than 30% involved in the cancer, urea treatment will not work, but if liver involvement is less than this, it is likely to be effective.

Other cell culture studies on a line of human cancer cells have shown that urea has cell-killing effects (cytotoxicity).[131] According to a report from India, the use of urea injections directly into the tumor, along with localized application of urea ointment, produced a 75% reduction in inoperable cancer of the uterine cervix. About 60% of these patients responded favorably to the orally administered urea, only 25% percent showed little or no response, and patients with liver metastases experienced significant symptomatic relief.[132]

The findings of Vincent Speckhart, M.D. (see Chapter 20) indicate milder benefits, but suggest that urea may be well worth investigating as an adjunctive cancer treatment. "When I began using urea, the response rate was not as good as Danapoulos', but still impressive," says Dr. Speckhart. "The best response rate we have been able to get [with urea] is about 15%." Urea is best taken orally, he adds, because it reaches the liver directly from the intestines (via the portal vein), and in such high concentrations as to have a significant therapeutic effect. Delivered intravenously, urea becomes too diluted in the blood before it reaches the liver.

Dr. Speckhart once reported the results of urea treatment for a female patient diagnosed with breast cancer that had metastasized to the lung and liver. The patient had experienced a complete remission between May and October of 1993, using only urea therapy. "Once again, this report seemed to fall on deaf ears because urea was an orphan drug," Speckhart says. "There's no patent on it, so there's no money in it. And yet, urea had definite biological activity against a variety of tumors."

Chapter 31

# New Approaches to Immune Stimulation for Reversing Cancer

**The human immune system itself, naturally charged with the defense of the body against all foreign, harmful substances, may be enlisted as a therapeutic agent against cancer. Using the principle of vaccines but with nontoxic substances, innovative physicians can provoke stronger than usual immune responses which in turn can help reverse the cancer process.**

In any discussion of cancer, either its cause or reversal, the immune system must be regarded as a central factor. Immunotherapy—therapies specifically designed to support, enhance, or restore optimal immune function—can enable the body to effectively subdue and reverse the cancer without the adverse side effects associated with conventional therapies. In short, immunotherapy enlists the human immune system itself and its system of defenses as a potent anticancer agent.

### In This Chapter



A strong immune system can stop cancer in its tracks by identifying cancer cells and mounting an effective attack against tumors and small groups of renegade cells that have spread from the original or primary tumor. Natural killer cells, macrophages, and cancer cell-killing T cells are the main types of immune cells involved in the body's protection against cancer. Their anticancer effects are particularly strong in the early stages of disease. The body's lymphatic system, including thymus, spleen, and lymph nodes, is the primary route, along with arteries and veins, whereby these immune cells travel to and identify cancer cells for destruction and removal.

Surgery, radiation, and chemotherapy each strongly suppress and weaken the immune system, sometimes producing irreversible damage. Blood transfusions, which often accompany surgery, will markedly suppress the immune system for 1-2 months on average and may actually elevate the risk of contracting cancer later on. When the immune-suppressing effects of these toxic treatments are placed upon an immune system already weakened by chronic stress, pollution, faulty nutrition, and aging, it is easy to see why many cancer patients have a difficult time surviving orthodox cancer treatments. Author W. Lee Cowden, M.D., has found that taking 3-5 g of vitamin C orally or intravenously immediately after each unit of blood is transfused can lessen the negative effect of transfused (foreign) blood.

In conventional medicine, if immunotherapies are used, it is typically only after surgery, radiation, or chemotherapy, and little or no effort is made to reduce the toxic effects produced by these therapies. Administering these conventional treatments without detoxifying the body and protecting the immune system, is, we believe, a form of medical malpractice.

# Coley's Toxins

**In the 1920s, New York physician William B. Coley, M.D., found that certain infectious diseases—notably, from bacteria—might stimulate a therapeutic effect against malignancies when introduced into the body in the form of a sterilized vaccine. Dr. Coley found his "toxins" could give the body's anticancer defenses a nonspecific "kick" against the cancer cells by mobilizing their defenses against an easier opponent.**

The first major discovery related to immunotherapy was made toward the end of the 19th century by William B. Coley, M.D., who developed a sterile vaccine. Dr. Coley was a surgeon at Memorial Hospital in New York City (the predecessor of Memorial Sloan-Kettering, one of the leading conven-

A **vaccine** is a preparation containing a weakened (attenuated) or "killed" solution of a specific bacterium or germ believed to produce a disease. After it is injected into the body, the immune system wages a protective response, developing antibodies to the disease organism's foreign proteins. The theory is that the antibodies "remember" how to respond and neutralize the vaccine antigen in the future, thereby bestowing immunity to this illness. The word vaccine derives from *vacca*, which is Latin for "cow," because the first vaccination in 1796 was for cowpox.

tional cancer treatment centers in the U.S.) from 1892 to his death in 1936, and he refused to believe that cancer was incurable. At the time, surgical methods typically involved amputation of the body parts affected by the cancer; understandably, surgeons who had to perform such operations were more than willing to explore alternatives. Bear in mind that in 1900, radiation therapy and chemotherapy had not yet been conceived.

Observing that erysipelas, a dangerous skin infection caused by the bacteria *Streptococcus pyogenes*, was followed by a dramatic tumor regression in a cancer patient with advanced sarcoma, Dr. Coley reasoned that certain infectious diseases might stimulate a therapeutic effect on malignancies. Dr. Coley developed a mixture of sterile bacteria, which became known as "mixed bacterial vaccine," or "Coley's Toxins." Specifically, Dr. Coley used *Streptococcus* pyogenes (the causative agent for erysipelas) and the bacterium *Serratia marcescens*, which he cultured in beef broth; the product contained the toxins produced by these 2 heat-killed bacteria and the dead bacteria themselves.

His idea was that the bacteria would give the body's anticancer defenses a nonspecific "kick" in the right direction—that is, against the cancer cells—by mobilizing their defenses against an easier opponent, namely, the bacteria. Technically, some work on this approach and the development of a sterile vaccine based on these components had been completed as early as 1884 by other researchers.

## Coley's Toxins: Immune Vaccine Predating Chemotherapy

Dr. Coley injected his patients with the bacterial mixture (usually at the site of the tumor or nearby) and claimed success with both partial and complete tumor regression for a number of different types of cancer. If the injection was given in the morning, the patient would typically experience a chill followed by a fever, but would feel normal again by the afternoon. For patients receiving the vaccine for sarcoma (cancer of connective tissue and bone), Dr. Coley reported 41% complete cures. He generally recommended a minimum of 5 months treatment for effective results; treatments lasting only 4-6 weeks often failed.

At the time, Dr. Coley was regarded as a dedicated and respected physician. Dr. Coley's death in 1936 coincided with the explosive growth of chemotherapy; as a consequence, his research was buried in the decade that followed. However, during his lifetime, about 50 physicians in the U.S., including one at the Mayo Clinic, as well as Europe, treated cancer patients with Coley's Toxins, as prepared by Parke Davis and Company, a major pharmaceutical firm.

His work would have remained permanently obscure had it not been for the diligent efforts of his younger daughter, Helen Coley Nauts. Although Nauts had no scientific background, she was encouraged by Kanematsu Sugiura, Ph.D., a long-time friend of her father and an eminent chemist at Memorial Sloan-Kettering. In 1953, after collecting nearly 1,000 case reports, Nauts founded the New York-based Cancer Research Institute; later, with the help of physicians and researchers, she wrote and published 18 monographs and several peer-reviewed articles on the treatment of malignant tumors with Coley's vaccine.[1]

Unfortunately, regulatory changes in 1962 (the passage of the Kefauver-Harris Amendment to the Pure Food and Drug Act) made it impossible to use the product in the U.S. The American Cancer Society lobbied to prevent Coley's Toxins from being exempted from these regulations by way of a "grandfather" clause which would have permitted its use based on prior proof of efficacy. As a result, the FDA declared the vaccine a "New Drug" making it subject to the usual hyper-expensive testing associated with new drugs.

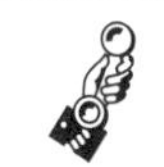

For more information about **Coley's Toxins**, contact: Innovative Therapeutics, 2020 Franklin Street, P.O. Box 512, Carlyle, IL 62231: tel: 618-594-8244 or 888-688-9922; fax: 618-594-7712. Also contact: People Against Cancer, 604 East Street, P.O. Box 10, Otho, IA 50569; tel: 515-972-4444; fax: 515-972-4415. For a clinic using Coley's vaccines, contact: GenesisWest Research Institute for Biological Medicine, Del Agua #256 Secc. Jardines, Fracc., Playas de Tijuana, Baja California, Mexico 22700; U.S. address: P.O. Box 3460, Chula Vista, CA 91909; tel: 619-424-9552; fax: 619-424-7593.

Five-year survival rates after treatment with Coley's vaccine based on data collected by Nauts in the 1970s showed the following: 65% for patients with inoperable breast cancer; 69% for patients with inoperable ovarian cancer; and 90% for those with bone cancer.[2] Research conducted at Memorial Sloan-Kettering Cancer Center in New York City in 1976 showed that patients with advanced non-Hodgkin's lymphoma experienced a 93% remission rate using Coley's Toxins, versus 29% for those in the control group who had only chemotherapy.[3] In 1990, Nauts and her colleagues reported that this approach significantly improved the outcome of a great number of advanced-cancer patients.[4]

After reviewing the mixed bacterial vaccine for 9 months,

***In general, Coley's Toxins are not used in conventional cancer treatment, not because they are judged ineffective or experimental, but mostly because they are inexpensive and unpatentable.***

Charles Starnes, Ph.D., an immunologist at Amgen, Inc., in Thousand Oaks, California, declared that it is among the most promising cancer treatments in existence. According to Dr. Starnes' review, Dr. Coley accomplished an impressive cure rate using his bacterial vaccine to treat primarily inoperable sarcoma. For soft tissue sarcomas, 40 out of 84 patients (48%) were free of disease after at least 5 years; 17 of these survived for up to 20 years. In another group, 19 out of 33 cases (58%) of lymphoma were cancer free after 5 years; 8 of these patients survived for up to 20 years.[5]

According to Dr. Starnes, "It just could be that the results achieved by Coley are the best results we will ever achieve in the treatment of cancer."[6] After Dr. Coley's death, the original mixture was diluted by Parke Davis and Company in order to minimize the chance of a lethal reaction and thus reduce the physician's liability; *S. pyogenes*, after all, are powerful bacteria, capable of causing serious illness when administered full strength. This diluted version, however, proved to be too weak. Innovative Therapeutics, Inc., of Carlyle, Illinois, introduced a more accurate representation of Coley's original vaccine.[7]

Coley's mixed bacterial vaccine can cause some disconcerting side effects, beginning with a shaking chill that lasts 10 to 15 minutes and typi-

## 5-Year Survival Rates of Advanced Cancer Patients Receiving Coley's Mixed Bacterial Vaccine

| TYPE OF CANCER | PERCENT SURVIVING 5 YRS. AFTER TREATMENT |
|---|---|
| Inoperable breast cancer | 65% |
| Inoperable ovarian cancer | 69% |
| Osteosarcoma | 90% |
| Soft tissue sarcomas | 48% |
| Lymphomas | 58% |

cally followed by the development of a fever in the range of 102°F to 105°F. The transient fever is simply the body reacting to the bacterial toxins in the vaccine and the fever's heat has therapeutic benefit to the body. This means the temporarily elevated temperature may be considered a positive sign that the vaccine is working. Unfortunately, most conventional doctors mistakenly insist that any fever reaction should be suppressed rather than carefully monitored and supported. In general, Coley's Toxins are not used in conventional cancer treatment, not because they are judged ineffective or experimental, but mostly because they are inexpensive and unpatentable.

# Immuno-Augmentative Therapy

**Lawrence Burton, Ph.D., a biologist and cancer researcher at the California Institute of Technology, isolated blood protein components in mice capable of crossing the species barrier and producing cancer remissions in humans. When 4 key blood protein components are balanced, the body should be able to subdue cancer cells as part of its normal activity.**

Immuno-Augmentative Therapy (IAT) is the alternative cancer therapy that has received the greatest amount of attention from the U.S. Congress. According to cancer historian Ralph Moss, Ph.D., it was the controversy surrounding IAT that triggered the Office of Technology Assessment's landmark 1990 report on unconventional cancer therapies. In the 1980s, cancer patients who had benefited from IAT pressured Congress to investigate the closing of an IAT clinic in the Bahamas.

IAT was developed during the 1960s by Lawrence Burton, Ph.D., a biologist and cancer researcher at the California Institute of Technology and St. Vincent's Hospital in New York City. Working first with fruit flies then mice, Dr. Burton identified and isolated a tumor-inhibiting factor capable of crossing the species barrier and producing cancer remissions in humans. In fact, so fast were the experimental cancer remissions that a Los

SUCCESS STORY

## Reversing Uterine Cancer

Roberta, aged 78, credits her long-term survival to Dr. Lawrence Burton's IAT. In 1968, Roberta was diagnosed with uterine cancer. Her physician recommended a hysterectomy (removal of the uterus) which she underwent; she also received radiation therapy. However, 11 years later, however, Roberta was diagnosed with infiltrating ductile carcinoma of the breast, which had spread to her lymph nodes. Although the breast tumor was very large, she refused to undergo a mastectomy; she received further radiation therapy, with minimal results. Two years later, she began IAT treatments with Dr. Burton and achieved complete remission of her condition; 12 years later, she was still cancer free.

Angeles newspaper reportedly trumpeted the results in this headline: "15-Minute Cancer Cure for Mice: Humans Next?"[8]

More specifically, Dr. Burton identified and isolated blood protein components that he suspected were associated with the development of cancer. These consisted of tumor complement, a substance derived from the blood clots of patients with many types of cancer. This factor, also described by immunologists as the C3 complement, activates 2 tumor antibodies, TA1 and TA2.[9] A fourth protein, called the deblocking protein factor (DPF), is derived from the blood serum of healthy donors. A fifth protein, called blocking protein factor (BPF), is not given as part of the IAT regimen since, according to Dr. Burton, it blocks the antitumor effects of TA1 and TA2. The DPF is said to interfere with this blocking mechanism.

According to Dr. Burton's theory, when the 4 blood protein components are balanced, the body should be able to subdue cancer cells as part of its normal activity; but if any of the components are out of balance, the body cannot adequately defend itself. For example, if there is too much of the blocking protein, the tumor antibody will be inhibited and unable to neutralize cancer cells. "All cells, when they die, release a blocking protein," Dr. Burton explained. "This prevents further activation of the [tumor] antibody."

Dr. Burton discovered that by injecting certain amounts of these components into his patients, he could bring about remissions in many forms of cancer, including those that supposedly were terminal. He was quick to point out that his treatment was not a cure for cancer: "It is like using insulin for diabetes. It controls the cancer and the patient can live a normal life span." Dr. Burton claimed that IAT achieved tumor reduction and even complete remission in 40 to 60% of patients who received it. Particularly impressive were the recoveries of patients with advanced colon cancer and cancer of the abdomen; according to standard statistics, the 5-year survival rate with conventional therapies for both of these diseases is zero.

"We are the court of last resort," Dr. Burton once joked, noting that the patients who came to him had tried everything else first, with their conditions only becoming worse. "Yet, on an overall basis, we are still sending 4-6 out of every 10 people home improved." One of his patients who suffered from abdominal cancer, for example, received IAT treatments for 4 years; 3 years after he had finished his treatments, his cancer remained in complete remission.

According to Dr. Burton's records, IAT has shown good results as a treatment for cancers of the bladder, prostate, pancreas, and lymphomas; since IAT builds on the body's anticancer immune function, it is virtually nontoxic. Dr. Burton reported on the favorable results of treating 11 patients with abdominal cancer (mesothelioma),[10] but since this asbestos-related cancer is said to be incurable and deadly, Dr. Burton's claims were considered outrageous and he was promptly dismissed as a "quack" by the American Medical Association.

Although the Office of Technology report on *Unconventional Cancer Treatments* stated that Dr. Burton's IAT method had not definitively been shown to shrink human tumors, it acknowledged the results of another important study. Here, of 79 advanced cancer patients receiving IAT, 50 patients (63%) were alive an average of 65 months (longer than 5 years) after diagnosis. The 29 deceased patients survived an average of 59 months, or nearly 5 years.[11] These findings are remarkable, given that the expected survival for the majority of these patients was 36 months or less.

***Dr. Burton claimed that IAT achieved tumor reduction and even complete remission in 40 to 60% of patients who received it.***

Thus, the survival rate of Dr. Burton's patients approximately doubled the maximum survival rate of conventionally treated patients. As all patients had metastatic cancers, these IAT-induced survival results were particularly impressive. Furthermore, the findings are all the more noteworthy given that the study's coordinator, Dr. Barrie Cassileth (now based at the University of North Carolina School of Medicine), is a long-time critic of alternative cancer therapies and an ardent spokesperson for the American Cancer Society (ACS).

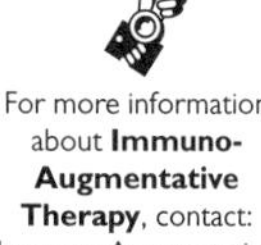

For more information about **Immuno-Augmentative Therapy**, contact: Immuno-Augmentative Therapy Center, P.O. Box F-42689, Freeport, Grand Bahama, tel: 242 352-4755.

*The survival rate of Dr. Burton's patients approximately doubled the maximum survival rate of conventionally treated patients. Had these findings pertained to a chemotherapy drug instead of IAT, massive amounts of funding would have been allocated to investigate the drug. Once again, the politics of cancer barred a potentially valuable treatment from reaching the public.*

It is significant that the National Cancer Institute, for which ACS serves as the public relations arm, has repeatedly declined to conduct a study of IAT, despite the obviously compelling nature of Dr. Cassileth's report. Had these findings pertained to a chemotherapy drug instead of IAT, massive amounts of funding would have been allocated to investigate the drug. Once again, the politics of cancer barred a potentially valuable treatment from reaching the public. Although Dr. Burton died in 1993, IAT is still offered today at the clinic he founded in Freeport on Grand Bahama Island.

# TVZ-7 Lymphocyte Treatment

**In this new therapy, particular components of the immune system called lymphocytes are targeted and activated for a more precise response to cancer. The solution is usually administered intravenously in the course of 44-50 treatments over a 14-day period.**

While Coley's Toxins and Burton's Immuno-Augmentative Therapy are examples of nonspecific immunotherapy, TVZ-7 is an example of a specific immunotherapy. While the concept of using cell cultures for immunological enhancement had been in circulation for some years, it was only in the late 1980s that a Canadian physician developed a manufacturing process capable of producing a uniformly effective TVZ-7. In TVZ-7, particular components of the immune system are targeted and activated for a more precise response.

The central component of this anticancer strategy relies on B Lymphoid

Supernatant Technology (BLST), a technique of culturing and harvesting B lymphocytes. The process involves extracting a mixture of cytokines and other immune-activating chemicals from the lymphocytes. As mentioned previously, cytokines are specific immune molecules (proteins) involved in the body's defense processes, and they include interferons, interleukins, and tumor necrosis factor.

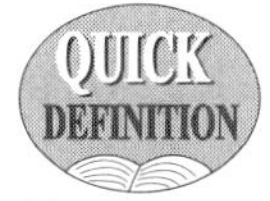


A **lymphocyte** is a form of white blood cell, representing 25% of the total count, whose numbers increase during infection. Lymphocytes, produced in the bone marrow, come in two forms: B cells, which produce antibodies to neutralize foreign and potentially dangerous matter in the blood; and T cells, matured in the thymus gland (behind the breastbone) and having many functions in the body's immune response.

The extracted material, or supernatant mixture, is called TVZ-7, and is presently classified as a biological response modifier (BRM).[12] TVZ-7 is usually administered intravenously in 44-50 treatments over a 14-day period. A limited number of Canadian physicians are legally allowed to use TVZ-7. Doctors in Mexico, Holland, Belgium, Korea, and China, however, enjoy a wider scope of application.

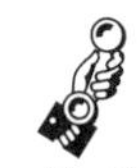

**Roscoe Van Zandt, M.D.**, can be contacted at: 801 Road to 6 Flags, Suite 101, Arlington, TX 76012; tel: 817-265-6221; fax: 817-460-4250. **Ravi Devgan, M.D.**, 42 Redpath Avenue, Toronto, Ontario, Canada M4S 2J6; tel: 416-487-0882; fax: 416-487-9164.

One of the prominent practitioners of TVZ-7 therapy is Roscoe Van Zandt, M.D., a board-certified gynecologist who practices in Arlington, Texas, and in various cancer clinics in Mexico. Dr. Van Zandt regards nutrition, botanicals, and energy medicine as essential to the treatment program of any chronic disease, including cancer. "We have yet to see a hormonally responsive tumor—including tumors of the prostate, breast, uterus, ovary, and melanoma—which has not responded well to this therapy. We don't know whether the B lymphocytes are producing something with direct antitumor activity, or whether these substances, the cytokines, are a switch which gets the immune system to function more optimally."

In 1996, the FDA granted TVZ-7 IND (Investigational New Drug) status, permitting its limited use for relieving pain from bone cancer.

Dr. Van Zandt treated a man with advanced prostate cancer that had metastasized to the bone. Under Dr. Van Zandt's supervision, the TVZ-7 treatment enabled the man to wean himself from a large dose of morphine (400 mg daily) within 5 weeks. Another patient with advanced pancreatic cancer was on 200 mg of morphine but was off it in 17 days after starting TVZ-7. "That man is now walking 10 miles a day without pain," says Dr. Van Zandt. A third case involved a woman with breast cancer that had metastasized to both hips; after 10 weeks on TVZ-7, bone scans showed no trace of cancer.

The encouraging clinical experiences reported by Dr. Van Zandt in-

***Dr. Devgan has seen positive results with TVZ-7 as a cancer treatment. "It's among the most potent immune modulators I know of. In addition, TVZ-7 has shown great promise in alleviating pain in cancer patients, reducing the side effects of chemotherapy and radiation treatments, and halting the growth of tumors."***

dicate that many types of cancer can be effectively reversed with this experimental treatment. "We've seen all kinds of cancer respond, including primary liver cancer, colon cancer, brain tumors, and cancers of the gallbladder and bile ducts. In every case, the patient came in with an advanced-stage cancer, and in most cases extensive metastases were involved."

Another physician using TVZ-7 is Ravi Devgan, M.D., of Toronto, Canada, who remarks: "So far, TVZ-7 has been used alone and in combination with chemotherapy and radiation. Although more research is needed, we have seen definite evidence that it can be used alone with considerable success for a variety of cancers." Drs. Van Zandt and Devgan both agree that TVZ-7 can work well on its own, but that it seems to be most effective when combined with intensive detoxification as well as nutritional and botanical support, as described elsewhere in this book.

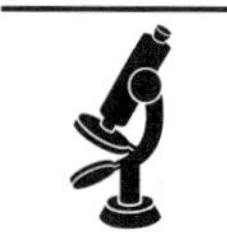

The therapeutic use of TVZ-7 represents a promising area of research. A multicenter clinical trial is presently being developed in the U.S, which will form the basis for an FDA Investigational New Drug application. The National Academy of Science in China has assigned 10 research teams to investigate IB-700. Several biomedical centers are using it in Mexico, Costa Rica, Holland, and Switzerland. In Canada, trials are expected to begin in 1997 under the auspices of the government-run Cancer Research and Treatment Foundation.

The product is a kind of "cytokine soup," says Dr. Devgan. In addition, TVZ-7 has shown great promise in alleviating pain in cancer patients, reducing the side effects of chemotherapy and radiation treatments, and halting the growth of tumors.

Dr. Devgan has seen impressive results with TVZ-7 as a cancer treatment. "It's among the most potent immune modulators I know of. It seems to work through the cytokines, which are the crux of the immune system. Based on records obtained from Mexican cancer clinics, all the hormone-sensitive cancers have been highly responsive to TVZ-7." The formula is also reportedly effective against malignant melanoma, primary liver cancer, glioblastomas and astrocytomas, stomach and esophageal cancers, and colon cancer with metastases to the liver.

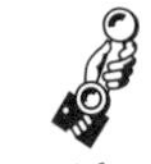

For more information about **TVZ-7**, contact: Integrated Biologics, Ltd., Biotechnology Research & Development, 130 Commerce Way, Woburn, MA 01801; tel: 617-938-9088, ext. 114; fax: 617-933-2731.

# T/Tn Antigen Breast Cancer Vaccine

**Georg Springer, M.D., showed that 2 antigens, called T and Tn, play a vital role in the immune system's ability to respond to cancer and are present in 90% of all cancers. Through the use of a specially developed vaccine, Dr. Springer demonstrated that the immune system's reaction to T and Tn antigens results in strong cancer cell-killing activity .**

Cancer cells have proteins, or antigens, on their surfaces that can be recognized by the immune system. The identification of certain cancer-related antigens forms the basis for the exciting approach embraced by Georg Springer, M.D. Dr. Springer is an immunologist who founded the Heather Bligh Cancer Research Laboratories at the Chicago Medical School. This pioneering German scientist-physician has shown that 2 antigens, called T and Tn, play a vital role in the immune system's ability to respond to cancer. Since the early 1980s, Dr. Springer has repeatedly shown that the immune system's reaction to T and Tn antigens results in strong cancer cell-killing activity in both animal and human studies.[13]

Using various biochemical tests, Dr. Springer has detected the T and Tn antigens in over 90% of all cancers. The less aggressive cancers (meaning they are well differentiated) produce a higher proportion of the T antigen, while the Tn antigen predominates in the more aggressive cancers (meaning they are poorly differentiated).[14] The overall concentrations of the T and Tn antigens correlate specifically with the aggressiveness of breast cancer.[15]

In 1974, Dr. Springer had his first opportunity to test his experimental vaccine when his wife, Heather Bligh, developed breast cancer and was told she had only a year to live. After receiving the T/Tn vaccine, however, she lived a full 6 years. Encouraged, Dr. Springer began a pilot study with 19 breast cancer patients, all of whom went on to survive at least 5 years on the T/Tn vaccine; 16 of these women (84%) are still alive, 11 of them af-

***"A great number of our patients have had no recurrence of breast cancer for 10 years and some have been out over 18 years," says Dr. Springer. These results should have prompted the National Cancer Institute to conduct large-scale clinical trials, but no such efforts have been made, despite the fact that his findings have been well-publicized.***

ter a decade or more of their supposedly terminal diagnosis.

In another study, 26 women with advanced breast cancer (10 with Stage IV, 6 Stage III, 10 Stage II cancers) were given the T/Tn vaccine after undergoing an operation for their primary cancer or after the first recurrence. All survived over 5 years, and only 5 out of the 26 patients died within 5-10 years from the time of vaccination; 14 of 18 patients (78%) who were vaccinated over 10 years ago are still alive, and half of these long-term survivors have lived longer than 18 years since their operation.[16] An additional 49 breast cancer patients have been vaccinated since 1994 and are being closely monitored by Dr. Springer and his colleagues.

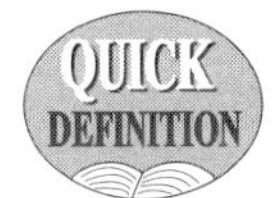


**Staging** in cancer terminology is a relative index of how much cancer exists in the body, its size, location, and containment or metastasis. *Stage I*, the earliest, most curable stage, shows local tumor involvement. *Stage II* indicates some spreading of cancer to the surrounding tissues and perhaps to nearby lymph nodes; *Stage III* involves metastasis to distant lymph nodes; *Stage IV*, the most advanced and least easily cured, means the cancer has spread to distant organs.

Once breast cancer has spread to the bone or to a distant organ (Stage III or Stage IV cancer), only 10% of cancer patients on conventional treatment survive 5 years. In contrast, breast cancer patients who receive Dr. Springer's T/Tn vaccine have shown a clearly superior survival advantage. "A great number of our patients have had no recurrence of cancer for 10 years and some have been out over 18 years, but we cannot say that they are 'cancer free,'" says Dr. Springer. These results should have prompted the National Cancer Institute to conduct large-scale clinical trials, but no such efforts have been made, despite the fact that his findings have been well-publicized.[17]

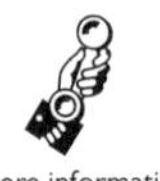

For more information about the **T/Tn vaccine**, contact: The Heather Bligh Clinic, Georg Springer, M.D., 3333 Green Bay Road, North Chicago, IL 60064; tel: 847-578-3435; fax: 847-578-3432.

Dr. Springer emphasizes that nutritional support is also important. He advises his patients to take, once daily, a multivitamin, vitamin C (3-4 g), beta carotene (20,000 IU) and vitamin E (1600 IU). Maurice Black at New York Medical College's Institute of Breast Diseases found that Stage II patients with compromised immune systems cut their five-year risk of a recurrence from 38% to 6% by taking vitamin E.[18] "The nutritional component is extremely important because nutrients have been shown to influence both cell-mediated and antibody facets of the immune response," says Dr. Springer. "I recommend that my patients consume a wholesome, high-fiber diet that includes fish and liver to obtain the beneficial nutrients from these foods."

In theory, says Dr. Springer, his immune-stimulating vaccine could be used for the treatment of all cancers. "Breast cancer serves as our model for treating all carcinomas, which make up about 85% of all lethal cancers. Most importantly, we may be able to prevent all these cancers using the vaccine." However, since the T antigen has not been found in brain tumors or in sarcomas (bone and muscle), the vaccine is unlikely to have any therapeutic impact on these cancers.

# Bacillus Calmette-Guérin (BCG) Vaccine

**This vaccine uses highly weakened tuberculosis microbes to evoke a strong immune response against cancer and gets results often superior to chemotherapy when used against certain types of cancer.**

A good example of immunotherapy as applied to cancer treatment is the vaccine called Bacillus Calmette-Guérin (BCG) commonly used against tuberculosis since its introduction in 1921. When used against a highly aggressive form of bladder cancer called transitional-cell carcinoma in situ, the BCG vaccine evokes a strong immune response to the presence of the highly weakened tuberculosis microbes in the vaccine. Introduced into the bladder by way of a catheter, BCG produces an inflammatory response—in effect, a curative fever. The immune cells, thereby activated, destroy all preexisting cancer cells in the bladder, thus lowering the recurrence of bladder cancer.[19]

## Using a Tuberculosis Vaccine to Boost the Immune System

The BCG vaccine was found to be considerably superior to chemotherapy in dealing with this cancer. Whereas chemotherapy resulted in complete reversal of the disease in 50% of patients, with fewer than 20% still disease free after five years, BCG had a response rate of 87%, with more than 80% of patients still disease free after 5 years.[20] In other words, this immunotherapy approach led to a 4-fold improvement in 5-year survival. BCG's effectiveness is even better when used with specific interferons[21] and biological response modifiers.[22]

The main advantage of BCG and other immunotherapies may be the ability to prevent recurrences or secondary cancers. Burton A. Waisbren, Sr., M.D., a cancer vaccine researcher and head of the Waisbren Clinic in Milwaukee, Wisconsin, has treated cancer patients with the combination of BCG and other vaccines and other immune-modulating substances such as Mixed Bacterial Vaccine (formerly called Coley's Toxins), Lymphoblastoid Lymphocytes, and Transfer Factor (TF). TF, derived from the immune system of healthy donors, has been shown to improve the clinical response of breast cancer patients,[23] possibly by enabling the cancer patient's body to recognize and target cancer cells.

One of Dr. Waisbren's studies found that combinations of these vaccines could help postpone recurrences of lung cancer. This study compared 22 lung cancer patients receiving vaccines to a control group receiving only conventional treatment and no vaccine. Cancer patients in the vaccine group lived, on average, 9 months longer than those in the control group.[24] Other vaccine treatments have shown some effectiveness against colon cancer, breast cancer, lymphoma, leukemia, and melanoma.[25]

Although surgery can halt about 90% of new skin cancers (melanomas), when the cancer reoccurs or spreads to a new site, surgery is ineffectual and death generally follows within a year. Researchers found that they could use monoclonal antibodies—molecules engineered to bind only to certain cancer cells—to attack tumors directly or to carry toxins se-

An **antigen** is any biological substance (a toxin, virus, fungus, bacterium, amoeba, or other protein) that the body comes to regard as foreign and dangerous to itself. As such, an antigen induces a state of cellular sensitivity or immune reaction that seeks to neutralize, remove, or destroy the antigen by dispatching antibodies against it. An antibody is a protein molecule containing about 20,000 atoms, made from amino acids by B lymphocyte cells in the lymph tissue and set in motion by the immune system against a specific foreign protein, or antigen. An **antibody** is also referred to as an immunoglobulin and may be found in the blood, lymph, colostrum, saliva, and the gastrointestinal and urinary tracts, usually within 3 days after the first encounter with an antigen. The antibody binds tightly with the antigen as a preliminary for removing it from the system or destroying it. An **immunoglobulin** is one of a class of specially designed antibody proteins produced in lymph tissue and involved in the immune system's defense response to foreign substances. There are 5 main types of immunoglobulins, grouped according to their concentration in the blood: IgG, IgA, IgM, IgD, IgE.

**CAUTION**

When used for bladder cancer, BCG tends to produce side effects in 50% of cases, along with a burning sensation and increased urgency and frequency of urination; and occasional blood upon urination; fever and fatigue have also been reported.

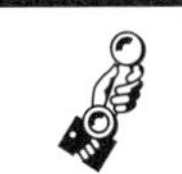

For more information about **BCG**, contact: Burton A. Waisbren, Sr., M.D., 2315 North Lake Drive, Suite 815, Milwaukee, WI 53211; tel: 414-272-1929. BCG is approved by the FDA for use in the treatment of carcinoma in situ of the bladder, but it is not advised for patients with immune deficiencies. BCG is available as TICE® from Organon, Inc., 375 Mt. Pleasant Ave., West Orange, NJ 07052; tel: 201-325-4500; fax: 201-325-4576.

lectively to the cancer cells. Twenty-five patients with recurrent melanoma were injected directly with monoclonal antibodies that were designed to respond to certain *features* of cancer cells. The researchers examined the tumor to determine which marker the cancer cells bore; after then injecting the appropriate antibody to match the cancer cells, all the tumors disappeared.[26]

# Autogenous Bacterial Vaccine

**Research by Virginia C. Livingston, M.D., indicated that a form-changing microbe called *P. cryptocides* exists in very high concentrations in cancer patients, which is why she labeled it "the ancestral hidden killer" and "a silent but lethal bloodstream infection." Dr. Livingston then administered a vaccine made from the patient's own bacteria to fight the cancer microbe.**

Virginia C. Livingston, M.D., who was in her 80s when she died in 1990, was one of the few women physicians of her time. Graduating from New York University in 1936, she became the first woman resident at a New York hospital and went on to develop a germ theory of cancer and vaccines which she successfully used on patients to eliminate cancer. In addition, she was an associate professor of biological sciences at Rutgers University, director of the Laboratory of Proliferative Diseases at Newark Presbyterian Hospital, research associate at the San Diego Biomedical Institution, and with her husband, Afton Munk Livingston, M.D., founder of the Livingston Medical Clinic of San Diego in 1971, which specializes in the outpatient treatment of immunodeficiency diseases.

Dr. Livingston's theory arose out of her experience with tuberculosis, leprosy, and scleroderma (a skin disease) among her patients. She began to see them as related to each other and to cancer as well. Already a researcher, she discovered certain organisms in scleroderma which were similar to those in tuberculosis and leprosy and set out to discover if they were also found in cancer. She writes, "I reasoned that perhaps scleroderma was a kind of slow cancer. I decided to begin examining cancer tissues with the same method.... Upon examining all kinds of cancerous tissues ... I found that a similar microorganism was present in all of them."[27]

In further research as part of a team Dr. Livingston herself brought together, she proved through recognized scientific principles that a bacterium called *Progenitor cryptocides* fuels the development of cancer. According to Dr. Livingston, *P. cryptocides* is present in everyone (and animals) from birth, but is held in check by the immune system. When immunity becomes suppressed by poor diet, chemical toxins, emotional distress, and other factors, the dormant microbe can multiply and promote the growth of tumors.[28] Dr. Livingston's research indicated that *P. cryptocides* exists in very high concentrations in cancer patients. In fact, Dr. Livingston labeled *P. cryptocides* "the ancestral hidden killer" and "a silent but lethal bloodstream infection."

Even more intriguing, Dr. Livingston discovered that *P. cryptocides* is actually a pleomorphic organism, capable of changing its shape and evolving through a series of forms, from simple to complex, from latent to active, depending on the health of the individual, or "host." For example, Dr. Livingston reported that *P. cryptocides* can exist as virus-sized bodies, as larger elementary bodies, as still larger coccoidal forms, but it may also appear less distinctly shaped, as rods or filaments of different lengths without cell walls called mycoplasma.

For more information about **pleomorphic theory**, see Chapter 25: What Causes Cancer?, pp. 633-637; and this chapter, pp. 905-909.

Of these varying forms, Dr. Livingston identified the virus stage as the "causative agent in human and animal cancers ... When our immune systems are weakened, either by poor diet, infected foods, or old age, this microbe gains a foothold and starts cancer cells growing into tumors." In effect, Dr. Livingston suggests that *P. cryptocides* acts similarly to an oncogene, a term oncologists use to denote a gene believed to start the cancer process. It is normally dormant within the cells, but when the immune system becomes unable to control it (a condition generated, in part, by nutritional deficiencies), then it starts producing neoplastic, or cancerous, cells.

With a microorganism identified as the source of cancer, a vaccine was the likely solution to treatment because, as she explained, "autogenous vaccines are prepared and used all over the world in the treatment of chronic, ongoing infections in the sick." Her theories and clinical results were met with opposition in the conventional medical community. According to Dr. Livingston, pressure exerted by researchers at Memorial Sloan-Kettering Cancer Center in New York forced her to close her laboratory.[29] She continued her research in San Diego, California, and developed vaccines for treatment of cancer after successfully treating a man with malignant lymphoma of the thymus gland with an autogenous vaccine (a vaccine cultured from his own blood or urine).

The concept was to use the bacteria in a person's body to fight that same bacteria; in this way, the vaccine was tailored precisely to match each individual. The vaccines Dr. Livingston developed also included vitamins and minerals to strengthen the immune system.[30] Doses are typically given every 3-5 days, depending on a patient's reaction, which may include soreness or redness at the site of injection, hypersensitivity, mild fever, and muscle or joint pains.

## Success Rate Is High with Livingston Vaccine

According to the Livingston Foundation, for people whose tumors are localized, such as in the prostate or the breast, the remission rate ranges from 70% to 95%. If the cancers have moved into the bone, local lymph nodes or other areas considered signs of metastasis, the remission rate drops down to 40% to 50%. In cases considered terminal, the patient may have 3 months to live according to conventional standards, but remission rates of 20% are reported with the Livingston approach.[31]

Dr. Livingston designed a complete treatment protocol which, in addition to a number of vaccines, included a largely vegetarian raw foods diet, gamma globulin, vitamin and mineral supplements, attention to dental problems, heat therapy, and detoxification. More specifically, the Livingston therapy calls for eliminating  from the diet all poultry and egg products, sugars, white flours, and processed foods. Tobacco, and alcohol are also to be avoided. Spleen glandular extracts, the BCG vaccine (to stimulate the patient's immune system), and sometimes hydrochloric acid (to acidify the patient's blood and urine) are administered. However, in her view, the protocol is aimed less at cancer than at reversing a state of immunological dysfunction. Dr. Livingston once had to justify her approach to an FDA official. "I assured him that I was not treating *cancer* with vaccines, but that I am using autogenous vaccines obtained from the patient's own tissues and body fluids to treat an underlying chronic infection."

The cancer treatment center, the Livingston-Wheeler Medical Clinic in San Diego, which she founded in 1968, "became one of the landmark

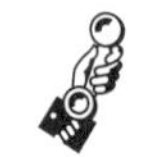

For more information about **Livingston therapy** and to order her books *The Conquest of Cancer: Vaccines and Diet* (1984), *The Microbiology of Cancer Compendium* (1977), and *Cancer: A New Breakthrough* (1972), contact: The Livingston Foundation Medical Center, 3232 Duke Street, San Diego, CA 92110; tel: 619-224-3515; fax: 619-224-6253.

For more information about **Dr. Speckhart** and his cancer protocols, see Chapter 20: Vincent Speckhart, M.D.

alternative therapy clinics in the United States."[32] The clinic still operates today. Dr. Livingston reported success in treating individuals with many forms of advanced cancer, and presented numerous case histories involving remission of metastatic disease, but she never conducted controlled studies or statistically valid research on humans.

Other researchers have reported positive results with the Livingston vaccines. One of the doctors in this book, Vincent Speckhart, M.D., (see Chapter 19), along with Alva Johnson, Ph.D., a microbiologist at the East Virginia School of Medicine, conducted a study of Dr. Livingston's therapy. They found the vaccine useful in reversing the immune-suppressed condition of cancer patients. In a study of 40 patients, Dr. Speckhart observed several cases of tumor regression, ranging from partial to complete, and no adverse reactions except for an occasional rash.[33] Three patients with advanced cancers showed complete remission, while 4 others showed dramatic improvement, including shrinkage or disappearance of tumors.[34]

"The autogenous vaccines, when included as part of a comprehensive immune-enhancing approach, seemed to result in tumor reduction and stabilization," says Dr. Speckhart. "Based on our preliminary studies, the remission rates seemed most favorable for people whose tumors were localized, such as in the prostate or breast."[35] However, Dr. Speckhart notes that the Livingston vaccines are expensive to produce and are not cost-effective for most practitioners.

# Anti-Mycoplasma Auto-Vaccine

**When a special vaccine, cultured from a patient's own cancer disease organisms, is cultured, purified, and reintroduced into the body, it helps the immune system recognize the cancer-producing agents and take steps to reverse the cancer process. A complete detoxification program, including ultraviolet filtration of the blood, nutritional and**

**herbal supplementation, colonics, and removal of all dental toxins are also part of the program.**

Another approach involves the culturing of a patient's blood for a cell-wall-deficient bacterium called mycoplasma, found in the blood of all cancer patients. The process produces a vaccine, called the anti-mycoplasma auto-vaccine, for reintroduction into the patient's system. Originally developed in Germany, the anti-mycoplasma auto-vaccine technique is now practiced in North America by Filibert Muñoz, M.D., and Fernando C. Ramirez del Rio, M.D., at the Instituto Medico Biologico (IMB) in Tijuana, Mexico. When this mycoplasma vaccine is given to the patient from whom it was made, the cancer often arrests or regresses.

IMB physicians are qualified in the handling of different biological medicine modalities for the nontoxic treatment of chronic degenerative conditions, including cancer. Drs. Muñoz and Ramirez use the anti-mycoplasma vaccine as part of a multifaceted cancer treatment program that involves ultraviolet photophoresis of the patient's blood, detoxification, dietary change, and nutritional supplementation. It is best explained in the context of a patient case, as follows.

## SUCCESS STORY

### Reversing Metastatic Prostate Cancer

Manuel, aged 73, was a retired engineer diagnosed with Stage IV prostate cancer with metastases to the lumbar spine that were dangerously compressing the spinal cord and its nerve roots. Manuel refused chemotherapy, radiation, and surgery, and was willing to try the vaccine protocols used by Dr. Muñoz.

First, Dr. Muñoz had to study Manuel's blood. Specifically, he used a darkfield microscope to study a living sample of Manuel's blood for platelet shape. Platelets are disc-shaped cellular elements in blood that are essential for clotting. By studying their shape and activity and their rate of dying off, Dr. Muñoz gained valuable information about the state of Manuel's cancer and, to an extent, the amount and nature of toxins present in his blood. Blood platelets can be compromised by bacteria, mycoplasmas, viruses, and parasites such that their shape and ability to clump together (clot-

## What is Mycoplasma?

It takes about 2 months to grow the vaccine in the laboratory from the cancer "germs" or mycoplasma, and other blood-borne cancer factors, says Dr. Ramirez. A mycoplasma is a tiny biological life-form without a cell wall, normally harmless, but capable of becoming harmful in a cancer process.

Mycoplasma is also known as a cell-wall deficient organism. According to Dr. Muñoz, mycoplasma is a bacteria that grows on the surface of the cells such as platelets, lymphocytes, red blood cells, and on malignant cells. "When we take a sample of blood, we separate the serum, then culture the mycoplasma. After 4-6 weeks or so, the mycoplasma is separated from the culture and broken down into its biochemical components. We use the polysaccharide portion of it to develop the vaccine."

ting) may be impaired, Dr. Muñoz explains.

"These changes may be observed during a period of platelet cultivation for several days using darkfield microscopy. The culture allows for the identification of platelet forms typical of many illnesses, particularly of malignant cancers; these typical forms can be observed from the initial states of the illness." As a result, very early detection of tendencies to develop malignant neoplastic (cancerous) processes can be made, such that a skilled physician may know the type of tumor that would likely appear up to several years later. "It should be noted that any type of radiation, as well as any type of cytotoxic [cell-killing] medication or anesthetic, will make it impossible to observe the shape changes of the platelets," Dr. Muñoz notes. The platelet test also enables the physician to evaluate the effectiveness of the particular course of treatment in a given patient, as the pathological forms of platelets appear decreasingly less as the patient's condition improves.

Dr. Muñoz examined the platelet activity on the same blood slide once every 24 hours for 3 days. "This test confirmed that there was a prostate cancer with metastasis to the bones, and that Manuel had a high amount of toxins in his blood coming from bacterial infections in a root canal tooth and from his dental amalgams," explains Dr. Ramirez.

Next, Dr. Muñoz drew 120 ccs of Manuel's blood as the basis for preparing the anti-mycoplasma vaccine. Generally, the results of the platelet test indicate if it is appropriate to prepare an anti-mycoplasma vaccine from the patient's blood, says Dr. Muñoz. This vaccine will help to eliminate the pathogenic mycoplasma that acts as a causative factor of different illnesses, especially cancer. Dr. Muñoz explains that a single blood culture from the patient is sufficient to produce enough vaccine to last 4-5 months at the rate of 2-3 injections weekly. He also notes that this therapy has been used successfully in Germany since the 1950s, mainly by Dr. B. Freitag, former director of the Institute of Bacteriology of Bavaria. Today, the anti-mycoplasma auto-vaccine is also used by physicians in Barcelona, Spain, and Buenos Aires, Argentina.

Dr. Ramirez adds that "once the germs are grown, they get deactivated and detoxified so the patient can have the vaccine reintroduced into his body as a subcutaneous injection, given 2-3 times weekly." The purpose of the anti-mycoplasma vaccine is to enhance and strengthen the immune system, he says. "It helps the immune system be able to *recognize* the 'germs' that were formerly blocking its own immune response creating a condition in which the body did not act against the mycoplasma, viruses, and other cancer-related factors."

Manuel received the anti-mcyoplasma vaccine 3 times weekly for several months, then as his cancer began to reverse itself and he became healthier, the injections were gradually reduced to twice then once weekly to eventually once monthly when the disease was completely out of his system and his immune system was restored to proper working order. According to Dr. Ramirez, Manuel will need to receive the anti-mycoplasma injection about once every month for the rest of his life as a precaution against any further cancer activity.

***"The purpose of the anti-mycoplasma vaccine is to enhance and strengthen the immune system," Dr. Ramirez says. "It helps the immune system be able to*** **recognize** ***the 'germs' that were formerly blocking its own immune response."***

During the 2 months culturing time for the anti-mycoplasma vaccine, Dr. Muñoz drew a pint of Manuel's blood and ran it through an ultraviolet photophoresis machine. The process of ultraviolet light therapy killed viruses and bacteria and neutralized toxins in the blood; ozone, a form of oxygen, was also introduced into the blood sample to further purify it, then the blood was reinfused into Manuel. "For patients with advanced cancers, we do this once daily for the first 1-2 weeks," says Dr. Ramirez. Photophoresis and ozone treatments were only part of the detoxification program than Manuel underwent.

There was also chelation therapy, sauna, massage, and supplements, including *L. acidophilus*, enzymes, glutathione, N-acetyl cysteine, and both herbal and synthetic antiviral substances, says Dr. Muñoz. These included *Echinacea*, goldenseal, interferon, Pranosine, and Zovirax. In addition,

Manuel's diet underwent significant changes, based on a modified macrobiotic approach. He was to eat only fresh fruits and vegetables and fish, and to avoid red meats and minimize his poultry consumption. He also started a regular exercise program to induce sweating and the discharging of toxins through the skin, and he received regular intestinal colonics. "When the patients are very toxic, they receive colonics every day," says Dr. Ramirez. "Sometimes we introduce ozone rectally as another way to detoxify a patient, usually twice weekly, then eventually once weekly until the intestines are detoxified."

A prime source of Manuel's toxins was his teeth, specifically a toxic substance called di-methylsulphite released from several root canals. Di-methylsulphite is a by-product of the interaction of bacteria and heavy metals placed in the mouth by dental procedures such as amalgam fillings and root canals, says Dr. Ramirez. "This substance will depress the immune system and can even weaken the heart." As part of his cancer treatment program, Manuel had his root canal teeth extracted.

Finally, Manuel required spinal surgery for the nerve compression produced by the bony metastases. "Once his cancer was completely controlled and the cancer markers and antigen factors were down to zero, meaning there was no cancer activity, we still had to deal with Manuel's spinal cord compression at the lumbar nerve roots," says Dr. Ramirez, who is an orthopedic surgeon. This operation was necessary to allow Manuel to regain the use of his lumbar nerves and the ability to walk again without pain or fatigue. "The important fact here is that when we did the spinal surgery, Manuel's vertebral bone was quite strong thanks to a substance called pamidronate [known by the brand name of Aredia] that we used to treat the metastasis of the cancer to the bones. This

For more information about **ultraviolet light therapy**, or photophoresis, see Chapter 34: Energy Support Therapies, p. 1050.

**Chelation therapy** refers to a method of binding ("chelating") an organic substance known as a chelating agent to a metallic ion with a positive electric charge (e.g., a heavy metal) and removing it from the body. One type of chelation therapy involves the chelating agent disodium EDTA given as an intravenous infusion over a 3-$^1/_2$ hour period. Usually 20 to 30 treatments are administered at the rate of 1 to 3 sessions per week. Chelation therapy is especially beneficial for all forms of atherosclerotic cardiovascular disease including angina pectoris and coronary artery disease.

**Macrobiotics** is a specialized diet and food philosophy roughly based on Chinese medicine and filtered through contemporary Japanese culture and American representatives such as Georges Ohsawa and Michio Kushi. The diet emphasizes balancing the energy qualities of fresh, whole foods to maximize their delivery of *Qi*, or vital life force, to the body. The diet comprises cooked whole grains, beans and bean products, vegetables, fruits, nuts, seeds, small amounts of saltwater fish (salmon), fermented soybean products (miso), seaweeds, shiitake mushrooms, and special pickles and condiments. Macrobiotics has been used successfully when clinically prescribed as a curative and restorative diet in treating chronic and serious illness, including cancer; as a health maintenance diet, it has produced excellent results for many people.

QUICK DEFINITION

A **cancer marker** refers to any of a variety of blood tests that measure the level of a protein material or other chemical produced by cancer cells. These numbers become elevated in the presence of a cancer or tumor. There are different cancer markers for different kinds of cancer; CEA (carcino-embryonic antigen) test for colon cancer, AFP (Alpha fetoprotein) test for liver cancer (primary hepato-cellular carcinoma), PSA (prostate specific antigen) for prostate cancer, CA (carcinoma) 15-3 or 27.29 for breast cancer, and CA 125 for ovarian cancer, to name a few.

substance allows the bones to regrow the part that was destroyed by the cancer. It also enhances calcification by getting the osteoblasts to start rebuilding bone cells." Pamidronate was given to Manuel by intravenous infusion.

In less than 1 year of receiving the anti-mycoplasma vaccine, Manuel's cancer markers were down to zero. Two years later, Manuel remained healthy and active, and had taken to traveling all over Mexico, "happy, with no pain," says Dr. Ramirez. Success of this caliber requires that the patient be "willing to follow all the steps in the program," he adds.

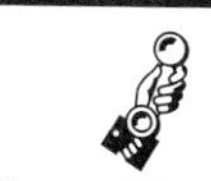

For more information about the **anti-mycoplasma vaccine**, contact: Filibert Muñoz, M.D. or Fernando C. Ramirez del Rio, M.D., Instituto Binacional de las Californias de Traumatologia Ortopedia, Rehabilitacion y Ciencias Afines A.C., Edificio Allen W. Lloyd, Paseo Tijuana 406, Suite 203, Segundo Piso, Zona del Rio, Tijuana, Baja California, Mexico C.P. 22310; tel: 52-6683-2944 or 52-6683-6225. Or write Dr. Ramirez at: P.O. Box 451, Bonita, CA 91908. Also contact both Drs. Muñoz and Ramirez at: Instituto Medico Biologico, Paseo Tijuana 406-203, Tijuana, Baja California, Mexico: fax: 526-6824030. U.S. address: P.O. Box 431697, San Ysidro, CA 92143; tel: 619-216-1455; fax: 619-482-4394.

# Immuno-Placental Therapy (IPT)

**According to Russian immunologist Valentine I. Govallo, M.D., Ph.D., cancer has a unique immunologic character that, in most cases, enables it to evade attack by the human immune system. Dr. Govallo, discovering that this special factor is found in the placenta surrounding fetuses, developed a vaccine from placental blood obtained after a live human birth to empower the immune system to overpower the cancer and its "cloaking" device.**

Cancer immunologists have long proposed that by stimulating the immune system in specific ways they could stop and possibly reverse cancer. The use of vaccines and interleukin-2 (an immune system stimulator) has worked well with malignant melanoma and to some extent with kidney cancer (renal cell carcinoma).[36] Dr. Springer's vaccine has repeatedly shown effectiveness against breast cancer, but its potential usefulness in treating other cancers has yet to be evaluated. In treating bladder cancer, as mentioned earlier, the BCG vaccine has proved far superior to even the most aggressive forms of chemotherapy,[37] while monoclonal antibodies appear to be promising for the treatment of melanoma. For other cancers, however,

## Placental Blood Increases Leukemia Survival

Physicians at Duke University observed a 50% survival rate over a period of 7-32 months when 25 leukemia patients, mostly children, received infusions of blood from the placenta (which would otherwise be discarded) of newborn humans, according to the *New England Journal of Medicine* (July 1996). While all 25 patients required marrow to replace stem cells destroyed by the cancer, the use of placental blood produced a better survival rate than standard bone-marrow transplantation and made it easier to match donors with recipients.

BCG, monoclonal antibodies, and most other vaccines seem to have fallen short or yielded inconsistent results.

The main reason for this inconsistency, according to Russian immunologist Valentine I. Govallo, M.D., Ph.D., is that cancer has a unique immunologic character that, in most cases, enables it to evade attack by the human immune system. Dr. Govallo, author of over 250 scientific articles and 20 books, including *The Immunology of Pregnancy and Cancer*, is the director of the Moscow Medical Institute's Laboratory of Clinical Immunology.

Over the years, Dr. Govallo observed that a large number of the women who came to him indicated miscarriages as part of their health history. His observations led him to conclude that the problem was due to a general deterioration of the fetal-placental immune system as a result of environmental pollution. Dr. Govallo's approach is based on an understanding of the way a fetus relates to its mother on an immunological level.

The **placenta** is the disk-shaped organ responsible for metabolic exchange between a fetus and its mother; it is made partly from the fetal embryo and partly from the mother's uterine mucosa. The placenta receives nutrients and oxygen (and toxins, if present) through the mother's blood, and it can discharge carbon dioxide and nitrogen waste products back into the mother for elimination. The placenta is, on average, 1/6 the weight of the infant at birth; the umbilical cord of the fetus attaches to the middle of the placenta.

Although it is dependent on its mother for everything, the fetus has a primitive immune system with features individualized slightly different from its mother. The fetus and the mother actually have *competing* immune systems. It sounds strange but it is possible for the mother's immune system to regard the fetus as foreign protein and set out to eliminate it. Under normal, healthy circumstances, the fetus is not rejected because its placenta-based immunity manages to block the mother's local immune system.

In the case of miscarriage, the mother's immune system recognizes in the fetus the father's antigens (proteins from the father), and since her immune system perceives these as alien to her, the fetus is rejected.

Environmental pollution, which is quite fierce in Russia, further adds to the problem, because it gives the mother's immune system even more foreign proteins and materials to react against, and thus further jeopardizes the fetus.

Based on this medical insight, Dr. Gavallo was able to prevent miscarriages with a 91% success rate by stimulating the development of the placenta, thus strengthening placental immunity and protecting the fetus against rejection by the mother's immune system.

This discovery gave Dr. Govallo a key insight into the riddle of cancer. He reasoned that just as the placenta synthesizes "blocking factors" to keep it from being rejected as foreign by its mother, so might tumors have this ability to hamper the immune system using a kind of immunological "cloaking device" that shields it from the host. In a sense, the tumor uses the same technique as the fetus to avoid being rejected by the host's immune system.

Today, scientists know that tumors produce blocking factors[38] and that some of these blocking factors appear to be proteins that are "shed" from the tumor as it interacts with the host's immune system. For example, one type of tumor protein may shut down the tumor-killing activity of natural killer cells;[39] another is the immune system cytokine called "tumor necrosis factor" which in addition to its ability to cause tumor cells to die (necrose) may also turn off the body's immune response to foreign tissues.[40] The secretion of these blocking factors may be one mechanism by which the tumor cells gain advantage over the antitumor immune responses of the host. By these means, tumor cells seem to adapt in such a way as to evade or subvert the immunological response directed against them.

***"Cancers have figured out a way of turning off the host's immune system, like a burglar who first turns off the burglar alarm before he goes about stealing things," Dr. Govallo says. "If it is possible to breach the tumor's immunological shield, the organism should be in a position to neutralize the tumor growth and even destroy it."***

"Cancers have figured out a way of turning off the host's immune system, like a burglar who first turns off the burglar alarm before he goes about stealing things," Dr. Govallo says. "This is the true nature of tumors, the reason for their biological survivability, and this nature must be respected." Dr. Govallo adds, "If it is possible to breach the tumor's immunological shield, the organism should be in a position to neutralize the tumor growth and even destroy it." The healthy human placenta contains factors that appear to suppress the defense mechanism of malignant cells. Dr.

Govallo's placenta-derived vaccine basically provides a way to "decloak" the tumor.

The vaccine is produced from human placental tissue *after* a live human birth. "We select the most active preparations of placental extracts to neutralize the protective blocking factors [produced by the primary tumor] in the patient's blood serum," says Dr. Govallo. "We only use extracts derived from the fetal part of the placenta obtained after a live birth or Caesarean section."

Dr. Govallo called his approach "immuno-placental therapy," or IPT, but it is now known as VG-1000. The kinds of cancer for which IPT seems particularly effective include malignant melanoma as well as lung, breast, kidney, and colorectal cancers.[41] "The therapy works best with a smaller tumor mass, even if this reduction has to be obtained through surgical intervention." The VG-1000 vaccine is administered only after an evaluation of the status of the cancer patient's immune system the day before treatment is scheduled to begin. Usually tumor reduction becomes noticeable within a few weeks after beginning the injections; however, within minutes of the injection, most cancer patients report that they experience sensations in areas surrounding their tumors or lymph nodes affected by cancer. The explanation is that the vaccine components apparently migrate to the tumor sites and stimulate immune reactions there.

> ***Dr. Govallo's first pilot study in 1974 focused on 45 patients with advanced cancer; today, 29 of the original 45 remain alive—a 64.4% survival rate after 20 years. In a more recent study of advanced cancer patients, the survival was 77% after 5 years.***

"If the tumor is in the breast and the injection is in the leg, then soon the products of immunization migrate to the tumor site in the breast and a painful sensation occurs," says Frank Wiewel, executive director and founder of People Against Cancer, who traveled to Moscow to interview Dr. Govallo and evaluate his records. "The immune reaction is typically accompanied by flu-like symptoms and in some cases fever and malaise for 1-2 days, but this is neither dangerous nor life-threatening."

VG-1000 has been used effectively in the treatment of advanced cancers. Dr. Govallo's first pilot study in 1974 focused on 45 patients with advanced cancer; today, 29 of the original 45 remain alive—a 64.4% survival rate after 20 years. A more recent study of advanced-cancer patients compared their survival withVG-1000 to survival following other immunotherapy approaches; the survival in the IPT group was far superior—77% versus 6% after 5 years.

According to Wiewel's independent evaluation of Dr. Govallo's records over a 20-year span, 60% of VG-1000-treated patients with advanced cancer have survived at least 5 years, and many of them 10 years or longer. Importantly, "these patients are enjoying an excellent quality of life, with no health complaints," says Wiewel. "It is a remarkable outcome."

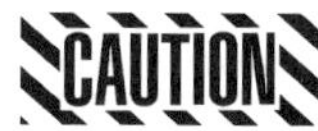


Dr. Govallo's immune therapy is contraindicated for liver cancer because it can destroy the liver tumor so quickly that the liver cannot adequately process and eliminate the dead cancer cells. Consequently, the person tends to develop a hepatitis-like condition.

Dr. Govallo notes that if the tumor is destroyed too suddenly, it can release massive amounts of toxins that can actually kill the patient. This is called "tumor lysis syndrome" because the dead tumor cells, once sloughed off, enter the blood and lymphatics and eventually must be eliminated from the body. In the process, however, they may overwhelm the body's detoxification capacities. For this reason, the body must be well-supplied with nutrients to accelerate its detoxification capacities. "Intensive nutritional support is needed during VG-1000 therapy and must be used afterwards because the body is certainly going to mount an attack on the tumor," says Wiewel. "In so doing you're going to destroy many, many tumor cells."

# Pleomorphism and SANUM Remedies

**According to German researcher Guenther Enderlein, M.D., Ph.D., human blood contains tiny components capable of changing shape and evolving from benign parasites to harmful pathogens according to changes in cell conditions. By reintroducing into the blood the earliest and purest form of these cellular components, balance is often restored and the cancer process reversed.**

The German researcher Guenther Enderlein, M.D., Ph.D. (1872-1968) opened up a new vista in understanding cancer and devising treatments through his use of darkfield microscopy. Observing living blood cells of his

**Darkfield microscopy** is a way of studying living whole blood cells under a specially adapted microscope that projects the dynamic image, magnified 1,500 times, onto a video screen. With a darkfield light condenser, images of high contrast are projected, so that the object appears bright against a dark background. The skilled physician can detect early signs of illness in the form of microorganisms in the blood known to produce disease. Blood cells live for about 20 minutes, so the amount of time the blood cell stays viable and alive indicates the overall health of the individual. Specifically, darkfield microscopy reveals distortions of red blood cells (which in turn indicate nutritional status), possible undesirable bacterial or fungal life forms, and blood ecology patterns indicative of health or illness.

patients, Dr. Enderlein detected living microorganisms in the blood, some of which are harmful to health, that were otherwise invisible to conventional means of study and analysis. The electron microscope only enables scientists to study dead matter, which is why they typically dismiss microorganisms picked up by the darkfield microscope as artifacts and organelles (cell component) or routine blood elements of unknown origin and function.[42]

In the course of studying live blood under the darkfield microscope for 6 decades, Dr. Enderlein observed protein-based microorganisms, which he called *protits*, that flourish in the blood cells, tissues, body fluids, and plasma. Protits appear to live in a mutually beneficial or symbiotic relationship with the body under *healthy* conditions, but when the body's internal environment—its cellular terrain—changes in terms of pH (acidity/alkalinity ratio), toxin load, or the availability of oxygen and/or nutrients, the protits pass through different stages of cyclic development, eventually reaching a disease-causing (pathogenic) form. The ability of fundamental life organisms (protits) to undergo sequential shape changes is a theory of bacteriology called pleomorphism, meaning, literally "many" (*pleo*) "shapes" (*morph*).

This idea, not surprisingly, has been heretical ever since French physician and pharmacist Antoine Béchamp (1816-1908), the intellectual rival to Louis Pasteur and his germ theory, first proposed it in the 1870s. Béchamp's theory, known as pleomorphism, says that a microbe—a bacterium, fungus, virus—can change shape and in fact take on many sequential shapes that are increasingly pathogenic. It can thereby produce illness from *within* the body. In contrast, Pasteur's monomorphism holds that bacteria do not ever change shape but maintain "one" (*mono*) "shape" (*morph*), and invade the body from outside, producing infection and illness. Of historical interest, on his deathbed Pasteur reportedly admitted, "The microbe is nothing, the terrain is everything," in essence confessing that he was wrong and Béchamp right.

Biochemical changes, such as alterations in pH and oxidation-reduction potential within the cells and blood, initiate this microbiological shape-shifting. Outside influences, such as faulty diet, inadequate nutrition, exposure to carcinogens, chronic organ toxicity, stress, or trauma provide the impetus to throw the cells out of balance.

The microbe that Dr. Enderlein linked with cancer is primarily *Mucor racemosus Fresen.* Under certain conditions, suitable biochemical conditions in the body fluids foster development of the protits into their more lethal forms, either the *Mucor* bacterial or fungal state. Dr. von Brehmer more specifically identified the blood parasite *Siphonospora polymorpha*—the most advanced stage of the *Mucor racemosus Fresen*, according to Dr. Enderlein—as a major cancer-promoting agent.[43]

Dr. Enderlein and his colleagues noted that a diet rich in animal fats and proteins seemed to promote these transient changes in pH and cause these normally harmless microbes to change into the harmful *Mucor* fungi. Thus, the typical American diet provides the ideal conditions for transforming *protits* into their harmful forms. This situation is made worse by carcinogenic substances—dietary factors (food additives, pesticides), viruses, alcohol, tobacco, radiation, etc.—which can damage cell membranes and mitochondria (the cell's energy-producing subunits) and thereby alter the cell's ability to metabolize proteins and fats and to make energy.

The protit, in its altered form, leads to faulty genetic mechanisms which, in turn, result in incorrect synthesis of proteins such as those used by the immune system.[44] This situation, combined with the "blocking factors" mentioned earlier, may help explain why the immune system often fails to respond appropriately to cancer cells.

Dr. Enderlein theorized that disease must be treated at the cellular level—where biochemical terrain is formed, or changed—and he formulated his remedies accordingly. His formulas, known as SANUM remedies, are dilutions of bacteria and fungi which, once injected into the cancer patient, work according to the principles of homeopathy. As such, the Enderlein remedies may be thought of as a type of vaccination, because the healthy form of the organism is given to the patient whose body may be carrying the unhealthy form. By injecting harmless forms of bacteria exemplifying the microorganism in its benign state, the

**Oxidation-reduction** refers to a basic chemical mechanism in the cell by which energy is produced from foods. Electrons (negatively charged particles in an atom) are removed from one atom, resulting in "oxidation" of this first atom, and then are added or transferred to another atom, resulting in "reduction" of this second atom. This continual process of energy metabolism is actually a flow of electrons, or a minute electrical current within the cell.

**SANUM remedies**, developed by Guenther Enderlein, M.D., Ph.D. (1872-1968), are produced by SANUM-Kehlbeck GmbH & Co. of Hoya, Germany. The line includes about 100 preparations of tiny, benign microorganisms or protein particles identified by pleomorphic practice. For example, "Mucokehl" is *Mucor racemosus*, a fungus, that regulates microorganisms affecting the thickness of blood. These remedies, injected around the tumor site, adjust the pH and cellular terrain and help the pathogenic microorganisms revert back to harmless forms. In effect, the SANUM remedies help the body restore the optimal cellular terrain for health.

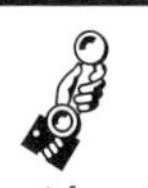

For more information about **SANUM remedies** and for the actual products, contact: Enderlein Sales Group, P.O. Box 2352, Santa Rosa, CA 95405; tel: 800-203-3775 or 707-537-9505; fax: 707-538-9179. Enderlein Sales Group "Pleo" remedies include Pleo-Muc (*Mucor racemosus*), Pleo-Not (*Penicillium notatum*), Pleo-Quent (*Penicillium frequentans*), and others. In contrast to homeopathic remedies, the *lower* the dilution of Pleo remedies, the stronger the dosage. Hence, a 3X dilution is 100 times more potent than a 5X dilution. The remedies are available as drops, tablets, capsules, suppositories, and ointments.

disease-causing protits revert to their benign form, which, in turn, promotes normal immune function.[45]

Most of the physicians trained in the United States fail to realize that blood pH balance is critical in determining whether or not tumor cells thrive or die. Whereas German physicians say that blood pH is slightly alkaline at 7.1, American physicians are taught to view a higher alkaline level, 7.4, as acceptable. However, some physicians following Dr. Enderlein's protocols observe that whenever a cancer patient's blood pH drops from an initial 7.6 to a range of 7.2-7.3, cancers often stop growing.

Overly alkaline blood can result from the body's attempt to balance the gastric acids produced after a person overeats, consumes too many high-protein or high-sugar foods, or fails to breathe normally or exercise in a regular, moderate fashion. On the other hand, the locally acid pH surrounding tumors (a result of lactic acid production) spurs the further development of the *Mucor* protits.

A German physician used Dr. Enderlein's methods to successfully treat more than 50 breast cancer patients. In each case, the tumors were completely eliminated. The injections administered to these women included *Mucor racemosus*, *Aspergillus niger*, and Sinuvis L(+) lactic acid.[46] Another German physician reports a success rate of greater than 90% in healing prostate disorders of various kinds with SANUM remedies.[47]

Erik Enby, M.D. of Gothenberg, Sweden, has carried forth the work of Dr. Enderlein and confirmed all his original findings. During Dr. Enby's initial 8-year experience with the darkfield microscope and Enderlein remedies, he successfully treated more than 100 cases of prostate and uterine cancer and effectively stabilized or reversed many cases of breast cancer and leukemia.[48] Dr. Enby notes that Enderlein remedies are most successful when used with an effective program of detoxification. "As long as the physician or practitioner ensures that the body can excrete toxins and other products released from dismantled tumors, the natural biological preparations work very well. To achieve success, the excretion systems of the body must be able to eliminate the neutralized cancer growth, which the body identifies as toxic wastes."[49]

Dr. Enby also recommends the following measures to maximize the effectiveness of Enderlein remedies: (1) remove metal fillings or mercury dental amalgams; (2) avoid or minimize the intake of animal proteins and fats; (3) eat pesticide-free raw vegetables and fresh fruits; (4) avoid chemotherapy and other anticancer drugs; (5) avoid unnecessary antibiotics and other synthetic infection-reducing drugs; (6) avoid steroid medications; (7) avoid taking medications that reduce fever during an illness, unless health is impaired; and (8) keep X rays to a bare minimum.

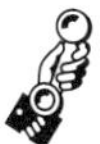

For information about **Enderlein medicine**, contact: Biological Medicine Institute, Avenida de la Paz, No. 16420 Colonia Mineral Sante Fe, Tijuana, B.C. 22360 Mexico; for mailing, Biological Medicine Institute, P.O. Box 433656, San Ysidro, CA 92173; tel: 52-66-240786, 52-66-240939, or 52-66-245110; fax: 52-66-240786. Dr. Govallo's placental vaccine which, prior to 1996 was virtually unknown outside Russia, is now available in North America at 2 alternative cancer clinics: Max Gerson Memorial Center Hospital in Tijuana, Mexico, and Immuno-Augmentative Clinic (IAT) in Freeport, Bahamas. The arrival of VG-1000 in North America was made possible by the efforts of medical historian Harris L. Coulter, Ph.D., director of the Center for Empirical Medicine in Washington, D.C. Dr. Coulter is the author of the landmark 4-volume *Divided Legacy*, a 3,000-page work documenting the history of and conflicts between conventional and alternative medicines. In 1994, Dr. Coulter traveled to Moscow, met with Dr. Govallo, and made arrangements to introduce VG-1000 in the West. For preliminary screening information, contact: People Against Cancer, Box 10, Otho, IA 50569; tel; 515-972-4444. To contact Dr. Coulter about licensing VG-1000 for other locales: Harris L. Coulter, Ph.D., Empirical Therapies, Inc., 4221 45th Street, N.W., Washington, D.C. 20016; tel: 202-362-3185 or 202-364-0898; fax: 202-362-3407.

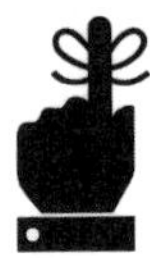

*The most powerful alternative cancer therapies are those aimed at strengthening all levels of a person's being at the same time—at reducing the body's toxic burden while also enhancing its multifaceted self-healing capacities and bringing the true character of the individual into focus and healthy expression.*

Chapter 32

# Enhancing Whole-Body Metabolism for Treating Cancer

**When you correct overall imbalances in how the body derives energy from foods and oxygen—biochemical processes at the heart of organic life—it makes it impossible for cancer cells to thrive because they depend on unbalanced conditions. Once metabolism is corrected, the energy becomes available again for healing.**

In this chapter, we examine different therapies, such as the use of hydrogen peroxide, ozone, enzymes, and glandular extracts, vital to the functioning of all systems of the body. Along with diet and nutritional factors, these make up what we call metabolic therapies.

**In This Chapter**



Metabolism is the sum total of all the biochemical processes going on inside the body, and metabolic therapies focus on ways to balance these chemical processes—enabling normal cells to thrive and cancer cells to become depleted and die, or revert back to normal. The therapeutic goal of metabolic therapies is to rebuild and revitalize all of the body's life-sustaining functions, thereby helping to stop and reverse cancer, or to prevent a recurrence.

## Making and Using Energy at the Cellular Level

First we need to briefly review the metabolism of healthy and cancerous cells as a background to understanding the need and mode of action for metabolic therapies. The primary goal of metabolic therapy is to alter the cancer cells' chemical processes and thereby promote their vulnerability or reversion to normal cells (cellular redifferentiation). Some of these processes—the metabolism of oxygen and glucose, for example—are directly aimed at the cancer cells. Others exert an indirect influence by boosting the patient's immune system, influencing cancer tissue damage by free radicals, and detoxifying the body. Most standard chemotherapy drugs, hydrogen peroxide, and ozone work by producing free-radical damage to cancer cells at greater rates than to noncancerous cells.

When it comes to understanding how healthy and cancerous cells make and use energy, the key is oxygen. The metabolism of cancer cells is similar

THE INSIDE STORY ON

# Metabolism: How We Get Energy From Foods

Metabolism is the biological process by which we extract energy from the foods we eat, producing carbon dioxide and water as by-products for elimination from the body. More generally, metabolism refers to any of the chemical reactions that take place in our cells. These chemical reactions are controlled by enzymes, which are specialized catalytic proteins produced by the cells. Enzymes initiate and regulate the speed of all chemical reactions; hence they are known as catalysts.

There are 2 kinds of metabolism: anabolic and catabolic. In anabolic metabolism, the upbuilding phase, larger molecules are constructed by joining smaller ones together; in catabolic metabolism, the deconstructing phase, larger molecules are broken down into smaller ones. The anabolic function produces substances for cell growth and repair, while the catabolic function controls digestion (called hydrolysis), disassembling food into forms the body can use for energy. For example, proteins are broken down into amino acids, fats into glycerol and fatty acids, and carbohydrates into monosaccharides or simple sugars.

Anabolic and catabolic metabolism are constantly underway in the cells. Here the anabolic phase is made possible or energized by the catabolic. Under healthy, normal conditions, both phases operate in balance with each other so that energy needs do not outstrip energy supply and energy reserves are not in excess of body requirements.

Biochemically, metabolism involves hundreds of different chemical reactions, necessitating the involvement of hundreds of different enzymes, each of which handles a specific reaction.

Some chemical reactions have a number of stages that must occur in a certain order. In this case, a different enzyme will be responsible for each stage and they must work together to ensure the proper sequence. This certain sequence of enzyme-controlled reactions is known as a metabolic pathway.

The carbohydrate pathway is one example of a metabolic pathway and also a good illustration of the interaction of anabolic and catabolic metabolism. When carbohydrates enter the body as food, amylase breaks them down into monosaccharides (the main one is glucose); this can then be immediately converted into energy via the catabolic pathway or converted via the anabolic pathway into glycogen or fat for storage in the liver and muscle cells as an energy reserve. Between meals, this action is reversed; now liver and muscle cells convert glycogen into glucose and release it into the blood to supply energy to the body.

Another metabolic process is called cellular respiration. This involves the breakdown of glucose and other substances and the release of energy from them. Through a sequence of chemical reactions occurring in the cytoplasm and mitochondria of cells, glucose is eventually converted to citric acid and energy is transferred to ATP (adenosine triphosphate), which is an energy-carrying molecule. At this point, the Kreb's cycle (also called the citric acid cycle) begins.

In this, during another series of chemical conversions, molecules of carbon dioxide and hydrogen atoms are released. The carbon dioxide is transported out of the cell into the blood and the hydrogen atoms are joined with oxygen. Again, the chemical reactions release energy, some of which is transferred to ATP molecules for use by the cell in other metabolic processes and the remainder is expended as heat. This completes the Kreb's cycle. The entire process represents the "breathing" of the cell.[1]

to that of normal cells in many respects, probably because most cancers originate from the host's normal tissues. But there are crucial differences. In normal cell metabolism, oxygen is used in the cell along with glucose (blood sugar) to produce energy for the cell to function. This aerobic (oxygen/air-dependent) form of energy production is about 18 times more efficient than its opposite, anaerobic metabolism, in which the cell burns glucose in the absence of oxygen.

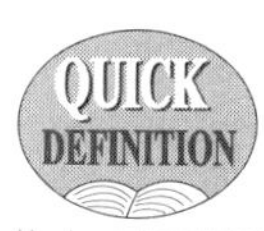

The term **pH**, which means "potential hydrogen," represents a scale for the relative acidity or alkalinity of a solution. Acidity is measured as a pH of 0.1 to 6.9, alkalinity is 7.1 to 14, and neutral pH is 7.0. The numbers refer to how many hydrogen atoms are present compared to an ideal or standard solution. Normally, blood is slightly alkaline, at 7.35 to 7.45; urine pH can range from 4.8 to 7.5, although normal is closer to 7.0. **Acid-base metabolism** refers to the metabolic processes that maintain the balance of acids and bases (alkalines) in body fluids. Acids release hydrogen ions, while bases accept them. The total number of these hydrogen ions present determines the pH of a fluid. Too many hydrogen ions (a pH below 7) produce an acidic state called acidosis, while too few hydrogen ions (a pH above 7) cause an alkaline excess called alkalosis; both can lead to illness. **Oxidation-reduction** refers to a basic chemical mechanism in the cell by which energy is produced from foods. Electrons (negatively charged particles in an atom) are removed from one atom, resulting in "oxidation" of this first atom, and then are added or transferred to another atom, resulting in "reduction" of this second atom. This continual process of energy metabolism is actually a flow of electrons, or a minute electrical current within the cell.

For this reason, anaerobic cells must work harder than aerobic cells to derive energy from the glucose they "consume" or metabolize. This means that anaerobic cells burn far more glucose to derive the same amount of energy as aerobic cells.

Cancer cells exhibit the anaerobic mode of metabolism, which means they are not dependent on oxygen, a characteristic that seems related to the fact that the mitochondria, or primary energy-producing components of cells, are defective in cancerous conditions.[2] Mitochondria are small structures in the cell's cytoplasm (the fluid space between the outer cell membrane and the nucleus) that are often called the cell's "powerhouses" because they generate energy. Mitochondria contain enzymes that help them break down fats and carbohydrates in the presence of oxygen.

Under normal conditions of aerobic metabolism, with healthy mitochondria, the cell takes in glucose and oxygen and releases carbon dioxide; with its defective mitochondria, the tumor cell is incapable of carrying out this elementary aspect of cell respiration. In the process of cellular respiration, oxygen is used to oxidize organic fuel molecules (such as sugars, fats, or protein metabolities [amino acids]), subsequently releasing energy, carbon dioxide, and water. Unlike normal cells, cancer cells only partially metabolize glucose, producing lactic acid rather than carbon dioxide in the process. Cancer cells thrive under the conditions of high-sugar low-oxygen associated with fermentation but fare poorly under low-sugar high-oxygen conditions.

As cancer cells begin to multiply, forming a tumor, the liver must expend a considerable amount of energy converting the toxic lactic acid back to glucose. Also, most cancer cells can function only at a low pH—that is, in a very acidic state—because of all the lactic acid they constantly produce. The combined effect of the tumor's metabolism is to tax the liver and acidify the body. This leads to frequent bouts of fatigue, which are among the early warning signs of cancer.

Over time, the cancer cell's highly inefficient use of energy places a huge burden on the host. As the cancer grows, ever more lactic acid is produced, creating an even larger energy drain. This has the effect of drawing amino acids such as glutamine and alanine (which can be used for energy) out of the muscles, thereby causing physical wasting or loss of lean tissue mass.

# Oxygen (Hydrogen Peroxide and Ozone)

**Cancer only grows in the absence of oxygen, which means if you introduce sufficient oxygen into the body's cells, this will help reverse the cancer process by suffocating the tumor with too much oxygen. Physicians working with oxygen therapy find that hydrogen peroxide and ozone can produce excellent results.**

Most health-minded people are aware of the harmful effects of free radicals caused by oxidation. What is not well known is that when produced under controlled circumstances, as in oxygen therapy, free radicals are deadly to bacteria, viruses, fungi, and their spores or L-forms. In addition, oxygen therapy stimulates the immune system and various enzyme systems, probably through increasing the production of cytokines, immunologically active proteins that directly and indirectly destroy or inhibit the growth of microorganisms and/or tumor cells.

The knowledge that oxygen therapies had strong antimicrobial, antiviral, and sterilizing capabilities was known very shortly after their discovery in the last century. Recent research has begun to show the precise immune changes that occur in oxygen therapy. German scientist Otto

*Dr. Warburg proposed that normalizing the metabolism of cancer cells was the key to effective treatment of cancer and that the prime means to accomplish this was through oxygen so that "all growing body cells be saturated with oxygen."*

Warburg, M.D., was the first to propose that a lack of oxygen at the cellular level may be the prime cause of cancer and that oxygen therapy could be an effective treatment for it. He showed that normal embryonic cells, when subjected to reduced oxygen concentrations, quickly adopt the fermentative metabolism typical of cancer cells. The *lack* of oxygen apparently alters the normal cell's respiration during growth, triggering the development of cancer cells. When oxygen levels surrounding the cells are raised, cancer cells do not form.

Dr. Warburg, who served for many years as director of the Max Planck Institute for Cell Physiology in Germany, reported his findings in *The Prime Cause and Prevention of Cancer*, published in 1967. Here, he proposed that normalizing the metabolism of cancer cells was the key to effective treatment of cancer, and that the prime means to accomplish this was through oxygen. Specifically, Dr. Warburg suggested as the first priority of treatment "that all growing body cells be saturated with oxygen."[3] The second priority was to avoid further exposure to toxins, as a way to help shift the enzyme balance of the cancer cell and thereby restore a normal cellular metabolism.

## Oxygen's Role in the Growth of Cancer Cells

According to Dr. Warburg, almost anything can cause cancer, but even for cancer there is only one prime cause: The replacement of the respiration of oxygen in normal cells by a fermentation of sugar. "All normal body cells meet their energy needs by respiration of oxygen, whereas cancer cells meet their energy needs in great part by fermentation. Oxygen gas, the donor of energy in plants and animals, is dethroned in the cancer cells and replaced by an energy-yielding reaction of the lowest living forms, namely, a fermentation of glucose."[4]

Oddly, even as cancer research struggles to explain how and why the normal controls over cell growth and differentiation sometimes become deranged, medical textbooks on cancer rarely acknowledge Dr. Warburg's pioneering insights, even though he was awarded the Nobel Prize in Medicine in 1931 for his discovery of the oxygen-transferring enzyme of cell respiration.

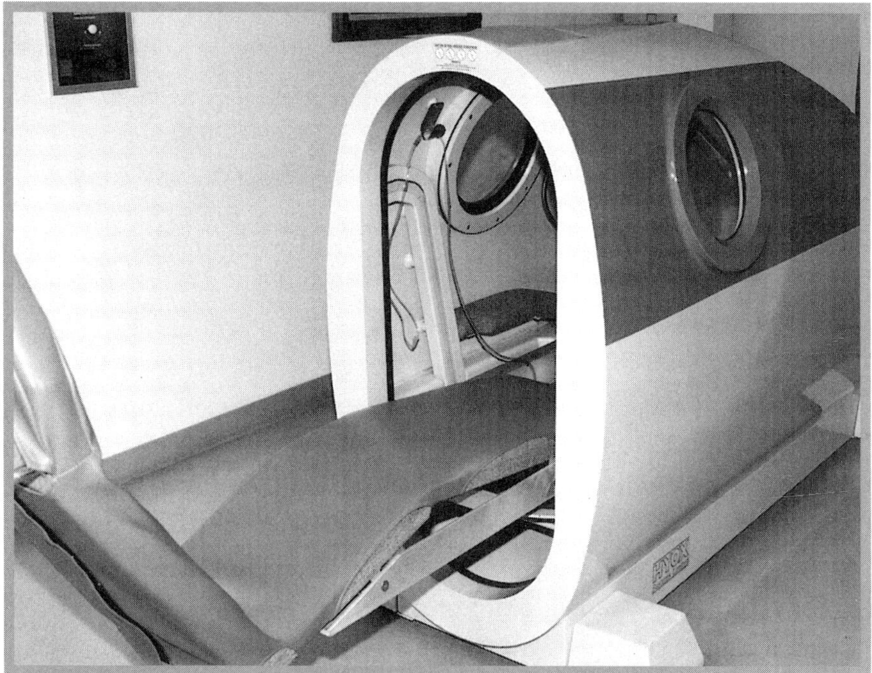

**A hyperbaric oxygen chamber, somewhat resembling a miniature submarine, delivers pure oxygen under pressure to all the cells of the body, including the brain.**

The metabolic approach originally proposed by Dr. Warburg entails exposing the cancer cell to high levels of oxygen. Since the cancer cell can participate only in fermentative (anaerobic) metabolism, oxygen at high levels is toxic to the cancer cell. The cancer cell has a very low production of the superoxide dismutase (SOD), an antioxidant enzyme that protects normal cells from high oxygen concentrations.[5] This lack of SOD may make cancer cells particularly vulnerable to high oxygen concentrations. Also of interest is the observed fact that tumors produce harmful superoxide free radicals that can be neutralized by SOD.[6]

Oxygen can be used in various forms to promote healing and to destroy pathogens (disease-producing microorganisms and toxins) in the body. These therapies have been used to treat a wide variety of conditions, including cancer, infections, circulatory problems, chronic fatigue syndrome, arthritis, allergies, and multiple sclerosis.

There are 2 principal types of oxygen therapy, classified according to the chemical process involved: oxygenation and oxidation.

**Oxygenation—**This is the process of enriching the oxygen content of the blood or tissues. Using oxygen as a safe selective "chemotherapy" for cancer patients has been studied thoroughly by Manfred von Ardenne in Germany and was found to be most effective when used in combination with regular aerobic exercise, hyperthermia (heat therapy) induced by infrared light projected onto the skin, intermittently induced hyperglycemia (high blood sugar, by giving glucose intravenously once every 18 days), and daily administration (just before exercise) of 30 mg of vitamin B1, 100 mg of magnesium orotate, and 75 mg of dipyridamol (a drug that prevents blood clotting).[7]

**Hyperbaric oxygen therapy** refers to pure oxygen delivered for 30-60 minutes to patients inside sealed chambers at high pressure (hence "hyperbaric" as in high barometric pressure), usually at 2.5 times higher than the atmospheric pressure at sea level. A monoplace chamber accommodates a single patient who absorbs the concentrated oxygen through the skin as well as through inhalation. A multiplace chamber services several people at once; patients wear oxygen masks.

One oxygenation therapy is called hyperbaric oxygen therapy, which introduces oxygen to the body in a pressurized chamber. All human cells, tissues, and organs need oxygen to function. A clinical process called hyperoxygenation saturates the body with oxygen through the use of gas, sometimes at high pressure. The application is based on the principle that insufficient oxygenation promotes the growth of pathogens whereas excessive (hyper) oxygenation damages normal tissues. Oxygenation employed under strictly controlled conditions (not too much or not too little) can have positive therapeutic effects.

**Oxidation—**Oxidation is a chemical reaction occurring when electrons (electrically charged particles) are transferred from one molecule to another. Oxygen molecules are frequently, but not always, involved in these reactions. (Oxidation refers to the chemical reaction and not to oxygen itself.) The molecules that give up their electrons are referred to as oxidized. The molecules that accept electrons are referred to as oxidants.

Although uncontrolled oxidation can be destructive—as is the case when free radicals are produced in excess—it can also be therapeutic when carefully used on weak and devitalized cells as the targets. These old weak cells are metabolically broken down. Destroying these sick cells permits the formation of new, healthy cells that are better able to resist disease.[8] Oxidation therapy may help by "jump-starting" the body's oxidative processes and returning them to normal, according to Charles Farr, M.D., Ph.D., a leading researcher in oxygen therapy.

## Hydrogen Peroxide as a Metabolic Cancer Therapy

Hydrogen peroxide ($H_2O_2$) is a natural substance made by normal healthy human cells in the body to regulate metabolism and act as a poison to destroy invaders. In 1920, the prestigious British journal, *Lancet*, reported the use of intravenous hydrogen peroxide by British Army doctors in India treating troops suffering from influenza. It reduced their death rate from 90% to 50%. In the 1950s, hydrogen peroxide was approved by the FDA as a food additive and was used by farmers to retard spoilage in animal feed. Following this, farmers noted an unexpected health benefit in the livestock and started using hydrogen peroxide themselves as a folk remedy for arthritis and other chronic problems.

***The American Cancer Society and FDA still dispute claims for the therapeutic value of $H_2O_2$, although neither agency has attempted to investigate this modality. Again, their laxity is not surprising, since the use of $H_2O_2$ represents a potentially grave threat to the chemotherapy and drug industry: the substance is inexpensive, easily produced, and can be bought without a prescription.***

Since that time, physicians have experimented with intravenous hydrogen peroxide treatment in a number of conditions including poor circulation, heart disease, angina, emphysema, bronchitis, asthma, influenza, Lyme disease, chronic fatigue, *Candida*, parasitic infections, arthritis, and more, with excellent results. Research indicates that $H_2O_2$ stimulates natural killer cells, which attack cancer cells throughout the body.[9]

Hydrogen peroxide is a simple compound made up of a molecule of water ($H_2O$) with an extra atom of oxygen (O) attached. It is produced in all mammalian cells during normal metabolism by enzymes called oxidases. The potent antioxidant activity of the enzyme superoxide dismutase (SOD) generates $H_2O_2$ as a by-product. This process would be destructive were it not for the protection afforded by another enzyme, catalase, also found in human cells. Hydrogen peroxide also occurs naturally in rain and snow, in fruits and vegetables, and in mother's milk, with particularly high concentrations found in colostrum.[10]

Hydrogen peroxide, when given at the correct dosage, can have an oxidizing or cleansing effect, although excessive amounts can be harmful. In previous decades, conventional doctors typically warned of the potential harm that could result from ingesting concentrated $H_2O_2$. The American Cancer Society and FDA still dispute claims for the therapeutic value of $H_2O_2$, although neither agency has attempted to investigate this modality.[11] Again, their laxity is not surprising, since the use of $H_2O_2$ represents a potentially grave threat to the chemotherapy and drug industry: the substance is inexpensive, easily produced (forms when ozone gas comes into contact with water), and can be bought without a prescription.

Oxygen or oxidative therapies today are based on *dilute* $H_2O_2$ which is relatively harmless, particularly when the individual is taking antioxidant supplements that help protect the body's normal cells. Many metabolic practitioners alternate the use of intravenous $H_2O_2$ with intravenous vitamin C, often with excellent results.[12]

Modern biology is well aware of the central role played by $H_2O_2$ in human health. Macrophages and other immune cells generate $H_2O_2$ to help kill bacteria, parasites, viruses, and other pathogens. Research indicates $H_2O_2$ helps enzymes remove toxins and can directly destroy invading microbes;[13] the $H_2O_2$ produced by these immune cells has also been shown to have antitumor properties.[14] In the lungs, for example, the macrophages' cell-killing ability is largely dependent on $H_2O_2$.[15]

According to Dr. Farr, oxidation achieved through $H_2O_2$ therapy regulates tissue repair, cellular respiration, growth, immune and energy functions, most hormone systems, and the production of cytokines (chemical messengers that are involved in the regulation of almost every system in the body). Some cytokines, such as interferon and interleukin-2, play key roles in helping the immune system destroy cancer cells, and the anticancer effect of interferon seems to depend on the $H_2O_2$ generated by immune cells.[16]

Hydrogen peroxide provides an additional boost to the anticancer defenses by stimulating natural killer cells which are needed to stop the spreading of cancer cells.[17] Intravenous. $H_2O_2$ also stimulates the oxidative enzymes in the body, helping them remove toxins and exert a direct cancer-killing effect on tumor cells.[18] Dr. Farr discovered that these intravenous $H_2O_2$ infusions almost doubled the metabolic activity of various detoxifying enzymes.[19] Taken together, these effects could account for the positive clinical results observed when oxygen therapies are used to treat cancer patients.

Most of the studies that have examined the ability of $H_2O_2$ to improve the survival rates in cancer patients are based on animal research. A study of rats implanted with tumors found that when their standard drinking water was replaced by a dilute $H_2O_2$ solution, the tumors completely disappeared within 2 to 8 weeks.[20] When oral $H_2O_2$ was given to mice preinjected with cancer cells, death rates declined and onset of palpable tumors was delayed.[21] Researchers at Rockefeller University in New York concluded that $H_2O_2$ could exert a "direct antitumor effect and thereby prolong the survival of the host [cancer patient]."[22]

Further proof of the effectiveness of $H_2O_2$ was published in the *British Journal of Cancer*. Researchers injected catalase, superoxide dismutase, and glucose oxidase (all enzymes) directly into the brain tumors of laboratory animals. The $H_2O_2$ generated by enzyme combination was toxic to the tumor and significantly halted the growth of the tumor. "Oxidation therapy ... is a promising area which warrants further investigation,"[23] the researchers concluded, adding that antioxidant supplementation may be necessary to ward off potential side effects of excessive $H_2O_2$ production.

Many studies have documented the value of combining $H_2O_2$ with conventional cancer treatments. In one, $H_2O_2$ improved the outcome of chemotherapy (vinblastine);[24] in another, $H_2O_2$ injected into the arteries for 10 days, followed by mitomycin C (an antibiotic showing antitumor activity), enhanced the effectiveness of the anticancer drug.[25] $H_2O_2$ has also been shown to make cancer cells more sensitive to the effects of radiation therapy. The use of $H_2O_2$ diluted in water led to increased oxygenation in the area of the tumor. This finding led the researchers to claim an "increased therapeutic ratio" in malignant tumors subjected to irradiation (radiotherapy) when oxygen levels of the affected area are increased with $H_2O_2$.[26] More recently, doctors proposed that $H_2O_2$ could aid in the treatment of Hodgkin's lymphoma.[27]

***Patients frequently report a heightened sense of well-being, including increased mental clarity and energy levels. These responses may be related to $H_2O_2$'s releasing pure oxygen, thereby saturating all the body cells and tissues, including those of the brain.***

Other beneficial effects of $H_2O_2$ are of a subjective nature. Patients frequently report a heightened sense of well-being, including increased mental clarity and energy levels. These responses may be related to $H_2O_2$'s

## Glyoxylide—A New Way to Deliver Oxygen to the Cells

In the 1940s, the talented chemist and physician William F. Koch, M.D., Ph.D., a physiology professor at Detroit Medical College (later part of Wayne State University) reasoned that cells become cancerous because the blood's oxygen levels get depleted. If sufficient oxygen were continually delivered to the body's tissues, cancer pathology would be virtually impossible.

Dr. Koch proposed to supply oxygen by means of carbonyl and ethylene, a compound he called glyoxylide.[28] Rather than use the intravenous methods of delivery, Dr. Koch preferred to give glyoxylide only once or twice in the form of intramuscular injections in a solution diluted to 6X, a mild homeopathic level containing only 1 part of glyoxylide in 1 million parts of water.[29] Dr. Koch also experimented with parabenzoquinone (a form of quinone) for its antitumor potential.

Harold R. Stark, M.D., a physician who studied with Dr. Koch, explains that glyoxylide, the catalyst used in the chemical treatment of cancer, promotes vigorous oxygenation and oxidation activity in spite of its great dilution. The cell is literally forced to take on oxygen through aerobic metabolism and give up the waste products. In other words, glyoxylide stimulates metabolism. With the Koch remedies, the cancer cell gradually dies and becomes an encumbrance to the body until it is digested and eliminated.[30]

Dr. Koch monitored the patient's diet and drug intake, attempting to minimize the latter. Because of his desire to keep cancer patients off anticancer drugs that might interfere with metabolism, Dr. Koch was harassed and eventually sued by the FDA. He was exonerated, but he decided to continue his studies of glyoxylide elsewhere. He went to Brazil, where he died in 1967. Due to FDA obstruction, the substance is not available in the U.S.; however, physicians may import it from Germany for single patient use.

releasing pure oxygen, or stimulating greater uptake of oxygen from the air by the lungs, thereby saturating all the body cells and tissues, including those of the brain, with this life-giving element. Since cancer cells thrive in an oxygen-poor (anaerobic) environment, the new oxygen-rich conditions would favor immune cell activity and disfavor tumor growth.

There are cautions to observe regarding hydrogen peroxide. Ross Pelton, Ph.D., reports that the medical staff at the Hospital Santa Monica in Mexico administered over 30,000 infusions of dilute hydrogen peroxide without a serious or life-threatening reaction.[28] On some occasions, however, a stinging or burning sensation occurred at the infusion site; patients with smaller veins tended to experience more of this discomfort, which is transitory and otherwise appears harmless. In rare cases, inflammation of the veins at the site of injection will occur. Dr. Pelton states that slowing down the rate of the infusion usually is sufficient to reduce the inflammation and attendant discomfort.

Hydrogen peroxide should not be taken orally as it causes nausea and vomiting, and rectal administration can lead to inflammation of the lower intestinal tract. Other effects can include temporary faintness, fatigue, headaches, and chest pain. However, most problems stem from the use of either an inappropriate administration route, administration above the individual's tolerance level, mixing oxidative chemicals with other substances, or using oxidative chemicals in too great a concentration, states Dr. Charles Farr, who has developed a protocol for IV administration of hydrogen peroxide.[32]

## HYDROGEN PEROXIDE IN THE TREATMENT OF METASTATIC BONE AND BRAIN CANCERS

Alternative cancer physician and certified oncologist Vincent Speckhart, M.D. (see Chapter 20) reported satisfactory preliminary results with hydrogen peroxide to treat cancer. In his research, Dr. Speckhart recorded impressive results in treating metastatic bone and brain cancers with intravenous $H_2O_2$. At the First International Conference on Bio-Oxidative Medicine, he reported that this treatment enhanced the therapeutic effects of the radiation.[33]

"There did seem to be a benefit for patients who were undergoing radiotherapy," Dr. Speckhart says. "My impression was that there was a protective effect on normal tissue and an accelerated effect on tumor tissue." In addition, the sick tissue around the cancer appeared to recover more rapidly after the radiation treatment.

Prior to the radiation treatment, Dr. Speckhart had given his patients a solution of 0.03% peroxide (very low concentration), and found that the high oxygen content was maintained even during the radiation treatment. Today, he believes that the dosages commonly used for hydrogen peroxide may be too high. "Lower doses may be equally as effective," he says. The more Dr. Speckhart manages people with chronic illness, the lower his recommended dosage levels tend to be. He has discontinued the $H_2O_2$ modality, not for therapeutic reasons but because of pressure exerted on him by the Virginia State Medical Board which does not approve of this modality.

## The Ozone Story

Around 1900, interest began to focus on the uses of ozone in medical therapy. It is estimated that more than 10 million ozone treatments have been given over the last 40 years worldwide and more than 1,000 articles on the subject have been published in medical and scientific journals, mostly in German, Russian, and Spanish.

Used primarily to kill viruses, destroy bacteria, and eliminate fungi, ozone produces important benefits in the human body, including the oxygenation of blood, improved blood circulation, and stimulation of the immune system. The range of human health problems that respond favorably to ozone therapy is broad and includes AIDS, arthritis, asthma, cancer, fungal diseases, gangrene, hepatitis, sinusitis, atherosclerosis, and more. Medical-grade ozone is made from pure oxygen. Ozone has been used clinically to increase local oxygen supply to lesions, improve and accelerate wound healing, deactivate viruses, bacteria, and fungi increase local tissue temperature, thus enhancing local metabolic processes.

## Ozone Can Stimulate Energy-Producing Activity

Another oxygen therapy uses ozone and relies on both oxidation and oxygenation pathways. Approximately 20% of the air we breathe is comprised of oxygen, which has 2 atoms ($O_2$). Ozone ($O_3$) contains 3 oxygen atoms and is a less stable form of oxygen. Due to this added molecule, ozone is more reactive than oxygen and readily oxidizes other chemicals. During oxidation in the body, the extra oxygen molecule in ozone can break away, leaving a normal $O_2$ molecule. Often it does this by combining with water to form hydrogen peroxide and oxygen. The net result is to increase the oxygen content of the blood or tissues. Thus ozone therapy is a combination of both oxygenation therapy and oxidation therapy.

In nature, oxygen released from plants floats upward into the atmosphere. Some of the oxygen is converted to ozone when ultraviolet energy from the sun or lightning temporarily recombines the oxygen into groups of 3 atoms. This is what gives air its fresh fragrance after a rainstorm.

Many Americans think of ozone as an air pollutant, present, for example, in the Los Angeles smog. Although it is true that high concentrations of ozone may be irritating to the lungs and cause free radical damage, controlled use of ozone may be beneficial for many purposes, such as the purification of air and water. Ozone air purification devices are used in bowling alleys, bars, and homes to cleanse the air of smoke and other pollutants. The City of Los Angeles uses ozone to purify its water system and many swimming pools are now kept clean with an ozone water purification system rather than with chlorine. This is much healthier for the swimmer. What is generally not known is that ozone has many medical uses as well.

Ozone can be administered intravenously, intra-arterially, intramuscularly (within the muscle), intra-articularly (into the joint), and subcutaneously (just beneath the skin). In the case of intravenous use of ozone, this is usually done by incrementally removing up to 1 quart of the patient's blood from a vein, mixing it with ozone gas, then reinjecting it into the body. Ozone may be applied topically as a gas or dissolved in water or olive oil, then applied to the skin. As a gas, it may be blown in vaginally or rectally; it may also be taken orally, rectally, or vaginally in the form of ozonated water. One of the most effective methods is to inject humidified ozone into the rectum, getting it directly into the bloodstream; this is ozone saturated with water, thereby dissolved in water vapor.[34] This facilitates getting therapeutic ozone concentrations easily and rapidly into the bloodstream.

***Ozone therapy can enhance the tumor-fighting ability of standard cancer drugs. Ozone seems to stimulate the activity of cytokines, natural cancer-killing proteins.***

Evidence shows that ozone has strong therapeutic value. It can selectively inhibit cancer cell growth in tissue culture for cancers of the lung, breast, and uterus when given in doses of as little as 0.3 to 0.8 parts per million (ppm) over a period of 8 days.[35] Exposure to the 0.8-ppm dose inhibited cancer cell growth more than 90%. The growth of normal cells was not inhibited, which suggested that "cancer cells are less able to compensate for the oxidative burden of ozone than normal cells."[36] At sea level (atmospheric pressure), ozone bubbled into drinking water or enema water will concentrate ozone in the water only up to 52 ppm which is still nontoxic to healthy human cells provided it is complemented daily with adequate antioxidant nutrients. However, the ozone content in ozonated water decreases rapidly after the ozonation bubbling of the water ceases.

Ozone therapy can also enhance the tumor-fighting ability of standard cancer drugs.[37] Test doses of ozone were found to selectively block the division of cancer cells (but not normal cells); this positive effect increased as the ozone doses got stronger until all cancer-cell activity was virtually halted at high doses.[38] Ozone seems to stimulate the activity of cytokines, natural cancer-killing proteins.[39]

To date, no controlled studies of ozone therapy have been conduct-

***Test doses of ozone were found to selectively block the division of cancer cells (but not normal cells); this positive effect increased as the doses got stronger until all cancer-cell activity was virtually halted at high doses.***

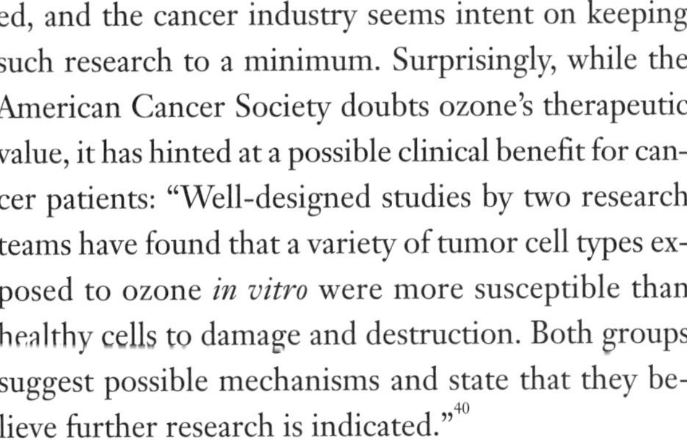

ed, and the cancer industry seems intent on keeping such research to a minimum. Surprisingly, while the American Cancer Society doubts ozone's therapeutic value, it has hinted at a possible clinical benefit for cancer patients: "Well-designed studies by two research teams have found that a variety of tumor cell types exposed to ozone *in vitro* were more susceptible than healthy cells to damage and destruction. Both groups suggest possible mechanisms and state that they believe further research is indicated."[40]

Until such further research is carried out, clinical case records provide the best evidence for the efficacy of ozone. For example, practitioners at the Hospital Santa Monica in Mexico have reported a 3-year remission rate of 70% with advanced cancer patients who were treated with ozone, botanicals, nutrition, DMSO, hyperthermia, and other natural modalities. Three years may not sound like a long time, but the official prognosis for the majority of these patients was less than one year. Similarly impressive results have been reported by Dr. Horst Kief of Germany; Dr. Kief integrates oxygen therapies into his specialized form of immune enhancement.[41]

For more information about oxygen therapy protocols, see Chapter 18: Michael B. Schachter, M.D., p. 348.

German surgeon Joachim Varro, M.D., has worked with hundreds of cancer patients, most of whom had received chemotherapy and radiation. Dr. Varro found that ozone therapy greatly reduces pain while increasing energy levels and appetite. Dr. Varro noted the following: (1) patients were free of metastases and recurrences for remarkably long periods of time; (2) the survival time could be prolonged, far exceeding the usual dubious prognoses of conventional treatment; and (3) most patients who had undergone ozone therapy shortly after surgery and radiation could return to full-time work.[42]

Jonathan Wright, M.D., medical director of the Tahoma Clinic in Kent, Washington, successfully used ozone therapy to treat a patient with a goose-egg-sized tumor on her right ear. Her conventional doctor said it could not be treated and gave her 6 months to live. Dr. Wright applied ozone topically at the site of the tumor, and then injected ozone directly into the tumor. The tumor regressed in size, and although a small lump remained, the patient recovered.

As with hydrogen peroxide, the prudent physician will observe caution with ozone therapy. Any time oxygen therapies are used, the possibility of generating excess free radicals must be guarded against by taking dietary antioxidants. "You can't use ozone alone," says Dr. Wright. "You need to combine it with a proper diet, [nutritional] supplements, herbs, botanicals, acupuncture, and chiropractic." Antioxidants (chemicals or substances that can neutralize free radicals or oxidizing agents) such as vitamin C should be given to all patients who are receiving any form of oxygen therapy since they prevent uncontrolled oxidation which is detrimental to the body.

Adverse effects associated with intravenously administered ozone can include phlebitis (inflammation of a vein), circulatory depression, chest pain, shortness of breath, fainting, coughing, flushing, cardiac arrhythmias, and gas bubbles. Rectal administration of ozone can lead to inflammation of the lower intestinal tract. Although it is easily tolerated in other tissues, ozone in high concentrations can cause severe inflammation of the lung tissues and even coughing up of blood.

## Ozone and the Politics of Medicine

This is a quietly inflammatory documentary about oxygen and its role in healing and the political aspect of product licensing by the FDA that is keeping ozone out of American doctors' offices.

Ozone, which is an energized form of oxygen, is now used in 2000 cities worldwide to disinfect public water supplies. For the last 30 years, physicians in Germany have used ozone therapy (oxygen is mixed with a patient's drawn blood then reinfused into the body) to successfully treat cancer, stroke, gangrene, eczema, burns wounds, pain, herpes, hepatitis, and now AIDS—40 medical conditions in all.

In fact, a 1980 study revealed that, of 1000 German therapists who gave ozone treatment to 5 million patients, 90% said the approach was effective and that it produced the lowest level of side effects of any existing medical treatment.

So why does the FDA condemn ozone therapy as untested, undocumented, and unsafe, and want somebody to shell out $231 million to prove them wrong? That's the politics of ozone. Meanwhile, Americans are flying to Germany or Mexico to get the healing benefits of oxygen. "Ozone is inexpensive, very potent, and if it works even one-half as well as the Germans claim, everyone in the world should be using it," says one prominent American physician who endorses it. "Ozone is the most important drug in the world," says another. Find out why in this excellent, clearly argued, and persuasive triple award-winning video.

These claims are valid assuming one consults a qualified, practitioner experienced in ozone therapy and that the techniques are properly used.

Source: Geoffrey Rogers, producer/director; Threshold Film, #301-356 E. 6th Avenue, Vancouver, V5T 1K1, Canada (tel: 800-216-4403); 1994, 30 minutes, VHS-color, $39.

# Enzymes

**Enzymes are crucial for digestion of all foods, especially protein, but when protein is inadequately broken down, due to enzyme deficiencies, it putrefies in the intestinal tract and tends to form ammonia, a highly toxic compound and a known carcinogen. Enzyme therapy gets the appropriate enzymes back into the body.**

One of the factors that can impede the body's ability to ward off cancer is a lack of enzymes. These are molecules that cause key transformations of organic substances, speed up or catalyze biochemical reactions, and keep metabolism running smoothly and efficiently. Diseases result when enzymes are inadequately produced or when essential elements are lacking in the diet; when minerals or trace elements are missing, the enzymatic action can be seriously upset.

For example, the trace element selenium is needed for the enzyme glutathione peroxidase, one of the body's essential antioxidant enzymes; manganese, copper, and zinc are required by another important antioxidant system, called superoxide dismutase (SOD). When these trace elements are inadequately supplied or unavailable, the resulting enzyme dysfunction can increase the body's vulnerability to toxins and harmful free radicals which, in turn, can help promote the growth of tumors.

The problem of enzyme dysfunction manifests at 2 fundamental levels: digestive and systemic. At the level of digestion, the body's inability to effectively metabolize protein may promote cancer. This inability may be linked to improper amounts of proteolytic (protein-digesting) enzymes such as pepsin from the stomach and proteases from the pancreas which, along with hydrochloric acid (HCl) in the stomach, are the body's first defense against cancer development.

## The Nature and Work of Enzymes

As people age, they tend to lose their capacity to produce sufficient amounts of digestive enzymes, as well as HCl. Protein is normally broken down into smaller nutritive units, called amino acids, which are then absorbed in the small intestine to be synthesized into proteins; these eventually become neurotransmitters (chemical messengers in the brain), functional hormones, antibodies, metabolic and digestive enzymes, cell membrane receptors, and myriad other structural components the body needs for healthy functioning. Approximately 50% of the daily utilization of protein by the living organism goes into producing enzymes, a major share of which is digestive enzymes.[43]

When protein is inadequately broken down, it putrefies in the intestinal tract and tends to form nitrosamines and ammonia, highly toxic compounds and known carcinogens. Although the extent to which ammonia may contribute to the development of cancer is unknown, some researchers speculate that it may significantly increase one's susceptibility to colon cancer. The effective action of digestive juices is critical not only for protein digestion, but also for processing of essential micronutrients—both vitamins and minerals.

Many of these micronutrients are bound up within protein complexes in food. To make these micronutrients available to the body, digestive enzymes and HCl must be secreted in adequate amounts. A lack of such secretions in later life is one of the reasons older people are more prone to mineral deficiencies and vitamin B12 deficiency, for example, regardless of the presence of these in their food. The absorption of many other vitamins and essential nutrients (like coenzyme Q10) can be similarly impeded by a lack of hydrochloric acid and digestive enzyme activity.

The human body makes approximately 22 different types of digestive enzymes, capable of digesting protein, carbohydrates, sugars, and fats. People digest food in stages: beginning in the mouth, moving to the stomach, and finally through the small intestine. At each step, specific enzymes break down dif-

## An Enzyme Primer

The following are some of the health conditions commonly associated with shortages of each of the 4 basic enzymes:

- **Protease (digests proteins)**

Anxiety; low blood sugar; kidney problems or disease; water retention; depressed immunity; bacterial and viral infections; cancer; appendicitis; bone problems, such as osteoporosis, arthritis, and bone spurs.

- **Amylase (digests non-fiber carbohydrates)**

Skin problems such as rashes, hives, fungal infections, herpes, and canker sores; lung problems such as asthma, bronchitis, and emphysema; liver or gallbladder disease.

- **Lipase (digests fats)**

High cholesterol; obesity; diabetes; "hardening" of the artery linings and other cardiovascular problems; high blood pressure; chronic fatigue; spastic colon; dizziness.

- **Cellulase (digests fiber)**

Gas and bloating; acute food allergies; facial pain or paralysis; candidiasis (bowel and vaginal yeast infections).

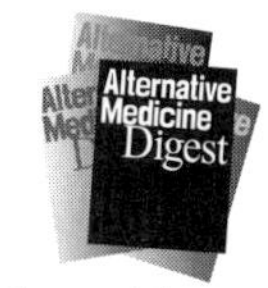


For more information on enzymes, see "Reversing Asthma, Seizures, and Colon Problems with Enzymes," Lita Lee, Ph.D., #14, pp. 40-43.

ferent types of food. An enzyme designed to digest protein, for example, has no effect on starch, and an enzyme active in the mouth will not be active in the stomach. This process is balanced through acidity; each site along the digestive tract has a different degree of acidity that allows certain enzymes to function while inhibiting others. Ideally, these enzymes work together, digesting food and delivering nutrients to cells to maintain their health. Protocols in enzyme therapy are based on this sequence of events.

Most of the digestive enzymes are produced by the pancreas and include proteases, amylases, and lipases. Pancreatic enzymes function in both the intestine and in the blood. Supplemental pancreatic enzymes from animal sources can aid digestion in the intestine, sharing the workload of the body's own pancreatic enzymes that are active there; however, they do not digest food in the stomach, or contribute to the important step of predigestion.

***The use of anticoagulants and proteolytic enzymes can effectively reduce the invasive or metastatic potential of cancer cells.In other words, by removing the "sticky" coating found on tumor cells, enzymes reduce the risk of tumors adhering to other areas of the body (i.e., prevent metastasis).***

Enzyme therapy can be an important first step in restoring health and well-being by helping to remedy digestive problems. Plant enzymes and pancreatic enzymes are used in complementary ways to improve digestion and absorption of essential nutrients and to enhance the immune system's ability to recognize and destroy cancer cells. Both plant-derived enzymes and animal-derived pancreatic enzymes are used in enzyme therapy, independently or in combination.

Plant enzymes are prescribed primarily to enhance the body's vitality by strengthening the digestive system, while pancreatic enzymes have historically been used to benefit both the digestive system and immune system. As proper digestive functioning is restored, many acute and chronic conditions are usually improved. For strict vegetarians (vegans) and those persons allergic to beef and pork, plant enzymes can be used efficiently to aid the immune system as well as to support food digestion.

Depending on the situation, some enzymes are given with meals to facilitate the breakdown and assimilation of protein, while some are given between meals to act as a "scavenger" of abnormal protein found in the bloodstream (the latter function is explained in the next section). Enzymes that may be given with meals include the proteases, amylases, or lipases.

Those usually given between meals include primarily the proteases and lipases, since those are the scavengers.

Pancreatic enzymes can help in the treatment of cancer in several ways. Enzymes help expose foreign antigens on the surface of cancer cells so they can be recognized as foreign and be destroyed by the immune system. They also help destroy CICs (circulating immune complexes) produced when cancerous cells shed their antigens into the blood, seemingly to avoid detection by the immune system. Pancreatic enzymes can stimulate natural killer cells, T cells, and tumor necrosis factor (anticancer agents), all toxic to cancer cells.

***Enzyme therapy improves the immune system's responsiveness to cancer by uncovering the cancer cell's surface receptors and by reducing the stickiness of tumor cells.***

While the protective role of enzymes against tumors is not widely appreciated in the United States, many European physicians know that enzymes play an invaluable role in keeping cancers from spreading or developing into "terminal tumors"—those capable of spreading and killing their host. The metastatic potential of a tumor depends, in part, on the adhesiveness of the cancer cells, i.e., their capacity to adhere to cell walls. Adhesiveness, in turn, seems to depend on the blood's "stickiness" or ability to coagulate. The greater this adhesive quality, the greater the capacity of the tumor to develop metastases.[44]

The use of anticoagulants and proteolytic enzymes can effectively reduce the invasive or metastatic potential of cancer cells.[45] In addition, it is now thought that the cancer cell uses a protein called fibrin (or sometimes fats and lipids) to mask its identity, effectively hiding it from recognition by the immune system. A logical therapeutic strategy would involve selectively degrading the cancer cell's fibrin and lipid coating, thus allowing the true cancer cell component (antigen) to be identified by the immune system, which could then mount an effective, full-scale attack and halt the progression of a potential metastasis.[46]

In other words, by removing the "sticky" coating found on tumor cells, enzymes reduce the risk of tumors adhering to other areas of the body (i.e., prevent metastasis). Pancreatic enzymes can enter cancer cells in their reproductive phase, when they are not completely formed and arc more susceptible to destruction, and start deactivating them. Vitamin A, incidentally, increases these effects, as it releases enzymes contained in lysosomes (components of the intracellular "digestive" system that consumes bacteria and other extraneous materials in white blood cells). In Germany, some physicians dissolve tumors by injecting pancreatic enzyme solutions directly into them.

At the First International Conference on Systemic Enzyme Therapy in 1990, Professor H. Wrba, a renowned Austrian physician and researcher, reported that systemic enzyme therapy improves the immune system's responsiveness to cancer by uncovering the cancer cell's surface receptors and by reducing the stickiness of tumor cells.[47]

Enzymes also play a therapeutically vital role in the relationship between digestion and immune overload. Protein molecules that are only partially digested in the small intestine can be absorbed in this state into the bloodstream. The immune system treats these substances as invaders, causing antibodies to form and couple with these antigens and create circulating immune complexes (CICs). In a healthy person, CICs (as complexes of antibodies and food or tumor antigens) may be neutralized in the lymphatic system, but in a person with cancer, CICs tend to accumulate in the blood where they burden the detoxification pathways or initiate an allergic reaction.

If too many CICs accumulate, the kidneys cannot excrete enough of them. The CICs then accumulate in soft tissues, causing inflammation and bringing unnecessary stress to the immune system. Enzyme expert Howard Loomis, D.C. comments: "I always wonder why the diets for cancer and AIDS include such high amounts of protein when an excess of undigested protein can so obviously lead to demands on the immune system." It is here that pancreatic enzymes come into play. Pancreatic enzymes break down CICs enabling them to pass through the kidneys for excretion.

Enzymes given as supplements can help cancer patients by reducing the level of circulating immune complexes (CICs) in the body. In many cases, CICs become more numerous with advanced cancer because each tumor releases large amounts of antigens. Over time, an accumulation of CICs can impose a serious burden on the immune system. High concentrations of CICs are associated with poorer prognoses in cancer patients.[48] In 75% of patients with acute leukemia in remission, for example, no CICs could be found.[49]

Research has shown that enzyme combinations can effectively reduce the numbers of CICs; in addition, the rate of degradation of CICs increases as the enzyme dosage increases.[50] As the level of CICs in the blood diminishes, many cancer patients experience marked improvements in their well-being.[51] Among the signs of this rejuvenating potential are improved appetite, weight gain, and increased vitality.[52] Many patients also report a decrease in depression and anxiety, as well as an increased ability to move or exercise.[53]

When too much of the enzyme production is allotted for digestion of food in the gut, less may be available for systemic protection against cancer (such as reducing CIC levels). "Ideally, you want to make it unnecessary for the digestive system to have to produce so many digestive enzymes," says Jack Taylor, D.C., who uses enzymes in his anticancer program (see Chapter 22). "If you assist in the process of digestion by providing food enzymes such as those found in papaya or pineapple, you can divert the body's overall enzyme production so that it has a greater capacity to make and channel more metabolic enzymes to the site of malignancy and normalize its enzyme chemistry."

Also, if a patient eats a lot of dairy products, meats, and cooked foods (whose own enzymes are destroyed in the cooking), then most of their pancreatic enzymes will be used up digesting foods, but if mostly raw fruits and raw vegetables are eaten, the active enzymes in these foods can assist in their own digestion, leaving more of the patient's pancreatic enzymes available to digest CICs and coatings on their cancer cells.

Some European physicians addressing cancer and other illnesses use special enzyme formulations called Wobenzyme® and Wobe-Mugos®, first developed in Germany. These formulas contain pancreatin, papain, bromelain, trypsin, chymotrypsin, lipase, amylase, and rutin (a bioflavonoid), and are administered variously in the form of injection, tablets, or suppositories.

The German physician Max Wolf, M.D., started using Wobe-Mugos and other multi-enzyme formulas in 1949. He treated over 1,000 patients using oral doses of 200 mg daily, then raising it to 2-4 g daily. Surveying the results of his work in 1972, Dr. Wolf explained that Wobenzyme appeared to curtail the spread of cancer and moderately prolong survival. For

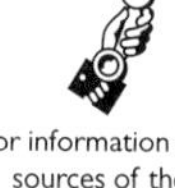

For information and sources of the **Chirozyme enzymes** developed by Howard Loomis, D.C., contact: 21st Century Nutrition, 6421 Enterprise Lane, Madison, WI 53719; tel: 800-662-2630 or 608-273-8100; fax: 608-273-8110. For information on the **Intenzyme Forte** and **Retenzyme Forte** brand of enzymes (used by Dr. Victor A. Marcial-Vega, see Chapter 13), contact: Biotics Research Corp., P.O. Box 36888, Houston, TX 77236; tel: 713-240-8010; fax: 713-240-2304. For information about **Gastroprotective Enzymes** (a plant enzyme combination) or the individual enzymes protease, lipase, amylase, and cellulase, contact: Health Restoration Systems, P.O. Box 832267, Richardson, TX 75083; tel: 972-480-8909; tel: 972-238-0327.

## Enzymes' Anti-cancer Benefits

By providing enzyme supplements that aid in protein digestion, the person with cancer has more enzyme power to run the body properly and to prevent cancer or perhaps even reverse the course of cancer. In summary, the 3 primary effects of using enzymes are (1) to expose the cancer cell's antigens by removing the fibrin coating, thus making the cancer cell an easier target for the immune system; (2) to reduce the adhesiveness of cancer and other cells, thus making it harder for cancer cells to adhere to cell walls; and (3) to reduce the levels of circulating immune complexes, which tend to weaken the immune system's ability to respond to the cancer.

107 women who had undergone mastectomies, their 5-year survival rate was 84% under Wobenzyme therapy compared to 43% to 48% with conventional therapy, reported Dr. Wolf. Localized application produced better results than systemic uses, and long-term use of the enzyme formula produced the best results in stopping the spread of cancer.

Research reported by the product's manufacturer indicated that pancreatic cancer responded well to this treatment, with 30 patients still alive 2 years after receiving the enzymes; some of these patients survived 5-9 years. All of this must be seen in contrast to the "standard" survival expectation of 7 months for pancreatic cancer. For post-surgical breast cancer patients with stage I and III cancers, the use of Wobe-Mugos produced 5-year survival rates of 91% and 58% respectively, compared to 78% and 42% under conventional treatment.[54] Wobe-Mugos® and other anticancer enzyme mixtures pioneered in Germany can help restore the immune system and attack cancer cells. One way it does this is by degrading tumor antigens and antibodies (known as "pathogenic immune complexes") that may disable the immune system over time.

Enzymes produced by the pancreas also prevent cancer from gaining a foothold in the body by digesting fibrin, a protein component necessary for blood clotting and cancer cell formation. This degradation of fibrin prevents the attachment of pre-cancerous cells to body tissues, thus releasing these cells into the blood where they are normally destroyed. Finally, the enzymes degrade the fibrin layer over cancer cells, which is about 15 times thicker than that of normal cells, according to Dr. Etienne Callebout (see Chapter 4). As mentioned earlier, this fibrin coating would otherwise hide the tumor antigens from the immune system, so that the system would fail to mount an attack against the tumor. There is evidence that enzyme therapy can increase T cell counts.[55] In other research, protein-digesting enzymes (proteases such as bromelain) induced the transformation of cancer cells into normal cells.

# Glandular and Organ Extracts (DHEA, Melatonin, Thymosin, T3 Thyroid)

**Purified extracts from the endocrine glands of animals can have considerable clinical benefit in helping to restore a cancer patient's overall metabolism, especially when a physician knows that the patient's own endocrine levels are low. Key glandulars frequently used are thyroid, thymus, and adrenal.**

Glandular and organ extracts usually taken from animals (known clinically as protomorphogens) can be an important component of a complete nutritional program. These substances provide immediate help as well as long-term benefits, so are particularly useful to the nutritional practitioner. Typical extracts drawn from animal sources include extracts from the pituitary, thyroid, adrenals, pancreas, heart, liver, kidney, thymus, and other glands and organs; they are called for when a patient's endocrine system is underproducing or undersecreting a specific hormone or when an organ is weakened or diseased. The efficacy of these extracts is generally recognized, yet they are all too often overlooked in conventional medicine.

Prior to the 1940s and the advent of "modern" technological medicine, glandular extracts were in wide use, and a considerable amount of research was in progress to support their use. World War II sparked a shift in priority to the development of antibiotics such as Sulfa drugs. Government funding by the United States and other nations soon resulted in the discovery of penicillin and other antibiotics. As drug companies launched their lucrative ventures into the drug business, research in glandular therapy came to a halt. However, the fact that the glandular approach was set aside does nothing to diminish the validity of its therapeutic value.

Glandulars are used nutritionally for 3 reasons:

## The Thyroid's Role in Cancer Resistance

From 1930 to 1980, Broda Barnes, M.D., Ph.D., a researcher at the University of Chicago, sought to uncover the thyroid's role in cancer. According to this physiologist-physician's shocking estimates, approximately 40% of the U.S. population suffers from chronically low thyroid function, or hypothyroidism. Most doctors would consider this figure absurd until they understand that the manifestation of this problem is quite different from that of an acute thyroid problem.

Dr. Barnes' pioneering research indicated that a low thyroid function may manifest simply as a relatively constant (basal) body temperature of less than 97.8° F. Among the many symptoms of low-thyroid function identified by Dr. Barnes are coldness, constipation, easy weight gain, heavy periods, regular miscarriages, elevated blood fats (lipids), mental confusion, depression, and hypoglycemia, as well as an increased risk for both diabetes and cancer.[56] Given that thyroid hormones affect the metabolism of cells and tissues throughout the body, this list should not necessarily be considered an improbable hodgepodge.

To test for suboptimal thyroid function, take your body temperature (by placing a thermometer under the tongue) first thing in the morning on several consecutive days before getting out of bed. If your temperature is below 97.8° F, you may benefit by taking an iodine or kelp supplement. Other alternatives for reviving normal thyroid function include ginseng, chromium, and L-carnitine.[57] If the patient is deficient in various nutrients that support the thyroid (iodine, chromium, copper, L-carnitine, and selenium, for example[58]), this gland's function becomes depressed, and the functioning of the immune system declines accordingly. If one's temperature is consistently less than 98.2° F, the immune system is suboptimal and thyroid medication may be indicated.

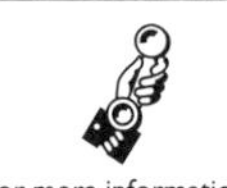

For more information about **glandular extracts**, contact: Innovative Therapeutics, 2020 Franklin Street, Carlyle, IL 62231-0512; tel: 888-688-9922 or 618-594-7711; fax: 618-594-7712. Also contact: Professional Health Products, P.O. Box 80085, Portland, OR 97280; tel: 503-245-2720 or 800-952-2219; fax: 503-452-1239.

**1. Active components**—These are the biochemical substances particular to the glandular tissue being administered. The effect of the biochemical compound often is one of "substituting" an exogenous (externally generated) source to make up for the endogenous (internally generated) deficiency. Examples include thymosin from the thymus and thyroid hormone from the thyroid gland.

**2. Associated nutritional factors**—Numerous nutrients are naturally present in glandular tissue, including vitamins, minerals, amino acids, fatty acids, polypeptides, enzymes, and many other substances. These can supply essential nutritional needs in a highly efficient manner.

**3. Adaptogenic effect—**This is the "support" role. For a tissue cell to repair or replace itself, it must have the raw materials necessary. "Like supports like" is the concept here: failing organs, glands, and tissues should be treated biologically with material corresponding in its entirety to these organs, glands and tissues.

Biochemist Jeffrey Bland, Ph.D., proposes a rational explanation for how these products work. "Glandular-based food supplements may contain small polypeptide, protein-like substances which have specific messenger activity and which act on target tissues."[59] Many of the hormones found in the glandular tissues, even at low concentrations, still have potent tissue-specific activities, according to Dr. Bland. "A small polypeptide material present in one tissue can have selective effects in encouraging another tissue at a different site in the body to produce hormonal materials, which may then affect a final target tissue and change its physiological function."[60]

The thyroid gland regulates metabolism by releasing hormones that control energy production in all the body's cells; thyroid extract helps cells eliminate cellular waste and speeds up their restorative functions. In this way, a healthy thyroid increases the body's cancer-resisting ability.

The raw materials for the glandular products come preferentially from lambs raised on the south island of New Zealand. "Lamb is preferred over other animals because of their resistance to disease," says Jack Taylor, D.C., (see Chapter 22) who uses them as part of his cancer treatment protocols. "The sheep of New Zealand are considered disease-free. Moreover, there's a low incidence of patient intolerance to lamb." The New Zealand lambs are raised on pesticide-free range lands and do not receive antibiotics or steroids.

Sheep can manufacture their own vitamins, and since they eat almost anything growing on their range land, their tissue contains a wide variety of nutrients. Dr. Taylor notes that the sheep digestive system produces enzymes more similar to human than either cows or pigs, the usual source of most glandular extracts. In addition, sheep tissue contains 2

An **antigen** is any substance (a toxin, bacteria, amoeba, or protein) that the body comes to regard as foreign and dangerous to itself. As such, an antigen induces a state of cellular sensitivity or immune reaction that seeks to neutralize, remove, or destroy the antigen by dispatching antibodies against it. An **antibody** is a protein molecule containing about 20,000 atoms, made from amino acids by B lymphocyte cells in the lymph tissue and set in motion by the immune system against a specific foreign protein, or antigen. An antibody is also referred to as an immunoglobulin and may be found in the blood, lymph, colostrum, saliva, and the gastrointestinal and urinary tracts, usually within 3 days after the first encounter with an antigen. The antibody binds tightly with the antigen as a preliminary for removing it from the system or destroying it.

A **glandular extract** is a purified nutritional and therapeutic product derived from one of several animal glands including the adrenal, thymus, thyroid, pancreas, pineal, and pituitary, and prescribed by a physician for a person whose own corresponding gland is underfunctioning and not producing enough of its own hormone. The various glands are part of the endocrine system which, along with the nervous system, coordinates the functioning of all of the body's functional systems.

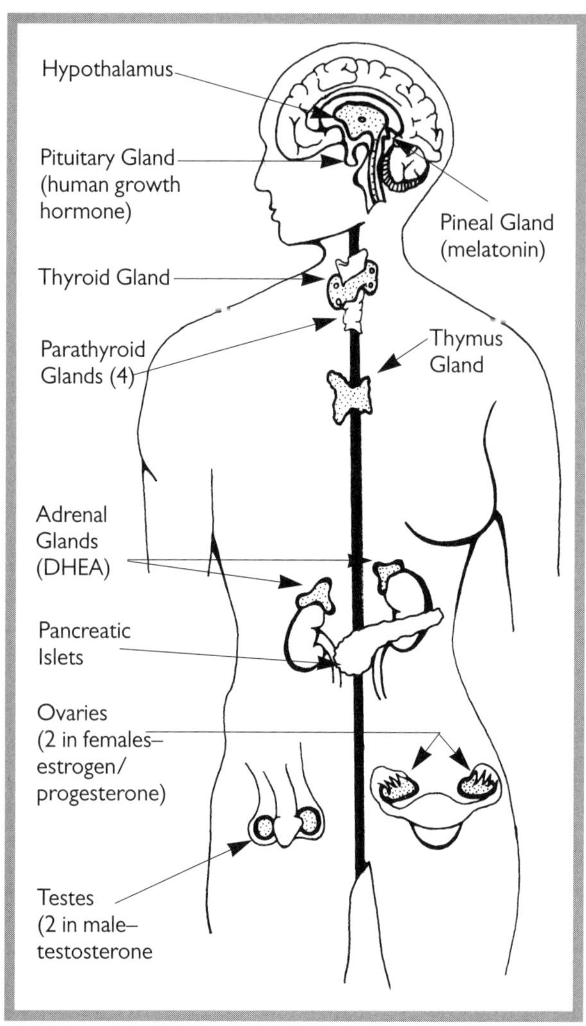


**Figure 32.1—The glandular system**

enzymes found in only one other living organism—the human body. These enzymes are (1) aldose reductase, an enzyme for sugar breakdown, and (2) steroid 17-20 lyase, an enzyme for both producing steroidal hormones and for the subsequent detoxification of those hormones from the body.

All New Zealand lambs must be certified by licensed veterinarians as healthy and free of disease, including scrapie, the presumed cause of mad cow disease. Processing begins immediately after the organs are obtained to prevent enzymatic breakdown of the tissue. The glandular extracts are prepared by a special low heat or "cold" process called lyophilization (freeze drying), which preserves intact the vitamins, minerals, enzymes, amino acids, and other tissue factors naturally present in the whole gland. After freeze drying, the glands are milled into a powder ready for placement in capsules.

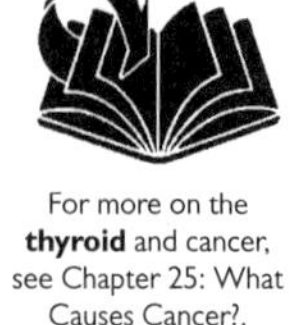

For more on the **thyroid** and cancer, see Chapter 25: What Causes Cancer?, p. 619-621.

Does the human body digest the glandular extracts as it would any protein? "Apparently not," Dr. Taylor notes. "The concept that proteins undergo absorption and enter cells whole is a difficult one, but recently it has been demonstrated that they can pass through cell membranes intact." Various antigens, or foreign proteins, can pass through the intestinal wall without first being broken down or degraded by the digestive juices.[61]

Dr. Taylor cautions that glandular extracts are not intended as a "cure" for any specific disease or condition of any organ: "The [extracts] provide nutritional support to assist normal cellular function and repair. Specific supplementation advice for glandular extracts should be made only after a determination of need. If you experience difficulty with any glandular concentrate or any other product, consult your physician."

**CAUTION**

DHEA has been shown to promote liver cancer in laboratory animals[62] and may also promote breast cancer in postmenopausal women.[63] Many uncertainties remain concerning the use of DHEA in cancer therapy; for example, hormone-sensitive cancers such as prostate cancer may actually be promoted by the compound.[64] Those people diagnosed with hormone-sensitive cancers should generally avoid taking DHEA. Most physicians who use DHEA recommend frequent measurements and careful monitoring of circulating levels of DHEA-sulfate.

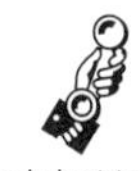

Licensed physicians may order 24-hour **urine or blood tests for DHEA levels** in patients by contacting: Meridian Valley Clinical Laboratory, 515 W. Harrison, Suite 9, Kent, WA 98032; tel: 206-859-8700; fax: 206-859-1135. **DHEA** is available in a prepared supplement called Endogen™. Actual dosages will vary with the individual or according to a physician's prescription, but can range from 25 mg to 3000 mg/day per person. For more information, contact: LifePlus, P.O. Box 3749, Batesville, AR 72503; tel: 800-572-8446. For another source, contact: Nature's Plus Company (which makes a sublingual DHEA spray), 548 Broadhollow Road, Melville, NY 11747. Only 1-2 sprays daily are required (as it contains 12.5 mg per spray).

## A Brief Glossary of Useful Hormones and Glandular Extracts

### DHEA (DEHYDROEPIANDROSTERONE)

DHEA is a naturally occurring hormone produced in the adrenal glands. In fact, it is the most abundant hormone found in the human bloodstream until the normal course of aging depletes it dramatically. If you live to be 80, your body will probably have only 10-20% of the DHEA it had when you were 20 years old. The healthiest older humans usually have the highest DHEA levels, while the sickest individuals have the lowest levels.

Low DHEA levels can leave one vulnerable to breast, prostate, and bladder cancer, atherosclerotic plaque, nerve degeneration, and other age-related conditions. Shoring up one's dwindling reserves of DHEA, according to medical research, can help prevent these conditions and improve memory, treat lupus and osteoporosis in women, and even help prevent diabetes, Parkinson's, and Alzheimer's.

DHEA is called the "mother of all hormones" because not only does it have many functions in the body pertaining to health and longevity, but it is the substance from which other important hormones, such as estrogen, progesterone, and testosterone, are made. Evidence (4,000 medical papers, so far) strongly suggests that DHEA hormone replacement therapy can work wonders for your health as you age.

**CLINIC HIGHLIGHT:**

## Metabolic Therapies at American Biologics Hospital

One of the largest metabolic treatment centers in operation today is the American Biologics Hospital in Tijuana, Mexico, headed by Robert Bradford, D.Sc., and Rodrigo Rodriguez, M.D. The elimination of dietary sugar, excess animal protein, refined carbohydrates, and stimulants such as caffeine, and the use of amygdalin (laetrile) as well as nutritional supplements, such as vitamin C and other antioxidants (to scavenge free radicals) are emphasized.

In addition, the clinic uses embryonic live cell therapy to bolster the patient's endocrine system; for example, embryonic brain and adrenal tissue are used to replenish DHEA, a hormone necessary for the proper function of the immune system. Detoxification therapy in the form of enemas and colonic irrigation is also important.

In 1987, American Biologics Hospital (ABH) presented an overview of its first 5000 cancer cases to the Office of Technology Assessment of the U.S. Congress. Among these cases, of which more than 90% were supposedly terminal, ABH achieved a 5-year survival rate of about 20% with few or no symptoms reported by patients.

For more information about ABH, contact: American Biologics, Azucena #15 La Mesa, T.J., B.C., Mexico; fax: 52-66-816435; for mailing: AB-Mexico, 1180 Walnut Avenue, Chula Vista, CA 91911; tel: 800-227-4458 or 619-429-8200; fax: 619-429-8004.

For more information about the link between **depressed thyroid condition** and cancer, see Chapter 25: What Causes Cancer? p. 619.

For example, a male engineer had bone cancer of the thigh, with a tumor the size of a bowling ball. According to Michael Culbert, D.Sc., information director for ABH, "His doctors told him he would have to have his leg and part of his groin removed and undergo radiation. We placed him on a metabolic program, and infused ozone gas directly into the tumor on alternate days; we also applied herbal poultices. Over a couple of months, the tumor became soft, then it popped open and oozed out. That was 10 years ago. At last report, the patient is still doing well."

A 1986 landmark study of 242 men, aged 50-79, based on 12 years of research, stated that a small supplementation of DHEA (100 mcg/ml) corresponded to a 48% reduction in death from heart disease and a 36% reduction in death from any cause, other than accidents. A Temple University medical researcher reports that DHEA can help you lose weight by blocking an enzyme known to produce fat tissue and promote cancer cell growth. In one study, DHEA supplementation enabled men to lose 31% of mean body fat with no change in body weight in 28 days. Another study involving 16 middle-aged to elderly men showed that taking DHEA for 1 year led to a 75% increase in their sense of overall well-being. The men said they coped better with stress, felt more physically mobile, and slept better.

"This common, powerful steroid hormone is clearly important in cancer prevention," states naturopathic physician Eileen Stretch, N.D., of the Institute of Complementary Medicine in Seattle, Washington. Dr. Stretch notes that premenopausal women with low circulating levels of DHEA tend to have a higher incidence of breast cancer, while postmenopausal women who with breast cancer have higher than normal DHEA levels.[65]

DHEA can inhibit the proliferation of cancer cells by blocking an enzyme called G6PD which, in turn, halts the synthesis of nucleic acids required for cell division.[66] Many physicians state that DHEA is effective in treating premenopausal breast cancer, but the only controlled studies in support of this claim have been done with animals.[67]

Laboratory studies in animals shows that DHEA can increase life span by 50%, which is why scientists believe DHEA replacement therapy can have a life-extending effect on humans. Other studies suggest that DHEA enhances the activity of the immune system, enabling it to better protect the body from bacteria and viruses, including EBV (Epstein-Barr Virus, associated with mononucleosis) and HIV (the virus associated with AIDS).[68]

According to Davis W. Lamson, M.S., N.D., of Tacoma Clinic, in Kent, Washington, in 80% of cases of ulcerative colitis for which he has used DHEA he has seen "extremely positive responses." Dr. Lamson strongly cautions physicians against *over*-prescribing DHEA, recalling the way cortisone was initially handled by overly enthusiastic doctors. DHEA levels can be increased by taking herbal Mexican yam (also called wild yam or *Dioscorea villosa*). This vegetable contains the nutritional precursors from which the body produces DHEA. A sublingual spray form of DHEA has merits since in this delivery mode DHEA is not deactivated by first passing through the liver as with orally ingested and intestine-absorbed DHEA.

## MELATONIN

Melatonin is a potent immune-enhancing hormone produced by the human pineal gland, a tiny cone-shaped gland inside the brain. Although known mainly as a sleep promoter—brain melatonin levels rise dramatically at night—melatonin also appears to have substantial cancer-repelling power. In addition to boosting the activity of key immune cells called T helper cells,[69] melatonin stimulates the tumor-killing action of natural killer cells by increasing the white blood cell production of the cytokine Interleukin-2 (IL-2).[70]

CLINIC HIGHLIGHT

## Metabolic Therapies at International Medical Center

The International Medical Center (IMC) in El Paso, Texas, a major metabolic treatment center, was the brainchild of H. Ray Evers, M.D., a pioneering alternative physician who died in 1990.

According to former medical director Francisco R. Soto, M.D., "Treatments rest on a foundation of nutrition, oxidative therapy (hyperbaric oxygen and ozone), Koch vaccination, and antioxidant chelation therapy. The Koch vaccine derives from work originally done by German bacteriologist Robert Koch (1843-1910) who developed it in 1883 as a medical response to typhoid and tuberculosis. IMC uses the Koch vaccine, based on the bacillus *Mycobacterium* (*M. tuberculosis*) as a preventive inoculation to enhance the immune system. It acts as an antibody, targeting diseased (cancerous) cells.

IMC also employs cell therapy administered in the form of frozen live cell and whole cell injections; in addition, magnetic field therapy, amygdalin, shark cartilage, and detoxification are also important."

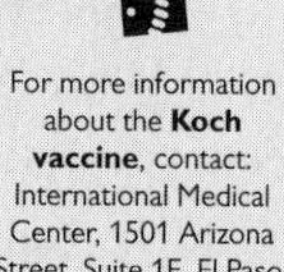

For more information about the **Koch vaccine**, contact: International Medical Center, 1501 Arizona Street, Suite 1E, El Paso, TX 79902; tel: 800-621-8924 or 915-543-5621; fax: 915-543-5625.

In one case, William, a retired commercial banker, was diagnosed with Stage IV bladder cancer. A biopsy showed that the tumor was growing directly on the lining of his bladder and there was strong indication that it had invaded the muscle wall of the bladder. William's urologist advised him to have his bladder removed within the next 2 weeks; instead, he went to Dr. Evers' IMC. There he received chelation therapy, megadoses of vitamin C, and hyperbaric oxygen to increase the oxygen content of his blood and enhance the effectiveness of the chelation. William's bladder cancer went into a complete remission within 20 days, and 6 years later, he was still cancer free.

A recent study of 60 cancer patients found that melatonin combined with synthetic Interleukin-2, produced by recombinant DNA technology, may be more effective than chemotherapy in treating patients diagnosed with non-small-cell carcinoma of the lung, an aggressive form of lung cancer. Whereas only 19% of those receiving chemotherapy were still alive after one year, 45% of those receiving the melatonin/IL-2 therapy survived the year.[71]

Melatonin treatment also appears to give certain cancer patients a survival advantage—those with inoperable brain tumors,[72] metastatic gastric cancer,[73] and metastatic colon cancer.[74] Other cancers that may benefit from melatonin treatment include metastatic breast cancer[75] and advanced endocrine (carcinoid) tumors.[76] Aside from the improved survival among patients taking melatonin, these patients also report consistent improvement in quality-of-life issues and a reduced frequency of cancer-related complications.

lated complications.

Melatonin has sedative qualities and helps reduce anxiety, panic disorders, and migraines as well as inducing sleep. It is also a powerful antioxidant (free-radical fighter) and is a primary regulator of the immune system.[77] Researchers have found that when a person ignores the 24 hour dark-light cycle and keeps irregular hours of work and rest, the body's internal rhythms go awry. The number of hours one sleeps is less important than *when* one sleeps in respect to daylight. Going to bed before midnight and getting up at dawn is the healthiest pattern for optimal melatonin production.

People who work in rotating shifts or at night have been shown to experience a higher incidence of heart disease, back pain, respiratory problems, ulcers, and sleep disorders. These people also have a higher rate of error and accidents and often experience a significant loss of alertness and ability to make decisions. Researchers are using high-intensity bright lighting (5-10 times brighter than ordinary room level) as well as the administration of melatonin to help shift workers adjust to their schedules.[78]

Travel between time zones often results in jet lag, a less serious, but often debilitating and disorienting condition caused by the upset of the body's internal clock. Melatonin and full spectrum bright-light therapies are being explored as useful antidotes. Some airports are now considering the installation of full-spectrum lights in their first class lounges to help passengers adjust to their destination time zones.

People over age 50 may benefit from regular melatonin supplementation. The tablets should be taken at the same time every evening to help regulate the pineal gland's production. MIT scientist Richard Wurtman, Ph.D., found that a mere 0.1 to 0.3 mg was sufficient for inducing sleep. This appears to be a good benchmark for starting supplementation. Since most melatonin tablets contain 10 to 30 times this amount (3 mg), breaking the tablets into smaller pieces is advised. This practice could help avert some of the side effects that have been observed in melatonin supplement users, such as sluggishness, fatigue or even nausea.

If you take melatonin tablets that also contain vitamin B6, you may find yourself more "hyper" than sleepy at night. This is because vitamin B6 tends to raise the metabolism in certain individuals. Also, people with altered circadian cycles may require special timing of melatonin supplements. Factors that are known to lower the brain's melatonin production include high-protein diets, overeating, chronic stress, alcohol, "street" drugs and various medications, tobacco, caffeine, lack of natural lighting exposure during the daytime, sleep deprivation (or sleeping during the day and not at night), electromagnetic fields, geopathic fields, and sleeping in a room that is not pitch black (because of a night-light, streetlight, or even the Moon shining through the window).

## THYMOSIN

Moderate success has been reported with this active ingredient from the thymus. In animal research focusing on lung cancer, a combination of thymosin and interferon caused a "dramatic and rapid disappearance of tumor burden."[79] Animals treated with the thymosin had more vigorous natural killer (NK) cell activity—a measure of the body's ability to repel cancer—and significantly longer survival compared to those that received chemotherapy. Similarly, in trials involving people with lung cancer, patients receiving thymosin had "significantly prolonged survival times relative to the other treatment groups."[80] Lung cancer patients treated with thymosin had "significantly prolonged survival times relative to the other treatment groups."[81] Trials with isolated thymus hormones have found enhanced survival of patients with melanoma and lung cancer and reduced immunosuppression in patients with breast cancer and other cancers.[82] Clinical trials in Poland found that immune-suppressed patients receiving TFX, a semipurified calf thymus extract, showed significant improvements in immune function as well as reductions in disease symptoms.[83]

## T3 THYROID HORMONE

In the 1990s, E. Dennis Wilson, M.D., described a medical concept he called Wilson's Syndrome. Dr. Wilson had treated hundreds of patients with low body temperatures (and a multitude of other symptoms) using a sustained-release form of active thyroid (T3) hormone (made by combining pharmaceutical grade T3 with methylhydroxycellulose in a custom-compounding pharmacy). Dr. Wilson used the custom-compounded sustained-release form of T3 hormone rather than the commercially available prescription Cytomel, because Cytomel has a short half-life of only 3 to 4 hours. In contrast, the custom-compounded form has a half-life of 12 hours and therefore only needs to be taken twice rather than 6 times a day.

Dr. Wilson documented significant improvement in symptoms and normalization of temperatures in the majority of patients treated in this fashion. Dr. Wilson is not an oncologist and did not pursue the relationship between the treatment with active T3 hormone and any cancer conditions. However, if Dr. Barnes and fellow researchers were correct in their observations about the relationships among depressed thyroid, goiter, and cancer, this type of difficult-to-detect thyroid condition should be looked for and possibly treated in cancer patients who are undergoing either conventional or alternative therapies.

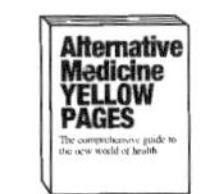


See "Enxyme Therapy," p. 124, and "Oxygen Therapy," p. 200.

It is important to note that standard T3 and T4 thyroid blood tests will not detect this condition. The only way to detect the condition is by measuring the temperature under the arm for 10 minutes every morning with a glass thermometer, before the person gets out of bed; if the temperature is consistently below 97.8°F, the physician should assume that the person may deserve a short trial of thyroid medication while following morning temperatures and symptoms. (An exhaustive search for a laboratory that will measure reverse T3 levels in the United States has yielded none.) Reverse T3 is a form of T3 that has no positive action in the body and is capable of blocking the activity of T3.

The second best thyroid medication to use after active T3 is a glandular thyroid hormone derived from beef, pork, or sheep thyroid glands. Giving T4 either has no effect on this condition or makes the condition worse presumably by causing more production of reverse T3. Persons taking T4 should measure their morning temperatures and discuss their findings with a health practitioner who understands this reverse T3 condition.

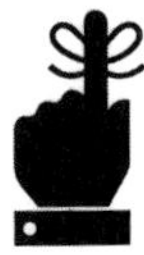

*Making adjustments in one's attitude and emotional life is just one factor in healing. How one lives also needs to be looked at closely. This includes the quality and dynamics of one's job, major relationships, living situation, and sexual habits. The entire lifestyle must be reoriented to one that supports the immune system and total body healing.*

Chapter 33

# Physical Support Therapies for Reversing Cancer

**Flushing toxins out of the body is a prime task of any cancer therapy, and to achieve this alternative physicians draw upon a variety of techniques from dentistry to massage, colon cleansing to heat therapy, combining them according to the needs of the individual patient.**

The successful approach to reversing cancer and preventing its future recurrence is always multimodal. No single therapy, technique, or substance can prevail against the complexity of this disease. The exact combination of therapies and substances depends entirely on the individuality of the patient and the skill and knowledge of the physician. In this chapter, we present detailed information regarding several highly useful therapies that provide physical support to the body as it struggles to overcome cancer.

Specifically, we will discuss detoxification, or ways of getting the toxins out of the body; biological dentistry, or the crucial role your teeth play in both contributing to and reversing the cancer process; hydrotherapy and hyperthermia, how the basic process of water and heat can fortify the body; therapeutic massage and exercise, which can relax the tension and stress associated with serious illness; and Qigong, a form of relaxed, meditative movement that weaves together body and mind, organism and energy, for therapeutic benefit.

**In This Chapter**

# Detoxification

**One of the most essential practices in any cancer-reversal program, and for prevention, too, is to detoxify the body, down to the level of its cells, of a myriad of toxins, chemicals, parasites, and foreign substances, and to open up clogged elimination channels to move them out of the body.**

Each year, people are exposed to thousands of toxic chemicals and pollutants in air, water, food, and soil. People living today carry within their bodies a "chemical cocktail" made up of industrial chemicals, pesticides, food additives, heavy metals, general anesthetics, and the residues of therapeutic pharmaceuticals, as well as of legal (alcohol, tobacco, caffeine), and illegal drugs (heroin, cocaine, marijuana).

Today people are exposed to chemicals in far greater concentrations than were previous generations. For example, over 70 million Americans live in areas that exceed smog standards; most municipal drinking water contains over 700 chemicals, including excessive levels of lead. Some 3,000 chemicals are added to the food supply; and as many as 10,000 chemicals in the form of solvents, emulsifiers, and preservatives are used in food processing and storage, which can remain in the body for years.[1]

To make matters worse, food and product labels do not always list every ingredient. When people consume these foods—especially seafood, meat, and poultry—they ingest *all* the chemicals and pesticides that have remained as accumulated contaminants in the food chain.

## Detoxification Therapy Can Rid the Body of Poisons

These pollutants lodge in the body and manifest in a variety of symptoms, including decreased immune function, nerve cell toxicity, hormonal dysfunction, psychological disturbances, environmental illness and chronic fatigue, degenerative diseases, and cancer. "The current level of chemicals in the food and water supply and the indoor and outdoor environment has lowered our threshold of resistance to disease and has altered our body's metabolism, causing enzyme dysfunction, nutritional deficiencies, and hormonal imbalances," says Marshall Mandell, M .D., a pioneer of environmental medicine.

***Since 1945, toxins have accumulated in the human system faster than they can be naturally eliminated, which means the body now needs assistance in detoxifying.***

Where do all the toxins come from? They come from a polluted environment (air, water, and food), lack of water, overconsumption of food, a faulty, nutritionally inadequate diet, lack of exercise, accumulated stress, excess antibiotic use, and chronic constipation and poor elimination. Bioaccumulation (a buildup in the body of foreign substances) seriously compromises physiological and psychological health. Since 1985, hundreds of studies have demonstrated the dangers to health from toxic bioaccumulation.[2] Since 1945, toxins have accumulated in the human system faster than they can be naturally eliminated, which means the body now needs assistance in detoxifying.

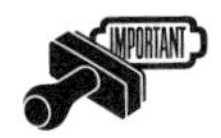


People with cancer should almost always assume that a detoxification program is necessary; however, any effort at detoxifying should be planned and executed under direct supervision of a physician. Those recovering from substance abuse, alcoholics, diabetics, people with eating disorders, and those who are underweight or physically weak or who have a hypothyroid or hypoglycemic condition should not detoxify without strict medical supervision.

"A body with a healthy immune system, efficient organs of elimination and detoxification, and a sound circulatory and nervous system can handle a great deal of toxicity," states Leon Chaitow, N.D., D.O., of London, England. "But if a person's immune system has been damaged from chronic exposure to environmental pollutants, restoring these functions, organs, and systems can be accomplished only through detoxification therapies, including fasting, chelation, and nutritional, herbal, and homeopathic methods, which accelerate the body's own natural cleansing processes."

Most alternative physicians agree that detoxification is essential and that it brings many benefits to the person undertaking it. "The process of detoxification through special cleansing diets as well as juice and water fasts is the missing link to rejuvenating the body and preventing such chronic diseases as cancer, cardiovascular problems, arthritis, diabetes, and obesity," says Elson Haas, M.D., director of the Marin Clinic of Preventive Medicine and Health Education in San Rafael, California. "The modern diet with animal proteins, fats, caffeine, alcohol, and chemicals inhibits the optimum functioning of our cells and tissues. The cleansing of toxins and waste products will restore optimum function and vitality."

One of the most important and longest lasting effects of detoxification therapy is the reduction of stress on the immune system, says Dr. Haas. Other benefits can include increased vitality, reduced blood pressure and blood fats (cholesterol and triglycerides), improved assimilation of vitamins and minerals, and mental clarity.

Everyone has a natural, specific level of tolerance for toxins that cannot be exceeded if good health is to be maintained. When the system gets overwhelmed with toxins, the immune system mechanisms malfunction, and fatigue, confusion, aggression, or mental disorder may occur. Symptoms indicating that you may need detoxification are headaches, joint pain, recurrent respiratory problems, back pain, nasal or sinus inhalant allergy symptoms, insomnia, mood changes, and food allergies. Conditions such as arthritis, constipation, hemorrhoids, ulcers, psoriasis, and acne can also indicate the need for detoxification.

***"If a person's immune system has been damaged from chronic exposure to environmental pollutants, restoring these functions can be accomplished only through detoxification therapies, including fasting, chelation, and nutritional, herbal, and homeopathic methods, which accelerate the body's own natural cleansing processes," says Leon Chaitow, N.D., D.O.***

## 7 General Precautionary Steps to Improve Intestinal Health

There are 7 steps anyone can adopt starting today to improve their intestinal health as a way of preventing illness.

**First,** make some dietary changes. Start eating a diet that is high in fiber, fresh raw vegetables and fruits, and very low in mucus-producing foods. It would be wise to completely stop eating all milk products from cows and all refined white flour products, such as pastas, breads, and baked goods. At least for the duration of this program, it is also advisable to reduce your intake of sugar, eggs, meats, fowl, most fish, nuts, seeds, and unsprouted beans and grains.

**Second,** reduce your stress load. Practice stress-reduction techniques before each meal. These might include muscle relaxation, deep breathing, or the visualization of a favorite and pleasant natural setting. Listening to a stress-reduction audiotape before the meal can be helpful. It is also advisable to eat in a calm, pleasant environment, either by yourself or with a companion whose presence does not produce stress or discomfort in you.

**Third,** practice lymphatic drainage. It is important to take steps to clean out your lymphatic system, especially the lymph vessels that attach to the intestines. You can do this by gently bouncing on a mini-trampoline or rebounder for 5-15 minutes once daily. This will stimulate the numerous lymph nodes in your neck, chest, and groin to start draining toxins into the bloodstream for removal from the body.

**Fourth,** brush your skin. In the early morning, soon after you get up, take a wooden brush with stiff natural bristles and lightly brush your skin. Move the brush across the skin towards the middle end of the collarbones on each side of the body, as important lymph drainage sites are located here. Spend 8-10 minutes dry brushing your entire body.

This procedure will mechanically aid your lymph system in its detoxification efforts. Do the dry brushing before taking the bath, but be aware that skin brushing just before bedtime can make it difficult to fall asleep. (See p. 971 in this chapter for more information on skin brushing.)

**Fifth,** try ozonated bathing. Many of the toxins that build up in the body are fat soluble and gather in the fatty tissues. If you immerse yourself in a tub of warm ozonated water for 30 minutes once daily for 2-3 weeks this will aid in removal of the toxins from your body.

Ozone is used in this program to purify the bath water by killing living viruses, bacteria, fungi, and parasites. It will also oxidize the water-insoluble toxins on the skin, turning them into water-soluble toxins. Once water soluble, they may be flushed from the system.

Here's how to do it. Purify the tapwater by running it through a KDF solid charcoal showerhead filter as you fill the tub. A KDF solid charcoal showerhead filter can remove up to 99% of the toxic substances found in tap water. Next, bubble ozone ($O_3$, a form of oxygen) into the water using an ultraviolet ozone generator and an ozone-diffusing bath bubbler. Do not use an electric spark ozonating system because this produces more nitrates and other harmful chemical substances. This converts the ozone that is accumulating in the air above the bubbling water back into oxygen so that it is not irritating to the lungs. While you remain in the bath, scrub your entire skin surface with a loofa sponge or natural fiber brush 3 times during the 30-minute soak. Bubble the ozone for 15 minutes before you get into the tub and also during your 30-minute soak.

Adding to your bath water ½ cup of Body Soak Gold, increasing this amount to 1 cup over 2-3 weeks, will usually produce a faster removal of toxins from the body than ozonated water alone. After you have used one full bottle of Body Soak Gold, you may gain additional detoxification benefit by switching to 1/4 cup of Liquid Needles Foot Soak added to the bath water; over a period of several days, increase this amount to 1 cup for each 30-minute bath. Best results are obtained if both Soaks are added to KDF charcoal-filtered water. As a variation on skin brushing, use a loofa sponge to brush your skin.

**Sixth,** fortify yourself with nutrients. It is important to take at least 400 IU of vitamin E, 25,000 IU of beta carotene and/or mixed carotenoids, 2000 mg vitamin C, and 100 mg of grape seed extract (pycnogenol) 30-40 minutes before your ozonated bath or 10-15 minutes after it.

**Seventh,** take 1 lozenge of superoxide dismutase (SOD) and 100 mg of L-glutathione powder (an amino acid). Dissolve both substances under your tongue before each bath; this enables it to be absorbed faster and more completely. These nutrients will facilitate toxin removal from your system. SOD is an antioxidant enzyme that protects the system against free-radical damage from chemicals or radiation. L-glutathione is a sulfur-containing peptide (made of amino acids, which are protein building blocks) and antioxidants essential to the body's toxic waste disposal system.

## Instructions for 5-Month Detoxification Program

Author W. Lee Cowden, M.D., often recommends a 5-month gentle detoxification program. Here, you are required to maintain a diet low in foods known to produce mucus while taking herbs and fiber that help to break up the intestine's mucoid lining. This program, which takes 3-5 months to clean out the intestine's false lining, is effective for people with allergies, irritable bowel syndrome, yeast and fungal overgrowth, parasites, severe liver or kidney disease, or for anyone seeking an improved state of health.

**Preliminaries—**Begin a low-mucus-forming diet (described on page 951) and practice dry skin brushing once daily for 3 months, then twice weekly afterwards.

**Herbal Fiber—**Take an herbal fiber product as a bowel-bulking agent 2 times daily at first, building up to 3-4 times daily after a week. Dr. Cowden developed the NatureSpring Friendly Flora and Fiber formula specifically for this purpose. This product may be taken daily for maintenance after the 3-5 month cleanse.

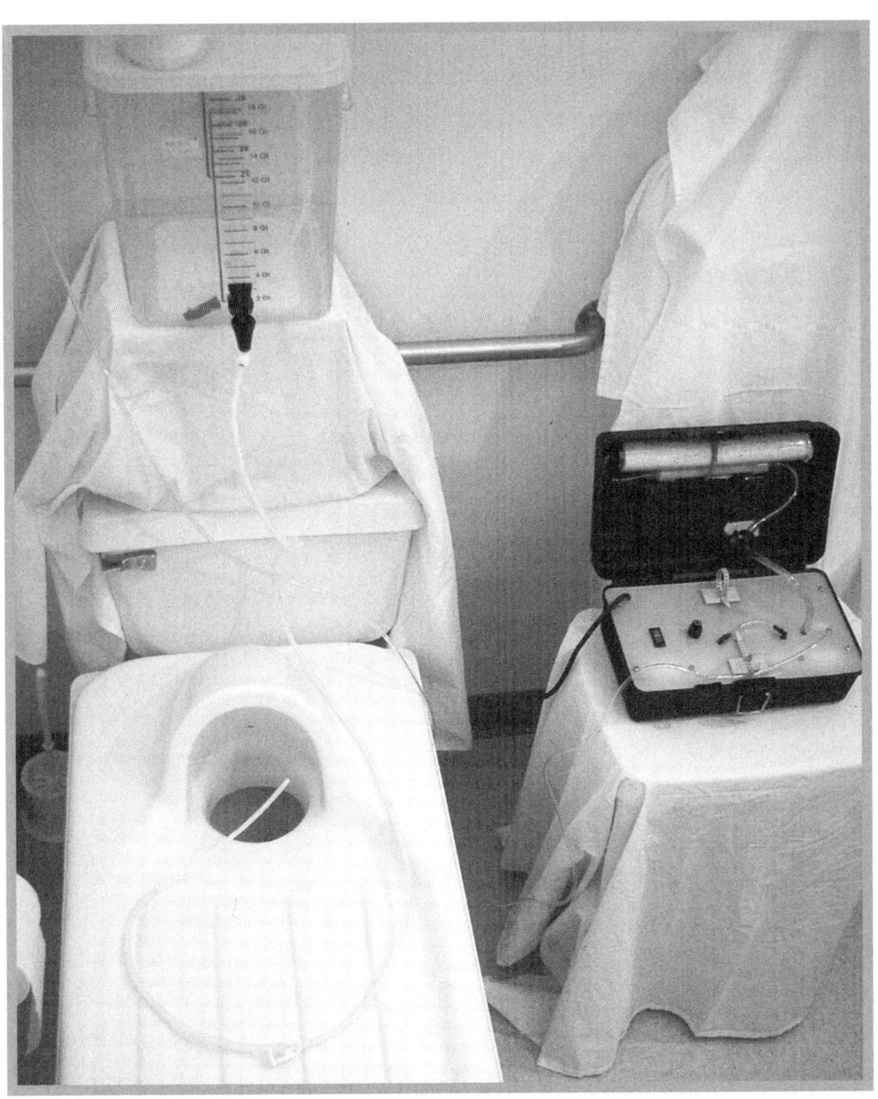

**The essential equipment for the 7-Day Rapid Colon Cleanse includes an ultraviolet ozone generator (right), an ozone diffusing bubbler (top left), and colema board (bottom left).**

Along with this, start taking an herbal product called NatureSpring Intestinal Cleanse at the rate of 1 capsule twice daily, building up gradually to 1-2 tablets taken 3-4 times daily. The goal is to have 2-3 bowel motions daily. Its herbs—slippery elm, cascara sagrada, papain, cayenne, ginger—will help to break down the mucoid lining of the intestines and stimulate the intestines to push toxic feces out. Some may find this product unnecessary, and most should taper off after 4-5 weeks.

**Mucoid remover**—On the third day, add NatureSpring Bowel, Blood and Body Cleansing Formula starting with ½ to 1 tablet, 2 times daily; build gradually to 3 tablets taken 3-4 times daily. This formula has 30 ingredients that break down the mucoid lining, cleanse the blood, drain the lymphatics, and stabilize the function of various organ systems. Based on transient symptoms that you notice once you begin this program—toxin release, frequency and size of bowel movements—you, the user, are able to decide the rate of advancement in terms of dosage. Be sure to drink copious amounts of pure water (nonchlorinated but not distilled) while on this program.

An **antioxidant** (meaning "against oxidation") is a natural biochemical substance that protects living cells against damage from harmful free radicals. Antioxidants work against the process of oxidation—the robbing of electrons from substances. If unblocked or left uncontrolled, oxidation can lead to cellular aging, degeneration, arthritis, heart disease, cancer, and other illnesses. Antioxidants in the body react readily with oxygen breakdown products and free radicals, and neutralize them before they can damage the body. Antioxidant nutrients include vitamins A, C, and E, beta carotene, selenium, coenzyme Q10, pycnogenol (grape seed extract), L-glutathione, superoxide dismutase, and bioflavonoids. Plant antioxidants include *Gingko biloba* and garlic. When antioxidants are taken in combination, the effect is stronger than when they are used individually.

## 7-Day Rapid Colon Cleanse

This approach works rapidly and involves semi-fasting in conjunction with taking fiber, nutritional supplements, and ozonated water delivered directly to the intestines. This program is helpful for people with cancer that is rapidly spreading, chemical toxin overload, and women with silicone implant toxicity.

This 7-day program requires the following equipment: a colema board, an ultraviolet ozone generator, an ozone diffusing bath bubbler, a 5-gallon bubbler bucket, and tubings.

**Preliminaries**—The night before beginning this program, take 2 tablets of cascara sagrada herbal laxative to get the colon stimulated to begin detoxifying. If you have a history of chronic constipation (less than 1 bowel movement daily), use 4 tablets.

**Special Diet**—During the 7 days you will be on this program, it is necessary that you eat nothing except 2-5 servings of vegetable broth daily; be sure the broth contains no beans or grains.

**Antioxidants**—Melt 10 mg of superoxide dismutase (SOD) powder under the tongue, along with 100 mg of L-glutathione powder (NatureSpring SOD L-glutathione) each morning and again each evening just before the ozonated colemics, described below.

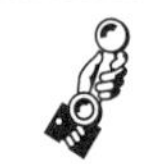

For information and sources of **NatureSpring products**, all brand-named products, generic products, and the equipment described in this article, contact: Health Restoration Systems, Inc., P.O. Box 032267, Richardson, TX 75083-2267; tel: 972-480-8909; fax: 972-480-8807. HRS offers a 6-day residential educational/detoxification intensive program with professional medical supervision in Dallas, Texas. This program is helpful for people with cancer that is rapidly spreading, chemical toxin overload, and women with silicone implant toxicity. **Body Soak Gold**, (containing water, sea minerals, and glycerin) and **Liquid Needles Foot Soak** (containing electrolytes from mineral particles in a clear solution) are also available from HRS. For a source of **SOD** as Opti-Guard™ (Antioxidant/S.O.D. Enzyme Enhancer), contact: Optimal Nutrients, 1163 Chess Drive, Suite F, Foster City, CA 94404; tel: 415-525-0112 or 800-966-8874; fax: 415-349-1686. For information about **A.M./P.M. Ultimate Cleanse**™, contact: Nature's Secret, 4 Health, Inc., 5485 Conestoga Court, Boulder, CO 80301; tel: 303-546-6306; fax: 303-546-6416. For information about **Nature's Pure Body Program**™, contact: Pure Body Institute of Beverly Hills, 423 East Ojai Avenue, #107, Ojai, CA 93023; tel: 800-952-7873; (orders); 805-653-5448 (customer service); 805-653-0373 (fax).

**Special Drinks—**Immediately following this, mix and consume the following two drinks. Drink No. 1 contains cool purified water (10 oz), pure organic apple juice (4 oz), psyllium seed husk powder (1 tbsp), and 1-3 tablets of NatureSpring's small bowel and tissue cleanser.

Drink No. 2 contains 10 oz hot pure water (but not heated by a microwave), organic apple cider vinegar or fresh lemon or lime juice (1 tbsp), and raw unfiltered honey (1 tbsp). Consume this drink immediately after Drink No. 1. The pair of drinks is mixed and consumed in rapid sequence 5 times daily during the 7-day program.

**Ozonated Colemics—**Twice daily, shortly after the first and fourth pairs of drinks are consumed, the next step is to combine ozonated water with the use of a colema board. This is a device (also called a colonic board or home enema board) that enables one to use an enema and empty one's bowels while lying on a sanitary plastic board stretched between a chair and the toilet bowl. Feces, spontaneously voided from the colon, flow through a girded hole in the board into the toilet.

The colema differs from both an enema, which typically uses gravity flow to move 2 quarts to 1 gallon of water into the colon, and a colonic, which administers up to 25 gallons by pressure. The name means, in essence, colon enema, and as a device, the colema board has been in use for nearly a century.

First, run 5 gallons of warm, body-temperature water through a KDF solid charcoal showerhead filter into the 5-gallon bucket that has a special top to prevent ozone from escaping into the room. Next, bubble ozone for 15 minutes into the water in the bucket with the top closed securely. The ozone generator sits on top of the toilet tank, while the 5-gallon bucket stands on a high stool or platform so that its contents can flow by gravity into the person's colon.

Place the business end of the colema board over the toilet and the other on a chair or stool so that the end furthest from the toilet bowl is 2 inches higher than the end over the bowl.

The person about to receive the ozonated colemic lies down on the colema board with the buttocks centered over the end of the board over the toilet bowl. Lubricate the tip of the plastic tube from the water drain on the 5-gallon bucket with coconut, grape seed, or olive oil. Then gently insert the tube about 3 inches into the rectum.

Next, push one finger deep into the abdomen for 3 minutes at a point that is 1 inch above and 1 inch to the left of the belly button. This will help relax the small intestine before running water into it; this point is usually tender if the small intestine is stressed.

Open the valve on the tube coming from the 5-gallon bucket so that the ozonated water can run slowly into the colon for 30-45 minutes. For this to happen, set the bucket so that the bottom is 3 feet higher than the level of the colema board. The ozone continues to bubble into the 5-gallon bucket as the water continues to flow into the rectum.

**Ozone** ($O_3$) is a less stable, more reactive form of oxygen, containing 3 oxygen atoms. This extra atom enables ozone to more readily oxidize other chemicals. In oxidation, the extra oxygen atom breaks off, leaving ordinary oxygen ($O_2$), thereby favorably increasing the oxygen content of body tissues or blood. Ozone is a commonly occuring natural substance. Medical-grade ozone is used as part of oxygen therapy to increase local oxygen supply to lesions, speed wound healing, reduce infections, and stimulate metabolic processes. Ozone may be administered by physicians intravenously, by injection, or applied topically as a gas or dissolved in water or in olive oil; it may also be taken orally or rectally as ozonated water.

**Ileocecal Block**—While the ozonated water is running into your colon, it is important to manually keep the ileocecal valve closed. This valve controls the passage of material from the small into the large intestine. Use one or both hands to press firmly on your right lower abdomen.

**Let It Flow**—Periodically, the water inflow hose may be clamped off. Then push the water out of the intestines into the toilet by contracting the abdominal muscles; only after this should you release the hand that is blocking the ileocecal valve. Then massage your abdomen, especially around the belly button, to stimulate movement of the false lining in the small intestine through the ileocecal valve into the large intestine.

When you restart the flow of colema water, the false lining may be flushed into the toilet. Be sure to hold the ileocecal valve closed as the hose clamp is opened and colema water runs into the colon again.

**Ozonated Bath**—After each ozonated colemic, take a 30-minute bath in ozonated water. Prepare the bath by running very warm water through the KDF showerhead filter to a depth of 8-10 inches. Next, bubble ozone into

# The Mayr Intestinal Detoxification Program

Various methods are used to purge the small intestine of a pasty layer of mucus under which most parasites originate and propagate. This "false lining," a product of refined white flour products, inhibits nutrient absorption. Parasites and pathogenic yeasts that produce toxins live between this lining and the true lining of the intestine itself, producing ill health for their human host.

Helpful in eliminating this false lining is the digestive system detoxification program of Dr. med. Franz Xavier Mayr (1875-1965), an Austrian physician who lived to be 90 and attributed this in part to his intestinal health. Dr. Mayr explained that if the digestive system and particularly the intestines are not "clean," that is, unobstructed and free of toxins, they cannot operate efficiently and then become a breeding ground for disease. Working at the world-famous Karlsbad spa in Czechoslovakia, Dr. Mayr applied his intestinal detoxification program to aid European luminaries in improving their health.

Dr. Mayr's program does not involve colonics or enemas, but cleans out the intestines through dietary changes. The program calls for a diet based on avoiding whole grains, margarine, decaffeinated coffee, and alcohol. Other aspects of his diet include eating only cooked food, chewing thoroughly, eating only when hungry, not drinking beverages with meals, drinking pure water, and not eating again after dinner. The Mayr program calls for taking natural products such as the Bittersalz drink (usually including magnesium sulfate or Epsom salts) that acts as a natural laxative, taken only in the morning, plus homeopathic remedies and botanicals. Dr. Mayr's program (in use today by hundreds of physicians worldwide) includes a 15-minute abdominal treatment technique to be manually performed on patients to increase intestinal activity and improve circulation throughout the abdomen.

The Mayr diet is designed to help move excessive accumulations of mucus out of the intestinal tract. The goal is to slough off the small intestine's layer of mucus, the false lining. When this happens, 3 benefits accrue: (1) nutrient absorption is increased by as much as 4-5 times; (2) the buildup of toxins is reduced; and (3) antiparasite medicines work more effectively.

A "tea fast" requires the patient to consume only herbal tea (typically chamomile, mint, sage, or peppermint), honey and mineral water, and a small amount of clear vegetable broth for 1-2 weeks. This is usually followed by a diet consisting of a teaspoon of yogurt or milk and a single hard, stale wheat roll taken in the morning; the purpose of the old, crusty rolls is to force the patient to thoroughly chew the food (70-80 times) so that it becomes liquified. Other than the wheat rolls and ½ cup daily of uncooked rice, most cereal grains are avoided because grains are directly converted into sugar (glucose), which can be used by tumor cells to stimulate tumor growth, Dr. Mayr explained. The sugar also stimulates the release of the hormone insulin, which in turn activates a set of hormone-like substances (called PGE2 prostaglandins) that trigger tumor growth and inflammatory processes.

In the absence of a blood sugar surge, the body produces more of another kind of hormone, glucagon, which stimulates another set of hormone-like substances (the PGE1 prostaglandins). This group of prostaglandins are the "good guys" because they tend to inhibit tumor formation and clot formation which, in turn, increases oxygenation of the tissues, thereby promoting the aerobic conditions that inhibit cancer growth.

For more information about **Mayr therapy,** active practitioners, and training seminars, contact: Occidental Institute Research Foundation, P.O. Box 100, Penticton, B.C. V2A 6J9 Canada; tel: 604-497-6020; fax: 604-497-6030.

this water for 15 minutes before and continually during immersing yourself. Scrub your skin all over with a loofah 3 times during the bath.

**Nutrient Fortification**—About 15 minutes before the morning colema, take niacin (100 mg) and flaxseed oil (3 capsules). Before the first colema, consume Drinks No. 1 and 2 and dissolve under your tongue 100 mg of L-glutathione powder and 10 mg of SOD powder.

After the morning ozonated bath, take the following nutritional supplements:

- Vitamin C (2000 mg)
- Protease (an enzyme: 2 capsules)
- NatureSpring Gastro-Protective enzyme
- NatureSpring Essential Nutrients (1 capsule)
- Cracked chlorella (6 capsules; 335 mg per capsule)
- Nature's Sunshine CA-ATC (a mixture of herbs high in calcium; 2 capsules)
- Dulse (2 tablets or 1 dropperful)
- Colloidal minerals (1 tbsp)
- Magnesium malate or magnesium citrate (2 capsules)
- Potassium (200 mg)
- EPA fish oil (1 capsule)
- Beet crystals (5 tablets; 400 mg per tablet)

Take this group of supplements again, either late in the morning or early afternoon, then again just before receiving the second colema in the late afternoon. You may complement the nutrients with warm vegetable broth.

Before the afternoon ozonated colema, melt 10 mg of SOD and 100 mg of L-glutathione powder under the tongue, and take 3 capsules of flaxseed oil and 100 mg of vitamin B3 as niacin.

**Program Review**—Just after the morning ozonated colemic and ozonated bath, you take all remaining nutrients that were not taken earlier.

About 90 minutes after this first set of supplements, consume Drinks No. 1 and 2. Then, 90 minutes after that, take the nutrients again; 90 minutes later, consume the 2 drinks again; after another 90 minutes, consume the warm vegetable broth; 90 minutes later, have the 2 drinks again; after another 90 minutes, it's time for the supplements. Following this, take the ozonated colema again followed by the ozonated bath. End the day with the final set of drinks. Follow this schedule for 7 days.

If you find at bedtime that you are too hungry to sleep, have a serving of vegetable broth. As an alternative to preparing your own vegetable broth, Nature's Sunshine powdered Vegetable Seasoning Broth is suitable.

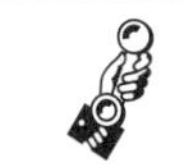

For a source of **friendly bacteria**, or probiotics, Nature's Biotics™ are available from Life Science Products, Inc., 321 North Mall Drive, Building F-201, St. George, UT 84790; tel: 801-628-4111 or 800-713-3888; fax: 801-628-6114. ***L. plantarum*** is available from: Health Restoration Systems, P.O. Box 832267, Richardson, TX 75083; tel: 972-480-8909; fax: 972-238-0327.

**Friendly Bacteria**—When you have completed the 7-day program, it's advisable to restock your intestines with friendly bacteria, or probiotics, such as Nature's Sunshine Bifidophilus Flora Force (3 capsules, 3 times daily) and NatureSpring Lactobacillus Plantarum (3 capsules, 3 times daily). Take both for the next 10 days.

For more information about **toxic chemicals**, see Chapter 25: What Causes Cancer? pp. 568-577.

## Additional Detoxification Programs for Intestines, Lymph, and Circulation

If there is one thing that most alternative medicine doctors agree on, it is that too many toxins in the body produce illness. Increasingly, toxicity is being identified as the predisposing factor in a long list of acute and chronic, degenerative illnesses. Signs and symptoms of the toxic body can include being overweight, bloating and intestinal gas, insomnia, nausea, bad breath, asthma, constipation, tension, headaches, depression, stress, allergies, menstrual problems, and many others. In addition to the commercial products mentioned above, there are several others available over the counter, enabling anyone to start a self-care detoxification program.

**A.M./P.M. Ultimate Cleanse™**—"When was the last time you cleaned your liver, your heart, your lungs, or your body's sewage system?" asks nutritionist Lindsey Duncan, C.N., chief nutritionist for Home Nutrition Clinic in Santa Monica, California. Duncan offers a practical way to accomplish this, a series of inner detoxification products, including Super Cleanse™, Ultimate Fiber™, and A.M./P.M. Ultimate Cleanse™.

Regarding the latter, this program is set up as a 2-part vegetarian detoxification formula. It involves 29 cleansing herbs, amino acids, antioxidants, digestive enzymes, vitamins, and minerals, and 5 kinds of fiber.

Both Multi-Herb™ and Multi-Fiber™ formulas are taken in the morning and evening in gradually increasing dosages, for several weeks. Positive signs that the detox program is working include flu-like sensations, runny nose, transient pimples, headaches, "brainfog," or fatigue, all of which will pass in 1 to 2 days. "The goal is to stimulate, feed, and detoxify the complete internal body, not just the bowel," states Duncan. "My objective was to address all 5 channels of elimination, as well as all of the vital organs and tissues in the body." At the end of the program, a person should be having 2 to 3 bowel movements every day.

Once the internal system is cleaned out, nutrient absorption can proceed much more efficiently. The key to the effectiveness of the Ultimate Multi™ formula, Duncan explains, is that of timing: the morning formula stimulates; the evening formula relaxes. Following your body's natural digestive and cleansing cycles is the key to proper detoxification and supplementation, says Duncan.

One user, who had endured chronic constipation and bloating for 25 years and as few as 2 to 3 bowel movements a week, lost 16 pounds on the program and started moving her bowels up to 3 times daily after being on the formula for 3 weeks. Another user reported that persistent acne—for 38 years—fatigue, and depression cleared up by the time he completed the internal cleansing program. Another client with lifelong migraine headaches learned that her chronic constipation was a major factor; both were resolved as a result of taking A.M./P.M. Ultimate Cleanse™.

For more information on **detoxification**, see Chapter 4: Etienne Callebout, pp. 100-107; Chapter 23: Lawrence W. Taylor, pp. 492-499; and Chapter 18: Michael B. Schachter, M.D., pp. 354-357.

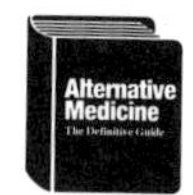


See "Colon Therapy," pp. 143-148; "Detoxification Therapy," pp. 156-166.

CAUTION

All protocols are for adult dosage only and are generalized; that is, dosages and conditions will vary with the individual. Listen to your body; build up the dosage slowly and carefully and only go at a rate you can tolerate. Before beginning any treatment, consult a qualified health-care professional. This is especially important in the case of treating children or if you are pregnant.

**Nature's Pure Body Program™**—Another inner cleansing herbal formula is called Nature's Pure Body Program™ made by Pure Body Institute of Beverly Hills, California. The program is a blend of 27 herbs specifically chosen for their ability to flush toxins out of the organs and old fecal matter from the intestines. For example, buckthorn bark stimulates bile secretion; chickweed and black cohosh root combat blood toxicity; cascara sagrada bark promotes intestinal peristalsis (the intestine's natural contraction rhythms); yarrow flower regulates liver function; peach leaves are

## How to Detoxify Your Fruits and Vegetables

Here's how to get the pesticides and poisons off your foods, according to the late naturopathic physician Hazel Parcells, N.D., of the Parcells Center in Santa Fe, New Mexico. This technique will rid the food items of harmful toxins, chemicals, sprays, and poisons, and it will noticeably improve the flavor and shelf life of the foods.

Before cooking with them, soak all your fruits, eggs, meats, and vegetables in a bath of Clorox and water, at the rate of 1/2 teaspoon Clorox to 1 gallon water. Make sure it is the old-fashioned, pure Clorox; this is hydrochloric acid, not chlorine. Divide your foods into the following categories and soak no longer than the time listed: leafy vegetables (10-15 minutes); root vegetables (15-30 minutes), thin-skinned berries (10-15 minutes), heavy-skinned fruits (15-30 minutes), eggs (20-30 minutes), thawed meats (5-10 minutes per pound).

Prepare a fresh batch of Clorox water for each category of foods; dispose of baths after use. Soak all Clorox-water treated foods in a fresh water bath for 5-10 minutes before using. "This treatment has been used for the last 30 years by many families, saving them untold expenses for illness with no unfavorable reports," said Dr. Parcells.

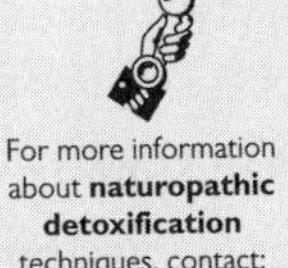

For more information about **naturopathic detoxification** techniques, contact: Parcells Center, 112 W. San Francisco Street, Suite 308B, Santa Fe, NM 87501; tel: 800-811-6784.

a natural laxative; and licorice root stimulates the adrenal glands.

The program consists of 2 sets of pills: colon and whole-body blends. Users start with one colon and 3 whole-body pills taken twice daily with water, 30 minutes before breakfast and 30 minutes before dinner. The colon pills can be increased to 3 pills twice daily, or more, until the bowels move twice daily; the whole-body pills are increased to 4-7, taken 2 times daily. Users need to double their intake of pure water (to at least 64 ounces daily), take one day off from the pills every week, and take a daily multivitamin.

The key here is to go slowly and be patient. The program is designed to last about 30 days although first-time users may find that 3 courses are required for complete inner cleansing and detoxification. Even if you consider yourself healthy, given the degree of toxins in our outer and inner environments, an inner cleansing is beneficial for everyone. "When poor diet, stress, or lack of exercise tax the body beyond its natural abilities to digest, absorb, and eliminate wastes, it is time for a general, internal 'house-cleaning,'" says company president, Ken Wright.

**Restoring the Intestine's Friendly Bacteria**—Under the best of conditions, the estimated 100 trillion bacteria that live in the human intestines do so in a delicate balance. Certain bacteria such as *Lactobacilli* and *Bifidobacteria* are beneficial "friendly" bacteria that support numerous vital physiological processes. Other bacteria, such as *E. coli*, *Staphylococcus*, and *Clostridrium* may be present in smaller numbers, but they are considered "unfriendly," even dangerous bacteria.

For more information about **FOS** and **NutraFlora**®, contact: GTC Nutrition Company, 1400 W. 122nd Avenue, Suite 110, Westminster, CO 80234; tel: 303-254-8012; fax: 303-254-8201.

A healthy intestine maintains a balance of the various intestinal flora, but with current lifestyles and the use of antibiotics, drugs, and processed foods, this balance is often upset. For example, people who eat a high-fat, low-fiber diet have reduced *Bifidobacteria* populations in their intestines. Practitioners of alternative medicine often recommend using probiotics, which means deliberately introducing live "friendly" bacteria into the system through food products (yogurt, *Acidophilus* milk) or through special supplements.

***FOS acts like an intestinal "fertilizer," selectively feeding the friendly microflora in the large intestine so their numbers can usefully increase.* Bifidobacteria *work to lower the pH (acidity/alkalinity balance) in the large intestine to a slightly more acidic condition; this discourages the growth of unfriendly bacteria.***

A new approach, developed in Japan in the mid-1980s, is called *prebiotics*. Here you introduce nutrients that directly feed the beneficial bacteria already in place in a person's large intestine, most typically, *Bifidobacteria* and *Lactobacilli*. In infancy, *Bifidobacteria* account for 95-99% of all intestinal flora, but this percentage declines with age. Japanese researchers determined that a naturally occurring form of carbohydrate called fructo-oligosaccharides (FOS), found in certain foods in minute amounts could be a perfect food for *Bifidobacteria*. FOS acts like an intestinal "fertilizer," selectively feeding the friendly microflora in the large intestine so their numbers can usefully increase. *Bifidobacteria* work to lower the pH (acidity/alkalinity balance) in the large intestine to a slightly more acidic condition; this discourages the growth of unfriendly bacteria.

Studies have demonstrated that taking 1/4 teaspoon (1 g) of NutraFlora® FOS powder daily for 4 weeks led to a 5-fold increase in the total count of beneficial bacteria. A Japanese study found that when 23 hospital patients, aged 50-90, took 8 g of FOS daily for 2 weeks, their *Bifidobacteria* levels increased by 10 times. Benefits from increasing *Bifidobacterium* levels include relief of constipation or diarrhea, promotion of regularity, serum cholesterol reduction, control of blood sugar levels, immune function enhancement, improved calcium absorption and B vitamin synthesis, better digestibility of milk proteins, and a reduction of the detoxification load on the liver, among others. FOS also has been shown to lower blood pressure by 9% when taken at 11.5g daily by people with high blood pressure.

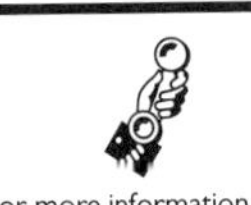

For more information on **FOS**, see Robert Crayhon, *Health Benefits of FOS*, A Keats Good Health Guide (1995), Keats Publishing, 27 Pine Street, P.O. Box 876, New Canaan, CT 06840.

NutraFlora® contains 95% pure FOS in dry powder form or as a syrup to be used as a dietary supplement. While FOS is found in garlic, honey, Jerusalem artichokes, soybeans, burdock, chicory root, asparagus, banana, rye, barley, tomato, onions, and triticale, according to nutrition expert Robert Crayhon, M.S., C.N., "There is not enough FOS in foods in the average diet to get an optimal or therapeutically significant dose."

Technically, you would have to eat 429 garlic gloves to get the same amount of FOS in 1 teaspoon of Nutraflora power. Recognizing this, in Japan today, over 500 commercially prepared foods contain FOS (known there as "neosugar") with the endorsement of Japan's Minister of Health. FOS, which is made by fermenting sucrose with a fungus called Aspergillus niger, is about 30% as sweet as sucrose.

**Coffee enema—**Many alternative cancer physicians use the coffee enema as part of their detoxification program. One of the first to do so was Max Gerson, M.D., founder of the Gerson Diet Therapy for cancer. The following is a review of the procedure, according to Howard Straus, vice president of the Gerson Institute in Bonita, California.[3]

First, it is essential to start with organically raised coffee beans to avoid introducing pesticides, fungicides, and other toxic agricultural chemicals into the intestines. Second, the water used for the enema must be free of chlorine and fluoride; to be completely sure that the water is pure, Straus recommends using distilled water. Straus suggests mixing 3 rounded tablespoonsful of drip-grind coffee to 1 quart of water. The coffee is boiled for 3 minutes, simmered for 15-20 minutes, then strained and cooled to body temperature. This produces enough coffee for a single enema.

As a shortcut to repeating this procedure 5 times each day (for 5 enemas), Straus suggests preparing a "concentrate or instant enema" mix. He suggests boiling 2 quarts of water to which 3 cups of organic drip-grind coffee is added; this boils for another 3 minutes, then is simmered for 12-15 minutes, then strained. If the resulting product is less than 2 quarts, add enough distilled water to bring the volume back to 2 quarts. Straus then advises using 4 ounces of this concentrate mixed with 3 1/2 cups of water for each enema. Refrigerate the unused amounts of prepared coffee. "Do not prepare the enema coffee as though you were brewing coffee," Straus says. Otherwise the potassium normally present in coffee, and which is of considerable benefit to the body as a nutrient, is lost.

***When the lymph-collecting terminals become blocked, it's like a bottleneck: lymph starts backing up in the system creating a toxic, oxygen-deprived environment conducive to degeneration. It can develop into a tumorous condition.***

## Deciphering the Link between Lymph Circulation and Cancer

The cells of the immune system, called lymphocytes or white blood cells, have 2 ways of circulating through the body: the circulatory system and the lymphatic system. The latter comprises a network of lymph ducts or channels and transports lymph fluid. Lymph is a clear fluid that accumulates in the tissue spaces between cells and in the tiniest blood vessels (capillaries) to eventually enter the lymphatic network.

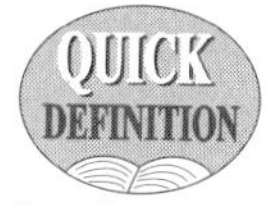


**Lymph nodes** are clusters of immune tissue that work as filters or "inspection stations" for detecting foreign and potentially harmful substances in the lymph fluid. The body has many dozens of lymph nodes, but most are clustered in the chest, groin, armpits, neck, and abdomen.

Interspersed throughout the lymph channels are tight clusters of cells called lymph nodes, which act as primary filters protecting the bloodstream from numerous foreign and toxic substances. Each lymph node contains various scavenger cells (macrophages and reticuloendothelial cells) that help break down toxins and microbes. In this way, the lymphatic system serves primarily as a highly efficient filter for the bloodstream.

Since the lymph carries essential nutrients and various immune components, any interference with its flow can adversely affect the body as a whole. Unlike the blood, which is moved primarily by the pumping action of the heart, the lymphatic system lacks a pump. Its movement depends entirely on the body's own movements, including contractions of the diaphragm in the act of breathing and muscular contractions during physical activity. During physical inactivity, the fat droplets can form in the large lymph channels in the chest and abdomen and float to blood vessels where they may impede blood circulation.

The lymphatic system and digestive system share an intimate relationship. A person consuming a low-fiber, heavy meat diet will tend to

## How to Limit Your Exposure to Toxins in the Home

It is highly advisable to be wary of carcinogenic chemicals and contaminants found in common consumer items, including household products, cosmetics, processed foods, beverages, paints, paint thinners, furniture polishes, car interior cleaners, and the like. They all contain carcinogens ranging from formaldehyde to crystalline silica. Although none of these products alone may present a critical carcinogenic exposure, when many little exposures are added together, they present a *cumulative* toxic load, that stresses the body's immune system and damages cells until eventually, over time, cancer can set in.[4]

For example, avoiding electromagnetic exposure (especially while you are asleep) by measuring your environment with a gauss meter and unplugging all electric appliances that have high gauss readings (a basic unit of electromagnetic energy) reduces your cancer risk. Avoiding geopathic exposure (again, especially while you are asleep) by measuring your immediate environment with a geomagnetometer (or using copper or brass dowsing rods) also significantly reduces cancer risk. Radiation exposures from televisions, computer monitors, microwave ovens, and fluorescent lights should also be minimized or avoided altogether.

Generally, it is wise to be cautious about nearly all products. Many chemicals used in cosmetics, pesticides, and other products do not require full safety testing before they are allowed to be marketed and used by millions of consumers. For example, among 2 brands of kitchen cleansers, Ajax™ contains high amounts of crystalline silica while its competitor, Comet™, does not.[5]

Therefore, one must become a prudent, wary, and skeptical shopper. "This sort of conscientious buying will enable people to vote with their dollars for an environmental clean-up of all carcinogenic substances used in manufacturing and industry, including those found in pesticides," according to Samuel Epstein, M.D. Dr. Epstein recommends boycotting all consumer products containing known carcinogens, then finding healthy, natural substitutes. "For example, a combination of plain water mixed with distilled white vinegar and a small amount of baking soda, Borax, and lemon juice can clean the home and bathroom as effectively as many higher-priced cleaners."

accumulate carcinogens and toxic matter in the intestine. These products can form a potentially lethal mixture of intestinal bacteria, parasites, toxins, and blood-derived products which can then enter the circulation via the intestinal lymphatics or by absorption from the peritoneal cavity. (Also called the peritoneum, this is the membrane that covers the entire abdominal wall on the inside of the body and envelops the organs in that area.)[6] This situation, in turn, can lead to blood toxicity (toxemia) and eventually to the immune-related changes that predispose a person to cancer and other diseases.

The lymphatic system may be likened to an efficient plumbing system. If the plumbing's clogged, the bathroom isn't worth much. That's the same situation with the lymphatics. The system has to be capable of flowing freely and filtering out the toxins. Otherwise, the liver, kidneys, and lungs have to work much harder to keep the system clean. Eventually, these other organs themselves become weakened by the constant flow of toxins from the polluted lymph nodes and channels.

Few people actually die of cancer. Rather, they die of toxemia, produced by an excessive buildup of toxins. This is where the lymph system comes into play. As people grow old or become less physically active, the flow of lymph fluid is impaired; muscle tension from chronic stress can further promote accumulations of toxins. Proteins begin to concentrate in the lymph vessels and nodes, which become clogged, stagnated, and inflamed; the result is a kind of "traffic jam" in the lymph channels.

> ***The lymph system is the beginning and end of all disease. Once you get the lymph circulating freely again, this enhances recovery from any illness by reversing the slow, possibly lifetime, poisoning your body has endured.***

The functional integrity of the lymphatic system is intimately linked with 2 factors that have generally eluded modern medicine: a person's psychological state and the electromagnetic energy surrounding and permeating the body. First, chronic muscular tensions created from stressful emotional experiences can constrict the lymphatic system and lead to increased accumulations of toxins. Second, the body's electromagnetic energies can be affected by the state of one's psyche.

The flow and distribution of the body's electromagnetic energy is automatically responsive to the psychological state of the individual and acts as a bridging influence, linking the psyche to the body. Problems in metabolism appear to be influenced by a toxic chemical environment, but these problems become amplified when the person is experiencing some form of extreme distress.

In addition, many important lymphocytes, including natural killer (NK) cells, are formed in the lymph nodes. The lymphatic system is thus responsible not only for moving waste and microbes from body tissue, but also for forming lymphocytes. Taken together, these points highlight important links between the lymphatic system, stress, toxemia, and cancer.

When the lymph fails to function properly, it becomes stagnant. The clear lymph fluid becomes cloudy and thick, progressively changing from its watery condition to the consistency of milk, then yogurt, then cottage cheese. Thickened, stagnant lymph overloaded with toxic wastes is the ideal condition for the development of numerous illnesses, including cancer. When the collecting terminals become blocked, it's like a bottleneck: lymph starts backing up in the system creating a toxic, oxygen-deprived environment conducive to degeneration. It can develop into a tumorous condition. Toxic lymph can be stored for a long time in the system, just the way the intestines "store" fecal matter, often for years. This is not a healthy condition. The pivotal point here is that when the lymph circulation is impeded, the entire body tends to become more toxic and oxygen deprived. When the lymph fluid backs up because of blockage, pressure builds up in the lymph channels, and, subsequently, in the cell bed. At this point, the system becomes toxic due to waste disposal failure. This is when cancer and other degenerative ailments can accelerate.

There are many interlinked conditions that contribute to sluggish lymph circulation and that get improved during lymphatic treatment. These include hormonal imbalances; chronic constipation and intestinal blockages; muscle and tissue tension including structural misalignment in the neck and shoulders; mental confusion and emotional disorder. The lymph system is the beginning and end of all disease. Once you get the lymph circulating freely again, this enhances recovery from any illness by reversing the slow, possibly lifetime, poisoning your body has endured.

A primary goal of lymph therapy, then, is to break up the lymph congestion—all the waste debris, toxins, and fatty acids that the lymphatics *should be* eliminating from the body.

## How Lymphatic Therapy Works

The equipment used for lymphatic therapy resembles a flashlight with a long, extensible housing. Noble gases such as argon and neon are stimulated by an electrical current to emit a diffuse orange light through the treatment "flashlight" head. The physician projects the light upon the skin, first concentrating on opening up the 2 drainage sites in the upper chest and neck where lymph dumps into the bloodstream.

Specifically, the practitioner directs the light on the exit points of the subclavian vein at the clavicle and this, in turn, breaks up stagnation and creates rapid improvements in health. Lymph enters into the blood at the subclavian vein. It is most important to open up the exit area during the treatment protocol. Then it is important to continue the treatment in a systematic way, closely following the lymphatic flow, using the light emissions and hand-delivered lymph-draining procedures. Lymphatic decongestion and blockages are charged with incoherent light, creating separation by allowing molecules to repel each other. Trapped blood protein clusters are thus broken up and unobstructed lymph flow is reestablished. This effect significantly enhances the body's efficiency in dealing with pathological conditions.

As for its effects on cancer specifically, lymphatic therapy may enhance the immune system's capacity for cell-eating [phagocytosis] of the metastatic cancer cell or it may make establishment of the cancer cell at a new site much more difficult by significantly increasing the negative charges present on the walls of the fluid system. In this way, the use of lymphatic therapy should actually lower the risk of early metastatic disease.

Lymph therapy is a whole-body approach. After these sites are opened, the natural flow of the lymph throughout the body is stimulated. The light breaks up the protein congestion in the lymph, turning it from "cottage cheese" back to "milk;" then precise hand-delivered massage gets the lymph moving again, draining into the bloodstream with its toxic wastes. Thus the treatment detoxifies the tissues by freeing up the lymph circulation.

Detoxification in this way, by reestablishing free lymphatic circulation throughout the body, is a vital part of any healing process. Once you clear up the lymph flow, which is an essential component of the immune

## The Negative Health Impact of Bras

The lymph channels and nodes of the armpit tend to become congested from wearing bras and from lack of exercise. This observation has recently been confirmed by Sidney Singer and Soma Grismaijer, who present compelling evidence for a connection between bras and breast cancer in *Dressed to Kill* (Avery, 1995). The authors conducted a 3-year study of 4,700 women living in cities throughout the U.S.

Women who wore their bras over 12 hours daily but not to bed—the majority—were 21 times more likely to develop breast cancer compared with women who wore their bras less than 12 hours a day. On extreme ends of the bra-wearing spectrum, women who also wore bras to bed had a 125-fold greater chance of getting breast cancer than did women who refrained from wearing bras altogether.[7]

system, you enhance the body's natural healing ability to help clear up nearly *any* illness. Even after a single treatment, the patient's complexion and skin tone begin to acquire a healthy glow. Breast cancer patients in particular show rapid benefits from lymphatic therapy treatment as a clinical focus on the lymphatics in the armpit area and subclavian vein help detoxify the breast tissues.

A related system called manual lymph drainage developed in the 1930s by a Danish scientist, Emil Vodder, Ph.D., working in France as a masseur is also of value. This consists of specific massage movements performed by a trained practitioner that enable the lymph to begin draining. Dr. Vodder described these as "circular pumping and draining movements" of sufficiently light pressure so as to prevent blood congestion. "We employed gentle stationary circles on the lymph nodes, an area that no one had previously dared to massage, palpating with the tips or the entire length of the fingers," Dr. Vodder explained.

"Massaging was always in the direction of the clavicular fossa, the terminus of all lymph pathways in the body." Dr. Vodder noted that the method had benefits not only for cosmetic and preventive measures, but also "to cure illnesses," and that it was capable of producing "surprising and rapid results." Providing slow and rhythmic movements, Dr. Vodder obtained positive results for conditions such as skin rejuvenation, hematomas produced by accidents, eczema, varicose veins, and ulcerous legs.

He noted that an average of 35 billion lymphocytes enter the blood every day through the lymph nodes that empty into veins in the neck, but during stress, this number can climb to 562 billion. "One thing, however, is certain, said Dr. Vodder. "The lymph system not only serves to clean tissues through the drainage, but is also a protection, a defense mechanism, and carries out vital functions."[8]

**Light Beam Generator (LBG)—**To free up a clogged lymphatic system as part of a detoxification program, devices called the Light Beam Generator™ and Lymph-Pho Laser™ are highly effective. The devices radiate photons (light) to help restore the cells' normal energy state, allowing the body to heal itself more readily. The equipment used resembles a flashlight with a long, extensible housing. Noble gases such as argon and neon are stimulated by an electric current to emit a diffuse purple light through its "flashlight" head. The practitioner projects the light onto the skin, often focusing on lymph nodes and channels, such as the 2 drainage sites in the upper chest and neck where lymph flows into the bloodstream.

"The Light Beam Generator can be used anywhere on the body where there is a problem," says Robert Jacobs, N.M.D., D.Hom. (Med), of London, England, "and because of its deep penetration, it can help heal organs and structures deep within the body, as well as skin problems." Dr. Jacobs also points out that since healthy cells are in a stable energetic state, there are no adverse effects when the LBG is used in 30-45 minute sessions. The effectiveness of the LBG is due to its stimulation of the lymphatic system, the intricate network of vessels and ducts that filter toxins out of the bloodstream.

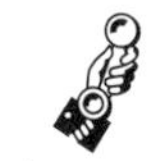

For information about lymph detoxification equipment such as the **Lymph Pho/Laser**®, contact: Marika von Viczay, Ph.D., N.M.D., 16 Arlington Street, Asheville, NC 28801; tel: 704-253-8371; fax: 704-258-1350. For information about the **Light Beam Generator**, contact: ELF Teslar, Star Route 1, Box 21, St. Francisville, IL 62460; tel: 618-948-2393; fax: 618-948-2650.

## Dry Skin Brushing Helps the Lymph System Remove Toxins

The skin is the largest eliminative organ of the body which is why it is sometimes called the third kidney. The skin can eliminate more than a pound of waste products in the form of sweat throughout the day. It is also an absorptive organ, capable of absorbing oxygen, vitamins, minerals, even protein; but it can also absorb toxic substances (such as through air and water contact), which can find their way into internal organs.

Dry skin brushing is based on concepts from acupuncture which states that there are an estimated 3 million nerve points spread over the surface of the skin, 700 of which are nodal, meaning they can serve as treatment nodes in acupuncture. For example, a point in the web between the thumb and forefinger of the right hand connects to the liver. Dry skin brushing, by applying friction to these acupuncture nodal points, can take advantage of these energy connections, stimulating and invigorating the entire nervous system, such that every organ, gland, muscle, and ligament benefits.

Dry skin brushing, if done in the correct fashion, also helps to physically move toxic lymph fluid through the lymph vessels toward the central venous circulation so that the toxins in the lymph fluid and in the tissue can be cleared from the body by other toxin clearing organs including the kidneys, liver, intestines, and lungs. This dumping of toxins significantly improves the function of the immune system and most other organ systems.

You will need a moderately soft natural vegetable fiber bristle brush, preferably with a removable wooden handle. Nylon or synthetic fibers build up undesirable static electromagnetic energy, in addition to being too sharp and possibly hurting the skin. Brush gently at first; some parts of the body are more sensitive than others. Within a few days, your skin will become conditioned. As you become accustomed to dry brushing, the process should take no more than 10 minutes daily. It would be a good idea to brush your skin daily for 3 months then twice weekly as a lifetime practice. Every 2 weeks or so, wash your brush with soap and water and dry it in the sun or in a warm place. Your brush will rapidly fill with impurities and should be washed regularly. For hygienic reasons, each member of the family should have a separate brush.

**Summarizing the benefits of dry skin brushing:**

- Blood circulation is stimulated and increased in all organs and tissues, skin is toned, tightened, and given a warm, rosy glow.
- Brushed skin is better able to eliminate toxins from the body, relieving the burden on kidneys, liver, lungs and colon.
- Metabolism of all tissues is improved thus helping to relieve mental and muscular fatigue.
- Nerve endings are stimulated, rejuvenating the entire nervous system.
- Cellulite is reduced, which is toxic material stored in the body's fat cells.
- Stress is released, which can relieve chronic headaches.
- The lungs and circulation are stimulated which increases oxygen to the brain.

## The Removal of Internal Parasites Is Essential in Detoxification

Most conventional doctors are unaware of the connection between parasites and health and thus fail to recognize the clinical symptoms. These include joint and muscle aches, anemia, allergy, skin conditions, nervousness, diarrhea, bloating, constipation, chronic fatigue, and immune dysfunction, among others. In fact, members of the same family can have the same species of parasites yet show completely different symptoms—emotional upsets, food allergies, fatigue, bowel discomfort—or no symptoms. That is why nutrition educator Ann Gittleman states, "If these symptoms and feelings

## Chelation Removes Heavy Metals and Reduces Cardiovascular Disease

Chelation therapy refers to a method of binding ("chelating") an organic substance known as a chelating agent to a metallic ion with a positive electric charge (e.g., a heavy metal) and removing it from the body. One type of chelation therapy involves the chelating agent disodium EDTA given as an intravenous infusion over a 3-1/2 hour period. Usually 20 to 30 treatments are administered at the rate of 1 to 3 sessions per week.

In addition to removing heavy metals from the body, chelation has other therapeutic benefits. For example, infusions of EDTA are extremely beneficial for all forms of atherosclerotic cardiovascular disease including angina pectoris and coronary artery disease, intermittent claudication and gangrene, atherosclerotic cardiovascular disease of the legs and feet, and strokes in cardiovascular disease of the neck and brain arteries.

Chelation reduces abnormal tissue calcification, enhances and stimulates a variety of enzymes for healing purposes, improves circulation to all tissues throughout the body, and reduces free-radical damage—one of the major common denominators of cancer and all other degenerative diseases. By reducing the body's free-radical burden (which would otherwise promote tumor growth), chelation probably enhances one's ability to fight cancer.[9]

Chelation therapy produced health improvements in up to 91% of patients, according to a 1993 Danish study of 470 people with heart problems. Of 92 patients recommended for surgery, only 10 still needed it after chelation. In addition to the savings in human suffering, avoiding these surgeries amounted to a savings of $3 million in insurance payments. "We conclude that EDTA chelation therapy is safe, effective, and cost-saving," said C. Hancke, M.D., and K. Flytlie, M.D., in the *Journal of Advancement in Medicine*.

When researchers L. Terry Chappell, M.D., and John P. Stahl, Ph.D., reviewed the results of 19 studies evaluating the effectiveness of EDTA chelation therapy on 22,765 patients, they found that 87% registered clinical improvement according to objective tests. In one study, 58 out of 65 coronary bypass candidates and 24 of 27 people scheduled for limb amputation were able to cancel their surgery. The analysis provides "very strong evidence that EDTA is effective in the treatment of cardiovascular disease," state Chappell and Stahl in *Questions from the Heart* (Virginia Beach, VA: Hampton Roads Publishing, 1996).

sound familiar, then you may be an unsuspecting victim of the parasite epidemic that is affecting million of Americans."

With this information in mind, here are practical steps often employed to start detoxifying one's system of presumed parasites.

**1. Cleanse the Intestines:** Parasites tend to embed themselves in the intestinal wall, but over the course of several weeks, you can flush them out by using some of these natural substances (preferably in combination): psyllium husks, agar-agar, citrus pectin, papaya extract, pumpkin seeds, flaxseeds, comfrey root, beet root, and bentonite clay (take bentonite only in combination with another substance, such as psyllium). You might also take extra amounts of vitamin C (minimum 2g daily, but higher amounts up to individual bowel tolerance are more useful) to help flush out your intestine. Note, however, that vitamin C taken at the same time as wormwood makes wormwood ineffective.

**2. Do a Colon Irrigation:** Irrigate the colon with 2-16 quarts of water. To the water you may add black walnut tincture or extract, garlic juice, vinegar (2 tablespoons per quart of water), blackstrap molasses (1 tablespoon per quart of water), or organically raised coffee. Use filtered or distilled water for the enema; further sterilize it by boiling or ozonating it for 10-15 minutes before use, including before using it to prepare the coffee.

**3. Prepare Your System:** It is prudent to give your gallbladder and liver a week to prepare for the parasite program. To flush the gallbladder of its toxins, take lime juice in warm water or Swedish Bitters before each meal. Eliminate all refined and natural sugars, meats, and dairy products during the parasite program; even better, start cutting back on them during this preparatory week. Take barberry bark capsules, dandelion, or a similar herbal extract to help cleanse the liver. The amount depends on health and the strength or composition of the specific substance or brand-name product used.

**CAUTION**

Individuals with Chronic Fatigue and Immune Dysfunction Syndrome (CFIDS), multiple chemical sensitivity, or fibromyalgia, using Dr. Clark's program (with the added components of the amino acid ornithine and the daily use of an electronic "zapper" to kill parasites) have reported severe CFIDS relapses, infectious processes, sleep disorders, weight loss, severe fatigue anxiety, and fluctuating emotional states. Source: Meyer, Adrianna, R.N. "Iatrogenic Exacerbation of CFS Symptoms in Three Patients Who Used Hulda Clark's Methods in Cure for All Diseases," *Townsend Letter for Doctors & Patients* (November 1996), 97-100.

**4. The Herbal Cleanout:** Naturopathic physician Hulda Regehr Clark, N.D., Ph.D., recommends using a blend of 3 herbs to flush the parasites out of your system: black walnut hull tincture, wormwood capsules, and fresh ground cloves (to kill the parasites' eggs). The following protocol is a composite prepared for this book from the typical (independent) recommendations of Dr. Clark and author W. Lee Cowden, M.D. Do the program for 10-14 days, take 5-7 days off, then repeat for another 10-14 days.

**Black Walnut Hulls—**If you take liquid extract, make sure the extract is made from fresh whole green hulls of black walnut. You may also use black walnut capsules. Take with water 15-20 minutes before meals. This is a typical recommendation for black walnut hull capsules:

**Day 1:** 1 capsule 2X daily

**Day 2:** 2 capsules 2X daily

**Day 3:** 2 capsules 3X daily

**Day 4:** 3 capsules 3X daily

**Day 5:** 4 capsules 3X daily

**Day 6:** 5 capsules 3X daily

**Day 7:** 6 capsules 3X daily

Continue at 6 capsules 3X daily through day 14. During the second 10-day round, take 6 capsules 3X each day, but without repeating this gradual buildup in dose.

For black walnut hull extract, build up as follows:

**Day 1:** 2 drops 4X daily, mixed in water. Space the drops 4 hours apart, starting in the morning.

**Day 2:** 4 drops 4X daily

**Day 3:** 6 drops 4X daily

Work up to 20 drops taken 4 times daily and continue at this rate until the treatment program is finished.

CAUTION

Expect to feel uncomfortable during the first 10-14 days of the herbal cleanout. You may experience achiness, malaise, bloating, intestinal discomfort, gas, even diarrhea for 1 or more days. You may experience slight but odd shifts in your psychological state and you may experience a variety of temporary sensations, such as heat in your ears, activity behind your eyes, a momentary sense of dizziness or imbalance, or a transient loss of appetite. If you tend to have low blood sugar, this may temporarily worsen before it improves.

These are signs that parasites lodged in various body systems (eyes, or ears, for example) are being killed off. You may also have a day in which you feel completely rotten. It simply means that your body is temporarily toxic from the dead parasites your system is struggling to flush clear. You will feel fine—and possibly exceptional—the next day.

**Wormwood (or Artemisia Combination)**—This herb works best when the full day's dosage is taken at one time, 15-20 minutes before a meal. This is a typical recommendation for wormwood:

**Day 1:** 2 capsules

**Day 2:** 4 capsules

**Day 3:** 6 capsules

**Day 4:** 8 capsules

**Day 5:** 10 capsules

**Day 6:** 12 capsules

**Day 7:** 14 capsules

**Day 7:** 14 capsules

**Day 9:** 14 capsules

**Day 10:** 14 capsules

On days 11-14, take 14 capsules.

Stay off wormwood during the same 5-7 days you're off black walnut, Dr. Cowden advises; then resume at 14 capsules of wormwood daily for another 10-14 days.

**Cloves**—Crush fresh cloves in a coffee grinder and fill gelatin capsules

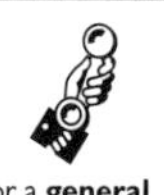

For a **general intestinal cleanser**, try Colon Enhancer from The Vitamin Shoppe, 4700 Westside Avenue, North Bergen, NJ 07047; tel: 800-223-1216. For the **black walnut, wormwood, and cloves** you need to start the parasite detoxification program as formulated by Dr. Hulda Clark, contact Self-Health Resource Center, 757 Emory Street, No. 508, Imperial Beach, CA 91932; tel: 619-429-4408. Another option is to use **Parasite Out**®, a blend of 2 kinds of wormwood, black walnut seeds, and grapefruit seed extract, available from Carotec, Inc., P.O. Box 9919, Naples, FL 33941; tel: 800-522-4279. For **Wormwood Combination** capsules, containing wormwood, quassia, cloves, male fern, and black walnut leaves, contact Hanna's Herb Shop, 5684 Valmont Road, Boulder, CO 80301; tel: 800-206-6722. Physicians may contact Kroeger Herb Products, 805 Walnut Street, Boulder, CO 80302; tel: 303-443-0261.

(size "00") with the ground substance. Fill the capsules at once and discard any leftover clove powder as it loses its potency quickly when exposed to the air. You will need 171 clove capsules for two 10-day regimens, or 243 for two 14-day regimens:

**Day 1:** 1 capsule 3X daily

**Day 2:** 2 capsules 3X daily

**Day 3:** 3 capsules 3X daily

Then 3 capsules 3X daily through day 10 or 14.

Take capsules 15-20 minutes before meals. Stay off cloves the same days you are off wormwood and black walnut, then resume at 3 capsules, 3X daily for another 10-14 days. You might also use Proseed Grapefruit Seed Extract during the first 3 days of this program for an extra germicidal boost.

**5. Children:** If you have children, they must be treated at the same time as the adults in the household. Children who can swallow capsules can take doses of the above-described herbs reduced according to their body weight. Typically, a 50-pound child would take 1/3 of the adult dose; a 75-pound child would take 1/2 the adult dose; and a 100-pound child would take 2/3 of the adult dose.

**6. Pets:** If you have pets, you must treat them at the same time as you treat yourself, otherwise the chance of your getting reinfected from them is high.

**7. Maintenance:** After you finish your second 10-day round, wait 7 days then take, before your largest meal of the day, 2 doses a week of: 3 capsules black walnut, 14 capsules wormwood, 3 capsules cloves. Take this dose once on Monday, then once on Thursday, and maintain for 2-3 months.

**8. Vitamin C:** The individual must drink extra pure water and take extra vitamin C to flush the toxins out of the blood. For adults, take 2000-4000 mg of vitamin C every 1-2 hours until bowel movements turn to water. This will indicate the toxins are being flushed out of your body. Do this over a 24-hour period, then reduce your vitamin C intake to 4000 mg daily.

**9. Oxygen Supplements:** It is advisable to take oxygen supplements to help flush the toxins out of your system and to oxygenate the blood during this process of killing parasites. Useful here are Oxyflex capsules (see below) which consist of super-oxygenated magnesium plus ascorbic acid and bioflavonoids. Take 2 capsules, 3 times daily, 1 hour before meals at one time.

**10. Drink Extra Water:** It is important to drink much more pure water (not from the tap) than usual during this process to help your body flush the now dead parasites from your system; at least 64 ounces of water per day for a 150-pound adult.

**11. Sanitize Your Environment:** When you have almost finished the 10-day round, wash all pajamas, bedclothes, and sheets before using them again.

**12. Eat Anti-Parasitic Foods:** According to Gittleman, these include pineapple and papaya, either as fresh juice or in supplement form, in combination with pepsin and hydrochloric acid. Avoid all meats and dairy products for at least 1 week. You can also use pomegranate juice (four 8-ounce glasses daily), papaya seeds, finely-ground or roasted pumpkin seeds (1/4 to 1/2 cup daily), and 2 cloves of raw garlic daily. Do not use the pomegranate juice for more than 4-5 days.

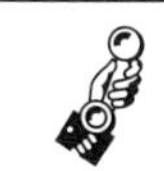

For **Oxyflex**, contact AMERIflex, Inc., 232 N.E. Lincoln, Suite I, Hillsboro, OR 97124; tel: 800-487-5463 or 503-640-0810. **Grapefruit Seed Extract** is available as ProSeed™ as Liquid Concentrate, Vegicaps® (vegetarian capsules), Feminine Rinse, Ear Drops, Gum Cleanser, Herbal Cleansing Spray, and Foot Powder. A similar line called Seed-a-Sept™, is formulated for physicians. For both, contact: Imhotep, Inc., P.O. Box 183, Ruby, NY 12475; tel: 800-677-8577.

**13. Modify Your Diet:** For bodies ridden with parasites, nutritionist Gittleman recommends a diet comprising 25% fat, 25% protein, and 50% complex carbohydrates. You also need a regular intake of unprocessed flaxseed, safflower, sesame, or sunflower oil (2 tablespoons daily), and higher than RDA amounts of vitamin A. Flaxseed oil is preferable because it has much higher levels of alpha linolenic acid (commonly deficient in many people) than the other oils.

**14. Recolonize Your Intestines:** You need to reintroduce beneficial, friendly bacteria (probiotics) into your intestinal system now that you have flushed out the parasites, Gittleman advises. The bacterial strains most helpful here are *Lactobacillus plantarum*, *salvarius*, *acidophilus*, *bulgaris*, and *bifidus*, and *Streptococcus faeceum*, which are available as nutritional supplements. *L. plantarum* is the most effective of these in combating parasite problems.

## Detoxifying the Mind and Emotions of the Cancer Patient

Fear and depression often follow the standard diagnosis of cancer. The continued presence of these emotions and other chronic toxic emotions such as anger, grief, guilt, or perceived lack of self-worth (any or all of which may be present only at the subconscious level) stimulates the production of potentially destructive neurotransmitters or hormones such as cortisone which, in turn, can cause the cancer to spread. People who tend to be overly accommodating or passive, particularly those who carry around a lot of unexpressed fear and anger, are the ones who generally don't do as well after a cancer diagnosis," says Lawrence Taylor, M.D. (the subject of Chapter 23). "The research I've seen on the psychosomatic basis for cancer survival suggests that these types of people may be 6 times more vulnerable to cancer and cancer mortality."[10]

***Women with breast cancer who participated in a weekly support group lived twice as long as those who did not. These women were given the opportunity to express their feelings about their condition, their doctors and anything else they were experiencing. It seems that this freedom to give vent to emotions gave support to the immune system.***

Success in reversing cancer requires getting rid of the negative thinking, says Dr. Taylor. "If you have anger or fear, you tend to stimulate a cascade of hormonal reactions that lead to immune system dysfunction." These anxiety-related emotions stimulate the production of ACTH (adrenocorticotropic hormone), which in turn stimulates the adrenal gland to produce cortisone and adrenaline. This so-called "fight or flight" reaction is desirable when you face a physical threat, such as an attacker. However, when neither fight nor flight occurs, the hormones produced are to no purpose, in which case they can suppress the anticancer defenses.

"People need to realize that they can alter the course of their cancer by the way they think about themselves and the world around them," says Dr. Taylor. "When you have feelings of joy and happiness, you produce more endorphins, which make you feel good." The endorphins, he adds, contribute to the synthesis of the hormone DHEA by the adrenal glands, which stimulates the thymus gland to carry out its immune functions more effectively. In other words, says Dr. Taylor, the immune system is bolstered by faith, hope, and happiness.

To win the battle against cancer, Dr. Taylor asserts that a total change in attitude is needed. The ideal anticancer attitude, he says, has two primary components: (1) it is hopeful, optimistic or life-affirming; and (2) it is assertive regarding one's own needs—asking a friend or loved one to turn the music down if it is disturbing.

Making adjustments in one's attitude and emotional life is just one factor in healing. "A person can have a perfectly great attitude and fairly balanced emotional disposition," says Dr. Taylor. "But if they eat an imbalanced diet, rich in high-fat and high-sugar foods, they're just going to reduce their chances of surviving a cancer diagnosis." In other words, the entire lifestyle must be reoriented to one that supports the immune system and total body healing.

How one lives also needs to be looked at closely. This includes the quality and dynamics of one's job, major relationships, living situation, and sexual habits. "There is overwhelming evidence that people who have few social contacts are more likely to get sick and less likely to recover from an illness," says Erik Peper, Ph.D., Associate Director of the Institute of Holistic Healing Studies at San Francisco State University. People with the fewest social ties are 2 to 3 times more likely to die of all causes than those with the most social connectedness.[13]

These lifestyle factors seem to be especially important when the diagnosis is cancer. David Spiegel, M.D., a psychiatrist at Stanford University, demonstrated that women with breast cancer who participated in a weekly support group lived twice as long as those who did not.[14] These women were given the opportunity to express their feelings about their condition, their doctors and anything else they were experiencing. It seems that this freedom to give vent to emotions gave support to the immune system. In a 30-year study, medical students characterized as "loners" who suppressed their emotions beneath a bland exterior were 16 times more likely to develop cancer than those who gave vent to emotions and, at times, took active measures to relieve anger or frustration.[15]

## Coping Style and Cancer Survival

The research evidence suggests that coping style can also help prevent the recurrence of cancer. A study of women with recurrent breast cancer found that joy, levity, and happiness are associated with longer periods of being free of symptoms;[11] a study of over 2,000 men, followed for 17 years, revealed that those who score highest on depression tests have twice the incidence of cancer-related deaths.[12] The high cancer rate among the more depressed men in this study cannot be explained on the basis of their drinking and smoking habits.

***"People need to realize that they can alter the course of their cancer by the way they think about themselves and the world around them," says Dr. Taylor.***

Taking a more assertive view toward one's personal needs may also have its advantages in curbing the development of cancer. Much research suggests a connection between the progression of certain cancers—breast cancer and malignant melanoma—and passivity in coping with stressful situations.[16] In this context, it is interesting to note that the body's response to repression—the "conservation-withdrawal" reaction—involves neuroendocrine mechanisms different from those involved in the body's fight-or-flight reaction.[17]

In addition, feeling a sense of control seems vital to health and resistance to all disease. The greater the perceived impact of a stressful event—a hurricane versus a thunderstorm—the lower one's sense of control tends to be. When people feel that some major life upheaval is overwhelming, they are more inclined to feel hopeless and such hopelessness increases their risk of cancer.[18] Research in breast cancer patients indicated that when a stressful life event was felt to be beyond the woman's control, the likelihood of relapse was greater.[19]

***Disease does not arise solely from external effects on the body; it is the interaction between these effects and the body's immune system that counts. By all indications, we should consider the mind to be an integral part of the immune system.***

It is crucial to understand here that the cause of cancer is not the presence of a carcinogen alone, but in combination with the body's weakened capacity to destroy cancer cells and tumors as they arise from the *influence* of carcinogens. Disease does not arise solely from external effects on the body; it is the *interaction* between these effects and the body's immune system that counts. By all indications, we should consider the mind to be an integral part of the immune system.

# Biological Dentistry

**Biological dentists work to remove these sources of dental toxins and to correct all dental problems potentially associated with cancer. Mercury that leaches from dental fillings and migrates to body tissues and root canals with hidden, untreated infections can contribute to the development of cancer.**

Biological dentistry stresses the use of nontoxic restoration materials for dental work and focuses on the unrecognized impact that dental toxins and hidden dental infections can have on overall health.

Typically, a biological dentist will emphasize the safe removal of mercury dental amalgams; in many cases, the avoidance or removal of root canals; the investigation of possible jawbone infections as a "dental focus" or source of bodywide illness centered in the teeth; and the health-injuring role of misaligned teeth and malformed jaw structures.

There is a slowly building recognition among dentists and physicians practicing alternative medicine that dental health has a tremendous impact on the health and illness of the body. European researchers estimate that perhaps as much as 50% of all chronic degenerative illness can be linked either directly or indirectly to dental problems and the techniques of modern dentistry.

***European researchers estimate that perhaps as much as 50% of all chronic degenerative illness can be linked either directly or indirectly to dental problems and the techniques of modern dentistry.***

## Eliminate the "Silent Toxins" of Infected Teeth and Tonsils

One of the first Western practitioners to address the hidden dental connection to cancer was the German physician, Josef Issels, M.D., who understood that in a person who has lung cancer, the *entire* body is involved, not merely the lung or breast. Therapeutic attention must be directed at healing the whole organism and changing the biochemical milieu that enables cancer cells to thrive. To reverse the cancer, the body needs to be detoxified, nourished, and biochemically rebalanced, said Dr. Issels.

In the late 1940s, Dr. Issels proposed that a healthy body would not develop cancer and that the best way to attack cancer was not to attack the tumor alone but to strengthen the individual's metabolism. In his words, "[T]he tumor is merely a late-stage symptom, accidentally triggered off, but able to exist and grow only in a bed already prepared for it."[20] Like other chronic illnesses, cancer can lie dormant and be activated only when the metabolism is altered to a point where the defense mechanisms are no longer capable of destroying the malignant cells.

***One of the first steps in WBT is the removal of infected, dead teeth and mercury fillings, a tremendous source of toxic stress on the body.***

From this realization Dr. Issels developed his *Ganzheitstherapie*, or whole-body therapy (WBT), which integrates many different modalities into a single protocol aimed at improving the body's natural defense systems. Wolfgang Wöppel, M.D., an associate of Dr. Issels, states that WBT focuses much attention on the contributions of "genetic traits, microbes, dental amalgams and infections, abnormal intestinal flora, faulty diet, neural interferences, chemical toxins, and radiation." One of the first steps in WBT is the removal of infected, dead teeth and mercury fillings, a tremendous source of toxic stress on the body.

Regarding the cancer-promoting potential of an infected tooth and root canal, Dr. Issels states, "Even after the most precise preparation of the main root canal, protein will always remain in the tiny interconnecting canals.... If this protein becomes infected, toxic products will be produced, and conveyed into the organism.... The toxins produced by the microbes in a tooth with a root filling can no longer be evacuated into the mouth, but ... are conveyed to the tonsils, and thus the flow systems of the body." A root canal procedure can "literally convert a tooth into a toxin-producing 'factory.'"[21]

The primary toxin generated by dead, infected teeth is dimethyl sulfide, a major carcinogen. According to Dr. Issels, 98% of his adult cancer patients have 2-10 teeth whose root canal fillings have become sources of toxins—"which means that they have just as many of the toxic factories in their bodies."[22] Unless these teeth are removed, the dental toxins are released continuously in tiny amounts into the blood circulation and, from there, adversely affect the liver, heart, brain and nervous system, endocrine glands, and much of the lymph system.[23]

Removal of the infected, dead tooth—including its roots—means drilling thoroughly through the tooth socket and up to the healthy bone. Dr. Issels then advises his patients to forgo putting in a crown or bridge anchorage, however unappealing this advice may seem. "This is really the only alternative. Empirically, the chance of recovery for cancer patients, as well as for any other patient with chronic disorders, can thereby become considerably improved."[24]

As with infected teeth, Dr. Issels notes that silent toxins generated by degenerated tonsils probably existed for years *prior* to the onset of cancer. Patients with this condition often have never been ill with tonsillitis nor can they recall any pain or swelling in their tonsils. Yet, these clinically unremarkable tonsils prove to be foci of the most dangerous kind whose toxins are drained into the bloodstream, thereby lowering immune function.

Based on Dr. Issels' sophisticated tests, he is able to show that the diseased tonsils represent a chronic source of toxins. Dr. Issels and his colleagues conclude that there is a definite correlation between tumor growth and the extent of tonsil degeneration and infection. Upon removing this obvious source of toxins, tumor growth is either halted or markedly depressed. As Dr. Issels says, "Many tumors appear to become responsive to our other therapies only after removing the diseased tonsils and [dead] teeth."[25]

***Based on Dr. Issels' sophisticated tests, he is able to show that the diseased tonsils represent a chronic source of toxins. Dr. Issels and his colleagues conclude that there is a definite correlation between tumor growth and the extent of tonsil degeneration and infection.***

A typical example of the success of this strategy concerns a man diagnosed with lymphoma who had tried many remedies. None of them worked until he met Dr. Issels who examined his mouth and teeth. Dr. Issels told the man there were 2 things wrong; he had too many mercury fillings in his mouth and his tonsils needed to be removed. As soon as the fillings and tonsils were removed, the toxins in the man's body began to drain again and his lymph nodes, which had been the size of eggs, began to shrink. Today, the patient is much improved and continues to work.

Dr. Issels' program uses botanical and homeopathic remedies to encourage cell regeneration and to stimulate the body's anticancer defenses. The body's detoxification system—which includes the liver, kidneys, intestines, and skin—is thus stimulated to start eliminating the toxins associated with the tumor. Patients are encouraged to drink plenty of water and herb tea to irrigate the kidneys, and to take mild herbal purgatives to cleanse their colon. The approach also uses hyperthermal techniques to re-energize

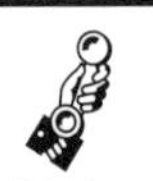

**Dr. Issels** is the senior consulting physician at the Max Gerson Memorial Cancer Center of CHIPSA, located at 670 Nubes, Playas de Tijuana, Mexico; U.S. address: Gerson Research Organization, 7807 Artesian Road, San Diego, CA 92127-2117; tel: 800-759-2966; fax, 619-759-2967. Naima Abdul-Ghany, M.D., Ph.D., uses Issels' therapy as part of a multimodal approach. To contact Dr. Abdul-Ghany: Amal Medical Center, 340 West 23rd Street, Suite E, Panama City, FL 32405; tel: 904-763-7689.

the immune system. By provoking a fever by mixed bacterial vaccines, Dr. Issels can increase the number of disease-destroying leukocytes in the bloodstream.

He also employs vaccines for specific types of cancer, using ultrafine filtrates of cancer tissues in much the same way as modern vaccines use infectious agents to stimulate antibody production. Dr. Issels also uses oxygen therapy such as hematogenic oxidation. Here, blood is drawn from the patient, oxygen is bubbled through it, and it is exposed to ultraviolet rays; the blood is left to settle for up to an hour, then returned to the patient by intravenous drip. This procedure activates the blood, in turn sparking an aggressive immune response.

As early as the 1950s, Dr. Issels realized that this approach gave cancer patients a valuable survival advantage over those treated conventionally alone.[26] In one long-term study, Dr. Issels' treatment protocol was applied to 252 terminal patients who had previously undergone conventional surgery and radiation therapy. These patients were considered "terminal" when they came to him for help; i.e., they were not expected to live more than 1 year. After 5 years, 16.6% were still alive and functioning, compared to a worldwide average cure rate of 2%; after 15 years on the program, over 92% of the original survivors were still alive and showed no signs of cancer.[27]

In another study, 370 cancer patients, with various types and in various stages of the disease, followed Dr. Issels' program; after 5 years, 322 patients (87%) were still alive and showing no sign of the cancer recurring. Further research showed the relapse rate to be only 13% with Dr. Issels' therapy.[28] Ahmed Elkadi, M.D., of Panama City, Florida, employed Dr. Issels' program but added his own refinements, such as the use of the herbal compound *Nigella sativa*, or black seed spice. With this herb Dr. Elkadi, has observed a 55% enhancement of helper T cells and suppressor T cells and a 30% enhancement of natural killer cell activity.

## The Advantages and Methods of Mercury Amalgam Removal

Colorado biological dentist Hal Huggins, D.D.S., recommends that people who choose to have their amalgams removed ask their dentists to use a rubber dam, a thin sheet of rubber that slips over the teeth. "Dams prevent over 95% of the mixture of mercury and water produced by the drilling out of old fillings from going down your throat. They also reduce the amount of mercury that you might absorb from your cheeks and under your tongue."

Dr. Huggins suggests that people consider early morning appointments for amalgam removal, rather than later in the day, because the mercury vapor from other patients' sessions can linger in the air for hours and be absorbed by breathing. Some dentists use mercury vapor filter systems, he points out, but those who do are rare.

Charles Gableman, M.D., of Encinitas, California, who is a leader in the field of environmental medicine, always advises the removal of his patients' amalgam fillings. According to Dr. Gableman, patients with chronic fatigue syndrome, or with a lack of resistance to infections, allergies, and thyroid destruction, all improve after their fillings are properly removed. He believes it is possible that these patients have suffered from basic allergies all their life and that the mercury toxicity from the fillings adds to the body's toxic load and "pushes them over the edge," resulting in chronic medical problems.

Once mercury toxicity has been demonstrated, by tests such as high electrogalvanism (electrical conductivity in the metals of the teeth), high mercury vapor emissions, and/or high mercury body burden (tissue deposits), mercury amalgam removal and replacement with alternate, nontoxic materials is the recommended step, advises Dr. Daniel Royal, D.O.S., of Las Vegas, Nevada.

QUICK DEFINITION

**Electrogalvanism**, the amount of positive or negative charges emitted by various metals, is measured by a device called a galvanometer. In biological dentistry, the metals are those in a patient's teeth. For measuring mercury vapor emissions from the teeth, biological dentists use the **Jerome Mercury Vapor Analyzer**, the same device used by the Environmental Protection Agency to check the mercury levels in dental offices.

To contact **Daniel F. Royal**, D.O.: The Nevada Clinic, 3663 South Pecos McLeod Road, Las Vegas, NV 89121; tel: 702-732-1400; fax: 702-732-9661.

For more information on the health hazards of **mercury toxicity** and other **dental factors**, see Chapter 25: What Causes Cancer? pp. 594-602.

While removal of amalgam fillings stops any further source of poisoning from mercury fillings, you still need to detoxify the body to eliminate the *residual* effect from mercury that remains behind in the body. After all, it has been accumulating for as long as you have had amalgam fillings. First you "turn off the faucet" by removing the fillings; then you "pull the plug" through oral detoxification; and lastly, you "drain the bathtub" (your body) of all traces of mercury.

Even if the fillings are removed, the negative influence of mercury will continue unless it is appropriately detoxified and eliminated from your body. The following guidelines for detoxifying mercury come from the clinical practice of Dr. Royal.[29]

Ideally, for those who are about to have amalgams removed and replaced, this detoxifying program should be initiated at least 2 weeks before amalgam removal and continued for at least 3 months after the last amalgams are removed, Dr. Royal says. If you have already had your amalgams removed, then start today. The usual length of time required for body elimination of mercury is 3-6 months.

**Chlorella**—This is a medicinal green algae that helps detoxify the body. Specifically, chlorella helps move mercury out of connective tissue so that substances such as DMPS (discussed later) can then remove it from the body. Begin with only one chlorella capsule daily for the first few weeks after amalgam removal, then gradually increase to 3 daily.

**L-glutathione**—This natural detoxifying substance (made from the amino acid cysteine) improves liver function and metabolism, thereby helping the body detoxify. Take 150 mg once daily.

**Kyolic Garlic Extract**—Garlic's high sulfur and cysteine content enable it to bind up (chelate) toxic metals and chemicals, and to work against harmful microbes. Take one capsule with meals 3 times daily.

**Silymarin**—Also known as milk thistle seed, silymarin has long been used as a liver purifying agent. Take one capsule twice daily.

**Vitamin C**—Ascorbic acid has a protective effect against free radical damage which can occur as heavy metals are being removed and excreted through the kidneys. On the day before amalgam removal, take your bowel tolerance of vitamin C (the amount your system can tolerate before producing diarrhea, usually 8,000-16,000 mg daily, divided into hourly doses of about 2000 mg for a 150-pound person), but decrease the dosage if you get diarrhea. My recommended daily dosage is 2000-8000 mg.

**Vitamin B complex**—Take 25-100 mg daily to help replenish nutrients lost when heavy metals are bound up and excreted.

**DHEA**—This is an adrenal hormone precursor. The adrenal glands of patients with mercury toxicity are often weak, contributing to an inability to handle stress. My recommended daily dosage is 5 mg for men and 2.5 mg for women, to be taken daily with pregnenolone.

On the day of amalgam removal, vitamin C should not be taken until *after* the procedure; otherwise, it may interfere with the anesthesia.

**Pregnenolone**—This substance (a steroid building block made from cholesterol, usually extracted from soybeans or wild yam) aids in the formation of key brain chemicals associated with memory and thinking. The recommended daily dosage is 10 mg for men and 30 mg for women. This dosage should initially be taken daily and may be decreased as symptoms improve.

**DMSA**—DMSA (2,3-dimercaptosuccinic acid) is an effective agent for binding up heavy metals because it crosses the blood-brain barrier and thus helps remove the remaining toxic residues from the central nervous system. On the day of amalgam removal, take three 100-mg capsules in the morning on the day of amalgam removal and the same dosage in the morning on the day after removal. Take 30 minutes before or after eating. Once the amalgams have been removed and after you have been on this supplement program for 3 months, on *one occasion only*, take 2 capsules (100 mg each) 3 times daily for 3 days.

**DMPS**—DMPS (2,3-dimercaptopropane-1-sulfonate) is the chelating (binding-up) agent of choice for the removal of elemental mercury from the human body. This agent was first developed in China, then introduced in Russia where it was used for workers injured by exposure to heavy metals. DMPS has since been researched for over 40 years in Japan, Germany, and the former Soviet Union, and, for the past 25 years, has been used as a treatment for humans in these countries.

DMPS can be given orally, intravenously, or intramuscularly with a maximum dose of 3 mg/2.2 pounds of body weight, with 250 mg being the typical dose. I recommend a single 250-mg capsule taken once a month or the same amount by injection, also once monthly. On the day of the last amalgam removal, the first DMPS treatment may be given.

People who have had exposure to amalgam through their fillings will usually require 3-5 injections. Those who have never had amalgam fillings,

CAUTION

Heavy metal-related symptoms, such as joint pains, depression, burning sensations, digestive-related problems, and fatigue can be temporarily aggravated as DMPS removes toxins from the cells. This is a transient occurrence. The routine use of intravenous DMPS is not advisable for patients who still have mercury amalgam fillings. This is because DMPS may appear in the saliva and act to dissolve the surface of the existing amalgam fillings. The potential outcome is acute toxicity from heavy metal injury to the lining of the gut.

but show evidence or suspicion of heavy metal toxicity through other sources, may require only 1-2 injections. An injection every 4-6 months thereafter is recommended for patient maintenance. Usually, the patient will begin to notice improvement within 3-4 weeks following the DMPS injections.

**Essential minerals**—As DMPS and DMSA remove vital nutrients from the body, zinc, copper, magnesium, and manganese should be taken in addition to the other vitamin supplements.

**Homeopathic amalgam drops**—This is a combination of homeopathically prepared elements found in amalgam fillings given for the purpose of enhancing the removal of heavy metals from the body. Beginning one week prior to amalgam removal, take 10 drops, 3 times daily; continue this dosage for one week after amalgam removal.

Once all the amalgams have been removed, begin taking homeopathic mercury (*Mercurius Solubilis* 30C) at the rate of 30 drops, 2-3 times weekly for the duration of the oral detoxification program or until you feel improved.

**Selenium**—Take 50 mcg 3 times daily between meals and, whenever possible, 2 hours before or after you have taken vitamin C, to help bind up mercury.

***Acidophilus***—As a final note, removing mercury-based fillings without intestinal cleansing can accomplish only 40% of the total detoxification. A toxic bowel can repollute the mouth through the acupuncture meridians that connect both the intestines and the teeth. Therefore, a complete bowel cleansing program must be undertaken around the same time as any removal of mercury fillings from the teeth and body tissues.

*Acidophilus* helps to restore the microflora of the intestine which can be adversely affected by the presence of mercury. Take one teaspoon daily, or more if diarrhea or constipation are present.

**Psyllium husk**—This acts as a bulk fiber laxative to absorb toxins and facilitate the removal of fecal debris from the intestines. Drink at least 6-8 glasses of water daily and slowly build up the amount of psyllium consumed.

Begin with one teaspoon in liquid once daily and gradually increase to 3 teaspoons once daily (3 times daily if constipation is present). Take psyllium separately from vitamin and mineral supplements as the fiber will reduce their effectiveness.

**Dietary changes—**A high-fiber diet, consisting primarily of fruits, vegetables, and legumes, will tend to decrease fecal transit time, reducing the amount of time that liquids containing heavy metals remain in the colon and thus reduce the quantity reabsorbed from the colon. Decrease consumption of refined carbohydrates. These include simple sugars, white flour, and saturated fats because they may reduce the availability of essential enzymes and nutrients required for more beneficial purposes.

Avoid fish. This is the largest dietary source of mercury. While some fish have comparatively lower mercury content (e.g., sardines, herring, pollack, mackerel, cod, redfish, and Greenland halibut), most tuna and shellfish have a fairly high content of mercury. Individuals who are sensitive to mercury usually have some type of adverse reaction to shellfish.

Reduce chicken/egg consumption. Fish meal has become a major source of feed for chickens. Depending on the mercury content of the fish products used to make the fish meal, chickens and eggs have the potential of containing a significant mercury content.

# Water Therapy

**The therapeutic use of water can be of great benefit to cancer patients, as water can stimulate the immune system, help increase the body's white blood cell count, aid the body in purging itself of accumulated toxins, and produce a state of general relaxation essential to the healing process.**

Water therapy, also called hydrotherapy, is the use of water, vapor, ice, steam, and water at hot and cold temperatures to maintain and restore health. Treatments include full-body immersion, steam baths, saunas, sitz baths (in which the pelvis is immersed in hot and/or cold water for the purposes of providing a heat contrast to the pelvis and genital area), colonic irrigation, and the application of hot and/or cold compresses. Hydrotherapy is effective for treating a wide range of conditions and can easily be used in the home as part of a self-care program.

## Water Therapy for Detoxification and Rejuvenation

Today, many alternative practitioners prescribe baths, Jacuzzi, steam, saunas, mineral tubs, mud baths, wraps, rubs, flushes, fasts, enemas, colonic irrigations, douches, sitz baths, and wet compresses to remedy a great variety of health conditions. Hot or cold water administered externally or internally can be effective in treating conditions ranging from stress and pain to the many toxins, parasites, bacteria, and viruses that can cause disease. Compresses and packs are particularly effective for applying hot or cold to specific parts of the body. According to Tori Hudson, N.D. (profiled in Chapter 11), they stimulate the immune system and help increase the body's white blood cell count.

### HYDROTHERAPY METHOD #1: HOT BLANKET PACKS

A hot blanket pack involves the use of a hot water bottle or nonelectric heating pad.[30] The purpose is to produce a mild increase in body temperature, the pack serving as a form of hyperthermia, or heat therapy, for immune stimulation or detoxification. It may also be used to prepare for cold applications.

The following guidelines are for the health practitioner. In a typical application, you assemble a dry cotton sheet, 2 wool blankets, 2 hot water bottles (or a nonelectric heating pad), and a cold compress. Lay out the 2 blankets and cover them with a dry sheet. Have patients undress and wrap themselves in the sheet. Place one hot water bottle on the abdomen and one at the feet, or place the heating pad on the abdomen. Wipe the face with the cold compress as needed. Leave the patient in the pack for 20-60 minutes depending on the amount of heating desired. The goal is to heat the body and induce sweating.

Where it is desirable to heat only the lower half of the body a hot half-pack may be used. In this case, wrap the body only from the waist to the feet with a hot water bottle or heating pad between the legs. This treatment is milder than the hot foot bath and may be used with people who have peripheral vascular diseases or loss of peripheral sensations.

Take care not to overheat the patient with the hot water bottles or heating pad and always follow the hot blanket pack with a cool rinse.

## HYDROTHERAPY METHOD #2: SELF-APPLIED HYPERTHERMIA

This local or whole-body treatment can be used by an individual in home treatment to raise the temperature of the tissues, a medical process also called artificial fever. The purpose is to destroy heat-sensitive organisms (viruses, bacteria, etc. that are sensitive to increases in temperature), to enhance immune function, and to encourage elimination of toxic material from the body.

The technique may also be useful as an adjunctive treatment of the upper respiratory infections that are a common complication of many different types of cancer including advanced cases of lung cancer. It is also useful in helping to eliminate toxic material from the body by encouraging sweating.

Materials required include a hot tub or deep bath with water at 103-104° F; a basin of ice water and terry cloth towel; and pure drinking water. A typical treatment may be performed by immersing the body in hot water (103-104° F) for up to 60 minutes at a time. Maintain this bath temperature for the entire time. To prevent a headache, apply a cold compress to the head early in the treatment and maintain it throughout. Check oral temperature every 10-15 minutes; if it exceeds 104° F, cool the bath and apply more cold to the head. Following the treatment, rinse in a cool shower with glycerin soap and KDF (charcoal) showerhead-filtered water, then wrap up and stay warm.

If a bath or hot tub are not available, heat the body in a steam bath or sauna. A hot blanket pack may also be used to raise body temperature. Local hyperthermia may be achieved by the use of hot packs or through the inhalation of steam. When inhaling steam for upper respiratory illness, avoid inhaling the steam deeply into the lungs.

**Precautions/Special Considerations—**Take the following precautions when using hyperthermia treatment.

1) Consult your physician before doing this treatment if you have any of the following: high or low blood pressure, serious illness, diabetes mel-

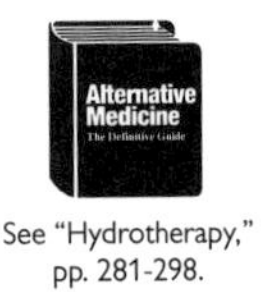

See "Hydrotherapy," pp. 281-298.

litus, multiple or muscular sclerosis. Do not use this treatment if you are or may be pregnant.

2) Watch for signs of hyperventilation. These include numbness and tingling in the lips, hands, or feet. If hyperventilation occurs, reduce the bath temperature; breathe from the abdomen, not the chest; or breathe into a paper bag until the tingling passes.

3) Hotter water can generally be tolerated for short periods, but it may cause an increase in body temperature that occurs too quickly. Then the treatment may have to be ended abruptly which may leave the patient feeling uncomfortable.

4) Stand slowly after finishing the treatment and be especially careful during the cool rinse in the shower so as not to faint. It is advisable to have an attendant at hand for the first few treatments.

## HYDROTHERAPY METHOD #3: WET SHEET PACKS

As implied, this procedure begins with a full-body wrap in a cold wet sheet. Typically, the treatment progresses in 3 phases; cold or cooling, neutral, and heating. The purposes are to stimulate, relax, and detoxify, respectively. The cold phase is stimulating and tonifying if it is stopped after the sheet loses its cool temperature. There are easier ways to achieve this stimulation and therefore it is rarely used this way. However, the cold application is useful to control a fever that is rising too rapidly or is too high.

The neutral temperature phase is useful to relax and sedate. The final phase, heating, is commonly used to promote sweating and elimination and is therefore useful in detoxifying from environmental or chemical exposure or from drug, alcohol, or tobacco use.

Materials for this treatment include a bed or treatment table, wool blankets (1-3 may be needed), 2 pillows (one for the head and one for under the knees), a cotton (polyester or cotton) sheet soaked in ice water, a terry cloth bath towel, and a terry cloth hand towel.

The procedure (again, written for the health-care practitioner) is typically done this way: Lay out 1 blanket placing a pillow at the head and another to support the knees under the blanket. The blanket should be large enough to fold over the shoulders of the patient. Thoroughly wring out the ice water sheet and lay it out over the blanket. Have patients undress and lie down on the center of the wet sheet and, standing beside the patient, pull the far half of the wet sheet toward you. Arrange the sheet by pulling the far half under the arms and around the far leg. Have patients place their arms in a comfortable position across the abdomen. (If the patient is claustrophobic, one arm may be left out.) Wrap the near half of the sheet over the shoulders, arms, and around the near leg.

Next, bring the blanket across the patient, draping it over the shoulders. Any extra length of wet sheet should be folded up over the blanket. Add extra layers of blanket over the patient to hold in the heat produced by the patient to warm the sheet. If the treatment is used to reduce fever, extra blankets are not needed. If general detoxification is desired, leave the patient in the wet sheet until profuse sweating occurs and for as long as can be tolerated. This may take 2-4 hours or more. The heating/detoxifying stage will be reached sooner if the patient has undergone some sort of heating activity before getting into the wet sheet pack, such as exercise or taking a hot shower or hot tub.

If relaxation is the primary goal, remove the patient from the pack before perspiration begins; then follow with a warm (not hot) wet sheet wrap. If tonifying, fever-reducing effects are sought, remove the patient as soon as the sheet begins to heat up. It may be necessary to restore the cold wet sheet one or more times to reach the desired effect.

**Precautions/Special Considerations—**Take the following precautions when using wet sheet packs:

1) Hot drinks such as ginger tea will promote sweating. However, don't burn the patient (test the temperature of the drinks first). Don't give too much fluid because the need to urinate could end the treatment too soon. Have the patient drink ample purified or spring water during subsequent elimination/perspiration phase.

2) The bath towel may be used to cover the patient's head and eyes to enhance the heating phase and shade the eyes. The hand towel may be used as a cold compress and to mop the patient's face once perspiration begins in the elimination phase.

## Detoxify, Relax Muscles, and Enhance Immunity with an Aromatherapy Spa

Physicians have long known of the many therapeutic benefits of steam heat,

## Aromatherapy Aids Cancer Treatment

Researchers at Memorial Sloan-Kettering Cancer Center in New York City used aromatherapy to ease the anxiety attacks of patients who received magnetic resonance imaging (MRI), a high-tech diagnostic procedure that involves being fully enclosed inside a large machine. Before their MRIs, some patients were exposed to the fumes of heliotropin essential oil, a scent often prescribed by aromatherapists for relaxation. Compared with those who received no aromatherapy, the heliotropin group experienced significantly less anxiety during the MRI.[31]

also known as hyperthermia or heat stress detoxification. Similarly, the benefits of aromatherapy—the inhalation of the vapors of essential plant oils—are widely recognized among alternative practitioners. Now Variel Health International has combined both modalities in the form of the aromaSpa™ aromatic steam capsule suitable for home use as a portable health spa. In the self-contained aromatherapy and steam heat diffuser, soothing aromatic mists envelop the *entire* body surface for maximum absorption and benefit.

The unit stands 5'6", weighs about 68 pounds, may be easily disassembled, and plugs into any standard 115-volt socket. Its walls and sliding door are made of the transparent polycarbonate used for airplane windows. The steam generator and aroma diffuser are located on the floor of the unit. Any of at least 250 aromatherapy oils may be used, singly or in combination, to support muscle relaxation, detoxification, or immune system stimulation, or to eliminate fatigue, lift mood, or revitalize skin. Other self-care benefits include general mind and body relaxation, stress reduction, energization, emotional cleansing, general rejuvenation, and "customized personal pampering," depending on the aromatherapy formula used, says Variel's Cathy Dammann.

The aromaSpa uses one quart of distilled water (preferable to chlorinated tap water) for a 40-minute steam heat session and can reach inside temperatures of 115° and 120°F within about 10 minutes. These temperatures are necessary as hyperthermia provides its benefits by temporarily raising the body temperature to between 101° and 103°F and inducing perspiration. Clinical information suggests that steam heat may have therapeutic advantages over the dry heat associated with saunas, says Variel's Cathy Dammann.

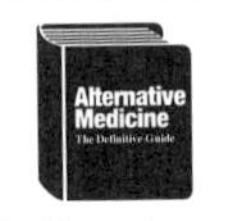


See "Aromatherapy," pp. 53-62.

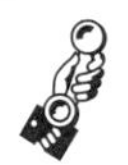

For more information about **aromaSpa™** aromatic steam capsule, contact: Variel Health International, 9618 Variel Avenue, Chatsworth, CA 91311; tel: 818-407-4717; fax: 818-407-0738. The single-seater "Serene" unit sells for about $1500; the two-seater "Gemini" model sells for about $2300.

For more information on the clinical use of **aromatherapy** as part of a cancer treatment program, see Chapter 13: Victor Marcial-Vega, M.D.

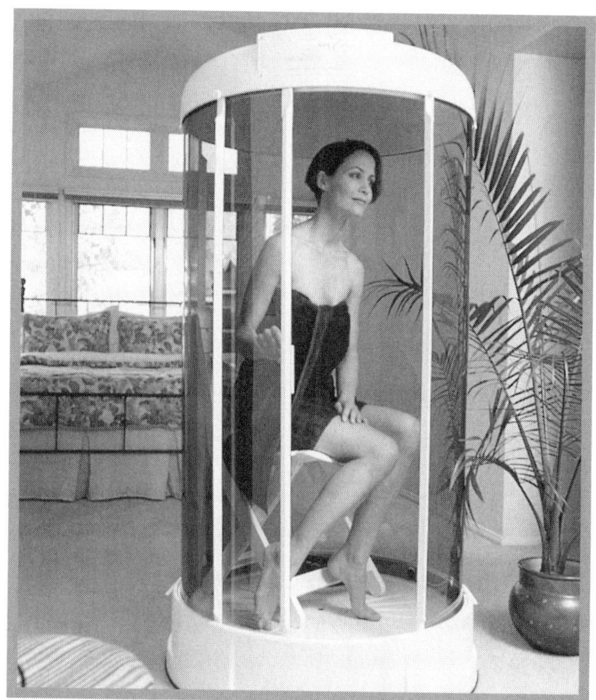
The aromaSpa

The aromaSpa was tested in 1994 by Jerry Schindler, Ph.D., director of the Sports Health Science Human Performance Lab at Life College School of Chiropractic in Marietta, Georgia. Dr. Schindler reported that the unit was effective in decreasing the risk of everyday and athletic injuries, primarily by increasing muscle flexibility, and blood flow and oxygen delivery to the muscles. Dr. Schindler demonstrated these benefits by way of thermographic studies (which register nerve sensory pathways) comparing the left and right sides of a test subject's body. Individuals whose thermographic readings are asymmetrical (indicating imbalances and sensory interference) are prone to injury, says Dr. Schindler. Symmetrical patterns were achieved after 30 minutes in the aromaSpa.

According to Cathy Dammann, aroma steam therapy can also reduce lactic acid buildup in muscles following exercise, thereby preventing soreness. The approach may be effective in reducing cellulite (lumpy fat areas in the skin), especially when used with rosemary, sandalwood, juniper, geranium, or lemon essential oils. These can produce detoxifying and water-draining effects in only 10 minutes compared to standard hot body wraps which require 60 minutes, says Dammann.

Steam heat therapy may increase blood circulation and heighten immune response by stimulating white blood cell production, Dammann says. The aromaSpa is now being used experimentally by patients with chronic fatigue syndrome, says Dammann. Heat therapy is also one of the most effective ways to remove fat-stored toxins from the body and the use of the essential oils of clove, cinnamon, melissa, or lavender have been clinically shown to benefit bronchial conditions as effectively as antibiotics, especially when delivered by steam heat, Dammann says.

# Heat Therapy

**The secret of hyperthermia, or heat therapy, is that cancer cells are vulnerable to high temperatures. Heat the cancer cells and they can be easily destroyed, especially if the tumor lies close to the skin surface. In the process, patients can reduce or even eliminate the need for radiation therapy.**

Hippocrates, the father of Western medicine, wrote: "Those diseases which medicines do not cure, iron [surgery] cures; those which surgery cannot cure, fire cures; and those which fire cannot cure, are reckoned wholly incurable." The ancient Greek physician was evidently onto something. Since the late 1970s, considerable research has shown that heating the body may aid in the treatment of cancer.

The principle behind hyperthermia is simple: heat cancer cells and they can be killed easily. Direct killing of cancer cells begins to occur when the cancerous tissue reaches about 104° F to 105.8° F.[32] "Only a relatively small rise in body temperature can make a huge difference," says Robert Atkins, M.D. (see Chapter 1), who includes it in his cancer protocols.

## Heat Therapy as a Detoxification Method

Though the principle sounds simple, the technique is far more complicated, thanks to the body's ability to regulate its internal temperature. As any sauna enthusiast will attest, the human body likes heat only to a point. When the body temperature rises, blood flow increases to dissipate the excess heat. One way to circumvent the body's ability to regulate its temperature is to apply the heat locally, targeting a specific tumor. This can be done with the use of microwaves and ultrasound, which can be directed at parts of the body with great precision.

Unlike normal tissue, tumors have poor blood flow relative to their metabolic needs and cannot dissipate the heat, so they tend to get hotter than the surrounding area. Rapidly dividing cells (i.e., cancer cells) are more vulnerable to the effects of heat. Normally, part of the damage caused by radiation is repaired by the cancer cells, enabling some to survive; however, heat foils this self-repair ability. Taken together, these facts tend to make tumors more vulnerable to heat treatment than normal tissues.

At the Duke Hyperthermia Program of the Duke University Medical Center in Durham, North Carolina, considerable success has been reported in using hyperthermia to treat soft-tissue sarcomas and often deadly recurrences of breast cancer. One recent study found that radiation combined with hyperthermia was 30% more effective against breast cancer than radiation treatment alone.[33] Tumors located near the surface of the body appear to be more amenable to treatment than deep-tissue tumors.

"I try never to use radiation treatment—which is even more dangerous than most forms of chemotherapy—without also using hyperthermia," says Dr. Atkins. "Thanks to hyperthermia, we can shrink tumors with far less radiation today to get the same therapeutic outcome in cancer patients, and our patients' immune systems and overall health are faring much better as a result." Hyperthermia is now approved in the U.S. for treatment of breast cancer recurrence, and it is covered by insurance.

Let's examine how heat therapy works. Heat results when atoms and molecules vibrate and move around at a higher rate or frequency. The body uses its own internally generated heat to protect itself from viruses, bacteria, and other harmful substances. A fever is the body's highly evolved attempt to destroy invading organisms and to sweat impurities out through the skin. Fever is an effective natural process of curing disease and restoring health; heat therapy, or hyperthermia, represents a way to *create* fever to call out this natural healing process.

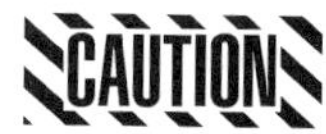


Patients with temperature regulation problems, especially the old and the very young, should not use hyperthermia. Microwave diathermy can burn tissue around the eyes; it should never be used by people with pacemakers. People with peripheral vascular disease (poor blood flow to the legs and feet) or loss of sensation should not use hyperthermia because of the risk of burns. Caution is advised with patients who have cardiovascular disease, in particular arrhythmia (irregularity or loss of rhythm in the heartbeat) and tachycardia (abnormally rapid heart rate), or severe hypertension or hypotension.

***Practitioners of alternative medicine have long recognized hyperthermia as a useful technique in detoxification therapy because it releases toxins stored in fat cells. Hyperthermia can be used to remove fat-stored chemicals such as pesticides, PCBs, and drug residues from the body.***

> ***"Thanks to hyperthermia, we can shrink tumors with far less radiation today to get the same therapeutic outcome in cancer patients, and our patients' immune systems and overall health are faring much better as a result," says Dr. Atkins.***

A state of natural hyperthermia exists when body temperature rises above its normal level of 98.6° F. An increase in body temperature causes many physiological responses to occur. For one, by increasing the production of antibodies and interferon (a protein substance produced by virus-invaded cells that prevents reproduction of the virus), it stimulates the immune system. Practitioners of alternative medicine have long recognized hyperthermia as a useful technique in detoxification therapy because it releases toxins stored in fat cells. Hyperthermia can be used to remove fat-stored chemicals such as pesticides, PCBs, and drug residues from the body. Only recently has conventional medicine caught up with this practice and begun to incorporate hyperthermia in the orthodox treatment protocols for cancer.

## Methods of Inducing Hyperthermia

Body temperature can be swiftly increased by the external application of heat. This approach causes blood vessels to temporarily enlarge (dilate) and the body to perspire in an attempt to prevent an increase in temperature. An increase in body temperature may be accomplished by immersing the body in hot water, sitting in a sauna or steam bath, or wrapping oneself in blankets with a hot water bottle, as described previously in the section on water therapy.

Other approaches, more commonly found in hospital and medical centers, include the use of shortwave or microwave diathermy, ultrasound, radiant heating, and extracorporeal heating. Diathermy raises body temperature by applying radio-frequency electromagnetic energy. Ultrasound causes an increase in body temperature as a result of friction produced at the molecular level as the high-energy sound waves strike different body tissues. (For whole-body or large-area treatments, multiple ultrasound applicators may be used.) Radiant heating devices produce infrared heat that is applied to the body. Extracorporeal heating involves removing blood from the body (via plastic tubes placed into the veins), heating it, and returning it to the body at a higher temperature.

As indicated previously, hyperthermia can be produced either locally or over the whole body. Locally applied hyperthermia is most often employed to treat infections such as upper respiratory infections (with inhalation of steam or a local application of diathermy), but is also used to treat infected wounds in a hand or foot (generally by immersion of the hand or foot in a hot water bath). Whole-body hyperthermia, on the other hand, is used when there is a general infection, when a local application is impractical, or when a general whole-body response is desirable or needed.

For whole-body moderate hyperthermia, practitioners normally rely on full-immersion baths, saunas, steam, and/or blanket packs. For localized applications, immersion baths, steam, or, occasionally, diathermy are used. In conventional medical settings, whole-body treatment usually involves diathermy, ultrasound, radiant and extracorporeal heating; for localized treatments, diathermy and ultrasound are used.

## Hyperthermia in the Treatment of Cancer

Studies have shown that hyperthermia treatment modifies cell membranes in such a way as to protect healthy cells and make tumor cells more susceptible to chemotherapy and radiation.[34] For this reason, hyperthermia is a useful adjunct in cancer therapy, largely because it enables the use of lower doses of chemotherapy and radiation. As suggested, hyperthermia treatments play a role in stimulating the immune system, as evidenced by the drop in white cell counts immediately following treatment and the rise that occurs within a few hours. Not only do the number of white cells increase, but their ability to destroy target cells appears to increase as well.[35] Siberian ginseng may be able to blunt the initial drop in white blood cells following hyperthermia.

A recent study has shown an increase in the production of interleukin-1 (a compound produced by the body in response to infection, inflammation, or other immunologic challenges) with whole-body hyperthermia.[36] These studies indicate that increased body temperature plays a positive role in the healing process of the body. According to A. C. Guyton, M.D., an authority in the field of medical physiology, the metabolic rate is increased 100% for every 10° C rise in temperature.[37] An increase in temperature from 98.6° F to 104° F should increase metabolism by about 30%. This increased metabolic rate no doubt accounts for some of the increased immune activity and thus hyperthermia's contribution to cancer reversal.

Alternative Medicine
The Definitive Guide

See "Hyperthermia," pp. 299-305.

When used knowledgeably and with care, hyperthermia is a safe and effective treatment for many conditions. Ill effects of hyperthermia usually appear only when body temperatures exceed 106° F. However, certain individuals are sensitive to the effects of heat, such as those with anemia, heart disease, diabetes, seizure disorders, or tuberculosis, and women who are or may be pregnant;[38] as noted earlier, individuals with these conditions should take great care and always consult with a doctor before embarking on self-administered treatments.

Other reported risks associated with the use of hyperthermia include herpes outbreaks[39] (including herpes zoster), liver toxicity,[40] and nervous system injury. Some substances used to induce hyperthermia are not recommended, including blood products, vaccines, pollens, and benign forms of malaria.[41] A secondary infection can occur from the injection of blood products and these other substances can be extremely dangerous. Hyperthermia used for detoxification should be performed only under medical supervision.

# Bodywork/ Therapeutic Massage/ Exercise

**It is essential to involve the physical body and its musculoskeletal system in the cancer-reversal process. A variety of physically-oriented techniques can help a person deeply relax, stimulate blood and lymphatic circulation, enhance the activity of the body's anticancer defenses, even clear emotions and attitudes "trapped" in the tissues.**

The term "bodywork" refers to hands-on therapies such as massage, deep tissue manipulation, movement awareness, and energy balancing, among others, which are variously employed to soothe injured muscles, stimulate blood and lymphatic circulation, reduce pain, and promote deep relaxation as well as to improve the structure and physical functioning of the body.

Movement therapies help realign the body by correcting postural imbalances and thereby promoting more efficient functioning of the nervous and musculoskeletal systems. A form of movement therapy known as Authentic Movement (AM) has been used therapeutically for breast cancer patients. In a study of 33 breast cancer patients, women attending regular support group sessions were encouraged to share their feelings and concerns. The women were also invited to move spontaneously with their feelings, all the while being observed impartially by a trained AM therapist, called the "witness."

In the act of witnessing, the therapist attends respectfully and sensitively to the other's experience. "The witness is in relationship with the mover yet has a clear sense of herself at the same time," says Tina Stromstead of the San Francisco-based Authentic Movement Institute. "A good witness is insightful, impartially attentive, and has the willingness and maturity to claim her own projections. Over time, she develops a deep respect and empathy for the mover."

After a movement session, witness and mover share their feelings, thoughts, and impressions regarding the session. The study's coordinator, psychologist Sandy Dibell-Hope, Ph.D., reports that the AM sessions improve mood, body image, and self-esteem, as well as decrease depression, anxiety, and a sense of social isolation.[42] Such changes translate into an improved quality of life for breast cancer patients, and this shift can help promote long-range survival.

Since the mid-1980s, considerable scientific evidence has supported the claim that massage therapy is beneficial.[43] According to John Yates, Ph.D., author of *A Physician's Guide to Therapeutic Massage*, massage can benefit such conditions as muscle spasm and pain, spinal curvatures (lordosis, scoliosis), soreness related to injury and stress, headaches, whiplash, temporomandibular joint syndrome (TMJ), and even tension-related respiratory disorders such as bronchial asthma or emphysema. Massage can also help reduce swelling, correct posture, improve body motion, and facilitate the elimination of toxins from the body.[44]

Lymphatic massage, for example, can move metabolic waste through the body to promote a rapid recovery from illness or disease. Other studies show that massage can be used as an adjunct in the treatment of cardiovascular disorders and neurological and gynecological problems, and

## The Therapeutic Effects of Massage

Gertrude Beard, R.N., R.P.T., former associate professor of physical therapy at Northwestern University Medical School, summarizes the findings of numerous research studies on the therapeutic effects of massage. Studies indicate that massage helps to:

- sedate the nervous system and promote voluntary muscle relaxation
- promote recovery from fatigue produced by excessive exercise
- break up scar tissue and lessen fibrosis and adhesions that develop as a result of injury and immobilization
- relieve certain types of pain
- provide effective treatment of chronic inflammatory conditions by increasing lymphatic circulation
- reduce swelling from fractures
- improve circulation through the capillaries, veins, and arteries, and increase blood flow through the muscles
- loosen mucus, promote drainage of sinus fluids, and increase drainage of mucus from the lungs (using percussive and vibratory techniques)
- increase peristaltic action (muscular contractions that move waste through the intestines to promote fecal elimination)[47]
- trigger reflex actions in the body to stimulate organs.

Beard adds that these uses of massage should be applied only under the direction of a knowledgeable physician or physical therapist.



can often be used in place of pharmacological drugs.[45]

According to the Quebec Task Force on Spinal Disorders, massage is the most frequently used therapy for musculoskeletal problems, and is particularly useful in controlling pain.[46]

However, in our view, for toxic patients muscle massage should *never* be done until *after* the lymphatic system is working well; this would be after manual lymph drainage and/or dry skin brushing (see above, this chapter) plus the use of homeopathic or herbal lymph stimulators. It is important to emphasize that if lymph work is done *before* other immune-stimulating and cancer-fighting therapies are performed, lymph work theoretically might cause existing cancer to spread.

Massage is useful for simply relaxing muscle tension and reducing stress. People who face a diagnosis of cancer, particularly for the first time, are often overwhelmed by a sense of anxiety and impending doom. This anxiety triggers the "fight or flight" response in the body, notably the release of adrenalin) and leads to heightened muscular tension, elevated blood pressure, and other characteristic signs of being "under stress."

Muscle tension, whether from normal activity or awkward movement or stress, contributes to muscle fatigue and pain by compressing nerve fibers in the muscle. Prolonged contraction interferes with the elimination of chemical wastes in the muscles and surrounding tissues, and can cause frequent nerve and muscle pain. If not properly addressed, these body tensions have a tendency to build into chronic patterns of stress.

Prolonged tension can often cause pain in other parts of the body. For example, headaches are often caused by overly tense muscles in the neck, shoulders, and lower back; even contracted abdominal muscles can trigger headaches—a common complaint of women with menstrual difficulties.

For these tension-related conditions, headache expert Robert D. Milne, M.D., of Las Vegas, Nevada, coauthor of *An Alternative Medicine Definitive Guide to Headaches*,[48] finds that massage can break up muscular waste deposits and stimulate circulation. Accumulated metabolic wastes often form "trigger points" within muscles; these are specific areas that are painful to the touch. "They feel like knots or ropes within the muscle and perpetuate muscle tension," explains Dr. Milne. By applying deep pressure to these points, the tension or spasm can often be eliminated. Sometimes this deep pressure will even release the assorted toxins from the tissues.

## The Therapeutic Benefits of Exercise

The benefits of exercise extend far beyond cardiovascular fitness and the prevention of obesity and heart disease. Exercise aids in detoxification, digestion, weight control, and immune processes and can do wonders for mood and attitude. Advanced-cancer patients treated conventionally often end up spending many hours in a hospital bed, in contrast to those who undergo alternative cancer therapies who typically engage in regular exercise or physical activity. A brisk walk several times a week is a good start for any exercise program; low-impact aerobics, calisthenics, Qigong, yoga, stretching and flexing exercises, and gardening, among others, are all ways of strengthening the body's self-healing system.

Among the anticancer benefits of physical exercise, well-documented by clinical research are the following:

- Aerobic activities increase oxygen supply to tissues; because cancer tends to flourish in an oxygen-poor environment, the well-exercised body is more likely to repel cancer cells.
- Any form of physical activity, because it involves muscle contractions, stimulates the lymphatic system, which filters toxins from the blood and supports the body's immune system.
- Exercise stimulates the activity of natural killer cells and other

## Exercise Helps Prostate Cancer

A study of 12,975 men, average age 44 and tracked over a 19-year period, showed that moderate to high amounts of regular aerobic exercise reduced the risk of prostate cancer. High levels of exercise that burned off at least 3,000 calories weekly reduced the prostate cancer risk by 70%, while moderate levels, burning off at least 2,000 calories weekly, reduced the risk by 25%, according to *Medicine and Science in Sports and Exercise,* (January 1996).

components of the body's anticancer defenses.[49]

- Exercise causes an elevation of body temperature and increases the production of pyrogen, a special substance (lymphokine) that enhances the function of white blood cells (lymphocytes).[50]

People who maintain regular activity are less likely to develop colon cancer, the second leading cause of cancer-related death in the U.S.[51] In helping to ward off colon cancer, exercise tends to benefit men more than women.[52] Female college athletes, when compared to their nonathletic counterparts, have a lower incidence of cancers of the breast, ovary, cervix, vagina, and uterus.[53] In the same study, the risk of developing cancers of the reproductive system was 2.5 times lower for the athletes than it was for the sedentary women.

Keith I. Block, M.D., (the subject of Chapter 2), notes that exercise also helps cancer patients maintain normal muscle mass, which can increase significantly their chances of recovery. "Patients who are overweight or who lose lean tissue or muscle during therapy tend to have poorer prognoses," Dr. Block says. He recommends finding a form of exercise that can be carried out consistently, without causing strain. Russian researchers found that anaerobic exercise weakened the immune system for up to 24 hours after the exercise; but they also demonstrated that this immune suppression could be prevented by taking Siberian ginseng orally 30-60 minutes before the anaerobic exercise.

In a study, men who burned as few as 500 calories a week in exercise—the equivalent to about an hour's worth of brisk walking—had death rates about 20% lower than men who rarely exercised.[54] More avid exercisers experienced fewer cancer-related deaths: men who walked about 4 hours each week (about 2,000 calories burned) died of all cancers about 35% less frequently than their less active counterparts. A recent report from the Cooper Clinic in Dallas indicates that even moderate exercise—5 hours of walking per week—significantly reduces the risk of developing prostate cancer.[55]

# Qigong

**This ancient Chinese slow-movement therapy has been used successfully in China with thousands of cancer patients not only to develop greater peace of mind, deep relaxation, and enhanced oxygen and lymph circulation, but in many cases to control tumor growth and reduce the numerous symptoms associated with cancer, such as pain.**

Among the more systematized programs of movement therapy that can be applied to treating serious illness is qigong (pronounced chee-GUNG), developed centuries ago in China. In China, it is estimated that nearly 100 million people, from the healthy to the severely ill, practice qigong every day. Qigong plays a central role in the Chinese doctor's anticancer arsenal and is used in almost all hospitals in China today. Thousands of qigong institutes provide qigong instruction, while major research centers in Beijing, Shanghai, and Guangzho, train qigong teachers and carry out government-sponsored research.

Qigong movements are gentle and unhurried; the slow rate tends to synchronize with the rate of breathing. People engaged in these activities experience a sense of deep relaxation and heightened alertness. In fact, many derive an immediate positive sensation from the practice, and this gives them an incentive to continue practicing on a regular basis, even long after recovering from cancer.

Qigong literally means to work with or cultivate the *qi* (pronounced CHEE), or the vital life force energy that flows through the body like a river. The Chinese consider the existence of qi to be a fundamental truth. In one laboratory demonstration performed by a qigong master upon a group of patients, researchers measured the following results: a 30% reduction in cervical cancer cells; a 50% reduction in flu viruses; and a 60-80% reduction in bacteria.[56]

*Qi* is a naturally occurring, internally produced, self-healing resource, says Roger Jahnke, O.M.D., an acupuncturist practicing in Santa Barbara, California, who uses Qigong as part of his support treatment for patients with serious illness, including cancer. "Qigong can facilitate the free flow of energy throughout the body, which supports and promotes blood and lymph flow and even the flow of neurological impulses necessary for good health," says Dr. Jahnke. "The primary benefit is to activate the bioelectrical currents that flow along the energy channels through breathing regulation, deep relaxation, and gentle movement."

One advantage of this kind of exercise is the lack of strain on the body's joints and organ systems, a problem associated with high-impact aerobic activities. "Qigong is simple and easy to learn," says Dr. Jahnke. "My goal as a physician is to teach and inspire my patients to learn these techniques for themselves, so they can play an active role in their recovery."

## How Qigong Helps You Resist Cancer

Qigong's medical applications have been studied in great depth—most of the research comes from major cancer treatment facilities in China. For example, immunologists have observed that qigong stimulates the activity of lymphocytes, neutrophils, and other immune cells that play a role in fighting cancer.[57] Research conducted at the Beijing Lung Cancer Research Institute has shown that qigong exercises increase the immune function of lung cancer patients, as indicated by studies of their white blood cells.

A study of 122 cancer patients found that the practice of qigong resulted in better control of tumor growth and that those patients who practiced longer had better reductions in their tumors.[58] Most of these patients reported an enhanced quality of life as well as reductions in pain and other forms of discomfort, right up until the time of their deaths. In one study, 2,873 terminal cancer patients practiced qigong for 6 months. The outcome: 12% of the patients were cured while 47% showed significant improvement.[59] It is worth noting that these are considerably better outcomes than are achieved through chemotherapy.

In Chinese medicine, cancer exists in two ways: either as "accumulations" (tumorous form in which the cancer is localized) or as a whole-body toxicity problem (metastatic, blood, or lymph forms, in which cancer has spread from one part of the body to another). As Dr. Jahnke explains: "Tumors and toxicity that contribute to cancer are caused by a severe derangement of the function of the *qi* in its ability to maintain and support the body's overall functioning. The *qi* has become disordered in its ability to function optimally, which shows up in numerous ways, such as pain, accumulations of toxins, and immune system deficiency."

From Dr. Jahnke's perspective, the practice of qigong has the 3 following beneficial effects on the individual with cancer.[60]

***Studies of patients with advanced cancer have found that qigong helped improve the condition of the immune system, stimulated appetite, and reduced adverse side effects of chemotherapy, such as nausea and vomiting.***

### 1. Improved Oxygen Supply

Under healthy conditions, body cells and tissues receive oxygen as needed and this helps repel cancer since cancer cells cannot thrive in a high-oxygen environment. During qigong, the body becomes deeply relaxed and oxygen is absorbed from the blood by the tissues. But unlike more vigorous physical activities in which this oxygen is utilized by the muscles, during qigong, oxygen is distributed throughout the body, including those areas that may be harboring cancer cells.

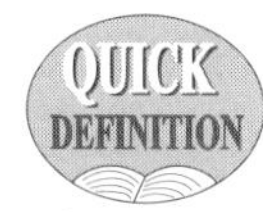


**Acupuncture meridians** are specific pathways in the human body for the flow of life force or subtle energy, known as *qi* (pronounced **CHEE**). In most cases, these energy pathways run up and down on both sides of the body, and correspond to individual organs or organ systems, designated as Lung, Small Intestine, Heart and others. There are 14 principal meridians and 8 secondary channels. Numerous points of heightened energy, or *qi*, exist on the body's surface along the meridians and are called acupoints. There are an estimated 1,000 such acupoints, each of which is potentially a place for acupuncture treatment.

"Qigong accelerates oxygen distribution in the body at a time when your muscles are not rapidly using it as they would be in running and other high-stress forms of exercise," says Dr. Jahnke. "The higher the oxygen supply, the more readily your body can reverse a cancerous condition." At the same time, there is an increased efficiency of cell metabolism and tissue regeneration through increased circulation of oxygen and nutrient-rich blood to the brain, organs and tissues.

### 2. Improved Balance of Autonomic Nervous System

The second major effect of qigong on the cancer patient involves the person's psyche and its effect on the autonomic nervous system (ANS). The ANS, which controls most of our basic body functions, contains 2 branches: the sympathetic and parasympathetic systems. The sympathetic nervous system is associated with arousal and stress; this system prepares us physically when we perceive a threat or challenge, by increasing our heart rate, blood pressure and muscle tension. The hormones released in this process tend to suppress the immune system, however, which is why a calm or centered way of responding to potentially difficult situations is more desirable.

During qigong practice, the individual can achieve a state of deep

**SUCCESS STORY**

## Helping to Reverse Breast Cancer

When Janice, aged 50, was diagnosed with breast cancer, she decided to explore the options of alternative medicine. She sought the guidance of Roger Jahnke, O.M.D., a practitioner of traditional Chinese medicine for 20 years. Dr. Jahnke encouraged Janice to pursue a therapeutic program that included a mainly vegetarian diet, herbal medicine, acupuncture, and qigong, a self-healing system that combines conscious regulation of the body, breath, and mind to enhance the flow of vital energy, or *qi*, through the body.

Janice learned an exercise focused on storing the *qi* in the bone marrow. "According to the Chinese tradition, the practice of qigong is believed to support the bone marrow's ability to produce immune cells," says Dr. Jahnke. "Anyone with a cancer diagnosis can benefit from the practice of qigong." These benefits include enhancing immune function and increasing blood and lymph circulation, as well as cultivating inner strength, calming the mind, and restoring the body to its natural state of health.

When Janice began qigong practice, she noticed that the tumor in her breast would actually feel hot, then would cool off when she stopped practicing. In the following weeks, her energy level increased noticeably. She felt that the practice, as an addition to other natural healing methods and conventional medicine, was helping to restore her health. Janice's health continued to improve and, 8 years after her diagnosis, Janice was doing well, living symptom free with cancer in apparent remission.

relaxation, enabling the parasympathetic nervous system to neutralize the stress response, says Dr. Jahnke. Qigong tends to reduce the sympathetic system's functioning to ensure that a balance exists between the 2 branches of the autonomic nervous system. This, in turn, decreases heart rate and blood pressure, dilates the blood vessels (enhancing the oxygen supply further), and supports optimal immune function.

"When the 2 parts of the autonomic nervous system are in balance, the immune system is more highly activated," says Dr. Jahnke. "There's a tremendous benefit to this deep relaxation state, and qigong is one of the most effective methods among the body-centered practices under investigation." A related benefit, Dr. Jahnke adds, is a reduction in depression and anxiety. "One of the most striking features of qigong is the optimism and cheerfulness of the practitioners."

**3. Improved Lymphatic Function—** Qigong exerts a powerful influence on the lymphatic system, which Dr. Jahnke regards as the "garbage disposal system" of the body. "People who are not well are generally not mobilizing their lymphatic systems. This system is moved by a kind of composite heart, including all the body's muscles, the breath, the cells' production of water, gravity, and an automatic contraction of the ends of the lymph vessels. Qigong practice stimulates circulation of the lymph fluid through the system, carrying the immune cells to key areas and eliminating toxins from the tissue spaces." One way to see the impact of this qigong-induced detoxification is by the improved skin condition of people who have practiced regularly for 1-2 months.

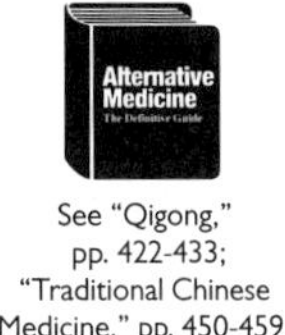


See "Qigong," pp. 422-433; "Traditional Chinese Medicine," pp. 450-459.

The combined effects of improving the oxygen supply, balancing the nervous system, enhancing mood and relaxation, and strengthening the lymphatic system make up qigong's main therapeutic benefits for cancer patients. "The beauty of qigong is that you can literally feel the sensation of the activation of the natural healing response internally," says Dr. Jahnke. "The Chinese call this '*qi* sensation.' We might call it the sensation of naturally occurring self-healing resources."

***"There's a tremendous benefit to this deep relaxation state, and qigong is one of the most effective methods among the body-centered practices under investigation," says Dr. Jahnke.***

He notes that the medical situation of bedridden cancer patients is complicated by accumulated metabolic by-products and medications that are not eliminated because of the inactivity of the lymph system. In most cases, a lot is done to medically neutralize the disease, but nothing is done to enhance health. "Just when cancer patients *need* gentle movement the most, they are told to just lay back and hope for the best," observes Dr. Jahnke.

## How Qigong Works as an Adjunctive Cancer Therapy

The cancer patients who come to Dr. Jahnke for guidance and medical care are typically already receiving some form of conventional treatment. Traditional Chinese doctors regard qigong not as an exclusive form of therapy; rather, they emphasize using it in combination with conventional treatment, Chinese herbal remedies, a healing diet, psychotherapy, and regular group activity.[61] Qigong appears to work more effectively when all of these components are addressed.

One study compared cancer patients treated with this integrated approach for half a year to those receiving *only* conventional therapy. Compared to the conventional group, the group treated with the qigong-integrated approach experienced clear benefits: the antitumor activity of immune cell counts increased, their DNA repair ability improved (a measure of the body's ability to reverse cancer), and the rate of cancer recurrence was reduced. At the same time, patients in the qigong group showed improved confidence and optimism, and in a few cases, tumors went into complete remission.[62]

Studies of patients with advanced cancer have found that qigong helped improve the condition of the immune system, stimulated appetite, and reduced adverse side effects of chemotherapy, such as nausea and vomiting.[63] The response rate to chemotherapy in the qigong-treated group was nearly 5 times better than that of the group that received chemotherapy without qigong. The substantial improvement in mood and attitude is no small feat: cancer is an emotionally devastating disease.

***A study of 122 cancer patients found that the practice of qigong resulted in better control of tumor growth and that those patients who practiced longer had better reductions in their tumors. In one study, 2,873 terminal cancer patients practiced qigong for six months. The outcome: 12% of the patients were cured while 47% showed significant improvement. It is worth noting that these are better outcomes than are achieved through chemotherapy.***

Dr. Jahnke notes that patients practicing qigong appear not to suffer from the side-effects of radiation treatments and, in addition, maintain their lean tissue mass—a significant factor since a loss of lean tissue mass can greatly worsen the cancer patient's prognosis. At least 25% of cancer patients lose lean tissue mass, usually when they are in the final stages of the disease. Qigong appears to raise the cancer patient's energy levels and improve muscle tone and coordination. According to Liu Guo Long, M.D., Ph.D., of the Beijing College of Traditional Chinese Medicine, the qigong-treated body can heal more effectively because of the increased blood and lymph flow and the greater supply of nutrients regenerating the cells.[64]

## A How-to Introduction to Qigong Practice

This section contains detailed instructions from Dr. Jahnke on a specific set of therapeutic qigong practices. The act of reading can interfere with the fluidity of the practice, so we advise that you tape record the entire section as you read so that you will be able to listen as you practice qigong movements in subsequent sessions.

## TRACING ACUPUNCTURE MERIDIANS TO CIRCULATE VITAL LIFE ENERGY

The goal of this practice is to move the *qi* along the meridians. Rub your hands together to build up heat and increase *qi*. They will become warmer if you are relaxed and your environment is comfortable. As if washing your face, stroke your palms upward across the cheeks, eyes, and forehead; continue over the top and side of your head, down the back of the neck, and along the shoulders to the shoulder joint (see Figure 33.1).

Continue under the arm and down the sides to the rib cage. At the lower edge of the rib cage, move the palms around to the back, across the buttocks, down the back and sides of the legs, and out the sides of the feet. Trace up inside the feet and the inner surface of the legs, up the front side of the torso and onto the face again, beginning the second round. You may rub the palms together before each round. Imagine that you are standing in a pool of healing water and that you are bathing your whole body in a profound medicine.

## DIRECTING VITAL LIFE ENERGY TO INTERNAL ORGANS

Again, rub your hands together to build up heat. Apply the right hand to the area over the liver at the lower right edge of your rib cage. Visualize the liver—the largest, most complex organ in the body—receiving the *qi* and its benefits (see Figure 33.2).

Apply the left hand to the area over the spleen and pancreas at the lower left side of the ribs. The spleen—a blood-

### Qigong Proven to Improve Cancer Outcomes

At the Kuangan Men's Hospital in Beijing, China, 93 cases of advanced malignant cancer were treated with a combination of drugs and qigong exercises, while a control group of 30 patients was treated by drugs alone. 81% percent of the qigong group gained strength, 63% experienced improved appetite, and 33% were free from diarrhea compared to comparable control group improvements of 10%, 10%, and 6%, respectively.[65]

***Traditional Chinese doctors regard qigong not as an exclusive form of therapy; rather, they emphasize using it in combination with conventional treatment, Chinese herbal remedies, a healing diet, psychotherapy, and regular group activity.***

storing and lymphatic organ—is the producer of white blood cells and the pancreas produces digestive enzymes as well as insulin and glucagon (the hormone that regulates blood sugar level and energy metabolism). Move your hands in a circular way, continuing to create heat, breathing restful breaths, and relax. Feel the heat, or *qi*, moving through the surface of the skin and penetrating the organs as the entire metabolic process becomes more efficient.

Still holding the hands over the organs, continue to feel the heat penetrate. On exhalation, visualize the *qi* circulating from the center of the body out along the arms, and into the hands, to finally penetrate into the organs.

Now, move your left palm to cover the navel and your right palm to cover the breastbone. The navel is the human's original connection to life and nourishment, and the Chinese feel that in adulthood it still connects, energetically, to the whole body. The breastbone protects several vital organs—the heart and the thymus. The heart pumps the blood, of course,

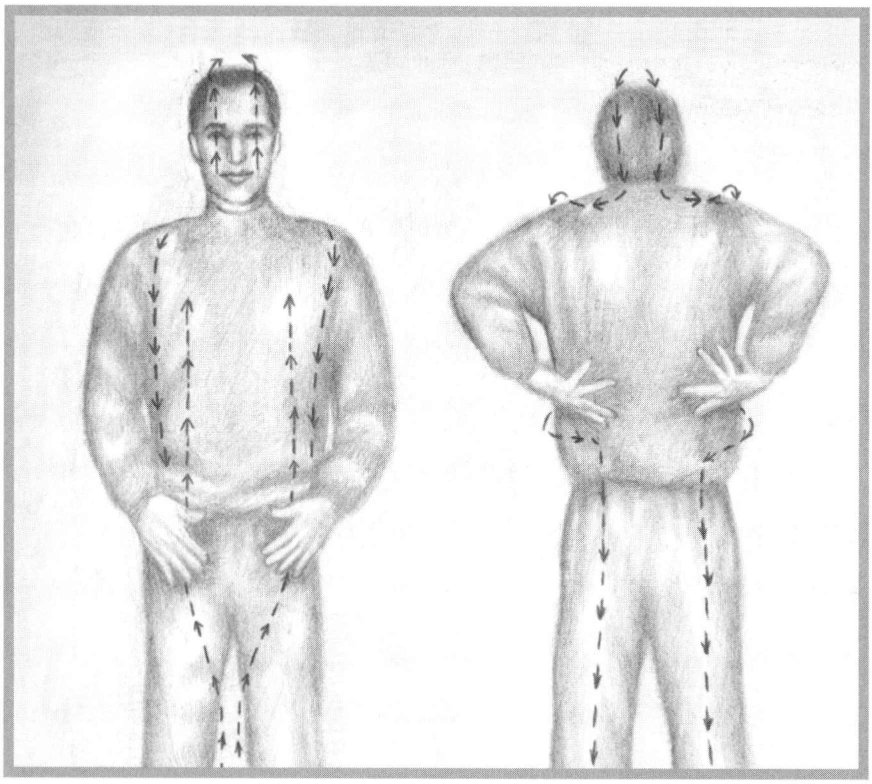

**Figure 33.1—Tracing acupuncture meridians to circulate vital life energy**

but the Chinese believe it is the resting place of one's emotional and spiritual self. The thymus is the original source of T cells, some of the most powerful immune agents. Visualize them benefiting from the warmth, the *qi*, pouring into the navel, heart and thymus, gathering strength to carry out their essential functions.

Move the palms around to cover the lower back. In traditional Chinese medicine, this area is thought to be directly connected to the kidneys, which not only remove toxins from the blood, but also are the storehouse of vital life energies. The adrenal glands rest on top of the kidneys, and control much of what the Chinese associate with the regulation of our energy. Rub these areas penetrating the *qi* deep into the body to improve the ability of the kidneys and adrenals to do their work. Visualize the kidneys and adrenals receiving the *qi* and being empowered to efficiently eliminate waste products, produce energy, and activate healing throughout the whole body.

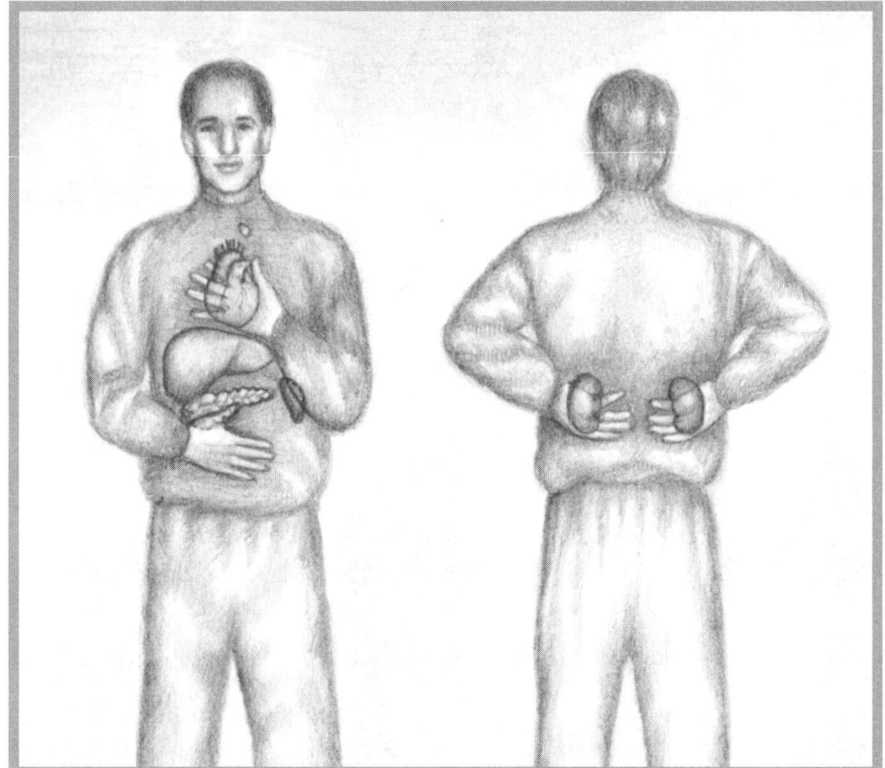

**Figure 33.2—Directing vital life energy to internal organs**

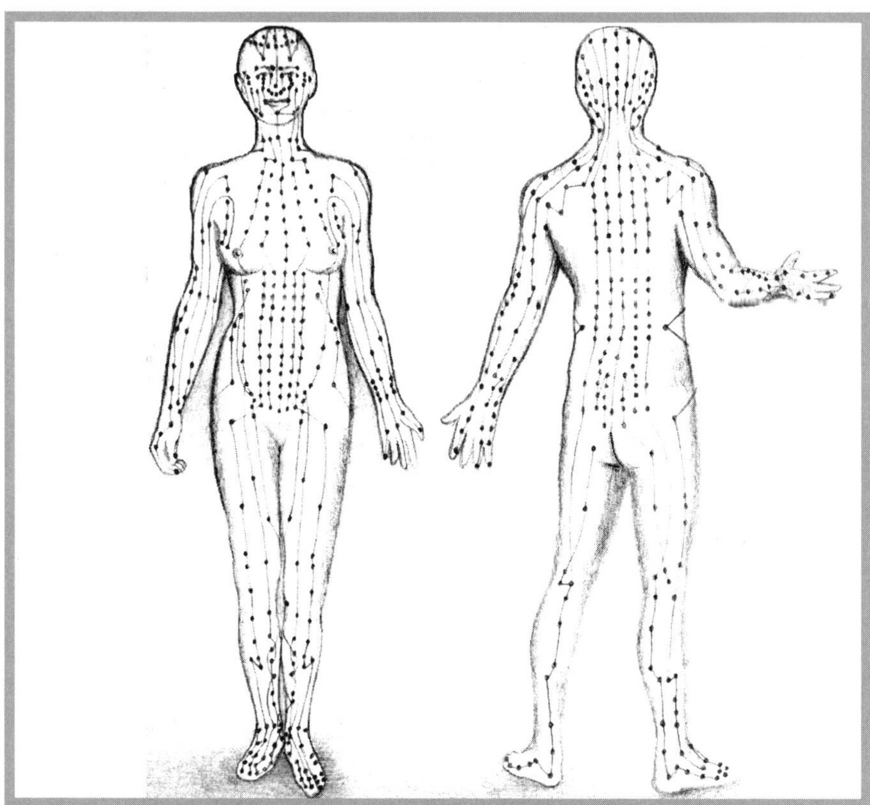

**Figure 33.3—Front and back view of acupunture meridians**

## MASSAGING THE ACUPUNCTURE MICROSYSTEMS

In modern Chinese medical terminology, the hands, feet, abdomen, and ears are called reflex microsystems. Pressure properly applied to these areas, usually with the thumbs, can stimulate *qi* throughout the body.

With your thumbs, vigorously press all areas of the palms and the soles of the feet. Find sore points and concentrate pressure on them several times. Press out along each segment of the fingers and toes. At the tips of the fingers and toes press on the lateral sides of the base of the finger or toenails (feel for an indentation). Continuing to press, roll the receiving finger or toe under the pressure of the thumb and forefinger of the working hand. Return to give additional pressure to those hand or foot points that were particularly tender.

Now using the thumbs and forefingers, massage both ears simultaneously. Begin with moderate pressure and work over the entire ear on both sides, until the ears begin to feel hot. Notice any areas of discomfort and rub the uncomfortable areas vigorously a second or third time.

## BUILDING UP VITAL LIFE ENERGY WITH BREATHING

Sit or stand, keeping your eyes lightly closed or just slightly open with your attention focused inward. Try to feel anything you can about your physical body or emotional state. Relax your shoulders and allow your head to rests directly on top of the shoulders and spine. Hold your hands with palms facing upward, fingertips pointing toward each other 2 inches below the navel.

Slowly inhaling, bring the hands upward to the lower edge of the breastbone. Then, take in 3 additional short puffs of breath to maximally fill the lungs, raising the hands a bit with each puff to the level of the center of the heart. Hold for a movement. Turn the palms face down and exhale slowly, gradually lowering the hands to the navel. Exhale 3 additional puffs of breath, to empty the lungs completely. Lower the hands a bit to the beginning level. Hold for a moment. Turn the palms upward and repeat.

On the exhalations you may feel a warm or tingling sensation spreading outward from the center of your body toward your hands. On inhaling, visualize the *qi* accumulating deep inside the pelvic and abdominal cavities (known as "the sea of energy").

## CONTRACTING AND RELAXING WHILE BREATHING

In this exercise, the body musculature contracts on exhalation and deeply relaxes on each inhalation. The breath and the contraction together help to cleanse the tissues of the body.

While sitting or standing, bring the hands in front of the heart/breastbone, inhale and relax. Begin to exhale, pressing the hands forward as if pushing something heavy. Contract as many of the body's muscles as possible. Grip the floor or ground with the toes and, while the hands slowly push forward, contract the perineal muscles (located on the pelvic floor between the genital and anal area, the muscles used to curtail the flow of urine).

When the hands are extended, all muscles contracted, the breath is completely exhaled. Now relax, release tension from all muscles and float

***"One factor makes qigong an inevitable innovation in Western culture: the staggering cost of postsymptomatic medical intervention," says Dr. Jahnke. "With qigong, individuals learn to heal themselves and maintain their health—this is a profoundly cost-effective feature."***

the hands back toward the heart with a deep inhalation. Release the toes, the perineum, and the abdomen.

Repeat the same cycle, pressing the hands upward as high as possible, as if lifting a great weight off yourself, exhaling and contracting. Then relax completely, inhale slowly, and return the hands to the position before the heart.

Next, repeat, pushing out to the sides then repeat, pressing downward. Continue for several rounds, pressing forward, then up, then to the sides and finally downward. Contraction and release of the muscles pumps large volumes of lymphatic fluid away from the tissues, carrying metabolic byproducts and pollutants through the lymph to the bloodstream, for elimination through the liver and kidneys.

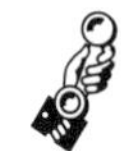

For more information about **qigong**, contact: Roger Jahnke, O.M.D., Health Action, 243 Pebble Beach Drive, Santa Barbara, CA 93117; tel: 805-685-4670; fax: 805-685-4710. Dr. Jahnke has practiced clinical acupuncture, herbal medicine, and Chinese physical therapy since 1976.

### QIGONG CONCENTRATION

This practice can be done standing, sitting, or lying down. In the severely ill, it can mobilize important healing resources; in a healthy person, it can help maintain health and coordinate body, mind, and spirit.

In this practice, natural forces accelerate through breath, relaxation, intention, and visualization. On inhalation, visualize a concentration of *qi* in the abdominal area. On exhalation, visualize these resources circulating out from the center to all the parts of the body: extremities, organs, tissues, and glands. Continue, through thought and visualization, to circulate healing energy with deep breathing and deep relaxation. On the inhalations, powerful healing *qi* gathers; on the exhalations, these healing resources circulate throughout the body.

## Maintaining the Therapeutic Practice of Qigong

If able, one should practice qigong for 30-60 minutes daily, says Dr. Jahnke. For those with cancer, if they feel they have the resources and energy to carry out qigong practice more aggressively, then they should practice it several times a day.

Cancer patients using qigong to treat advanced or "end-stage" cancer need to apply themselves on a vigilant, yet gentle basis, until they begin to experience some benefits. "There is great value in a continuing practice to ensure long-term healing and the increase of vitality," says Jahnke. Practicing qigong with other people, as is commonly done in China, provides positive reinforcement and makes the practice easier to maintain.

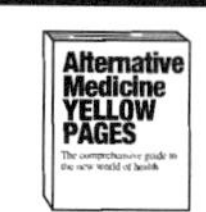


See "Chelation," p. 54; "Colon Therapy," p. 96; "CranioSacral Therapy," p. 98; "Dentistry—Biological and Neural," p. 115; "Detoxification Therapy," p. 119; "Heavy Metal Toxicity," p. 153; "Hydrotherapy," p. 166; "Hyperthermia," p. 167; and "Qigong," p. 235.

Some physicians recommend qigong to their patients as a "last resort," when other therapies fail. Dr. Jahnke considers this a grave mistake, since qigong aids in the recovery process by enhancing the immune system function. "Qigong should be incorporated into every cancer treatment approach from day one. It is better as a *first* resort," he says. "It is an excellent way to improve the cancer patient's appetite and sleep as well as increase their overall immune resistance, energy level, and emotional well-being. Why would anyone want to experience these benefits as a last resort?"

Although qigong exercises are increasingly practiced in the United States, the conventional medical community has been resistant to its use in a medical context. "Yet," says Dr. Jahnke, "one factor makes qigong an inevitable innovation in Western culture: the staggering cost of postsymptomatic medical intervention. With qigong, individuals learn to heal themselves and maintain their health—this is a profoundly cost-effective feature."

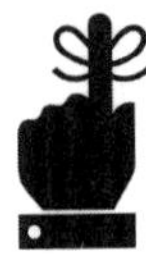

*Each year, people are exposed to thousands of toxic chemicals and pollutants in air, water, food, and soil. Increasingly, toxicity is being identified as the predisposing factor in a long list of acute and chronic degenerative illnesses. Most alternative physicians agree that detoxification is essential.*

Chapter 34

# Energy Support Therapies

**At the forefront of new alternative clinical approaches to cancer is recognition of the role of energy, both as a means of diagnosis and treatment. Acting at an even deeper cellular level than biochemicals, energy can make or break health.**

The realm of energy is at the forefront of new alternative approaches to cancer diagnosis and treatment. By energy, we mean a somewhat subtler level of bodily functioning than what is reflected in biochemistry and immunology. Traditional Chinese medicine and its acupuncture, for example, talk of *qi*, a basic flow of energy or life force through the body; homeopathy speaks of the *dynamis*, the fundamental self-healing vitality of the human organism. In this concluding chapter, we explore the diagnostic and therapeutic role of energy in addressing cancer, as exemplified in electrodermal screening and the applied energies of magnets and light.

**In This Chapter**

# Electrodermal Screening

**According to energy medicine theory, every disease state is preceded by and indicated by an energy signal, detectable by electrodermal screening (EDS) devices which gather information through the acupuncture meridian system. EDS can indicate the degree of stress that is affecting an organ and it can monitor the progress of therapy, avoiding trial and error and general guesswork.**

Imagine that you are sitting in a doctor's office. The doctor takes a small, handheld probe connected to a meter, and with no further questions, gently presses certain points on your hands or feet while noting the figures displayed on the meter. From this, she can tell you which parts of your body are functioning correctly and which organs are causing problems. Next, she places small glass vials containing colorless liquids into a container, which is also connected to the device. The doctor then remeasures some of the points on your hands.

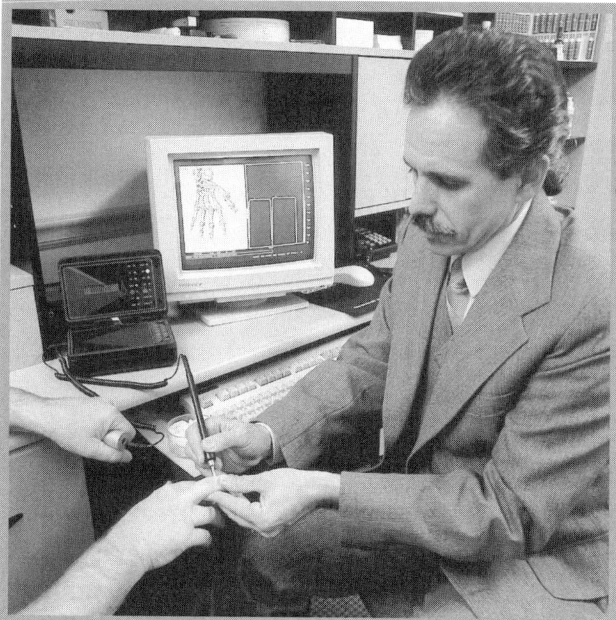

James H. Clark, the "Father of Computerized Electrodermal Screening (CEDS)" technology, takes a reading using the portable LISTEN System connected to a desktop computer.

***Through energy medicine, and particularly with electrodermal screening, you can see disease coming* before *it manifests, and thereby stop it early. At the same time, energy medicine provides proof that therapies are working and that no further traces of illness remain at the end of treatment because energy changes precede physical ones.***

On this basis, the doctor can tell you, in lucid terms, why you are not feeling well or whether you are likely to have a problem in the near future. By way of remedy, the physician gives you a few drops of a tasteless medicine (usually a homeopathic remedy), and before long you begin to feel better. This description is not a futuristic fantasy. It is a factual narrative of what practitioners of energy medicine using electrodermal screening are presently doing in medical clinics in the U.S., Europe, and Asia.

## The Growing Importance of Energy Medicine in Cancer Treatment

It may surprise you to note that many of the most sophisticated diagnostic systems used today in conventional medicine—EKG (electrocardiogram, to measure heart activity), EEG (electroencephalogram, to measure brain waves), EMG (electromyogram to measure electrical properties of skeletal muscle), MRI (magnetic resonance imaging, to "picture" internal organs)— employ the principles of energy medicine. Energy medicine, or bioenergetic medicine as it is sometimes called, refers to diagnostic procedures and therapies that use an energy field—electrical, magnetic, sonic, acoustic, microwave, infrared—to screen for health conditions by detecting imbalances in the body's energy fields, and then correct them.

The detection of energy imbalances in the body provides an early warning system for potential disruptions in biochemical balance and function that may lead to disease. Balance can be restored using a variety of alternative therapies, or with treatment devices that rebalance the energy levels of the various fields before the actual biochemical or structural disturbances can occur. Through energy medicine, and particularly with electrodermal screening (EDS), you can see disease coming *before* it manifests and thereby stop it early. At the same time, energy medicine provides proof that therapies are working and that no further traces of illness remain at the end of treatment, because energy changes precede physical ones.

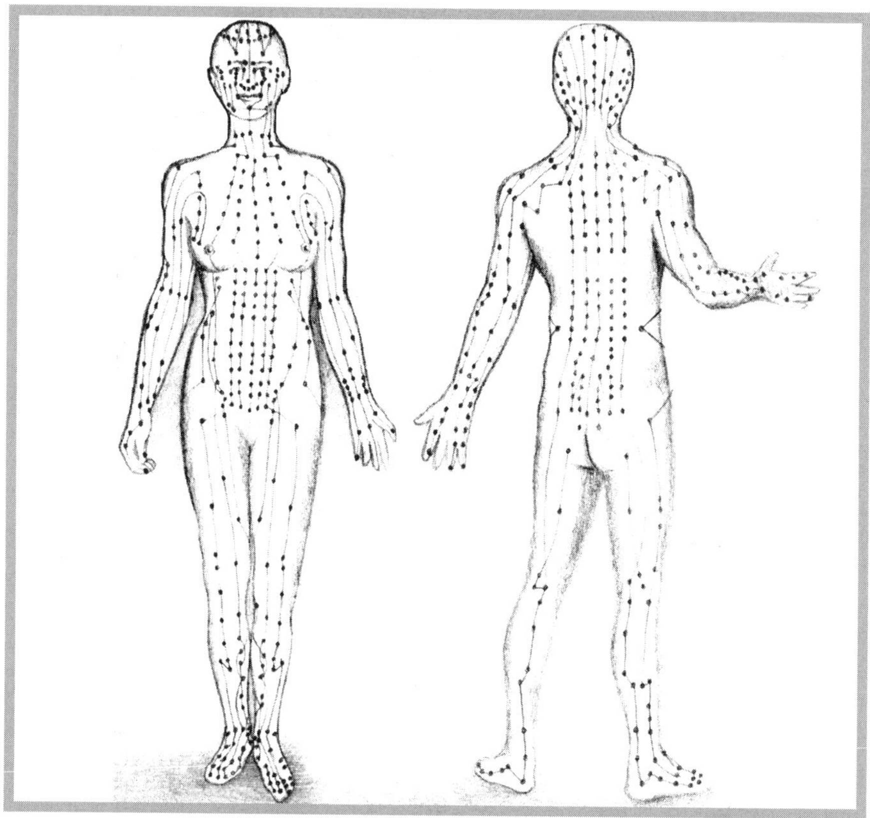

**Figure 34.1—Acupuncture meridians are specific pathways in the human body for the flow of life force or subtle energy, known as *qi* (pronounced CHEE). In most cases, these energy pathways run up and down both sides of the body, and correspond to individual organs or organ systems, designated as Lung, Small Intestine, Heart, and others. There are 12 principal meridians and 8 secondary channels. Numerous points of heightened energy, or *qi*, exist on the body's surface along the meridians and are called acupoints. There are more than 1,000 acupoints, each of which is potentially a place for acupuncture treatment.**

Most energy medicine devices are based on the acupuncture meridian system. Acupuncture works on the principle that there is a network of energy channels or pathways called *meridians*, running throughout the body. According to acupuncture theory, different organs are associated with different energy meridians, and health problems in various organs show up as disturbances of energy in the associated meridians. Acupuncture points, or acupoints, are the points along these meridians where energy flow can be measured and manipulated.

Although orthodox oncologists have trouble accepting the existence of

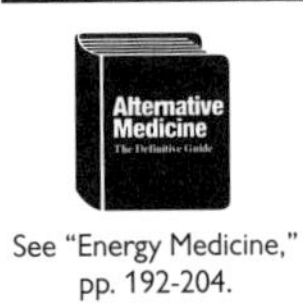

See "Energy Medicine," pp. 192-204.

energy meridians, the effectiveness of acupuncture treatment itself is now beyond dispute, particularly in the realm of pain relief for cancer patients. Its validity has been demonstrated by isotope tracings by both Korean and French researchers, demonstrating the location of acupuncture meridians. For example, in a study of 183 cancer patients attending a London clinic and receiving acupuncture, 82% of the patients reported experiencing pain relief in the early stages, and 52% reported benefits in the later stages.[1] Another study found that cancer patients treated with acupuncture showed a significant elevation in their natural killer cell activity, which, as you now know, are an integral part of the body's anticancer defenses.[2]

***The key idea is that an energetic event transfers its signal through an acupuncture meridian to the nervous system, with the end result being a cellular pathology. "Every inflammatory alteration of a cell starts with an increased energy production," says James Clark.***

Since the 1940s, research has established that acupuncture points possess electrical conductivity. Earlier, German doctors, led by Reinhold Voll, M.D., measured changes in electrical conductivity at many of the body's acupuncture points and discovered that the electrical resistance of the skin decreases dramatically at the acupuncture points compared to the surrounding skin, meaning the electrical current is conducted more efficiently at these points. They also found that each point appeared to have a standard measurement for anyone who is in good health, where there is a steady flow of energy in the meridians. This measurement changes when health deteriorates. For this reason, EDS researcher William A. Tiller, Ph.D., of Stanford University in Palo Alto, California, calls the conductance points "information-access windows." Comparing values before and after treatment provides useful information about a patient's condition.

In the original research, Dr. Voll measured the body's energy using skin resistance. More technically put, he measured changes in electrical conductivity at each of the body's acupuncture points then estimated at 1,000 points; doctors today have identified more than 1,000. Skin conductance can indicate or register physiological changes in the body. According to James Hoyt Clark of Orem, Utah, an EDS inventor and educator, "Research has shown that skin generally has a resistance of about 2 to 4 million ohms, but at the conductance points, the resistance is 100,000 ohms in a healthy, balanced person. They [investigators] were also surprised when these points corresponded to the acupuncture points."[3]

The impetus for Dr. Voll's research into electronic information-gathering systems was an attempt to reverse his own bladder cancer; he integrated this new research with his own medical training in acupuncture and came up with EAV point testing (Electro-Acupuncture according to Voll).[4] Specifically, Dr. Voll established a scale of 0 to 100, with 45-55 being "normal" or "balanced." Readings above 55 are interpreted as indicating an inflammation of the organ associated with the meridian tested, while readings below 45-50 suggest organ stagnation and degeneration.[5]

A homeopathic **miasm**, as originally described by Samuel Hahnemann, the 19th-century German founder of homeopathy, is a subtle taint or energy residue of previous illness, even across the generations. As an inherited predisposition for chronic disease that is far more subtle than anything genetic, miasms are broad-focused, predisposing individuals and families to specific illnesses, such as tuberculosis or cancer. According to Hahnemann, 3 miasms underlie all chronic illness and parallel broad stages in the history of human experience with primary disease states. They are the Psoric miasm (from psora, meaning "itch"), the Syphilitic miasm (deriving from syphilis), and the Sycotic miasm (arising as a residue of gonorrhea). Some homeopaths add a fourth Cancer miasm, and a fifth Petroleum miasm.

The key idea is that an energetic event transfers its signal through an acupuncture meridian to the nervous system, with the end result being a cellular pathology. "Every inflammatory alteration of a cell starts with an increased energy production," says James Clark. He adds that EDS is a "data acquisition process" in which the trained practitioner conducts an "interview" with the patient's organs and tissues, gathering information about the basic functional status of those systems and their energy pathways. As such, EDS is an investigational, not diagnostic, device because it requires the physician's knowledge of acupuncture, physiology, and therapeutic substances to interpret the energy imbalances, establish their precise focus, and select the most appropriate therapeutic response.

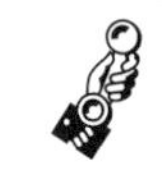

For more information about **EDS**, **Computronix**, and **Acupro**, contact: Doug Lieber, Computronix Electro-Medical Systems, 145 Canyon Oaks Drive, Argyle, TX 76226; tel: 817-241-2768; fax: 817-455-2605.

EDS can indicate the degree of stress that is affecting an organ and can monitor the progress of therapy, avoiding trial and error and general guesswork. Another way of explaining it, says Clark, is that EDS "like a thermometer, measures energy. The thermometer measures heat while the typical electrodermal screening device measures electric flow. The system measures the energy that is allowed to flow through each meridian. In either case, if the optimal reading is not measured, an energy imbalance has been detected."

Research by Voll, Tiller, and others has established that ion flow and concentration is a major factor in skin conductance. An organ inflammation (indicated by a reading above 55) increases ion concentrations and

## The Electrodermal Screening Product Library of Energy Signals

The more sophisticated EDS devices, such as the LISTEN system from Biosource (developed by James Hoyt Clark), the Omega Acubase from Digital Health, Inc., and the Acupro from Computronix, contain an inventory of energy signals corresponding to several thousand different substances. This inventory is called the Product Library.

Among the categories of products and substances found in an EDS Product Library are:

- alcohol products
- amino acids
- animal danders
- Ayurvedic herbs
- bacteria nosodes
- blossoming flowers
- cacti and succulents
- chemicals
- Chinese/Japanese herbs
- cleaners
- colors
- dental products
- detoxification list
- digestive enzymes
- endocrines
- environmentals
- essential oils
- flower essences
- food list
- gems/minerals
- geopathic list
- grasses, weeds
- habit drugs
- homeopathics-combinations
- homeopathics-drainage
- homeopathics-polychrest
- homeopathics-singles
- hormones
- insects
- metals
- miasms
- minerals
- molds/fungi
- nosodes
- parasites
- pesticides
- phenolics
- sarcodes
- shrubs
- snakes
- spiders
- tree pollens
- veterinary viruses
- vitamins[6]

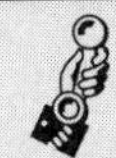

For more information about the **LISTEN System** and EDS seminars, contact James Hoyt Clark, Biosource, Inc., 1388 West Center Street, Orem, UT 84057; tel: 801-226-1117. For more information about the **Omega Acubase** system and seminars, contact: Vaughn Cook, L.Ac., Digital Health, Inc., 1770 East Fort Union Blvd., No. 101, Salt Lake City, UT 84121; tel: 801-944-4070; fax: 801-944-4067.

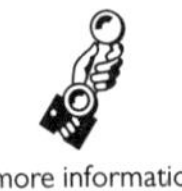

For more information about **electrodermal screening**, energy medicine, and devices, contact: Occidental Institute Research Foundation, P.O. Box 100 Penticton, British Columbia, Canada V2A 6J9; tel: 604-497-6020; fax: 604-497-6030.

electron flow, leading to a drop in resistance and a rise in conductance. Organ degeneration (indicated by a reading lower than 45-50) decreases ion concentrations, leading to a rise in resistance and a drop in conductance. Higher readings correlate with higher conductance, lower readings with lower conductance.[7]

More specifically, initial readings above 60 can indicate an inflammation somewhere in the body, while readings below 45 can often indicate physiological changes brought about by a degenerative process. Of even keener interest to EDS operators is a phenomenon called the Indicator Drop (ID). Soon after the initial reading is registered, the value may suddenly drop off; this is interpreted as indicative of an imbalance in the system while a reading that does not include an ID is taken as a sign of energy balance.

"When an ID is present, it is considered the most important part of the reading," explains EDS researcher Julia J. Tsuei, Ph.D., founder of the Foundation for East-West Medicine in Taipei, Taiwan. Through a process called medicine testing, the EDS operator can use the ID to determine the nature and cause of an imbalance, Dr. Tsuei explains. Various substances—"virtually any sort of biological reagent" especially homeopathic remedies—can be tested against the points that produced an ID.

The physician's task is to find a single substance or combination of substances that will balance the point, which means, bring its EDS reading back close to 50 without an Indicator Drop. For example, Dr. Tsuei explains that the pancreas readings for a person with diabetes will become balanced when the correct and appropriate dose of insulin is placed within the EDS circuit; put refined sugar there, however, and a large ID is likely to appear, Dr. Tsuei says. "With its solid theoretical foundation in modern physics and quantum mechanics, [EDS] is perhaps the most 'modern' medical methodology available today," she states.[8]

According to Douglas Lieber, L.Ac., director of Computronix Electro-Medical Systems in Argyle, Texas, and the inventor of the Computronix EDS hardware and accompanying Acupro software, Dr. Voll identified approximately 1,050 electrodermal screening points during his 35 years of research. Lieber reports that he has identified more than 400 additional points which are valuable EDS testing nodes. Since 1983, Lieber has performed EDS testing on thousands of individuals with cancer. He finds that there are 7 basic underlying contributors to the development and perpetuation of cancer.

According to Lieber, these are: 1) geopathic stress deriving from either where the cancer patient's bed or daytime chair is located; 2) parasites of many types present in the body; 3) degenerative toxic focuses, most commonly from chronic low-grade dental infections in the jaw where teeth have been extracted or root canals have been installed, but sometimes also in the tonsils, fallopian tubes, appendix, gallbladder, liver, or pancreas; 4) unresolved emotional trauma, often involving unrecognized subconscious issues from childhood; 5) miasmic influences passed from parent to child for several generations, usually the tuberculosis miasm (as in lung cancer)

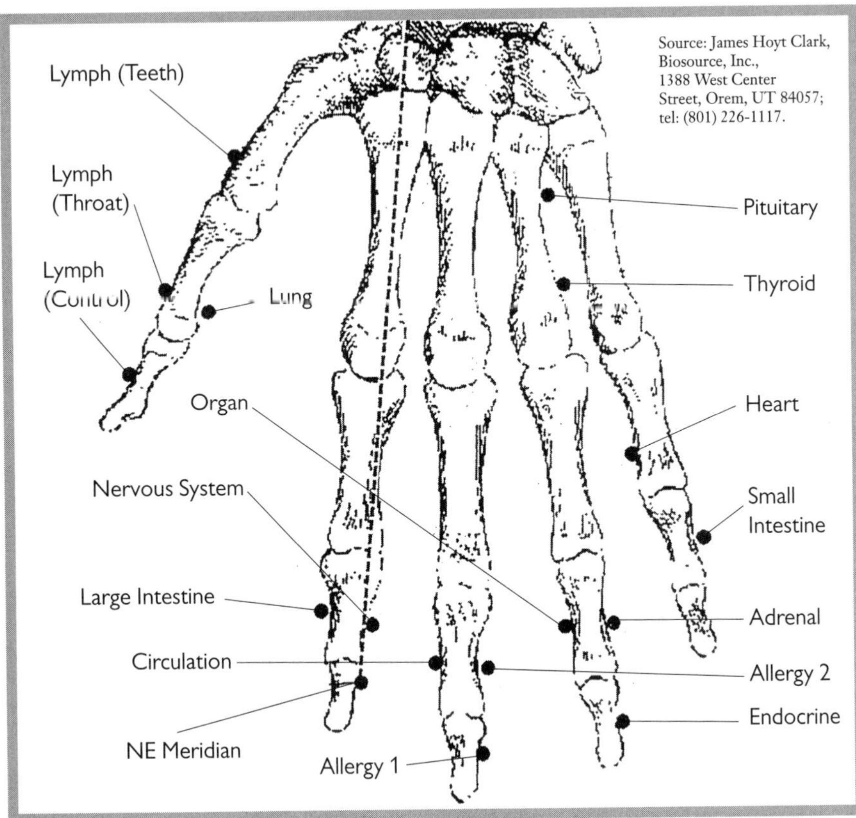


**Figure 34.2—EDS hand exam points**

and the syphilitic miasm in other cancers; 6) radiation and/or electromagnetic exposure; and 7) chemical toxins exposure, especially to nickel, cadmium, mercury, aflatoxins (from molds and fungi), pesticides, benzene, toluene, xylene, formaldehyde, isopropyl alcohol, and certain other solvents and autotoxins (produced mostly from toxic intestines).

In conducting follow-up EDS research on cancer patients who have identified and removed these cancer-contributing factors from their bodies and environment, Lieber has usually found dramatic improvement in the general condition of the patients, according to subsequent medical history, conventional tests, and EDS indicators.

## Electrodermal Screening Identifies a Hidden Dental Problem

As mentioned previously, the acupuncture meridian system and its proven energy flows are the basis for electrodermal screening. Researchers at the University of California at Los Angeles and the University of Southern California demonstrated an 87% correlation between an electrodermal screening biofeedback diagnosis of lung cancer and a standard X-ray diagnosis.[9]

Here is a case from Anthony J. Scott-Morley, H.M.D. (honorary), Ph.D., D.Sc., of Dorset, England, a pioneer in the use of EDS for diagnosing illness. Judy, aged 58, consulted with Dr. Scott-Morley regarding small tumors on her right breast. At the time of her initial visit, Judy did not know if the rumors were malignant. Instead of taking a biopsy of the breast tissue, which could perhaps spread any existing cancer cells in the region, he performed an EDS analysis on Judy.

During the course of Dr. Scott-Morley's EDS assessment, a chronic dental focus became evident. This means that somewhere in Judy's teeth or jaw a source of untreated infection was disturbing the energy and thus the structure and function of the body, in this case Judy's breast. EDS practitioners call this a "focal point" of toxicity (a toxic focus). Specifically in Judy's case, it was detected in the lower right second premolar. Troubles in this tooth "focused" toxicity and imbalanced energy through the acupuncture meridians to her breast. Subsequent EDS indicated that the cause of this toxic focus was a mercury amalgam filling in this tooth. At this point, Judy became irritated and told Dr. Scott-Morley that she felt this was wasting her time and money. "I do not have any teeth of my own. I am wearing full dentures, so there cannot be any filling material in my teeth."

This was potentially confusing, even for an EDS expert such as Dr. Scott-Morley. He had never physically looked inside her mouth. He rechecked the EDS results, and again concluded that it was amalgam toxicity. At this point, he suggested to Judy that she receive a dental X ray of the tooth socket. He trusted in the outcome so much that, he told her he would pay for it if nothing was found. She remained skeptical but agreed to see a dentist.

After chastising Judy for seeing an "alternative physician," the dentist agreed to take the X ray if only to confirm what he deemed to be nonsense. But when the X ray was processed, he apologized to Dr. Scott-Morley and congratulated him on the diagnosis. "There was a large amalgam fragment embedded in the socket which he thought must have fallen into the

For more information on **dental factors**, see Chapter 25: What Causes Cancer?, pp. 600-602; Chapter 33: Physical Support Therapies, pp. 980-989; for more on **parasites**, see Chapter 25: What Causes Cancer?, pp. 624-626; Chapter 33: Physical Support Therapies, pp. 972-977.

socket when the tooth was extracted," says Dr. Scott-Morley. "He estimated that this had been there for at least 10 years." Arrangements were made to have the amalgam fragment carefully removed and Dr. Scott-Morley prescribed appropriate homeopathic medicines to desensitize Judy against the amalgam and also to support her immune system. "Within 10 weeks of taking these steps, all breast nodules had disappeared and no further treatment was necessary," Dr. Scott-Morley reports.

Here is another case from his files that shows how EDS can work in identifying hidden factors in serious illness. Fred, aged 36, had constant pain in the region of his liver. Three extensive medical exams had found no evidence of pathology, after which the physician suggested that Fred seek psychiatric treatment. Using EDS, Dr. Scott-Morley measured Fred's liver points and confirmed inflammation and possible pathological damage. The test further revealed aflatoxin toxicity (frequently caused by a mold found on stale peanuts or stored grains).

Dr. Scott-Morley asked Fred if stale peanuts had any significance for him. Fred responded that he had been a truck driver and had transported peanuts from Italy to England, eating handfuls of them while en route. Upon arrival, these shipments were found to be stale and condemned as unhealthy. Dr. Scott-Morley prescribed a homeopathic remedy to eliminate the effects of aflatoxin from Fred's system, and recommended other remedies. Within a few weeks, Fred fully recovered.

Francine came to Dr. Scott-Morley with pains in her abdomen and digestive disorders. Dr. Scott-Morley's EDS test indicated liver malfunction along with an impaired right kidney. The toxic agent appeared to be *Bilharzia*, a parasite common in the Nile and irrigation canals of Egypt. But when Dr. Scott-Morley asked the woman when she had last been to Africa, she replied that she had never been outside of England.

A second EDS test again showed the presence of *Bilharzia*, leaving both Dr. Scott-Morley and the woman puzzled. Later, the woman phoned back to report that her mother had been born in Egypt and had fallen into an irrigation ditch when she was 18 months old. Somehow the negative effects of this very early contamination were transmitted to Francine when she was born. Dr. Scott-Morley was then able to eliminate the effect of the parasite by using a homeopathic remedy specific for that pathogen.

## Other Energy Medicine-Based Devices Useful in Diagnosis

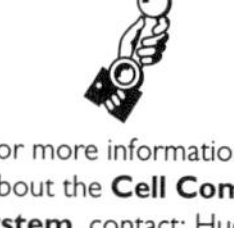

For more information about the **Cell Com System**, contact: Hugo Nielsen, Kirkealle 14, 6510 Gram, Denmark; tel: 45-74-822233; fax: 45-74-822065.

**TENS**—This device is commonly used for pain relief. The Transcutaneous Electrical Nerve Stimulator, or TENS, is widely used in doctors' offices and physiotherapy clinics, and can be used at home as well. It works by applying an electrical current to the affected nerves, causing nerve conduction to be blocked and pain to be relieved. TENS units are also believed to stimulate the productions of endorphins (a type of brain chemical or neurotransmitter), the body's natural painkillers. Many physicians have found TENS useful in pain reduction for cancer. Cancer patients typically respond positively after 2-3 TENS treatments; a considerable reduction in pain and discomfort is often reported within 2 weeks of regular TENS use.

**Cold Laser Therapy**—According to Marvin Prescott, D.M.D., of Los Angeles, California, cold laser therapy uses a beam of low-intensity laser light to initiate a series of enzymatic reactions and bioelectric events that stimulate the natural healing process at the cellular level. "Cold laser therapy has been successfully applied to pain control, orthopedic myofascial syndrome (inflammation of the muscles and their surrounding membranes), neurology, trauma, dermatology, and dentistry," says Dr. Prescott. "The effects on microcirculation, increased synthesis of collagen in the skin, production of neurotransmitters, and pain relief have all been documented."

"Cold laser therapy," he adds "is often used with patients who do not like acupuncture needles. Cold laser therapy has been used successfully at our W. John Diamond, M.D. Triad Medical Center in Reno, Nevada, to treat pain, particularly in children, who are often afraid of acupuncture. We have found it useful for back pain, bursitis, tendinitis, and chronic problems, especially when used in conjunction with homeopathy, herbs, and nutritional supplements."

**Cell Com System**—Hugo Nielsen, a Danish acupuncturist, spent 25 years investigating alternative treatments for cancer. On the basis of his research, he devised a cell energy communication system that enhances communication among the cells. It is a form of cellular biofeedback called the Cell Com System.

Nielsen's Cell Com System uses a small instrument run by a 9-volt battery to measure the energies represented on the surface of the skin at a given time; the amount of energy detected is transferred to the instrument, where it is displayed digitally. The instrument uses electrodes that are connected to acupuncture points on the skin enabling the physician to locate the exact position of these points on the body. Once the information is recorded by the instrument, it is altered and fed back to the brain. The brain then reads the altered signals, and controls and maintains the resulting pain-free situation.

Following operations for lung, kidney, and other cancers, patients visiting the Hugo Nielsen Institute in Gram, Denmark, have reported significant pain relief from Cell Com. "Nielsen believes that the electrical status of each cell's sodium/potassium balance controls overall health and enables the body to regulate its production of natural painkillers, such as the endorphins," says Dr. Etienne Callebout, M.D. (see Chapter 4). Moreover, the benefits may extend beyond pain relief to include direct therapeutic effects: when used in conjunction with conventional acupuncture needle treatment, a regression in lung cancer has been achieved. Since the potential toxicity of pain-killing drugs or medications is avoided, the individual's cancer-fighting resources can be more readily strengthened.

"Nielsen's system definitely works in pain reduction, and there may be some therapeutic usefulness as well," says Dr. Callebout. "With this device we may be able to achieve a specific, measurable transmission of energy from the acupoints and redirect this energy toward the healing process."

# Magnetic Field Therapy

**The use of magnets and electrical devices to generate controlled magnetic fields has many medical applications and has proven to be one of the most effective means available for diagnosing human illness and disease. Clinical evidence shows that cancers, subjected to a negative magnetic field, can start to reverse as the magnetic energy helps restore oxygen levels and reduce acidity.**

Electromagnetic energy is an integral part of the human body. It can help produce illness and help bring healing, depending on its type and strength. The world is surrounded by magnetic fields: some are generated by the Earth's magnetism, others are generated by solar storms and changes in the weather. Magnetic fields are also created by everyday electrical devices: motors, televisions, office equipment, computers, electrically heated water beds, electric blankets, microwave ovens, the electrical wiring in homes, and the power lines that supply them.

The human body produces subtle magnetic fields that are generated by the chemical reactions within the cells and the ionic currents of the nervous system.[10] The catalytic reactions of enzymes are all driven by magnetic fields and produce magnetic fields themselves.[11]

Recently, scientists have discovered that external magnetic fields can affect the body's functioning in both positive and negative ways, and this observation has led to the development of magnetic field therapy. The use of magnets and electrical devices to generate controlled magnetic fields has many medical applications and has proven to be one of the most effective means available for diagnosing human illness and disease. In addition to its diagnostic power, magnetic field therapy can be used to treat physical and emotional disorders.

Magnets and electromagnetic therapy devices are now being used to relieve symptoms and reverse degenerative diseases, eliminate pain, facilitate the healing of broken bones, counter the effects of

## A Quick Review of Magnet Basics

Magnets have 2 poles, positive and negative. There are conflicting methods of naming the pole of a magnet, so a magnetometer should be used as a standard method of determining which side of the magnet is negative (north) or positive (south). If you're using a compass to locate the poles, the arrowhead of the needle marked "N" or "North" will point to the magnet's negative pole. A magnetometer reads magnetic poles as negative and positive, which is the electromagnetic definition and identification of magnetic polarity (and also of electric polarity).

Many researchers claim that the negative pole generally has a calming effect and helps to normalize metabolic functioning. The positive pole, on the other hand, has a stressful effect. In fact, prolonged exposure interferes with metabolic functioning, produces acidity, reduces cellular oxygen supply, and encourages the replication of latent microorganisms.

The strength of a magnet is measured in units of gauss (a measurement of the intensity of magnetic flux) or Tesla (1 tesla=10,000 gauss), and every magnet or magnetic device carries a manufacturer's gauss rating. The actual strength of the magnet at the skin surface, however, is less than this number. For example, a 4000-gauss magnet transmits only about 1200 gauss to the patient. Magnets placed in bed pads will render even lower amounts of field strength at the skin surface, because a magnet's strength quickly decreases with the distance from the subject.

***The therapy is based on the fact that the body is surrounded by a magnetic field and is comprised of numerous smaller magnetic fields, which become disturbed in the course of illness. Clinical research indicates that magnetic therapy can restore the body's normal, healthy magnetic fields and thereby promote recovery from cancer, says Dr. Philpott.***

stress, and address the reversal of cancer. In 1974, researcher Albert Roy Davis noted that positive and negative magnetic energies have different effects upon the biological systems of animals and humans. He found that magnets could be used to arrest and kill cancer cells in animals, and could also be used in the treatment of arthritis, glaucoma, infertility, and diseases related to aging.[12] Davis concluded that negative polarity magnetic fields have a beneficial effect on living organisms, whereas positive polarity magnetic fields have a stressful effect.

See "Magnetic Therapy," pp. 330-338.

In a study designed to evaluate the risk to cancer patients of exposure to magnetic fields, tissue cultures were exposed to a positive magnetic field for a prolonged period. The cancer grew. With prolonged exposure to a negative magnetic field, the cancer receded.[13]

For more on **electromagnetic energy**, see Chapter 25: What Causes Cancer?, pp. 552-556.

## Magnetic Field Therapy as a Primary or Adjunctive Cancer Treatment

According to Wolfgang Ludwig, Sc.D., Ph.D., Director of the Institute for Biophysics in Horb, Germany, "Magnetic field therapy is a method that penetrates the whole human body and can treat every organ without chemical side effects." At Dr. Ludwig's Institute for Biophysics, magnetic field therapy has been effective in the treatment of cancer and numerous other disorders. Robert Becker, M.D., an orthopedic surgeon and prime researcher of magnetic energy, found that weak electric currents promote the healing of broken bones. Dr. Becker also brought national attention to the fact that electromagnetic interference from power lines and home appliances can pose a serious hazard to human health. "The scientific evidence leads to only one conclusion: The exposure of living organisms to abnormal electromagnetic fields results in significant abnormalities in physiology and function."[14]

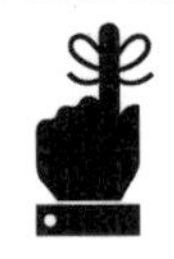

*Positive* magnetic energy possesses no capacity for regeneration or cancer reversal.

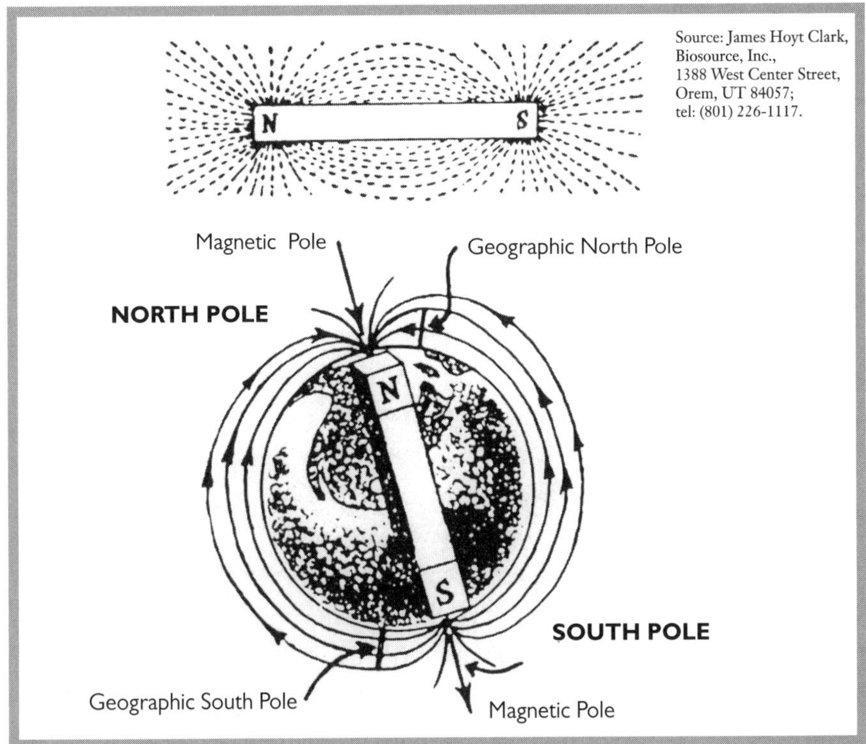


**Figure 34.3—Negative and positive magnetic fields**

## Magnetic Field Therapy: Changing Energy at the Cellular Level

"The healing potential of magnets is possible because the body's nervous system is governed, in part, by varying patterns of ionic currents and electromagnetic fields," reports John Zimmerman, Ph.D., president of the Bio-Electro-Magnetics Institute in Reno, Nevada. There are numerous forms of magnetic field therapy, including static field magnets and pulsating magnetic fields generated by electrical devices. The magnetic fields produced by magnets or electromagnetic generating devices are able to penetrate the human body and therapeutically affect the functioning of the nervous system, organs, and cells.

According to William Philpott, M.D., a magnetic therapy pioneer of Choctaw, Oklahoma, when used properly, magnetic field therapy has no known harmful side effects. Dr. Philpott has found that the "negative magnetic field" can even reverse cancer. (A compass or magnetometer is used to identify the positive and negative magnetic poles.[15]) "Whether it is a cut,

The term **pH**, which means "potential hydrogen," represents a scale for the relative acidity or alkalinity of a solution. Acidity is measured as 0.1 to 6.9, alkalinity is 7.1 to 14, and neutral is about 7.0. The numbers refer to how many hydrogen atoms are present compared to an ideal or standard solution. Normal blood is slightly alkaline, at 7.35 to 7.45; urine pH can range from 4.8 to 7.5, although normal is closer to 7.0.

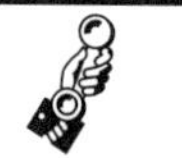

For more information about **magnetic therapy**, contact: William H. Philpott, M.D., 17171 SE 29th Street, Choctaw, OK 73020; tel: 405-390-3009. For information about Dr. Philpott's *Magnetic Health Quarterly*, contact: P.O. Box 50655, Midwest City, OK 73140; tel: 405-390-1444; fax: 405-390-2968

bruise, broken bone, infection or cancer, it is the negative magnetic energy that heals," Dr. Philpott states. He also points out that the same magnetic energy is capable of countering the toxic effects of poisonous chemicals, addictive drugs, and other potentially harmful substances.

The therapy is based on the fact that the body is surrounded by a magnetic field and is composed of numerous smaller magnetic fields, which become disturbed in the course of illness. Clinical research indicates that magnetic therapy can restore the body's normal, healthy magnetic fields and thereby promote recovery from cancer, says Dr. Philpott.

Positive magnetic energy possesses no capacity for regeneration or cancer reversal. When this positive magnetic energy is stronger than the negative magnetic energy in a biological system or living organism, the system has a tendency to develop acidity, lack of cellular oxygen, accumulation of toxins, increased microbial growth, and the uncontrolled, excessive cell division that leads to full-blown cancer.[16] "The body, through the cells that surround the nervous system, concentrates the negative electromagnetic field at the site of injury for healing," says Dr. Philpott. "It must maintain the negative magnetic field in order for healing to occur."

***"The human bio-oxidative energy system is able to defeat the biological life energy system of cancer cells. This is because our oxidative method is 10 times more efficient and effective than the fermentation method used by cancer cells," Dr. Philpott explains.***

The key to how magnetic fields can stimulate healing, and help in reversing cancer, has to do with its effect on oxygen, says Dr. Philpott. Magnetic fields can stimulate metabolism and increase the amount of oxygen available to cells. "I have concluded that oxygen deficiency, coupled with acidity, are unique characteristics of all cancer cells, and are actually the 2 main causes of cancer. In fact, from the standpoint of the physics and chemistry of life, the difference between normal cells and cancer cells is so great that one can hardly picture a greater contrast."

The more alkaline pH produced by a negative magnetic field is necessary for healing as cancer cannot grow in an alkaline environment, Dr.

Philpott explains. "It is the negative field that maintains the alkaline state. You can take an external magnetic field, place it over the body area, and get a bodily response as if the energy came from itself." These observations underscore Dr. Philpott's summary definition of the common denominator involved in cancer.

This common denominator is called acid-hypoxia, and refers to a cellular condition of acidity and low oxygen status. According to Dr. Philpott, cancer *only* develops in acid-hypoxia cellular tissue. Numerous precipitating factors, such as carcinogens, excess free radicals, maladaptive reactions to foods, geopathic stress, aberrant electromagnetic energy, and 60-cycle per second electrical pulsing frequency, can produce acid-hypoxia. From here, the conversion of normal cells to cancerous cells is the next step.

***"The way we can defeat cancer is to change the cellular conditions so that cancer cannot exist under them," says Dr. Philpott. "To do this, raise the alkalinity and oxygen level of the cells with a negative magnetic field." Cancer cells cannot thrive in an area dominated by negative magnetic fields.***

A normal cell is alkaline, he explains, because otherwise oxygen could not be there for the cell to make its energy. A key chemical called adenosine triphosphate (ATP) is made by cells as a biological energy source through the use of oxygen; it is central to the way in which energy is released and transported. This process is called oxidative phosphorylation and involves the addition of phosphate to adenosine, thereby creating high-energy phosphate bonds. Normal, healthy human cells use oxygen to produce ATP as an energy source. Oxidative phosphorylation depends on conditions of alkalinity and high levels of molecular oxygen to function properly, says Dr. Philpott.

Infectious microorganisms (bacteria, fungi, and some intestinal parasites) and cancer cells have a different way of producing energy; it is called fermentative phosphorylation. Here, under conditions of acidity and low or no oxygen, ATP is made through the fermentation of glucose (blood sugar) instead of through the use of oxygen. "In fact, if there were a lot of oxygen present, it would not work. Oxygen and the alkaline pH would inhibit this fermentation process, which requires a condition of acidity and no or low oxygen," explains Dr. Philpott.

Healthy human cells have the ability to make ATP by either method just described. However, fermentative phosphorylation cannot sustain life for humans but it will sustain the life of cancer cells, bacteria, fungi, and certain parasites, Dr. Philpott says. These 2 mechanisms of making energy are incompatible and thus are never working at the same time. They work under directly opposite and conflicting conditions, Dr. Philpott explains. In fact, *oxidative* phosphorylation actually blocks the fermentative. "The human bio-oxidative energy system is able to defeat the biological life energy system of cancer cells," he says. "This is because our oxidative method is 10 times more efficient and effective than the fermentation method used by cancer cells." The normal human cell (running on oxidative phosphorylation) has a lot of molecular oxygen and a normal alkaline pH, but the cancer cell (running on fermentation phosphorylation) has an acid pH and lack of oxygen. Here is how Dr. Philpott explains it:

"How do we get acidic states? We maladaptively react to foods, chemicals, inhalants, toxins. These produce acid states locally, where the symptom is. Anything that makes the area acidic is predisposition to the development of cancer over the long run. This means your food reactions (immunologic allergies, nonimmunologic maladaptive reactions, addictions) potentially predispose you to the development of cancer. Further, we get an estimated 10,000 injuries to our genetic material, or DNA, every day from carcinogenic chemicals. DNA can be repaired as long as the cells have plenty of oxygen and are alkaline; but if it is in an acid state it doesn't repair."

The cancer cells rapidly reproduce, consuming large stores of glucose; this process produces lactic acid as a by-product, and lactic acid lowers the cellular pH to a more acidic condition. With an acidic pH, it is even harder for human cells to use oxygen normally; molecular oxygen gets bound up in this acidic medium, and more oxygen-free radicals are produced (including hydrogen peroxide), further weakening the system and leaving it vulnerable.

There is yet another link, this one involving a crucial series of enzymes, explains Dr. Philpott. These enzymes help revert oxygen back to its normal molecular state where it can once again be active in the normal oxidative phosphorylation process. Dr. Philpott explains that a positive magnetic field blocks the catalytic function of these enzymes; further, without sufficient negative magnetic energy acting as a kind of energy nutrient, these enzymes cannot do their work of reversing the conditions leading to cancer. "Thus, in addition to acid-hypoxia (oxygen shortage in acid conditions), a lack of negative magnetic energy can also be considered a major cause of cancer," Dr. Philpott states.

"The way we can defeat cancer," says Dr. Phillpott, "is to change the cellular conditions so that cancer cannot exist under them. To do this, raise the alkalinity and oxygen level of the cells with a negative magnetic field. When the negative magnetic field, from a static field permanent magnet, is applied to the human body, it has the amazing ability to remove the cancerous conditions of acid-hypoxia and replace them with a favorable alkaline-hyperoxia (a condition of excess oxygen) environment." Cancer cells cannot thrive in an area dominated by negative magnetic fields.

The same principle also makes this approach an ideal preventive measure. "Perhaps the most effective method of preventing cancer is through the daily application of negative magnetic energy to the body. More specifically, negative magnetized oxygen is the most rewarding method of prevention as well as reversal of cancer." In light of these points, Dr. Philpott calls his approach Magnetic Resonance Bio-oxidative Therapy.

Dr. Philpott relates the following cases from his clinical file to demonstrate how magnetic therapy works in treating cancer.

- **Melanoma:** Roberta, aged 75, suddenly developed a rapid-growing invasive melanoma on her forehead. "This had the clinical appearance of a serious malignant melanoma," Dr. Philpott says. However, after 3 months of continuous treatment with a negative magnetic field, the melanoma dried up and peeled off and new skin appeared. Following 3 more weeks of negative magnetic field exposure, the depressed area in Roberta's forehead (where the melanoma had been situated) filled in, leaving no evidence of a scar. "There is now no way to tell where the tumor was," Dr. Philpott notes.
- **Prostate cancer:** After Thomas was diagnosed as having prostate cancer with bone metastasis (in the sacrum), he underwent magnetic treatment. "He was treated continuously over the sacral and lower abdominal areas, so that the magnetic energy would radiate into the pelvic area," Dr. Philpott says. Three months later there was no evidence of bone cancer on Thomas' X ray and his

**SUCCESS STORY**

## Brain Tumor Treated with Magnetic Energy

Here is a case from Michael B. Schachter, M.D. (see Chapter 18) of the Schachter Center for Complementary Medicine, in Suffern, New York, where magnetic therapy is used as part of a multimodal cancer treatment program.

At 31, Rafael's left cheek began to tingle. Soon after, he lost his ability to talk and his left arm moved uncontrollably. This episode lasted for about a minute. EEG and a CT scan of the brain were both negative. Doctors informed Rafael that the episode was probably migraine related. Five months later, he had a similar episode except this time he lost consciousness. It was now clear that Rafael was experiencing seizures. An MRI showed a tumor on the right side of his brain, which a biopsy revealed to be a malignant oligodendroglioma (oligodendroglia are supportive connective tissue cells in the brain).

The expected survival for individuals with malignancies of the brain is from 6 to 18 months. Due to its location, the tumor was considered inoperable. A cancer specialist offered Rafael immediate radiation therapy or the option of waiting until he became more symptomatic before undergoing radiation. Rafael decided to wait because of the risks associated with radiation to the brain, which include stroke and radiation-induced tumors. Instead, he sought alternative cancer therapy with Dr. Schachter. His neurologists and his sister, who was a nurse, thought this decision was a mistake.

After conducting a comprehensive laboratory evaluation to measure immune system function and check for vitamin and mineral deficiencies, hormonal imbalances, and toxic metabolite exposure, among others, Dr. Schachter started Rafael on intravenous vitamin C and amygdalin, intravenous hydrogen peroxide on different days, and a host of oral agents including shark cartilage, amygdalin, antioxidant and immune-enhancing vitamins, minerals, and natural herbs.

Magnetic energy therapy was also incorporated into the treatment protocol throughout this time period. Here, a small, but powerful magnet (more than 12,000 gauss) was placed on Rafael's head, the negative pole against the skin, over the area of the tumor and kept in place with a headband for several hours each day. The only conventional treatment Rafael continued was anti-seizure medication to treat the epileptic episodes that accompanied the tumor.

Over 4 1/2 years later, Rafael is doing well. He has a new baby and has worked almost continuously during this period. Repeated MRIs have revealed no further growth in the tumor. Rafael's sister and neurologists were so impressed by the results of the alternative treatment that they wrote letters on his behalf to keep his insurance company from ending compensation for these therapies. The insurance company continued to pay for his treatment, including weekly intravenous infusions. Rafael has survived well beyond the expected 6 to 18 months and looks forward to many more years with his family.

prostate specific antigen (PSA, a marker for prostate cancer) had reverted from an abnormal 28 to a normal 2.

- **Brain Cancer:** Bill, in his late 20s, was brought to Dr. Philpott with an inoperable glioblastoma of the brain. "This had rendered him unconscious and completely unresponsive to the environment," Dr. Philpott says. Yet this cancer was reversed by a continuous negative magnetic field applied to Bill's head.
- **Spinal Cancer:** After Patricia had a benign tumor removed from her spine, she could not walk without dragging her feet. When Dr. Philpott placed a positive magnetic pole over the area where the tumor had been removed, Patricia could walk perfectly. Practicing walking while the positive magnetic field was being applied to her spine restored her ability to walk. These practice sessions were 3 minutes each, followed by application of the negative magnetic field. The positive field stimulated the nonfunctioning neurons while the negative field restored oxygenation and alkalinity to the tissues after each use of the positive field which caused acid-hypoxia in addition to nerve stimulation.

In addition, magnetic field therapy can reduce the side effects of chemotherapy. Mark had been treated with chemotherapy for his cancer prior to seeing Dr. Philpott. Two years later, as the cancer was still present, Mark's oncologist advised a second course of chemotherapy. During his first chemotherapy treatment, Mark had lost his hair, fingernails and toenails; during the second course, he did not lose his hair, fingernails or toenails. The oncologist asked Mark what he had done differently this time. Mark told him he was sleeping on a negative-poled magnetic bed pad. "It may be that the entrance of magnetic therapy into oncology will be furthered by this example, in which a patient's exposure to a negative magnetic field reduced the harsh side effects of chemotherapy," says Dr. Philpott.

Magnetic energy also positively influences the activity of enzymes, says Dr. Philpott. We already know, from the considerable clinical discussion in this book, that enzymes play a crucial role in the generation and reversal of cancer. Enzymes are the body's "spark plugs," providing extra energy to speed up or "catalyze" the myriad chemical reactions in the body. A negative mag-

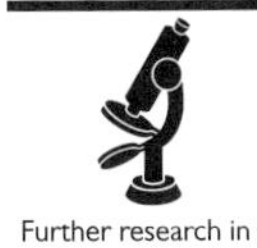

Further research in the application of magnetic field therapy to cancer would be beneficial.

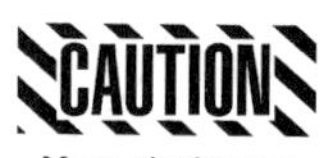


**Magnetic therapy** should be administered only by a trained physician or by a patient under the close supervision of a trained physician. In each case, only the negative magnetic field should contact the subject's skin. For research purposes, the monitoring physician should record the initial status of the subject and prepare additional reports 3 times a year during treatment, and the subject should keep a detailed diary of the type and degree of magnet exposure, and any changes in health and well-being that occur in the interim.

netic field directly supports enzyme function by minimizing acidic pH and enhancing alkalinity, thereby favoring oxygen utilization.

Dr. Philpott says that a negative magnetic field provides the ideal pH and energy conditions for efficient enzyme action, which in turn frees up organic acid-bound oxygen, aldehyde-bound oxygen, peroxides, and superoxides, enabling these forms of oxygen to revert back to functional molecular oxygen. The negative magnetic field energy activates the oxidoreductase system, which is a highly efficient enzyme system that aids in detoxification. According to Dr. Philpott, "These systems turn harmful toxic acids into harmless and biologically necessary alkali substances. This then provides body cells with an abundance of necessary molecular oxygen for biological energy production."

## Clinical Guidelines for Treating Cancers with Magnetic Therapy

Dr. Philpott states, "I do not claim a cure for any degenerative disease or even guarantee relief of pain or insomnia by means of magnetics. My only claim is that there is evidence justifying a definitive controlled research project following FDA guidelines to determine the value and limitations of Magnetic Resonance Bio-oxidative Therapy." These guidelines require a physician's diagnosis and physician monitoring under the supervision of a Scientific Institutional Review Board. The application of magnetic fields to humans has been approved by the FDA and, based on toxicity studies, classified as "not essentially harmful."

Magnetic therapy for cancer must still be considered an experimental approach warranting controlled studies, Dr. Philpott advises. The rationale for this therapy is that a negative magnetic field has been observed in both animals and humans to reverse neoplastic lesions. The theoretical basis for this effect seems to involve improved oxygenation of tissues and a normalization of the pH of these tissues under the influence of the applied magnetic field, explains Dr. Philpott. The clinical guidelines that follow are based on protocols that produced recoveries from cancer in patients treated by Dr. Philpott.

**Prostate Cancer—**Always use a negative magnetic field, negative pole side facing the body. For local treatment in sitting, sit on a comfort chair pad (containing $1\frac{7}{8}$" x $\frac{7}{8}$" x $\frac{3}{8}$" magnets placed $1\frac{1}{2}$" apart throughout the seat and back of the pad) with a 4" x 6" x $\frac{1}{2}$" ceramic magnet (3950 gauss) under the pad directly under the genital-rectal area. The more hours of treatment, the better.

For systemic treatment in sleeping, use a magnetic bed pad (containing $1\frac{7}{8}$" x $\frac{7}{8}$" x $\frac{3}{8}$" magnets, 3950 gauss placed $\frac{1}{2}$" apart throughout the pad). Place a 5" x 12" multi-magnet (2450 gauss) flexible mat crosswise on the lower abdomen-pubic area. In the center of this, place a 4" x 6" x $\frac{1}{2}$" ceramic magnet lengthwise on the pubic-lower abdomen area. This can be held in place with a 4" x 52" body band. Also use 4 magnets (6" x 4" x 1", 5000 gauss) at the crown of the head, placed $\frac{3}{4}$" apart in a wooden carrier on the headboard. The holder can be raised or lowered depending on the height of the pillow. The magnets should be slightly lower than the back of the head and no closer than 3 inches to the top of the head.

***"It may be that the entrance of magnetic therapy into oncology will be furthered by this example, in which a patient's exposure to a negative magnetic field reduced the harsh side effects of chemotherapy," Dr. Philpott says.***

**Squamous Cell Carcinoma of the Lips and Mouth—**Always use a negative magnetic field, negative pole side facing the body. Place a 5" x 6" multi-magnet (2450 gauss) flexible mat across the mouth to cover the lips, chin, and the area between the upper lip and the nose. Place a 4" x 6" x $\frac{1}{2}$" ceramic magnet (3950 gauss) on each side of the face, extending sufficiently forward for the magnetic field to cover the nose. This local treatment is a necessity and should be kept in place continuously, except for the brief periods of washing or eating. The minimum duration is 3 months.

The systemic treatment of sleeping on a magnetic pad is optional. For this, use a magnetic bed pad (containing $1\frac{7}{8}$" x $\frac{7}{8}$" x $\frac{3}{8}$" magnets, 3950 gauss, placed $1\frac{1}{2}$ apart throughout the pad). Also use 4 magnets (6" x 4" x 1", 5000 gauss) at the crown of the head, placed $\frac{3}{4}$" apart in a wooden carrier on the headboard. The holder can be raised or lowered depending on the height of the pillow. The magnets should be slightly lower than the back of the head and no closer than 3 inches to the top of the head.

**Malignant Melanoma—**Always use a negative magnetic field, negative pole side facing the body. Tape a cushion (with a hole in the middle, as those used for corns or bunions) over the malignant mole to prevent pressure on it. Use dermoclear or hypoallergenic tape. Tape a 1" x 1/4" superneodymium disc magnet (12,300 gauss) on the cushion. The magnet needs to be larger than the lesion being treated. If the lesion is more than 1" but less than 1 1/2" in width, use a 1 1/2" x 3/8" ceramic disc magnet (3950 gauss). For larger lesions, use an appropriate-sized flexible magnet (2000 gauss) with a neodymium or ceramic disc magnet on top. Do not depend on the flexible magnet alone. The only reason for using it is to spread the magnetic field to be larger than the lesion.

For systemic treatment in sleeping, see Squamous Cell Carcinoma above. In addition, sleep with magnets on the front and back of the chest. Use a 5" x 12" x 1/8" multi-magnet (2450 gauss) flexible mat held in place with a 4" x 52" body wrap supported by shoulder straps. This accomplishes negative magnetic poling of the oxygen in the lungs which then circulates throughout the body and prevents metastatic spread.

During waking hours, wear a 5" x 6" multi-magnet (2450 gauss) flexible mat over the heart with the negative pole facing the heart. Eliminating a malignant melanoma may take 3 to 4 months of these treatments.

## MAGNETIC THERAPY FOR PAIN RELIEF

Pain is the body's signal of injury. It registers both locally and in the brain as a positive magnetic field. Therefore, the solution for pain is to provide a negative magnetic field both at the site of pain and to the brain.

Place a magnet of suitable size over the pain site, negative pole side facing the body. The magnetic field must be larger than the site since the opposite pole is around the edge of the magnet. Pain is frequently relieved in 10-15 minutes, only occasionally taking up to 30 minutes. However, the longer the period of exposure the better, since the negative magnetic field also governs the healing process. Some common magnets used are: the 1 1/2" x 3/8" ceramic disc magnet (3950 gauss); 1 x 1/4" neodymium magnet (12,300 gauss); 4" x 6" x 1/2" ceramic magnet (3950 gauss), often used for treatment of body organs; flexible plastiform magnets (2450 gauss) in 2-4" widths and as long as needed; and 5" x 6" or 5" x 12" multi-magnet flexible mats to fit

## Science Demonstrates How Magnetic Therapy Can Reverse Cancer

In March 1965, the French Academy of Sciences published a report on the magnetic treatment of mice with lymphosarcoma. Every mouse in the untreated or "control" group died within 15 to 18 days. In 3 other groups, mice began magnetic treatment at different points in time, but with the same strength and duration of magnetic treatment: 620 gauss for 2 hours a day.

The first group received magnetic treatment within 5 days of starting the test and recovered quickly; all tumors and metastases disappeared. The second group began treatment on day 7 and showed the same recovery as the first group; a third group of mice was treated from the 10th day on, but did not recover. These mice all died in 19 to 22 days, just after the untreated mice had died.[17]

These findings were compelling enough to encourage the French Academy of Sciences to conduct another experiment, this time testing the effect of the daily dosage given. In the first group, the mice were treated from the 5th day, with 620 gauss 1 hour a day; in the second group, the mice were treated with 620 gauss 2 hours a day, also from the 5th day. Once again, the results were striking. As expected, all the mice in the untreated (control) group died within 15 days; all the mice in the first test group died after 19 days. Meanwhile, the mice in the second test group—they received twice the magnetic treatment per day as the first group—all survived and showed no signs of cancer.[18]

By this point, the reader will not be surprised to learn that the results of these studies were not reported with jubilation on the front pages of newspapers in the United States. The cancer industry is opposed to the use of magnetic fields, probably because magnets are inexpensive and can be handled by a layperson and their widespread use would siphon money and control from the cancer establishment.

The cancer industry's attitude toward energy medicine as a category is typified in a 1994 article in *CA: A Cancer Journal for Clinicians* in which scientists reported they had "found no evidence that treatment with the devices mentioned in this review results in objective benefit in the treatment of cancer in human beings."[19]

the curves of the body. Placing a 1½" x ⅜" ceramic disc magnet on top of the flexible mat over the painful area creates deeper penetration.

To treat the brain, place 1½" x ⅜" ceramic disc magnets on each temple along with a 5" x 6" x ⅛" multi-magnet flexible mat both held in place by a 2" x 16" adjustable elastic headband. This is valuable in treating brain lesions or increasing depth of sleep.

The systemic treatment when sleeping (see Squamous Cell Carcinoma above) is particularly helpful for people with generalized body pain.

### MAGNETS AND SOUND SLEEP

Using the procedure for systemic treatment while sleeping (see Squamous Cell Carcinoma above) promotes deep, energy-restoring sleep. The magnets at the crown of the head are especially effective in producing sound sleep. In addition, it is important to clear your bedroom of any 60-cycle per second pulsing frequencies emitted by electric clocks, nightlights, and other electrical devices. As mentioned earlier, this frequency cuts off the production of melatonin which regulates sleep.

# Light Therapy

**Light is a nutrient essential to health, which means light deficiencies and lack of exposure to full-spectrum light—called malillumination—may negatively affect the immune system, open the body to infection, and be linked to certain forms of cancer, especially melanoma. The restoration of the proper kinds and amount of natural light to the body is the basis of light therapy.**

Many health disorders can be traced to problems with the daily night-and-day rhythms called circadian. These rhythms are the body's inner clock and govern the *timing* of sleep, hormone production, body temperature, and many key biological functions. Disturbances in circadian rhythm can lead to health problems such as depression and sleep disorders. Natural sunlight and various forms of light therapy can help reestablish the body's natural rhythms. The ability of light to activate certain chemicals has become the basis of treatment for skin disorders such as psoriasis and for certain forms of cancer.

***Most artificial lighting, both incandescent and fluorescent, lacks the complete balanced spectrum of sunlight and, as Dr. Ott discovered, interferes with the body's optimal absorption of certain nutrients. He calls this condition "malillumination"—malnutrition of the nutrient called light.***

## Light Therapy: Restoring the Missing Nutrient for Cancer Patients

Here is how light can be therapeutic. When light enters the eye, millions of light and color-sensitive cells called photoreceptors convert it into electrical impulses. These impulses travel along the optic nerve to the brain where they trigger the hypothalamus gland to send chemical messengers called neurotransmitters to regulate the autonomic (automatic) functions of the body. The hypothalamus is part of the endocrine system whose secretions govern most bodily functions, including blood pressure, body temperature, breathing, digestion, sexual function, moods, the immune system, the aging process, and circadian rhythms. Full-spectrum light (containing all wavelengths) sparks the delicate impulses that regulate these functions and maintain health.

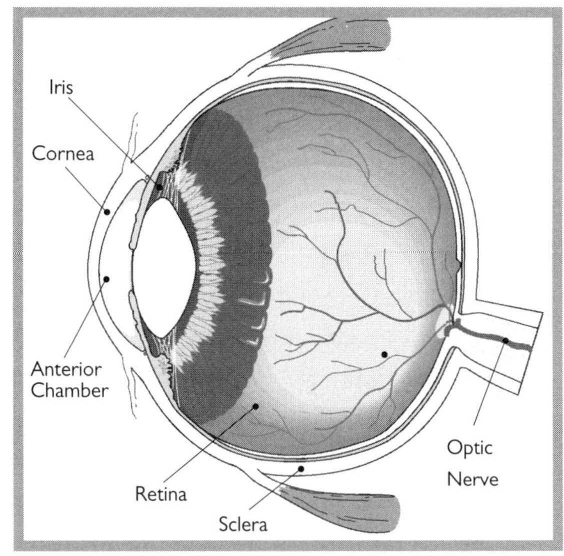


**Figure 34.4—The eye and the optic nerve**

Poor light poses a serious threat to health, according to the numerous published studies of photobiologist John Nash Ott, D.Sc.[20] He contends that the kind of light adequate for maintaining health must contain the full wavelength spectrum found in natural sunlight. In contrast, most artificial lighting, both incandescent and fluorescent, lacks the complete balanced spectrum of sunlight and, as Dr. Ott discovered, interferes with the body's optimal absorption of certain nutrients. He calls this condition "malillumination"—malnutrition of the nutrient called light.

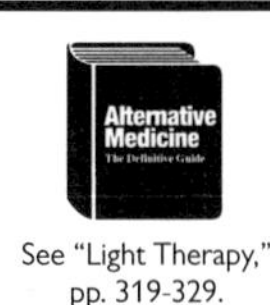


See "Light Therapy," pp. 319-329.

Many products we commonly rely on in daily life—windows, windshields, eyeglasses, suntan lotions—filter out parts of the light spectrum (as does smog) and contribute to malillumination. Research reveals that if certain wavelengths are absent in light, the body cannot fully absorb all dietary nutrients.[21] Malilllumination contributes to fatigue, tooth decay, depression, hostility, suppressed immune function, strokes, hair loss, skin damage, and, ultimately, cancer.[22] A study at the Clinical Pathology Department of the National Institutes of Health also linked malillumination to a loss of muscle tone and strength.[23]

According to John Zimmerman, Ph.D., most offices, even those with uncovered windows and with the lights on, have a light level of only 500 lux (the international unit of illumination: one lumen per square meter), as compared to outdoor light, which has about 50,000 lux, or approximately 100 times more. To put this in perspective, night-shift workers are usually exposed to a light level of only 50 lux.

According to John Downing O.D., Ph.D., of Santa Rosa, California, "By spending 90% of our lives indoors, under inadequate lighting conditions, we cause or worsen a wide range of health problems, including depression, heart disease, hyperactivity (in children), osteoporosis (in the elderly), and lowered resistance to infection."[24] To maintain health it is important to be exposed to light containing the full wavelength spectrum found in natural sunlight, says Dr. Downing. While many people associate an overexposure to sunlight with melanoma (a malignant, darkly pigmented skin moire, or tumor) or other skin cancers, the research of Drs. Downing, Ott, and others suggests that an underexposure to sunlight may also be involved in producing cancer.

***While many people associate an overexposure to sunlight with melanoma, or other skin cancers, the research of Drs. Downing, Ott, and others suggests that an underexposure to sunlight may also be involved in producing cancer. In a study by the U.S. Navy, personnel holding indoor occupations had the highest rate of melanoma while workers in occupations that required spending time both indoors and outdoors had the lowest rate.***

A recent study carried out by the U.S. Navy compared the risk of melanoma for different naval occupations. It was discovered that personnel holding indoor occupations had the highest rate of melanoma while workers in occupations that required spending time both indoors and outdoors had the lowest rate. In addition, a higher rate of melanoma occurred on the trunk (covered by clothes) of the body as opposed to the head and arms which are commonly exposed to sunlight. The authors of the study theorized that the anatomical site of melanoma suggests a "protective role for brief, regular exposure to sunlight."[25] On the other hand, an excess of sunlight leading to frequent sunburns, particularly for fair-skinned people on imbalanced and/or antioxidant-poor diets, probably makes people *more* vulnerable to melanoma.

These findings by the U. S. Navy are in keeping with recent laboratory studies showing that vitamin D (whose production is stimulated by ultraviolet light) suppresses the growth of malignant melanoma cells. These studies also call into question the belief that indoor occupations can provide safety for fair-skinned, freckled individuals who are at a high risk for skin cancers. It appears that an occupational deprivation of sunlight can lead to a vitamin D deficiency, which in turn may favor the development of melanoma.[26]

Here is a quick look at several promising applications of light therapy.

## FULL-SPECTRUM LIGHT THERAPY

Sunlight and full-spectrum light can be applied to the skin to relieve hypertension, depression, insomnia, premenstrual syndrome, migraines, and carbohydrate cravings associated with metabolic imbalances.[27] A 10-year epidemiological study conducted at Johns Hopkins University Medial School in Baltimore, Maryland, showed that exposure to full-spectrum light (including the ultraviolet frequency) is positively related to the prevention of breast, colon, and rectal cancers.[28]

***A 10-year epidemiological study conducted at Johns Hopkins University Medical School in Baltimore, Maryland, showed that exposure to full-spectrum light (including the ultraviolet frequency) is positively related to the prevention of breast, colon, and rectal cancers.[30]***

In Russia, a full-spectrum lighting system was installed in factories where colds and sore throats had become commonplace among workers. This system lowered the bacterial contamination of the air by 40 to 70%. Workers who did not receive the full-spectrum light were absent twice as many days as those who did,[29] strongly suggesting that the lights performed a health-protective role in the factory worker's life.

In a recent study undertaken by Dr. Ott and his associates, Lewis Mayron, Ph.D., Rick Nations, Ph.D., and Ellen L. Mayron, M.S., the effect of full-spectrum lighting was tested on first-grade students in Sarasota, Florida. Using 4 classrooms, 2 as a control with standard fluorescent lighting, and 2 outfitted with full-spectrum lights, the researchers tracked the students' behavior for a full semester, using a hidden camera. Their results demonstrated conclusively that the students exposed to the full-spectrum lighting had less absenteeism and a higher academic achievement record when compared with classes conducted under ordinary fluorescent lighting.[31]

For more information on the clinical use of **photophoresis** in a cancer treatment program, see Chapter 31: New Approaches to Immune Stimulation, pp. 896-901.

## ULTRAVIOLET LIGHT THERAPY

Nobel Prize winner and Danish physician Niels Finsen, M.D., observed that tubercular lesions occurred commonly during the winter but only rarely in the summer. Dr. Finsen suspected a lack of sunlight to be the cause of the lesions and successfully treated skin tuberculosis with ultraviolet light. Today, ultraviolet light therapies are used to treat diseases ranging from high cholesterol to premenstrual syndrome and cancer.

Hemo-irradiation or photophoresis involves the removal of up to a pint of a patient's blood from the body, irradiating it (particularly the hemoglobin component) with ultraviolet light, and reinfusing it back into the patient's circulation. William Campbell Douglass, M.D., of Clayton, Georgia, a practitioner of photophoresis, reports that irradiating blood with ultraviolet light produces the following results: calcium metabolism improves, body toxins become inert, bacteria are killed either directly or indirectly (by increased systemic resistance), biochemical balances are restored, and oxygen absorption is increased. He has successfully used ultraviolet light therapy to treat asthma and various immune-related disorders.[32]

## PHOTODYNAMIC THERAPY FOR CANCER

Photodynamic therapy (PDT) has been demonstrated effective as a cure for early-stage cancers of the lung, esophagus, stomach, and cervix.[33] *Business Week* described the case of a man diagnosed with esophageal cancer. The usual treatment for this form of cancer entails an operation so mutilating that the person cannot eat, and in 95% of cases the outcome is death. First the man was injected with Photofrin, a photosensitive drug that accumulates in cancerous cells. Three days later, doctors exposed the man's tumor to a low-power red laser light for 30 minutes. This triggered a reaction—the release of a free-radical form of oxygen—which killed the cancer cells without burning surrounding skin.

In Japan, PDT has resulted in complete remission in 90% of patients who had early-stage lung cancer and in more than 90% of those with cancers of the stomach, esophagus, and cervix.[34] Denis Cortese, M.D., of the Mayo Clinic in Jacksonville, Florida, found that 43% of early-stage lung cancer patients treated with PDT stayed disease free for at least 5 years.[35] In PDT, dyes or medications that absorb light are absorbed by tumors then exposed to specific types of light. "Light photons are absorbed by the pigment of the dye, which becomes chemically reactive and causes the cancer cells to die," says Meyrick Peak, Ph.D., a senior scientist at the Center of Mechanistic Biology and Biotechnology at Argonne National Laboratory in Argonne, Illinois. "This therapy has been used in China for over 20 years and has been successful in eliminating some types of tumors."

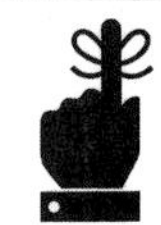

With the use of anti-malignin antibody screen (AMAS) and other early detection strategies, PDT could become a powerful form of medicine. Particularly with respect to lung cancer, the combination of aggressive AMAS screening and PDT could reduce mortality in one of the nation's top killers.

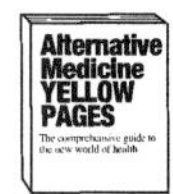


See "Energy Medicine," p. 117, and "Magnetic Field," p. 158.

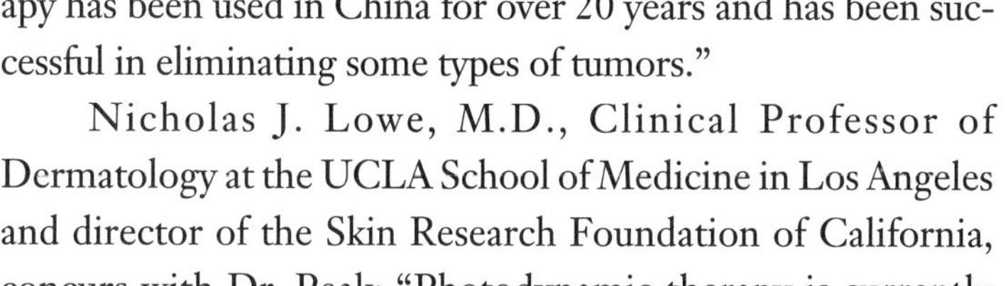

Nicholas J. Lowe, M.D., Clinical Professor of Dermatology at the UCLA School of Medicine in Los Angeles and director of the Skin Research Foundation of California, concurs with Dr. Peak: "Photodynamic therapy is currently being tested on basal and squamous cell cancer (skin cancers). However, the concern with some of these treatments is unwanted phototoxicity—some treatments are likely to make the patient sensitive to sunlight for long periods of time."

Warren Grundfest, M.D., of Cedars-Sinai Medical Center in Los Angeles, is using a type of photodynamic therapy called light-activated chemotherapy to treat patients with lung and bladder cancer. "We're using light to cause a chemical change in the drug. Because it is located only in the cancer tissue, or predominantly in the cancer tissue, it causes only the cancer cells to die." Dr. Grundfest reports that, after 18 months of treatment, bladder tumors showed an 85% successful response.

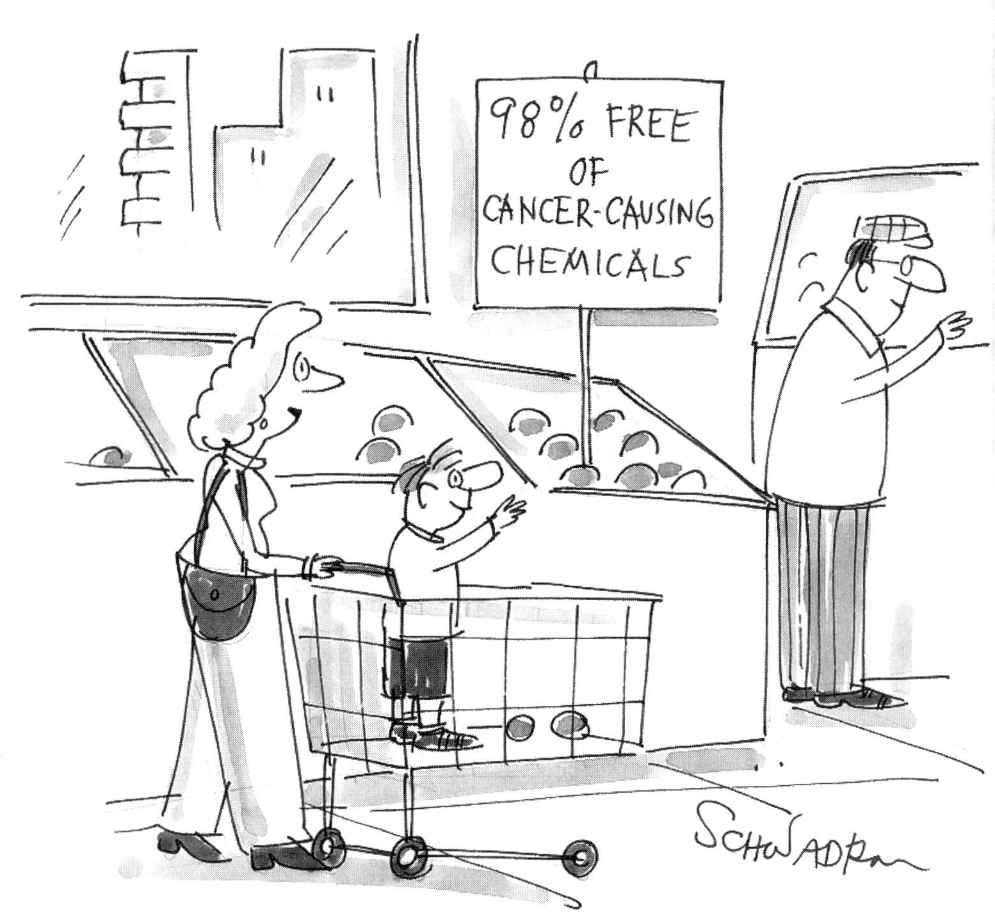
98% FREE
OF
CANCER-CAUSING
CHEMICALS
SCHWADRON

# Endnotes

# Introduction

1. Eisenberg, David M. et al. "Unconventional Medicine in the United States: Prevalence, Costs, and Patterns of Use."*The New England Journal of Medicine* 328:4 (January 28, 1993), 246-252.
2. "Government Data Proves It: Alternative Medicine Is Growing." *Alternative Medicine Digest* 9 (1995), 42.
3. "Patients Want Alternative Medicine: Their Office Visits Prove It." *Alternative Medicine Digest* 6 (1995), 32.
4. "Alternative Medicine Thrives in Bay Area." *San Francisco Chronicle* (May 17, 1995). See also: "Acceptance of Acupuncture Grows." *Marin Independent Journal* (July 3, 1995).
5. Kennedy, B.J. "Use of Questionable Methods and Physician Education." *Journal of Cancer Education* 8:2 (1993), 129-131.
6. Hauser, S.P. "Unproven Methods in Cancer Treatment." *Current Opinions in Oncology* 5:4 (1993), 646-654.
7. Office of Alternative Medicine. *Office of Alternative Medicine Workshop on the Collection of Clinical Research Data Relevant to Alternative Medicine and Cancer* (Bethesda, MD: Office of Alternative Medicine, 1994).
8. McGinnis, L.S. "Alternative Therapies, 1990. An Overview." *Cancer* 67:Suppl 6 (1991), 1788-1792.
9. Guzley, G.J. "Alternative Cancer Treatments: Impact of Unorthodox Therapy on the Patient with Cancer." *Southern Medical Journal* 85:5 (1992), 19-23.
10. Boik, John. "Cancer & Natural Medicine." *A Textbook of Basic Science and Clinical Research* (Princeton, MN: Oregon Medical Press, 1995), 3.
11. Downer, S.M., M.M. Cody, P. McCluskey and P.L. Wilson. "Pursuit and Practice of Complementary Therapies by Cancer Patients Receiving Conventional Treatment." *British Medical Journal* 9309:6947 (1994), 86-89.
12. Sawyer, M.G., A.F. Gannoni, I.R. Toogood, G. Antoniou, and M. Riew. "The Use of Alternative Therapies by Children with Cancer." *Medical Journal of Australia* 160:6 (1994), 323-324.
13. Van Der Zouwe, N., F.S. Van Dam, N.K. Aaronson and G.J. Hanewald. "Alternative Treatments in Cancer: Extent and Background of Utilization." *Nederlands Tijdscrift Voor Geneeskunde* 138:6 (1994), 300-306.
14. Pawlicki, M., J. Rachtan, J. Rolski and E. Sliz. "Results of Delayed Treatment of Patients with Malignant Tumors of the Lymphatic System." *Polski Tygodnik Lekarski* 46:48/49 (1991), 922-923.
15. Morant, R., W.F. Jungi, C. Koehli and H.J. Senn. "Why Do Cancer Patients Use Alternative Medicine?" *Schweizerische Medizinische Wochenschrift* 121:27/28 (1991), 1029-1034.

# Part I: Successful Cancer Treatment Plans of 23 Alternative Physicians

## Chapter 1

## Robert C. Atkins, M.D.

1. Atkins, R.C. *Dr. Atkins' Health Revolution: Cancer Therapy* (Boston: Houghton Mifflin, 1988), 311.
2. Nowicky, J.W. et al. "Ukrain as Both an Anti-cancer and Immunoregulatory Agent." *Drugs Under Experimental Clinical Research* XVIII:Suppl (1992), 51-54.
3. Musianowycz, J. et al. "Clinical Studies of Ukrain in Terminal Cancer Patients (Phase II)." *Drugs Under Experimental Clinical Research* XVIII:Suppl (1992), 45-50.
4. Atkins, R. Personal communications (1996). Despite Ukrain's ability to kill most cancer cell types, the NCI has denied further research funding for investigating Ukrain. The reason, Dr. Atkins suspects, is that this substance threatens to destroy the chemotherapy industry. Ukrain may be too *unlike* chemotherapy in the sense that chemotherapy's effective dose is the same as its toxic dose, while Ukrain's effective dose is many times lower than its toxic dose.
5. Moss, R.W. *The Cancer Industry: Unraveling the Politics* (New York: Paragon House, 1989). Ralph Moss, the author, was discharged by Memorial Sloan-Kettering Cancer Center when he revealed an apparent cover-up by authorities at the Center of positive findings about Amygdalin. According to Moss, subsequent research findings on Amygdalin have been consistently suppressed by the pharmaceutical industry, presumably because the substance is non-patentable.
6. Rubin, D. "Dosage Levels for Laetrile." *Choice* 3:6 (1977), 8-9.
7. Kidd, P. "Germanium-132: Homeostatic Normalizer and Immunostimulant: A Review of its Preventive and Therapeutic Efficacy." *International Clinical Nutrition Review* 7:1 (1987), 11-20.
8. Altman, N. "Hydrogen Peroxide in Medicine." *Oxygen Healing Therapies* (Rochester, VT: Healing Arts Press, 1995), 42-43.
9. "Common Denominators in Cancer Non-remedies and In Human Longevity." *Townsend Letter for Doctors & Patients* (January 1992), 48-50.
10. Garaci, E. et al. "Combination Treatment Using Thymosin Alpha 1 and Interferon after Cyclophosphamide Is Able to Cure Lewis Lung Carcinoma in Mice." *Cancer Immunology and Immunotherapy* 32 (1990), 154-160.
11. Cohen, M.H. et al. "Thymosin Fraction V and Intensive Combination Chemotherapy. Prolonging the Survival of Patients with Small-cell Lung Cancer." *Journal of the American Medical Association* 241 (1979), 1813-1815.
12. Cameron, E., and L. Pauling. *Proceedings of the National Academy of Sciences USA* 75:9 (1978), 4538. Dr. Pauling offers several reasons why subsequent studies have not found such positive results. First, the dosages were too low. Second, the supplements were

discontinued prematurely. Third, patients who had been heavily pretreated with chemo– and radiation therapy were beyond the point of recovery. Biological limits need to be recognized—there's a point where terminal cancer patients can no longer respond to even the best therapies.

13. Editorial. "The Effect of Vitamin E on Immune Responses." *Nutrition Reviews* 45:1 (1987), 27.

14. Schrauzer, G.N. "Selenium for the Cancer Patient." Supplements lecture delivered at the Adjuvant Nutrition in Cancer Treatment symposium. Tampa, Florida (September 29, 1995). Dr. Schrauzer is based at the Biological Trace Element Research Institute, San Diego, CA.

15. Schachter, M.S. Personal communications. Amygdalin is generally safe, but cancer patients on a sulfur-deficient diet may experience some discomfort or a lack of benefit from taking amygdalin, unless cysteine is added to the program.

16. Palermo, M.S. et al. "Immunomodulation Exerted by Cyclophosphamide Is Not Interfered by N-acetyl cysteine."*International Journal of Immunopharmacology* 8:6 (1986), 651-655. See also: Schmitt-Graff, A., and M.E. Scheulen. "Prevention of Adriamycin Cardiotoxicity by Niacin, Isocitrate or N-acetyl cysteine in Mice: A Morphological Study." *Pathology Resident Practice* 181:2 (1986), 168-174. See also: Kim, J.A. et al. "Topical Use of N-acetyl cysteine for Reduction of Skin Reaction to Radiation Therapy." *Seminars in Oncology* 10:Suppl 1 (1983), 86.

17. Kuroda, M. et al. "Decreased Serum Levels of Selenium and Glutathione Peroxidase Activity Associated with Aging, Malignancy and Chronic Hemodialysis." *Trace Elements in Medicine* 5:3 (1988), 97-103.

18. Yoshida, M. et al. "The Effect of Quercetin on Cell Cycle Progression and Growth of Human Gastric Cancer Cells." *FEBS Letters* 260 (1990), 10-13.

19. Thomas, R. *The Essiac Report* (Los Angeles: The Alternative Treatment Information Network, 1993).

20. The Burton Goldberg Group. *Alternative Medicine: The Definitive Guide* (Tiburon, CA: Future Medicine Publishing, 1995), 583.

21. Atkins, R.C. *Dr. Atkins' Health Revolution: Cancer Therapy* (Boston: Houghton Mifflin, 1988), 324.

## Chapter 2

## Keith I. Block, M.D.

1. Greer, S. et al. "Psychological Response to Breast Cancer and 15-year Outcome." *The Lancet* (1990), 49-50.

2. Sakamoto, G. et al. "Comparative Clinicopathological Study of Breast Cancer among Japanese and American Females." *Japanese Journal of Cancer Clinics* 25 (1979), 161-170.

3. Holm, L.E. et al. "Treatment Failure and Dietary Habits in Women with Breast Cancer." *Journal of the National Cancer Institute* 85:1 (1993), 32-36.

4. Office of Technology Assessment Report. "Dietary Treatment: An Example of an Adjunctive Nutritional Approach to Cancer Treatment." *Unconventional Cancer Treatments* (1990), 43.

5. Wei, H. et al. "Antioxidant and Antipromotional Effects of the Soybean Isoflavone Genistein." *Proceedings of the Society for Experimental Biology and Medicine* 208:5 (1995), 124.

6. Ibid.

7. Kuroda, M. et al. "Decreased Serum Levels of Selenium and Glutathione Peroxidase Activity Associated with Aging, Malignancy and Chronic Hemodialysis." *Trace Elements in Medicine* 5:3 (1988), 97-103.

8. Boik, J. "Amino Acids." *Cancer and Natural Medicine: A Textbook of Basic Science and Clinical Research* (Princeton, MN: Oregon Medical Press, 1995), 139-140.

9. Palermo, M.S. et al. "Immunomodulation Exerted by Cyclophosphamide Is Not Interfered by N-acetyl cysteine."*International Journal of Immunopharmacology* 8:6 (1986), 651-655. See also: Schmitt-Graff, A., and M.E. Scheulen. "Prevention of Adriamycin Cardiotoxicity by Niacin, Isocitrate or N-acetyl cysteine in Mice: A Morphological Study." *Pathology Resident Practice* 181:2 (1986), 168-174. See also: Kim, J.A. et al. "Topical Use of N-acetyl cysteine for Reduction of Skin Reaction to Radiation Therapy." *Seminars in Oncology* 10:Suppl 1 (1983), 86.

10. Emerit, I. et al. "Radiation-induced Clastogenic Factors: Anti-clastogenic Effects of *Gingko Biloba* Extract." *Free Radical Biology and Medicine* 18:6, 985-991.

11. Spiegel, D. et al. "Effect of Psychosocial Treatment on Survival of Patients with Metastatic Breast Cancer." *The Lancet* (1989).

12. Fawzy, F.I. et al. "Malignant Melanoma: Effects of an Early Structured Psychiatric Intervention, Coping and Affective State on Recurrence and Survival 6 Years Later." *Archives of General Psychiatry* 50 (1993), 681-689.

## Chapter 3

## Douglas Brodie, M.D.

1. Steinmetz, K., and J. Potter. "Vegetables, Fruit and Cancer: Epidemiology I." *Cancer Causes and Control 2* (1991), 325-357. See also: Ziegler, R.G. "Vegetables, Fruits and Carotenoids and the Risk of Cancer." *American Journal of Clinical Nutrition* 53:Suppl (1991), 251S-259S. See also: Negri, E. et al. "Vegetable and Fruit Consumption and Cancer Risk." *International Journal of Cancer* 48 (1991), 350-354.

2. Block, G. et al. "Fruit, Vegetables and Cancer Prevention: A Review of the Epidemiological Evidence." *Nutrition and Cancer* 18 (1992), 1-29.

3. Blair, S.N. et al. "Physical Fitness and All-cause Mortality." *Journal of the American Medical Association* 262:17 (1989), 2395.

4. Lee, I.M. et al. "Physical Activity and Risk of Develop-

ing Colorectal Cancer among College Alumni." *Journal of the National Cancer Institute* 83:18 (1991), 1324-1329.

5. Ballard-Barbash, R. et al. "Physical Activity and Risk of Large Bowel Cancer in the Framingham Study." *Cancer Research* 50:12 (1990), 3610-3613.

6. Goldfarb, R.H., and R.B. Herberman. "Natural Killer Cell Reactivity: Regulatory Interactions among Phorbol Ester, Interferon, Cholera Toxin and Retinoic Acid." *Journal of Immunology* 126 (1981), 2129.

7. Dennert, G., and R. Lotan. "Effects of Retinoic Acid on the Immune System: Stimulation of T-killer Cell Induction." *European Journal of Immunology* 8:23 (1970).

8. Dennert, G. et al. "Retinoic Acid Stimulation of the Induction of Mouse Killer T-cell in Allogeneic and Syngeneic Systems." *Journal of the National Cancer Institute* 62 (1979), 89.

9. Dartigues, J. et al. "Dietary Vitamin A, Beta-carotene and Risk of Epidermoid Lung Cancer in Southwestern France." *European Journal of Epidemiology* 6 (1990), 261-265.

10. Riordan, N.H. et al. "Intravenous Ascorbate as a Tumor Cytotoxic Chemotherapeutic Agent." *Medical Hypotheses* 44:3 (1995), 205.

11. Vojdani, A., and M. Ghoneum. "*In Vivo* Effect of Ascorbic Acid on Enhancement of Human Natural Killer Cell Activity." *Nutrition Research* 13 (1993), 753-754.

12. Maurer, H.R. et al. "Bromelain Induces the Differentiation of Leukemic Cells *In Vitro*: An Explanation for its Cytostatic Effects?" *Planta Medica* (1988), 377-381.

13. Aso, H. et al. "Induction of Interferon and Activation of NK Cells and Macrophages In Mice by Oral Administration of Ge-132, an Organic Germanium Compound." *Journal of Microbiology and Immunology* 29 (1985), 65-74. See also: Kumano, N. et al. "Antitumor Effect of Organogermanium Compound Ge-132 on the Lewis Lung Carcinoma (3LL) in C57 BL (B6) Mice." *Tohoku Journal of Experimental Medicine* 146 (1985), 97-104.

14. Panush, R.S., and J.C. Delafuente. "Vitamins and Immunocompetence: Group B Vitamins." *World Review of Nutrition and Diet* 45 (1985), 97-132.

15. Posner, B.M. et al. "Nutrition in Neoplastic Disease." *Advances in Modern Human Nutrition and Dietetics* 29 (1980), 130-169.

16. Ibid.

17. Basu, T.K. "Significance of Vitamins in Cancer." *Oncology* 33 (1976), 183.

18. Steinmetz, K., and J. Potter. "Vegetables, Fruit and Cancer." *Cancer Causes and Control* 2 (1991), 325-357, 427-442.

19. Ibid.

20. Nowicky, J.W. "New Immuno-stimulating Anti-cancer Preparation: Ukrain." Proceedings of the 13th International Congress of Chemotherapy. Vienna, Austria (August 28-September 2, 1983).

21. Nowicky, J.W. et al. "Ukrain as Both an Anti-cancer and Immunoregulatory Agent." *Drugs Under Experimental and Clinical Research* XVIII:Suppl (1992), 51-54.

22. Musianowycz, J. et al. "Clinical Studies of Ukrain in Terminal Cancer Patients (Phase II)." *Drugs Under Experimental and Clinical Research* XVIII:Suppl (1992), 45-50.

23. Gilewski, T.A., and H.M. Golomb. "Design of Combination Biotherapy Studies: Future Goals and Challenges." *Seminars in Oncology* 17 (1990), 3-10.

## Chapter 4

## Etienne Callebout, M.D.

1. Patterson, B.S.D. "A Comparison Between Conventional and Biodynamic Farming Systems as Indicated by Yields and Quality." Proceedings of the International Research Conference of the International Federation of Organic Agricultural Movements. Topsfield, Massachussetts (1978). Cited in: Knorr, D. "Quality of Ecologically-grown Foods." *Cereal Foods World* 27:4 (1982), 165-167.

2. Schuphan, W. "Nutritional Value of Crops as Influenced by Organic and Inorganic Fertilizer Treatments—Results of 12 Years of Experiments with Vegetables." *Qualitas Plantarum, Plant Foods for Human Nutrition* 23 (1974), 333. Cited in: Knorr, D. "Quality of Ecologically-grown Foods." *Cereal Foods World* 27:4 (1982), 165-167.

3. Smith, B. "Organic Foods vs. Supermarket Foods: Element Level." *Journal of Applied Nutrition* 45:1 (1993). See also: Bear, F.E. *Variations in Mineral Content in Vegetables* (New Brunswick, NJ: Rutgers University, 1984).

4. Whitfield, J.F. *Calcium, Cell Cycles, and Cancer* (New York: CRC Press, 1990).

5. Barnes, S. et al. "Soybeans Inhibit Mammary Tumors in Models of Breast Cancer." *Mutagens and Carcinogens in the Diet,* edited by Pariza, M. (New York: Alan R. Liss, 1990), 239-257.

6. Quillan, P. "Cancer Is a Sugar-feeder." *Beat Cancer with Nutrition* (Tulsa, OK: Nutrition Times Press, 1994), 122.

7. Maugh, T.H., II. "Experts Downplay Cancer Risk of Chlorinated Water." *The Los Angeles Times* (July 2, 1992).

8. Hildenbrand, G. "How the Gerson Therapy Heals." *Healing Newsletter* 6:3/4 (1990), 37.

9. Dr. Callebout bases this recommendation on the work of Dr. Kousmine at the Association Medicale Kousmine Internationale, 40 Bis, Rue Amiral Roussin, 21000 Dijon, France.

10. Lam, L.K.T. et al. "Isolation and Identification of Kahweol Palmitate and Cafestol Palmitate as Active Constituents of Green Coffee Beans that Enhance Glutathione-S-transferase Activity in the Mouse." *Cancer Research* 42 (1982), 1193-1198.

11. Spiegel, D. et al. "Effect of Psychosocial Treatment on Survival of Patients with Metastatic Breast Cancer." *The Lancet* ii (1989), 888-891.

12. Fawzy, F.I. et al. "Malignant Melanoma: Effects of an Early Structured Psychiatric Intervention, Coping and Effective State on Recurrence and Survival 6 Years Later." *Archives of General Psychiatry* 50 (1993), 681-689.

13. Ezzell, C. "Power-Line Static. Debates Rage Over the Possible Hazards of Electromagnetic Fields." *Science News* 140 (September 1991), 202-203.

14. Holmberg, B. "Magnetic Fields and Cancer: Animal and Cellular Evidence—An Overview." *Environmental Health Perspectives* 3:Suppl 2 (1995), 63-67. See also: Decker, C. "ELF-zapped Genes Speed DNA Transcription." *Science News* (April 14, 1990), 229.

15. Goldberg, R.B., and W.A. Creasey. "A Review of Cancer Induction by Extremely Low-frequency Electromagnetic Fields: Is There a Plausible Mechanism?" *Medical Hypotheses* 35:3 (1991), 265-274.

16. Oliveria, S. et al. "The Association between Cardiorespiratory Fitness and Prostate Cancer." *Medicine and Science in Sports and Exercise* 28:1 (1996), 97.

17. Lee, I.M. et al. "Physical Activity and Risk of Developing Colorectal Cancer among College Alumni." *Journal of the National Cancer Institute* 83:18 (1991), 1324-1329.

18. Frisch, R.E. et al. "Lower Prevalence of Breast Cancer in Cancers of Reproductive System among Former College Athletes Compared to Non-athletes." *British Journal of Cancer* 52 (1985), 885-891.

19. Boik, J. "Conducting Research on Natural Agents." *Cancer and Natural Medicine: A Textbook of Basic Science and Clinical Research* (Princeton, MN: Oregon Medical Press, 1995), 177.

20. Moss, R.W. *The Cancer Industry: Unraveling the Politics* (New York: Paragon House, 1989). Ralph Moss, the author, was discharged by Memorial Sloan-Kettering Cancer Center when he revealed an apparent cover-up by authorities at the Center of positive findings about amygdalin. According to Moss, subsequent research findings on amygdalin have been consistently suppressed by the pharmaceutical industry, presumably because the substance is non-patentable.

21. Rubin, D. "Dosage Levels for Laetrile." *Choice* 3:6 (1977), 8-9.

22. U.S. Patent No. 4,844,901. Oxindole alkaloids (from Uña de Gato) have properties that stimulate the immunologic system.

23. Fritsche, K.L., and P.V. Johnston. "Effect of Dietary Alpha-linolenic Acid on Growth, Metastasis, Fatty Acid Profile, and Prostaglandin Production of Two Murine Mammary Adenocarcinomas." *Journal of Nutrition* 120 (1990), 1601-1609.

24. Boik, J. "Chinese Herbs that Exhibit Antitumor Activity." *Cancer and Natural Medicine: A Textbook of Basic Science and Clinical Research* (Princeton, MN: Oregon Medical Press, 1996), 121.

25. Pitard, C.E. Protocol for combined immunologic/pharmacologic therapy: Indocin. Personal communications to Etienne Callebout. Knoxville, Tennessee (1996).

26. Boit, J. "Amino Acids." *Cancer and Natural Medicine: A Textbook of Basic Science and Clinical Research* (Princeton, MN: Oregon Medical Press, 1995), 139-140.

27. Palermo, M.S. et al. "Immunomodulation Exerted by Cyclophosphamide Is Not Interfered by N-acetyl cysteine." *International Journal of Immunopharmacology* 8:6 (1986), 651-655. See also: Schmitt-Graff, A., and M.E. Scheulen. "Prevention of Adriamycin Cardiotoxicity by Niacin, Isocitrate or N-acetyl cysteine in Mice: A Morphological Study." *Pathology Resident Practice* 181:2 (1986), 168-174. See also: Kim, J.A. et al. "Topical Use of N-acetyl cysteine for Reduction of Skin Reaction to Radiation Therapy." *Seminars in Oncology* 10:Suppl 1 (1983), 86.

28. Garaci, E. et al. "Combination Treatment Using Thymosin Alpha 1 and Interferon after Cyclophosphamide Is Able to Cure Lewis Lung Carcinoma in Mice." *Cancer Immunology and Immunotherapy* 32 (1990), 154-160.

29. Quillan, P. "Cancer is a Sugar-feeder." *Beat Cancer with Nutrition* (Tulsa, OK: Nutrition Times Press, 1994), 117.

30. As Dr. Callebout explains, "One has to take into account that an excess of glucagon, thyroxin, adrenaline, or corticosteroids (adrenal stress hormones) inhibits delta-6-desaturase, an enzyme without which the polyunsaturated fats (w-3, w-6) cannot be transformed into their more complex active compounds. Numerous studies on fats, especially those conducted by Dr. Caroline Mountford of Australia, noted that swirling spheres of triglycerides in the live cell membranes of cancer cells, again indicating their importance in the cancer question."

31. Meares, A. "Regression of Cancer of the Rectum after Intensive Meditation." *Medical Journal of Australia* 2 (1979), 539-540. See also: Meares, A. "Remission of Massive Metastasis from Undifferentiated Carcinoma of the Lung Associated with Intensive Meditation." *Journal of the American Society of Psychosomatic Dentistry and Medicine* 27 (1980), 40-41. See also: Meares, A. "Regression of Recurrence of Carcinoma of the Breast at Mastectomy Site Associated with Intensive Meditation." *Australian Family Physician* 10 (1981), 218-219. See also: Meares, A. "Meditation: A Psychological Approach to Cancer Treatment." *Practitioner* 222 (1979), 119. See also: Meares, A. "Regression of Osteogenic Sarcoma Metastases Associated with Intensive Meditation." *Medical Journal of Australia* 2:9 (1978), 433.


## Chapter 6

## W. John Diamond, M.D.


1. Prescott, D.M., and A.S. Flexer. "Cancer: The Misguided Cell." *Viruses and Cancer* (Sunderland, MA: Sinauer Associates, 1986), 192-222.

2. Shenker, B. et al. "Immunotoxic Effects of Mercuric Compounds on Human Lymphocytes and Monocytes. II. Alterations in Cell Viability." *Immunopharmacology and Immunotoxicology* 14:3 (1992), 555-557.

3. Shenker, B. et al. "Immunotoxic Effects of Mercuric Compounds on Human Lymphocytes and Monocytes. IV. Alterations in Cellular Glutathione Content." *Immunopharmacology and Immunotoxicology* 15:2/3 (1993), 273-290.

4. Dosch, Peter, M.D. *Manual of Neural Therapy According to Huneke* (Heidelberg, Germany: Karl F. Haug, 1984).

# Chapter 7

## Patrick Donovan, N.D.

1. Stanwyck and Anson. "Is Personality Related to Illness? Cluster Profiles of Aggregated Data." *Advances* 3:4 (Georgia State University, 1986).
2. Jaffe, R. "Immune Defense and Repair Systems: Clinical Approaches to Immune Function Testing and Enhancement." *Clinical Chemistry and Nutrition Guidebook: Physicians Desk Reference, Vol. 1*, edited by Yanick, R., and R. Jaffe. (Ariel, NY: T and H Publishing, 1988).
3. Dr. Donovan bases his nutritional and botanical program largely on the recommendations outlined by Dr. Patrick Quillan, Ph.D., a nutrition researcher, educator and author of *Beating Cancer With Nutrition* (Tulsa, OK: Nutrition Times Press, 1994).
4. Editorial. "The Effect of Vitamin E on Immune Responses." *Nutrition Reviews* 45:1 (1987), 27.
5. Prasad, K.N. et al. "Vitamin E Increases the Growth Inhibitory and Differentiating Effects of Tumor Therapeutic Agents on Neuroblastoma and Glioma Cells in Culture." *Proceedings of the Society for Experimental Biology and Medicine* 164:2 (1980), 158-163.
6. Svingen, B.A. et al. "Vitamin E Deficiency Accentuates Adriamycin Cardiotoxicity." *Cancer Research* 41 (1981), 3395.
7. Quillan, P. "Vitamin K." *Beating Cancer With Nutrition* (Tulsa, OK: Nutrition Times Press, 1994), 216-217.
8. Gridley, D.S. et al. *Nutrition Research* 8 (1988), 201.
9. Petrie, H.T. et al. *Journal of Leukocyte Biology* 45 (1989), 215.
10. Schrauzer, G.N. "Selenium for the Cancer Patient." Supplements lecture delivered at the Adjuvant Nutrition in Cancer Treatment Symposium. Tampa, Florida (September 29, 1995). Dr. Schrauzer is based at the Biological Trace Element Research Institute, San Diego, CA.
11. Erasmus, U. "Oil of Evening Primrose." *Fats and Oils: The Complete Guide to Fats and Oils in Health and Nutrition* (Vancouver, Canada: Alive Books, 1986), 254.
12. Palermo, M.S. et al. "Immunomodulation Exerted by Cyclophosphamide Is Not Interfered by N-acetyl cysteine."*International Journal of Immunopharmacology* 8:6 (1986), 651-655. See also: Schmitt-Graff, A., and M.E. Scheulen. "Prevention of Adriamycin Cardiotoxicity by Niacin, Isocitrate or N-acetyl cysteine in Mice: A Morphological Study." *Pathology Resident Practice* 181:2 (1986), 168-174. See also: Kim, J.A. et al. "Topical Use of N-acetyl cysteine for Reduction of Skin Reaction to Radiation Therapy." *Seminars in Oncology* 10:Suppl 1 (1983), 86.
13. Ibid.
14. Leibovitz, B. et al. "Dietary Supplements of Vitamin E, Beta-carotene, Coenzyme Q10, and Selenium Protect Tissues against Lipid Peroxidation in Rat Tissue Slices." *Journal of Applied Nutrition* 120 (1990), 97-104.

# Chapter 8

## Stephen B. Edelson, M.D.

1. Abrams, M.B. et al. "Early Detection and Monitoring of Cancer with the Anti-malignin Antibody Test." *Cancer Detection and Prevention* 18:1 (1994), 65-78.
2. Ibid.
3. Edelson, S. Personal communications (1995). Photopheresis is a Yale therapy which separates the nucleated blood cells from the red blood cells in the plasma, and irradiates all the patient's blood. This is far more expensive than UBI, about $2,000 per treatment, and photo-active drugs are used as well. Edelson questions the potential availability of photopheresis and notes that the long-range potential dangers of this therapy are unknown.
4. Edelson, S. Personal communications (1995). Most of the work with this therapy, from 1930 to 1950, was related to improving immune system function when dealing with acute and chronic infections.
5. "The Role of Haelan Nutrition in Enhancing the Anticancer Effect of Chemotherapeutic Drugs in Mice with HAC Cell Liver Cancer." Report #110. *The Therapeutic of Soybean Phytochemicals* (Metairie, LA: U.S. Research Reports, 1995).
6. Lam, L.K.T. et al. "Isolation and Identification of Kahweol Palmitate and Cafestol Palmitate as Active Constituents of Green Coffee Beans that Enhance Glutathione-S-transferase Activity in the Mouse." *Cancer Research* 42 (1982), 1193-1198.
7. Hildenbrand, G. "How the Gerson Therapy Heals." *Healing Newsletter* 6:3/4 (1990), 37.
8. Brockmeyer, N.H. et al. "Cimetidine and the Immune Response in Healthy Volunteers." *Journal of Investigative Dermatology* 9 (1989), 348-349.
9. Hast, R. et al. "Cimetidine as an Immune Response Modifier." *Medical Oncology and Tumor Pharmacotherapy* 6 (1989), 111-113.
10. Gold, J. "Hydrazine Sulfate: A Current Perspective." Nutrition & Cancer 9:2/3 (1987), 59-66.
11. Filov, V. et al. "Results of Clinical Evaluation of Hydrazine Sulfate." *Voprosy Onkologii* 36 (1990), 721-726.
12. Clarkson, T. "Overview of Mercury Vapor Toxicity, Toxicokinetics, and Critical Target Organs" and "Symposium Overview: Toxicity Assessment of Mercury Vapor from Dental Amalgams." edited by Goering, P. et al. *Fundamentals in Applied Toxicology* 19 (1992), 319-329.
13. Mosbacken, H. et al. "Oral Lichen Planus: Hypersensitivity to Dental Restoration Material." *Contact Dermatitis* 10 (1984), 11-15.

# Chapter 10

## Abram Hoffer, M.D.

1. Hoffer, Abram, M.D., Ph.D., and Morton Walker, D.P.M. *Putting It All Together: The New Orthomolecular*

*Nutrition* (New Canaan, CT: Keats Publishing, 1996), 166-167.

2. Hoffer, Abram. "One Patient's Recovery from Lymphoma." *Townsend Letter for Doctors & Patients* (November 1996), 50-51.
3. Hoffer, A., and L. Pauling. "Hardin Jones biostatistical analysis of mortality data for cohorts of cancer patients with a large fraction surviving at the termination of the study and a comparison of survival times of cancer patients receiving large regular oral doses of vitamin C and other nutrients with similar patients not receiving those doses." *Journal of Orthomolecular Medicine* 5 (1990), 143-154.
4. Hoffer, A., and L. Pauling. "Hardin Jones biostatistical analysis of mortality data for a second set of cohorts of cancer patients with a large fraction surviving at the termination of the study and a comparison of survival times of cancer patients receiving large regular oral doses of vitamin C and other nutrients with similar patients not receiving those doses." *Journal of Orthomolecular Medicine* 8 (1993), 1547-1670.
5. Cameron, E., and L. Pauling. *Proceedings of the National Academy of Sciences USA* 75:9 (1978), 4538. Dr. Pauling offers several reasons why subsequent studies have not found such positive results. First, the dosages were too low. Second, the supplements were discontinued prematurely. Third, patients who had been heavily pretreated with chemo– and radiation therapy were beyond the point of recovery. Biological limits need to be recognized—there's a point where terminal cancer patients can no longer respond to even the best therapies.
6. Riordan, N.H. et al. "Intravenous Ascorbate as a Tumor Cytotoxic Chemotherapeutic Agent." *Medical Hypotheses* 44:3 (1995), 205.
7. Pelton, R., and L. Overholser. "Vitamin C: Side Effects." *Alternatives in Cancer Therapy* (New York: Fireside, 1994), 62.
8. Hoffer, A., and L. Pauling. "Hardin Jones biostatistical analysis of mortality data for a second set of cohorts of cancer patients with a large fraction surviving at the termination of the study and a comparison of survival times of cancer patients receiving large regular oral doses of vitamin C and other nutrients with similar patients not receiving those doses." *Journal of Orthomolecular Medicine* 8 (1993), 1547-1670.
9. Hoffer, A. "Vitamin B-3: Niacin and its Amide." *Townsend Letter for Doctors & Patients* (October 1995), 35.
10. Panush, R.S., and J.C. Delafuente. "Vitamins and Immunocompetence: Group B Vitamins." *World Review of Nutrition and Dietetics* 45 (1985), 97-132.
11. Goldfarb, R.H., and R.B. Herberman. "Natural Killer Cell Reactivity: Regulatory Interactions among Phorbol Ester, Interferon, Cholera Toxin and Retinoic Acid." *Journal of Immunology* 126 (1981), 2129.
12. Dennert, G., and R. Lotan. "Effects of Retinoic Acid on the Immune System: Stimulation of T killer Cell Induction." *European Journal of Immunology* 8 (1978), 23.
13. Dennert, G. et al. "Retinoic Acid Stimulation of the Induction of Mouse Killer T-cell in All Ogeneic and Syngeneic Systems." *Journal of the National Cancer Institute* 62 (1979), 89.
14. Rotruck, J.T. et al. "Selenium: Biochemical Role as a Component of Glutathione Peroxidase." *Science* (1973), 588-590.
15. Good, R.A. et al. "Nutrition, Immunity and Cancer—A Review." *Clinical Bulletin* 9:3-12 (1979), 63-75.
16. Gershwin, M.E. et al. "The Potential Impact of Nutritional Factors on Immunological Responsiveness." *Nutrition and Immunity* (Orlando, FL: Academic Press, 1985), 222.
17. Morrow, W.J. et al. "Dietary Fat and Immune Function." *The Journal of Immunology* 135:6 (1985), 3857.
18. Bernstein, J. et al. "Depression of Lymphocyte Transformation Following Oral Glucose Ingestion." *American Journal of Clinical Nutrition* 30 (1977), 613.
19. Palmblad, J. "Lymphomas and Dietary Fat." *The Lancet* (January 15 1977), 142.
20. McWhorter, W.P. "Allergy and Risk of Cancer: A Prospective Study Using NHANES-I Follow-up Data." *Cancer* 62 (1988), 451-455.

## Chapter 11

## Tori Hudson, N.D.

1. Morra, M., and E. Potts. "Cancer of the Female Reproductive Organs." *Choices: Realistic Alternatives in Cancer Treatment* (New York: Avon, 1987), 566-574.
2. Hudson, T. "Consecutive Case Study Research of Carcinoma In Situ of Cervix Employing Local Escharotic Treatment Combined with Nutritional Therapy." *Journal of Naturopathic Medicine* 2:1 (1991), 6-10.
3. Hudson, T. "Escharotic Treatment of Cervical Dysplasia and Carcinoma." *Journal of Naturopathic Medicine* 4:1 (1993), 23.
4. Morra, M., and E. Potts. "Cancer of the Female Reproductive Organs." *Choices: Realistic Alternatives in Cancer Treatment* (New York: Avon, 1987), 573
5. The Burton Goldberg Group. *Alternative Medicine: The Definitive Guide* (Tiburon, CA: Future Medicine Publishing, 1995), 670.
6. Ibid.

## Chapter 13

## Victor A. Marcial-Vega, M.D.

1. Born, G.R. "The Scientific Rationale of Nutrition in the Cancer Patient." Clinical applications lecture delivered at the Adjuvant Nutrition in Cancer Treatment symposium. Tampa, Florida (September 30, 1995).
2. Vojdani, A., and M. Ghoneum. "*In Vivo* Effect of Ascorbic Acid on Enhancement of Human Natural Killer Cell Activity." *Nutrition Research* 13 (1993), 753-754.
3. Hildenbrand, G. "How the Gerson Therapy Heals." *Healing Newsletter* 6:3/4 (1990), 37.

# Chapter 14

## Martin Milner, N.D.


1. Patterson, B.S.D. "A Comparison Between Conventional and Biodynamic Farming Systems as Indicated by Yields and Quality." Proceedings of the International Research Conference of the International Federation of Organic Agricultural Movements. Topsfield, MA (1978). Cited in: Knorr, D. "Quality of Ecologically-grown Foods." *Cereal Foods World* 27:4 (1982), 165-167.
2. Schuphan, W. "Nutritional Value of Crops as Influenced by Organic and Inorganic Fertilizer Treatments—Results of 12 Years of Experiments with Vegetables." *Qualitas Plantarum, Plant Foods for Human Nutrition* 23 (1974), 333. Cited in: Knorr, D. "Quality of Ecologically-grown Foods." *Cereal Foods World* 27:4 (1982), 165-167.
3. Smith, B. "Organic Foods vs. Supermarket Foods: Element Level." *Journal of Applied Nutrition* 45:1 (1993). See also: Bear, F.E. *Variations in Mineral Content in Vegetables* (New Brunswick, NJ: Rutgers University, 1984).
4. Sternfeld, B. "Cancer and the Protective Effect of Physical Activity: The Epidemiological Evidence." *Medicine and Science in Sports and Exercise* 24 (1992), 1195-1209.
5. Frisch, R.E. et al. "Lower Lifetime Occurrence of Breast Cancer and Cancers of the Reproductive System among Former College Athletes." *American Journal of Clinical Nutrition* 45 (1987), 328-335.
6. Nieman, D.C. et al. "The Effects of Moderate Exercise Training on Natural Killer Cells and Acute Upper Respiratory Tract Infections." *International Journal of Sports Medicine* 11 (1990), 467-473.
7. Nieman, D.C. "Immune Function in Marathon Runners Versus Sedentary Controls." *Medicine and Science in Sports and Exercise* (1995), 986-992. See also: Pedersen, B.K. et al. "Natural Killer Cell Activity in Peripheral Blood of Highly Trained and Untrained Persons." *International Journal of Sports Medicine* 10 (1989), 129-131.
8. Crist, D.M. et al. "Physical Exercise Increases Natural Cellular-mediated Tumor Cytotoxicity in Elderly Women." *Gerontology* 35 (1989), 66-71. See also: Nieman, D.C. et al. "Physical Activity and Immune Function in Elderly Women." *Medicine and Science in Sports and Exercise* 25 (1993), 823-831.
9. Cannon, V., and J. Kluger. "Endogenous Pyrogen Activity in Human Plasma after Exercise." *Science* 220 (1983), 617-9. See also: Cannon, V., and C. Dinarello. "Interleukin I Activity in Human Plasma." *Federation Proceedings* 43 (1984), 462.
10. Mellion, M.B. "Exercise Therapy for Anxiety and Depression." *Postgraduate Medicine* 77:3, 59-66. See also: Carek, P.J., and T.C. Namey. "Include Exercise in Treatment for Anxiety." *Your Patient & Fitness* 6:2 (1992), 10-16.
11. Boutcher, S.H., and D.M. Landers. "The Effects of Vigorous Exercise on Anxiety, Heart Rate, and Alpha Activity of Runners and Nonrunners." *Psychophysiology* 25:6 (1988), 696-702. See also: Raglin, J.S., and W.P. Morgan. "Influence of Exercise and Quiet Rest on State Anxiety and Blood Pressure." *Medicine and Science in Sports and Exercise* 19:5 (1987), 456-463.
12. Shavit, Y. et al. "Opioid Peptides Mediate the Supressive Effect of Stress on Natural Killer Cell Cytotoxicity." *Science* 223 (1984), 188-223. See also: Kraut, R., and A. Greenberg. "Effects of Endogenous and Exogenous Opioids on Splenic Natural Killer Cell Activity." *Natural Immunity and Cell Growth Regulation* 5 (1986), 28-40.
13. Jamner, L. et al. "The Relationships between Repressive and Defensive Coping Styles and Monocyte, Eosinophil, and Serum Glucose Levels: Support for the Opioid Peptide Hypothesis of Repression." *Psychosomatic Medicine* 50 (1988), 567-575.
14. Levy, S. et al. "Persistently Low Natural Killer Cell Activity and Circulating Levels of Plasma Beta Endorphin Risk Factors for Infectious Disease." *Life Sciences* 48 (1991), 107-116. See also: Chiappelli, F. et al. "Differential Effect of Beta-endorphin on Three Human Cytotoxic Cell Populations." *International Journal of Immunopharmacology* 13 (1991), 291-297. See also: Kastin, A. et al. "Failure of Met-enkephalin to Enhance NK Cell Activity." *Immunobiology* 183 (1991), 55-68.
15. Greer, S. "Psycho-oncology: Its Aims, Achievements, and Future Tasks." *Psycho-Oncology* 3 (1994), 87-101.
16. Greer, S., and T. Morris. "Psychological Attributes of Women Who Develop Breast Cancer: A Controlled Study." *Journal of Psychosomatic Research* 19 (1975), 147-153.
17. "Uña de Gato: Its Therapeutic Characteristics, History and Clinical Effectiveness." *Wellness Advocate* 5:1 (1995), 1-5.
18. Gold, J. "Hydrazine Sulfate: A Current Perspective." *Nutrition & Cancer* 9:2/3 (1987); 59-66.
19. Biser, L. "Study Indicates Castor Oil Improves Immune System." *The Layman's Course on Killing Cancer 4* (Charlottesville, VA: University of Natural Healing, 1992), 6
20. "The Effect of Vitamin E on Immune Responses." *Nutrition Reviews* 45:1 (1987), 27.
21. Goldfarb, R.H., and R.B. Herberman. "Natural Killer Cell Reactivity: Regulatory Interactions among Phorbol Ester, Interferon, Cholera Toxin and Retinoic Acid." *Journal of Immunology* 126 (1981), 2129.
22. Dennert, G., and R. Lotan. "Effects of Retinoic Acid on the Immune System: Stimulation of T-killer Cell Induction." *European Journal of Immunology* 8 (1978), 23.
23. Dennert, G. et al. "Retinoic Acid Stimulation of the Induction of Mouse Killer T-cell in Allogeneic and Syngeneic Systems." *Journal of the National Cancer Institute* 62 (1979), 89.
24. Panush, R.S., and J.C. Delafuente. "Vitamins and Immunocompetence: Group B Vitamins." *World Review of Nutrition and Dietetics* 45 (1985), 97-132.
25. Posner, B.M. et al. "Nutrition in Neoplastic Disease." *Advances in Modern Human Nutrition and Dietetics* 29 (1980), 130-169.
26. Basu, T.K. "Significance of Vitamins in Cancer." *Oncology* 33 (1976), 183.

27. Gershwin, M.E. et al. "The Potential Impact of Nutritional Factors on Immunological Responsiveness." *Nutrition and Immunity* (Orlando, FL: Academic Press, 1985), 222.

28. Good, R.A. et al. "Nutrition, Immunity and Cancer—A Review." *Clinical Bulletin* 9 (1979), 3-12, 63-75.

29. Lane, I. William. "Shark Cartilage Therapy Results and Research Today." Physician Information Package. (Cartilage Consultants, March 4, 1995). Contact LaneLabs at 201-391-8601. See also: Moses, M.A. et al. "Identification of an Inhibitor of Neovascularization from Cartilage." *Science* 248 (1990), 630-634. See also: Oikawa, T. et al. "A Novel Angiogenic Inhibitor Derived from Japanese Shark Cartilage: Extraction and Estimation of Inhibitory Activities toward Tumor and Embryonic Angiogenesis." *Cancer Letters* 51 (1990), 181-186. See also: Britto, Fernandez J., and I.W. Lane. "Angiogenesis Modulation in Peritumor or Connective Tissue by Cartilage from Shark, The Cuban Experience." XVII World Congress of Anatomic and Clinical Pathology. Mexico (1993).

30. Blumberg, N., "Tumor Angiogenesis Factor. Speculations on an Approach to Cancer Therapy." *Yale Journal of Biology and Medicine* 47 (1974), 71-81. See also: Folkman, J. "Tumor Angiogenesis: A Possible Control Point in Tumor Growth." *Annals of Internal Medicine* 82 (1975), 96-100. Also: Folkman, J. "The Vascularization of Tumors." *Scientific American* 234:5 (1976), 58-64, 70-73. Also: Langer, R. et al. "Isolation of a Cartilage Factor that Inhibits Tumor Neovascularization." *Science* 193:4247 (1976), 70-72. Also: Sadove, A.M. et al. "Inhibition of Mammary Carcinoma Invasiveness with Cartilage-derived Inhibitors." *Surgical Forum* 28 (1977), 499-501. Also: Pauli, B.U. et al. "Regulation of Tumor Invasion by Cartilage-derived Anti-invasion Factor *In Vitro*." *Journal of the National Cancer Institute* 67 (July 1981), 65-73. Also: Folkman, J. "How Blood is Regulated in Normal and Neoplastic Tissue" *Cancer Research* 48 (February 1986), 467-473. Also: Folkman, J., and M. Klagnbrun. "Angiogenic Factors." *Science* 235 (January 1987), 235-247. Also: D'Amore, P.A. "Anti-angiogenesis as a Strategy for Anti-metastasis." *Seminars in Thrombosis & Hemostasis* 14:1 (1988), 73-78. Also: Folkman, J. et al. "Induction of Angiogenesis During the Transition from Hyperplasia to Neoplasia." *Nature* 339:6219 (1989), L58-61. Also: Weidner, N. et al. "Tumor Angiogenesis and Metastasis-correlation in Invasive Breast Carcinoma." *New England Journal of Medicine* 324 (1991), 1-8. Also: Wilson, J. "Shark Cartilage: A Review of Background Literature & Research." *Townsend Letter for Doctors & Patients* 133-134 (August/September 1994), 864-872.

31. Milner, Martin, N.D. "Follow-up of Cancer Patients Using Shark Cartilage." *Alternative & Complementary Therapies* 2:2 (March/April 1996), 99-109.

32. Gardener, M.L.G. "Gastrointestinal Absorption of Intact Proteins." *Annual Review of Nutrition* 8 (1988), 329-350.

# Chapter 15

## Emanuel Revici, M.D.

1. Revici, E. *Research in Physiopathology as the Basis for Guided Chemotherapy with Special Application to Cancer* (Princeton, NJ: Van Nostrand, 1961). A project sponsored by the American Foundation for Cancer Research.

2. Office of Technology Assessment Report. *Emanuel Revici and Biologically Guided Chemotherapy* (Washington, DC: U.S. Government Printing Office, 1990). The report notes that this leads to a reduction in cell membrane permeability and an inhibiton of the cells' oxidative processes, which in turn reduces the availability of intracellular oxygen, interferes with the breakdown of carbohydrates, and results in lactic acid buildup in the extracellular fluids.

3. Mangum, T. Personal communications (1996). In more classical biochemical terms, the catabolic reactions correspond to oxidation processes manifested either as fixation of oxygen, loss of hydrogen, or loss of electrons, while the anabolic reactions correspond to reduction reactions, loss of oxygen, fixation of hydrogen, or the gain of electrons.

4. McKee, D.L. *Emanuel Revici, M.D.: A Review of His Scientific Work* (New York: Institute of Applied Biology). Unpublished manuscript.

5. Ibid.

6. Ibid.

7. Walters, R. "Revici Therapy." *Options: The Alternative Cancer Therapy Book* (Garden City, NY: Avery Publishing Group, 1993), 39-40. Walters writes: "Revici's research has demonstrated that lipids (fats) have an affinity for tumors and other abnormal tissues. Because of this, the lipids or lipid-like synthetic compounds administered to the patient, either by mouth or injection, travel directly to the tumor or lesion. Cancerous tissue is abnormally rich in free lipids, and the lipidic agents introduced into the bloodstream are readily taken up by the tumor."

8. Mangum, T. Personal communications (1996). This situation, in turn, leads to an electrolyte imbalance, notably an increase in sodium in the extracellular fluids, and an alkaline environment in the tumor.

9. Office of Technology Assessment. *Emanuel Revici and Biologically Guided Chemotherapy* (Washington, DC: U.S. Government Printing Office, 1990).

10. McKee, D.L. *Emanuel Revici, MD: A Review of His Scientific Work* (New York: Institute of Applied Biology). Unpublished manuscript.

11. Moss, R. "Selenium." *Cancer Therapy: The Independent Consumer's Guide* (New York: Equinox Press, 1992), 112-113

12. Office of Technology Assessment. *Emanuel Revici and Biologically Guided Chemotherapy* (Washington, DC: U.S. Government Printing Office, 1990).

13. Eidem, William Kelley. *The Man Who Cures Cancer* (Bethesda, MD: Be Well Books, 1996), 177-181.

14. Subcommittee of the Committee on Appropriations. "Special Hearing on Alternative Medicine." U.S.

Senate (June 24, 1993), 180-182.

15. Office of Technology Assessment. *Emanuel Revici and Biologically Guided Chemotherapy* (Washington, DC: U.S. Government Printing Office, 1990).

16. Eidem, William Kelley. *The Man Who Cures Cancer* (Bethesda, MD: Be Well Books, 1996).

17. Ravich, RA. "Revici Method of Cancer Control: Evaluation of 1,047 Patients with Advanced Malignancies Treated from 1946-1955." (New York: Institute for Applied Biology). Unpublished manuscript.

18. Schrauzer, G.N. Letter to the Board of Regents, Department of Education, State of New York (February 14, 1996). This letter was written as an appeal to discourage the State of New York from taking away Revici's license to practice medicine.

## Chapter 16

## Robert C. Rountree, M.D.

1. Hutchison, G.B. "Carcinogenic Effects of Medical Irradiation." *Origins of Human Cancer* (Cold Spring Harbor, NY: Cold Spring Harbor Laboratory, 1977), 501-509.

2. *Journal of the National Cancer Institute* (May 1995).

3. Simone, C.B. "Carcinogens in Tobacco Smoke." *Breast Health* (Garden City, NY: Avery, 1995), 134.

4. Abramson, R. "EPA Officially Links Passive Smoke, Cancer." *The Los Angeles Times* (January 12, 1993), A27.

5. Steinman, David, and Samuel Epstein. *The Safe Shopper's Bible: A Consumer's Guide to Nontoxic Household Products, Cosmetics, and Food* (New York: Macmillan, 1995).

6. "Diet and Malignant Melanoma." *American Journal of Epidemiology* 139:9 (1994), 869.

## Chapter 18

## Michael B. Schachter, M.D.

1. Prasad, K.N. et al. *Proceedings of the Society for Experimental Biology and Medicine* 164 (1980), 158.

2. Myers, C.E. et al. *Annals of the New York Academy of Sciences* 393 (1982), 376.

3. Good, R.A. et al. "Nutrition, Immunity and Cancer—A Review." *Clinical Bulletin* 9 (1979), 3-12, 63-75.

4. Gershwin, M.E. et al. "The Potential Impact of Nutritional Factors on Immunological Responsiveness." *Nutrition and Immunity* (Orlando, FL: Academic Press, 1985), 222.

5. Stevens, R.G. et al. "Body Iron Stores and the Risk of Cancer." *New England Journal of Medicine* 319 (1988), 1047-1052. See also: *Nutrition Reviews* 47:6 (1989), 176.

6. Goyer, R.A. et al. "Role of Chelating Agents for Prevention, Intervention and Treatment Exposures of Toxic Metals." *Environmental Health Perspectives* 103:11 (1995), 1048-1052.

7. Clarkson, T. "Overview of Mercury Vapor Toxicity, Toxicokinetics, and Critical Target Organs. Symposium Overview: Toxicity Assessment of Mercury Vapor from Dental Amalgams." *Fundamentals in Applied Toxicology* 19 (1992), 319-329.

8. Mosbacken, H. et al. "Oral Lichen Planus: Hypersensitivity to Dental Restoration Material." *Contact Dermatitis* 10 (1984), 11-15.

9. Royal, Daniel F., D.O. "Health Hazard in Your Teeth." *Alternative Medicine Digest* 13 (1996), 40-44.

10. Palermo, M.S. et al. *International Journal of Immunopharmacology* 8:6 (1986), 651. See also Schmitt-Graff, A., and M. E. Scheulen. "Prevention of Adriamycin Cardiotoxicity by Niacin, Isocitrate or N-acetyl cysteine in Mice: A Morphological Study." *Pathology Resident Practice* 181:2, 168. And also: Kim, J.A. et al. "Topical Use of N-acetyl cysteine for Reduction of Skin Reaction to Radiation Therapy."*Seminars in Oncology* 10:1 Suppl 1 (1983), 86.

11. Meydani, et al. *Drug-Nutrient Interactions* 2 (1984), 217.

12. Schachter, M. Personal communications (1995). Combinations of enzymes are available in the form of Wobenzym®, Wobemugos®, and Polyzym® (021, 022, 023).

13. Esber, H.J. et al. "Specific and Nonspecific Immune Resistance Enhancement Activity of Staphage Lysate." *Journal of Immunopharmacology* 3 (1981), 79-92.

14. Aoke, T. et al. "Staphage Lysate and Lentinan as Immunomodulators and Immunopotentiators in Clinical and Experimental Systems." *Augmenting Agents in Cancer Therapy*, edited by Hirsh, E.M. et al. (New York: Raven Press, 1981), 101-111.

15. Manning, C.A., and L.J. Vanrenen. *Bioenergetic Medicines East and West: Acupuncture and Homeopathy* (Berkeley, CA: North Atlantic Books, 1988).

16. Danopoulos, E.D. et al. "Eleven Years of Oral Urea Treatment in Liver Malignancies." *Clinical Oncology* 7 (1981), 281-289.

17. Ott, J. *Health and Light* (Old Greenwich, CT: Devin-Adair, 1973), 72-75.

## Chapter 19

## Charles B. Simone, M.D.

1. Nelson, Nancy J. "Is Chemoprevention Overrated or Underfunded?" *Journal of the National Cancer Institute* 88:14 (July 17, 1996).

2. Wasserman, M. et al. "Organochlorine Compounds in Neoplastic and Adjacent Apparently Normal Breast Tissue." *Bulletin of Environmental Contaminants and Toxicology* 15 (1976), 478-484.

3. Dreher, H. *Your Defense Against Cancer* (New York: Harper & Row, 1988), 202-204.

4. Hersey, et al. "Effects of Cigarette Smoking on the Immune System." *Medical Journal of Australia* 2:9 (1983), 425-429. See also: Ginns et al. "Alterations in Immunoregulatory Cells in Lung Cancer and Smoking." *Journal of Clinical Immunology* 3:Suppl (1982), 90S-94S.

5. Simone, C.B. *Breast Health* (Garden City, NY: Avery Publishing, 1995), 141.

6. Schatzkin, et al. "Alcohol Consumption and Breast Cancer in the Epidemiologic Follow-up Study of the First NHANES." *New England Journal of Medicine* 316 (1987), 1169-1173. See also: Willet, W. et al. "Moderate Alcohol Consumption and the Risk of Breast Cancer." *New England Journal of Medicine* 316 (1987), 1174-1180. See also: Longnecker, et al. "A Meta-analysis of Alcohol Consumption in Relation to Risk of Breast Cancer." *Journal of the American Medical Association* 260 (1988), 652-656.

7. Simone, C.B. *Breast Health* (Garden City, NY: Avery Publishing, 1995), 143.

8. Simon, D. et al. "Coffee Drinking and Cancer of the Lower Urinary Tract System." *Journal of the National Cancer Institute* 54:3 (1975), 587.

9. Mulvihill, J. "Caffeine as a Teratogen and Mutagen." *Teratology* 8 (1973), 69. See also: Weinstein, D. et al. "The Effects of Caffeine on Chromosomes of Human Lymphocytes." *Mutation Research* 16 (1972), 391.

10. Brown, P. "Unnecessary X rays Blamed for Cancer Deaths." *New Scientist* (September 8, 1990), 27.

11. Simone, C.B. Personal communications (1996). See also: Simone, C.B. "Mammography." *Breast Health* (Garden City Park, NJ: Avery Publishing, 1995), 215-223.

12. National Cancer Institute. Personal communications with biostatisticians (1996). The NCI statisticians estimate that, for every 100,000 women over age 40 who are screened, mammography causes 10 more cancers than would normally be seen.

13. Feychting, M., and A. Ahlbom. "Childhood Leukemia and Residential Exposure to Weak Extremely Low Frequency Magnetic Fields." *Environmental Health Perspectives* Suppl 2 (1995), 59-62. See also: Savitz, D.A. "Overview of Epidemiologic Research on Electric and Magnetic Fields and Cancer." *American Industrial Hygiene Association Journal* 54:4 (1993), 197-204.

14. Savitz, D.A., and D.P. Loomis. "Magnetic Field Exposure in Relation to Leukemia and Brain Cancer Mortality among Electric Utility Workers." *American Journal of Epidemiology* 141:2 (1995), 123-134. See also: Loomis, D.P., and D.A. Savitz. "Mortality from Brain Cancer and Leukemia among Electrical Workers." *British Journal of Industrial Medicine* 47:9 (1990), 633-638.

15. Loomis, D.P. et al. "Breast Cancer Mortality among Female Electrical Workers in the United States." *Journal of the National Cancer Institute* 86:12 (1994), 921-925.

16. Savitz, D.A. et al. "Magnetic Field Exposure from Electric Appliances and Childhood Cancer." *American Journal of Epidemiology* 131:5 (1990), 763-773.

17. Tomasi, et al. "Immune Parameters in Athletes before and after Strenuous Exercise." *Journal of Clinical Immunology* 2 (1982), 173-178. See also: Soppi, et al. "Effect of Strenuous Physical Stress on Circulating Lymphocyte Number and Function Before and After Training." *Journal of Clinical and Laboratory Immunology* 8 (1982), 43-46.

18. Cannon, V., and J. Kluger. "Endogenous Pyrogen Activity in Human Plasma after Exercise." *Science* 220 (1983), 617-619. See also: Cannon, V., and C. Dinarello. "Interleukin I Activity in Human Plasma." *Federation Proceedings* 43 (1984), 462.

19. Fox, B.H. "Epidemiologic Aspects of Stress, Aging, Cancer and the Immune System." *Annals of the New York Academy of Sciences* 521 (1988), 16. See also: Fox, B.H. "Premorbid Psychological Factors as Related to Cancer Incidence." *Journal of Behavioral Medicine* 1 (1978), 45-133. See also: Fox, B.H. "Psychosocial Factors and the Immune System in Human Cancer." *Psychoneuroimmunology*, edited by Ader, R. (New York: Academic Press, 1981). See also: Borysenko, J.Z. "Behavioral-physiological Factors in the Development and Management of Cancer." *General Hospital Psychiatry* 4 (1982), 69-74. See also: Goodkin, K., M.H Antoni and P.H. Blaney. "Stress and Hopelessness in the Promotion of Cervical Intraepithelial Neoplasia in Invasive Squamous Cell Carcinoma of the Cervix." *Journal of Psychosomatic Research* 30:1 (1986), 67-76.

20. Simone, C.B. Personal communications (1996). See also: Simone, C.B. "Mammography." *Breast Health* (Garden City Park, NJ: Avery Publishing, 1995), 194.

21. Burish, T.G., and R.A. Jenkins. "Effectiveness of Biofeedback and Relaxation Training in Reducing the Side Effects of Cancer Chemotherapy." *Health Psychology* 11:1 (1992), 17-23. See also: Newton-Bernauer, W. "The Use of Hypnosis in the Treatment of Cancer Patients." *American Journal of Clinical Hypnosis* 25 (1982), 104-113. See also: Shapiro, A. "Psychotherapy as Adjunct Treatment for Cancer Patients." *American Journal of Clinical Hypnosis* 25 (1982), 150-155.

22. Decker, T.W. et al. "Relaxation Therapy as an Adjunct in Radiation Oncology." *Journal of Clinical Psychology* 48:3 (1992), 388-393. See also: Vasterling, J. et al. "Cognitive Distraction and Relaxation Training for the Control of Side Effects Due to Cancer Chemotherapy." *Journal of Behavioral Medicine* 16:1 (1993), 65-80. See also: Burish, T.G. et al. "Preparing Patients for Cancer Chemotherapy: Effect of Coping Preparation and Relaxation Interventions." *Journal of Consulting and Clinical Psychology* 59:4 (1991), 518-525. See also: Larsson, G., and B. Starrin. "Relaxation Training as an Integral Part of Caring Activities for Cancer Patients: Effects on Well-being." *Scandinavian Journal of Caring Sciences* 6:3 (1992), 179-185.

23. Spiegel, D. "Effect of Psychosocial Treatment on Survival of Patients with Metastatic Breast Cancer." *Lancet* ii (1989), 888-891.


## Chapter 20

## Vincent Speckhart, M.D.


1. The Burton Goldberg Group. *Alternative Medicine: The Definitive Guide* (Tiburon, CA: Future Medicine Publishing, 1995), 130.

2. Ibid.

3. McDonagh, E.W. et al. "The Clinical Change in Patients Treated with EDTA Chelation Plus Multivitamin/Trace Mineral Supplementation." *Journal of Orthomolecular Psychiatry* 14:1 (1985), 61-65.

4. Moss, R. "Essiac." *Cancer Therapy: The Independent Consumer's Guide* (New York: Equinox Press, 1992), 146-147. Moss reviews the technical cancer-related research on Essiac; many substances isolated from the herbs in Essiac show specific kinds of anticancer activity.

5. Ullman, Dana. *The Consumer's Guide to Homeopathy* (New York: Jeremy P. Tarcher/G.P. Putnam's Sons, 1995), 299 (Footnote 4).

6. Ibid.

7. Ibid.

## Chapter 21

## Jesse Stoff, M.D.

1. Leroi, A., and R. Leroi. "The Causes and Treatment of Cancer." *The Anthroposophical Approach to Medicine*, edited by Wolf, O. (Hudson, NY: Anthroposophic Press, 1989), 47.

2. Ibid., 46.

3. Heiligtag, H.R. "Biographical Work in Connection with Cancer." *Anthroposophical Medicine and Cancer Therapy*, edited by Heiligtag, H.R. (Spring Valley, NY: Mercury Press, 1994), 70.

4. Heiligtag, H.R. "Anthroposophical Viewpoints on Mistletoe." *Anthroposophical Medicine and Cancer Therapy*, edited by Heiligtag, H.R. (Spring Valley, NY: Mercury Press, 1994), 27-29.

5. Mueller, E.A., and F.A. Anderer. "A Viscum album Oligosaccharide Activating Human Natural Cytotoxicity Is an Interferon-Y Inducer." *Cancer Immunology and Immunotherapy* 32 (1990), 221-227.

6. Hu, S.Y. "The Genus *Panax* (Ginseng) in Chinese Medicine." *Economic Botany* 30:1 (1976), 11-28.

7. Kim, H. et al. "Quercetin as an Inhibitor of Lactate Transport and Hyperthermic Sensitizer of Hela Cells." *Cancer Research* 44:1 (1984), 102-106.

8. Elia, G., and M.G. Santoro. "Regulation of Heat Shock Protein Synthesis by Quercetin in Human Erythroleukemia Cells." *Biochemical Journal* 15:300 Part 1 (1994), 201-209.

9. Agullo, G. et al. "Quercetin Exerts a Preferential Cytotoxic Effect on Active Dividing Colon Carcinoma HT29 and Caco-2 Cells." *Cancer Letters* 87 (1994), 55-62.

10. Boik, J. "Effects of pH on Neoplasia: Hyperthermia." *Cancer and Natural Medicine: A Textbook of Basic Science and Clinical Research* (Princeton, MN: Oregon Medical Press, 1995), 55.

11. Tomasi, et al. "Immune Parameters in Athletes before and after Strenuous Exercise." *Journal of Clinical Immunology* 2 (1982), 173-178. See also: Soppi, et al. "Effect of Strenuous Physical Stress on Circulating Lymphocyte Number and Function before and after Training." *Journal of Clinical Laboratory Immunology* 8 (1982), 43-46.

12. Cannon, V., and J. Kluger. "Endogenous Pyrogen Activity in Human Plasma after Exercise," *Science* 220 (1983), 617-619. Also: Cannon, V., and C. Dinarello. "Interleukin I Activity in Human Plasma." *Federation Proceedings* 43 (1984), 462.

13. Spiegel, D. et al. "Effect of Psychosocial Treatment on Survival of Patients with Metastatic Breast Cancer." *Lancet* ii (1989), 888-891.

14. Richardson, J.L. et al. "The Effect of Compliance with Treatment on Survival among Patients with Hematologic Malignancies." *Journal of Clinical Oncology* 8 (1990), 356-364.

15. Fawzy, F.I. et al. "Malignant Melanoma: Effects of an Early Structured Psychiatric Intervention, Coping and Affective State on Recurrence and Survival 6 Years Later." *Archives of General Psychiatry* 50 (1993), 681-689.

16. Greer, S., and T. Morris. "Psychological Attributes of Women Who Develop Breast Cancer: A Controlled Study." *Journal of Psychosomatic Research* 19 (1975), 147-153. See also: Greer, S. "Psycho-oncology: Its Aims, Achievements, and Future Tasks." *Psycho-Oncology* 3 (1994), 87-101.

17. Levy, S. et al. "Survival Hazards in First Recurrent Breast Cancer Patients: Seven-year Follow-up." *Psychosomatic Medicine* 50 (1988), 520-528.

18. Achterbeg, J., and G.F. Lawlis. *Imagery of Cancer: A Diagnostic Tool for the Process of Disease* (Champaign, IL: Institute for Personality and Ability Testing, 1978). Cited by Pelton, R., and L. Overholser. "Visualization and Meditation." *Alternatives in Cancer Therapy* (New York: Fireside/Simon & Schuster, 1994), 235.

19. Heiligtag, H.R. "Artistic Therapies: String Instruments." *Anthroposophical Medicine and Cancer Therapy*, edited by Heiligtag, H.R. (Spring Valley, NY: Mercury Press, 1994), 56.

20. "Asthma." *Alternative Medicine Digest* 6 (1996), 29-30.

## Chapter 22

## Jack O. Taylor, D.C.

1. Editorial. "The Effect of Vitamin E on Immune Responses." *Nutrition Reviews* 45:1 (1987), 27.

2. Good, R.A. et al. "Nutrition, Immunity and Cancer: A Review." *Clinical Bulletin* 9:3-12 (1979), 63-75.

3. Gershwin, M.E. et al. "The Potential Impact of Nutritional Factors on Immunological Responsiveness." *Nutrition and Immunity* (Orlando, FL: Academic Press, 1985), 222.

4. Morazzoni, P., and S. Malandrino. "Anthocyanins and their Aglycons as Scavengers of Free Radicals and Antilipoperoxidant Agents." *Pharmacology Res Comms* 20:2 Suppl (1988), 254.

## Chapter 23

## Lawrence H. Taylor, M.D.

1. Serraino, M., and L. Thompson. "The Effect of Flaxseed Supplementation on the Initiation and Promotional Stages of Mammary Tumorigenesis." *Nutrition and Cancer* 17 (1992), 153-159.

2. Pienta, K.J. et al. "Inhibition of Spontaneous Metastases in a Rat Prostate Cancer Model by Oral Administration of Modified Citrus Pectin." *Journal of the National Cancer Institute* 87:5 (1995), 348-353.

3. Watanabe, K. et al. "Effect of Dietary Alfalfa, Pectin, and Wheat Bran on Azoxymethane- or Methylnitrosourea-induced Colon Carcinogenesis in F344 Rats." *Journal of the National Cancer Institute* 63 (1979), 141-145.

4. Blair, S.N. et al. "Physical Fitness and All-cause mortality." *Journal of the American Medical Association* 262:17 (1989), 2395.

5. Goyer, R.A. et al. "Role of Chelating Agents for Prevention, Intervention and Treatment Exposures of Toxic Metals." *Environmental Health Perspectives* 103:11 (1995), 1048-1052.

6. Trowbridge, J.P., and M. Walker. "Free Radical Pathology." *Chelation Therapy* (Stamford, CT: New Way of Life, 1985), 20-31.

7. Cranton, E.M., and J.P. Frackelton. "Free Radical Pathology in Age-associated Diseases: Treatment with EDTA Chelation, Nutrition and Antioxidants." *Journal of Holistic Medicine* 6:1 (1984), 6-36.

8. Clarkson, T. "Overview of Mercury Vapor Toxicity, Toxicokinetics, and Critical Target Organs. Symposium Overview: Toxicity Assessment of Mercury Vapor from Dental Amalgams." *Fundamentals in Applied Toxicology* 19 (1992), 319-329.

9. Mosbacken, H. et al. "Oral Lichen Planus: Hypersensitviity to Dental Restoration Material." *Contact Dermatitis* 10 (1984), 11-15.

10. Goldfarb, R.H., and R.B. Herberman. "Natural Killer Cell Reactivity: Regulatory Interactions among Phorbol Ester, Interferon, Cholera Toxin and Retinoic Acid." *Journal of Immunology* 126 (1981), 2129.

11. Dennert, G., and R. Lotan. "Effects of Retinoic Acid on the Immune System: Stimulation of T-killer Cell Induction." *European Journal of Immunology* 8 (1978), 23.

12. Dennert, G. et al. "Retinoic Acid Stimulation of the Induction of Mouse Killer T-cell in Allogeneic and Syngeneic Systems." *Journal of National Cancer Institute* 62 (1979), 89.

13. "The Effect of Vitamin E on Immune Responses." *Nutrition Reviews* 45:1 (1987), 27.

14. Prasad, K.N. et al. "Vitamin E Increases the Growth Inhibitory and Differentiating Effects of Tumor Therapeutic Agents on Neuroblastoma and Glioma Cells in Culture." *Proceedings of the Society for Experimental Biology and Medicine* 164:2 (1980), 158-163.

15. Myers, C.E. et al. "Effect of Tocopherol and Selenium on Defenses against Reactive Oxygen Species and their Effect on Radiation Sensitivity." *Annals of the New York Academy of Sciences* 393 (1982), 419-425.

16. Rotruck, J.T. et al. "Selenium: Biochemical Role as a Component of Glutathione Peroxidase." *Science* (1973), 588-590.

17. Schrauzer, G.N. "Selenium in Nutritional Cancer Prophylaxis: An Update." *Vitamins, Nutrition and Cancer*, edited by Prosad, K.N. (Basel, Switzerland: Karger, 1984).

18. Yoshida, M. et al. "The Effect of Quercetin on Cell Cycle Progression and Growth of Human Gastric Cancer Cells." *FEBS Letters* 260 (1990), 10-13.

19. Sears, B. *The Zone: A Dietary Road Map* (New York: HarperCollins/ReganBooks, 1995).

20. Good, R.A. et al. "Nutrition, Immunity and Cancer—A Review." *Clinical Bulletin* 9:3-12 (1979), 63-75.

21. Gershwin, M.E. et al. "The Potential Impact of Nutritional Factors on Immunological Responsiveness." *Nutrition and Immunity* (Orlando, FL: Academic Press, 1985), 222.

22. Garland, et al. "Dietary Vitamin D and Calcium and Risk of Colorectal Cancer: A 19-year Prospective Study in Men." *The Lancet* i (1985), 307.

23. Prudden, J. "Use of Cartilage in Cancer Treatment." Lecture at the 1995 Adjuvant Nutrition for Cancer Treatment Symposium. Tampa, Florida (September 30, 1995).

24. Contreras, Francisco, M.D. Personal communication to Dr. Taylor.

25. Weinstein, I. et al. "Molecular Biology and Epidemiology of Cancer." *Cancer Prevention and Control*, edited by Greenwald, Peter et al. (National Cancer Institute/Marcel Dekker, 1995), 83-103.

26. Because it protects the cell DNA, Dr. Garnett's medicine is called a nucleotide reductase. Garnett-McKeen Laboratories: Nucleotide reductase. U.S. Patent No. 557,637 (October 31, 1995).

27. Weinstein, I.B., R.M. Santella and F. Perera. "Molecular Biology and Epidemiology of Cancer." *Cancer Prevention and Control*, edited by Greenwald, Peter et al. (National Cancer Institute, 1995), 83-86.

28. Taylor, L.H. Dr. Taylor was arrested, jailed, and held at $1 million bail in 1993; his offices and home were raided by the police and medical records and equipment were confiscated. In August of 1995, however, all 130 charges against Dr. Taylor were thrown out of court as being without legal merit, and his medical practice was restored. Even so, California medical authorities continue to seek grounds to revoke his license. Personal communications (1996).


## Part II: Criteria for Successful Cancer Treatment

### Chapter 24
### What Is Cancer?


1. Zajicek, G. "A New Cancer Hypothesis." *Medical Hypotheses* 47 (1996), 111-115.

2. Dr. Zajicek suggests that carcinogens deplete a vital metabolic substance, as yet not precisely identified; this depletion induces a state of progressive wasting and deterioration (called cachexia) and eventually the emergence of a tumor. Dr. Zajicek further suggests that the tumor arises as a self-protective mechanism of the body to replenish the missing substance; over

time, the tumor worsens and begins to seriously compromise the entire organism.

3. Dermer, G.B. "Contradictions of Stability and Differentation." *The Immortal Cell* (Garden City Park, NY: Avery Publishing, 1994), 47.

4. Blackburn, G. et al. "Developing Strategies for Intervention/Prevention Trials of Individuals at Risk of Hereditary Colon Cancer." *Journal of the National Cancer Institute Monographs* 17 (1995), 107-110.

5. Nash, J. Madeleine. "The Enemy Within." *Time* (Fall 1996), 20.

6. American Cancer Society. *Facts about Cancer* (Atlanta, GA: American Cancer Society, 1996).

7. Bailar, J.S., and E.M. Smith. "Progress Against Cancer?" *New England Journal of Medicine* 314 (1986), 1226.

8. Hankey, B. Chief of the Cancer Statistics Branch, National Cancer Institute. Personal communications (1994). The incidence of all cancers combined for the total population increased 13% from 1975 to 1989, from 332 per 100,000 to 376 per 100,000. The mortality rate rose 7%, from 162 deaths per 100,000 to 173 per 100,000.

9. National Cancer Institute. *Cancer Statistics Review, 1973-1989* (Washington, DC: National Institutes of Health, Office of Cancer Communications, 1992).

10. Henderson, B.E. et al. "Toward the Primary Prevention of Cancer." *Science* 254 (1991), 1131-1138. Cited in: McAllister, R.M. et al. *Cancer: What Cutting-Edge Science Can Tell You and Your Doctor about the Causes of Cancer and the Impact of Diagnosis and Treatment* (New York: HarperCollins, 1993), 3-4.

11. Meredith, Nikki. "Medical Dilemma." *Pacific Sun* (July 24-30, 1996), 11.

12. Nash, J. Madeleine. "The Enemy Within." *Time* (Fall 1996), 20.

13. Hankey, B. Chief of the Cancer Statistics Branch, National Cancer Institute. Personal communications (1994).

14. Beardsley, Tim. "A War Not Won." *Scientific American* (January 1994), 130-138.

15. Hankey, B. Chief of the Cancer Statistics Branch, National Cancer Institute. Personal communications (1994).

16. Schuette, et al. "The Costs of Cancer Care in the United States: Implications for Action." *Oncology* 9:11S (1995), 19-22.

17. Ibid. These costs include the estimates of the value of lost days of work due to illness, as well as the costs reflected in premature death of workers.

18. Hankey, B. Chief of the Cancer Statistics Branch, National Cancer Institute. Personal communications (1994).

19. Page, H.S., and A.J. Asire. *Cancer Rates and Risks* 3rd Edition. (Washington, DC: National Institutes of Health, 1985), 11. Cited by: Prescott, D.M., and A.S. Flexer. *Cancer: The Misguided Cell* 2nd Edition. (Sunderland, MA: Sinauer Associates, 1986), 224.

20. Rennie, John, and Ricki Rusting. "Making Headway Against Cancer." *Scientific American* (September 1996), 56-58.

21. Wilkens, Cheryl. "Daring to Heal My Cancer with Nutrition." *Alternative Medicine Digest* 6 (1995), 4-7.

22. Foster, H. "Lifestyle Changes and the Spontaneous Regression of Cancer: An Initial Computer Analysis." *International Journal of Biosocial Research* 10:1 (1988), 17-33.

## Chapter 25

## What Causes Cancer? Its Origin Is Multifactorial

1. Gerson, Max, M.D. *A Cancer Therapy. Results of Fifty Cases* (Bonita, CA: Gerson Institute, 1958), 102.

2. Becker, Robert O., M.D. *Cross Currents: The Promise of Electromedicine, The Perils of Electropollution* (Los Angeles: Jeremy P. Tarcher, 1990), 206.

3. Pizzorno, Joseph, N.D. *Total Wellness: Improve Your Health by Understanding the Body's Healing Systems* (Rocklin, CA: Prima Publishing, 1996), 24.

4. Weinberg, Robert A. *Racing to the Beginning of the Road. The Search for the Origin of Cancer* (New York: Harmony Books, 1996), 252.

5. Macek, C. "Of Mind and Morbidity: Can Stress and Grief Depress Immunity?" *Journal of the American Medical Association* 248:4 (1982), 405-407.

6. Havlik, R.J., A.P. Vukasin and S. Ariyan. "The Impact of Stress on the Clinical Presentation of Melanoma." *Plastic and Reconstructive Surgery* 90:1 (1992), 57-61.

7. Greene, M.H., T.I. Young and W.H. Clark. "Malignant Melanoma in Renal Transplant Recipients." *The Lancet* 1 (1981), 1196.

8. Herberman, R.B., and J.R. Ortaldo. "Natural Killer Cells: Their Role in Defenses Against Disease." *Science* 214 (1981), 24.

9. Calabrese, J.R. et al. "Alterations in Immunocompetence during Stress, Bereavement, and Depression: Focus on Neuroendocrine Regulation." *American Journal of Psychiatry* 144 (1987), 1123.

10. Adams, D.O. "Molecular Biology of Macrophage Activation: A Pathway Whereby Psychosocial Factors Can Potentially Affect Health." *Psychosomatic Medicine* 56 (1994), 316-327.

11. Boik, J. "The Immune System: Monocyte-macrophages." *Cancer and Natural Medicine* (Princeton, MN: Oregon Medical Press, 1996), 63.

12. Leffell, David J., and Douglas E. Brash. "Sunlight and Skin Cancer." *Scientific American* (July 1996), 52-59.

13. Mugh, T.H., II. "Studies Stir Fears over Cancer Risks for Children." *The Los Angeles Times* 111 (November 8, 1992), A1.

14. Holmberg, B. "Magnetic Fields and Cancer: Animal and Cellular Evidence—An Overview." *Environmental Health Perspectives* 103:Suppl 2 (1995), 63-67.

15. The Burton Goldberg Group. *Alternative Medicine: The Definitive Guide* (Tiburon, CA: Future Medicine Publishing, 1995), 332.

16. Ibid.

17. Pierpaoli, W., and W. Regelson. "A Powerful Protector and Treatment against Cancer." *The Melatonin Miracle* (New York: Simon & Schuster, 1995), 113-129.

18. Smith, Cyril W., and Simon Best. *Electromagnetic Man: Health and Hazard in the Electrical Environment.* (London: J.M. Dent & Sons, 1990), 172.

19. Knave, B. "Electric and Magnetic Fields and Health Outcomes—An Overview." *Scandinavian Journal of Work, Environment, and Health* (1994), 20 Spec No 78-89 Ref 136.

20. Ezzell, C. "Power-Line Static: Debates Rage over the Possible Hazards of Electromagnetic Fields." *Science News* 140 (September 1991), 202-203.

21. The Burton Goldberg Group. *Alternative Medicine: The Definitive Guide* (Tiburon, CA: Future Medicine Publishing, 1995), 332.

22. Ibid.

23. Savitz, D.A., and W.T. Kaune. "Childhood Cancer in Relation to a Modified Residential Wire Code." *Environmental Health Perspectives* 101:1 (1993), 76-80.

24. Feychting, M., and A. Ahlbom. "Childhood Leukemia and Residential Exposure to Weak Extremely Low Frequency Magnetic Fields." *Environmental Health Perspectives* 103:Suppl 2 (1995), 59-62.

25. Raloff, J. "EPA Suspects ELF Fields Can Cause Cancer." *Science News* 137 (June 30, 1990), 2-3.

26. Loomis, D.P. et al. "Breast Cancer Mortality among Female Electrical Workers in the United States." *Journal of the National Cancer Institute* 86:12 (1994), 921-925.

27. Pool, R. "Electromagnetic Fields: The Biological Evidence." *Science* 249 (1990), 1378-1381.

28. Ibid.

29. The Burton Goldberg Group. *Alternative Medicine: The Definitive Guide* (Tiburon, CA: Future Medicine Publishing, 1995), 332.

30. Ibid.

31. Ibid.

32. Ibid.

33. Ibid.

34. Edwards, R. "Leak Links Power Lines to Cancer." *New Scientist* 4 (October 7, 1995), 4.

35. Ezzell, C. "Power-Line Static: Debates Rage over the Possible Hazards of Electromagnetic Fields." *Science News* 140 (September 1991), 202-203.

36. Holmberg, B. "Magnetic Fields and Cancer: Animal and Cellular Evidence—An Overview." *Environmental Health Perspectives* Suppl 2 (1995), 63-67. See also: Decker, C. "ELF-zapped Genes Speed DNA Transcription." *Science News* (April 14, 1990), 229.

37. Goldberg, R.B., and W.A. Creasey. "A Review of Cancer Induction by Extremely Low-frequency Electromagnetic Fields: Is There a Plausible Mechanism?" *Medical Hypothesis* 35:3 (1991), 265-274.

38. Tenforde, T.S. "Biological Interactions and Potential Health Effects of Extremely Low-frequency Magnetic Fields from Power Lines and Other Common Sources." *Annual Review of Public Health* 13 (1992), 173-196.

39. Feychting, M., and A. Ahlbom. "Childhood Leukemia and Residential Exposure to Weak Extremely Low Frequency Magnetic Fields." *Environmental Health Perspectives* Suppl 2 (1995), 59-62. See also: Savitz, D.A. "Overview of Epidemiologic Research on Electric and Magnetic Fields and Cancer." *American Industrial Hygiene Association Journal* 54:4 (1993), 197-204.

40. Savitz, D.A., and D.P. Loomis. "Magnetic Field Exposure in Relation to Leukemia and Brain Cancer Mortality among Electric Utility Workers." *American Journal of Epidemiology* 141:2 (1995), 123-134. See also: Loomis, D.P., and D.A. Savitz. "Mortality from Brain Cancer and Leukemia among Electrical Workers." *British Journal of Industrial Medicine* 47:9 (1990), 633-638.

41. Loomis, D.P. et al. "Breast Cancer Mortality among Female Electrical Workers in the United States." *Journal of the National Cancer Institute* 86:12 (1994), 921-925.

42. Edwards, R. "Leak Links Power Lines to Cancer." *New Scientist* (October 7, 1995), 4.

43. The Burton Goldberg Group. *Alternative Medicine: The Definitive Guide* (Tiburon, CA: Future Medicine Publishing, 1995), 332.

44. von Pohl, Gustav Freiherr. *Earth Currents: Causative Factor of Cancer and Other Diseases* (Stuttgart, Germany: Frech-Verlag, 1983).

45. Nieper, Hans A., "Modern Medical Cancer Therapy Following the Decline of Toxic Chemotherapy." *Townsend Letter for Doctors & Patients* (November 1996), 88-89.

46. U.S. Department of Health, Education, and Welfare. *Geomagnetism, Cancer, Weather, and Cosmic Radiation* (Salt Lake City, UT: 1979).

47. Hodgson, Michael, M.D., M.P.H. "The Medical Evaluation" and "The Sick Building Syndrome: Effects of the Indoor Environment on Health." Cited in *Occupational Medicine: State of the Art Reviews* 10:1 (January-March 1995), 167-194.

48. Steinman, D. *Diet for a Poisoned Planet* (New York: Ballantine, 1992), 265.

49. Simone, C. B., M.D. *Cancer and Nutrition* (Garden City Park, NY: Avery Publishing, 1992), 20-21.

50. Beir, V. *Health Effects of Exposure to Low Levels of Ionizing Radiation.* Committee on the Biological Effects of Ionizing Radiations and the National Research Council (Washington, DC: National Academy Press, 1990).

51. Gofman, John W., M.D., Ph.D., and Egan O'Connor. *X Rays: Health Effects of Common Exams* (San Francisco: Sierra Club Books, 1985), 18.

52. Reid, W. Personal communications (1995). William Reid, M.D., is an oncologist-hematologist at the Biological Therapy Institute in Franklin, TN.

53. Wing, S. et al. "Mortality among Workers at Oak Ridge National Laboratory: Evidence of Radiation Effects in Follow-up Through 1984." *Journal of the American Medical Association* 265:11 (1991), 1397-1402.

54. Cancer Prevention Coalition. *Breast Cancer Deaths Linked to Nuclear Emissions* (New York: Cancer Prevention Coalition, 1994). This press release cites a 1991 article in the *Journal of the American Medical Association*, which claims "if...any excess cancer risk was present in U.S. counties with nuclear facilities, it

was too small to be detected with the methods employed." This study raises serious questions about the particular statistical methods used by NCI in that they used inappropriate controls based on small populations that were also exposed to nuclear emissions.

55. Sternglass, Ernest J., M.D. "Low-Level Radiation and the Deterioration of Human Health." Speech at the American Association of Naturopathic Physicians Conference (September 7-11, 1994).

56. Sternglass, E.J., and J.M. Gould. "Breast Cancer: Evidence for a Relation to Fission Products in the Diet." *International Journal of Health Services* 23:4 (1993), 783-804.

57. Holden, C. "Entomologists Wane as Insects Wax." *Science* 246 (1989), 754-756.

58. "Changing Profile of Pesticide Poisonings." *New England Journal of Medicine* 316:13 (1987), 807-809.

59. Wong-Anan, Nopporn. "Thai Horror Stories: Pesticide Misuse Taints Domestic and Export Produce." *The Wall Street Journal* (October 3, 1996).

60. Stewart, John Cary. *Drinking Water Hazards: How to Know if There are Toxic Chemicals in Your Water and What to Do If There Are* (Hiram, OH: Envirographics, 1990), 152.

61. Ibid., 158.

62. Wasserman, M. et al. "Organochlorine Compounds in Neoplastic and Adjacent Apparently Normal Breast Tissue." *Bulletin of Environmental Contaminants and Toxicology* 15 (1976), 478-484.

63. Westin, J., and E. Richter. "Israeli Breast Cancer Anomaly." *Annals of the New York Academy of Sciences* 609 (1990), 269-279.

64. Wolff, M.S. et al. "Blood Levels of Organochlorine Residues and Risk of Breast Cancer." *Journal of the National Cancer Institute* 85:8 (1993), 648-652. Cited in: Epstein, S., and D. Steinman. "Foods and Beverages." *The Safe Shopper's Bible: A Consumer's Guide to Nontoxic Household Products, Cosmetics, and Food* (New York: Macmillan, 1995), 296.

65. Rae, W. J., and H.C. Liang. "Effects of Pesticides on the Immune System." *Journal of Nutritional Medicine* 2 (1991), 399-410.

66. Associated Press. "Dirt with DDT from San Francisco Bay to be Buried at Arizona Site." *Marin Independent Journal* (August 30, 1996), A4.

67. The Burton Goldberg Group. *Alternative Medicine: The Definitive Guide* (Tiburon, CA: Future Medicine Publishing, 1995), 168.

68. Ibid.

69. "Risky Business: Has the Danger of Cancer from Pesticides Been Underrated?" *Scientific American* (May 1989), 35-36.

70. Sewell, B.H. "The Littlest Consumers: Exposure to Pesticide Residues in Childhood May Pose Lifelong Risks." *American Health* (May 1988).

71. Raloff, J. "Pesticides: The Human Body Burden." *Science News* (September 24, 1983), 199.

72. Falck, F., Jr. et al. "Pesticides and Polychlorinated Biphenyl Residues in Human Breast Lipids and their Relation to Breast Cancer." *Archives of Environmental Health* 47:2 (1992), 143-146.

73. Wolff, M.S. et al. "Blood Levels of Organochlorine Residues and Risk of Breast Cancer." *Journal of the National Cancer Institute* 85:8 (1993), 648-652.

74. Krieger, N. et al. "Breast Cancer and Serum Organochlorines: A Prospective Study Among White, Black, and Asian Women." *Journal of the National Cancer Institute* 86:8 (1994), 589-599.

75. *National Academy of Sciences 1984 Report on Pesticides and Cancer*. Note: These findings are based on the highest pesticide levels found in produce and assumes that consumers will not wash or cook their food.

76. Schechter, D. "Pesticides and Cancer." *Physicians Weekly* 5:9 (1988), 1.

77. Cantor, K.P. et al. "Pesticides and Other Agricultural Risk Factors for Non-Hodgkin's Lymphoma among Men in Iowa and Minnesota." *Cancer Research* 52:9 (1992), 2447-2455.

78. Hoar, S.K. et al. "Agricultural Herbicide Use and Risk of Lymphoma and Soft-tissue Sarcoma." *Journal of the American Medical Association* 256:9 (1986), 1141-1147.

79. Wiklund, K. et al. "Risk of Cancer in Pesticide Applicators in Swedish Agriculture." *British Journal of Industrial Medicine* 46:11 (1989), 809-814.

80. Lowengart, R. A. et al. "Childhood Leukemia and Parents' Occupational and Home Exposures." *Journal of the National Cancer Institute* 79:1 (July 1987), 39-46.

81. Davis, J. R. et al. "Family Pesticide Use and Childhood Brain Cancer." *Archives of Environmental Contamination and Toxicology* 24:1 (1993), 87-92.

82. "No Pest Strip Insecticide Poses an Unacceptably High Risk of Cancer in People and Pets." *Journal of Pesticide Reform* (Spring 1988), 29.

83. Ibid.

84. Fletcher, John. "More States Cracking Down on Use of Home Pesticides." *The Wall Street Journal* (October 18, 1996).

85. Arnold, Steven F. et al. "Synergistic Activation of Estrogen Receptor with Combinations of Environmental Chemicals." *Science* 272 (June 7, 1966), 1489.

86. Colborn, Theo, Dianne Dumanoski and John Peterson Wyers. *Our Stolen Future: Are We Threatening Our Fertility, Intelligence, and Survival?—A Scientific Detective Story* (New York: Dutton, 1996).

87. Nation, Nancy Isles. "Many With Breast Cancer Blame Marin." *Marin Independent Journal* (October 29, 1996).

88. Trichopoulos, Dimitrios, Frederick P. Li and David J. Hunter. "What Causes Cancer?" *Scientific American* (September 1996), 84.

89. Simone, Charles B., M. D. *Cancer & Nutrition* (Garden City Park, NY: Avery Publishing Group, 1992), 18, 21.

90. The Burton Goldberg Group. *Alternative Medicine: The Definitive Guide* (Tiburon, CA: Future Medicine Publishing, 1995), 186.

91. Ibid.

92. Stewart, John Cary. *Drinking Water Hazards: How to Know If There Are Toxic Chemicals in Your Water and What to Do If There Are* (Hiram, OH: Envirographics, 1990), 98, 107.

93. Lappenbusch, William L., Ph.D., *Contaminated Drinking Water and Your Health* (Alexandria, VA: Lappenbusch Environmental Health, 1986), 133.

94. "Stay Vigilant, MMWD." *Marin Independent Journal* (September 1, 1996).

95. Benson, Mitchel. "State EPA Study Finds PCE in Many Wells." *The Wall Street Journal* (October 2, 1996).

96. Maugh, T.H., II. "Experts Downplay Cancer Risk of Chlorinated Water." *The Los Angeles Times* (July 2, 199?).

97. Cousins, Gabriel, M.D. "Health Today." *New Frontier* (May 1994). See also: Valerian, Val. "On the Toxic Nature of Fluorides, Part 2: Fluorides and Cancer." *Perceptions* (September/October 1995), 30-37. See also: Glasser, George. "Dental Fluorosis: A Legal Time Bomb." *Health Freedom News* (July 1995), 40-46. See also: Yiamouyiannis, John, Ph.D. *Fluoride: The Aging Factor* (Delaware , OH: Health Action Press, 1993), 72-93.

98. Judd, G.J. "Mass Fluoridation Causes Alarming Rise in Cancer Deaths." *Health Freedom News* (May 1995), 10.

99. Yiamouyiannis, John, Ph.D. *Fluoride: The Aging Factor* (Delaware , OH: Health Action Press, 1993), 61. Dr. Yiamouyiannis also states: "It is quite clear that fluoride causes genetic damage... Most evidence indicates that fluoride acts on the DNA repair enzyme system... Furthermore, fluoride-induced genetic damage may also result from the general metabolic imbalance caused by fluoride selectively inhibiting certain enzymes."

100. Trichopoulos, Dimitrios, Frederick P. Li and David J. Hunter. "What Causes Cancer?" *Scientific American* (September 1996), 80-87.

101. American Cancer Society. *Cancer Facts & Figures* (Atlanta, GA: ACS. 1993). See also: Dreher, H. *Your Defense against Cancer* (New York: Harper & Row, 1988), 149-150.

102. Abramson, R. "EPA Officially Links Passive Smoke, Cancer." *The Los Angeles Times* (January 12, 1993), A27.

103. Trichopoulos, Dimitrios, Frederick P. Li and David J. Hunter. "What Causes Cancer?" *Scientific American* (September 1996), 85.

104. Simone, C.B. "Carcinogens in Tobacco Smoke." *Breast Health* (Garden City, NY: Avery Publishing, 1995), 134.

105. Dreher, H. *Your Defense against Cancer* (New York: Harper & Row, 1988), 200.

106. Hersey, et al. "Effects of Cigarette Smoking on the Immune System." *Medical Journal of Australia* 2:9 (1983), 425-429. See also: Ginns, et al. "Alterations in Immunoregulatory Cells in Lung Cancer and Smoking." *Journal of Clinical Immunology* Suppl 3 (1982), 90S-94S.

107. Simone, C.B., M.D. *Cancer and Nutrition* (Garden City Park, NY: Avery Publishing, 1992), 15.

108. Dreher, H. *Your Defense against Cancer* (New York: Harper & Row, 1988), 200.

109. Stout, David. "Direct Link Found Between Smoking and Lung Cancer." *The New York Times* (October 18, 1996). See also: Bishop, Jerry E., and Milo Geyelin. "Researchers Show How Smoking Causes Cancer." *The Wall Street Journal* (October 18, 1996).

110. Kushi, M. *The Cancer Prevention Diet* (New York: St. Martin's Press, 1983).

111. Hilts, Philip J. *Smokescreen: The Truth Behind the Tobacco Industry Cover-up* (Reading, MA: Addison-Wesley, 1996), 1-7.

112. Levy, Clifford J. "New York City Sues Big Tobacco Companies to Recover Billions in Health Costs." *The New York Times* (October 18, 1996).

113. Weinstein, A.L. et al. "Breast Cancer Risk and Oral Contraceptive Use: Results from a Large Case-Control Study." *Epidemiology* 2:5 (September 1991), 353-358.

114. Seaman, Barbara. *The Doctors' Case Against the Pill* (Alameda, CA: Hunter House, 1995), 124-134.

115. "Tranquilizers, Antidepressants Linked to Ovarian Cancer." *Medical Tribune for the Family Physician* 36:8 (April 20, 1995). See also: Goleman, Daniel. "Use of Antidepressant in Children at Issue." *The New York Times* (December 15, 1993).

116. Gilbert, Susan. "No Link is Found Between Pill and Cancer." *The New York Times* (September 25, 1996).

117. Minkin, Mary Jane, M.D., and Carol V. Wright. *What Every Woman Needs to Know about Menopause* (New Haven, CT: Yale University Press, 1996), 111-112.

118. Lee, John R., M.D. with Virginia Hopkins. *What Your Doctor May Not Tell You About Menopause* (New York: Warner Books, 1996), 223.

119. Epstein, Samuel S., M.D. "Unlabeled Milk from Cows Treated with Biosynthetic Growth Hormones: A Case of Regulatory Abdication." *International Journal of Health Services* 26:1 (1996), 173-185. See also: Jones, Suzanna. "BGH Meets Strong Opposition." *Food and Water Journal* (Winter 1996), 12-13.

120. Pizzorno, Joseph, N.D. *Total Wellness: Improve Your Health by Understanding the Body's Healing Systems* (Rocklin, CA: Prima Publishing, 1996), 55.

121. The Burton Goldberg Group. *Alternative Medicine: The Definitive Guide* (Tiburon, CA: Future Medicine Publishing, 1995), 170.

122. Rosenberg, B. "A Diner's Guide to Irradiation." *Science Digest* (September 1986), 30.

123. Mayell, M. "Zapping Your Daily Diet: The Risks of Irradiated Foods." *EastWest: The Journal of Natural Living* (February 1986), 36.

124. Ibid.

125. The Burton Goldberg Group. *Alternative Medicine: The Definitive Guide* (Tiburon, CA: Future Medicine Publishing, 1995), 170.

126. Ibid.

127. Dreher, H. *Your Defense Against Cancer* (New York: Harper & Row, 1988), 113.

128. Isaac, K., and S. Gold. "Some Chemicals Found in Food." *Eating Clean: Overcoming Food Hazards* (Washington, DC: Center for the Study of Responsive Law, 1990), 16.

129. Croce, P. "Think before You Sweeten." *Eating Clean: Overcoming Food Hazards* (Washington, DC: Center for the Study of Responsive Law, 1990), 52.

130. Jacobson, M. F. "Undoing Delaney: FDA Allows Free Use of Dangerous Additives." *Eating Clean: Overcoming Food Hazards* (Washington, DC: Center for

the Study of Responsive Law, 1990), 48-49.

131. Kudsk, F. "Uptake of Hg Vapors in Blood *In Vivo* and *In Vitro* from HG-containing Air." *Acta Pharmacologica et Toxicologica* 27 (1969), 49.

132. Meinig, George E., D.D.S. *Root Canal Cover-up* (Ojai, CA: Bion Publishing, 1994).

133. Royal, Daniel F., DO. "Health Hazard in Your Teeth." *Alternative Medicine Digest* 13 (1996), 40-44.

134. Ibid.

135. Shan, X. et al. "Glutathione-dependent Protection against Oxidative Injury." *Pharmacology and Therapeutics* 47 (1990), 61-71.

136. Hanson, M. "Effects of Inorganic Mercury on the Nervous System." Presented at the First Nordic Neuroscience Meeting. Hemsdal, Norway (1988).

137. Levine, S., and P. Kidd. *Antioxidant Adaptation: Its Role in Free Radical Pathology* (San Leandro, CA: Biocurrents Division, Allergy Research Group, 1986). Cited in: Strong, G.A. *Does Mercury from Dental Amalgam Contribute to Free Radical Pathology?* (Billings, MT: Strong Health Publications, 1995), 30-33.

138. Ibid.

139. The Burton Goldberg Group. *Alternative Medicine: The Definitive Guide* (Tiburon, CA: Future Medicine Publishing, 1995), 4.

140. Ibid., 5.

141. Ibid., 6.

142. Ibid., 7.

143. Ibid., 8.

144. Ibid., 9.

145. Ibid., 10.

146. Ibid., 14.

147. Blesius, C.K., M.D. "Dental Amalgam and Mercury." *Townsend Letter for Doctors & Patients* (October 1996), 86-91.

148. Thomsen, Joachim, D.D.S. "The Frequent Involvement of 'Vital' Teeth in Focal Disturbances." *American Journal of Acupuncture: Special EAV Issue* (1989), 94-99.

149. Bessen, Richard A. "Neurodegenerative Prion Diseases." *Science & Medicine* (September/October 1996), 13.

150. Klinghardt, Dietrich, M.D., Ph.D. "Neural Therapy." *Journal of Neurological Orthopedic Medical Surgery* 14 (1993), 109-114.

151. Committee on Diet, Nutrition and Cancer. Assembly of Life Sciences, National Research Council. *Diet, Nutrition and Cancer* (Washington, DC: National Academy Press, 1982).

152. Toniolo, P. et al. "Consumption of Meat, Animal Products, Protein and Fat and Risk of Breast Cancer: A Prospective Cohort Study in New York." *Epidemiology* 5:4 (1994), 391.

153. Giovannucci, E. et al. "A Prospective Study of Dietary Fat and Risk of Prostate Cancer." *Journal of the National Cancer Institute* 85:19 (1993), 1571.

154. Giovannucci, E. et al. "Intake of Fat, Meat and Fiber in Relation to Risk of Colon Cancer in Men." *Cancer Research* 54:9 (1994), 2390.

155. The Burton Goldberg Group. *Alternative Medicine: The Definitive Guide* (Tiburon, CA: Future Medicine Publishing, 1995), 171.

156. Ibid.

157. Ibid.

158. Campbell, T.C. Cornell University, Department of Nutrition. Personal communications (1995).

159. Committee On Diet, Nutrition and Cancer. Assembly of Life Sciences, National Research Council. *Diet, Nutrition and Cancer* (Washington, DC: National Academy Press, 1982).

160. "Breast Cancer Victims Unite." *San Francisco Examiner* (August 12, 1995). See also: "Energy Department Faces Vast Toxic-Waste Cleanup." *Marin Independent Journal* (September 18, 1995). See also: "Breast Health Update." *Energy Times* (July/August 1995).

161. The Burton Goldberg Group. *Alternative Medicine: The Definitive Guide* (Tiburon, CA: Future Medicine Publishing, 1995), 173.

162. "Is Our Fish Fit to Eat?" *Consumer Reports* (February 1992), 103-114.

163. Committee On Diet, Nutrition and Cancer. Assembly of Life Sciences, National Research Council. *Diet, Nutrition and Cancer* (Washington, DC: National Academy Press, 1982).

164. Simone, C.B., M.D. *Cancer and Nutrition* (Garden City Park, NY: Avery Publishing, 1992), 15.

165. Enig, M.G. et al. "Dietary Fat and Cancer Trends." *Federation Proceedings* 37 (1978), 2215-2220.

166. Alavanja, Michael, C.R., et al. "Estimating the Effect of Dietary Fat on the Risk of Lung Cancer in Nonsmoking Women." *Lung Cancer* 14:Suppl 1 (1996), S63-S74.

167. The Burton Goldberg Group. *Alternative Medicine: The Definitive Guide* (Tiburon, CA: Future Medicine Publishing, 1995), 185.

168. Ibid.

169. Simone, C.B. *Cancer and Nutrition* (Garden City Park, NY: Avery Publishing, 1992), 99.

170. Boik, J. "Humoral Factors that Affect Neoplasia: Eicosanoids." *Cancer and Natural Medicine* (Princeton, MN: Oregon Medical Press, 1995), 46-49.

171. Bougnoux, P. et al. "Alpha-linolenic Acid Content of Adipose Breast Tissue: A Host Determinant of the Risk of Early Metastasis in Breast Cancer." *British Journal of Cancer* 70:2 (1994), 330-334.

172. Horobin, D.F. "The Regulation of Prostaglandin Biosynthesis." *Medical Hypothesis* 6 (1980), 687-709.

173. Jones, W.B. "The Effects of Aspirin on Gastric Prostaglandins." *Annals of Internal Medicine* 121 (1994), 72.

174. Thun, M.J. "Aspirin, NSAIDs, and Digestive Tract Cancers." *Cancer and Metastasis Reviews* 13 (1994), 269-277.

175. Tamari, G.M. "To Prevent CHD and Cancer: ASA or EFA?" *Townsend Letter for Doctors & Patients* (May 1995), 71-74.

176. Bristol, J.B. "Colorectal Cancer and Diet: A Case-Control Study with Special Reference to Dietary Fibre and Sugar." *Proceedings of the American Association of Cancer Research* 26 (March 1985), 206. See also: Bristol, J.B. et al. "Sugar, Fat and the Risk of Colorectal Cancer." *British Medical Journal* Clinical Research

Edition 291:6507 (November 1985), 1467-1470.

177. Pizzorno, Joseph, N.D. *Total Wellness: Improve Your Health by Understanding the Body's Healing Systems* (Rocklin, CA: Prima Publishing, 1996), 39-40.

178. Quillan, P. "Bioenergetics." *Beating Cancer With Nutrition* (Tulsa, OK: Nutrition Times Press, 1994), 112.

179. Hsing, A.W. et al. "Cancer Risk Following Primary Hemochromatosis: A Population-based Cohort Study in Denmark." *Journal of Cancer* (1995), 160-162.

180. Knekt, P. et al. "Body Iron Stores and Risk of Cancer." *International Journal of Cancer* 56 (1994), 379-382. See also: Sevenes, R.G. et al. "Moderate Elevation of Body Iron Level and Increased Risk of Cancer Occurrence and Death." *Journal of Cancer* 56 (1994), 364-369.

181. Giovannucci, E., and W.C. Willett. "Dietary Lipids and Colon Cancer." *PPO Updates: Principles and Practice of Oncology* 9:5 (1995), 1-12.

182. Sandler, R.S. "Diet and Cancer: Food Additives, Coffee, and Alcohol." *Nutrition and Cancer* 4:4 (1983), 273-278. See also: "Beer Drinking and the Risk of Rectal Cancer." *Nutrition Reviews* 42:7 (July 1984), 244-247. See also: Potter, J.D., and A.J. McMichael. "Alcohol, Beer and Lung Cancer: A Meaningful Relationship?" *International Journal of Epidemiology* 13:2 (June 1984), 240-242.

183. Simone, C.B. *Breast Health* (Garden City Park, NY: Avery Publishing, 1995), 143.

184. Simon, D. et al. "Coffee Drinking and Cancer of the Lower Urinary Tract System." *Journal of the National Cancer Institute* 54:3 (1975), 587.

185. Mulvihill, J. "Caffeine as a Teratogen and Mutagen." *Teratology* 8:69 (1973). See also: Weinstein, D. et al. "The Effects of Caffeine on Chromosomes of Human Lymphocytes." *Mutation Research* 16 (1972), 391.

186. Schellhardt, Timothy D. "Company Memo to Stressed-Out Employees: 'Deal With It'." *The Wall Street Journal* (October 2, 1996).

187. Marx, J.L. "The Immune System 'Belongs to the Body'." *Science* 277 (1985), 1190-1192.

188. Schleifer, S.J., S.E. Keller and M. Stein. "Central Nervous System Mechanisms and Immunity: Implications for Tumor Reponse." Cited in: Levy, S.M. *Behavior and Cancer* (San Francisco: Jossey-Bass, 1985), 130-133. See also: Borysenko, M., and J. Borysenko. "Stress, Behavior and Immunity." *General Hospital Psychiatry* 4 (1985), 59-67.

189. Pettingale, K.W. "Towards a Psychobiological Model of Cancer: Biological Considerations." *Social Science & Medicine* 20 (1985), 179-187. See also: Lippman, M.E. "Psychosocial Factors and the Hormonal Regulation of Tumor Growth." *Behavior and Cancer*, edited by Levy, S.M. (San Francisco: Jossey-Bass, 1985), 134-147.

190. Forsen, A. "Psychosocial Stress as a Risk for Breast Cancer." *Psychotherapy and Psychosomatics* 55 (1991), 176-185.

191. Schleifer, S.J. et al. "Suppression of Lymphocyte Stimulation Following Bereavement." *Journal of the American Medical Association* 250 (1983), 374.

192. Arnetz, B.B. et al. "Immune Function in Unemployed Women." *Psychosomatic Medicine* 49 (1987), 3.

193. Adler, R. *Psychoneuroimmunology* (New York: Academic Press, 1981).

194. Bloom, B.L., S.J. Asher and S.W. White. "Marital Disruption as a Stressor: A Review and Analysis." *Psychological Bulletin* 85:4 (1978), 867-894.

195. Ibid. See also: LeShan, L.L. "An Emotional Life History Pattern Associated with Neoplastic Disease." *Annals of the New York Academy of Sciences* 125:3 (1966), 780-793. Also: Ernster, B.L. et al. "Cancer Incidence by Marital Status: U.S. Third National Cancer Survey." *Journal of the National Cancer Institute* 63:3 (1979), 567-585.

196. Greer, S., and T. Morris. "Psychological Attributes of Women Who Develop Breast Cancer: A Controlled Study." *Journal of Psychosomatic Research* 19:2 (1975), 147-153.

197. Rogentine, G.N., Jr. et al. "Psychological Factors in the Prognosis of Malignant Melanoma: A Prospective Study." *Psychosomatic Medicine* 41 (1979), 647-655. See also: Greer, S., and T. Morris. "Psychological Attributes of Women Who Develop Breast Cancer: A Controlled Study." *Journal of Psychosomatic Research* 19 (1975), 147-153.

198. Northrup, Christiane, M.D. *Women's Bodies, Women's Wisdom* (New York: Bantam, 1994), 35-40.

199. Greer, S. "Psycho-oncology: Its Aims, Achievements and Future Tasks." *Psycho-Oncology* 3 (1994), 87-101. Eight prospective studies are cited: Schmale and Iker, 1971. Wiesman and Worden, 1977. Greer, et al., 1979. Di Clemente and Temoshok, 1985. Goodkin, et al., 1986. Jensen, 1987. Wirsching, et al., 1988. Morris, et al., 1992.

200. Ader, R. et al. *Psychoneuroimmunology* 2nd edition. (San Diego, CA: Academic Press, 1991), xxv.

201. Ader, R., and N. Cohen. "Behaviorally Conditioned Immunosuppression." *Psychosomatic Medicine* 37 (1975), 333.

202. Borysenko, M., and J. Borysenko. "Stress, Behavior and Immunity." *General Hospital Psychiatry* 4 (1985), 59-67.

203. Shakin, E.J. et al. "Psychiatric Complications of Cancer." *Complications of Cancer Management*, edited by Plowman, P.N., T. McElwain and A. Meadows. (Oxford: Butterworth-Heineman, 1991), 423-435.

204. Grossarth-Maticek, R. et al. "Interpersonal Repression as a Predictor of Cancer." *Social Science & Medicine* 16 (1982), 493-498.

205. Dattore, P. et al. "Premorbid Personality Differentiation of Cancer and Non-cancer Groups." *Journal of Counseling and Clinical Psychology* 48:3 (1980), 388-394.

206. Shaffer, J.W. et al. "Clustering of Personality Traits in Youth and the Subsequent Development of Cancer among Physicians." *Journal of Behavioral Medicine* 10:5 (1987), 441-448. See also: Graves, P.L. et al. "Familial and Psychological Predictors of Cancer." *Cancer Detection and Prevention* 15:1 (1991), 59-64.

207. Goodwin, J.S. et al. "The Effect of Marital Status on Stage, Treatment and Survival of Cancer Patients." *Journal of the American Medical Association* 258:21 (1987), 3125-3130.

208. Greer, S., and T. Morris. "Psychological Attributes of

Women Who Develop Breast Cancer: A Controlled Study." *Journal of Psychosomatic Research* 19 (1975), 147.

209. Bower, B. "Hopelessness Tied to Heart, Cancer Deaths." *Science News* 149:15 (April 13, 1996).

210. Petet, J.R. et al. "Emotional Support for Patients with Cancer Who Are Undergoing CT; Semistructured Interviews of Patients at a Cancer Institute." *Radiology* 182:1 (1992) 99-102.

211. Mehl, L. "Mind and Breathing." *Mind and Matter* (Berkeley, CA: Mindbody Press, 1986), 196.

212. Schimmel and Utiger. "Thyroid and Peripheral Production of Thyroid Hormones."*Annals of Internal Medicine* 87 (1970), 760-768. Apparently there are 2 key enzymes in the body which can act on and convert 4 thyroid hormones by cleaving off 1 of the 4 iodines from the T4 molecule. If the correct enzyme acted upon the T4 and the correct iodine was cleaved off, then active T3 thyroid hormone was formed that would bind to a receptor on a cell and have a significant action within the cell. If the wrong enzyme was activated by emotional or physical stress or by infections, then the incorrect iodine was cleaved off the T4 hormone and an inactive reverse T3 hormone would be formed. If the reverse T3 hormone became bound to the cell receptor site where T3 should bind, then no action would occur inside the cell and T3 would be competitively blocked from binding to that receptor site. In addition, the reverse T3 would also bind to the normal enzyme that is supposed to cleave the correct iodine off the T4 hormone and prevent T4 from binding to that enzyme, thus preventing the formation of active T3 hormone.

213. Davies, Daniel T., and James T.G. Illtyd. "An Investigation into the Gastric Secretion of a Hundred Normal Persons over the Age of Sixty." *Quarterly Journal of Medicine* 24 (1930), 1-4. See also: Rafsky, Henry A., and Michael Weingarten. "A Study of Gastric Secretory Response in the Aged." *Gastroenterology* 8 (1947), 348-352. See also: Montgomery, R.D. et. al. "The Aging Gut: A Study of Intestinal Absorption in Relation to Nutrition in the Elderly." *Quarterly Journal of Medicine* 47 (1978), 197-211.

214. Guyton, Arthur C., M.D., and John E. Hall, M.D. "Secretory Functions of the Alimentary Tract" *Textbook of Medical Physiology* (Philadelphia, PA: W.B. Saunders, 1996), 825.

215. The hydrochloric acid and pepsin production in the stomach can usually be restored by eliminating these causes of parietal cell damage and by doing different types of stress reduction techniques and taking herbs that help to heal the lining of the stomach (cabbage, aloe vera, licorice, etc.). If the hydrochloric acid and pancreatic function are both impaired, usually restoring the hydrochloric acid function of the stomach will help to restore the pancreatic function unless there are parasites in the pancreas or stones or a tumor in the pancreatic duct. By using this approach to restore the function of the stomach lining and pancreas, the individual often needs supplemental enzymes or betaine hydrochloride for a period of only 4 to 12 months rather than for life.

216. Gittleman, Ann Louise. *Guess What Came to Dinner: Parasites and Your Health* (Garden City, NY: Avery Publishing, 1993).

217. Clark, Hulda Regehr, Ph.D., N.D. *The Cure for All Cancers* (San Diego, CA: ProMotion Publishing, 1993), 1-20.

218. Trichopoulos, Dimitrios, Frederick P. Li, and David J. Hunter. "What Causes Cancer?" *Scientific American* (September 1996), 82-83.

219. Pizzorno, Joseph, N.D. *Total Wellness: Improve Your Health by Understanding the Body's Healing Systems* (Rocklin, CA: Prima Publishing, 1996), 93-94.

220. Haseman, J.K. "Issues in Carcinogenicity Testing: Dose Selection." *Fundamental and Applied Toxicology* 5 (1985), 66-78.

221. Munro, I.C. "Considerations in Chronic Toxicity Testing: The Chemical, the Dose, the Design." *Journal of Environmental Pathology and Toxicology* 1 (1977), 183-197.

222. Kinsella, A.R., and M. Radman. "Tumor Promoter Induces Sister Chromatid Exchanges." *Proceedings of the National Academy of Sciences* 75 (1978), 6149-6153.

223. Issels, J. "More Cures for Cancer." Transl. from German. (Bad Homburg, Germany: Helfer Publishing, 1995), 19.

224. Quoted in: Weinberg, Robert A. *Racing to the Beginning of the Road: The Search for the Origin of Cancer* (New York: Harmony Books, 1996), 11.

225. Warburg, O. "On the Origin of Cancer Cells." *Science* 123 (1956), 309-315.

226. Walters, R. "Enderlein Therapy: A Cancer Therapy that Promotes Gentle Self-healing." *Raum & Zeit* 3:1 (1991), 24.

227. Thomas, Gordon. *Dr. Issels and His Revolutionary Cancer Treatment* (New York: Peter H. Wyden, 1973), 137-138.

228. Walters, R. "Enderlein Therapy: A Cancer Therapy that Promotes Gentle Self-healing." *Raum & Zeit* 3:1 (1991), 24.

229. Ibid.

230. Ibid.

231. McAllister, Robert M., M.D., Sylvia Teich Horowitz, Ph.D., and Raymond V. Gilden, Ph.D. *Cancer* (New York: Basic Books, 1993), 39-43.

232. Govallo, Valentin, M.D. *Immunology of Pregnancy and Cancer* (Comack, NY: Nova Science Publishers, 1993), 140.

233. McAllister, Robert M., M.D., Sylvia Teich Horowitz, Ph.D., and Raymond V. Gilden, Ph.D. *Cancer* (New York: Basic Books, 1993), 68-69.

234. Zakour, R.A., T.A. Kunkel and L.A. Loeb. "Metal-Induced Infidelity of DNA Synthesis." *Environmental Health Perspectives* 40 (August 1981), 197-205.

235. Kiecolt-Glaser, J.K. et al. "Distress and DNA Repair in Human Lymphocytes." *Journal of Behavioral Medicine* 8 (1985), 311-320.

236. Boik, J. Personal communications (1996).

237. Travis, J. "Putting Tumor Suppressor Back to Work." *Science News* (August 31, 1996), 134.

238. Perera, F.P. "Uncovering New Clues to Cancer Risk." *Scientific American* (May 1996), 54-62.

239. Angier, Natalie. "Surprising Role Found for Breast Cancer Gene." *The New York Times* (March 5, 1996).

240. Kolata, Gina. "2nd Breast Cancer Gene Found in Jewish Women." *The New York Times* (October 2, 1996).

241. Vithoulkas, George. *The Science of Homeopathy* (New York: Grove Press, 1980), 121.

## Chapter 26

## How Cancer Politics Have Kept You in the Dark Regarding Successful Alternative Treatments

1. American Cancer Society. *Cancer Facts & Figures* (Atlanta, GA: ACS. 1988).

2. Ibid., 26.

3. Schuette, H.L. et al. "The Costs of Cancer Care in the United States: Implications for Action." *Oncology* 9:11 Suppl (1995), 19-22.

4. Brown, M.L.. "Special Report: The National Economic Burden of Cancer: An Update." *Journal of the National Cancer Institute* 82 (1990), 1811-1814.

5. Moss, R. "Relative Values of Cancer Treatments." *Questioning Chemotherapy* (Brooklyn, NY: Equinox Press, 1995), 78. See also: Tattersall, M.H.N., and M.L. Frielander. "Cost Considerations in Cancer Chemotherapy." *Aust Health Rev* 5 (1982), 21-24.

6. Kolata, G. "Women Resist Trials to Test Marrow Transplants." *The New York Times* (February 15, 1995).

7. Riley, GF, et al. "Medicare Payments from Diagnosis to Death for Elderly Cancer Patients by Stage of Diagnosis." *Medical Care* 33 (1995), 828-841.

8. Brown, M.L., and L. Fintor. "The Economic Burden of Cancer." *Cancer Prevention and Control* (New York: Marcel Dekker, 1995).

9. Moss, R. "The Cancer Establishment." *The Cancer Industry* (Brooklyn, NY: Equinox Press, 1996), 389-419.

10. Ibid.

11. Yergin, Daniel. *The Prize: The Epic Quest for Oil, Money, and Power* (New York: Simon & Schuster, 1991).

12. Griffin, G. Edward. *World Without Cancer: The Story of Vitamin B17* (Westlake Village, CA: American Media, 1974). Much of the documentation for the I.G. Farben and Rockefeller involvement comes from Griffin's research.

13. Starr, Paul, *The Social Transformation of American Medicine* (New York: Basic Books, 1982).

14. Coulter, H. L. *Divided Legacy: A History of the Schism in Medical Thought, Vol. IV. Twentieth-Century Medicine: The Bacteriological Era* (Berkeley, CA: Center for Empirical Medicine and North Atlantic Books, 1994).

15. American Cancer Society. *Cancer Facts & Figures: The American Cancer Society Profile* (Atlanta, GA: ACS. 1992), 21.

16. American Cancer Society. *Cancer Facts & Figures: Allocation of American Cancer Society Funds* (Atlanta, GA: ACS, 1992), 22.

17. Chowka, P.B., "Cancer Research: The $20 Billion Failure." *EastWest: The Journal of Natural Living* (March, 1981), 45.

18. Bennett, J. T., and T. DiLorenzo. *Unhealthy Charities: Hazardous to Your Health and Wealth* (New York: Basic Books, 1994).

19. Moss, R. "The Cancer Establishment." *The Cancer Industry* (Brooklyn, NY: Equinox Press, 1996), 405.

20. Colby, M. "Losing the War on Cancer after 20 years. Cancer Establishment Makes False Claims; Massive Reforms Urged by Scientists, Doctors." Food & Water Inc., news release (February 4, 1992).

21. Ibid.

22. Moss, R. "The Cancer Establishment." *The Cancer Industry* (Brooklyn, NY: Equinox Press, 1996), 406.

23. Ibid., 407.

24. Epstein, S. *Evaluation of the National Cancer Program and Proposed Reform* (Chicago: University of Illinois Medical Center/School of Public Health). In press.

25. Ibid., 10.

26. Seoud, M.A. et al. "Gynecologic Tumors in Tamoxifen-Treated Women with Breast Cancer." *Obstetrics and Gynecology* 82 (1993), 165.

27. Fugh-Berman, A. *Alternative Medicine: What Works* (Tucson, AZ: Odonian Press, 1996), 18.

28. Brown, R. K., M.D. *AIDS, Cancer, and the Medical Establishment* (New York: Trizoid Press, 1993).

29. Moss, R. "The Cancer Establishment." *The Cancer Industry* (Brooklyn, NY: Equinox Press, 1996), 415.

30. Lynes, Barry. *The Healing of Cancer* (Wilmington, DE: Marcus Books, 1992).

31. Sharaf, M. "Medical Effects of the Orgone Accumulator." *Fury on Earth* (New York: St. Martin's Press, 1983), 302-310.

32. Anson, S. "Ozone therapy." *LA Village View* (June 16, 1995), 33.

33. Ibid., 34.

34. Wilkes, M.S., M.D. et al. "Pharmaceutical Advertisements in Leading Medical Journals: Expert's Assessments." *Annals of Internal Medicine* 116 (1992), 912-919.

35. Holt, S. "Cartilage and Nutriceutical Update." *Alternative & Complementary Therapies* 1:6 (1995), 51-54.

36. Coulter, Harris L. *Divided Legacy: The Conflict between Homoeopathy and the American Medical Association. Science and Ethics in American Medicine, 1800-1914* (Richmond, VA: North Atlantic Books, 1973).

37. Wolinsky, H., and T. Brune. *The Serpent on the Staff: The Unhealthy Politics of the American Medical Association* (New York: Jeremy P. Tarcher/G.P. Putnam's Sons, 1994).

38. Kamen, J. "From Russia with Love: Stonewalled in the U.S.A." *Penthouse* (July 1994), 31.

39. Ibid.

40. Kamen, J. "Hope, Heartbreak, and Horror." *Omni* (September 1993).

41. Sugiura, K. Unpublished taped interview (July 1974). Cited in: Moss, R. "Laetrile at Sloan-Kettering." *The Cancer Industry* (New York: Equinox Press, 1996), 158.

42. Ibid.

43. This model is characterized by a focus on the organic mechanisms and physiological causes of disease, and the indispensability of medical intervention following the onset of a disease.

44. Editorial. "Burzynski's Antineoplastons Increase Activity of Tumor Suppressor Genes." *Options* (June 1995), 2. 86th Annual Meeting of the American Assocation for Cancer Research (March 1995).

45. Burzynski, S.R. et al. "Antineoplaston A in Cancer Therapy (I)." *Physiological Chemistry and Physics* 6:9 (1977), 485-500.

46. Smith, M.E.G. "The Burzynski Controversy in the United States and in Canada: A Comparative Case Study in the Sociology of Alternative Medicine." *Canadian Journal of Sociology* 17:2 (1992), 133-159.

47. Ibid.

48. Scheer, J. F. "Burzynski Angered by NCI Discredibility Attempts." *Health Freedom News* (February 1996), 16-18.

49. Ibid.

50. NCI minutes of the Decision Network Committee meeting. A copy of the minutes appears in *Health Freedom News* (February 1996), 16-18.

51. Dermer, Gerald B., Ph.D. *The Immortal Cell: Why Cancer Research Fails* (Garden City Park, NY: Avery Publishing, 1994).

52. Culbert, Michael L., D.Sc. *Medical Armageddon: Behind the Healthcare Calamity of the Western World and How to Fix It* (San Diego, CA: C and C Communications, 1995).

53. Bird, C. "What Has Become of the Rife Microscope?" *NAJ* 43 (1984). See also: "Filtrable Bodies Seen with the Rife Microscope." *Science* Suppl (December 11, 1931).

54. "Questionable Methods of Cancer Management: Electronic Devices." *CA: A Cancer Journal for Clinicians* 44 (1994), 115-127. This was a public relations report for the American Cancer Society.

55. Colby, M. "Losing the War on Cancer after 20 Years. Cancer Establishment Makes False Claims; Massive Reforms Urged by Scientists, Doctors." Food & Water Inc., news release (February 4, 1992).

56. Edell, D. "Declare War on Cancer Quackery" *The Edell Health Letter* (February 1992), 2.

57. The articles in question are: "On Fringes of Health Care, Untested Therapies Thrive." *The New York Times* (June 17, 1996); "In Quests Outside Mainstream, Medical Projects Rewrite Rules." *The New York Times* (June 18, 1996); "Doctor's Cancer 'Cure' Attacked by FDA." *The New York Times* (July 24, 1996).

58. Aulas, Jean-Jacque. "Alternative Cancer Treatments." *Scientific American* 275:3 (September 1995).

59. Proctor, R.N. *Cancer Wars: How Politics Shapes What We Know and Don't Know about Cancer* (New York: Basic Books, 1995).

60. Whitaker, J. "Everyone's Health Is at Stake If We Lose This Therapy." *Health & Healing Supplement* (February 1996), 4.

61. Ibid., 5.

62. Best, B. "A Chemotherapy Runaway Alive and Well on Essiac and 714-x." *Options* (October 1995), 8.

63. Associated Press. "Cancer Patient, 6, Seized in Contra Costa." (1995).

64. McGrady, Patrick M. "The Revocation of Dr. Glenn Warner's License Is Unjust and Cruel." *Townsend Letter for Doctors & Patients* (August/September 1996).

65. Klotter, Jule. "Glenn Warner." *Townsend Letter for Doctors & Patients* (November 1996), 14.


## Chapter 27

# Early Detection and Prevention of Cancer


1. Morra, M., and E. Potts. "Diagnostic Tests." *Choices: Realistic Alternatives in Cancer Treatment* (New York: Avon, 1987), 97.

2. Scardino, P.T. "Early Detection of Prostate Cancer." *Urologic Clinics of North America* 16 (1989), 635-655.

3. McDonagh, E.W. "Detecting Cancer." *Townsend Letter for Doctors & Patients* (February/March 1996), 108-110.

4. Waterbor, J.W., and A.J. Bueschen. "Prostate Cancer Screening." *Cancer Causes and Control* 6 (1995), 267-274.

5. American Cancer Society. *Prostate Cancer Information* (Atlanta, GA: ACS, 1995).

6. Skerrett, P.J. "Screening for Prostate Cancer." *Technology Review* 8-9 (1994), 16-17.

7. Editorial. "The PSA Debate Continues." *John Hopkins Medical Letter* (February 1995), 3.

8. Garnick, M.B. "The Dilemmas of Prostate Cancer." *Scientific American* (April 1994), 72.

9. Editorial. "The PSA Debate Continues." *Johns Hopkins Medical Letter* (February 1995), 2.

10. Waterbor, J.W., and A.J. Bueschen. "Prostate Cancer Screening." *Cancer Causes and Control* 6 (1995), 267-274.

11. Skerrett, P.J. "Screening for Prostate Cancer." *Technology Review* 8-9 (1994), 16-17.

12. American Cancer Society. *Prostate Cancer Information* (Atlanta, GA: ACS, 1995).

13. Baran, G.W. et al. "Biological Aggressiveness of Palpable and Nonpalpable Prostate Cancer: Assessment with Endosonography." *Radiology* 178 (1991), 201-206.

14. Skerrett, P.J. "Screening for Prostate Cancer." *Technology Review* 8-9 (1994), 16-17.

15. Catalona, W.J. "Management of Cancer of the Prostate." *New England Journal of Medicine* 331:15 (1994), 996-1003.

16. Fowler, F.J. "Prostate Conditions, Treatment Decisions, and Patient Preferences." *Journal of the American Geriatrics Society* 43:9 (1995), 1058-1060.

17. Schardt, D. "The Cancer Men Don't Talk About." *Nutrition Action* 20:1 (1993), 1-6.

18. Whittemore, A. S. et al. "Prostate Cancer in Relation to Diet, Physical Activity, and Body Size in Blacks, Whites, and Asians in the United States and Canada." *Journal of the National Cancer Institute* 87:9 (1995), 652-661.

19. Mills, P.K. et al. "Cohort Study of Diet, Lifestyle and Prostate Cancer in Adventist Men." *Cancer* 64 (1989), 598-604. See also: Oishi, K. et al. "A Case-Control Study of Prostatic Cancer with Reference to Dietary Habits." *The Prostate* 12 (1988), 179-190.

20. "Tomatoes Prevent Cancer." Associated Press (December 6, 1995). Commentary on a report that appeared in the *Journal of the National Cancer Institute.*

21. Wynder, E. L. "Research on Omega 3 Fatty Acids." Cited by: Challem, J. "Prevent Prostate Cancer and Other Male Problems" *Let's Live* (July 1995), 14-26.

22. Karmah, R. et al. "The Effects of Dietary Omega-3 Fatty Acids on DU-145 Transplantable Human Prostate Tumors." *Antioxidant Research* 7 (1987), 1173-1179.

23. Webber, M.M. "Inhibitory Effects of Selenium on the Growth of DU-145 Human Prostate Carcinoma Cells *In Vitro*." *Biochemical and Biophysical Research Communications* 130:2 (1985), 603-609.

24. Webber, M.M. "Selenium Prevents the Growth Stimulatory Effects of Cadmium on Human Prostatic Epithelium." *Biochemical and Biophysical Research Communications* 127:3 (1985), 871-877.

25. Aldercreutz, H. et al. "Plasma Concentrations of Phytoestrogens in Japanese Men." *The Lancet* 342:8881 (1993), 1209-1210.

26. Linehan, W. "Inhibition of Prostate Cancer Metastasis: A Critical Challenge Ahead." *Journal of the National Cancer Institute* 87 (1995), 348-352.

27. Oliveria, S.A. et al. "The Association between Cardiorespiratory Fitness and Prostate Cancer." *Medicine and Science in Sports and Exercise* 28:1 (1996), 97-104.

28. Nelson, et al. *Proceedings of the National Academy of Sciences USA* 91 (1994), 11733-11737.

29. Gann, P.H. et al. "Prospective Study of Plasma Fatty Acids and Risk of Prostate Cancer." *Journal of the National Cancer Institute* 86 (1994), 281-286.

30. NIH Publication 94-2079. *Eating Hints for Cancer Patients* (Washington, DC: U.S. Department of Health & Human Services, National Cancer Institute, 1994).

31. Kushi, L. Personal communications with Michael Lerner, Ph.D (January 24, 1991). See also: Lerner, M. *Healing Choices* (Boston: MIT Press, 1994), 344.

32. Brody, Jane. "Discovery on Prostate Cancer." *The New York Times* (October 15, 1996).

33. Parker, S.L. et al. "Cancer Statistics 1996." *CA: A Cancer Journal for Clinicians* 46 (1996), 5-27.

34. Licciardone, J.C. et al. "Cigarette Smoking and Alcohol Consumption in the Etiology of Uterine Cervical Cancer." *International Journal of Epidemiology* 18:3 (1989), 533-537.

35. Graham, I.T. et al. "Cigarette Smoking and the Incidence of Cervical Intraepithelial Neoplasia, Grade III, and Cancer of the Cervix Uteri." *American Journal of Epidemiology* 135:4 (1992), 341-346.

36. Szarewski, A. "Effect of Smoking Cessation on Cervical Lesion Size." *The Lancet* 347:9006 (1996), 941-943.

37. American Cancer Society. *Information on Smoking-Related Cancer Risks* (Atlanta, GA: ACS, 1996).

38. Rosenthal, Dorothy, M.D. et al. "Computer-assisted Rescreening of Clinically Important False Negative Cervical Smears Using the PAPNET Testing System." *Acta Cytologica* 40:1 (January-February 1996). See also: Koss, Leopold G., M.D. "Reducing the Error Rate in Papanicolaou Smears." *The Female Patient* 19:6 (June 1994).

39. Meyskens, F.L., and A. Manetta. "Prevention of Cervical Intraepithelial Neoplasia and Cervical Cancer." *American Journal of Clinical Nutrition* 62:Suppl (1995), 1417S-1419S.

40. Passwater, R.A. "Cervical Cancer." *Cancer Prevention and Nutritional Therapies* (New Canaan, CT: Keats Publishing, 1993). This conclusion is based on Dr. Passwater's assessment of 9 studies published in peer-review journals, all listed on page 184.

41. Butterworth, C.E. "Effect of Folate on Cervical Cancer: Synergism among Risk Factors." *Annals of the New York Academy of Sciences* 669 (1992), 293-299.

42. Delgado-Rodgriguez, M. et al. "Oral Contraceptives and Cancer of the Cervix Uteri: A Meta-Analysis." *Acta Obstetricia et Gynecologica Scandinavica* 71:5 (1992), 368-376.

43. Ibid.

44. Parker, S.L. et al. "Cancer Statistics 1996." *CA: A Cancer Journal for Clinicians* 46 (1996), 5-27.

45. Petrek, J.A., and A.I. Holleb. "The Foremost Cancer—Revisited." *CA: A Cancer Journal for Clinicians* 45:4 (1995), 197-243.

46. Kenny, E. et al. "Breast Self-examination among College Women: Predictors for Cancer Control." *American Journal of Preventive Medicine* 5 (1989), 27-33.

47. Kash, K.M. et al. "Psychological Distress and Surveillance Behaviors of Women with a Family History of Breast Cancer." *Journal of the National Cancer Institute* 84 (1992), 24-30.

48. Donoghue, Elizabeth. "BCA Reader Survey Results Are In." *Breast Cancer Action Newsletter* 38 (October/November 1996), 5.

49. McKeenna, R.J. "The Abnormal Mammogram Radiographic Findings, Diagnostic Options, Pathology, and Stage of Cancer Diagnosis." *Cancer* 74 (1994), 244-255. See also: Radford, D.M. et al. "Pathology and Treatment of Impalpable Breast Lesions." *American Journal of Surgery* 164 (1992), 427-431.

50. Pelton, R. et al. "Does Mammography Extend and Save Lives?" *How to Prevent Breast Cancer* (New York: Simon & Schuster, 1995), 39-40.

51. Block, K.I. "Dietary Impact on Quality and Quantity of Life in Cancer Patients." *Adjuvant Nutrition in Cancer Treatment* (CTCA/American College of Nutrition, 1993), 99-127.

52. Plotkin, D. "Good News and Bad News about Breast Cancer." *The Atlantic Monthly* (June 1996), 82.

53. Helvie, M.A. et al. "Mammographic Follow-up of Low-suspicion Lesions: Compliance Rate and Diagnostic

Yield." *Radiology* 178 (1991), 155-158.

54. Plotkin, D. "Good News and Bad News about Breast Cancer." *The Atlantic Monthly* (June 1996), 82.

55. Wright, C.J., and C.B. Mueller. "Screening Mammography and Public Health Policy: The Need for Perspective." *The Lancet* 346 (July 1995), 29-32.

56. Ibid.

57. Spratt, J.A. et al. "Mammographic Assessment of Human Breast Cancer Growth and Duration." *Cancer* 71 (1993), 2020-2026. See also: Spratt, J.S. et al. "Geometry, Growth Rates and Duration of Cancer and Carcinoma-in-situ of the Breast before Detection by Screening." *Cancer Research* 46 (1986), 970-974.

58. Gofman, J.W. *Preventing Breast Cancer* (San Francisco: Committee for Nuclear Responsibility, 1995).

59. Peterson, Norma. "Mammograms May Rupture In Situ Cysts, Causing Invasive Cancer." *Breast Cancer Action Newsletter* 38 (October/November 1996), 9.

60. Bogoch, S., and E.S. Bogoch. "A Checklist for Suitability of Biomarkers as Surrogate Endpoints in Chemoprevention of Breast Cancer." *Journal of Cellular Biochemistry* Suppl 19 (1994), 173-185.

61. Bogoch, S. et al. *Return of Elevated Antimalignin Antibody to Normal Indicates Remission of Breast Cancer.* (Boston: Foundation for Research on the Nervous System and Oncolab, 1996). Unpublished manuscript.

62. Sox, H. "Screening Mammography in Women Younger Than 50 Years of Age." *Annals of Internal Medicine* 122:7 (1995), 550-552.

63. For an excellent review of the literature on the relationship between low-fat diet and low breast cancer incidence, please refer to: Pelton, R. et al. "Dietary Fat—The 20 Percent Solution." *How to Prevent Breast Cancer* (New York: Simon & Schuster, 1995), 145-158.

64. Diamond, W.J., and W.L. Cowden. (1996.) Our survey of the literature indicates that studies that have not found high-fat diets to be a risk factor for breast cancer have had one or more critical limitations: (1) women's diets in early life were not evaluated (dietary fat may exert its cancer-initiating influence at this time); (2) women included in the study for comparison to high-fat consumers did not have fat intakes low enough to lower their cancer risk; (3) types of dietary fat were not considered, such as the use of omega-3 fatty acids, which are protective against breast cancer; and (4) women who may have consumed high-fat diets for long periods of time before switching to extremely lean (and probably imbalanced) diets for weight-loss purposes were included in the "low-fat diet" segments of the study populations.

65. Nordevang, E. et al. "Dietary Habits and Mammographic Patterns in Patients with Breast Cancer." *Breast Cancer Research and Treatment* 26 (1993), 207-215.

66. Pelton, R. et al. "The Pros and Cons of Hormone Replacement Therapy." *How to Prevent Breast Cancer* (New York: Simon & Schuster, 1995), 11-12.

67. Ibid., 104-116.

68. Wolff, M.S. et al. "Blood Levels of Organochlorine Residues and Risk of Breast Cancer." *Journal of the National Cancer Institute* 85 (1993), 648-652. See also: Falck, F. et al. "Pesticides and Polychlorinated Biphenyl Residues in Human Breast Lipids and Their Relation to Breast Cancer." *Archives of Environmental Health* 47 (1992), 143-146.

69. Krieger, N. et al. "Breast Cancer and Serum Organochlorines: A Prospective Study among White, Black, and Asian Women." *Journal of the National Cancer Institute* 86:8 (1994), 589-599.

70. Falck, F., Jr. et al. "Pesticides and Polychlorinated Biphenyl Residues in Human Breast Lipids and Their Relation to Breast Cancer." *Archives of Environmental Health* 47:2 (1992), 143-146.

71. Hayes, W.J., and E.R. Laws. *Handbook of Pesticide Toxicology* (San Diego, CA: Academic Press, 1991).

72. Raloff, J. "Pesticides May Challenge Human Immunity." *Science News* 149 (1996), 149.

73. Bock, S., and M. Boyette. *Stay Young the Melatonin Way* (New York: Dutton, 1995). Excellent discussion of factors affecting the body's melatonin supply, and possible health consequences. Many of these factors overlap with risk factors for breast cancer.

74. Morra, M., and E. Potts. "Diagnostic Tests." *Choices: Realistic Alternatives in Cancer Treatment* (New York: Avon, 1987), 86.

75. Giovannucci, E., and W. Willett. "Dietary Factors and Risk of Colon Cancer." *Annals of Medicine* 26 (1994), 443-452.

76. Ibid.

77. Steinmetz, K.A. et al. "Vegetables, Fruit, and Colon Cancer in the Iowa Women's Study." *American Journal of Epidemiology* 139 (1994), 1-15.

78. Sandler, R.S. et al. "Cigarette Smoking, Alcohol, and the Risk of Colorectal Adenomas." *Gastroenterology* 104 (1993), 1445-1451.

79. Flaten, T.P. "Chlorination of Drinking Water and Cancer Incidence in Norway." *International Journal of Epidemiology* 21 (1992), 6-15.

80. Springer, G.F. "Blood Group MN Antigens and Precursors in Normal and Malignant Human Breast Glandular Tissues." *Journal of the National Cancer Institute* 40 (1975), 183-192.

81. Springer, G.F. et al. "T/Tn Pancarcinoma Autoantigens: Fundamental, Diagnostic and Prediagnostic Aspects." *Cancer Detection and Prevention* 19 (1995), 173-182.

82. Cao, Y. et al. "Expression of Thomsen-Friedenreich-related Antigens in Primary and Metastatic Colorectal Carcinomas: A Reevaluation." *Cancer* 76:10 (1995), 1700-1708.

83. Langkilde, N.C. et al. "Nuclear Volume and Expression of T-antigen, Sialosyl-Tn-antigen and Tn-antigen in Carcinoma of the Human Bladder." *Cancer* 69 (1992), 219-227.

84. Namada, M. et al. "Expression of the Tn Antigen and T-Lymphoid Cell Line." *Biochemical and Biophysical Research Communications* 179 (1991), 762-767.

85. Studies reviewed in: Springer, G.F. "T and Tn Pancarcinoma Markers: Autoantigenic Adhesion Molecules in Pathogenesis, Prebiopsy Carcinoma Detection, and Long-term Breast Carcinoma Immunotherapy." *Critical Reviews in Oncogenesis* 6:1 (1995), 57-85.

86. Ibid.

87. Ibid.

88. Springer, G.F. "T/Tn Antigen: Two Decades of Experience in Early Immuno-Detection and Therapy of Human Carcinoma." *Jung Foundation Proceedings* (Stuttgart, Germany: G. Thieme, 1996).

89. Coulter, H.L. *Proposals for the Immunological Diagnosis and Treatment of Patients* (Washington, DC: V.I. Govallo Center for Empirical Medicine, 1996).


## Part III: A Complete Guide to Innovative Approaches to Cancer Treatment

# Chapter 28

# Nutrition as Cancer Medicine


1. The Burton Goldberg Group. *Alternative Medicine: The Definitive Guide* (Tiburon, CA: Future Medicine Publishing, 1995), 385.

2. Ibid.

3. Ibid.

4. Ibid.

5. Ibid.

6. Ibid.

7. Djuric, Z., and D. Kritchevsky. "Modulation of Oxidative DNA Damage Levels by Dietary Fat and Calories." *Mutation Research* 295 (1993), 181-190.

8. Colditz, G.A. et al. "Increased Green and Yellow Vegetable Intake and Lowered Cancer Deaths in an Elderly Population." *American Journal of Clinical Nutrition* 41:1 (January 1985), 32-36.

9. Aspry, K.E., and L.F. Bjeldanes. "Effects of Dietary Broccoli and Butylated Hydroxyanisole on Liver-Mediated Metabolism of Benzo[a]pyrene." *Food and Chemical Toxicology* 21:2 (1983), 133-142.

10. Malter, M. et al. "Natural Killer Cells, Vitamins, and Other Blood Components of Vegetarian and Omnivorous Men." *Nutrition and Cancer* 12:3 (1989), 271-278.

11. Ibid.

12. La Vecchia, C. et al. "Dietary Vitamin A and the Risk of Invasive Cervical Cancer." *International Journal of Cancer* 34:3 (1984), 319-322.

13. Menkes, M.S. et al. "Serum Beta-Carotene, Vitamins A and, Selenium and the Risk of Lung Cancer." *New England Journal of Medicine* 315 (1986), 1250.

14. "Dietary Aspects of Carcinogenesis." (September 1983).

15. Ramaswany, P., and R. Natarajan. "Vitamin B-6 Status in Patients with Cancer of the Uterine Cervix." *Nutrition and Cancer* 6 (1984), 176-180.

16. Stahelin, H. B. et al "Cancer, Vitamins, and Plasma Lipids: Prospective Basel Study." *Journal of the National Cancer Institute* 73 (1984), 1463-1468.

17. Ibid.

18. Willett, W.C., and B. MacMahon. "Prediagnostic Serum Selenium and the Risk of Cancer." *Lancet* 2:8342 (July 1983), 130-134.

19. Butterworth, C.E. et al. "Improvement in Cervical Dysplasia Assoiated with Folic Acid Therapy in Users of Oral Contraceptives." *American Journal of Clinical Nutrition* 35:1 (1982), 73-82.

20. Slattery, M. L., A.W. Sorenon and M.H. Ford. "Dietary Calcium Intake as a Mitigating Factor in Colon Cancer." *American Journal of Epidemiology* 128:3 (1988), 504-514.

21. Stadel, V.W. "Dietary Iodine and the Risk of Breast, Endometrial, and Ovarian Cancer." *The Lancet* 1:7965 (1976), 890-891.

22. Blondell, J. M. "The Anticarcinogenic Effect of Magnesium." *Medical Hypothesis* 6:8 (1980), 863-871.

23. Whelen, P., B.E. Walker and J. Kelleher. "Zinc, Vitamin A and Prostatic Cancer." *British Journal of Urology* 55:5 (1983), 525-528.

24. Kroning, F. "Garlic as an Inhibitor for Spontaneous Tumors in Mice." *Acta—Unio Internationalis Contra Cancrum* 20:3 (1964), 855.

25. You, W.C. et al. "Allium Vegetables and Reduced Risk of Stomach Cancer." *Journal of the National Cancer Institute* 81:2 (1989), 162-164.

26. Wynder, E.L. et al. "Diet and Breast Cancer in Causation and Therapy." *Cancer* 58:8 Suppl (1986), 1804-1831

27. Greenward, P., and E. Lanze. "Dietary Fiber and Colon Cancer." *Contemporary Nutrition* 11:1 (1986).

28. "Risk Reduction Objectives." *Health People 2000: National Health Promotion and Disease Prevention Objectives* (Washington, DC: U.S. Public Health Service, U.S. Dept. of Health and Human Services, 1990), 425.

29. The Burton Goldberg Group. *Alternative Medicine: The Definitive Guide* (Tiburon, CA: Future Medicine Publishing, 1995), 385.

30. Emerich, Monica. "Industry Growth: 22.6%." *Natural Foods Merchandiser* XVII:6 (June 1996).

31. Newberne, P.M., and M. Locniskar. "Roles of Micronutrients in Cancer Prevention: Recent Evidence from the Laboratory." *Progress in Clinical and Biological Research* 346 (1990), 119-134.

32. Petrie, H.T. "Differential Regulation of Lymphocyte Functional Activities by Selenium." University of Nebraska Medical Center Dissertation, 1988.

33. Aso, H. et al. "Induction of Interferon and Activation of NK Cells and Macrophages in Mice by Oral Administration of Ge-132, an Organic Germanium Compound." *Journal of Microbiology and Immunology* 29 (1985), 65-74. See also: Kumano, N. et al. "Antitumor Effect of Organogermanium Compound Ge-132 on the Lewis Lung Carcinoma (3LL) in C57 BL (B6) Mice." *Tohoku Journal of Experimental Medicine* 146 (1985), 97-104.

34. Vojdani, A., and M. Ghoneum. "*In Vivo* Effect of Ascorbic Acid on Enhancement of Human Natural Killer Cell Activity." *Nutrition Research* 13 (1993), 753-754.

35. Malter, M. et al. "Natural Killer Cells, Vitamins, and Other Blood Components of Vegetarian and Omnivorous Men." *Nutrition and Cancer* 12:3 (1989), 271-278.

36. Bougnoux, P. et al. "Alpha-linolenic Acid Content of Adipose Breast Tissue: A Host Determinant of the Risk of Early Metastasis in Breast Cancer." *British Journal of Cancer* 70:2 (1994), 330-334.

37. Baronzio, G.F. et al. "Adjuvant Therapy with Essential Fatty Acids (EFAs) for Primary Liver Tumors." *Medical Hypotheses* 44 (1995), 149-154.

38. Barnes, S. et al. "Soybeans Inhibit Mammary Tumors in Models of Breast Cancer." *Mutagens and Carcinogens in the Diet*, edited by Pariza, M. (New York: Alan R. Liss, 1990), 239-257.

39. Messina, M.J. et al. "Soy Intake and Cancer Risk: A Review of the *In Vitro* and *In Vivo* Data." *Nutrition & Cancer* 21:2 (1994), 113-131.

40. Haag, J.D. et al. "Enhanced Inhibition of Protein Isoprenylation and Tumor Growth by Perillyl Alcohol, an Hydroxylated Analog of d-limonene." *Proceedings of the American Association of Cancer Research* 33 (1992), 524.

41. Rhee, Y.H. et al. "Inhibition of Mutagenesis and Transformation by Root Extracts by Panax Ginseng *In Vitro*." *Planta Medica* 57 (1991), 125-128.

42. Klein S., and R.L. Koretz. "Nutrition Support in Patients with Cancer: What Do the Data Really Show?" *Nutrition in Clinical Practice* 9:3 (1994), 91-100. See also: *Nutrition in Clinical Practice* 9:3 (1994), 87-89.

43. Clifford, C., and B. Kramer. "Diet as Risk and Therapy for Cancer." *Medical Clinics of North America* 77:4 (1993), 725-744.

44. Istfan, N.W. et al. "Nutrition and Tumor Promotion: *In Vivo* Methods for Measurement of Cellular Proliferation and Protein Metabolism." *Journal of Parenteral & Enteral Nutrition* 16:Suppl 6 (1992), 76S-82S.

45. Harman, D. "Nutritional Implications of the Free-radical Theory of Aging." *Journal of the American College of Nutrition* 1:1 (1982), 27-34.

46. Grimble, R.F. "Nutritional Antioxidants and the Modulation of Inflammation: Theory and Practice." *New Horizons* 2:2 (1994), 175-185.

47. Chaitow, L., and N. Trenev. "The Role and Nature of Friendly Bacteria." *Probiotics* (Prescott, AZ: Hohm Press, 1995), 11-18.

48. Chaitow, L., and N. Trenev. "The Lactobacilli and Bifidobacteria." *Probiotics* (Prescott, AZ: Hohm Press, 1995), 24-25.

49. Goldin, B., and S.L. Gorbach. "Alterations in Fecal Microflora Enzymes Related to Diet, Age, Lactobacillus Supplements, and Dimethylhydrazine." *Cancer* 40 (1977), 2421-2426.

50. Gorbach, S. "The Intestinal Microflora and Its Colon Cancer Connection." *Infection* 10:6 (1982), 379-384.

51. Aso, Y. et al. "Preventive Effect of *Lactobacillus casei* Preparation on the Recurrence of Superficial Bladder Cancer in a Double-blind Trial." *European Urology* 27 (1995), 104-109.

52. Gogdanov, I.G. et al. "Antitumor Glycopeptides from *Lactobacillus bulgaricus* Cell Wall." *FEBS Letters* 57 (1975), 259-261. Cited by Moss, R. *Cancer Therapy* (New York: Equinox Press, 1992), 239.

53. Reynolds, J.V. et al. "Immunomodulatory Mechanisms of Arginine." *Surgery* 104:2 (1988), 142-151.

54. Akimoto, M. et al. "Modulation of the Antitumor Effect of BRM under Various Nutritional or Endocrine Conditions." *Gan To Kagaku Ryoho* 13 (1986), 1270-1276.

55. Tachibana, K. et al. "Evaluation of the Effect of Arginine-enriched Amino Acid Solution on Tumor Growth." *Japanese Journal of Parenteral and Enteral Nutrition* 9 (1985), 428-434.

56. Newberne, P.M. et al. "Inhibition of Hepatocarcinogenesis in Mice by Dietary Methyl Donors Methionine and Choline." *Nutrition and Cancer* 14 (1990), 175-181.

57. Palermo, M.S. et al. "Immunomodulation Exerted by Cyclophosphamide Is Not Interfered by N-acetyl cysteine." *International Journal of Immunopharmacology* 8:6 (1986), 651-655. See also: Schmitt-Graff, A., and M.E. Scheulen. "Prevention of Adriamycin Cardiotoxicity by Niacin, Isocitrate or N-acetyl cysteine in Mice: A Morphological Study." *Pathology Resident Practice* 181:2 (1986), 168-174. See also: Kim, J.A. et al. "Topical Use of N-acetyl cysteine for Reduction of Skin Reaction to Radiation Therapy." *Seminars in Oncology* 10:Suppl 1 (1983), 86.

58. Kuroda, M. et al. "Decreased Serum Levels of Selenium and Glutathione Peroxidase Activity Associated with Aging, Malignancy and Chronic Hemodialysis." *Trace Elements in Medicine* 5:3 (1988), 97-103.

59. Strong, Gary. *Does Mercury from Dental Amalgams Influence Systemic Health?* (Billings, MT: Strong Health Publications, 1995).

60. Boit, J. "Amino acids." *Cancer and Natural Medicine: A Textbook of Basic Science and Clinical Research* (Princeton, MN: Oregon Medical Press, 1995), 139-140.

61. Palermo, M.S. et al. "Immunomodulation Exerted by Cyclophosphamide Is Not Interfered by N-acetyl cysteine." *International Journal of Immunopharmacology* 8:6 (1986), 651-655. See also: Schmitt-Graff, A., and M.E. Scheulen. "Prevention of Adriamycin Cardiotoxicity by Niacin, Isocitrate or N-acetyl-cysteine in Mice: A Morphological Study." *Pathology Resident Practice* 181:2 (1986), 168-174. See also: Kim, J.A. et al. "Topical Use of N-acetyl cysteine for Reduction of Skin Reaction to Radiation Therapy." *Seminars in Oncology* 10:Suppl 1 (1983), 86.

62. Braverman, E.R., and C. Pfeiffer. *The Healing Nutrients Within* (New Canaan, CT: Keats Publishing, 1987), 149.

63. Boik, J. "Dietary Macronutrients and Their Effects on Cancer. " *Cancer and Natural Medicine* (Princeton, MN: Oregon Medical Press, 1995), 140.

64. Quillan, P. *Beating Cancer With Nutrition* (Tulsa, OK: Nutrition Times Press, 1994), 225.

65. Goldfarb, R.H., and R.B. Herberman. "Natural Killer Cell Reactivity: Regulatory Interactions among Phorbol Ester, Interferon, Cholera Toxin and Retinoic Acid." *Journal of Immunology* 126 (1981), 21-29.

66. Dennert, G., and R. Lotan. "Effects of Retinoic Acid on the Immune System: Stimulation of T-killer Cell Induction." *European Journal of Immunology* 8 (1978), 23.

67. Dennert, G. et al. "Retinoic Acid Stimulation of the Induction of Mouse Killer T-cell in All Ogeneic and Syngeneic Systems." *Journal of the National Cancer Institute* 62 (1979), 89.

68. Machlin, L.J., and A. Bendich. "Free Radical Tissue Damage: Protective Role of Antioxidant Nutrient." *FASEB Journal* 1:6 (1987), 441-445.

69. Bendich, A. "Carotenoids and the Immune Response." *Journal of Nutrition* 119:1 (1989), 112-115.

70. Bland, J., Ph.D. "The Beta Carotene Controversy in Perspective." *Townsend Letter for Doctors & Patients* (May 1996).

71. Garland et al. "Dietary Vitamin D and Calcium and Risk of Colorectal Cancer: A 19-year Prospective Study in Men." *The Lancet* i (1985), 307.

72. Wargovich, M.J. et al. "Modulating Effects of Calcium in Animal Models of Colon Carcinogenesis and Short-term Studies in Subjects at Increased Risk for Colon Cancer." *American Journal of Clinical Nutrition* 54 (1991), 202S-205S. See also: Wargovich, M.J. "New Dietary Anticarcinogens and Prevention of Gastrointestinal Cancer." *Diseases of the Colon and Rectum* 31 (1988), 72-75.

73. Schroeder, H. *The Poisons Around Us* (Bloomington, IN: Indiana University Press, 1974), 126.

74. Underwood, E. *Trace Elements in Human and Animal Nutrition* 4th ed. (New York: Academic Press, 1977), 267.

75. Todd, Gary P. "The Trace Elements." *Nutrition, Health, & Disease* (Norfolk, VA: Donning, 1985), 183.

76. Bliznakov, Emile, and Gerald Hunt. *The Miracle Nutrient Coenzyme Q10* (New York: Bantam, 1987).

77. Leibovitz, B. et al. "Dietary Supplements of Vitamin E, Beta-carotene, Coenzyme Q10, and Selenium Protect Tissues Against Lipid Peroxidation in Rat Tissue Slices." *Journal of Clinical Nutrition* 120 (1990), 97-104.

78. Folkers, K. et al. "Survival of Cancer Patients on Therapy with CoQ10." *Biochemical and Biophysical Research Communications* 192:1 (1993), 241-245.

79. Lockwood, K. et al. "Partial and Complete Regression of Breast Cancer in Relation to Dosage of Coenzyme Q10." *Biochemical and Biophysical Research Communications* 199 (1994), 1504-1508.

80. Lockwood, K. et al. "Progress on Therapy of Breast Cancer with CoQ10 and the Regression of Metastases." *Biochemical and Biophysical Research Communications* 212:1 (1995), 172-177.

81. Gershwin, M.E. et al. "The Potential Impact of Nutritional Factors on Immunological Responsiveness." *Nutrition and Immunity* (Orlando, FL: Academic Press, 1985), 222.

82. Beach, R.S. et al. "Zinc, Copper and Manganese in Immune Function and Experimental Oncogenesis." *Nutrition and Cancer* 3 (1982), 172-191.

83. Murray, Michael T., N.D. *Encyclopedia of Nutritional Supplements* (Rocklin, CA: Prima Publishing, 1996), 237-278. See also Barilla, Jean, ed. *The Nutrition Superbook* (New Canaan, CT: Keats Publishing, 1996) 261-263.

84. Sakaguchi, M. et al. "Reduced Tumor Growth of the Human Colonic Cancer Cell Lines COLO-320 and HT-29 *In Vivo* by Dietary n-3 Lipids." *British Journal of Cancer* 62:5 (1990), 742-747.

85. Reich, R. et al. "Eicosapentanoic Acid Reduces the Invasive and Metastatic Activities of Malignant Tumor Cells." *Biochemical & Biophysical Research Communications* 160:2 (1989), 59-564.

86. Burns, C.P., and A.A. Spector. "Effects of Lipids on Cancer Therapy." *Nutrition Reviews* 48:6 (1990), 233-240.

87. Man-Fan, W.J. et al. "Omega-3 fatty Acids and Cancer Metastasis in Humans." *World Review of Nutrition and Dietetics* 66 (1991), 477-487.

88. Yetiv, J.Z. "Clinical Applications of Fish Oils." *Journal of the American Medical Association* 260:5 (1988), 665-670.

89. Quillan, P. *Beating Cancer With Nutrition* (Tulsa, OK: Nutrition Times Press, 1994), 224.

90. Erasmus, U. "Fatty Degeneration: Cancer." *Fats and Oils: The Complete Guide to Fats and Oils in Health and Nutrition* (Vancouver, Canada: Alive Books, 1988), 303-304.

91. Murray, Michael T., N.D. *Encyclopedia of Nutritional Supplements* (Rocklin, CA: Prima Publishing, 1996), 266-267.

92. Fritsche, K.L., and P.V. Johnston. "Effect of Dietary Alpha-linolenic Acid on Growth, Metastasis, Fatty Acid Profile, and Prostaglandin Production of Two Murine Mammary Adenocarcinomas." *Journal of Nutrition* 120 (1990), 1601-1609.

93. Murray, Michael T., N.D. *Encyclopedia of Nutritional Supplements* (Rocklin, CA: Prima Publishing, 1996), 267.

94. Erasmus, U. "Fatty Degeneration: Cancer." *Fats and Oils: The Complete Guide to Fats and Oils in Health and Nutrition* (Vancouver, Canada: Alive Books, 1986), 303-304.

95. Budwig, Johanna. *Flax Oil as a True Aid Against Arthritis, Heart Infarction, Cancer, and Other Diseases* (Vancouver, Canada: Apple Publishing, 1992).

96. Erasmus, U. "Recommendations." *Fats and Oils: The Complete Guide to Fats and Oils in Health and Nutrition* (Vancouver, Canada: Alive Books, 1988), 321.

97. Van Der Merwe, C.F. et al. "Oral Gamma-linolenic Acid in 21 Patients with Untreatable Malignancy: An Ongoing Pilot Open Clinical Trial." *British Journal of Clinical Practice* 41:9 (1987), 907.

98. Van Der Merwe, C.F. "The Reversibility of Cancer." *South African Medical Journal* 65:18 (1984), 712.

99. Begin, M.E. et al. "Differential Killing of Human Carcinoma Cells Supplemented with n-3 and n-6 Polyunsaturated Fatty Acids." *Journal of the National Cancer Institute* 77:5 (1986), 1053-1062.

100. Erasmus, U. "Oil of Evening Primrose." *Fats and Oils: The Complete Guide to Fats and Oils in Health and Nutrition* (Vancouver, Canada: Alive Books, 1986), 251.

101. Ibid.

102. Kidd, P. "Germanium-132: Homeostatic Normalizer and Immunostimulant: A Review of Its Preventive and Therapeutic Efficacy." *Internationl Clinical Nutrition Review* 7:1 (1987), 11-20.

103. Itoh, K. and K. Kumagai. "Augmentation of NK Activity by Several Anti-inflammatory Agents." *Proceedings of the International Symposium on Natural Killer Cell*

*Activity and its Regulation, Fifth International Congress of Immunology* (1983).

104. Gerson, Max, M.D. *A Cancer Therapy: Results of Fifty Cases* (Bonita, CA: Gerson Institute, 1958), 7-10.

105. Ibid., 124.

106. Hildenbrand, G., and S. Cavin. "Five-Year Survival Rates of Melanoma Patients Treated by Diet Therapy after the Manner of Gerson: A Retrospective Review." *Alternative Therapies in Health and Medicine* 1:4 (1995), 29-37.

107. Ibid.

108. Steinmetz, K.A., and J.D. Potter. "Vegetables, Fruit and Cancer II Mechanisms." *Cancer Causes and Control* (1991), 427-442.

109. Murray, Michael T., N.D. *Encyclopedia of Nutritional Supplements* (Rocklin, CA: Prima Publishing, 1996).

110. Kutsky, R. "Iodine." *Handbook of Vitamins, Minerals, and Hormones* (New York: Van Nostrand Reinhold, 1981), 138.

111. Stadel, V.W. "Dietary Iodine and the Risk of Breast, Endometrial and Ovarian Cancer." *The Lancet* 1:7965 (1976), 890-891.

112. Langer, S.E. et al. *Solved: The Riddle of Illness* (New Canaan, CT: Keats, 1984).

113. Shoden, R.J. and S. Griffin. "Iodine." *Fundamentals of Clinical Nutrition* (New York: McGraw Hill, 1980), 97.

114. Quillan, P. "Nutrients Have a Profound Impact on the Immune System." *Beating Cancer with Nutrition* (Tulsa, OK: Nutrition Times Press, 1994), 214.

115. Kelley, William Donald, D.D.S. *One Answer to Cancer: An Ecological Approach to the Successful Treatment of Malignancy* (Grapevine, TX: Wedgestone Press, 1969), 14.

116. Personal Communications with Nicholas Gonzalez, M.D., New York, NY (1995).

117. Kutsky, R. "Iodine." *Handbook of Vitamins, Minerals, and Hormones* (New York: Van Nostrand Reinhold, 1981), 125.

118. Gershwin, M.E. et al. "The Potential Impact of Nutritional Factors on Immunological Responsiveness." *Nutrition and Immunity* (Orlando, FL: Academic Press, 1985), 201-204.

119. Kutsky, R. "Iodine." *Handbook of Vitamins, Minerals, and Hormones* (New York: Van Nostrand Reinhold, 1981), 167.

120. Todd, G.P. "The Trace Elements." *Nutrition, Health and Disease* (Norfolk, VA: Donning, 1985), 183.

121. The Burton Goldberg Group. *Alternative Medicine: The Definitive Guide* (Tiburon, CA: Future Medicine Publishing, 1995), 398.

122. Ibid.

123. Ibid.

124. Walters, R. "Gerson Therapy." *Options: The Alternative Cancer Therapy Book* (Garden City Park, NY: Avery Publishing, 1993), 197.

125. Schrauzer, G.N. "Selenium in Nutritional Cancer Prophylaxis: An Update." *Vitamins, Nutrition and Cancer*, edited by Prosad, K.N. (Basel, Switzerland: Karger, 1984).

126. Schrauzer, G.N. "Selenium for the Cancer Patient." Adjuvant Nutrition in Cancer Treatment Symposium. Tampa, Florida (September 29, 1995). Dr. Schrauzer is based at the Biological Trace Element Research Institute, San Diego, CA.

127. Petrie, H.T. "Differential Regulation of Lymphocyte Functional Activities by Selenium." (University of Nebraska Medical Center, 1988).

128. Ip, C. "Prophylaxis of Mammary Neoplasia by Selenium Supplementation in the Initiation and Promotion Phases of Carcinogenesis." *Cancer Research* 41 (1981), 4386- 4393.

129. Schrauzer, G.N. "Selenium in Nutritional Cancer Prophylaxis: An Update." *Vitamins, Nutrition and Cancer*, edited by Prosad, K.N. (Basel, Switzerland: Karger, 1984).

130. Schauzer, G.N. et al. "Cancer Mortality Correlation Studies—III; Statistical Associations with Dietary Selenium Intake." *Bioinorganic Chemistry* 7 (1977), 23-34.

131. Salonen, J.T. et al. "Association between Serum Selenium and the Risk of Cancer." *American Journal of Epidemiology* 120 (1984), 342-349.

132. Goldfarb, R.H., and R.B. Herberman. "Natural Killer Cell Reactivity: Regulatory Interactions among Phorbol Ester, Interferon, Cholera Toxin and Retinoic Acid." *Journal of Immunology* 126 (1981), 2129.

133. Dennert, G., and R. Lotan. "Effects of Retinoic Acid on the Immune System: Stimulation of T-killer Cell Induction." *European Journal of Immunology* 8 (1978), 23.

134. Dennert, G. et al. "Retinoic Acid Stimulation of the Induction of Mouse Killer T-cell in Allogeneic and Syngeneic Systems." *Journal of the National Cancer Institute* 62 (1979), 89.

135. Hong, W.K. et al. "Prevention of Second Primary Tumors with Isotreninoin in Squamous-cell Carcinoma of the Head and Neck." *New England Journal of Medicine* 323 (1990), 795-801.

136. Miscksche, M. et al. "Vitamin A in the Treatment of Metastatic Unresectable Squamous Cell Carcinoma of the Lung." *Oncology* 34 (1977), 234.

137. Meyskens, F.L. Jr. "Prevention and Treatment of Cancer with Vitamin A and the Retinoids." *Vitamins, Nutrition and Cancer*, edited by Prosad, K.N. (Basel, Switzerland: Karger, 1984), 266.

138. Panush, R.S., and J.C. Delafuente. "Vitamins and Immunocompetence: Group B Vitamins. World Review." *Nutrition Digest* 45 (1985), 97-132.

139. Posner, B.M. et al. "Nutrition in Neoplastic Disease." *Advances in Modern Human Nutrition and Dietetics* 29 (1980), 130-169.

140. Ibid.

141. Beisel, W.R. et al. "Single Nutrients and Immunity." *American Journal of Clinical Nutrition* 35 Suppl (1982), 417-468.

142. Basu, T.K. "Significance of Vitamins in Cancer." *Oncology* 33 (1976), 183.

143. Hoffer, A. "Vitamin B-3: Niacin and Its Amide." *Townsend Letter for Doctors & Patients* (October 1995), 35.

144. Shoden, R.J., and W.S. Griffin. "Niacin." *Fundamentals of Clinical Nutrition* (New York: McGraw-Hill, 1980), 56.

145. Gridley, D.S. et al. "*In Vivo* and *In Vitro* Stimulation of Cell-mediated Immunity by Vitamin B6." *Nutrition Research* 8:2 (1988), 201-207.

146. Posner, B.M. et al. "Nutrition in Neoplastic Disease." *Advances in Modern Human Nutrition and Dietetics* 29 (1980), 130-169.

147. DiSorbo, D.M., and G. Litwack. "Vitmain B6 Kills Hepatoma Cells in Culture." *Nutrition and Cancer* 3:4 (1982), 216-222.

148. Byar, D., and C. Blackard. "Comparisons of Placebo, Pyridoxine, and Topical Thiopepa in Preventing Recurrence of Stage I Bladder Cancer." *Urology* 10:6 (1977), 556-561.

149. Ladner, H.A. et al. *Nutrition, Growth & Cancer* (New York: Alan Liss, 1988), 273. Cited in: Quillan, P. *Beating Cancer With Nutrition* (Tulsa, OK: Nutrition Times Press, 1994).

150. Stahelin, H.B. et al. "Cancer, Vitamins and Plasma Lipids. Prospective Basel Study." *Journal of the National Cancer Institute* 73 (1984), 1463-1468. See also: Cameron, E., and L. Pauling. *Cancer and Vitamin C* (Menlo Park, CA: Linus Pauling Institute of Science and Medicine, 1979).

151. Cameron, E.T. et al. "Ascorbic Acid and Cancer: A Review." *Cancer Research* 39 (1979), 663-681.

152. Yonemoto, R.H. "Vitmain C and Immunological Response in Normal Controls and Cancer Patients." *Medico Dialogo* 5 (1979), 23-30.

153. Siegel, B.V., and J.I. Morton. "Vitamin C and the Immune Response." *Experientia* 33 (1977), 393-395.

154. Riordan, D. "Nutrition Therapy for Cancer Patients." Adjuvant Nutrition in Cancer Treatment Symposium. Tampa, Florida (September 30, 1995).

155. Tschetter, L. et al. "A Community-based Study of Vitamin C (ascorbic acid)—Therapy in Patients with Advanced Cancer." *Proceedings of the American Society of Clinical Oncology* 2 (1983), 92. See also: Cameron, E., and L. Pauling. "Vitamin C and Cancer." *International Journal of Environmental Studies* 75 (1977), 4538-4542.

156. Veltri, R.W. et al. "L-ascorbic acid (vitamin C) Augmentation of Anticancer Activity of Methoxy-substituted Benzoquinones, Adriamycin, and a Dihydroxyulated Amino Substituted Quinone (DHAQ)." Unpublished. Cited in: Pelton, R., and L. Overholser. *Alternatives in Cancer Therapy* (New York: Fireside/Simon & Schuster, 1994).

157. Koch, C.J., and J.E. Bigalow. "Toxicity Radiation Sensitivity Modification, and Metabolic Effects of Dehydroscorbate and Ascorbate in Mammalian Cells." *Journal of Cell Physiology* 94 (1978), 299-306. See also: Okunieff, P. "Ascorbic Acid: Biologic Functions and Relation to Cancer." Symposium in Bethesda, MD (September 1989). Cited in Pelton, R. and L. Overholser. *Alternatives in Cancer Therapy* (New York: Fireside/Simon & Schuster 1994).

158. Veltri, R.W. et al. "L-ascorbic acid (vitamin C) Augmentation of Anticancer Activity of Methoxy-substituted Benzoquinones, Adriamycin, and a Dihydroxyulated Amino Substituted Quinone (DHAQ)." Unpublished. Cited in: Pelton, R., and L. Overholser. *Alternatives in Cancer Therapy* (New York: Fireside/Simon & Schuster, 1994).

159. Riordan , N.H. et al. "Intravenous Ascorbate as a Tumor Cytotoxic Chemotherapeutic Agent." *Medical Hypotheses* 44:3 (1995), 205.

160. Poydock, M.E. "Effect of Combined Ascorbic Acid and B12 on Survival of Mice with Implanted Ehrlich Carcinoma and L1210 Leukemia." *American Journal of Clinical Nutrition* 54:Suppl 6 (1991), 1261S-1265S.

161. Cameron, E., and L. Pauling. *Proceedings of the National Academy of Sciences* 75:9 (1978), 4538.

162. The Burton Goldberg Group. *Alternative Medicine: The Definitive Guide* (Tiburon, CA: Future Medicine Publishing, 1995), 9.

163. Block, G. "Vitamin C and Cancer Prevention: The Epidemiologic Evidence." *American Journal of Clinical Nutrition* 53 (1991), 270S.

164. Pelton, R., and L. Overholser. "Vitamin C: Side-effects." *Alternatives in Cancer Therapy* (New York: Fireside/Simon & Schuster, 1994), 62.

165. Cameron, E. "Protocol for the Use of Vitamin C in the Treatment of Cancer." *Medical Hypotheses* 36 (1991), 190-194.

166. Park, C.H. "Vitamin C in Leukemia and Preleukemia Cell Growth." *Nutrition, Growth and Cancer,* edited by Tryfiates and Prasad. (New York: Alan R. Liss, 1988), 321-330.

167. Tsao, C.S., and S.L. Salimi. "Effect of Large Intake of Ascorbic Acid on Urinary and Plasma Oxalic Acid Levels." *International Journal of Vitamin and Nutritional Research* 54 (1984), 245-249. See also: Hoffer, A. "Vitamin C and Infertility." *The Lancet* 2:7838 (1973), 1146.

168. Henson, D.E. "Ascorbic Acid: Biological Functions in Relation to Cancer." *Journal of the National Cancer Institute* 83:8 (1991), 547. For a summary of symposium abstracts on vitamin C and cancer, write to: Donald E. Henson, M.D., Division of Cancer Prevention and Control, Executive Plaza Rm. 305, National Institute of Health, Bethesda, MD 20892.

169. Good, R.A. et al. "Nutrition, Immunity and Cancer—A Review." *Clinical Bulletin* 9 (1979), 3-12, 63-75.

170. Boik, J. "Conducting Research on Natural Agents: Vitamin D Metabolites." *Cancer and Natural Medicine* (Princeton, MN: Oregon Medical Press, 1995), 181.

171. Martin, Wayne. "Anti-Cancer Effect of Vitamin D." *Townsend Letter for Doctors & Patients* (October 1996), 111.

172. "The Effect of Vitamin E on Immune Responses." *Nutrition Reviews* 45:1 (1987), 27.

173. Benner, S.E. et al. "Regression of Oral leukoplakia with Alpha-tocopherol: A Community Clinical Oncology Program Chemoprevention Study." *Journal of the National Cancer Institute* 85:1 (1993), 44-47. Note: The subjects in this study were all in the early stages of oral cancer (premalignant oral leukoplakia lesions).

174. Cook, M.G., and P. McNamara. "Effect of Dietary Vitamin E on Dimethyl-hydrazine-induced Colonic Tumors in Mice." *Cancer Research* 40:4 (1980), 1329-1331.

175. Shklar, G. et al. "Regression by Vitamin E of Experimental Oral Cancer." *Journal of the National*

*Cancer Institute* 78:5 (1987), 987-992.

176. Prasad, K.N. et al. "Vitamin E Increases the Growth Inhibitory and Differentiating Effects of Tumor Therapeutic Agents on Neuroblastoma and Glioma Cells in Culture." *Proceedings of the Society for Experimental Biology and Medicine* 164:2 (1980), 158-163.
177. Svingen, B.A. et al. "Vitamin E Deficiency Accentuates Adriamycin Cardiotoxicity." *Cancer Research* 41 (1981), 3395.
178. Myers, C.E. et al. "Effect of Tocopherol and Selenium on Defenses Against Reactive Oxygen Species and Their Effect on Radiation Sensitivity." *Annals of the New York Academy of Sciences* 393 (1982), 419-425.
179. Quillan, P. "Vitamin K." *Beating Cancer With Nutrition* (Tulsa, OK: Nutrition Times Press, 1994), 216-217.
180. Ibid.
181. Good, R.A. et al. "Nutrition, Immunity and Cancer: A Review." *Clinical Bulletin* 9 (1979), 3-12, 63-75.
182. Boik, J. "Zinc: Dietary Micronutrients and Their Effects on Cancer." *Cancer and Natural Medicine* (Princeton, MN: Oregon Medical Press, 1995), 147.
183. Gershwin, M.E. et al. "The Potential Impact of Nutritional Factors on Immunological Responsiveness." *Nutrition and Immunity* (Orlando, FL: Academic Press, 1985), 222.

## Chapter 29

## Botanicals as Cancer Medicines

1. Duke, J.A. "Weeds? Or Wonder Drugs?" *Organic Gardening* (July/August 1994), 38-40.
2. Tyler, V.E. "Significant Anticancer Herbs." *Herbs of Choice: The Therapeutic Use of Phytomedicinals* (New York: Pharmaceutical Products Press, 1994), 178-179.
3. Pisha, E. et al. "Discovery of Betulinic Acid as a Selective Inhibitor of Human Melanoma that Functions by Induction of Apoptosis." *Nature Medicine* 10 (1995), 1046-1051.
4. Centofanti, M. "Birch Bark Has Anticancer Bite." *Science News* 148 (1995), 231. Original report appeared in *Nature Medicine* (October 1995).
5. Cook, B. "Tree of Life Helps in Advanced Cancer." *International Journal of Alternative & Complementary Medicine* (January 1992), 23.
6. "Cancer Patients Should Eat Pineapples." *International Journal of Alternative & Complementary Medicine* (January 1992), 23. Original report appeared in *Planta Medica* 54:5 (1988), 377-378.
7. Duke, J.A. "Weeds? Or Wonder Drugs?" *Organic Gardening* (July/August 1994), 39.
8. Tenney, L. "Gotu kola." *Today's Herbal Health: The Essential Reference Guide to Understanding Herbs Used for Medicinal Purposes* (Provo, UT: Woodland Books, 1992), 78.
9. Babu, T.D. et al. "Cytotoxic and Antitumor Properties of Certain Taxa of Umbelliferae with Special Reference to *Centella Asiatica*." *Journal of Ethnopharmacology* 48 (1995), 53-57.
10. Haag, J.D. et al. "Enhanced Inhibition of Protein Isoprenylation and Tumor Growth by Perillyl Alcohol, an Hydroxylated Analog of d-limonene." *Proceedings of the American Association of Cancer Research* 33 (1992), 524.
11. Brown, R. *Bee Hive Product Bible* (Garden City Park, NY: Avery Publishing, 1994), 47.
12. Ibid., 116-117.
13. Ibid., 49.
14. Johnson, T. "Herbs for Cancer." Personal communications (1996). See Overmind web page at http://www.hooked.net/users/overmind/.
15. Chang, M. Preface to *Anticancer Medicinal Herbs* (Hunan Changsha, China: Hunan Science and Technology Press, 1992), ii.
16. Zhuang, H. et al. "Effects of *Radix Slaviae Miltiorrhizae* Extract Injection on Survival of Allogenic Heart Transplantation." *Journal of Traditional Chinese Medicine* 10:4 (1990), 276-281.
17. Liu, F. "Application of Traditional Chinese Drugs in Comprehensive Treatment of Primary Liver Cancer." *Journal of Traditional Chinese Medicine* 10:1 (1990), 54-60. This study showed that TCM diagnosis could enhance the prognosticative accuracy of survival of patients with primary liver cancer and that Chinese herbal medicine enabled patients to recuperate to a point where they could successfully undergo surgery and complete regimens of chemotherapy, thus prolonging survival.
18. Dharmananda, S. *Chinese Herbal Therapies for Immune Disorders* (Portland, OR: Institute for Traditional Medicine, 1988), 9-25.
19. "Special Hearing on Alternative Medicine." *Report of the Subcommittee of the Committee on Appropriations, U.S. Senate* (June 24, 1993), 65.
20. Dharmananda, S. *Chinese Herbal Therapies for Immune Disorders* (Portland, OR: Institute for Traditional Medicine, 1988), 10.
21. Walters, R. "Chinese Medicine." *Options: The Alternative Cancer Therapy Book* (Garden City, NY: Avery Publishing, 1993), 311.
22. Liu, X.Y., and N.Q. Ang. "Effect of *liu wei di huang* or *jin gui shen qi* Decoction as an Adjuvant Treatment in Small Cell Lung Cancer." *Chung Hsi I Chieh Ho Tsa Chih* 10 (1990), 720-722.
23. Wang, R.L. et al. "Potentiation by *Rabdosia rubescens* on Chemotherapy of Advanced Esophageal Carcinoma." *Chung Hua Chung Liu Tsa Chih* 8 (1986), 297-299.
24. Cheng, J.H. "Clinical Study on Prevention and Treatment to Chemotherapy Caused Nephrotoxicity with *jian-pi yi-qi li-shui*." *Chung-Kuo Chung Hsi Chieh Ho Tsa Chih* 14:6 (1994), 331-333.
25. You, J.S. et al. "Combined Effects of Chuling (*Polyporous umbellatus*) Extract and Mitomycin C on Experimental Liver Cancer." *American Journal of Chinese Medicine* 22:1 (1994), 19-28.
26. Ji, Y.B. et al. "Effects of *buzhong yiqi* Decoction on the Anticancer Activity and Toxicity Induced by Cyclophosphamide." *Chung Kuo Chung Yao Tsa Chih* 14 (1989), 48-51.
27. Lin, P.F. "Antitumor Effect of Actinidia Chinensis Polysaccharide on Murine Tumor." *Chung Hua Chung*

*Liiu Tsa Chih* 10 (1988), 441-444. See also: Franz, G. "Polysaccharides in Pharmacy: Current Application and Future Concepts." *Planta Medica* 55 (1989), 493-497.

28. Chang, M. Preface to *Anticancer Medicinal Herbs* (Hunan Changsha, China: Hunan Science and Technology Press, 1992), ii.

29. Ibid.

30. Konoshima T. et al. "Antitumor Promoting Activities and Inhibitory Effects on Epstein Barr Virus Activation of *Shi-un-kou* and Its Constituents." *Yakugaku Zasshi* 109 (1989), 843-846.

31. Okamoto, T. et al. "Clinical Effects of *Juzen-taiho-to* on Immunologic and Fatty Metabolic States in Postoperative Patients with Gastrointestinal Cancer." *Gan To Kagaku Ryoho* 16 (1989), 1533-1537. See also: Kiyohara, H. et al. "Characterization of Mitogenic Pectic Polysaccharides from Kampo Medicine *Juzen-taiho-to.*" *Planta Medica* 57 (1991), 254-259.

32. Ikeuchi, T. "Clinical Studies on Chronic Prostatitis and Prostatitis-like Syndrome. The Kampo Treatment for Intractable Prostatitis." *Hinyokika Kihyo* 36 (1990), 801-806.

33. Nagatsu, Y. et al. "Modification of Macrophage Functions by Shosaikoto (Kampo Medicine) Leads to Enhancement of Immune Response." *Chemical and Pharmaceutical Bulletin* 37 (1989), 1540-1542.

34. Oka, H. et al. "Prospective Study of Chemoprevention of Hepatocellular Carcinoma with *Sho-saiko-to* (TJ-9)." *Cancer* 76:5 (1995), 743-749.

35. Ning, C. et al. "Therapeutic Effects of *jian pi yi shen* Prescription on the Toxicity Reactions of Postoperative Chemotherapy in Patients with Advanced Gastric Carcinoma." *Journal of Traditional Chinese Medicine* 8:2 (1988), 113-116.

36. Guo, Z.H. et al. "Chinese Herb Destagnation Series 1: Combination of Radiation with Destagnation in the Treatment of Nasopharyngeal Carcinoma (NPC), a Prospective Randomized Trial on 188 Cases." *International Journal of Radiation Oncology, Biology and Physics* 16 (1989), 297-300. See also: Sun, Y. "The Role of Traditional Chinese Medicine in Supportive Care of Cancer Patients." *Recent Results in Cancer Research* 108 (1988), 327-344.

37. Shiu, W.T.C. et al. "A Clinical Study of PSP on Peripheral Blood Counts during Chemotherapy." *Phytotherapy Research* 6 (1992), 217-218.

38. Swamy, B.V.K. "Ayurvedic Strategies of Cancer and Its Management and Relevance to Modern Oncology." World Congress on Cancer. Sydney, Australia (April 1994), 309-313.

39. Sharma, H.M. et al. "Marharish Ayur-veda: Modern Insights into Ancient Medicine." *Journal of the American Medical Association* 265 (1991), 2633-2634. Published erratum appears in *Journal of the American Medical Association* 266 (1991), 798.

40. Sharma, H.M. et al. "Antineoplastic Properties of Maharishi-4 against DMBA-induced Mammary Tumors in Rats." *Pharmacology, Biochemistry & Behavior* 35:4 (1990), 767-773.

41. Moss, R. "Ayur-veda." *Cancer Therapy: The Independent Consumer's Guide to Non-Toxic Treatment & Prevention* (New York: Equinox Press, 1992), 134.

42. Prasad, G.C. "The Use of Ayurvedic Drugs in the Management of Cancer." World Congress on Cancer. Sydney, Australia (April 1994), 315-319.

43. Ibid.

44. Ibid., 317.

45. "Greater Health and Longevity: Chlorella, the Green Algae Superfood, May be the Answer." *Alternative Medicine Digest* 12 (1996), 56.

46. Wilner, J. "Suggested Nutritional Supplements: Algae." *The Cancer Solution* (Boca Raton, FL: Peltec Publishing, 1994).

47. Beim, A. "Algae May Curb Mouth Cancer." *American Health* (June 1996), 29.

48. Yamamoto, I. et al. "Antitumor Effect of Seaweeds." *Japanese Journal of Experimental Medicine* 44 (1974), 543-546.

49. Yamamoto, I. et al. "Antitumor Effect of Seaweeds." *Japanese Journal of Experimental Medicine* 47:3 (1977), 133-140.

50. Teas, J. et al. "Dietary Seaweed (Laminaria) and Mammary Carcinogenesis in Rats." *Cancer Research* 44:7 (1984), 2758.

51. Hirayama, T. "Changing Patterns of Cancer in Japan." *Origins of Cancer in Humans*, edited by Hiatt, H.H. et al. (Cold Spring Harbor, NY: Cold Spring Harbor Laboratory, 1977), 55-75.

52. Tanaka, Y. et al. "Studies on Inhibition of Intestinal Absorption of Radioactive Strontium." *Canadian Medical Association Journal* 99 (1968), 169-175.

53. Ibid.

54. "The Super Vitamin: 2 Ways to Go Green." *Alternative Medicine Digest* 11 (1996), 58-59.

55. Ibid.

56. Kupchan, S.M., and A. Karim. "Tumor Inhibitors. Aloe Emodin: Antileukemic Principle Isolated from *Rhamnus Frangula L.*" *Lloydia* 39 (1976), 223-224.

57. Ralamboranto, L. et al. "Immunomodulating Properties of an Extract Isolated and Partially Purified from Aloe Vahombe. Study of Antitumoral Properties and Contribution to the Chemical Nature and Active Principle." *Archives de l' Institut Pasteur de Madagascar* 50 (1982), 227-256.

58. Grivel, N.V., and V.G. Pashinskii. "Antimetastatic Properties of Aloe Juice." *Voprosy Onkologii* 32 (1986), 38-40.

59. Harris, C. et al. "Efficacy of Acemannan in Treatment of Canine and Feline Spontaneous Neoplasms." *Molecular Biotherapy* 3:2 (1991), 207-213. Peng, S.Y. et al. "Decreased Mortality of Norman Murine Sarcoma in Mice Treated with Immunomodulator, Acemannan." *Molecular Biotherapy* 3:2 (1991), 79-87.

60. Boik, J. "Conducting Research on Natural Agents." *Cancer and Natural Medicine: A Textbook of Basic Science and Clinical Research* (Princeton, MN: Oregon Medical Press, 1995), 177.

61. Moss, R.W. *The Cancer Industry: Unraveling the Politics* (New York: Paragon House, 1989).

62. Rubin, D. "Dosage Levels for Laetrile." *Choice* 3:6 (1977), 8-9.

63. Tatsumura, T. et al. "Antitumor Effect of 4, 6 benzylidene-D-glucose in Clinical Studies." *Proceedings of the Annual Meeting of the American Society of Clinical Oncologists* 6 (1987), A559.

64. Kochi, M. et al. "Antitumor Activity of Benzaldehyde Derivative." *Cancer Treatment Report* 69:5 (1985), 533-537.

65. Zhang, Z.L. et al. "Hepatoprotective Effects of Astragalus Root." *Journal of Ethnopharmacology* 30 (1990), 145-149.

66. Chan, T. "Ancient Remedies Clues to Cancer Cures." *Health Freedom News* 3:5 (1984), 12-13.

67. Tani, T. et al. "Biphasic Action of Rikkunshi-to and Hochu-ekki-to (GAC)." *Japanese Journal of Allergy* 37:2 (1988), 107-114.

68. Oka, T. et al. "Studies on the Effects of Rikkunshi-to and Hochu-ekki-to (GAC) on Adrenal and Autonomic Nervous Function." *Japanese Journal of Oriental Medicine* 43:3 (1993), 439-446.

69. Sugiyama, K. et al. "Protective Effects of Kampo Medicine Against Cis-diaminedischloroplatinum Induced Nephrotoxicity and Bone Marrow Toxicity in Mice." *Wakan Iyaku Gakkaishi* 10:1 (1993), 76-85.

70. Yang, Y.Z. et al. "Effect of *Astragalus membranaceus* on Natural Killer Cell Activity and Induction of Alpha- and Gamma-interferon in Patients with Coxsackie B Viral Myocarditis." *Chinese Medical Journal* 103:4 (1990), 304-307.

71. Humphries, M.J. et al. "Augmentation of Murine Natural Killer Cell Activity by Swainsonine, a New Antimetastatic Immunomodulator." *Cancer Research* 48 (1988), 1410-1415.

72. Bertino, J.R. "Swainsonine Inhibition of Spontaneous Metastasis." *Journal of the National Cancer Institute* 81 (1989), 1024-1028.

73. U.S. Patent No. 4,844,901. Oxindole alkaloids, from uña de gato (cat's claw), have immune-stimulating properties.

74. "Uña de Gato: Its Therapeutic Characteristics, History and Clinical Effectiveness." *Wellness Advocate* 5:1 (1995), 1-5.

75. Ibid.

76. Steinberg, P.N. "Cat's Claw Update: Wondrous Herb from the Peruvian Rain Forest." *Townsend Letter for Doctors & Patients* (August/September 1995), 70-71.

77. Lersch, C. et al. "Simulation of Immunocompetent Cells in Patients with Gastrointestinal Tumors During an Experimental Therapy with Low-dose Cyclophophamide, Thymostimulin, and *Echinacea purpurea* Extract (Echinacin)." *Tumordiagen Therapy* 13 (1992), 115-120. Cited in: Werbach, M., and M. Murray. *Botanical Influences on Illness* (Tarzana, CA: Third Line Press, 1994), 94-95.

78. Lersch, C. et al. "Stimulation of the Immune Response in Outpatients with Hepatocellular Carcinomas by Low Doses of Cyclophopsphamide (LDCY), *Echinacea purpurea* Extracts (Echinacin) and Thymostimulin." *Arch Geschhwulstforsch* 60:5 (1990), 379-383.

79. Luettig, B. et al. "Macrophage Activation by the Polysaccharide Arabinogalactan Isolated from Plant Cell Cultures of *Echinacea purpurea*." *Journal of the National Cancer Institute* 81:9 (1989), 669-675.

80. Walters, R. "Essiac." *Options: The Alternative Cancer Therapy Book* (Garden City, NY: Avery Publishing, 1993), 110.

81. Ibid.

82. Thomas, R. *The Essiac Report* (Los Angeles: Alternative Treatment Information Network, 1993).

83. Moss, R. "Essiac." *Cancer Therapy: The Independent Consumer's Guide* (New York: Equinox Press, 1992), 146-147. Moss reviews the technical cancer-related research on Essiac; many substances isolated from the herbs in Essiac show specific kinds of anticancer activity

84. Chen, Q.H. et al. "Studies on Chinese Rhubarb XII. Effect of Anthraquinone Derivatives on the Respiration and Glycolysis of Ehrlich Ascites Carcinoma Cells." *Acta Pharmaceutica Sinica* 15 (1980), 65-70. See also: Kawai, K. et al. "A Comparative Study on Cytotoxicities and Biochemical Properties of Anthraquinone Mycotoxins Emodin and Skyrin from *Penicillium Islandium Sopp*." *Toxicology Letters* 20 (1984), 155-160.

85. Lu, M., and Q.H. Chen. "Biochemical Study of Chinese Rhubarb XXIX. Inhibitory Effects of Anthraquinone Derivatives on P338 Leukemia in Mice." *Journal of China Pharmacology University* 20 (1989), 155-157.

86. Morita, K. et al. "A Desmutagenic Factor Isolated from Burdock *(Arctium lappa linne)*." *Mutation Research* 129 (1984), 25-31.

87. Walters, R. "Essiac." *Options: The Alternative Cancer Therapy Book* (Garden City, NY: Avery Publishing, 1993), 112.

88. Ibid., 115.

89. Yoshida, M. et al. "The Effect of Quercetin on Cell Cycle Progression and Growth of Human Gastric Cancer Cells." *FEBS Letters* 260 (1990), 10-13.

90. Morazzoni, P., and S. Malandrino. "Anthocyanins and Their Aglycons as Scavengers of Free Radicals and Antilipoperoxidant Agents." *Pharmacology Rees Commission* 20:2 Suppl (1988), 254. See also: Meunier, M.T. et al. "Free Radical Scavenger Activity of Procyanidolic Oligomers and Anthocyanocides with Respect to Superoxide Anion and Lipid Peroxidation." *Plantes Medicinales et Phytotherapies* XXIII (1989), 267.

91. Lin, R.S. *Garlic and Health: Recent Advances in Research* (Irvine, CA: International Academy of Health and Fitness, 1994), 22.

92. Lau, B.H.S. et al. "*Allium sativum* (Garlic) and Cancer Prevention." *Nutrition Research* 10 (1990), 937-948.

93. Lin, R.S. *Garlic and Health: Recent Advances in Research* (Irvine, CA: International Academy of Health and Fitness, 1994), 23.

94. Bennett, S.A. et al. "Platelet Activating Factor, an Endogenous Mediator of Inflammation, Induces Phenotypic Transformation of Rat Embryo Cells." *Carcinogenesis* 14:7 (1993), 1289-1296.

95. Nigam, S. et al. "Elevated Plasma Levels of Platelet-activating Factor (PAF) in Breast Cancer Patients with Hypercalcemia." *Journal of Lipid Mediators and Cell Signalling* 1:6 (1989), 323-328. See also: Pitton, C. et al. "Presence of PAF-acether in Human Breast Carcinoma: Relation to Axillary Lymph Node Metastasis." *Journal of the National Cancer Institute*

81:17 (1989), 1298-1302.

96. Wilford, J.N. "Ancient Tree Yields Secrets of Potent Healing Substance." *The New York Times* (March 1, 1988), C3. Cited in: Murray, F. *Gingko Biloba* (New Canaan, CT: Keats Publishing, 1993).

97. Rong, Y. et al. "*Gingko Biloba* Attenuates Oxidative Stress in Macrophages and Endothelial Cells." *Free Radical Biology & Medicine* 20:1 (1996), 121-127.

98. Pincemail, J., and A.C. Deby. "The Antiradical Properties of *Ginkgo Biloba* Extract." *Rokan (Ginkgo Biloba): Recent Results in Pharmacology and Clinic* edited by Funfgeld, F.W. (Berlin: Springer-Verlag, 1988), 71-82.

99. *Ginkgo Biloba Extract* (EGb 761) *in Perspective* (Auckland, New Zealand: ADIS Press, 1990), 3. Cited in: Murray, F. *Gingko Biloba* (New Canaan, CT: Keats Publishing, 1993), 37-38.

100. Hu, S.Y. "The Genus Panax (Ginseng) in Chinese Medicine." *Economic Botany* 30:1 (1976), 11-28.

101. Hou, J.P. "Chemical Constituents of Ginseng Plants." *American Journal of Chinese Medicine* 5:2 (1977), 123-145.

102. Boik, J. "Effect of Panax Ginseng (ren shen)." *Cancer and Natural Medicine: A Textbook of Basic Science and Clinical Research* (Princeton, MN: Oregon Medical Press, 1995), 73.

103. Zhang, D. et al. "Ginseng Extract Scavenges Hydroxyl Radical and Protects Unsaturated Fatty Acids from Decomposition Caused by Iron-mediated Lipid Peroxidation." *Free Radical Biology and Medicine* 20:1 (1996), 145-150.

104. Ng, T.B., and H.W. Yeung. "Scientific Basis of the Therapeutic Effects of Ginseng." *Folk Medicine: The Art and the Science*, edited by Steiner, R.P. (Washington, DC: American Chemical Society, 1986), 139-151. See also: Zhang, D. et al. "Ginseng Extract Scavenges Hydroxyl Radical and Protects Unsaturated Fatty Acids from Decomposition Caused by Iron-mediated Lipid Peroxidation." *Free Radical Biology & Medicine* 20:1 (1996), 145-150.

105. Yun, Taik-koo et al. "Anticarcinogenic Effect of Long-term Oral Administration of Red Ginseng on Newborn Mice Exposed to Various Chemical Carcinogens." *Cancer Detection and Prevention* 6 (1983), 515-525.

106. Tode, T. et al. "Inhibitory Effects of Oral Administration of Ginsenoside Rh2 on Tumor Growth in Nude Mice Bearing Serous Cyst Adenocarcinoma of the Human Ovary." *Acta Obstetrica et Gynaecologica Japonica* 45 (1993), 1275-1282.

107. Wang, M. et al. "Effects of Ginseng Volatile Oil on Cytochemical Components of SGC-823 Gastric Carcinoma in Cell Culture." *China Journal of Chinese Materia Medica* 17:2 (1992), 110-112.

108. Yun, Taik-koo, and Soo-yong Choi. "Preventive Effect of Ginseng Intake against Various Human Cancers: A Case-control Study on 1987 Pairs." *Cancer Epidemiology, Biomarkers & Prevention* 4 (1995), 401-408.

109. Kim, J.Y. et al. "Panax Ginseng as a Potential Immunomodulator: Studies in Mice." *Immunopharmacology and Immunotoxicology* 12:2 (1990), 257-276.

110. Morazzoni, P., and S. Malandrino. "Anthocyanins and Their Aglycons as Scavengers of Free Radicals and Antilipoperoxidant Agents." *Pharmacology Rees Commission* 20:2 Suppl (1988), 254.

111. Meunier, M.T. et al. "Free Radical Scavenger Activity of Procyanidolic Oligomers and Anthocyanocides with Respect to Superoxide Anion and Lipid Peroxidation." *Plantes Medicinales et Phytotherapies* XXIII (1989), 267.

112. Chisaka, T. et al. *Chemical and Pharmaceutical Bulletin* (1988). Cited in: Wilner, J. "Green Tea." *The Cancer Solution* (Boca Raton, FL: Peltec Publishing, 1994), 75.

113. Bu-Abbas, A. et al. "Marked Antimutagenic Potential of Aqueous Green Tea Extracts: Mechanism of Action." *Mutagenesis* 9 (1994), 325-331.

114. Mukhtar, H. et al. "Green Tea and Skin—Anticarcinogenic Effects." *Journal of Investigative Dermatology* 102 (1994), 3-7.

115. Klaunig, J.E. "Chemopreventive Effects of Green Tea Components on Hepatic Carcinogenesis." *Preventative Medicine* 21 (1992), 510-519. See also: Gao, Y.T. et al. "Reduced Risk of Esophageal Cancer Associated with Green Tea Consumption." *Journal of the National Cancer Institute* 86 (1994), 855-858.

116. "The Role of Haelan Nutrition in Enhancing the Anti-cancer Effect of Chemotherapeutic Drugs in Mice with HAC Cell Liver Cancer." Report #110. *The Therapeutic of Soybean Phytochemicals* (Metairie, LA: U.S. Research Reports, 1995).

117. "Gastric Cancer *in vivo* Study." Report #112. "Anti-Lipid Peroxidation and Improvement of Lung Function." Report #108. "Relieving Leukopenia in Liver Cancer." Report #109. *The Therapeutic of Soybean Phytochemicals* (Metairie, LA: U.S. Research Reports, 1995).

118. "A Clinical Study of Haelan 851 Concentrated Nutritional Oral Liquid in Supporting Healthy Energy and Lowering Toxic Effects of Radiation and Chemotherapy on Cancer Patients." Report #103. *The Therapeutic of Soybean Phytochemicals* (Metairie, LA: U.S. Research Reports, 1995).

119. Pelton, R. Personal communications (1995).

120. Walker, Morton. "Anticancer Attributes of Modified Citrus Pectin." *Townsend Letter for Doctors & Patients* (August/ September 1996), 85.

121. Office of Technology Assessment. *Unconventional Cancer Treatments* (Washington, DC: U.S. Government Printing Office, 1990).

122. Kazuyoshi, M. et al. "A Desmutagenic Factor Isolated from Burdock. *Arctium lappa linne." Mutation Research* 129 (1984), 25-31.

123. Dhawan, B.N. et al. "Screening of Indian Plants for Biological Activity: VI." *Indian Journal of Experimental Biology* 15 (1977), 208. See also: Hoshi, A. et al. "Anti-tumor Activity of Berberine Derivatives." *Japanese Journal of Cancer Research* 67 (1976), 321-325.

124. Messina, M.J. et al. "Soy Intake and Cancer Risk: A Review of *in vitro* and *in vivo* Data." *Nutrition and Cancer* 21:2 (1994), 113-131.

125. Boik, J. "Conducting Research on Natural Agents: A Summary of Effects of *Glycyrrhiza uralensis*." *Cancer*

and Natural Medicine: A Textbook of Basic Science and Clinical Research (Princeton, MN: Oregon Medical Press, 1995), 179.

126. Pierson, H. "Designer Foods and Cancer." World Congress on Cancer. Sydney, Australia (April 1994), 25.

127. Austin, S. et al. "Long-term Follow-up of Cancer Patients Using Contreras, Hoxsey, and Gerson Therapies." *Journal of Naturopathic Medicine* 5:1 (1994), 74-76. Given the small size of this study, and the fact that many different cancers were involved, at different stages and with different treatments used for each cancer, it is impossible to draw statistically meaningful conclusions from this study. However, the results at least *suggest* a benefit for cancer patients receiving the Hoxsey formula. In no way should the reader assume that the Gerson or Contreras clinics are failing to help patients based on the results of this study. Remember, these were advanced-stage cancer patients, many of whom had undergone conventional therapies first.

128. Office of Technology Assessment. *Unconventional Cancer Treatments* (Washington, DC: U.S. Government Printing Office, 1990), 83. Iscador with copper is used for primary tumors of the liver, gallbladder, stomach, and kidneys; Iscador with mercury is used to treat tumors of the intestine and lymphatic system; Iscador with silver is used to treat cancers of the breast and urogenital tract; and Iscador without any added metals is used to treat most other cancers. The OTA report notes that this form,*Viscum album*, differs markedly from mistletoe found in the U.S.

129. Kiene, H. "Clinical Studies on Mistletoe Therapy for Cancerous Diseases: A Review." *Therapeutikon* 3:6 (1989), 347-350.

130. Hajito, T., and C. Lanzrein. "Natural Killer and Antibody-Dependent Cell-mediated Cytotoxicity and Large Granular Lymphocyte Frequencies in *Viscum album*-Treated Breast Cancer Patients." *Oncology* 43 Suppl 1 (1986), 93-97. See also: Hajito, T. "Immunomodulatory Effects of Iscador: A *Viscum album* Preparation." *Oncology* 43 Suppl 1 (1986), 51-65.

131. Nienhaus, J. "Tumor Inhibition and Thymus Stimulation with Mistletoe Preparations." *Elemente Naturowissenschaft* 13 (1970), 45-54. See also: Salzer, G., and H. Muller. "Local Treatment of Malignant Pleural Effusions with Mistletoe Preparation Iscador." *Praxix Pneumologia* 32 (1978), 721-729. See also: Linder, M. "Mistletoe Preparations Prevent Changes in Copper Metabolism." American Association of Cancer Researchers, Annual Meeting. Saint Louis, MO (1982).

132. Leroi, R. "Fundamentals of Mistletoe Therapy." *Krebsgeschehen* 5 (1979), 145-146.

133. Kiene, H. "Clinical Studies on Mistletoe Therapy for Cancerous Diseases: A Review." *Therapeutikon* 3:6 (1989), 347-533.

134. Studies on clinical effects of Iscador were all cited in *Journal of Anthroposophical Medicine* 11:2 (1994), 20-26; and in Heiligtag, R. *Anthroposophical Medicine and Therapies for Cancer* (Spring Valley, NY: Mercury Press, 1994).

135. *Unconventional Cancer Treatments; Herbal Treatments: Mistletoe* (Washington, DC: Office of Technology Assessment, U.S. Congress, 1990), 84.

136. "Ovarian Cancer and Mistletoe Treatment." *Journal of Anthroposophical Medicine* 13:3 (1996), 51-53.

137. Egert, D., and N. Beuscher. "Studies on Antigen Specificity of Immunoreactive Arabinogalactan Proteins Extracted from *Baptisia tinctoria* and *Echinacea purpurea." Planta Medica* 58:2 (1992), 163-165.

138. Ibid.

139. D'Adamo, P. "Larch Arabinogalactan is a Novel Immune Modulator." *Townsend Letter for Doctors & Patients* (April 1996), 42-46.

140. Kiyohara, H. et al. "Relationship between Structure and Activity of an Anti-complementary *Arabinogalactan* from the Roots of *Angelica Autiloba Kitagawa." Carbohydrate Research* 193 (1989), 193-200.

141. Gonda, R. et al. "Arabinogalactan Core Structure and Immunological Activities of Ukonana C, an Acidic Polysaccharide from the Rhizome of *Curcuma longa." Biological & Pharmaceutical Bulletin* 16:3 (1993), 235-238.

142. D'Adamo, P. "Larch Arabinogalactan is a Novel Immune Modulator." *Townsend Letter for Doctors & Patients* (April 1996), 42-46.

143. Hagmar, B. et al. "Arabinogalactan Blockade of Experimental Metastases to Liver by Murine Hepatoma." *Invasion Metastasis* 11:6 (1991), 348-355. See also: Beuth, J. et al. "Inhibition of Liver Metastasis in Mice by Blocking Hepatocyte Lectins with Arabinogalactan Infusions and D-galactose." *Journal of Cancer Research and Clinical Oncology* 113:1 (1987), 51-55.

144. Beuth, J. et al. "Inhibition of Liver Tumor Cell Colonization in Two Animal Tumor Models by Lectin Blocking with D-galactose or Arabinogalactan." *Clinical and Experimental Metastasis* 6:2 (1988), 115-120.

145. D'Adamo, P. Personal communications (April 1996).

146. Hauer, J., and F.A. Anderer. "Mechanism of Stimulation of Human Natural Killer Cytotoxicity by Arabinogalactan from *Larix Occidentalis." Cancer Immunology and Immunotherapy* 36 (1993), 237-244.

147. Note: In some of the blood donors, the lack of NK activity was likely traced to an increase in a "bad eicosanoid" (PGE2) from immune cells (monocytes). This undesirable effect could perhaps be inhibited by fish oils and certain other nontoxic agents, though this has yet to be studied.

148. Mueller, E.A., and F.A. Anderer. "A *Viscum album* Oligosaccharide Activating Human Natural Cytotoxicity Is an Interferon-y Inducer." *Cancer Immunology and Immunotherapy* 32 (1990), 221-227.

149. Hauer, J., and F.A. Anderer. "Mechanism of Stimulation of Human Natural Killer Cytotoxicity by Arabinogalactan from *Larix occidentalis." Cancer Immunology and Immunotherapy* 36 (1993), 237-244.

150. Wagner, H. "Low Molecular Weight Polysaccharides from Composite Plants Containing Arabinogalactan, Arabinoglucan and Arabinoxylan." German Patent No. DE 3,042,491 (July 15, 1982).

151. Chang, R. Personal communications (1995). New York-based Raymond Chang, M.D., formerly at Memorial Sloan-Kettering Cancer Center, is an expert on medicinal mushrooms.

152. Adachi, K. et al. "Potentiation of Host-mediated

Antitumor Activity in Mice by Beta-glucan Obtained from *Grifola frondosa* (Maitake)." *Chemical & Pharmacological Bulletin* 35:1 (1987), 262-270.

153. Nanba, H. "Maitake Mushroom: Immune Therapy to Prevent Cancer Growth and Metastasis." *Explore* 6:1 (1995), 17.

154. Nanba, H. "Antitumor Activity of Orally Administered 'D-fraction' from Maitake Mushroom (*Grifola frondosa*)." *Journal of Naturopathic Medicine* 1:4 (1993), 10-15.

155. Awang, D.V.C. "Commercial Taheebo Lacks Active Ingredient." *Canadian Pharmacology Journal* 121 (1991), 323-326.

156. Rao, K.V. "Quinone Natural Products. Streptonigrin (NSC-45383) and Lapachol (NSC-11905) Structure-activity Relationships." *Cancer Chemotherapy Reports* (Part 2) 4:4 (1974), 11-17. See also: Rao, K.V. et al. "Recognition and Evaluation of Lapachol as an Antitumor Agent." *Cancer Research* 28 (1968), 1952-1954.

157. Santana, C.F. et al. "Preliminary Observations with the Use of Lapachol in Human Patients Bearing Malignant Neoplasms." *Revista de Instituto de Antibioticos* 20 (1980/1981), 61-68. Cited in: Werbach, M.R., and M.T. Murray. *Botanical Influences on Illness* (Tarzana, CA: Third Line Press, 1994).

158. Linardi, M.D.C. et al. "A Lapachol Derivative Active against Mouse Lymphocyte Leukemia P-388." *Journal of Medicinal Chemistry* 18:11 (1975), 1159-1162.

159. Block, J.B. et al. "Early Clinical Studies with Lapachol (NSC-11905)." *Cancer Chemotherapy Reports* (Part 2) 4:4 (1978), 27-28.

160. Zollner, T.M. et al. "Induction of NK-like Activity in T cells by IL-s/anti-CD3 Is Linked to Expression of a New Antitumor Receptor with Specificity for Acetylated Mannose." *Anticancer Research* 13:4 (1993), 923-930.

161. Zhu, H.G. et al. "Activation of Human Monocyte/Macrophage Cytotoxicity by IL-2/IFN Gamma Is Linked to Increased Expression of an Antitumor Receptor with Specificity for Acetylated Mannose." *Immunology Letters* 38:2 (1993), 111-119.

162. Pienta, K.J. et al. "Inhibition of Spontaneous Metastases in a Rat Prostate Cancer Model by Oral Administration of Modified Citrus Pectin." *Journal of the National Cancer Institute* 87:5 (1995), 348-353.

163. Weiss, R.F. *Herbal Medicine* (Beaconsfield, England: Beaconsfield Publishers, 1988).

164. *Cardui Mariae Fructus: Silybum marianum*. Monograph of the German Health Authorities (BGA). *Bundesanzeiger* 13:3 (1986).

165. Hikino, H., and Y. Kiso. *Natural Products for Liver Disease*, edited by Wagner, H. (New York: Academic Press, 1988). See also: *Economic and Medicinal Plant Research* 2 (1988), 39-72.

166. Feher, H. et al. "Hepatoprotective Activity of Silymarin Therapy in Patients with Chronic Alcoholic Liver Disease." *Orvosi Hetil*ap 130 (1990), 51.

167. Nagabhushan, M., and S.V. Bhide. "Curcumin as an Inhibitor of Cancer." *Journal of the American College of Nutrition* 11:2 (1992), 192-198.

168. Polasa, K. et al. "Effect of Turmeric on Urinary Mutagens in Smokers." *Mutagen* 7:2 (1992), 107-109.

169. Mukundan, M.A. et al. "Effect of Turmeric and Curcumin on BP-DNA Adducts." *Carcinogenesis* 14 (1993), 493-496.

170. Azuine, M.A., and S.V. Bhide. "Protective Single/Combined Treatment with Betel Leaf and Turmeric Against Methyl (acetoxymmethyl) Nitrosamine-induced Hamster Oral Carcinogenesis." *International Journal of Cancer* 51:3 (1992), 412-415.

171. Kakar, S.S., and D. Roy. "Curcumin Inhibits TPA Induced Expression of C-fos, C-jun and C-myc Proto-oncogene Messenger RNAs in Mouse Skin." *Cancer Letters* 87:1 (1995), 85-89.

172. Kuttan, R. et al. "Turmeric and Curcumin as Topical Agents in Cancer Therapy." *Tumori* 73 (1987), 29-31.

173. Nagabhushan, M. and S.V. Bhide. "Curcumin as an Inhibitor of Cancer." *Journal of the American College of Nutrition* 11:2 (1992), 192-198.

174. Rao, C.V. et al. "Chemoprevention of Colon Carcinogenesis by Dietary Curcumin, a Naturally Occurring Plant Phenolic Compound." *Cancer Research* 55:2 (1995), 259-266.

175. Aruna, K., and V.M. Sivaramakrishnan. "Plant Products as Protective Agents against Cancer." *Indian Journal of Experimental Biology* 28:11 (1990), 1008-1111.

## Chapter 30

## The New Pharmacology for Treating Cancer

1. The exception to this statement concerns the use of hormones, which in any case may be deemed a different form of therapy.

2. Reich, R., and J. Metcalf. *Dealing with Side-Effects: The Facts About Chemotherapy* (Mount Vernon, NY: Consumer Reports Books, 1991), 161.

3. Greenwald, H. "Cancer Treatment: The Industry of Hope." *Who Survives Cancer?* (Berkeley, CA: University of California Press, 1992), 46.

4. Abel, U. *Cytostatic Therapy of Advanced Epithelial Tumors: A Critique* (Stuggart, Germany: Hippocrates Verlag, 1990).

5. Powles, T.J. "Failure of Chemotherapy to Prolong Survival in a Group of Patients with Metastatic Breast Cancer." *The Lancet* (March 15 1980), 580.

6. Lucien, I. *Conquering Cancer* (New York: Random House, 1978), 95.

7. Lazlo, J. *Understanding Cancer* (New York: Harper and Row, 1987).

8. Schmahl, D. "Experimental Development of Anticancer Drugs—Problems and Objectives, Strategies and Results." *Current Cancer Research* (New York: Springer, 1989), 157-243.

9. Ibid.

10. Shen, R.N. et al. "Bio-immunotherapy for Cancer in Experimental Studies and Clinical Applications." *In Vivo* 8:5 (1994), 643-652.

11. Hansen, H.H. "Lung Cancer." *Cancer: Chemotherapy and Biological Response Modifiers*, edited by Pinedo, H.M. et al. (Amsterdam: Elsevier, 1988), 222-240.

12. Reich, R., and J. Metcalf. *Dealing with Side-Effects: The Facts About Chemotherapy* (Mount Vernon, NY: Consumer Reports Books, 1991), 175.

13. Ibid.

14. Chlebowski, R.T. et al. "Late Mortality and Levamisole Adjuvant Therapy in Colorectal Cancer." *British Journal of Cancer* 69 (1994), 1094-1097.

15. Moertel, C.G. et al. "Levamisole and Fluorouracil for Adjuvant Therapy of Resected Colon Carcinoma." *New England Journal of Medicine* 322 (1990), 352-358.

16. Eidem, William Kelley. *The Man Who Cures Cancer* (Bethesda, MD: Be Well Books, 1996).

17. Moss, R. "Conclusions." *Questioning Chemotherapy* (New York: Equinox Press, 1995), 170.

18. Pace, J.C. "Oral Ingestion of Encapsulated Ginger and Reported Self-care Actions for the Relief of Chemotherapy-associated Nausea and Vomiting." *Dissertation Abstracts International* 8 (1987), 3297.

19. Kolata, G. "New Finding Offers Insights into How Cancer Develops: Why Tumors Resist Chemotherapy and Radiation." *The New York Times* (January 4, 1996).

20. Boice, J.D., and L.B. Travis. "Body Wars: Effect of Friendly Fire (Cancer Therapy)." *Journal of the National Cancer Institute* 87:10 (1995), 732-741.

21. Greenwald, H. "Cancer Treatment: The Industry of Hope." *Who Survives Cancer?* (Berkeley, CA: University of California Press, 1992), 45.

22. Abel, U. *Cytostatic Therapy of Advanced Epithelial Tumors: A Critique* (Stuggart, Germany: Hippocrates Verlag, 1990).

23. Silberstein, S. "German Biostatistician Cites Chemotherapy's Failures." *Health News & Views* 1:2 (1992), 1.

24. Malins, D.C. et al. "Progression of Human Breast Cancer to the Metastatic Stage Is Linked to Hydroxyl Radical Induced DNA Damage." *Proceedings of the National Academy of Sciences* 93:6 (1996), 2557-2563.

25. Lockwood, K. et al. "Apparent Partial Remission of Breast Cancer in "High Risk" Patients Supplemented with Nutritional Antioxidants, Essential Fatty Acids and Co-enzyme Q10." *Molecular Aspects of Medicine* 15 (1994), 231-240.

26. Lamm, D.L. et al. "Megadose Vitamins in Bladder Cancer: A Double-blind Clinical Trial." *Journal of Urology* 151 (1994), 21-26.

27. Boyar, A.P. et al. "Response to a Diet Low in Total Fat in Women with Postmenopausal Breast Cancer: A Pilot Study." *Nutrition and Cancer* 11 (1988), 3-99.

28. Newberne, P.M., and M. Locniskar. "Roles of Micronutrients in Cancer Prevention: Recent Evidence from the Laboratory." *Progress in Clinical and Biological Research* 346 (1990), 119-134.

29. Ning, C. et al. "Therapeutic Effects of *jian pi yi shen* Prescription on the Toxicity Reactions of Postoperative Chemotherapy in Patients with Advanced Gastric Carcinoma." *Journal of Traditional Chinese Medicine* 8:2 (1988), 113-116.

30. Guo, Z.H. et al. "Chinese Herb Destagnation Series 1: Combination of Radiation with Destagnation in the Treatment of Nasopharyngeal Carcinoma (NPC), a Prospective Randomized Trial on 188 Cases." *International Journal of Radiation Oncology, Biology and Physics* 16 (1989), 297-300. See also: Sun, Y. "The Role of Traditional Chinese Medicine in Supportive Care of Cancer Patients." *Recent Results in Cancer Research* 108 (1988), 327-344.

31. Shiu, W.T.C. et al. "A Clinical Study of PSP on Peripheral Blood Counts during Chemotherapy." *Phytotherapy Research* 6 (1992), 217-218.

32. Mohr, P.E. "Serum Progesterone and Prognosis in Operable Breast Cancer." *British Journal of Cancer* 73:12 (1996), 1552-1555.

33. Kostler, W. Personal communications. See also: Kostler, W. "Prevention of Recidives and Metastasis of Tumors by Immunotherapy: Activating the Immune System; Immune Modulation." World Congress on Cancer. Sydney, Australia (April 1994), 111.

34. Kostler, W. Personal communications (June 1996).

35. Ibid.

36. Brohult, A. "Effect of Alkoxyglycerols on the Frequency of Injuries Following Radiation Therapy for Carcinoma of the Uterine Cervix." *Acta Obstetrica et Gynecologica Scandinavica* 56:4 (1977), 441-448. See also: Brohult A. "Effect of Alkoxyglycerols on the Frequency of Injuries Following Radiation Therapy." *Experientia* 29 (1973), 81-82.

37. Hallgren, B., and S. Larsson. "The Glycerol Ethers in the Liver Oils of Elasmobranch Fish." *Lipid Research* 3 (1962), 31-38.

38. Ibid., 39-43.

39. Berdel, W.E. et al. "Antitumor Action of Alkyl-lysophospholipids." *Anticancer Research* 1:6 (1981), 345-352.

40. Diamoede, L. "Increased Ether Lipid Cytotoxicity by Reducing Membrane Cholesterol Content." *International Journal of Cancer* 49:3 (1991), 409-413.

41. Brohult, A. et al. "Regression of Tumor Growth after Administration of Alkoxyglycerols." *Acta Obstetrica et Gynecologica Scandinavica* 57 (1978), 79-83.

42. Brohult, A. "Alkoxyglycerols and Their Use in Radiation Treatment." *Acta Radiologica* 223 (1963), 7-99.

43. Daniel, L.W. et al. "Ether Lipids Inhibit the Effects of Phorbol Diesters Tumor Promoters." *Lipids* 22:11 (1987), 851-855. See also: Holub, B.J. et al. "Dietary Lipid Modification of Renal Disorders and Ether Phospholipid Metabolism." *Biochemistry and Cell Biology* 69:7 (1991), 485-489.

44. "Burzynski's Antineoplastons Increase Activity of Tumor Suppressor Genes." *Options* 2 (June 1995).

45. Pelton, R., and L. Overholser. "Antineoplastons." *Alternatives in Cancer Therapy* (New York: Simon & Schuster, 1994), 192.

46. Tsuda, H. et al. "The Inhibitor Effect of Antineoplaston A10 on Breast Cancer Transplanted to Athymic Mice and Human Hepatocellular Carcinoma Cell Lines." *Kurume Medical Journal* 37 (1990), 97-104.

47. "Antineoplastons: New Antitumor Agents Stir High Expectations." *Oncology News* 16:4 (1990), 1-6.

48. Ibid.

49. Wiewel, F. "Burzynski's Antineoplastons Increase Activity of Tumor Suppressor Genes." *Options* 1:4 (1995), 2.

50. Krishnaswamy, M., and K.K. Purushothaman. "Plumbagin: A Study of Its Anticancer, Antibacterial, and Antifungal Properties." *Indian Journal of Experimental Biology* 18 (1980), 876-877. See also: Chandrasekaran, B. et al. "New Methods for Urinary Estimation of Antitumor Compounds Echitamine and Plumbagin." *Indian Journal of Biochemistry and Biophysics* 19 (1982), 48-149.

51. Melo, A.M. et al. "First Observations on the Topical Use of Primin, Plumbagin, and Maytenin in Patients with Skin Cancer." *Revista de Instituto de Antibioticos* 14:1-2 (1974), 9-16.

52. Prudden, J. "The Treatment of Human Cancer with Agents Prepared from Bovine Cartilage." *Journal of Biological Response Modifiers* 4:6 (1985), 590-595.

53. Durie, B.G. et al. "Antitumor Activity of Bovine Cartilage Extract (Catrix-S) in the Human Tumor Stem Cell Assay." *Journal of Biological Response Modifiers* 4:6 (1985), 590-595.

54. Prudden, J. "Use of Cartilage in Cancer Treatment" Adjuvant Nutrition for Cancer Treatment Symposium. Tampa, Florida (September 30, 1995).

55. Prudden, J. "The Treatment of Human Cancer with Agents Prepared from Bovine Cartilage." *Journal of Biological Response Modifiers* 4 (1985), 551-584.

56. Lane, I. William. "Shark Cartilage Therapy Results and Research Today." Physician Information Package. Cartilage Consultants (Spring 1995). Contact LaneLabs at 201-391-8601.

57. Lane, I.W. *Shark Cartilage Update Newsletter* 1:3 (1994), 1.

58. Oikawa, T. et al. "A Novel Angiogenic Inhibitor Derived from Japanese Shark Cartilage. Extraction and Estimation of Inhibitory Activities toward Tumor and Embryonic Angiogenesis." *Cancer Letters* 51 (1990), 181-186.

59. Altman, L. "Tumor Growth Is Controlled by Substance Found in Sharks." *The New York Times* (May 1, 1996).

60. Moss, R. "Cesium and Rubidium." *Cancer Therapy: The Independent Consumer's Guide* (New York: Equinox Press, 1992), 91-95.

61. Sartori, H.E. "Nutrients and Cancer: An Introduction to Cesium Therapy." *Pharmacology, Biochemistry and Behavior* 1 (1984), 7-10.

62. Sartori, H.E. "Cesium Therapy in Cancer Patients." *Pharmacology, Biochemistry and Behavior* 1 (1984), 11-13.

63. Messha, F.S., and D.M. Stocco. "Effect of Cesium and Potassium Salts on Survival of Rats Bearing Novikoff Hepatoma." *Pharmacology, Biochemistry and Behavior* 1 (1984), 31-34.

64. El Domeiri, A. et al. "Effect of Alkali Metalsalts on Sarcoma I in A/J mice." *Journal of Surgical Oncology* 18 (1981), 423-429.

65. Moss, R. "Cesium and Rubidium." *Cancer Therapy: The Independent Consumer's Guide* (New York: Equinox Press, 1992), 91-95.

66. Neulieb, R. "Effects of Oral Intake of Cesium Chloride: A Single Case Report." *Pharmacology, Biochemistry and Behavior* 21 (1984), 15-16.

67. Moss, R.W. "DMSO." *Cancer Therapy: The Independent Consumer's Guide* (New York: Equinox Press, 1992), 301.

68. De la Torre, J.C. "Biological Actions and Medical Applications of Dimethyl Sulfoxide." *Annals of the New York Academy of Sciences* (1983). See also: Spremulli, E.N., and D.L. Dexter. "Polar Solvents: A Novel Class of Antineoplastic Agents." *Journal of Clinical Oncology* 2:3 (1984), 227-241.

69. Toren, A., and G. Rechavi. "What Really Cures in Autologous Bone Marrow Transplantation? A Possible Role for Dimethylsulfoxide." *Medical Hypotheses* 41:6 (1993), 495-498.

70. "DMSO Report." *Urology Times* (April 1987). Cited by: Walters, R. "DMSO Therapy." *Options: The Alternative Cancer Therapy Book* (Garden City Park, NY: Avery Publishing, 1993), 249.

71. Stanley, J.W., and R. Herschler. "Pharmacology of DMSO." *Cryobiology* 23 (1986), 14-27.

72. Pommier, R.F. et al. "Synergistic Cytotoxicity between DMSO and Antineoplastic Agents against Ovarian Cancer *In Vitro*." *American Journal of Obstetrics and Gynecology* 159 (1988), 848-852.

73. McCabe, D. et al. "Polar Solvents in the Chemoprevention of Dimethylbenzanthracene-induced Rat Mammary Cancer." *Archives of Surgery* 121 (1986).

74. Volden, D.G. et al. "Inhibition of Methyl-cholanthrene-induced Skin Carcinogenesis in Hairless Mice by Membrane-labelizing Agent DMSO." *British Journal of Dermatology* 109:225S (1983), 133-136.

75. Marks, P.A., and R.A. Rifkind. "Erythroleukemic Differentiation." *Annual Review of Biochemistry* 47 (1990), 419-448.

76. Wilner, J. "DMSO." *The Cancer Solution* (Boca Raton, FL: Peltec Publishing, 1994), 76.

77. Pommier, R.F. et al. "Cytotoxicity of DMSO and Antineoplastic Combinations against Human Tumors." *American Journal of Surgery* 155 (1988), 672-676.

78. Walters, R. "DMSO Therapy." *Options: The Alternative Cancer Therapy Book* (Garden City Park, NY: Avery Publishing, 1993), 249.

79. Walker, M. *DMSO Nature's Healer* (Garden City Park, NY: Avery Publishing, 1993), 177-207.

80. Neulieb, R.L., and M.K. Neulieb. "The Diverse Actions of Dimethyl Sulphoxide: An Indicator of Membrane Transport Activity." *Cytobios* 63:254-255 (1990), 139-165.

81. Wilner, J. "DMSO." *The Cancer Solution* (Boca Raton, FL: Peltec Publishing, 1994), 76.

82. Ranney, D.F. "Drug Targeting to the Lungs." *Biochemical Pharmacology* 35:7 (1986), 1063-1069.

83. Walker, M. *DMSO Nature's Healer* (Garden City Park, NY: Avery Publishing, 1993), 177-207.

84. Thuning, C.A. et al. "Mechanisms of the Synergistic Effect of Oral DMSO on Antineoplastic Therapy." *Annals of the New York Academy of Sciences* 411 (1983), 150-160. See also: Warren, J. et al. "Potentiation of Antineoplastic Compounds by Oral Dimethyl Sulfoxide in Tumor-bearing Rats." *Annals of the New York Academy of Sciences* 243 (1975).

85. Pommier, R.F. et al. "Cytotoxicity of DMSO and

Antineoplastic Combinations against Human Tumors." *American Journal of Surgery* 155 (1988), 672-676.

86. Pommier, R.F. et al. "Synergistic Cytotoxicity between DMSO and Antineoplastic Agents against Ovarian Cancer *In Vitro*." *American Journal of Obstetrics and Gynecology* 159 (1988), 848-852.

87. Mickey, D.D. et al. "Conventional Chemotherapeutic Agents Combined with DMSO or DFMO in Treatment of Rat Prostate Carcinoma." *Prostate* 15 (1989), 221-282.

88. Kuroda, M. et al. "Decreased Serum Levels of Selenium and Glutathione Peroxidase Activity Associated with Aging, Malignancy and Chronic Hemodialysis." *Trace Elements in Medicine* 5:3 (1988), 97-103.

89. Boit, J. "Amino Acids." *Cancer and Natural Medicine: A Textbook of Basic Science and Clinical Research* (Princeton, MN: Oregon Medical Press, 1995), 139-140.

90. Palermo, M.S. et al. "Immunomodulation Exerted by Cyclophosphamide Is Not Interfered by N-Acetyl cysteine." *International Journal of Immunopharmacology* 8:6 (1986), 651-655. See also: Schmitt-Graff, A., and M.E. Scheulen. "Prevention of Adriamycin Cardiotoxicity by Niacin, Isocitrate or N-acetyl cysteine in Mice: A Morphological Study." *Pathology Resident Practice* 181:2 (1986), 168-174. See also: Kim, J.A. et al. "Topical Use of N-acetyl cysteine for Reduction of Skin Reaction to Radiation Therapy." *Seminars in Oncology* 10:Suppl 1 (1983), 86.

91. Chlebowski, R.T. et al. "Hydrazine Sulfate's Influence on Nutritional Status and Survival in Non-small-cell Lung Cancer." *Journal of Clinical Oncology* 8:1 (1990), 9-15.

92. Filov, V.A. et al. "Results of Clinical Evaluation of Hydrazine Sulfate." *Voprosy Onkologii* 36:6 (1990), 721-726. See also: Gershanovich, M.L. et al. "Results of Clinical Study of Antitumor Action of Hydrazine Sulfate." *Nutrition and Cancer* 3 (1981), 7-12.

93. Chlebowski, R.T. et al. "Hydrazine Sulfate's Influence on Nutritional Status and Survival in Non-small-cell Lung cancer." *Journal of Clinical Oncology* 8:1 (1990), 9-15. Note: This was a randomized, prospective, placebo-controlled clinical trial—the gold standard of modern medical research.

94. Gold, J. "Hydrazine Sulfate: A Current Perspective." *Nutrition and Cancer* 9:2-3 (1987), 59-66.

95. Filov, V. et al. "Results of Clinical Evaluation of Hydrazine Sulfate." *Voprosy Onkologii* 36 (1990), 721-726.

96. Gold, J. "Hydrazine Sulfate: A Current Perspective." *Nutrition and Cancer* 9:2-3 (1987), 59-66.

97. Pitard, C.E. "Protocol for Combined Immunologic/Pharmacologic Therapy: Indocin." Personal communications with Etienne Callebout, M.D. Knoxville, TN (1996).

98. Pollard, M., and P. Luckert. "Indomethacin Treatment of Rats with Dimethylhydrazine-induced Intestinal Tumors." *Cancer Treatment and Research* 64 (1980), 1323-1327. See also: Kudo, T. et al. "Antitumor Activity of Indomethacin on Methylazoxy-methanol-induced Bowel Tumors in Rats." *Gann* 71 (1980), 260-264. See also: Pollard, M., and P. Luckert. "Treatment of Chemically-induced Intestinal Cancers with Indomethacin." *Proceedings of the Society for Experimental Biology and Medicine* 167 (1981), 161-164.

99. Beckman, M.D. "The Latest Buzz on Cancer Cures." *The Natural Way* (June/July 1995), 6.

100. Callebout, E., M.D. Personal communications (1996).

101. Patte, M. "Communication et Information Medicales." Twenty-one case histories in French (April 19, 1996). Contact: LaboLife, La Rambourgere Sainte Marie, 79160, La Chapelle Thireuil, France. Fax: 33-49-04-22-13.

102. Naessens, G. "Béchamp's Microzyma to the Somatid Theory: 714X, a Highly Promising Non-toxic Treatment for Cancer and Other Immune Deficiencies." (Unpublished manuscript.) Symposium. Quebec, Canada (1991).

103. Ibid.

104. Anger, G. et al. "Treatment of Multiple Myeloma with New Cytostatic Agent: Gamma-1-methyl-5-bis-(beta-chloroethyl)-amyino-benzimidazolyl-(2)-butyric acid hydrochloride." *Deutsche Medizinische Wochenschrift* 94 (1969), 2495-2500. See also: Finklestine, J.Z. et al. "Unorthodox Therapy for Murine Neuroblastoma with 6-hydroxydomapine (NSC-233898), Bretylium Tosylate (NSC-62164), Papaverine (NSC-35443), and Butyric Acid (NSC-8415)." *Cancer Chemotherapy Reports* 59 (1975), 571-574.

105. Marks, P.A., and R.A. Rifkind. "Differentiating Factors." *Biologic Therapy of Cancer*, edited by DeVita, V.T. et al. (Philadelphia: J.B. Lippincott, 1991).

106. Freeman, J.H. "Effects of Differing Concentrations of Sodium Butyrate on 1,2-dimethylhydrazine-induced Rat Intestinal Neoplasia." *Gastroenterology* 91 (1986), 596-602.

107. Pitard, C.E. "Protocol for Combined Immunologic/Pharmacologic Therapy." Personal communications to Etienne Callebout, M.D. Knoxville, TN (1996).

108. Pitard, C.E. "Cancer Combination Therapy Utilizing Licensed, Low-cost, Effective and Universally Available Members of That Class of Biologicals and Biological Response Modifiers Constituting the Fourth Conventional Modality of Cancer Treatment." University of Tennessee School of Medicine. Unpublished manuscript (1987), 1-18.

109. Esber, H.J. et al. "Specific and Nonspecific Immune Resistance Enhancement Activity of Staphage Lysate." *Journal of Immunopharmacology* 3 (1981), 79-92.

110. Aoke, T. et al. "Staphage Lysate and Lentinan as Immunomodulators and Immunopotentiators in Clinical and Experimental Systems." *Augmenting Agents in Cancer Therapy*, edited by Hirsh, E.M. et al. (New York: Raven Press, 1981), 101-111.

111. Tutton, P.J., and D.H. Barkla. "Cell Proliferation in Dimethylhydrazine-induced Colonic Adenocarcinomata Following Cytotoxic Drug Treatment." *Virchows Archiv A: Pathological Anatomy and Histology* 28 (1978), 151-156.

112. Hast, R. et al. "Cimetidine as an Immune Response Modifier." *Medical Oncology and Tumor Pharmacotherapy* 6:1 (1989), 111-113.

113. Brockmeyer, N.H. et al. "Cimetidine and the Immunoresponse in Healthy Volunteers." *Journal of Investigative Dermatology* 93 (1989), 757-761.

114. Pitard, C.E. "Protocol for Combined

Immunologic/Pharmacologic Therapy: Tagamet." Personal communications to Etienne Callebout, M.D. Knoxville, TN (1996).

115. Nowicky, J.W. et al. "Ukrain as Both an Anti-cancer and Immunoregulatory Agent." *Drugs Under Experimental and Clinical Research* XVIII:Suppl (1992), 51-54.

116. Lohninger, A., and F. Hamler. "*Chelidonium Majus L.* (Ukrain) in the Treatment of Cancer Patients." *Drugs Under Experimental and Clinical Research* XVIII:Suppl (1992), 73-77.

117. Staniszewski, A. et al. "Lymphocyte Subsets in Patients with Lung Cancer Treated with Thiophosphoric Acid Alkaloid Derivatives from *Chelidonium Majus L* (Ukrain)." *Drugs Under Experimental and Clinical Research* XVIII:Suppl (1992), 63-67.

118. Pengsaa, P. et al. "The Effect of Thiophosphoric Acid (Ukrain) on Cervical Cancer, Stage IB Bulky." *Drugs Under Experimental and Clinical Research* XVIII:Suppl (1992), 69-72.

119. Nowicky, J.W. "New Immuno-stimulating Anti-cancer Preparation: Ukrain." Proceedings of the 13th International Congress of Chemotherapy. Vienna, Austria (August 28-September 2, 1983).

120. Nowicky, J. "Cancer Treatment Using Anticancer Preparation Alkaloid Derivative Ukrain." Fourth Mediterranean Congress of Chemotherapy. Rhodos, Greece (October 1984). *Chemioterapia* 4:Suppl 2 (1985), 1169-1171. See also: Nowicky, J. et al. "Biological Activity of Ukrain *In Vitro* and *In Vivo*." Fifth Mediterranean Congress of Chemotherapy. Cairo, Egypt (January 26-November 1, 1986). *Chemioterapia* 6:Suppl 2 (1987), 683-685.

121. Hohenwarter, O. et al. "Selective Inhibition of *In Vitro* Cell Growth by the Anti-tumor Drug Ukrain." *Drugs Under Experimental and Clinical Research* 18:Suppl 1-4 (1992).

122. Liepins, A. "Ukrain as an Experimental Cytotoxic Agent." *Journal of Chemotherapy* 5:Suppl 1 (1992), 797-799.

123. Nowicky, J.W. et al. "Macroscopic UV-marking through Affinity." *Journal of Tumor Marker Oncology* 3:4 (1988), 463-465.

124. Ibid. Note: This journal was published by the American Academy of Tumor Marker Oncology until 1992.

125. Danopoulos, E.D., and I.E. Danopoulou. "The Results of Urea Treatment in Liver Malignancies." *Clinical Oncology* 1 (1975), 341.

126. Danopoulos, E.D. et al. "Eleven Years of Oral Urea Treatment in Liver Malignancies." *Clinical Oncology* 7 (1981), 281-289.

127. Pelton, Ross, and Lee Overholser. *Alternatives in Cancer Therapy* (New York: Fireside/Simon & Schuster, 1994), Chapter 20, Footnote 1.

128. Pelton, Ross, and Lee Overholser. *Alternatives in Cancer Therapy* (New York: Fireside/Simon & Schuster, 1994), Chapter 20, Footnote 5. Tumor cell surfaces contain large amounts of surfactants (glycoproteins and other large molecular surface-active agents), which have hydrophobic and hydrophilic properties at nonpolar and polar sites, respectively, producing a structured water matrix surrounding cancer cells that is markedly different from that surrounding normal cells.

129. Danopoulos, E.D., M.D., and I.E.Danopoulo. "Effects of Urea Treatment in Combination with Curettage in Extensive Periophthalmic Malignancies." *Opthalmogica* 179 (1979), 52-61.

130. Pelton, Ross, and Lee Overholser. *Alternatives in Cancer Therapy* (New York: Fireside/Simon & Schuster, 1994), Chapter 20, Footnote 2.

131. Ibid., Chapter 20, Footnote 7.

132. Ibid., Chapter 20, Footnote 6.

## Chapter 31:

## New Approaches to Immune Stimulation for Reversing Cancer

1. Nauts, H.C. et al. "The Treatment of Malignant Tumors by Bacterial Toxins, as Developed by the Late William B. Coley, M.D., Reviewed in the Light of Modern Research." *Cancer Research* 6 (1946), 205-216.

2. Wiewel, F. Personal communications with Charles Starnes (1995).

3. Ward, Patricia Spain. "History of BCG Vaccine (Bacillus Calmette-Guerin)." *Townsend Letter for Doctors & Patients* (October 1996), 72-77.

4. Nauts, H.C., and J.R. McLaren. "Coley's Toxins—The First Century." *Advances in Experimental Medicine and Biology* 267 (1990), 483-500.

5. Wiemann, B., and C.O. Starnes. "Coley's Toxins, Tumor Necrosis Factor and Cancer Research: A Historical Perspective." *Pharmacology & Therapeutics* 64:3 (1994), 536.

6. Wiewel, F. Personal communications with Charles Starnes (1995).

7. Wiewel, F. Personal communications (1996).

8. Anderson, Alan, Jr. "The Politics of Cancer: How Do You Get the Medical Establishment to Listen?" *The New York Times* (July 29, 1974).

9. U.S. Congress Office of Technology Assessment. "Burton's Theory of Cancer Control through Augmentation of the Immune System." *Unconventional Cancer Treatments* (September 1990), 130. See also: U.S. Congress Office of Technology Assessment. "The IAT Cancer Treatment Regimen." *Unconventional Cancer Treatments* (September 1990), 131.

10. Clement, R.J. et al. "Peritoneal Mesothelioma." *Quantum Medicine* 1 (1988), 68-73.

11. Cassileth, B.R. et al. *Report of a Survey of Patients Receiving Immunoaugmentative Therapy* (University of Pennsylvania Cancer Center, 1987), unpublished. Cited in: U.S. Congress Office of Technology Assessment. "Burton's Theory of Cancer Control through Augmentation of the Immune System." *Unconventional Cancer Treatments* (September 1990), 130.

12. Note: The Food and Drug Administration classifies IB 700 simply as a "biological," while some physicians

refer to it as a modulator of immune system function (immunomodulator).

13. Springer, G.F. "T and Tn General Carcinoma Autoantigens." *Science* 224 (1984), 1198-1206. See also: Avichezer, D.B. et al. "Immunoreactivities of Polyclonal and Monoclonal Antibodies Specific for Human Thomsen-Friedenriech (T) and Tn Antigens with Human Carcinoma Cells." Abstract from the 25th Israel Immunological Society Meeting (1995).

14. Springer, G.F. "T/Tn Antigen: Two Decades of Experience in Early Immuno-detection and Therapy of Human Carcinoma." *Jung Foundation Proceedings* (Stuttgart, Germany: G. Thieme) In press.

15. Springer, G.F. et al. "T/Tn Pancarcinoma Autoantigens: Fundamental Diagnostic and Prognostic Aspects." *Cancer Detection and Prevention* 19 (1995), 173-182.

16. Springer, G.F. "T/Tn Antigen: Two Decades of Experience in Early Immuno-detection and Therapy of Human Carcinoma." *Jung Foundation Proceedings* (Stuttgart, Germany: G. Thieme) In press. Note: Twelve of the 26 patients were over age 50 at the time of the operation.

17. Dowling, C.G. "Fighting Back Against Breast Cancer." *Life* (May 1994), 79-88.

18. Ibid.

19. Old, Lloyd J. "Immunotherapy for Cancer." *Scientific American* 275:3 (September 1996).

20. Lamm, D.L. "BCG Immunotherapy for Transitional-cell Carcinoma In Situ of the Bladder." *Oncology* 9:10 (1995), 947-952.

21. Glashan, R.A. "Randomized Study of Intravesical Alpha-2b Interferon in Carcinoma In Situ of the Bladder." *Journal of Urology* 144 (1990), 658.

22. Rios, A. et al. "Phase Study of 2-amino-5-bromo-6-phenyl 4(3H) pyrimidinone (ABPP): An Oral Interferon Inducer in Cancer Patients." *Journal of Biological Response Modifiers* 5 (1986), 330-338.

23. Oettgen, J.F. et al. "Effects of Dialyzable Transfer Factor in Patients with Breast Cancer." *Proceedings of the National Academy of Sciences* 71 (1974), 2319-2323.

24. Waisbren, B.A. "Observations on the Combined Systemic Administration of Mixed Bacterial Vaccine, (BCG), Transfer Factor, and Lymphoblastoid Lymphocytes to Patients with Cancer, 1974-1985." *Journal of Biological Response Modifiers* 6 (1987), 1-19.

25. Falcone, R. "Adjuvant Vaccine Therapies." *The Complete Guide to Alternative Cancer Therapies* (New York: Carol Publishing, 1994), 168.

26. Weiss, R. "Melanoma Shrinks from Human Monoclonals." *Science News* 137 (1990), 324.

27. Livingston-Wheeler, Virginia. *The Conquest of Cancer: Vaccines and Diet* (New York: Franklin Watts, 1984), 55-56.

28. Walters, R. "Livingston Therapy." *Options: The Alternative Cancer Therapy Book* (Garden City Park, NY: Avery Publishing, 1993), 72-81. The mechanism for this microbe-cancer interaction is unknown, but Livingston speculated that it might relate to an effect on the genetic material of the cell.

29. Lerner, Michael. *Choices in Healing* (Cambridge, MA: MIT Press, 1994), 322.

30. Walters, R. "Livingston Therapy." *Options: The Alternative Cancer Therapy Book* (Garden City Park, NY: Avery Publishing, 1993), 72-81. Dr. Livingston also used the Bacillus Calmette-Guerin (BCG) vaccine, a mild tuberculin vaccine that stimulates white blood cells to kill cancer cells.

31. Livingston-Wheeler, V., and Edmond G. Addeo. *The Conquest of Cancer* (New York: Franklin Watts, 1984). Also based on personal communications with Neal Nathan, M.D., Livingston Foundation in San Diego, CA. These case histories are available from the Livingston Foundation.

32. Walters, R. "Livingston Therapy." *Options: The Alternative Cancer Therapy Book* (Garden City Park, NY: Avery Publishing, 1993), 323.

33. U.S. Congress Office of Technology Assessment. *Unconventional Cancer Treatment* (Washington, DC: U.S. Congress Office of Technology Assessment, 1990).

34. Speckhart, V. Personal communication (1996).

35. Ibid. Dr. Speckhart reported his preliminary study of the Livingston vaccines to a number of groups, including the Office of Technology Assessment advisory group for the U.S. Congress. The OTA responded that more research was warranted; however, the East Virginia School of Medicine denied Speckhart's proposal to include the Livingston vaccine in his research.

36. Cheson, B.D. et al. "Tumor Vaccine Clinical Trials." *Oncology* 9:10 (1995), 929.

37. Lamm, D.L. "BCG Immunotherapy for Transitional-cell Carcinoma In Situ of the Bladder." *Oncology* 9:10 (1995), 947-952.

38. Scott, M.T. "Tumor-induced Specific Suppression: A Limitation to Immunotherapy." *Immunology Today* 3 (1982), 8-9. See also. Kamo, I., and H. Friedman. "Immunosuppression and the Role of Suppressive Factors in Cancer." *Advanced Cancer Research* 25 (1977), 271-321.

39. Serrano, R. et al. "Isolation of a Novel Tumor Protein That Induces Resistance to Natural Killer Cell Lysis." *Journal of Immunology* 145 (1990), 3516-3523.

40. Note: TNF seems to exert a dual, conflicting influence on the anticancer defenses. For more information regarding its negative role, see *Cell* 61 (1990), 361-370; or *Proceedings of the National Academy of Sciences* 87 (1990), 8781-8784.

41. Moss, R. "Russian Immunologist Reports Remarkable Results." *The Cancer Chronicles* (New York: Equinox Press, 1994), 4.

42. Note: As discussed in Chapter 27, "Early Detection & Prevention of Cancer," darkfield microscopy enables us to look at *living* blood for the first time, which is a different world entirely from the static conditions observed through orthodox forms of microscopy.

43. Enby, E. et al. "Hidden Killers: Causes of Cancer: A New Look." *The Revolutionary Medical Discoveries of Professor Gunther Enderlein* (Saratoga, CA: Sheehan Communications, 1990), 77.

44. Ibid.

45. Walters, R. "Enderlein Therapy: A Cancer Therapy that Promotes Gentle Self-healing." *Raum & Zeit* 3:1 (1991), 24-27.

46. Enby, E. et al. "Hidden Killers: Causes of Cancer: A New Look." *The Revolutionary Medical Discoveries of*

*Professor Gunther Enderlein* (Saratoga, CA: Sheehan Communications, 1990), 84.

47. Ibid., 89.
48. Walters, R. "Enderlein Therapy: A Cancer Therapy that Promotes Gentle Self-healing." *Raum & Zeit* 3:1 (1991), 24-27.
49. Enby, E. et al. "Hidden Killers: Causes of Cancer: A New Look." *The Revolutionary Medical Discoveries of Professor Gunther Enderlein* (Saratoga, CA: Sheehan Communications, 1990), 84.

## Chapter 32

## Enhancing Whole-Body Metabolism for Treating Cancer

1. Hole, John, Jr. *Human Anatomy and Physiology* (Dubuque, IA: William C. Brown, 1978).
2. Wallach, D.F.H. "Cellular Aspects of Tumor Thermobiology." *Proceedings of the International Congress on Chemotherapy, 13th* 18 (1983), 273.
3. Warburg, O. "Preface to the Second Edition of the Lindau Lecture." *The Prime Cause and Prevention of Cancer* (Wurzburg, Germany: Konrad Triltsch, 1967), 2. Translation by Dean Burk, Ph.D., National Cancer Institute, Bethesda, MD.
4. Ibid., 6.
5. Oberley, L.W., and G.R. Buettner. "Role of Superoxide Dismutase in Cancer: A Review." *Cancer Research* 39:4 (1979), 1141-1149.
6. Ibid.
7. Von Ardenne, Manfred. *Oxygen Multistep Therapy, Physiological and Technical Foundations* (New York: Thiene Medical, 1990).
8. Altman, N. "Hydrogen Peroxide." *Oxygen Healing Therapies* (Rochester, VT: Healing Arts Press, 1995), 51.
9. Helfland, S.L. et al. "Oxygen Intermediates Are Required for Interferon Activation of NK Cells." *Journal of Interferon Research* 3:2 (1983), 143-51.
10. Ibid.
11. Anonymous. "Questionable Methods of Cancer Management: Hydrogen Peroxide and Other 'Hyperoxygenation' Therapies." *CA: A Cancer Journal for Clinicians* 43:1 (1993), 47-56.
12. Douglass, W.C. *Hydrogen Peroxide: Medical Miracle* (Atlanta, GA: Second Opinion Publishing, 1992).
13. Dormandy, T.L. "In Praise of Peroxidation." *The Lancet* 2:8620 (1988), 1126-1128.
14. Yamazaki M., and S. Tsunawaki. "Anti-tumor Effect by Leukocyte-derived Active Oxygens." (Japanese) *Tanpakushitsu Kakusan Koso-Protein, Nucleic Acid, Enzyme* 33:16 (1988), 3031-3036.
15. Chung, T., and Y.B. Kim. "Two Distinct Cytolytic Mechanisms of Macrophages and Monocytes Activated by Phorbol Myristate Acetate." *Journal of Leukocyte Biology* 44:5 (1988), 329-336.
16. Nathan, C.F. et al. "Administration of Recombinant Interferon Gamma to Cancer Patients Enhances Monocyte Secretion of Hydrogen Peroxide." *Proceedings of the National Academy of Sciences* 82:24 (1985), 8686-8690.
17. Helfland, S.L. et al. "Oxygen Intermediates Are Required for Interferon Activation of NK Cells." *Journal of Interferon Research* 3:2 (1983), 143-151.
18. Apffel C.A. "Nonimmunological Host Defenses: A Review." *Cancer Research* 36:5 (1976), 1527-1537.
19. Farr, C.H. "The Therapeutic Use of Intravenous Hydrogen Peroxide." Monograph. (Oklahoma City, OK: Genesis Medical Center, 1987).
20. Holman, R.A. "A Method of Destroying a Malignant Tumor *In Vivo*." *Nature* 179 (1957), 1033.
21. Wirth, W. "The Effects of Hydrogen Peroxide on Ehrlich Carcinoma in Laboratory Mice." Lecture at St. Thomas Institute. Cincinatti, Ohio (November 15, 1982). Cited in: Pelton, R. *Hydrogen Peroxide: Alternatives in Cancer Therapy* (New York: Simon & Schuster, 1994), 113.
22. Nathan, C.F., and Z.A. Cohn. "Antitumor Effects of Hydrogen Peroxide *In Vivo*." *Journal of Experimental Medicine* 154 (1981), 1539-1553.
23. Ben-Yoseph, O., and B.D. Ross. "Oxidation Therapy: The Use of a Reactive Oxygen Species-generating Enzyme System for Tumor Treatment." *British Journal of Cancer* 70 (1994), 1131-1135.
24. Mealey, J. "Regional Infusion of Vinblastine and Hydrogen Peroxide in Tumor-bearing Rats." *Cancer Research* 25 (1965), 1839-1843.
25. Kaibara, N.T. et al. "Experimental Studies on Enhancing the Therapeutic Effect of Mitomycin-C with Hydrogen Peroxide." *Japanese Journal of Experimental Medicine* 41 (1971), 323-329.
26. Oliver, T.H., and D.V. Murphy. "Influenzal Pneumonia: The Intravenous Use of Hydrogen Peroxide." *The Lancet* (February 21, 1920), 432-433.
27. Farr, C.H. *Protocol for Intravenous Administration of Hydrogen Peroxide* (Oklahoma City, OK: International Bio-Oxidative Medicine Foundation, 1993), 32.
28. Altman, N. "Hydrogen Peroxide in Medicine." *Oxygen Healing Therapies* (Rochester, VT: Healing Arts Press, 1995), 42-43.
29. "Common Denominators in Cancer Non-remedies and in Human Longevity." *Townsend Letter for Doctors & Patients* (January 1992), 48-50.
30. Stark, H.R. "Cause and Treatment of Malignancy." *The Koch Treatment* (Asheville, NC: Christian Medical Research League, 1950), 103.
31. Pelton., R. "Hydrogen Peroxide." *Alternatives in Cancer Therapy* (New York: Simon & Schuster, 1994), 117.
32. Farr, C.H. *Protocol for Intravenous Administration of Hydrogen Peroxide* (Oklahoma City, OK: International Bio-Oxidative Medicine Foundation, 1993), 32.
33. Speckhart, V. "Hydrogen Peroxide in Malignancy with and without Radiation Therapy." *Proceedings of the First International Conference on Bio-Oxidative Medicine*, edited by Farr, Charles (Dallas, TX: International Bio-Oxidative Medicine Foundation, 1989), 35-38.

34. Donsbach, K.W. *Oxygen-Peroxides-Ozone* (Tulsa, OK: Rockland Corporation, 1993), 66.

35. Ibid.

36. Farr, C.H. *Oxidative Therapy* (Oklahoma City, OK: International Bio-Oxidative Medicine Foundation, 1993), 3.

37. Zanker, K.S. "*In Vitro* Synergistic Activity of 5-fluorouracil with Low-dose Ozone against Chemoresistant Tumor Cell Line and Fresh Human Cells." *International Journal of Experimental and Clinical Chemotherapy* 36 (1990).

38. Sweet, J. et al. "Ozone Selectively Inhibits Growth of Human Cancer Cells." *Science* 209 (1980), 931-933.

39. Bocci, V. "Ozonization of Blood for the Therapy of Viral Diseases and Immunodeficiencies: A Hypothesis." *Medical Hypotheses* 39:1 (1992), 30-34.

40. American Cancer Society (statement). Cited in: Falcone, R. "Oxygen Therapies." *The Complete Guide to Alternative Cancer Therapies* (New York: Citadel Press, 1994), 132.

41. Altman, N. "Cancer." *Oxygen Healing Therapies* (Rochester, VT: Healing Arts Press, 1995).

42. Varro, J. "Ozone Applications in Cancer Cases." *Medical Applications of Ozone*, edited by LaRaus, J. (Norwalk, CT: International Ozone Association Pan American Committee, 1983), 97-98.

43. Howell, E. *Enzyme Nutrition: The Food Enzyme Concept* (Garden City Park, NY: Avery Publishing, 1985), 130.

44. Wrba, H., and O. Pecher. *Enzyme: Wirkstoff der Zukunft Mitt der Enzymtherapie das Immunsystem Starken* (Vienna: Verlag Orac, 1993).

45. Cichoke, A.J. "The Effect of Systemic Enzyme Therapy on Cancer Cells and the Immune System." *Townsend Letter for Doctors & Patients* (November 1995), 30-32.

46. Wolf, M., and K. Ransberger. *Enzyme Therapy* (Los Angeles: Regent House, 1972), 156-166, 193-194.

47. Wrba, H. "New Approaches in Treatment of Cancer with Enzymes." Lecture at the First International Conference on Systemic Enzyme Therapy (September 12, 1990).

48. Nydegger, U.E., and J.S. Davis. "Soluble Immune Complexes in Human Disease." *Critical Reviews in Clinical Laboratory Sciences* 12 (1980), 123.

49. Ibid.

50. Steffen, C., and J. Menzel. "Basic Studies on Enzyme Therapy of Immune Complex Diseases." *Wiener klinische Wochenschrift* 97:8 (1985) 376-85. See also: Steffen, C., and J. Menzel. "*In Vivo* Degradation of Immune Complexes in the Kidney by Orally Administered Enzymes." *Wiener klinische Wochenschrift* 99:15 (1987), 525-31.

51. Kim, H.K. et al. "The Alteration in Cellular Immunity Following the Enzyme Therapy: The Influence of Wobe-Mugos on the Destructibility of NKMC (Natural Killer Cell Mediated Cytotoxicity)." 7th Korean Cancer Research Society. National University Hospital, Seoul, South Korea (October 4, 1980). See also: Kim, J.P. et al. "Effect on Rosette-forming T-lymphocyte Level in Immunochemotherapy Using Picabanil and Wobe-Mugos in Gastric Cancer Patients." *Journal of the Korean Surgical Society* 23 (1981), 44.

52. Wrba, H., and O. Pecher. *Enzyme: Wirkstoff der Zukunft Mitt der Enzymtherapie das Immunsystem starken* (Vienna: Verlag Orac, 1993).

53. Krueger, G.R.F. *Klinische Immunopathologe* (Stuttgart, Germany: 1985). Cited in: Cichoke, A.J. "The Effect of Systemic Enzyme Therapy on Cancer Cells and the Immune System." *Townsend Letter for Doctors & Patients* (November 1995), 30-32.

54. Boik, John. *Cancer & Natural Medicine: A Textbook of Basic Science and Clinical Research* (Princeton, MN: Oregon Medical Press, 1995).

55. Bube, F. et al. "Detection of Fibrinolytic Split Products in Patient Collections with Disordered Hemostasis. I. In Pathologically Verified Lung Cancer. II. In Thrombotic/Embolic Occurrences." *Folia Haematologica* 108:3 (1981), 447-54. Cited in: Wilner, J. "Enzyme Preparations." *The Cancer Solution* (Boca Raton, FL: Peltec Publishing, 1994), 79.

56. Langer, S.E. et al. *Solved: The Riddle of Illness* (New Canaan, CT: Keats, 1984).

57. Quillan, P. *Beating Cancer With Nutrition* (Tulsa, OK: Nutrition Times Press, 1994), 117.

58. Ibid.

59. Bland, J. *Glandular-based Food Supplements: Helping to Separate Fact from Fiction* (Tacoma, WA: Bellevue-Redmond Medical Laboratory, Department of Chemistry, University of Puget Sound, 1980), 20-21.

60. Ibid.

61. Herning, W.A. "Transmission of High Molecular Weight Protein Products across the Gut." *Antigen Absorption By the Gut* (Baltimore, MD: University Park Press, 1978).

62. Hayashi, F. et al. "Characteristics of Hepatocarcinogenesis Caused by DHEA, a Peroxisome Proliferator, in Male F-344 rats." *Carcinogenesis* 15:10 (1994), 2215-2219.

63. Ebeling, P., and V.A. Koivisto. "Physiological Importance of Dehydroepiandrosterone." *The Lancet* 343:8911 (1994), 1479-1481.

64. Labrie, F. et al. "Intracrinology: The Basis the Rational Design of Endocrine Therapy at All Stages of Prostate Cancer." *European Urology* 24:Suppl 2 (1993), 94-105.

65. Stretch, Eileen, N.D. "DHEA & Cancer Prevention in Women: Friend or Foe?" *Townsend Letter for Doctors & Patients* (October 1996), 144-145.

66. Pashko, L.L. "Cancer Chemoprevention with Adrenocortical Steroid Dehydroepiandrosterone and Structural Analogs." *Journal of Cell Biochemistry* Suppl 17G (1993), 73-79.

67. Li, S. et al "Prevention by Dehydroepiandrosterone of the Development of Mammary Carcinoma Induced by 7,12-dimethylbenzy(a)anthracene (DMBA) in the Rat." *Breast Cancer Research and Treatment* 29:2 (1994), 203-217.

68. Ward, Dean, M.D., and J. Morgenthaler. *Smart Drugs & Nutrients* (Santa Cruz, CA: B&J Publications, 1991). Information from Palm Springs Life Extension Institute, Palm Springs, CA. See also: Brody, J. "Restoring Ebbing Hormones May Slow Aging." *The New York Times* (July 18, 1995). See also: *Dr. Jonathan V. Wright's Nutrition & Healing* 2:1 (January 1995).

69. Caroleo, M. et al. "Melatonin as Immunomodulator in Immunodeficient Mice." *International Journal of*

*Immunopharmacology* 23 (1992), 81-89. See also: Hadden, J.W. "T-cell Adjuvants." *International Journal of Immunopharmacology* 16:9 (1994), 703-710.

70. Neri, B. et al. "Effects of Melatonin Administration on Cytokine Production in Patients with Advanced Solid Tumors." *Oncology Reports* 2 (1995), 45-47. See also: Del Gobbo, V. et al. "Pinealectomy Inhibits IL-2 Production and NK Activity in Mice." *International Journal of Immunopharmacology* 11 (1989), 567-577.
71. Lissoni, P. et al. "Immunotherapy wih Subcutaneous Low-dose Interleukin-2 Plus Melatonin vs. Chemotherapy with Cisplatin and Etoposide as First-line Therapy for Advanced Non-small-cell Lung Cancer." *Tumori* 80 (1994), 464-467.
72. Lissoni, P. et al. "A Randomized Study with the Pineal Hormone Melatonin Versus Supportive Care Alone in Patients with Brain Metastases Due to Solid Neoplasms." *Cancer* 73:3 (1994), 699-701.
73. Lissoni, P. et al. "Subcutaneous Therapy with Low-dose Interleukin-2 Plus the Neurohormone Melatonin in Metastatic Gastric Cancer Patients with Low-performance Status." *Tumori* 79:6 (1993), 401-404.
74. Barni, S. et al. "A Randomized Study of Low-dose Subcutaneous Interleukin-2 Plus Melatonin Versus Supportive Care Alone in Metastatic Colorectal Cancer Patients Progressing under 5-fluorouracil and Folates." *Tumori* 78:6 (1992), 383-387.
75. Blask, D.E. "Melatonin Modulates Growth Factor Activity in MCF-7 Human Breast Cancer Cells." *Journal of Pineal Research* 17:1 (1994), 25-32.
76. Lissoni, P. et al. "Immunoendocrine Therapy with Low-dose Subcutaneous Interleukin-2 Plus Melatonin of Locally Advanced or Metastatic Endocrine Tumors." *Oncology* 52:2 (1995), 163-166.
77. Pierpaoli, W., and W. Regelson. "A Powerful Protector and Treatment against Cancer." *The Melatonin Miracle* (New York: Simon & Schuster, 1995), 113-129.
78. The Burton Goldberg Group. *Alternative Medicine: The Definitive Guide* (Tiburon, CA: Future Medicine Publishing, 1995), 12.
79. Garaci, E. et al. "Combination Treatment Using Thymosin Alpha 1 and Interferon after Cyclophosphamide Is Able to Cure Lewis Lung Carcinoma in Mice." *Cancer Immunology and Immunotherapy* 32 (1990), 154-160.
80. Cohen, M.H. et al. "Thymosin Fraction V and Intensive Combination Chemotherapy. Prolonging the Survival of Patients with Small-cell Lung Cancer." *Journal of the American Medical Association* 241 (1979), 1813-1815.
81. Ibid.
82. Drozdova, T.S. et al. "Immunologic Correction Using Thymus Gland Preparation (T- activin) in the Programmed Treatment of Patients with Non-lymphoid Leukemia." *Gematologiia I Transfuziologiia* 35:1 (1990), 14-16. Cited in: Boik, J. "Thymostimulin." *Cancer and Natural Medicine: A Textbook of Basic Science and Clinical Research* (Princeton, MN: Oregon Medical Press, 1995), 76-77.
83. Skotnicki, A.B. "Therapeutic Application of a Calf Thymus Extract (TFX)." *Medical Oncology and Tumor Pharmacotherapy* 6:1 (1989), 32-43.

## Chapter 33

## Physical Support Therapies for Reversing Cancer

1. The Burton Goldberg Group. *Alternative Medicine: The Definitive Guide* (Tiburon, CA: Future Medicine Publishing, 1995), 3.
2. Ibid., 4.
3. Straus, Howard. "Coffee Corner." *Gerson Healing Newsletter* 11:5 (1996), 9-11.
4. Steinman, D., and S.S. Epstein. *The Safe Shopper's Bible* (New York: Macmillan, 1994).
5. Ibid.
6. Mayer, D.K. "Diagnosis and Management of Intestinal Obstruction in Individuals with Cancer." *Nurse Practitioner* 11:2 (1986), 36-46.
7. Singer, Sidney R., and Soma Grismaijer. *Dressed to Kill: The Link Between Breast Cancer and Bras* (New York: Avery Publishing, 1995).
8. Wittlinger, Gunther, and Hildegard Wittlinger. *Textbook of Dr. Vodder's Manual Lymph Drainage Vol. 1: Basic Course* 4th Edition (Brussels: Editions Haug International, 1992), 10-36.
9. Cranton, E.M., and J.P. Frackelton. "Free Radical Pathology in Age-Associated Diseases: Treatment with EDTA Chelation, Nutrition and Antioxidants." *Journal of Holistic Medicine* 6:1 (1984), 6-36.
10. Eysenck, H. "Psychosocial Factors, Prognosis and Prevention of Cancer." *Coping with Cancer and Beyond* (Berwyn, PA: Swets and Zeitlinger, The Helen Dowling Institute, 1991), 35.
11. Levy, S.M. et al. "Survival Hazards Analysis in First Recurrent Breast Cancer Patients: Seven-Year Follow-Up." *Psychosomatic Medicine* 50 (1988), 520-528.
12. Shekelle, R. B. et al. "Psychological Depression and 17-Year Risk and Death from Cancer." *Psychosomatic Medicine* 43 (1981), 117-125.
13. Berkman, L.F., and S.L. Syme. "Social Networks, Host Resistance, and Mortality: A Nine-Year Follow-Up Study of Alameda County Residents." *American Journal of Epidemiology* 109:2 (1979), 189-204.
14. Spiegel, D. et al. "Effect of Psychosocial Treatment on Survival of Patients with Metastatic Breast Cancer." *The Lancet* 2:8668 (1989), 888-891.
15. Shaffer, J.W. et al. "Clustering of Personality Traits in Youth and the Subsequent Development of Cancer among Physicians." *Journal of Behavioral Medicine* 10:5 (1987), 441-448. Cited in: Bower, B. "The Character of Cancer." *Science News* 131 (1987), 120-121.
16. Greer, S. et al. "Psychological Response to Breast Cancer: Effects on Outcome." *The Lancet* 2 (1979), 785-787. See also: Rogentine, G. et al. "Psychological Factors in the Prognosis of Malignant Melanoma: A Prospective Study." *Psychosomatic Medicine* 41 (1979), 647-655.
17. Kneier, W.W., and L. Temoshok. "Repressive Coping Reactions in Patients with Malignant Melanoma as

Compared to Cardiovascular Disease Patients." *Journal of Psychosomatic Research* 28 (1984), 145.

18. Goodkin, K. et al. "Stress and Hopelessness in the Promotion of Cervical Intraepithelial Neoplasia in Invasive Squamous Cell Carcinoma of the Cervix." *Journal of Psychosomatic Research* 30:1 (1986), 67-76. See also: Schmale, A.H., and H. Iker. "The Effect of Hopelessness in the Development of Cancer. I. Identification of Uterine Cervical Cancer in Women with Atypical Cytology." *Psychosomatic Medicine* 28 (1966), 714-721.
19. Ramirez, A.J. et al. "Stress and Relapse of Breast Cancer." *British Medical Journal* 298 (1989), 291-293.
20. Thomas, G. *Into the Unknown: Dr. Issels and His Revolutionary Cancer Treatment* (New York: Peter H. Wyden, 1973), 94.
21. Issels, J. *More Cures for Cancer* (Bad Homburg, Germany: Helfer Publishing, 1995), 5.
22. Ibid., 7.
23. Ibid., 11.
24. Ibid., 7.
25. Thomas, G. *Into the Unknown: Dr. Issels and His Revolutionary Cancer Treatment* (New York: Peter H. Wyden, 1973).
26. Ibid., 96.
27. Anonymous. *Cancer: A Healing Crisis* (Los Angeles: Cancer Resource Center, 1980), 13.
28. Ibid.
29. Royal, Daniel F., D.O. "Health Hazard in Your Teeth," *Alternative Medicine Digest* 13 (1996), 40-44.
30. Electric blankets and heating pads weaken immunity. As an alternative, a denim or cotton heating pad filled with sand can be heated carefully in the oven or microwave.
31. Castleman, M. "Aromatherapy." *Nature's Cures* (Emmaus, PA: Rodale Press, 1996), 39. Castleman notes that heliotropin is a close relative of vanilla oil.
32. Dewhirst, M., Professor of Radiation Oncology and Director of the Duke Hyperthermia Program at the Duke University Medical Center, Durham, North Carolina. Personal communications (1996).
33. Ibid.
34. The Burton Goldberg Group. *Alternative Medicine: The Definitive Guide* (Tiburon, CA: Future Medicine Publishing, 1995), 6.
35. Ibid., 7.
36. Ibid., 8.
37. Ibid., 10.
38. Ibid., 13.
39. Ibid., 14.
40. Ibid., 15.
41. Ibid., 16.
42. Dibell-Hope, S. "Moving toward Health: A Study of the Use of Dance-movement Therapy in the Psychological Adaptation to Breast Cancer." University of California School of Professional Psychology Dissertation (1989).
43. The Burton Goldberg Group. *Alternative Medicine: The Definitive Guide* (Tiburon, CA: Future Medicine Publishing, 1995), 1.
44. Ibid., 2.
45. Ibid., 3.
46. Ibid., 4.
47. Ibid., 5.
48. Milne, Robert D., M.D., and Blake More with Burton Goldberg. *An Alternative Medicine Definitive Guide to Headaches* (Tiburon, CA: Future Medicine Publishing, 1997).
49. Tomasi, et al. "Immune Parameters in Athletes before and after Strenuous Exercise." *Journal of Clinical Immunology* 2 (1982), 173-8. See also: Soppi, et al. "Effect of Strenuous Physical Stress on Circulating Lymphocyte Number and Function before and after Training." *Journal of Clinical and Laboratory Immunology* 8 (1982), 43-46.
50. Cannon, V., and J. Kluger. "Endogenous Pyrogen Activity in Human Plasma after Exercise." *Science* 220 (1983), 617-9. See also: Cannon, V., and C. Dinarello. "Interleukin I Activity in Human Plasma." *Federation Proceedings* 43 (1984), 462.
51. Ballard-Barbash, R. et al. "Physical Activity and Risk of Large Bowel Cancer in the Framingham Study" *Cancer Research* 50:12 (1990), 3610-3613.
52. Ibid.
53. Frisch, R.E. et al. "Lower Prevalence of Breast Cancer in Cancers of Reproductive System among Former College Athletes Compared to Non-Athletes." *British Journal of Cancer* 52 (1985), 885-891.
54. Blair, S.N. et al. "Physical Fitness and All-cause Mortality." *Journal of the American Medical Association* 262:17 (1989), 2395.
55. Oliveria, S. et al. "The Association between Cardiorespiratory Fitness and Prostate Cancer." *Medicine and Science in Sports and Exercise* 28:1 (1996), 97.
56. "Chinese Display Qigong Energy for U.S. Doctors." *Brain Mind Bulletin* 11:6 (March 3, 1986), 1. In addition, subjects showed measurable changes in brain states during Qigong practice. When a Qigong master directed his *qi* at a crystal for 15 minutes, light was diffracted differently through it afterward.
57. Yi, Y. et al. "The Effect of Self-controlling Qigong Therapy on the Immune Function of Cancer Patients." Second World Conference on Academic Exchange of Medical Qigong (September 15, 1993), 128.
58. Hongmei, A., and B. Jingnan. "Curative Effect Analysis of 122 Tumor Patients Treated by the Intelligence Qigong." Second World Conference on Academic Exchange of Medical Qigong (September 15, 1993), 130.
59. Chang, S. *The Complete System of Self-Healing: Internal Exercises* (San Francisco: Tao Publishing, 1986).
60. Jahnke, R. *The Most Profound Medicine* (Santa Barbara, CA: Health Action Books, 1990).
61. Yao, W. et al. "The Effect of Traditional Chinese Medicine on Cancer Rehabilitation." Fourth International Symposium on Qigong. Shanghai, China (September 1992), 76.
62. Ibid.
63. Shouzhang, W. et al. "A Clinical Study of the Routine Treatment of Cancer Coordinated by Qigong." Second

World Conference on Academic Exchange of Medical Qigong (September 15, 1993), 129.

64. Li-da, F. "The Effects of External Qi on Bacterial Growth Patterns." *China Qi Gong* 1 (1983), 36.

65. Lee, R.H. *Scientific Investigations into Chinese Qigong* (San Clemente, CA: China Healthways Institute, 1992).

# Chapter 34
# Energy Support Therapies

1. Filshie, J. et al. "Report on Acupuncture-induced Pain Relief for Cancer Patients." International Medical Acupuncture Conference. London, England (1986).

2. Wu, B. et al. "Effect of Acupuncture on Interleukin-2 and NK Cell Immunoactivity of Peripheral Blood of Malignant Tumor Patients." *Chung-Kuo Chung Hsi I Chieh Ho Tsa Chih* 14:9 (1994), 37-39.

3. Clark, James Hoyt, B.Sc., M.Sc. *Computerized Electro Dermal Screening & The Life Information System* (Orem, UT: Biosource, 1994), 34.

4. Dr. Voll reported 4 principles as a result of his research: 1) the body's resistance is not uniform; 2) meridians (energy pathways) show electrical fields; 3) meridians actually generate the body's energy; and 4) the skin is a semi-insulator with respect to the external environment. Dr. Voll's first instrument to measure body energy signals by point testing was called the *Diatherapuncteur* and was exhibited in 1955 as part of an electroacupuncture demonstration. A more sophisticated version was renamed *Dermatron* and released by the Pitterling Electronic Company of Munich, Germany, in the 1970s. Dr. Voll discovered that higher or lower readings than normal at a particular acupuncture point indicate a problem in the organ that corresponds to that acupoint; a higher reading generally means there is irritation or inflammation in the organ, while a lower reading usually indicates fatigue or degeneration.

5. Clark, James Hoyt, B.Sc., M.Sc. *Computerized Electro Dermal Screening & The Life Information System* (Orem, UT: Biosource, 1994), 27-33.

6. A related device is called the MORA. The MORA was created by Franz Morrel, M.D., a close colleague of Dr. Voll. Dr. Morrel contended that all biological processes are a matter of electromagnetic signals making complex wave forms. Healthy conditions make a smooth wave, while disease generates a wave with many variations, both higher and lower than the norm. Dr. Morrel's approach was to first register the electromagnetic signals from the body, then to correct the aberrant wave forms. These corrected waves are then fed from the MORA device back to the patient through the appropriate acupuncture points. The signals can be taken from any area of the body, modified, and then returned to that specific area. "The crucial point of the MORA is that disease is considered to be a question of 'wrong' electromagnetic information," says Dr. Scott-Morley. "The MORA instrument 'reads' the wave information of the patient and corrects it. There is no artificial electrical signal introduced. In this sense, it is an extremely pure form of treatment because it deals only with the wave information of the patient." The MORA's primary utility in cancer therapy is to alleviate aches and pains that may result as symptoms of advanced disease or from previous exposure to conventional treatment, and to increase vitality.

7. Tsuei, Julia J. "The Science of Acupuncture—Theory and Practice." *IEEE Engineering in Medicine and Biology* (May/June 1996), 52-57.

8. Clark, James Hoyt, B.Sc., M.Sc. *Computerized Electro Dermal Screening & The Life Information System* (Orem, UT: Biosource, 1994), 40.

9. The Burton Goldberg Group. *Alternative Medicine: The Definitive Guide* (Tiburon, CA: Future Medicine Publishing, 1995), 192.

10. Ibid., 330.

11. Fersht, Alan. *Enzyme Structure and Mechanism* 2nd Edition (New York: W.H. Freeman, 1994).

12. The Burton Goldberg Group. *Alternative Medicine: The Definitive Guide* (Tiburon, CA: Future Medicine Publishing, 1995), 330.

13. Trappier, A. et al."Evaluating Perspectives on the Exposure Risks from Magnetic Fields." *Journal of the National Medical Association* 82:9 (September 1990).

14. The Burton Goldberg Group. *Alternative Medicine: The Definitive Guide* (Tiburon, CA: Future Medicine Publishing, 1995), 330.

15. Philpott, W.H. "Cancer Prevention and Reversal." *Journal of the Bio-Electro-Magnetics Institute* 2:3 (1990), 12-16.

16. Ibid.

17. Riviere, M. et al. "Test with Lymphosarcoma on Mice." *Comptes Rendus de' l' Academie des Sciences* (March 1, 1965).

18. Troeng, I. Commenting on the study's results. Laholm, Sweden (July 1984). See: Riviere, M. et al. "Test with Lymphosarcoma on Mice." *Comptes Rendus de' l' Academie des Sciences* (March 1, 1965).

19. "Questionable Methods of Cancer Management: Electronic Devices." *CA: A Cancer Journal for Clinicians* 44 (1994), 115-127.

20. The Burton Goldberg Group. *Alternative Medicine: The Definitive Guide* (Tiburon, CA: Future Medicine Publishing, 1995), 319.

21. Ibid., 2.

22. Ibid., 3.

23. Ibid., 4.

24. Ibid., 5.

25. Ibid., 319.

26. Ibid., 7.

27. Ibid., 319.

28. Ibid., 9.

29. Ibid., 10.

30. Ibid., 9.

31. Ibid., 11.

32. Ibid., 16. See also: "Holistic Physician-Asthma." *Alternative Medicine Digest* 8 (1995), 13.

33. Symonds, W.C., and B. Bremner. "A Ray of Hope for

Cancer Patients: Photodynamic Therapy May Stop Early-stage Tumors." *Business Week* (June 10, 1996), 104-106.

34. Ibid.

35. Ibid.

# Index

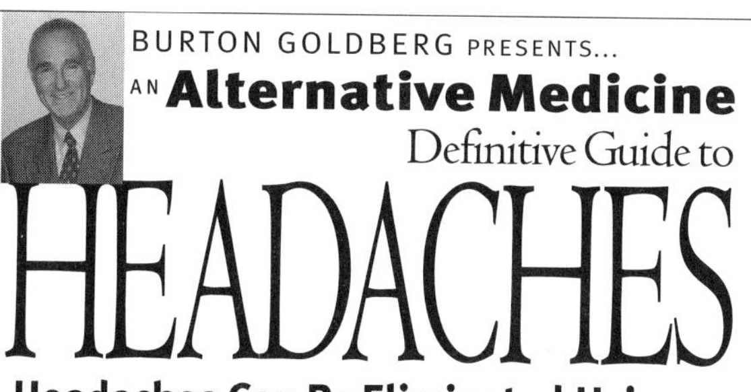


**Headaches Can Be Eliminated Using Natural Alternative Therapies.**

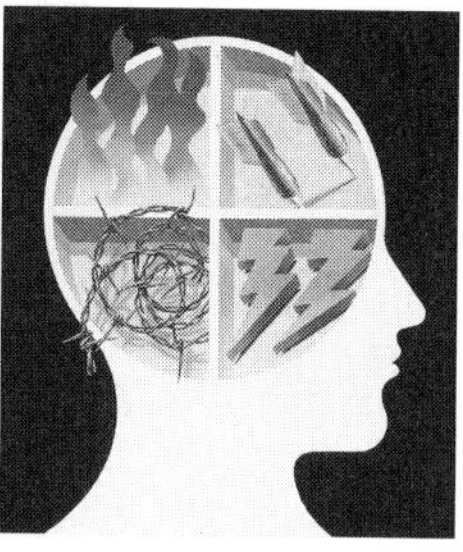

**Learn how proven alternative and natural therapies can help eliminate all types of headaches...**

- **MIGRAINE** ▪ **SINUS** ▪ **TENSION**
- **CLUSTER** ▪ **ALLERGY** ▪ **TRAUMA**
- **FOOD-RELATED** ▪ **EYESTRAIN**
- **CHEMICAL SENSITIVITY**

**ROBERT MILNE, M.D. AND BLAKE MORE**
**WITH BURTON GOLDBERG**

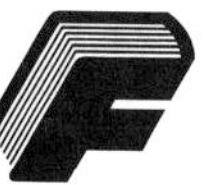

ISBN #1-887299-03-3
525 pages, Hardcover
Future Medicine Publishing
1640 Tiburon Blvd., Suite #2
Tiburon, California 94920

If you suffer from headaches, this book could change your life. It is entirely possible that with this invaluable practical information, you may well put headaches behind you as something you once suffered from, but no more.

Robert Milne, M.D., and Blake More expertly guide you through the root causes and multiple treatment options for 11 major types of headaches, from sinus to migraine, cluster to tension.

We have made every effort possible to make this book practical and user-friendly for you. For a quick reference to headache types, symptoms, and treatment options, use our Master Symptom Chart. If you suffer from tension headaches, turn directly to Chapter 6; if migraines are your millstone, see Chapter 7; and if you're not sure what type of headache you have, study the symptoms list in the Master Symptom Chart until you find the clinical term that best matches your condition.

No matter what kind of headache you *used* to have, after reading this book your head may never pain you again.

—BURTON GOLDBERG

# To Order, Call 800-333-HEAL

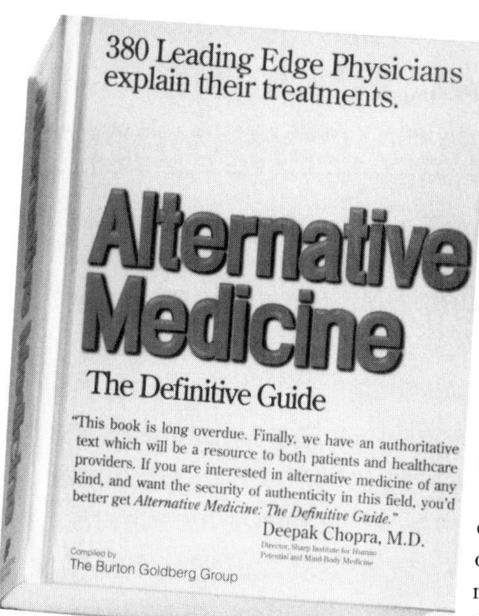


If you are one of the millions of people who are searching for a better way to health—this is the book for you. *Alternative Medicine: The Definitive Guide* is a must for anyone interested in the latest information on how to get healthy and stay that way. At 1100 pages, this encyclopedia puts all the schools of alternative medicine—50 different therapies—under one roof.

The Washington Post says "this is the book that's needed right now." The *Guide* is packed with life-saving information and alternative treatments from 380 of the world's leading alternative physicians.

Organized by type of therapy and health condition, each section clearly and succinctly outlines the steps you can take to get treatment for your health conditions. Not only that, but each section also provides information on further resources—books, organizations, and doctors. No wonder the *Guide* was selected as an "Outstanding Reference Source" by the American Library Association!

The *Guide* gives you the knowledge you need so that you can make intelligent choices about the future of your health. Order yours today! ISBN #0-963633-4-3-0

## o available, these books and videos—

### ural Medicine Chest and ne Remedies

This instructional videotape and concise, easy-to-read handbook puts natural healing at your fingertips. Learn how to make natural remedies with ingredients found in your home (video) and what to buy in your local h food store to treat com- conditions such as flu, ear- s, acne, and much more.

N #0-9636334-7-3

### Alternative Medicine Yellow Pages

Put a one-stop telephone directory of 17,000 practitioners of alternative medicine around the U.S. at your fingertips. Find the alternative specialist by state and city, type of practitioner, and health problem. Listings span back pain to weight management, arthritis to thyroid disorders. The Yellow Pages' resource lists guide you to further sources of information. Learn even more about how alternative medicine can help end your health problem by browsing the hundreds of informative display ads throughout the book.

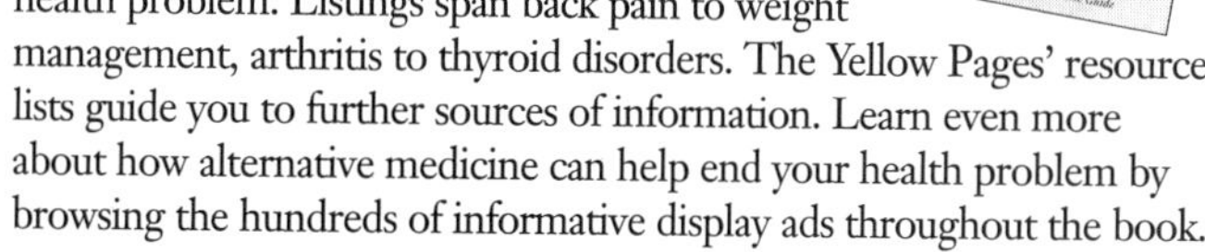

242 pages, ISBN #0-9636334-2-2

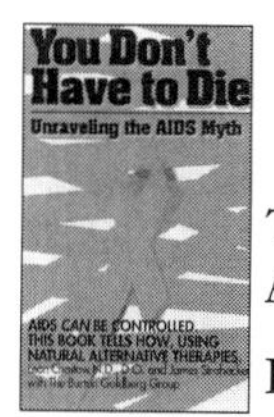


This is the indispensable book for successfully treating AIDS with alternative medicine.

ISBN #0-9636334-4-9

**TO PLACE YOUR ORDER, CALL 800-333-HEAL**
**OR VISIT OUR WEB SITE AT www.alternativemedicine.com**